Endodontic Therapy

Endodontic Therapy

Franklin S. Weine
B.S., D.D.S., M.S.D., F.A.C.D., F.I.C.D.

Professor Emeritus, Loyola University (Chicago);
Formerly Professor and Director, Post-Graduate Endodontics,
Loyola University School of Dentistry,
Maywood, Illinois;
Visiting Professor of Endodontics, Osaka Dental University,
Osaka, Japan

FIFTH EDITION

with 2241 illustrations

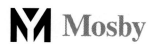 Mosby

St. Louis Baltimore Boston Carlsbad Chicago Naples New York Philadelphia Portland
London Madrid Mexico City Singapore Sydney Tokyo Toronto Wiesbaden

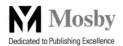

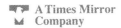

Publisher: Don Ladig
Executive Editor: Linda L. Duncan
Developmental Editor: Melba Steube
Project Manager: Deborah L. Vogel
Production and Editing: A-R Editions
Manufacturing Supervisor: Karen Lewis

Printed in the United States of America
Composition by A-R Editions
Printing/binding by Maple-Vail Book Mfg. Group

Mosby-Year Book, Inc.
11830 Westline Industrial Drive
St. Louis, Missouri 63146

Library of Congress Cataloging in Publication Data

Weine, Franklin S.
    Endodontic therapy / Franklin S. Weine. — 5th ed.
       p.   cm.
    Includes bibliographical references and index.
    ISBN 0-8016-7963-X
    1. Endodontics.   I. Title.
    [DNLM: 1. Endodontics. WU 230 W423e 1995]
  RK351.W44 1995
  617.6'342—dc20
  DNLM/DLC
  for Library of Congress   95-22054
                                               CIP

95 96 97 98 99 / 9 8 7 6 5 4 3 2 1

Contributors

Manuel A. Bustamante, D.D.S.

Private Practice Limited to Endodontics,
Los Angeles, California

James A. Dewberry, Jr., D.D.S.

Private Practice Limited to Endodontics,
Dallas, Texas

Susan J. Ellenz, D.D.S.

Private Practice Limited to Endodontics,
Rockford, Illinois

James C. Hagen, B.S., M.S., Ph.D.

Formerly Associate Professor of Microbiology,
Loyola University School of Dentistry,
Maywood, Illinois

Jerome V. Pisano, D.D.S., M.S., F.A.C.D., F.I.C.D.

Formerly Clinical Associate Professor,
Department of Endodontics,
Loyola University School of Dentistry,
Maywood, Illinois

Steven R. Potashnick, D.D.S.

Clinical Assistant Professor,
Department of Restorative Dentistry,
University of Illinois at Chicago,
School of Dentistry,
Chicago, Illinois

Steven M. Sieraski, D.D.S., M.S.

Private Practice of Endodontics,
Bloomington, Illinois

Marshall H. Smulson, D.D.S., F.I.C.D.

Professor Emeritus and Formerly Chairman,
Department of Endodontics,
Loyola University School of Dentistry,
Maywood, Illinois

Sherwin Strauss, B.S., D.D.S.

Private Practice of Dentistry,
Chicago, Illinois

Jeffrey L. Wingo, R.Ph., D.D.S.

Private Practice of Periodontics,
Memphis, Tennessee

Preface

Over 25 years ago, when I started to write the first edition of this textbook, endodontic therapy was much different than it is today. Canals were filed to the radiographic apex, silver points were often used in treatment of curved canals, and culturing was a mainstay of most endodontists and every undergraduate curriculum in the United States. When I wrote that there were more maxillary first molars with four canals than there were with three canals, that there were enormous differences between preparing curved canals and straight canals, and that hand modification of files was a good idea, I was deluged with uncomplimentary mail.

When any former dental student looks back on his or her endodontic education, it appears that just about everything that was taught prior to 1970 was totally wrong. If a clinician who graduated before that time is uncertain about the correct course of therapy in a specific case, it may be best to think of what was taught in school for this condition and then do exactly the opposite in order to gain best results!

If the previous four editions of my book have helped to promote this attitude, so be it. We must question constantly the ideas of the past. It wasn't that Grossman, or Coolidge, or Sommer, Ostrander, and Crowley were wrong—they just hadn't reached the best answers. My conclusions may not last very long, either, and just as I was laughed at by claiming the "ridiculously high" percentage of two-canaled mesiobuccal roots, I don't mind it. I believe that we are just reaching the edge of great progress in the field of endodontics, and I am proud of any contribution that I have made toward that position.

My teachers and colleagues who helped me learn so much, whom I have lauded in earlier editions—Healey, Patterson, Gerstein, Evanson, Frank, Kelly, Smulson, Arens—are all deceased or retired now. I have been privileged to learn from them and to be able to use their views in these pages. A new group has been forming that will continue the progress that has been started. I am privileged to be able to learn from them, too.

In this edition I have sought to include all of the new items useful during endodontic therapy. Because of the importance of canal preparation, the methods by which the new file systems work are emphasized. This edition also features a new, separate chapter on calculation of working length. The latest views on the treatment of avulsions and review of the most significant studies on canal configuration are presented. With the added importance of avoiding cross-contamination, Jerome Pisano has rewritten completely the chapter dealing with sterilization and the microbes most likely associated with endodontic disease.

Wherever possible, I have attempted to follow up my already published cases with recent films to indicate the present conditions. Remarkably, a great percentage of these long-time patients cooperated by returning to my office or having their radiographs forwarded. I have added approximately 400 new or additional figures (mostly radiographs) since the fourth edition to add to the ability of the readers to visualize all aspects of my treatment regimens.

Like its predecessors, this edition clearly is oriented toward the clinical aspects of endodontic treatment. Endodontic therapy has been ingrained deeply into every sophisticated dental practice. Considerable knowledge and awareness of the subject are necessary to every practitioner and dental student in order that proper treatment be undertaken or, if the dentist wishes to refer such therapy to another who is more clinically competent in the field, to understand the possible parameters available.

I wish to thank all the clinicians and educators who have accepted my views and principles, applying and promulgating them to save a lot of teeth. That has been the epitome of my professional career. I also thank my partners in practice, Chris Wenckus and Chuck Neach, for allowing me the latitude to contribute to our area of dentistry in methods other than by treating patients.

I wish all of my readers continued success in endodontics.

Franklin S. Weine

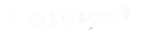

Contents

Endodontic Therapy

1 Basis for successful endodontics

As dentists became increasingly aware that natural teeth function more efficiently than any replacement, they found it worth additional effort to retain pulpally involved teeth. In the practice of dentistry the role of endodontics has greatly broadened in scope in the past decade. Although many factors are responsible, the most important reason behind this growth is the extremely high predictability of endodontic success.

Recent studies, compiling records of patients treated in dental schools and by general practitioners, indicate that 95% success is obtainable in endodontics. Increased experience, continued professional study, and training at the postgraduate level may further enhance this success ratio. Acceptance and the high predictability of endodontic therapy are often taken for granted by both practitioners and patients. To help one appreciate more fully the circumstances surrounding and the effort that has gone into the art and science of endodontics, a brief history will be presented.

HISTORY OF ENDODONTICS

Effect of Hunter's address. After the turn of the twentieth century, the finger of scorn and ridicule was pointed at the treated tooth, and routine extraction of such teeth was advocated in both dental and medical journals. The lowest point in the history of endodontics occurred shortly after an address by William Hunter, an English physician, at McGill University in 1910 on "The Role of Sepsis and Antisepsis in Medicine." Much of his subject matter came from an earlier relatively unnoticed paper by W.D. Miller, who in 1891 had expounded the intimate relationship between the dental and medical professions. Hunter vehemently criticized the prosthetic dentistry of the United States in particular, asserting that gold fillings, caps, bridges, and dentures were being built around and upon islets of frank infection and

that, instead of eliminating sepsis, these restorations were responsible for its perpetuation.

Hunter was really speaking of periodontal rather than periapical disease and even suggested scaling and debridement procedures that would be readily accepted by the periodontists of today as solutions to the problem. Despite the many hazards restricting their efforts, a number of dentists of that time were able to perform a high caliber of endodontic therapy. Without radiographic and bacteriologic control, however, a considerable number of endodontic cases ended in failure. Dentists who disagreed with the philosophy of endodontics or were unwilling to spend the greater time required for therapy (compared with extraction) eagerly publicized the failures. Billings and Rosenow applied Hunter's views to the pulpless tooth, and their animal experiments indicated a definite relationship between periapical and systemic disease.

Early use of x rays. Rhein soon adopted the roentgen ray for endodontic use to determine canal length and degree of filling. These initial radiographs were used by some as adjuncts to treatment, but they were used by others to evaluate previous therapy performed without such help. Even when x-ray guidance is coupled with present advanced knowledge, some cases are difficult to treat. Endodontic therapy performed in the nineteenth and early twentieth centuries without radiographs or the knowledge of bacteriology, and later evaluated by x-ray studies, was determined in general to be an abysmal failure. Rather than recognize the limitations that had forced earlier workers to have so many failures and attempt to organize a regimen that would increase chances for success, members of the health professions demanded extraction of pulpless teeth for their patients and, in fact, full-mouth extractions for patients with chronic diseases.

Not desiring criticism from physicians and happy to take the easier way out that tooth removal afforded, dentists subscribed to wanton extraction in preference to endodontic or periodontal therapy. The net result left many persons with impaired nutrition, since they were unable to masticate properly certain foods required in a balanced diet.

Reacceptance of endodontics.   Fortunately some pioneer endodontists—Coolidge, Prinz, Sharp, Blayney, Appleton, and others—launched a counterattack against the extractionists. By demonstration of successful cases based on sound biologic principles, these men illustrated methods by which strategic teeth could be saved without any danger to the patient's health—in fact, with improvement in health.

By the late 1930s the corner had been turned in endodontics, and treatment of the pulpless tooth had become an integral part of dentistry. Continued research on a clinical and laboratory basis developed techniques, methods of evaluation, and selection of materials to further increase the success ratio. The American Association of Endodontists was formed to disseminate interest and develop increased skill in the area. Under the direction of Dr. Louis Grossman of Philadelphia, international conferences on endodontics were held where interested persons from all over the world met and discussed mutual problems.

PRINCIPLES OF ENDODONTIC THERAPY

The results of these organizations and efforts by the pioneers of the field led to the development of basic principles of endodontic practice. Since research and clinical analysis have caused elimination or alteration of some earlier guidelines, I want to enumerate the principles and philosophies that are the basis for this text.

Objective.   The objective of endodontic therapy is restoration of the treated tooth to its proper form and function in the masticatory apparatus, in a healthy state.

Dentists must realize that initiation of endodontic therapy for a patient would not be a responsibility taken lightly. Although those who in the past decried endodontic treatment as a significant health hazard were surely incorrect in their basic premise, improper therapy may have an effect on a patient's systemic condition. By the same token, proper endodontic treatment may alleviate a systemic condition not thought to be related to a dental problem. Fig. 1-1 illustrates such a situation.

Basic phases of therapy.   There are three basic phases in endodontic treatment. First is the diagnostic phase, in which the disease to be treated is determined and the treatment plan developed. Second is the preparatory phase, when the contents of the root canal are removed and the canal prepared for the filling material. The third phase involves the filling or obliteration of the canal to gain a hermetic seal with an inert material as close as possible to the cementodentinal junction.

Endodontic therapy may be thought of as a tripod, with the perfectly treated tooth on a pedestal and every leg representing a basic phase. If any leg is faulty, the entire system may fail. Although every leg is a separate portion, in the overall situation each phase must be meticulously carried out to obtain success. Every facet of treatment must be performed in a predetermined manner, with every step having its definite position in the series of procedures. Therefore much of this book, as well as other clinically oriented endodontic literature, is presented in a carefully outlined form to emphasize the importance of following the same step-by-step procedure for every case.

Importance of debridement.   Endodontic therapy is essentially a debridement procedure that requires the removal of the irritants of the canal and periapical tissue if success is to be gained. The debridement may be carried out in various ways as the case demands and may include instrumentation of the canal, placement of medicaments and irrigants, and electrolysis or surgery. No cases lend themselves to successful treatment without some degree of debridement.

From time to time considerable emphasis in clinics or papers is given to various methods of canal filling, and the necessity for correct debridement is not always properly emphasized. Although preparation of the canal is often tedious and its results not immediately evident when a postoperative radiograph of a canal filling is viewed, there is no doubt that canal debridement is of paramount importance. When a canal is properly prepared, any of the accepted methods of filling will almost certainly produce a successful result.

Use of the rubber dam mandatory.   As complex dentistry has developed, with restorative techniques utilizing telescopes, splints, superstructures, copings, etc., endodontic access is often extremely difficult. For this reason it is frequently best to be sure of proper access to the canal before rubber dam application so that the structures can be used

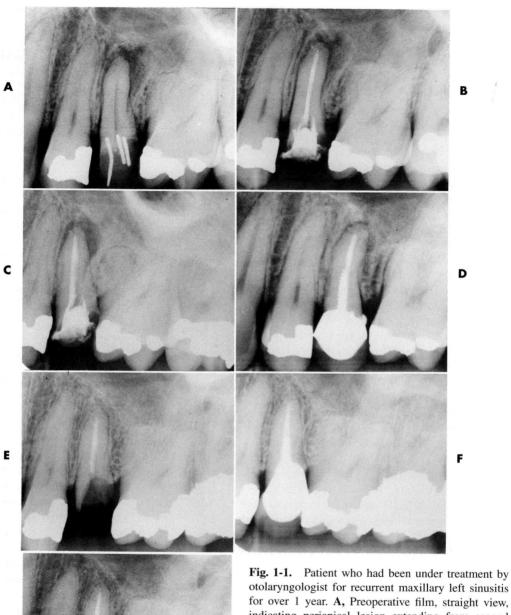

Fig. 1-1. Patient who had been under treatment by otolaryngologist for recurrent maxillary left sinusitis for over 1 year. **A,** Preoperative film, straight view, indicating periapical lesion extending from second bicuspid and eroding the floor of the left maxillary sinus. **B,** Immediate postoperative film, straight view. **C,** Angled view from the distal. As soon as the canals were prepared (Type II canal system), the sinusitis stopped. Canals were filled with laterally condensed gutta-percha and Wach's paste sealer. **D,** One year later, lesion had decreased in size considerably. **E,** Three years after original treatment, the crown and post had been dislodged. The entire wall of the sinus adjacent to the treated tooth had been reconstituted, according to the radiograph. **F,** Five years after original treatment; compare to **A. G,** Twelve years after original treatment, still perfect healing. (Restoration by Dr. James Discipio, Berwyn, Ill.)

as a guide. However, once access is obtained, the rubber dam should be placed immediately and under no circumstances should an enlarging instrument be used without its presence. Several excuses are given for avoiding the use of a rubber dam in endodontic therapy, but all are basically procrastinations and easily refutable. Some of the excuses offered are the additional time required for application (rarely more than a few seconds), plans for the tooth to be left open anyway, and lack of supragingival tooth structure (a crown-lengthening procedure may be performed).

The original use of the rubber dam was to aid in the gaining of an aseptic environment, and this is still a major purpose. Of equal importance is confinement of the irrigants, most of which are distasteful. The greatest need, however, is to prevent the aspiration of an instrument, a potentially grave matter. The mental anguish experienced by the dentist guilty of such an incident, plus the current attitudes of the courts in such matters, makes the placement of a rubber dam an extremely small premium for the excellent insurance it provides (Fig. 1-2).

The Kansas Supreme Court ruled that the general dentist performing endodontic treatment on a patient must apply the same precautions during therapy as those employed by an endodontic specialist. There is no question that whereas many general dentists do not utilize the rubber dam during endodontic therapy, virtually all endodontists keep the dam in place. If a patient aspirates an instrument due to the failure of the dentist to place the dam, the practitioner is considered negligent, according to the Kansas Supreme Court, since the precautions normally taken by the specialist were not applied.

Great respect due the periapical tissue during treatment. Although some techniques advocate intentional irritation of periapical tissue, many studies have indicated that all enlargement and filling procedures should be carried out within the canal. These studies have shown that even where there are large radiolucencies, when debridement and filling are carried out within the confines of the canal, healing will take place in most cases without surgery. Overinstrumentation is the most frequent cause of postoperative pain. Since the dentist should always be concerned with the elimination or reduction of pain, an accurate determination of canal length must be made and strictly adhered to during the enlargement and filling pro-

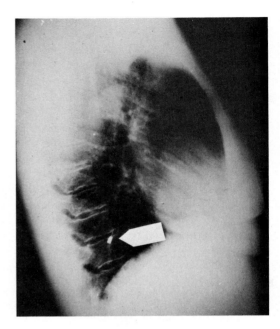

Fig. 1-2. Chest x-ray film showing aspirated file *(arrow)* in bronchial tree. Rubber dam was not used because dentist intended to leave the tooth open. (Courtesy Dr. Paul Hoffer, University of Chicago Hospitals.)

cedures. Proper treatment of periapical tissues also means that caustic drugs should not be used as medicaments.

Even though endodontic therapy involves working within the tooth, it is the surrounding structures and their response that determine success or failure.

Proper restoration the culmination of success. Sufficient confidence is warranted in the endodontic result to insist that a proper restoration be placed on the treated tooth as soon as possible. Nothing is more disheartening than to see a well-treated tooth require extraction because of fracture following the placement of a restoration that does not afford cuspal coverage. Equally discouraging is a fracture or secondary caries that develop when the posttreatment temporary filling is retained for an extended period to see if success has been gained (Fig. 1-3). A greater number of endodontically treated teeth are lost because of fracture due to improper restorations than because of poor endodontic result. Proper restoration of the treated tooth is an integral part of therapy and must be explained to the patient as a part of the treatment plan.

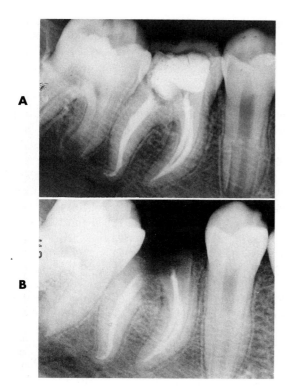

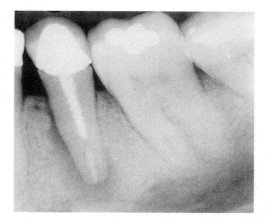

Fig. 1-4. Well-treated mandibular second bicuspid with proper post room prepared by the endodontist. The restorative dentist, however, did not match the specialist in skill and judgment. A tapered, serrated post was used, screwed into the tooth rather than cemented passively, and a fracture resulted. The restorative dentist wanted to take advantage of the extra retention that such a post system offered. Instead, an unnecessary failure resulted.

Fig. 1-3. **A,** Immediate postoperative film of mandibular first molar, slight angle from the mesial, in 14-year-old patient. The case was quite difficult due to the extreme curvature of the distal root, but the result was excellent. Canals were filled with laterally condensed gutta-percha and Wach's paste sealer. **B,** Eighteen months later, no permanent restoration had been placed, and decay had passed through the furcation. Despite the excellent treatment, the tooth was lost. Note the mesial tipping of the second molar is already present.

Other discouraging situations transpire when the restorative dentist places an inadequate or improper crown, onlay, or amalgam restoration; fails to provide cuspal protection when needed; or fabricates an inadequate or damaging post/core system (Fig. 1-4).

Postoperative obervation necessary. Despite the high degree of success, some failures will occur. Some of these may be successfully re-treated, and many will heal after surgery. Unless the patient is impressed with the necessity for recall, some of the initial failures that can be reversed will not be intercepted in time.

Case presentation to set the stage. A case presentation should be given to each patient for any phase of dental treatment, whether the treatment needed is only an oral prophylaxis or encompasses a full-mouth reconstruction. If endodontic procedures are required in an overall treatment plan, the reasons for such therapy should be explained. At the time that the endodontic portion is to be commenced, a further examination should be given. Case presentation for endodontics should briefly explain the responsibilities of the patient and the dentist, the time involved, the prognosis, and the fee (including restoration). Most patients prefer a brief description of the phases of therapy, and a suggested method of presentation will be found in Chapter 2.

At times a patient will be seen for the first appointment on an emergency basis when endodontics is required and a proper case presentation is difficult to perform. Correct procedure then is to make a brief explanation of the need to retain the involved tooth and utilize the available time to ensure the patient relief from pain. Time should be allowed at the next appointment for the presentation.

INDICATIONS AND CONTRAINDICATIONS

There are few true contraindications to endodontic therapy. Two frequent causes for the extraction of pulpally involved teeth are a patient's inability to afford the fee for endodontic work and a dentist's inability to perform the necessary service adequately. The few true contraindications include insufficient periodontal support, a canal unsuitable for instrumentation or for surgery, a tooth that is not restorable after therapy, the presence of massive resorption, a nonstrategic tooth, or a vertical fracture.

Contraindications

Patient unable to afford fee. The significance of this category is diminishing for two reasons, one economic and one educational. As society increases in affluence and as many employee fringe benefits are extended to include dental treatment, the fee for endodontic care is brought within the reach of a greater portion of the population than ever before, and this percentage is increasing. Also, with the dental IQ of the public increasing as a result of hygiene programs in schools, magazine articles, television programs and commercials, and other publicity, more patients are understanding the true value of each tooth as an integral part of the chewing mechanism and are able to realize that retention of the tooth in question is well worth the fee involved. On a purely economic basis the fee for endodontic therapy plus restoration is usually less than the fee for a replacement by a fixed partial denture, making the retention of the tooth a more reasonable undertaking than its loss and replacement.

Inability of the dentist. With improved instruments and filling materials, the performance of endodontic therapy has become much easier than it was only a few years ago. Continuing instructional courses are offered by most dental institutions and dental societies in an effort to increase the knowledge and skill of those interested. Some states are now making refresher courses mandatory for license renewal. The use of extracted teeth for practice in the procedures of endodontic treatment gives excellent exercise in improving technique. For these reasons the ability of the average dentist to perform routine treatment is enhanced. In addition, there is an excellent geographic distribution of enough specialists and general practitioners with great skill in endodontics who are able to retain all but the most complicated cases on a referral basis.

Insufficient periodontal support. In evaluating periapical and/or pulpal disease, the practitioner must make a complete periodontal evaluation. Unless sufficient support is present to ensure retention of the tooth, endodontic treatment is contraindi-

cated. Occasionally endodontic treatment is required to retain periodontally questionable teeth, as when an apparent periodontal lesion is due to pulpal involvement. Further guidance in making this periodontal evaluation will appear in Chapter 2.

Canal instrumentation not practical. This problem may be satisfactorily solved with surgical treatment. Three types of canal conditions are encountered that may contraindicate endodontic therapy.

Instruments broken within the canal can rarely be recovered or bypassed. In a study by Grossman there was a relatively good prognosis if the broken instruments were within the apical third of vital teeth with normal periapical tissue, whereas other situations involving broken instruments usually resulted in failure (Fig. 1-5).

A second type of inoperable canal occurs when irregular dentinal sclerosis closes portions of the canal so as to make the passage of the smallest enlarging instrument impossible (Fig. 1-6). Since this dystrophic calcification rarely completely obliterates the canal, careful exploring procedures often enable the apex to be reached. If the apex is not attainable, particularly when a periapical radiolucency is present, treatment is contraindicated.

The third type of inoperable canal occurs when the canal anatomy is such that a sharp dilaceration or a series of dilacerations makes enlargement impossible. Although on occasion such canals are successfully treated, unless the tooth has tremendous strategic value, the best advice is extraction. Teeth of this type require two or three times the normal working time for enlargement and filling, cause great frustration during treatment, and in the end often are failures. The same amount of time spent in replacement will usually afford a better final result.

Interestingly, two of the endodontic contraindications—sharp dilaceration and a calcified canal—frequently lead to the other contraindication mentioned, a broken instrument. In some of these cases the tooth may be saved by surgical intervention; however when that is impossible or impractical, extraction becomes inevitable.

Nonrestorable tooth. Since the objective of endodontics is to return the treated tooth to good form and function, it is necessary to place a proper restoration after completion of the root canal filling. The best canal filling is useless if it is impossible to place a restoration. With alveoloplasty, gingivoplasty, improved dowel procedures,

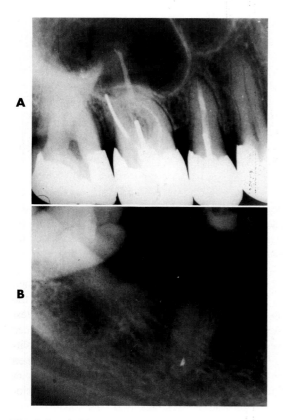

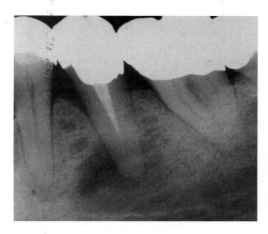

Fig. 1-6. Mandibular bicuspid with large radiolucency and dentinal sclerosis preventing preparation anywhere near apex. Tooth was symptomatic and required extraction.

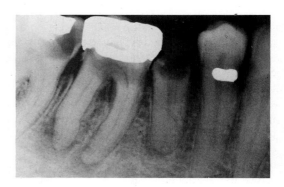

Fig. 1-7. Severe furcation caries in mandibular first molar and root caries in second bicuspid necessitated extractions.

Fig. 1-5. **A,** Four-year postoperative radiograph shows maxillary first molar with normal radiographic appearance. File was broken in mesiobuccal canal; however, since the tooth was asymptomatic with normal periapical tissue before treatment, the case was completed. Canal had been enlarged to size 25 before accident, and file is very close to apical foramen. **B,** Mandibular second bicuspid with what appears to be segments of two instruments near apex. Case has been symptomatic, and periapical tissue was not normal. Obstruction could not be bypassed, and tooth required extraction. (In **A,** restorations by Dr. Rod Nystul, formerly of Park Ridge, Ill.)

and other techniques, many more teeth are now restorable than with the limited techniques that were formerly available; however, some teeth still remain for which proper restoration is not possible. Among these are teeth with severe root caries, furcation caries, poor crown-root ration, and internally weakened root (Fig. 1-7).

Massive resorption. Resorption may be of either internal or external variety; if the resorption is of extremely large dimension, with perforations, therapy for the tooth is contraindicated. The resorptive process occurs because of phagocytic cells that destroy dentin. Unless all these cells are removed, either by surgery or by intracanal instrumentation, the process will continue. A large resorptive defect that is found on only one portion of the tooth may be surgically (Chapter 11) or nonsurgically (Chapter 16) correctable. Defects that have not perforated may respond to nonsurgical treatment. It is the severe defect involving large portions of the tooth structure that makes successful treatment impractical (Fig. 1-8).

Nonstrategic tooth. At the time that treatment is considered, a tooth may not appear to have great strategic value. However, before condemnation to extraction, thought should be given to possible future needs for the tooth. A good example for

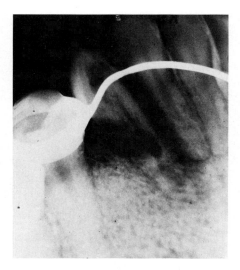

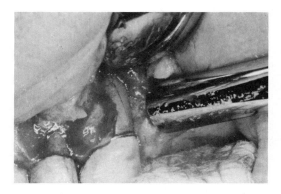

Fig. 1-9. Vertical fracture of maxillary cuspid. Area did not heal after routine endodontic therapy, and periapical surgery was suggested. When flap was raised, a defect to the apex was seen.

Fig. 1-8. Massive internal resorption of mandibular cuspid contraindicated endodontic therapy.

consideration would be an involved third molar in a patient with multiple missing teeth and a high caries incidence. Although the patient still retains other posterior abutments, the tooth probably should be retained if treatable because of possible further tooth loss. On the other hand, a pulpally involved third molar in a patient with full dental complement in a well-cared-for mouth is obviously better extracted than retained.

The use of root amputation to retain precarious teeth has aided immeasurably in allowing key abutments to avoid extraction. However, when a case for amputation presents a poor prognosis but the adjacent teeth appear to be good candidates for bridge abutments, loss of the involved tooth appears justified.

Vertical fractures. Vertical fractures through root structure have an almost hopeless prognosis (Fig. 1-9). Many exotic treatments have been suggested, including circumferential root wiring, "zipper" amalgam implants, and removal of the smaller fragment. Experience shows, however, that in only the rarest instance does any measure of success result. A related condition that often has symptomatology similar to that of teeth requiring endodontic treatment, but may have a hopeless prognosis, is the cracked-tooth syndrome (Chapter 2).

Indications

Any teeth not contraindicated are excellent candidates for successful endodontic therapy. Many of the supposed contraindications of the past have been proved false. These include the presence of severe disease, a number of previously treated teeth, advanced age of the patient, or large size of the radiolucency. A brief discussion of a few of these false contraindications follows. In the presence of serious illnesses (e.g., rheumatic fever, malignancies, coronary artery disease), endodontic treatment is definitely preferable to extraction. Bender and Seltzer have demonstrated that there is a lower incidence of bacteremia after endodontic treatment than after extraction. For patients with heart problems, endodontics requires no alteration of existing anticoagulant administration. Patients with malignancies may be undergoing radiation therapy that makes extraction sites conducive to osteoradionecrosis.

Some time ago it was contended that no patient should have more than five treated teeth and that extraction was indicated for any beyond that number having pulpal involvement. Of all the supposed contraindications to endodontic therapy, this is probably the most ridiculous. Many patients have two or three times that many successfully treated teeth; some reports show patients with all their teeth treated. In fact, if any patient has multiple successful cases, the prognosis for additional teeth is excellent. On the other hand, a patient with a history of endodontic failures should be evaluated cautiously if another tooth requires treatment, since this patient may have poor recuperative ability, unusual canal anatomy, or some rarely found condition that militates against successful treatment.

PROGNOSIS FOR ENDODONTIC THERAPY

One of the first questions asked by patients concerning treatment deals with the anticipated degree of success. Endodontics is extremely fortunate in that the degree of success enjoyed is probably the best found in any phase of dentistry, much higher than that in periodontics and other phases of reconstructive dentistry. This degree of predictability has been the factor most responsible for the acceptance of endodontics by the general practitioner, who is acutely aware that a treated tooth may be counted on to perform any function in the oral cavity that an untreated tooth performs in a tremendous preponderance of cases. Some of the factors that affect prognosis in endodontics will now be discussed.

Studies dealing with success ratios. Many studies have investigated the degree of success in endodontics, using certain variables for comparison. One of the most interesting was reported by Ingle and Beveridge, indicating that undergraduate students at the University of Washington were capable of obtaining 95% success. The significance of this study points out that when a carefully followed course of therapy is instituted, results are strongly in favor of success. Undergraduate students treating their initial cases have close supervision and little opportunity to deviate from predetermined patterns of therapy. The advisability of remaining within a regimen of this type is affirmed by the results.

Strindberg reported on degree of success, basing his criteria on the point to which the canal was filled—whether past the radiographic apex, exactly to it, or short of it. All types, even those teeth grossly overfilled, responded with success more than 90% of the time, although teeth that were filled slightly short of the apex had the highest ratio of success.

Results of filling after positive and negative cultures. Successes after positive and negative culture tests have been reported. Except for the study by Bender and Seltzer, in which the degree of success was the same for both groups, filling after negative cultures consistently gave a higher degree of success. In the seven studies surveyed, the average degree of success after a negative culture was 95%, whereas the degree of success was lowered to an average of 88% after a positive culture. In Bender and Seltzer's study, both groups showed 82% of cases still responding favorably. On the average for all the other studies, figures well into the 90% bracket were consistently reported. Even teeth that were filled after a positive reading (i.e., in the presence of active microorganisms) had many more favorable results than unfavorable results.

Most of the studies referred to were based on statistical information about teeth treated in the late 1950s or early 1960s. Since that time the emergence of important new endodontic materials, particularly standardized instruments and stainless steel instruments, as well as improved cleansing and lubricating agents and better understanding of the biologic basis for endodontic therapy, would undoubtedly raise the already impressive statistics to an even higher level.

Prognosis for older patients. The prognosis for older patients is actually better than that for the younger age group on a statistical basis. This is probably because of the tighter apical foramina, lack of completely patent auxiliary canals, and dense periapical bone, and because the teeth of patients who have reached advanced age usually are healthier specimens than those of patients whose teeth succumb at earlier ages.

Elderly patients rarely have painful exacerbations during treatment, with a tendency toward a chronic type of problem rather than acute fulmination. This means that intratreatment visits to relieve pain that disturb the normal day's scheduling of patients are infrequent. Although healing for older patients might be somewhat retarded, particularly if certain systemic problems are present, in general they heal satisfactorily (Fig. 1-10). In fact, reports of healing in many septagenarians and octagenarians are included in this text without specific comments because of their good healing potential (see Figs. 13-1 and 13-2, *A* and *B,* in particular).

Significance of large or longstanding radiolucencies. Large radiolucencies will usually heal extremely well, often without surgery (Fig. 1-11). Studies have been published to indicate that the success ratio for teeth with radiolucencies is lower than that for teeth with normal periapical bone. This is contrary to my clinical observation and certain unpublished findings of groups at Loyola University and Indiana University. Pulpless teeth are usually easier to treat than those that have vital tissue, since no anesthetic is required and the solvents used as intracanal irrigants are not resisted by vital tissue; the necrotic material that remains is highly susceptible to the solvent action.

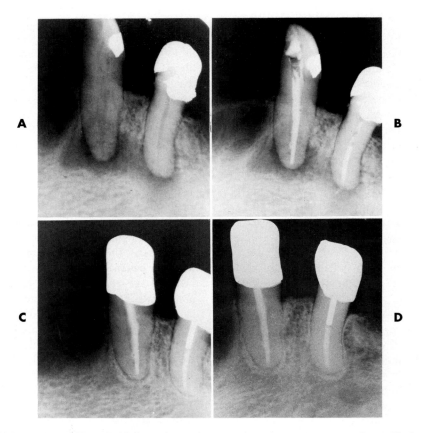

Fig. 1-10. Healing ability of elderly patients. **A,** Large periapical lesions around mandibular cuspid and bicuspid of 73-year-old patient. **B,** Canal fillings with laterally condensed gutta-percha. **C,** Perfect healing 18 months later, teeth are serving as partial denture abutments. **D,** Perfect healing still demonstrated 15 years after original treatment. (Restoration by Dr. Robert Wheeler, Chicago.)

The longer a periapical lesion is present, the better the chance that it will undergo cystic degeneration and convert from a granuloma, with excellent healing potential, to an apical periodontal cyst. There is considerable evidence that this type of cyst will heal after nonsurgical endodontic treatment, although in some cases surgery does become necessary. Even when a periapical lesion is known to have been present for a long time and there are the classic cystic appearances for a very radiolucent lesion with a sclerotic border, routine treatment should be undertaken with equanimity. An observation period should follow, during which radiographs are taken at 6-month intervals. Generally, healing will occur (Fig. 1-12). If the lesion persists or becomes larger, surgery may be performed (see Fig. 11-3).

Although the percentage is quite low, in some cases surgery must be utilized in order to achieve a successful result. Many such examples are presented in Chapter 11. Generally, a suitable observation period has indicated lack of healing before any attempt at surgical intervention.

In some instances, however, surgery must be instituted early in the treatment plan. Some radiolucent lesions may exhibit an aggressive or suspicious appearance. In these cases, the canal preparation and filling are performed in a minimal number of appointments. Periapical surgery follows at the same appointment, or at a subsequent sitting soon thereafter, to gain information from the biopsy. Depending upon the histologic diagnosis, the treatment is continued accordingly (Fig. 1-13).

The quality of healing of some radiolucencies might surprise even the operator on occasion. Fig. 1-14 illustrates a case where it was not certain if the lesion was of endodontic origin. However, since any subsequent surgery probably would

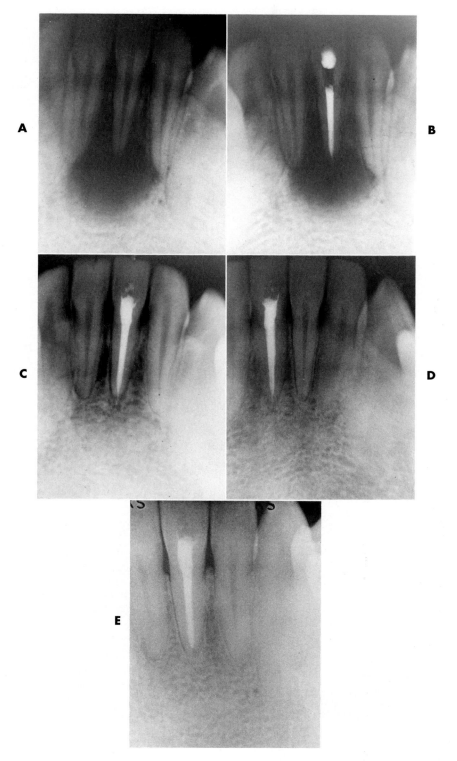

Fig. 1-11 **A,** Large periapical radiolucency associated with mandibular incisor. **B,** Canal filling with gutta-percha and lateral condensation. No surgery was performed. **C,** Excellent healing after 12 months. **D,** Complete healing at 30 months. Note that canal filling was just short of radiographic apex in **C,** but it now is several millimeters short of radiographic apex, indicating apposition of apical cementum. **E,** Healing is still perfect 17 years after original treatment. (Restoration by Dr. Morton Schreiber, Highland Park, Ill.)

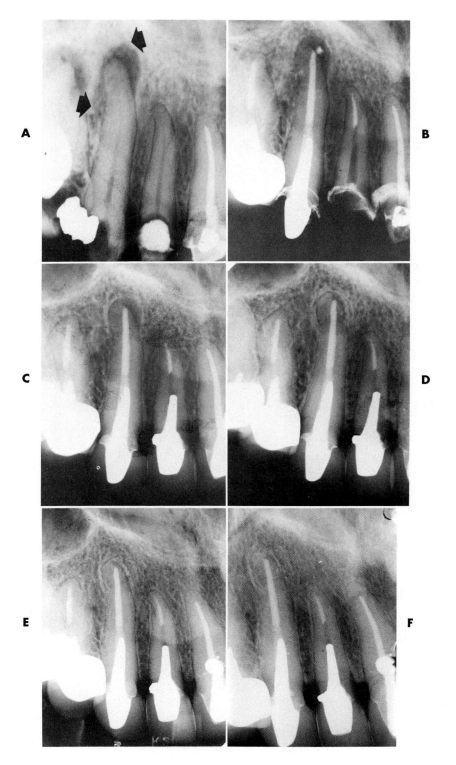

Fig. 1-12. **A,** Large periapical radiolucency associated with maxillary cuspid. Patient had been aware that the problem was present for several years before treatment. Lesion extended down the labial surface of the root for a considerable distance. Arrows indicate apical and cervical extents of the radiolucency. **B,** Three months after canal filling with gutta-percha and lateral condensation. No surgery was performed. **C,** One year after treatment, area is much smaller. **D,** Excellent healing 2 years after treatment. **E,** Area 14 years after treatment continues to look excellent. **F,** Twenty-three years after original treatment. Periapical lesion completely healed. Also, note canal filling is now several millimeters from the radiographic apex. Compare to **B** and **C,** where it was flush to the radiographic apex. (Restorations by Dr. Sherwin Laff, Chicago.)

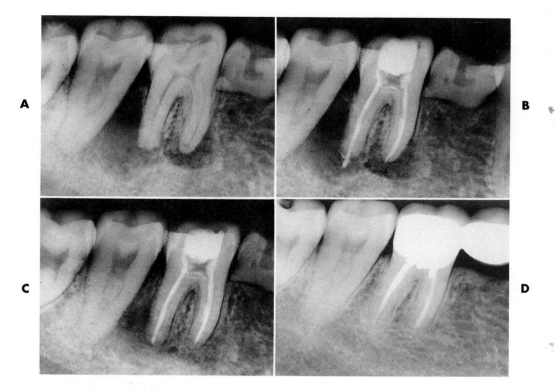

Fig. 1-13. **A,** Preoperative film of mandibular first molar. The periapical lesion did not appear typical to me, and I was afraid that it was other than purely endodontic in origin, although electric pulp testing gave no response. **B,** Accordingly, the canals were prepared and filled with laterally condensed gutta-percha and Tubliseal, followed by periapical curettage. Biopsy indicated periapical granuloma. **C,** Nine months later, advanced healing is noted. With favorable biopsy report, restoration was undertaken. **D,** Twelve years after original treatment, healing is perfect. The primary molar had loosened and was extracted, with the first molar serving as posterior bridge abutment. (Restoration by Dr. Sherwin Strauss, Chicago.)

jeopardize the vitality of the involved tooth, the canal was prepared and filled. The result was quite gratifying, but not entirely expected.

Significance of large, rapidly growing radio-lucencies. If large radiolucencies of a longstanding nature have healing ability, what is the reaction to treatment of large, rapidly growing lesions? Rapidly growing lesions that are not of endodontic origin may be very serious, and concern about a malignancy in such instances is justifiable. If, however, the lesion is definitely of endodontic origin, the prognosis is quite good for nonsurgical treatment.

Generally, if a lesion of endodontic origin grows very rapidly, it will heal very rapidly with proper treatment. Fig. 1-15 demonstrates such a case, in which a large, diffuse lesion was known to be less than 6 months in development. After correct ther-

apy, it healed perfectly in that amount of time.

Significance of periodontal disease. The periodontal condition of the involved tooth has an important bearing on the prognosis. As will be discussed in Chapter 13, necrotic teeth that simulate periodontal disease, but are not in fact periodontally involved, respond well to endodontic therapy. On the other hand, if a periodontal condition is present but untreated on an endodontically involved tooth, the prognosis is poor. Since the periapical area remains within the confines of the periodontal ligament space, the disease process from the periodontal condition will retard or prevent proper healing if endodontic treatment alone is performed.

Reaching the apex. Ability to reach the apical foramen has definite implications. Since the objective of filling is to seal this foramen, inability to

A   **B**   **C**

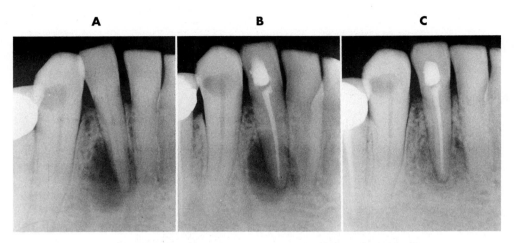

Fig. 1-14. Unusual healing of periapical lesion and realignment of affected tooth. **A,** Preoperative film of mandibular lateral incisor area. A large periapical lesion is present that seems to involve the lateral incisor, but no etiology was apparent. The alignment of the tooth was poor, with a large space between it and the adjacent central incisor and overlapping of the cuspid. The patient stated that the tooth had gradually taken this position over the previous several years after being straight originally. Electric pulp testing gave some, but not normal, response. However, it was decided that if surgery were employed to curette the lesion, the vitality of the pulp probably would be compromised, so endodontic therapy was instituted. **B,** After canal preparation and filling with laterally condensed gutta-percha and Wach's paste sealer in two appointments. The tooth was entered originally without anesthetic, but the patient could not tolerate the pain. A local anesthetic was administered, but it was impossible to tell the condition of the pulp upon extirpation. **C,** Eighteen months later, with excellent periapical healing. Even more surprising, the alignment of the tooth is greatly improved.

debride and fill this area may alter the prognosis. There are various reasons why an apical foramen may not be reachable, even by the most expert operator. Severe curvatures, broken instruments, miscalculation of canal length, development of ledges, and inadequate instrumentation are among the most common reasons. A preoperative radiograph can often indicate if the apex will be difficult to reach. If so, the patient should be informed about the chance of failure. When the pulp is vital and the periapical tissue normal before treatment, a good prognosis persists even if the root canal filling must be terminated a few millimeters short of the apex.

However, when a preoperative radiolucency is present, unless the apical portion of the canal is reachable with the cleansing instruments and the irritants responsible for apical inflammation can be removed, the prognosis is poor. In these cases, apical surgery should be instituted when possible; otherwise, extraction is necessary.

Many teeth have apical foramina located some distance short of the radiographic apex (Fig. 1-16).

Often this is revealed by the preoperative radiograph or by subsequent instrumentation and measurement radiographs. In these cases a favorable prognosis results when the canal is enlarged and filled to the true apical foramen. Any attempt at overinstrumentation to reach the radiographic apex will result in intratreatment pain and a diminished success ratio.

Re-treatment of failures. Analysis of failures will be discussed further in subsequent chapters, and suggestions will be made concerning re-treating these cases. When a failure by another practitioner makes re-treatment necessary, a careful diagnosis must be performed to ascertain the prognosis. The most common cause of failure is lack of apical seal, which may be diagnosed by radiograph in some instances. Typical of this kind of failure is the extremely short canal filling, the single cone "swimming" in the much larger canal, and the failure to follow root curvature. Another type of failure is seen when a canal has been left unfilled in a multicanaled tooth because it went unnoticed by the previous operator. When these

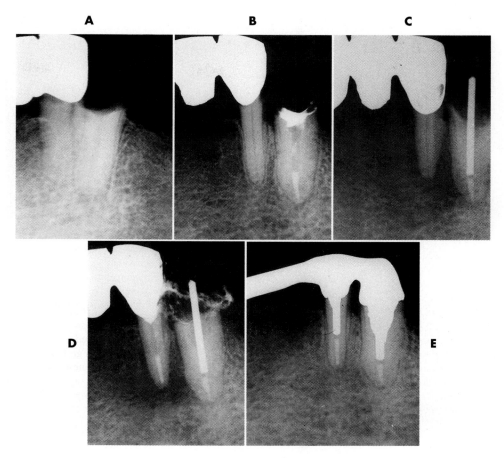

Fig. 1-15. Healing of a rapidly growing lesion of endodontic origin. **A,** Preoperative radiograph of mandibular cuspid, obviously requiring endodontic treatment because of massive caries. Deep decay under the adjacent lateral incisor is seen, as well as a failing bridge abutment. **B,** Treatment is completed easily on the cuspid; canal filled with laterally condensed gutta-percha and Wach's paste, with post room prepared. The patient was returned to the restorative dentist to remove the defective bridge and fabricate a temporary bridge. For several reasons, this took almost six months to accomplish. **C,** Patient developed a swelling and rushed to the endodontist to treat the lateral incisor. The preoperative film indicated a very large, diffuse radiolucency extending almost to the treated cuspid. **D,** After emergency treatment (Chapter 5), the patient did well and the tooth was completed similarly to the cuspid. **E,** Six months later, a splint has been fashioned over the two treated teeth together with the opposite cuspid to anchor an overdenture. The radiolucency is completely gone; compare to **D.** (Restoration by Dr. Edward LeMire, Chicago.)

obvious causes are determined to be present, the prognosis for re-treatment is good.

However, when treatment appears to have been adequate yet unsuccessful, the patient should be warned of the possible need for surgery (if practical) or continued failure (if re-treatment is undertaken).

ROLE OF ENDODONTICS IN RESTORATIVE DENTISTRY

The next segments of this chapter will discuss the role of endodontics in the three major areas of general practice: restorative, reconstructive, and prosthetic dentistry. Many dental practices include all three of these areas as well as other important phases of dentistry, whereas some practices are principally involved in only one of these fields.

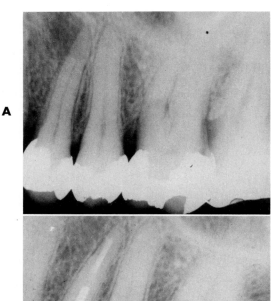

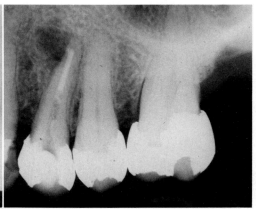

Fig. 1-16. **A,** Radiolucency on mesial surface of root of maxillary first bicuspid. **B,** Canal filling stops short of radiographic apex, but sealer extrusion seems to indicate exit site of apical foramen. **C,** Radiograph a year later shows complete resolution, indicating that canal was well filled. (Restoration by Dr. Jacob Lippert, Chicago.)

The importance of endodontics in any general practice is to be emphasized.

The restorative dentist is principally concerned with the placement of restorations in teeth with carious lesions and the replacement of restorations that show faults due to improper margins, contour, or function. This dentist is additionally interested in replacing missing teeth with bridges of short or medium span and avoiding the use of removable partial dentures.

Miller states that the goal of modern restorative dentistry is preservation of the masticatory apparatus for the life of the patient. Without endodontics, this goal becomes extremely difficult to attain in a significant number of patients. Some of the situations in which the use of endodontics is necessary will now be discussed.

Saving the irreplaceable tooth. The most posterior tooth in any dental arch cannot be easily replaced with a fixed prosthesis. Cantilever bridges, full-arch splints, and similar prostheses fall into the category of reconstructive rather than restorative dentistry. The most typical case to illustrate the importance of the posterior tooth can be demonstrated by the pulpal or periapical involvement of a mandibular second molar. Unless this tooth is retained by endodontic intervention (Fig. 1-17), supereruption of the maxillary second molar may occur and cause the extraction of that tooth as well.

In some patients a second molar already may be missing and the first molar involved. Unless this tooth is retained, fixed replacement becomes extremely difficult, and a removable partial denture is usually indicated.

If a single irreplaceable tooth is important to save, two irreplaceable teeth are twice as important to save, as demonstrated in Fig. 1-18, involving two maxillary molars. When two teeth are involved, treatment of both should be attempted rather than deciding which tooth would be better, then treating that one and extracting the other. If, from a financial standpoint or for another acceptable reason, only one may be saved, it is best to

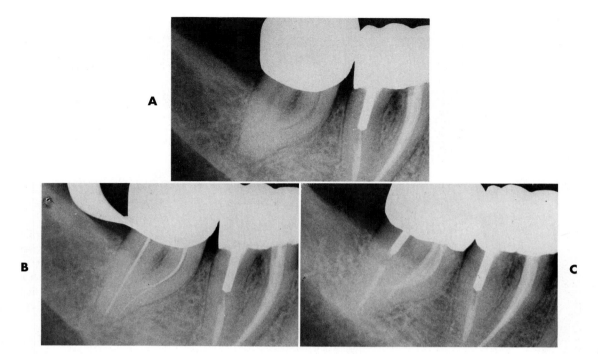

Fig. 1-17.   Endodontic treatment to retain the irreplaceable tooth. **A,** Mandibular second molar, tender to percussion and temperature changes, requiring endodontic therapy. **B,** Case is quite difficult due to curvature of the mesial canals; however, since the tooth is irreplaceable, therapy is continued. **C,** Three years later, tooth is symptom free and a desirable result is assured. (Restoration by Dr. Steve Labkon, Kenilworth, Ill.)

initiate treatment for both, ensure that at least one is salvageable, and then make a choice. If one is extracted first, the one retained may prove to be untreatable or unrestorable, and the other, already extracted tooth has been wasted. In this scenario, nothing is left.

Retaining the posterior bridge abutment.   One of the most important indications for endodontic treatment is a pulpally involved molar with an edentulous space anterior to it. If such a tooth is lost, the entire segment becomes edentulous, with no posterior abutment for a fixed partial denture available. Only a removable partial prosthesis can then be used to replace the missing teeth (Fig. 1-19).

Preserving enough remaining teeth for use with a fixed partial denture.   In addition to the absence of an abutment posterior to an edentulous area, removable partial dentures are indicated when the ratio between the number of missing teeth in an arch and the number of retained teeth in the same arch approaches one to one (Fig. 1-20).

The presence of multiple teeth requiring endodontic care in one arch should be no stumbling block. Many successful results are seen where quadrants are entirely composed of treated teeth (Fig. 1-21). If endodontic treatment were not performed, the number of teeth requiring extraction would force replacement by a removable partial denture only.

Lessening the length of bridge span.   When pulpal involvement has occurred in teeth adjacent to an edentulous area, some pracitioners have recommended extraction to use only uninvolved teeth as bridge abutments. Experience with treated teeth as abutments has now demonstrated their ability to serve as well as uninvolved teeth (Fig. 1-21). In fact, wherever it can be achieved, the reduction in length of bridge span made possible by using treated teeth as abutments reduces both periodontal strain and possible damage to the retainers.

Improving esthetic results in an arch with diastemas and involved anterior teeth.   The replacement of an anterior tooth with a fixed partial denture is usually a relatively simple procedure. However, when the involved arch has natural diastemas, the esthetic result is extremely poor

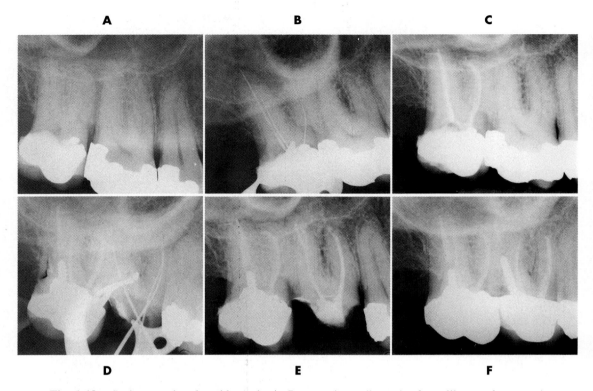

Fig. 1-18.   Saving two irreplaceable teeth. **A,** Preoperative radiograph of maxillary molar area. A porcelain fused to metal crown is present, but the patient reported that the dentist had placed a pulp capping over the exposed pulp (note area distal to the pulp horns). Pain became severe after the crown was seated. **B,** Initial files in place. **C,** Completion of treatment with filling of laterally condensed gutta-percha and Wach's paste. **D,** Several years later at a checkup appointment for the second molar, the patient complained of tenderness to percussion in the area, thinking that it was the treated tooth. A periapical radiolucency was noted on the mesiobuccal root of the first molar, and that tooth, not the second molar, responded to percussion. Accordingly, the first molar was treated. Files in place indicated two canals in a Type II configuration (Chapter 6) in the mesiobuccal root. **E,** The tooth was completed with laterally condensed gutta-percha and Wach's paste, with post room prepared. **F,** Twelve years after treatment of the first molar, 14 years after completion of the second molar. The filling of the mesiobuccal root of the first molar now appears to be 2 mm short of the radiographic apex, although it was flush in **E.** Radiolucency has healed, and both teeth look excellent. (Restoration by Dr. Peter Feimer, Chicago.)

because of the necessary overcontouring and excessive width of each tooth in the bridge. In such an arch the anterior tooth with endodontic involvement may be restored with a post-and-core jacket crown and excellent esthetic results obtained (Fig. 1-22).

Avoiding use of lower anterior teeth as abutments. Because of their anatomy and/or arch position, lower anterior teeth are difficult to use as bridge abutments. When lower anterior teeth have pulpal or periapical involvement, endodontic therapy avoids the necessity for cutting down or pin-

ledging narrow, frequently crowded adjacent teeth.

Limiting the extent of the problem. When a tooth in an intact quadrant requires endodontic treatment, adjacent teeth remain uninvolved in the subsequent restorative procedures. If the tooth is extracted, however, the adjacent teeth must be prepared as bridge abutments, with possible resultant problems. These adjacent teeth may be virgin but require considerable tooth reduction, or existing restorations in these teeth may be extensive and serviceable yet have to be discarded and new retainers fabricated. Endodontic care limits the

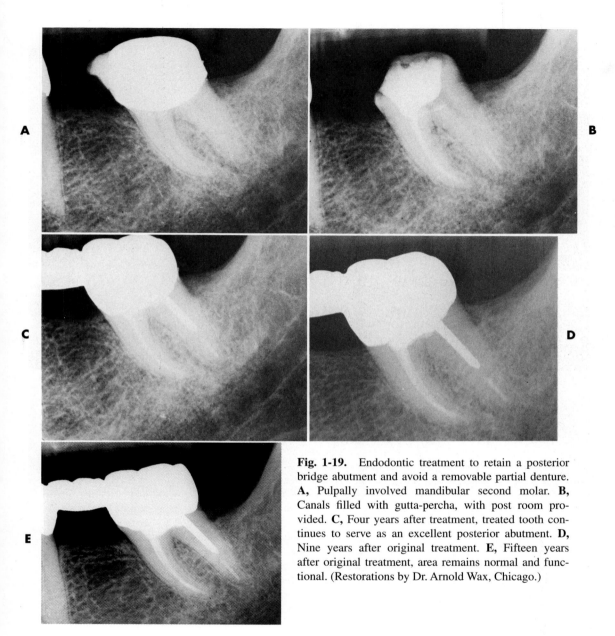

Fig. 1-19. Endodontic treatment to retain a posterior bridge abutment and avoid a removable partial denture. **A,** Pulpally involved mandibular second molar. **B,** Canals filled with gutta-percha, with post room provided. **C,** Four years after treatment, treated tooth continues to serve as an excellent posterior abutment. **D,** Nine years after original treatment. **E,** Fifteen years after original treatment, area remains normal and functional. (Restorations by Dr. Arnold Wax, Chicago.)

extent of the problem to only the involved tooth (Fig. 1-23).

Retaining involved teeth with large restorations. Operative dentistry has provided many complex procedures for successfully restoring badly broken-down teeth. Pins, indirect casting with impression materials of extremely low-dimensional change, high-speed cavity preparation, and other procedures have enabled dentists to restore rather easily teeth that formerly provided tremendous problems.

However, the use of any of these procedures may result in some irreversible pulpal damage; even when direct pulpal exposure is avoided, sufficient pulpal damage may accrue from the combinations of procedures to cause a severe pulpitis or pulpal death.

After considerable time, effort, and money have been expended in an effort to save a tooth, extraction is a step that is difficult for both the dentist and the patient. Endodontic treatment may be used

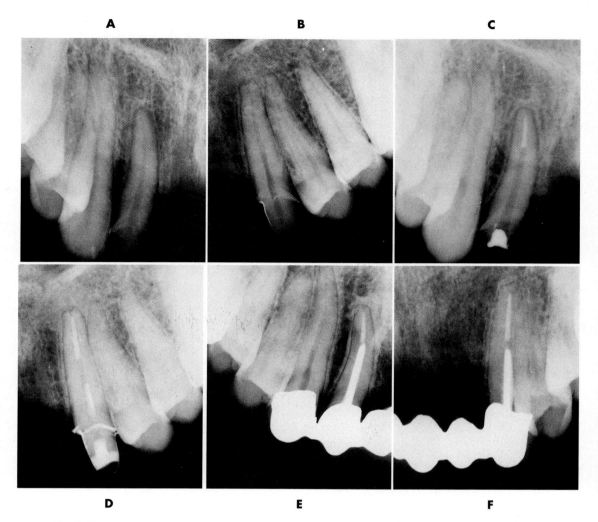

Fig. 1-20.   Patient was a 22-year-old female, badly injured in an automobile accident in a foreign country she visited as a present for graduating college. Two teeth had been avulsed but not replanted, and two teeth were fractured and extracted. The dentists in the foreign country also wanted to extract the maxillary lateral incisor (no. 7), but she was able to stop this despite severe pain in the area. **A,** Preoperative radiograph of no. 7 with obvious exposure, mobility, and tenderness to percussion. **B,** Preoperative film of opposite cuspid (no. 11) with temporary plastic crown and tenderness to percussion. **C** and **D,** Canal filling with laterally condensed gutta-percha and Wach's paste, with post room prepared. **E** and **F,** Areas 14 years after treatment, indicating excellently fabricated bridge, with normal bone associated with each treated tooth, avoiding the need for removable partial denture. (Restorations by Dr. Kerry Voit, Chicago.)

to retain such a tooth. Usually, access may be prepared directly through the existing restoration. If cuspal coverage is already present, after completion of endodontic therapy a reinforcing post or pin may be employed to utilize the previously placed restoration and thus not completely waste the earlier restorative efforts.

Avoiding loss of bridge and abutments.   Two-appointment bridge construction is relatively routine at present. The first appointment consists of tooth preparation with high-speed instruments, making impressions, and bite registration and temporization; the second appointment involves try-in, adjustment, and cementation. All these procedures

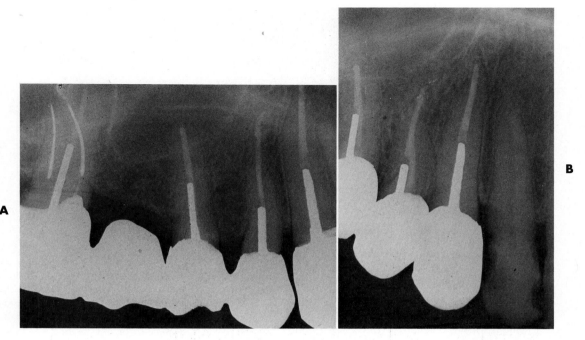

Fig. 1-21.   A, Case originally shown in the first edition with entire quadrant composed of endodontically treated teeth, avoiding the need for a complex maxillary partial denture. **B,** Fifteen years after therapy and restoration, area looks excellent. (Restorations by Dr. Arnold Wax, Chicago.)

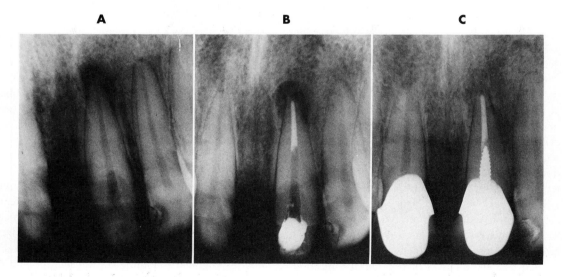

Fig. 1-22.   A, Maxillary anterior area. Note wide diastema and periapical involvement of a central incisor. **B,** Endodontic therapy completed and post space provided. **C,** Complete healing 1 year later, preventing the need for a fixed bridge that would have poor esthetic qualities. (Restorations by Dr. Sherwin Strauss, Chicago.)

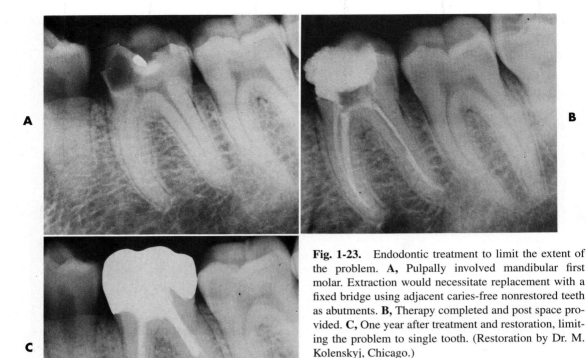

Fig. 1-23. Endodontic treatment to limit the extent of the problem. **A,** Pulpally involved mandibular first molar. Extraction would necessitate replacement with a fixed bridge using adjacent caries-free nonrestored teeth as abutments. **B,** Therapy completed and post space provided. **C,** One year after treatment and restoration, limiting the problem to single tooth. (Restoration by Dr. M. Kolenskyj, Chicago.)

may cause pulpal damage and even without actual pulpal exposure may result in a pulpitis or pulpal degeneration.

Continued pain after cementation usually indicates the need for endodontic intervention. As in treatment of a tooth with an extensive restoration, access may be prepared directly through the casting and a reinforcing pin or post utilized to retain the previously placed crown after completion of endodontic therapy. Loss of the bridge with the involved abutment is thus averted (Fig. 1-24).

Facilitating restoration after fracture of a tooth with insufficient supragingival structure for a crown. Traumatic or accidental fracture of a tooth located near the gingival margin and having minimal remaining supragingival structure offers a considerable restorative problem. To limit the extent of the problem, the dentist should avoid extracting the injured member and constructing a bridge.

A temporary tissue-borne partial denture (flipper or spring-plate) is constructed to give satisfactory esthetics during the endodontic and restorative procedures if an anterior tooth is involved. A post-and-core type of crown is fabricated after completion of canal filling and post preparation, and the problem is solved (Fig. 1-25).

ROLE OF ENDODONTICS IN RECONSTRUCTIVE DENTISTRY

Reconstructive dentistry involves the reshaping, repositioning, and frequently the replacing of teeth by the use of castings and other complex procedures. Although periodontal therapy is most intimately involved in reconstructive dentistry, endodontic treatment is required in a great number of cases. Many of the restorative dentist's needs for endodontics are shared by the reconstructive dentist, particularly the need to avoid removable prostheses. Whenever possible, fixed replacements are

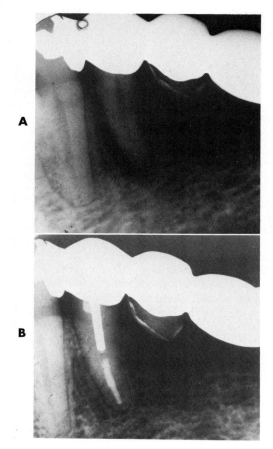

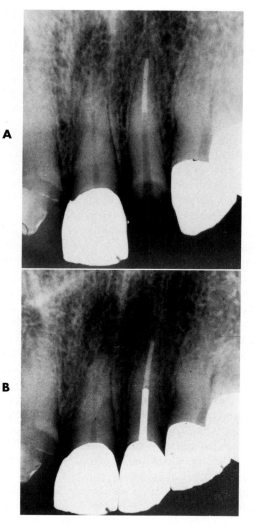

Fig. 1-24. **A,** Large radiolucency on mesial surface of mandibular first bicuspid acting as bridge abutment. **B,** After endodontic treatment area has healed, avoiding remaking of the bridge with an even larger span. Post has been used to reinforce crown after therapy. (Restoration by Dr. Edward LeMire, Chicago.)

Fig. 1-25. **A,** Maxillary lateral incisor fractured at gingival margin. Canal filled and post room prepared. **B,** Restored with veneer crown over cast core and dowel. (Restoration by Dr. Morton S. Rosen, Chicago.)

utilized. Endodontics is required by the reconstructive dentist in additional areas as well.

Preserving teeth after reshaping of crown contours. Although vertical and occlusal relationships may be altered by orthodontic treatment, these changes are most often obtained by reshaping the coronal contour of the tooth by using crowns or onlays. This may require considerable reduction of tooth structure to obtain sufficient thickness of material, and consequent pulpal exposure or irreversible damage may occur. Since reconstructive dentistry requires the most possible abutments with periodontal health, many reshaped teeth will require endodontic therapy if they are to be retained.

Problems are frequently seen in lower anterior teeth that were originally overcrowded and sustained periodontal damage. After necessary periodontal therapy, such teeth are splinted to gain a desired occlusal relationship and esthetic appearance. Preparation of the teeth requires considerable reduction of tooth structure in either the labial or the lingual direction, rarely both, to obtain the necessary parallelism for splint insertion and may cause considerable pulpal damage to these thin teeth. Through endodontic therapy and post-and-core types of crowns, retention of affected teeth is accomplished.

Accommodating an attachment, or key and keyway. Key and keyway attachments—Chayes, Sterns, and other types—are frequently used to avoid the use of clasps for partial dentures or to distribute forces of stress in fixed replacements. To accommodate the male attachment, which is usually placed on the partial denture or posterior segment of a fixed prosthesis, considerable tooth reduction for the female attachment must be performed, which may result in pulpal damage. On occasion the pulp of the tooth that will house the female attachment is purposely sacrificed, and endodontic procedures are performed so an attachment can be placed directly over the center of the root.

Anticipating the possibility of future pulpal damage. In certain cases it becomes advisable to perform endodontic therapy on teeth that have exhibited no pulpal exposure when there is considerable indication that endodontics will be required in the future. This is frequently seen in a case involving the splinting of anterior teeth after extensive periodontal therapy. Necessary root planning and scaling, considerable tooth reduction during preparation to gain parallelism and adequate width of finishing line, and other restoration procedures may cause irreversible pulpal damage. It is easier to perform endodontic therapy before the castings are cemented, and a wise treatment plan will allow this to be done.

Cases in which only minimal tooth structure remains after abutment preparation are often best served by performing endodontic treatments and restoring with a post-and-core type crown even if the tooth is unexposed. When one member of a splint is placed over a tooth with little structure available for retention, that abutment may pull off, exposing the tooth to massive carious activity. Meanwhile, the splint is still held in place by the other abutments, and neither the patient nor the dentist is aware of the damage that is developing. If endodontic therapy is performed on these marginal teeth, post-and-core crowns will afford superior retention and greater protection to the remaining root face.

Utilizing bicuspidized and amputated teeth. Any tooth or portion of a tooth with good periodontal health may be utilized by the reconstructive dentist as an abutment. Bicuspidized or hemisected mandibular molars, as well as maxillary molars with one or even two amputated roots, afford greater retentive qualities to the reconstruction than would the pontic needed if the entire

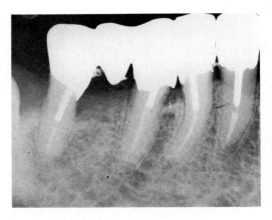

Fig. 1-26. Hemisected second molar and bicuspidized first molar, still in place and serving as excellent abutments more than 10 years after treatment. If I were treating this combination today, I probably would remove one root of the first molar as well or move the first molar distal root orthodontically. This combination allowed the patient to avoid a free-end removable partial denture with unilateral replacement of teeth. (Restorations by Dr. Arnold Wax, Chicago, and molar endodontics by Dr. Harold Gerstein, formerly of Chicago.)

tooth were extracted. These fractions of a tooth may be extremely valuable, since their presence in the posterior segment of the arch allows for added retention in that area. Endodontics provides the necessary initial step in any of these procedures (Fig. 1-26). (See Chapter 12.)

ROLE OF ENDODONTICS IN PROSTHETIC DENTISTRY

For many years a common philosophy in prosthetic dentistry was to extract any tooth with pulpal involvement in an arch in which a removable partial denture was to be used. The rationale was that a prosthesis was to be fabricated to replace missing teeth anyway and treated teeth could not be relied on. Experiences with treated teeth have indicated the fallacy of such an argument, and the need for endodontics has been well recognized by the prosthetic dentist for a number of purposes.

Limiting the number of teeth in the removable partial denture. Obviously, the greater the number of natural teeth in an arch, the fewer are the teeth required in the prosthesis. The higher the ratio of natural to replaced teeth in any involved arch, the better is the prognosis for the partial den-

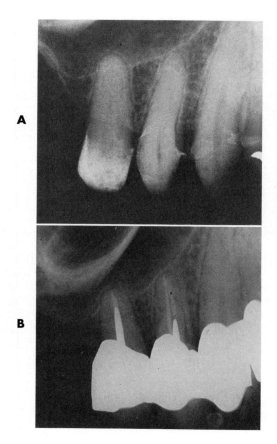

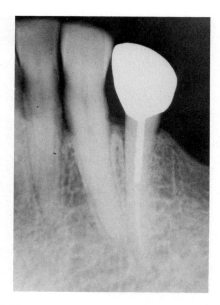

Fig. 1-28. Endodontic treatment retains the mandibular first bicuspid, a better partial denture abutment than the adjacent cuspid. (Restoration by Dr. Jacob Lippert, formerly of Chicago.)

Fig. 1-27. Limiting number of teeth in a removable partial denture by utilizing endodontic therapy. **A,** Maxillary area with pulpal involvement of bicuspids. **B,** Three years after treatment. Fewer teeth were needed in removable partial denture, since endodontic therapy retained the involved teeth. (Restoration by Dr. Henry Leib, formerly of Chicago.)

ture. Reasons include the following: (1) more abutments may be utilized, (2) less strain accrues to the abutments, and (3) there is a greater choice of available abutments (Fig. 1-27).

Allowing for retention of teeth with greater bulk as abutments. As a general rule, the more posterior any abutment is, the better it serves. This is because of the greater bulk, both coronal and root, found in posterior teeth. Thus molars are better than bicuspids, which in turn are better than cuspids, as partial denture abutments (Fig. 1-28).

If posterior teeth are pulpally or periapically involved, endodontic therapy must be utilized if the prosthetic dentist wishes to take advantage of the greater bulk available.

Avoiding free-end saddles. Any posterior abutment, even if only on one side in a bilateral case, is extremely valuable. A posterior tooth utilized as an abutment prevents the torquing or settling that bilateral free-end saddles frequently cause (Fig. 1-29).

Providing for splinted multiple abutments. Experience with partial denture clasps on non-splinted singly abutting teeth, particularly mandibular premolars, has indicated that a considerable degree of periodontal breakdown occurs. Many articles have reported on the need for two or even three abutting teeth with conically shaped roots to be used as partial denture abutments. Endodontics is necessary in retaining teeth to provide multiple splinted abutments if pulpal involvement has affected potential candidates.

Accommodating an attachment, or key and keyway. See p. 24.

Retaining alveolar bone. Shortly after an extraction, the alveolar bone in the vicinity begins a resorptive process. Only retention of the tooth can prevent this loss of bone. Therefore, when endodontic therapy is required, not only is the treated tooth retained, but the adjacent alveolar bone—important for retention of the tissue-borne portion of the partial denture—is also retained.

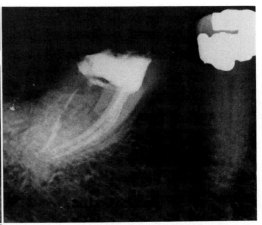

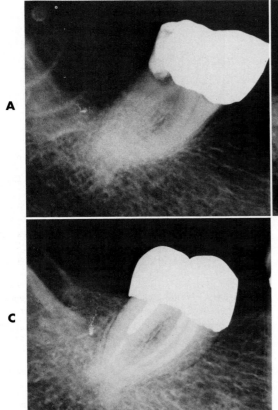

Fig. 1-29. Endodontic treatment to avoid a free-end saddle. **A,** Mandibular second molar is only molar on that side of arch. **B,** Endodontic treatment completed and post room provided. **C,** Two years after treatment, molar is serving as posterior abutment of a removable partial denture, avoiding the less desirable free-end saddle case. (Restoration by Dr. Mort Fireman, formerly of Chicago.)

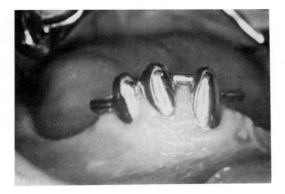

Fig. 1-30. Minimal number of remaining teeth, treated endodontically and restored with telescopes and bars. Note poor bone level of mandibular edentulous areas. Overdentures had excellent stability. (Reconstruction by Dr. Donald Cunningham, formerly of Indianapolis.)

Avoiding a full denture.   Even one or two periodontally healthy teeth are often sufficient to retain a partial denture. Although some controversies exist as to the advisability of preserving only a few maxillary teeth in preference to supplying a full denture, there is unanimity concerning the necessity for retaining mandibular teeth to hold a partial denture. Again, endodontics may be required if such teeth have pulpal or periapical involvement.

If a minimal number of abutments are available and they are judged to be rather weak for supporting a removable partial denture, the use of an overdenture may avoid the need for a full denture supported solely by tissue. The remaining teeth may be treated endodontically and restored with post, cores, and telescopes. A bar may be used between the abutments to provide further retention. The full denture fabricated to utilize such retained teeth has much greater retention than the routine denture (Fig. 1-30).

REFERENCES

Amsterdam M, Fox L: Provisional splinting—principles and techniques, *Dent Clin North Am,* March 1959, p 73.

Beaudreau DE: The role of the posterior fixed bridge in occlusion, *Dent Clin North Am,* March 1959, p 73.

Bender IB, Seltzer S: To culture or not to culture? In Grossman LI, editor: *Transactions of the Third International Conference on Endodontics,* Philadelphia, 1963, University of Pennsylvania.

Dumsha TC, Gutmann JL: The status and direction of endodontic research for the 1980's, *J Endod* 12:174, 1986.

Grossman LI: Rationale of endodontic treatment, *Dent Clin North Am,* Nov 1967, p 483.

Grossman LI: Guidelines for the prevention of fracture of root canal instruments, *Oral Surg* 28:746, 1969.

Grossman LI, Shepard LI, Pearson LA: Roentgenologic and clinical evaluation of endodontically treated teeth, *Oral Surg* 17:368, 1964.

Healey HJ: Endodontics: selection of cases and treatment procedures, *J Am Dent Assoc* 53:434, 1956.

Healey HJ: *Endodontics,* St Louis, 1960, Mosby.

Hirschfeld L: Tooth repositioning as an adjunct to oral rehabilitation, *Dent Clin North Am,* Nov 1962, p 737.

Ingle JI, Beveridge EE: *Endodontics,* ed 2, Philadelphia, 1976, Lea & Febiger.

Kornfeld M: *Mouth rehabilitation—clinical and laboratory procedures,* vol 1, ed 2, St Louis, 1974, Mosby.

Leavitt JM: Endodontic adjuncts to oral rehabilitation, *Dent Clin North Am,* Nov 1963, p 723.

Lin LM, Skribner JE, Gaengler P: Factors associated with endodontic treatment failures, *J Endod* 18:625, 1992.

McGivney GP, Castleberry DJ: *McCracken's removable partial prosthodontics,* ed 9, St Louis, 1995, Mosby.

Milas VB: *A history of the American Association of Endodontics, 1943-1968,* American Association of Endodontics, Chicago, 1983.

Miller CJ: *Inlays, crowns and bridges,* Philadelphia, 1962, Saunders.

Rosen H, Gitnick PJ: Integrating restorative procedures into the treatment of periodontal disease, *J Prosthet Dent* 14:343, 1964.

Rudolph CE Jr: Midtreatment triage in endodontics, *Dent Clin North Am* 13:757, 1969.

Schweitzer JM: *Oral rehabilitation problem cases,* vol 1, St Louis, 1964, Mosby.

Sharp GC: The historical and biological aspects of the pulpless tooth question, *J Am Dent Assoc* 24:1231, 1937.

Simring M, Thaller JL: Temporary splinting for multiple mobile teeth, *J Am Dent Assoc* 53:429, 1956.

Staffileno H Jr.: Furcation treatment in periodontics, *Dent Radiogr Photogr* 38:85, 1965.

Storms JL: Factors that influence the success of endodontic treatment, *J Can Dent Assoc* 35:83, 1969.

Strindberg LZ: The dependence of the results of pulp therapy on certain factors: an analytic study based on radiographic and clinical follow-up examinations, *Dent Abstr* 2:176, 1957.

Weine FS: Endodontic treatment for the geriatric patient, *J Am Soc Geriatr Dent* 2:2, 1967.

2 Diagnosis and treatment planning

Many excellent texts have been written on diagnosis and treatment planning. All emphasize that a thorough diagnosis, the determination of what is wrong, must be made before any definitive treatment may be considered. This chapter will deal with diagnosis and treatment planning as related to diseases of the pulp and periapical tissues. It will attempt to clarify the position of endodontics in an overall treatment plan.

IMPORTANCE OF A MEDICAL HISTORY

For many years the medical history was taken so that the patient could be treated in a manner most harmonious with maintenance of general health. Toward that end, it was important to know if a patient had a history of rheumatic fever so that antibiotics could be prescribed; if the patient were diabetic, appointments could be scheduled after meals; or medications already being taken by a patient would be considered when additional prescriptions were needed to prevent undesirable drug interactions.

At this time the dentist must consider not only the actions of treatment modalities on the patient's existing conditions, but also the potential impact of the patient's medical profile on the health of the entire dental operating team. Such conditions as hepatitis B, human immunodeficiency virus disease (HIVD), and other sexually transmitted diseases (STDs), as well as active oral infections, may be passed from the patient to the dentist or auxiliary. Dental personnel involved in a high number of surgical cases, such as oral surgeons, periodontists, some endodontists, general dentists with surgically oriented practices, and their surgical assistants, have been identified serologically as having a greater percentage of hepatitis B infections, even though some were unaware of actively having the disease.

Patients confined to hospital, nursing homes, and other medical institutions may have the poten-
tial for infecting a healthy dental team. Institutionalized patients with Down's syndrome also have a higher incidence of positive hepatitis B antigen than do mentally handicapped people without Down's syndrome. There surely are other serious communicable diseases that have similar proclivities for occurring along with conditions not normally considered dangerous.

Just as protecting patients from attacks of subacute endocarditis is extremely important, so must the dentist appreciate the seriousness of spread within the practice and self-protection when treating patients with these insidious conditions. Hepatitis is annoying and potentially debilitating; HIVD is assumed to be fatal.

As stated in Chapter 1, virtually no medical contraindications exist to routine endodontic treatment. However, multiple situations might arise in which the patient's medical condition, past history, or regimen of medications may have implications that could alter the usual course of treatment. Therefore a complete medical history must be taken before any diagnosis, treatment planning, or even emergency treatment for pain relief is contemplated.

In addition to the patient's name, address, and business and home telephone numbers, the name of the physician of responsibility should always be included on each individual's record. Usually an internist or general practitioner is listed who is responsible for the patient's general well-being. Some patients have a number of physicians, including, among others, a surgeon, an allergist, otolaryngologist, and (for a woman) a gynecologist. After the patient's initial visit, the office receptionist should look up and record the telephone number of each physician listed. If an emergency arises and a physician must be swiftly contacted, the few minutes that would have to be wasted in looking up a telephone number are saved.

Patients should be asked if they have had or presently have any of the following diseases. Both the diseases and their significance in endodontic therapy are listed here.

Rheumatic fever

Any patient with a history of rheumatic fever has the potential of suffering an attack of subacute bacterial endocarditis (SBE) after any bacteremia. Since almost every dental procedure, whether a simple prophylaxis, the extraction of a tooth, or an endodontic treatment, causes some degree of bacteremia, definite measures must be taken to avoid the possibility of SBE.

Bender et al.'s classic paper in 1963 on the degree of bacteremia after various dental procedures firmly established that certain phases of endodontic treatment will induce no bacteremia. The authors reported that pulp extirpation and filing beyond the apex did produce a bacteremia, which dissipated after 10 minutes. However, when enlarging procedures were carried out within the confines of the canal, no bacteremia was produced in most cases. Even the placement of a rubber dam causes gingival impingement, and a bacteremia may result. Therefore it is best to use the standard prophylactic procedures before any endodontic appointment.

On the basis of this report, it is strongly suggested that antibiotic premedication be given to any patient with a history of rheumatic heart disease—at the initial appointment for endodontic treatment, at any subsequent appointment if the possibility of going past the apex exists, whenever a periapical lesion is present, and at any surgical appointment.

The preferred antibiotic management of such a patient was changed in 1990 by the American Heart Association's (AHA) Committee on Rheumatic Fever and Infective Endocarditis. The Council on Dental Therapeutics of the American Dental Association (ADA) had representation on that committee; thus these current guidelines have carefully considered dental procedures to be covered and appropriate action to be taken as part of the report.

Conditions requiring the use of antibiotic coverage are as follows: prosthetic heart valves, including bioprosthetic and homograft valves; previous history of bacterial endocarditis, even without a history of heart disease; most congenital heart malformations; history of rheumatic heart disease and any other valvular disfunction, even after intervening cardiac surgery; hypertrophic cardiomyopathy; and mitral valve prolapse with valvular regurgitation and mitral valve prolapse without valvular regurgitation but with thickening and/or redundancy of the valve leaflets in men ages 45 years and older.

Antibiotic coverage is *not* necessary for the following: isolated secundum atrial defects; surgical repair without residua 6 months after repair of atrial septal defect, ventricular septal defect, or patent ductus arteriosus; previous coronary bypass graft surgery; mitral prolapse without regurgitation; physiologic, functional, or innocent heart murmurs; previous Kawasaki disease or previous rheumatic fever without valvular dysfunction; and cardiac pacemakers and implanted defibrillators.

Dental procedures requiring antibiotic prophylaxis include any treatment known to induce gingival or mucosal bleeding, including professional cleaning. Procedures for which antibiotic coverage is *not* recommended include treatment not likely to induce gingival bleeding, such as adjustment of orthodontic appliances or restorations completely supragingival, not requiring the use of a matrix retainer.

For many years the standard regimen for at-risk patients was to use intramuscular (IM) and, occasionally, intravenous (IV) injections of the antibiotics. Gradually, this was altered to make oral use acceptable for compliant patients. Now the oral route has become the preferred method, except for the few patients who are not reliable or cannot take antibiotics by the oral route. A huge proportion of patients would much rather take pills than IM or IV coverage.

The standard regimen for patients of 60 pounds (27 kg) and greater is 3.0 g amoxicillin (six tablets or capsules of 500 mg each) orally 1 hour before the dental procedure and then 1.5 g (three capsules of 500 mg each) 6 hours later. For patients with allergy to amoxicillin or penicillin, 800 mg erythromycin ethylsuccinate or 1.0 g erythromycin stearate is taken orally 2 hours before the procedure and then half that dose 6 hours later. Clindamycin may also be used with allergic patients, taking 300 mg (two 150 mg tablets) 1 hour before the procedure and then one 150 mg tablet 6 hours later. Clindamycin is a powerful antibiotic that may cause severe, or even fatal, colitis if taken for 1 week or more, which is very unlikely when being used for endocarditis prophylaxis.

For children, amoxicillin may be taken as a syrup, using 50 mg/kg of weight or, for those sensitive to amoxicillin, erythromycin at 20 mg/kg or clindamycin at 10 mg/kg. The total child's dose should not exceed the adult dose.

For those patients who are unable to take oral prophylaxis or who may not follow the oral dosage regimen, 2.0 g ampicillin is administered IV or IM 30 minutes before the procedure, followed by 1.0 g 6 hours later (or 1.5 g oral amoxicillin). For patients allergic to ampicillin, amoxicillin, or penicillin, 300 mg clindamycin is administered IV 30 minutes before the dental procedure and 150 mg (IV or oral) 6 hours later. For children, ampicillin is dispensed initially at 50 mg/kg or clindamycin initially at 10 mg/kg, with follow-up doses at half the initial dose and no total dose greater than the adult dose.

Some time ago the suggested method was to start the antibiotic therapy 1 day before the procedure. This schedule has been discarded, since it was found to allow more time for producing organisms resistant to the antibiotic.

Since the production of SBE is one of the most hazardous possibilities that may occur from any dental treatment, the regimen described must be followed whenever a prior episode of rheumatic fever is established in the taking of a medical history. In addition to merely asking a patient about the history of rheumatic fever, further questioning should be pursued with a patient who mentions having had any of the symptoms. These symptoms, usually appearing in childhood or early adolescence, include red, tender, and painful joints; small fibrous nodules on the extensor surfaces of the wrists or ankles; recurrent tonsillitis or other streptococcal diseases; and chorea, acute carditis, or rheumatic arthritis. If any question exists as to the possibility of this disease, it is much safer to prescribe the suggested antibiotic medication than to chance SBE. Consultation with the patient's physician is recommended in any cases of doubt.

Wahl published an excellent paper on the pros, cons, and "in-betweens" for the use of deterrents for SBE, describing some of the myths and truths that exist in relation to these procedures. Among the problems he discussed were that compliance by U.S. dentists and physicians to the AHA guidelines has been very poor and that attempting to err on the positive side of antibiotic use may cause serious conditions, including anaphylaxis (rare), allergy, buildup of resistant strains, fungal overgrowth, gastrointestinal (GI) tract upset, and interference with oral contraceptives.

Wahl also discussed the fact that the British Society of Antimicrobial Chemotherapy, a body similar to the AHA in promoting guidelines for endocarditis prophylaxis, only recommends antibiotic coverage for the dental procedures of extractions, scalings, or surgery involving gingival tissues. Endodontic treatment, most crown and bridge procedures, and periodontal examinations are excluded from coverages.

The latest AHA recommendations are the most simple and logical ever proposed in the United States, and compliance should be higher than accorded previously published guidelines. However, if studies currently underway and the experiences of health care workers in Great Britain indicate that some facets of prophylaxis are not necessary, further modifications may be forthcoming.

Artificial heart valves

Insertion of an artificial valve in the heart to replace a valve damaged by congenital defect or by systemic or local disease is no longer a rare surgical procedure. Artificial valves currently used are composed chiefly of Teflon or Teflon-like materials to diminish the possibility of adhesions. The danger of clumps of bacterial colonies collecting on these valves increases greatly after a bacteremia. Therefore any patient with artificial heart valves should receive the same prophylactic antibiotic administration as a patient with a history of rheumatic fever.

Coronary artery disease

The tremendous increase in life expectancy secured in the twentieth century has caused more people of advanced age to require dental treatment. Coronary occlusion and other cardiovascular diseases are most common after middle age (i.e., past 50 years), although they may be seen frequently in the 40s as well. Associated factors may include hypertension, angina pectoris, arteriosclerosis, stressful occupations, and smoking. Patients exhibiting these conditions may be suspected of tendency toward cardiovascular disease and should be treated accordingly.

Cardiovascular disease does not contraindicate endodontic therapy, but certain precautions should be observed when treating patients with such a history. Often the patient with a previous episode of coronary occlusion is receiving anticoagulant therapy. Nonsurgical endodontic treatment, including vital pulp extirpation, requires no alteration in the administration of anticoagulants. If surgery becomes mandatory, the patient's physician should be advised. It is up to the physician and not the dentist to alter the administration of the drug to secure a blood level compatible with the clotting required for a surgical procedure.

Because it is necessary to either remove or reduce the anticoagulant cover for a patient undergoing surgery, nonsurgical treatment is much preferred if a choice exists. Conditions such as the presence of a large radiolucency, failure to reach the apex, persistent postoperative tenderness, and other possible indications for endodontic surgery should be given every opportunity to heal without surgical intervention. Only when there is no other choice should surgery be considered. However, since endodontic surgery usually ends with the areas of incision apposed and sutured, it is still preferable to the extraction of an involved tooth.

Pain from any source may cause excitation and resultant heart strain in patients with a history of coronary occlusion. Therefore, during therapy, these patients should be given prescriptions for mild to moderate analgesics to diminish the effects of postoperative pain. As with any analgesic, the initial dose should be given while the local anesthetic (if one has been used) is still effective so that the drug's pain-relieving qualities have ample time to work before the anesthetic is dissipated. If a local anesthetic has not been used, the analgesic should be taken immediately at the conclusion of the appointment. If postoperative pain is anticipated and no local anesthetic is to be used, it is wise to have the patient take an analgesic before the placement of the rubber dam so that much of the drug's effect will be gained right at the conclusion of the appointment.

Most patients with a history of coronary occlusion require no premedication during therapy. If any doubt exists, the patient's physician should be consulted. When more than one tooth is to receive endodontic care at one appointment, a brief recess should be granted between applications of the rubber dam unless the time required for one of the treatments is brief. The use of multiple isolation and treatment of two or more teeth simultaneously, even when adjacent, should be avoided.

If the patient complains of substernal pain during an appointment, a dressing should be placed and the treatment terminated for that day. The patient should be sent to the physician for further investigation. The most common reasons for this symptom are GI disturbance or angina pectoris, but a mild coronary attack may be occurring.

Hypertension

High blood pressure may occur either as a separate disease entity or in conjunction with cardiovascular-renal disease or arteriosclerosis. Among the causative factors are an occupation causing tension and worry, familial tendency, overweight, unbalanced diet, and abnormal stimulation of the sympathetic nervous system, often on an emotional basis. Symptoms include shortness of breath, frequent and persistent headaches, poor vision, ringing ears, nosebleeds, and dizziness. Some patients, however, have no symptoms at all. Treatment is based on reduction of the symptoms by means of various drugs to lower the blood pressure.

The ADA has made a strong effort to organize dentists to aid in the detection of hypertension by routinely taking blood pressure of their patients. Many people visit the dentist at least once yearly but do not see their physician during that period. Screening of all dental patients may locate hypertensive individuals and allow for treatment before the occurrence of serious cardiovascular disease.

For many years, physicians advised dentists who were treating patients with hypertension to avoid the use of epinephrine in local anesthetic administrations. On occasion, patients with a history of coronary attack were also included. Unfortunately, the local anesthetics without vasoconstrictors have a less profound effect and shorter duration of action than those that contain epinephrine. Great depth of anesthesia is required in endodontics for pulp extirpation and surgery. Any pain felt by the patient would produce much more epinephrine within the individual's own system than would ever be included in the anesthetic solution. For that reason the epinephrine content of 1:100,000 available in many anesthetic solutions is considered safe. These solutions should be injected extremely slowly, at a rate no faster than 30 sec/ml, with frequent aspiration to avoid injection directly into a blood vessel. The caliber of the needle must be 27 gauge or larger to be wide enough for blood to back up into the syringe when aspirated.

It is wise to place the Carpules of anesthetic into the salt sterilizer for a few seconds before injection. This warms the solution from room temperature, at which it is stored, to slightly above body temperature and permits a less painful injection. This is a good practice to follow before any injection.

Since any anxiety induces an increased blood pressure, therapy should be developed to create as tranquil a mood as possible. Case presentation should be streamlined, with minimal mention of any complications or possible failure. The entire therapy must be performed with a firm and confident manner.

The patient's physician should be consulted concerning the need for premedication. Many of these patients may already be receiving some type of hypnotic or tranquilizer treatment. When the first appointment in a series is handled by the dentist smoothly, competently, and painlessly, the patient will experience more relief from psychogenic attack than could be accomplished by any premedicament. However, when it is anticipated that a particular appointment for endodontic treatment of a hypertensive individual will be long, difficult, and frustrating, suitable premedication should be employed.

In the treatment of known hypertensive patients, a general anesthetic should be avoided and no more than three Carpules of anesthetic solution should be used at each appointment. In addition, morning appointments are preferred so that the patient does not have all day to mull over the impending procedure. Early appointments may be preceded by a nighttime premedication. If possible, the total length of any single appointment should not exceed 1 hour; and if the dentist sees that the patient is being overstressed, the session should be terminated.

Diabetes

Regardless of the type of maintenance therapy necessary for control of blood glucose level, all diabetic patients present certain problems when undergoing endodontic treatment. Healing is usually retarded, which should be considered when evaluating periodic postoperative recheck radiographs. Radiolucencies are slower to fill with bone than in normal patients (Fig. 2-1). Therefore surgical procedures to save a case that appears to be failing should be delayed until it is certain that the radiolucency is really increasing in size rather than merely healing slowly. In a patient who had normal-appearing periapical bone before treatment, 6-month postoperative radiographs may demonstrate a small periapical radiolucency, particularly if the canal was overinstrumented or overfilled. This generally will reverse within a year, again illustrating the retarded healing of a diabetic patient.

Since diabetic patients are susceptible to infections and to slow healing, antibiotics should be employed in the presence of infection or if a surgical procedure is to be employed. In the case of an infection, penicillin V is the drug of choice, 1000 mg to start and then doses of 500 mg four times a day for 4 days. Diabetic patients, used to taking medication according to a specific schedule, generally cooperate sufficiently to employ the oral route for antibiotics. For surgery the diabetic patient is given penicillin prophylactically on the same schedule as previously discussed for patients with rheumatic heart disease. Erythromycin is used for those patients with a history of penicillin sensitivity.

Alteration in blood glucose level as a result of an acute infection or during and after a surgical procedure is a common finding among diabetic patients. In these circumstances the patient should be referred to his physician for any adjustment in medication or diet necessary to combat the change.

The choice of anesthetics for diabetic patients differs from that for other patients. As pointed out by Burket, epinephrine should not be used in the local anesthetic solution, since it increases the blood glucose level by stimulating the sympathetic nervous system. Additionally, since diabetic patients often suffer from capillary ischemia due to arteriosclerosis, the increased ischemia produced by the epinephrine may cause tissue sloughs after a surgical procedure. If a vasoconstrictor is desired, levonordefrin (Neo-Cobefrin) may be used, since it does not cause sympathetic stimulation (although it does elevate the blood pressure).

Mepivacaine and lidocaine are available without a vasoconstrictor, and both are effective for routine endodontic procedures of short duration. For longer appointments, as when considerable depth of anesthesia is required, and for surgical procedures, either mepivacaine with levonordefrin (2% Carbocaine HCl with Neo-Cobefrin) or a combination of propoxyphene (Ravocaine), procaine (Novocain), and levarterenol bitartrate (norepinephrine bitartrate; Levophed) is an excellent anesthetic solution for use with diabetic patients.

All general anesthetics cause considerable rise in the blood glucose level and should be administered to diabetic patients only with a physician present. When a choice of local or general anesthetic exists for a diabetic patient, local anesthetic should always be preferred.

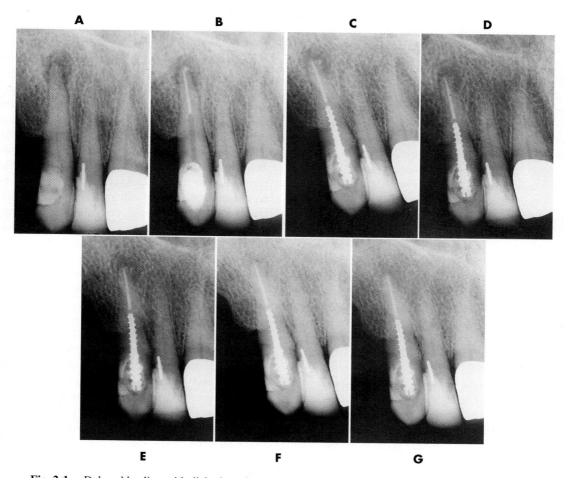

Fig. 2-1. Delayed healing with diabetic patients. **A,** Preoperative radiograph of maxillary cuspid with periapical lesion of moderate size, apical tenderness to palpation, nonvital pulp, and obvious pulpal involvement from the distal. **B,** Radiograph immediately after canal filling with laterally condensed gutta-percha and Wach's paste, with post room prepared and a slight excess of sealer apparent. A much larger lesion associated with a maxillary cuspid is shown in Fig. 1-12, considerably healed after 1 year and totally healed after 2 years. In Fig. 1-16, a lateral lesion, also larger, associated with a maxillary first bicuspid was completely healed after 1 year. Both these patients were healthy. In the diabetic patient, delayed healing is more common. **C,** Six months after treatment, lesion is still the same size, although the excess sealer has migrated slightly to the mesial and apical tenderness is totally absent. **D,** One year after treatment, lesion appears to be slightly smaller. On a healthy patient, you would expect to see considerable healing after 1 year. **E,** Eighteen months after treatment, lesion has decreased slightly and sealer almost gone. **F,** Two years after treatment, lesion has decreased considerably. **G,** Three years after treatment, complete repair. (Restoration by Dr. Steven Fishman, Chicago.)

The scheduling of appointments for diabetic patients requires some discussion. It is important for them to eat at certain specific intervals. Therefore it is best to schedule their appointments early in the morning or early in the afternoon, soon after their meals. In this way, neither running late in appointments nor encountering procedural difficulties that cause a longer appointment than anticipated will delay the mealtime and cause an alarming drop in blood glucose level.

It is well to keep a fresh candy bar in the office among emergency drugs for use in case a diabetic patient feels a coma coming on. Although coma may be due to either too little sugar or too little insulin, it is much safer to administer sugar than insulin in doubtful cases. If the patient does not respond to the sugar administration in a few minutes, a physician should be called. When hypoglycemia is present, the patient's face and clothing becomes wet and clammy while the pulse rate, blood pressure, and breathing remain normal. In hypoinsulinism the skin is cold, a severe pallor is present, and both blood pressure and pulse rate are diminished due to imminent circulatory collapse.

Since the healing needed to gain relatively complete bone filling after an extraction is greater than after any endodontic procedure, it is much better for diabetic patients to retain pulpally involved teeth when a satisfactory result seems obtainable. If the prognosis is highly questionable, particularly when a chronically infected tooth is involved, it may be better for the diabetic patient to have the tooth extracted than to chance the products of infection being constantly present.

Hepatitis

The microorganisms responsible for hepatitis, both serum and infectious, are highly resistant to the sterilization procedures normally used in endodontics. Additionally, these microorganisms may remain in the affected patient's blood for a considerable time after the active phase. Therefore, when a patient gives the history of having had hepatitis, all intracanal instruments, which may have picked up causative agents, should be discarded after use. Any files, reamers, broaches, probes, or other such instruments that do pick up potentially dangerous microorganisms, even through subsequently sterilized by dry heat or steam, might cause cross-contamination if used on another patient.

A history of hepatitis, jaundice, or other liver disease may indicate less-than-normal liver function. Any drugs that are detoxified by the liver should be avoided. Drugs typically used in dentistry and falling into this category include erythromycin and halothane (Fluothane), a nonexplosive general anesthetic agent.

Blood diseases

Although it is relatively rare, a patient with hemophilia may require endodontic therapy. The extraction of a hemophiliac's tooth, at one time a potentially lethal situation, may now be safely accomplished by using packs and prefabricated splints. Even so, using endodontic therapy to avoid an extraction is still more desirable.

Among the greatest hazards involved in treating a hemophiliac patient is the chance of internal bleeding caused by the injection of a local anesthetic, particularly for a mandibular block. If the tooth to be treated is necrotic, no injection is needed. However, if a vital pulp is involved, extirpation becomes too painful without an anesthetic. To accomplish pulp removal without chancing the possibility of severe internal bleeding caused by an injection, the dentist can gain access to the cavity by using a high-speed instrument with a very sharp bur, water spray, and a brush stroke. When pulp exposure has been gained, a cotton pellet dampened with formocresol is placed as a dressing and sealed with zinc oxide–eugenol (ZOE), and the patient is scheduled to return approximately a week later. The formocresol acts as a fixative on the pulpal tissue and aids in gaining a satisfactory clot by its caustic action.

At the second appointment the dressing is opened and any fixed pulpal tissue removed by sharp spoon excavators and broaches until pain becomes severe. Another formocresol dressing is placed; since much tissue has been removed, the medicament must be placed on a paper point to reach the vital tissue. This process is repeated until all the vital tissue has been removed, and the canals can be enlarged and filled with relatively little pain.

As in all endodontic procedures, the use of the rubber dam is mandatory. Care must be exercised to avoid placing the rubber dam clamp on the gingival tissues and causing severe bleeding. To avoid this possibility, notches may be placed on the labial and lingual surfaces of the treated tooth with a fissure bur, into which the clamp's prongs will tightly fit (Fig. 2-2).

Some patients give a history of periodic oral bleeding. This is usually due to a periodontal condition, will clear up after proper therapy, and has no real significance during endodontic therapy.

There are many disease states in which oral bleeding is a much more serious sign, however. Thinking that it falls into the dentist's province, patients may bring this symptom to the attention of their dentist rather than their physician. Among the diseases characterized by gingival hemorrhage are aplastic anemia, cyclic neutropenia, thrombocytopenia, leukemia, purpura, and macroglobu-

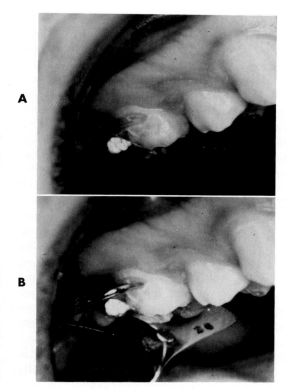

A

B

Fig. 2-2. A, In endodontic therapy for a hemophiliac patient, a groove is cut on both buccal and lingual surfaces of the tooth to be treated. **B,** Rubber dam clamp is placed into depressions so there will be no chance for impingement on gingival tissues.

linemia. Two other blood diseases, pernicious anemia and sprue, are accompanied by burning tongue, which might be revealed to the dentist.

If gingival bleeding is not halted by periodontal therapy, referral to a physician is mandatory to investigate for the possible presence of a systemic condition. Except for emergency treatment, endodontic therapy should not be instituted until the systemic condition is diagnosed and under treatment.

Small petechial hemorrhages near the junction of the hard and soft palate, coupled with weakness, fever, sore throat, chills, and severe lymphadenopathy, indicate the presence of infectious mononucleosis. Endodontic treatment of patients with this disease is exasperating, since it is characterized by severe intratreatment pain, exacerbations, and exaggerated responses to drugs. Since some of the symptoms of the disease are similar to those encountered during a severe dental infection, the dentist may be fooled into thinking that an

involved tooth is responsible for the condition. "Mono" usually attacks young persons, who normally pose no problems during therapy. Therefore the presence of these typical symptoms in a young patient should alert the dentist to the presence of mononucleosis.

After a regimen of bed rest, special diet, and antibiotics, in some patients the disease will run its course of 2 to 6 weeks. If the patient can be kept dentally comfortable while the disease is in its acute state, it is better to postpone the final canal enlargement and filling procedures until all the symptoms subside. At that time the patient's normal level of resistance is regained and a more favorable prognosis results.

Prostheses for total replacement of joints

According to Mulligan, patients who have had total replacement of joints with prostheses are also very susceptible to infections. The most common joint to be replaced is the hip, but knees, elbows, and shoulders may also become involved. If a bacteremia occurs, which may be initiated by dental treatment, the infection may lead to failure of the prosthesis.

Therefore Mulligan suggests that when such patients are being treated, antibiotic coverage is indicated in any dental procedure that might cause bleeding (e.g., vital extirpation or surgery). The patient's orthopedic surgeon should be contacted before the appointment to determine the desired antibiotic coverage, which may or may not coincide with that suggested for patients with a history of rheumatic fever. If a patient with a replaced joint develops a dental infection, culture and sensitivity testing should be instituted immediately to determine the most effective antimicrobial agent. If a joint becomes painful after dental treatment, the patient should consult the orthopedic surgeon immediately.

Other serious diseases

The foregoing diseases have the greatest implication in endodontics, and when the medical history is taken, patients should be asked specifically about them. They should be asked further if they have had other serious diseases, and any mentioned should be recorded.

Some infrequently present but often debilitating diseases (e.g., malignancy, nephritis, pemphigus) will indicate that treatment may take longer than usual to gain a desirable result; the delay is due to the alteration of local responses by the systemic condition.

Asthma, hay fever, hives, or skin rashes indicate hypersensitivity states. Only when necessary should drugs and medications be used for a patient with this type of problem. Unless a history of nonsensitivity is established, no new or unusual drugs should be prescribed.

HIVD, syphilis, and other sexually transmitted diseases

With changes in sexual attitudes in the 1960s, STDs have increased dramatically recently, and some symptoms of these illnesses may be manifested by lesions in the oral cavity that prompt patients to seek treatment from a dentist. With the advent of antibiotics, syphilis cases very significantly decreased, but now again are on the increase. Oral syphilitic lesions may resemble a chronic draining sinus tract (fistulous tract), poorly healed apicoectomy or periodontal surgery scar, fibroma, or draining periodontal pocket. As a result of decreased resistance, HIVD patients may succumb to Kaposi's sarcoma, which demonstrates oral lesions in approximately half its occurrences.

HIVD has become the scourge of those involved in public health. Much has been written and discussed about the subject, some factual and some speculative. As with the bubonic plague 400 years ago and poliomyelitis 45 years ago, some of the information concerning HIVD may be blown out of proportion or be incorrect.

HIVD does have two seriously insidious aspects that cannot be minimized. First, patients with HIVD have little to look forward to except probable death, perhaps not from the virus that causes the disease, but from associated illnesses that attack people whose immune systems have been seriously weakened. Second, for every person with active symptoms of HIVD, it is estimated that 10 times as many have precursors of the disease and as many as 50 times that number will test positive for the antibody to the virus responsible for the disease.

Originally called AIDS, or acquired immunodeficiency syndrome, this disease is now referred to in terms of the etiologic agent, the human immunodeficiency virus (HIV). Patients suffering from HIVD will test positive for HIV and thus are considered to be HIV positive. HIV is considered to be a lentivirus, or slow virus, indicating a long incubation period and slow progression of the disease. The mean incubation period, from first contact and infection to initial signs and clinical symptomatology, is approximately 10 years, but this time is extremely variable.

Because HIV progressively incapacitates the immune system, any diseases that thrive in this immunologically depressed atmosphere will fulminate in these patients. Because of the long period of latency, initially no deviation from normal may be noted by the patient or during cursory examination by a health professional. Eventually, however, opportunistic infections (persistent candidiasis, herpes simplex or zoster, *Mycobacterium* infections, pneumonia, *Salmonella* infections) or neoplasms (Kaposi's sarcoma, several types of lymphoma) eventually cause death. The symptoms of several types of these diseases may be revealed after examination or consultation with a dentist.

One of the major factors in the insidious attack of HIVD is that HIV is a retrovirus and therefore carries genetic material as ribonucleic acid (RNA) and reverse transcriptase, which may convert into the proviral deoxyribonucleic acid (DNA). The latter attaches and then enters into the infected host cell and is able to produce more viruses. The usually infected cell is the T4-helper lymphocyte, important in immune regulation and cellular response to infections. When infected by HIV, the T4-helper lymphocytes no longer perform their normal function and reduce significantly in number, from 700 to 1000 cells/mm^3 to less than 500 cells/mm^3 in adults. Thus the infections and other conditions previously listed have an enhanced environment in which to develop.

In the United States, 96% of HIV-positive patients are male homosexuals and bisexuals, IV drug users, or recipients of infected blood. Inner-city poor are overrepresented in these statistics, with blacks (12% of U.S. population) accounting for 25% of the cases and Hispanics (7% of population) 14% of cases.

It would appear that performing endodontic treatment, even for those at high risk for HIVD, can be made acceptably safe. The virus seems to be killed easily by 5% sodium hypochlorite, the dominant irrigant used during therapy. Contact with the patient's blood is very minimal, since most therapy is performed without surgery with a rubber dam and the major condition in which blood may flow in significant amounts is during the extirpation of a vital, inflamed pulp. Even at that time the dentist does not contact any of the blood, and the instruments used to extirpate the pulp and enlarge the bloody canal are disposed of according to those involved with possibly blood-borne pathogens. Chapter 17 will present the suggestions for barrier controls for HIVD and other possibly infected patients.

Those working in dental offices, including doctors, assistants, and auxiliaries, seem to be doing a very good job preventing transmission of HIVD from infected patients. At this writing, no documented case of HIV to dental workers has been reported. It is estimated that the risk of HIV to workers in the health care industry is very low, much less than the risk of hepatitis B. Most of the documented HIV transmissions have involved nurses or laboratory technicians infected by blood due to needle sticks or sharps accidents.

Similarly, studies concerning transmissions of HIV from HIV-infected health care workers to their patients indicate that the case involving the dentist from Florida is the only one on record. Recently an investigation by the Centers for Disease Control and Prevention indicated that 19,036 patients treated by 57 HIV-infected health care workers resulted in absolutely no HIV transmissions. This information should make all of us feel much better as to the scourge of HIV attacking us in our offices. Undoubtedly, this has resulted from the care and intensity applied to the aseptic techniques, barrier control practices, and sterilization procedures carried out in dental offices. However, this should not lead anyone to believe that these high standards need not be maintained. On the contrary, the success undoubtedly is due to the diligence thus far practiced.

Other STDs may be found in the general dental population with oral manifestations or the ability to be transmitted during dental treatment. Sexually transmitted herpes has struck 20 million heterosexual Americans. The disease is incurable, may be painful, may have oral lesions, but is never fatal. Gay males may be struck by hepatitis, which might be fatal but usually is not, and certain lower GI diseases, which fall under the umbrella term *gay bowel syndrome*, usually related to having sexual encounters with inhabitants from or visitors to tropical islands. Gonorrhea, as with syphilis, is easily treated with antibiotics.

Recent change in weight

Although not a disease in itself, a recent significant gain or loss of weight may indicate factors to be considered during endodontic therapy. If this symptom or any other symptom uncovered in the taking of the medical history is suggestive of systemic disease, the dentist should immediately contact the patient's physician, who would conduct further diagnostic examinations.

A common cause for significant loss of weight is intentional dieting. Many drugs—hypnotics, antibiotics, analgesics, and occasionally local anesthetics—may have increased action or possibly cause ordinarily rarely seen side effects, particularly in the GI system, when administered to a patient who is dieting. Also, if a surgical procedure is to be performed, optimal healing requires that correct amounts of vitamins, minerals, and proteins be present in the diet. If a diet is being followed under the advice and guidance of a physician, usually no problems arise. However, if the diet is self-imposed, an analysis of the foodstuffs ingested often reveals considerable lack of balance, and supplementation is required.

Loss of weight may be due to appetite decrease from drug ingestion, anxiety, pain, excessive smoking, or alcoholism. Neoplasms, diabetes, and Addison's disease also are accompanied by weight loss.

Weight gain generally is due to excessive eating, which may be stimulated by psychogenic reasons, hormonal disturbances, or pregnancy. This increased food ingestion usually is heaviest in carbohydrates and may be accompanied by increased caries incidence. If this is the case, restorations, particularly after endodontic therapy, must be fabricated to give the greatest possible protection to exposed tooth surfaces. Temporary crowns, splints, orthodontic bands, or other prostheses and appliances should be removed infrequently and the teeth examined for recurrent decay.

Weight gain may also result from water and salt retention due to renal or heart disturbances, which have already been discussed. Uchin states that the endodontic patient with water retention problems frequently suffers from intratreatment exacerbations when not receiving medications. Typically, this patient has swollen, edematous ankles or wrists. During the taking of the medical history, direct questioning about the condition will either confirm its presence or rule it out. Many patients with water retention problems take their medications only at certain times (e.g., women who take diuretics shortly before their menstrual period). If it is established that a patient falls into this category, a consultation with the patient's physician is indicated to prescribe necessary medication to avert the possibility of exacerbations.

Patients who give a history of recurrent acute exacerbations in relation to previous endodontic therapy and who appear to have the typical water retention problem should be referred to their physician for consultation before a new tooth is treated. Emergency treatment should be given, of course, but the patient should be evaluated before routine treatment is provided.

Psychologic problems

There is not sufficient space here for listing all the psychologic problems that may enter into the treatment of a patient in endodontics. The fact that a patient is under the care of a psychiatrist for an emotional difficulty does not indicate that a serious management problem will arise during dental treatment. In fact, a patient receiving treatment for an emotional condition may have come to grips with the disorders and be able to react normally to the phases of endodontic therapy. On the other hand, a patient with unsolved psychologic disorders who is not receiving professional help may prove to be difficult to manage.

Although it is helpful to know, it is difficult to ask the patient directly about emotional problems. Certain hints concerning a patient's emotional condition may be disclosed during the taking of the medical history. Some physical problems indicate a tendency toward anxiety, fears, and other emotional disorders. These include colitis, stomach and duodenal ulcers, asthma, hypertension, frequent severe headaches, and temporomandibular joint (TMJ) dysfunction syndrome. Persons taking tranquilizers or antidepressives probably have some type of emotional problem.

If the patient is referred by another dentist, the referring individual is usually aware of the problems and alerts a colleague by a phone call or note before the patient is seen to facilitate proper handling to avoid an initial disturbing conflict. Relatives may be a source of information by similarly advising the dentist of the prevailing situation. Some patients freely volunteer such information, including their psychiatrist, when asked for the names of their physicians or stating that they are receiving psychotherapy when disclosing what diseases they have had.

Some of the more frequent psychologic problems that might affect endodontic therapy will be briefly discussed. If more information is desired by the reader, the bibliography at the end of this chapter may act as a guide.

In general, two types of patients with emotional conditions must be considered in relation to endodontic therapy. One type is the patient who has converted a psychologic condition into a physical problem in or around the oral cavity. The other is the patient with such severe fears and anxieties that treatment becomes extremely difficult.

Conversion reactions are those in which a physical dysfunction is manifested from an emotional conflict without any organic pathosis. The physical symptom reduces the emotional pain and anxiety, attracts attention and concern from others (e.g., family and members of the medical professions), and provides a concrete condition to avoid treatment for the true problem. Because the oral cavity is the earliest site of pleasure for the infant and remains an area of pleasurable responses throughout life, it is only natural that diseases of emotional origin may be encountered in the vicinity.

Fortunately for those involved in endodontics, few disorders of this type stimulate a typical pulpal or periapical condition. However, occlusal problems, particularly bruxism, and such periodontal conditions as acute necrotizing gingivitis, desquamative gingivitis, lichen planus, glossodynia, and dental caries may have psychosomatic origins. Of these, only advanced dental caries causing pulpal involvements is likely to bring this type of emotionally disturbed patient directly in contact with an endodontic problem. However, here the symptoms of pulpal exposure are quite real and will respond favorably.

Problems arise for the endodontist when a patient is treated for a dental condition with a psychosomatic etiology. No relief is provided, and thus a pulpal problem is suspected. The patient may have several deep restorations or other suspicious elements, and endodontic treatment may be undertaken. When no change in symptoms is noted after seemingly correct treatment in a patient who is suspected of having emotional problems, the existence of a conversion reaction must be strongly considered.

Certain patients become extremely upset before and during dental treatment and are so physically and emotionally drained during even the briefest appointment that they are unable to function properly for at least the remainder of that day. These patients have a deep fear of dental pain and manipulation or treatment, to the extent that they are completely worked up before even entering the office.

Many state that they have had unfortunate dental experiences, such as severely painful injections; syncope after injections; poor reaction to an anesthetic or inability to be anesthetized; rough, inhumane, or sadistic treatment; dry sockets; or other severe postoperative pain. Any of these symptoms may occur to any patient who has had considerable dental treatment, but the patient with deep anxiety tells of the recurrences of these problems and greatly dramatizes the events. He or she is obviously fearful that the approaching appointment will lead to another traumatic experience. Because of this deep fear, regular dental visits are neglected; when finally forced to seek treatment for relief of pain or because of family pressures, the person may have an extremely advanced periodontal or carious condition requiring complex endodontic, periodontal, and restorative procedures.

In treating patients of this type, the practitioner must maintain a friendly but firm manner. The case presentation should be brief but confident. Instruments should be kept out of sight of the patient during the explanatory period. Booklets prepared by the ADA and the American Association of Endodontists (AAE) to give patients information concerning endodontics are excellent and supportive. They may be given to the anxious patient at the end of the appointment, to be read at home. Often a fearful patient is so tense that the case presentation is neither heard nor understood, and after appointment completion, he or she may conjure up incorrect assumptions. These would be dispelled by these brochures.

Many researchers have documented that as the degree of anxiety is increased, the tolerance for pain decreases and the response to pain increases. Anxiety, which is reflected as a psychologic stress in certain individuals, causes the same kind of physiologic changes that occur when there is direct physical assault to the tissues. Beacher and Sweet reported on the effects of anxiety in two groups of 150 young men. One group required surgery after injuries at the Anzio beachhead during World War II. The other group was composed of surgery patients in a civilian hospital. Of the soldiers, only 32% required a narcotic for pain relief, whereas 83% of the civilians needed a narcotic. For the soldiers, leaving the field of battle reduced their anxieties, since the war was a greater threat than was surgery. The civilians were removed from their normal comforting environment and subjected to surgery. Their anxieties were increased, as was their pain.

Applications of this information in treating the patient with anxiety about approaching endodontic therapy are apparent. One must emphasize that endodontics is preferable to extraction. The patient should be told that the treatment saves the tooth and prevents drilling of adjacent teeth, that no bleeding results, and that any pain after the appointment is minimal. When treating a tooth with necrotic pulp, the dentist should point out that no injection is needed.

If a choice of teeth to treat at the initial visit exists, the easiest should be chosen (preferably not a mandibular molar, where the greatest anesthetic problems occur). All the anesthetic administration precautions discussed in the segment on hypertension should be observed. By all means, some treatment, even if only perfunctory, should be performed at the first visit. A smooth, relatively painless initial visit is the best medicine to indicate that further treatment will be uneventful.

For long or potentially painful appointments, hypnotics should be prescribed if someone is available to accompany the patient when he or she leaves the office. Under no circumstances should these premedicaments be used if the patient cannot be so chaperoned.

A highly emotional state that may be encountered in endodontics is seen in patients suffering from cancerophobia. Great care must be exercised in the case presentation to avoid even the mere suggestion that a growth is present, since a problem in the periapical area might be carelessly described. A chronic draining sinus, chronic alveolar abscess, or endodontic-periodontal pocket might be thought of as malignant by such a patient. If a cancerophobic patient has a periapical area disorder and is concerned about its implication, surgery with biopsy of the lesion may be the best method by which to set the patient's mind to rest. The time required for a radiolucency to demonstrate healing after nonsurgical treatment may cause too much anxiety.

Drug and medication therapy

In addition to illnesses, the medical history must include information concerning the patient's past and present drug and medication therapy. This information is important in clarifying any questions about a patient's physical condition and the possible effects expected from any medications that might be needed for the present dental problem. This segment of the history must also include any adverse reactions that the patient has had to any drugs, particularly to those used in connection with dental therapy.

Some dentists prefer to take a medical history directly rather than by having the patient fill out a form. However, because of the long list of drugs presently in common use, the patient's history of medications must be obtained by using a prepared list or by having the patient fill out a questionnaire. If a form is used, it should include the following:

Have you taken or are you now taking any of the following drugs or medications? Indicate any unusual reactions you have had to any of them.
Penicillin
Sulfonamides
Other antibiotics
Aspirin or aspirin substitutes
Other pain relievers, such as Darvon or Tylenol
Antihistamines
Sedatives or sleeping pills
Tranquilizers
Cortisone or other steroids
Anticoagulants or blood thinners
Digitalis, nitroglycerin, or other drugs for heart trouble
Medicines to reduce blood pressure
Medicines to reduce excessive fluids (diuretics)
Insulin or other medications for diabetes
Others (please list)

A patient may be taking a medication but be unaware of its action or its major ingredients. Through the *Physician's Desk Reference (PDR)*, the drug may be determined by matching with the product identification section, which has full-color reproductions of most products. The type and action of most drugs may be explained by other sections of the *PDR*. Consultation with the patient's physician is advisable if further clarification is needed.

Before prescribing any drugs for a patient, the dentist must be certain that previous administration has not resulted in an allergic reaction or idiosyncrasy. This is particularly true for antibiotics or analgesics, which are frequently prescribed during endodontic treatment but have considerable allergic potential. Allergic reactions to penicillin or tetracyclines have been reported with some frequency. Some patients experience gastric distress after taking aspirin, and others have unusual reac-

tions to codeine, Darvon, or other pain relievers. Sulfonamide may be used as an intracanal medication, but only when there is no history of allergy.

Patients with general allergies, as opposed to those solely caused by specific medications, may offer some problems during the course of endodontic therapy. Although no hard facts are available, many clinicians have observed that allergenic patients suffer from flare-ups more frequently than nonallergic patients. This should be considered when treating conditions that are more prone to intratreatment problems in patients with a history of allergies. When treating patients with periapical lesions, time set between appointments should be kept to the minimum when using the tables in Chapter 19. Such patients should be well monitored during treatment and seen quickly if an incipient sign of exacerbation is noted. Merely putting these patients under antibiotic coverage may not solve the problem. The antibiotic may be ineffective or, worse still, cause an allergic response. The flare-up might be immunologic (Chapter 4) rather than bacterial.

Just as no contraindications exist to endodontic therapy for any specific illnesses, no regimens of medication suggest avoidance of such treatment. However, patients taking heavy dosage of steroids often experience intratreatment pain and exacerbations due to the suppression of the inflammatory response. Steroids are prescribed for patients with pemphigus, rheumatoid arthritis, scleroderma, lupus erythematosus, and other collagen diseases. The mildest type of infection may become serious in patients receiving steroid therapy. Also, many signs and symptoms of inflammation that aid a physician or dentist in making a diagnosis are suppressed.

When performing endodontic treatment on patients receiving steroid therapy, the dentist should ensure that the appointments are scheduled a maximum of 48 to 72 hours apart. The usual separation of appointments by a week or more stretches out the period of therapy too greatly and increases the possibility for microorganisms to be attracted to the site of irritation and gain a foothold for an exacerbation. Therapy for teeth with vital pulps should be completed in two sittings, even if each appointment requires considerable time. Necrotic cases are completed in three appointments whenever possible, preferably in a 1-week period. Rapid sealing of the apical areas prevents microbes from finding an excellent breeding area. If indications of an infection appear or if surgery is required, antibiotic therapy plus increased dosage of steroids must be instituted by the patient's physician. Stressful conditions for these patients, as in surgery, infections, or trauma, might produce adrenal insufficiency unless the steroid dose is raised.

Patients who consume large and frequent doses of aspirin may experience bleeding problems after periapical surgery or extraoral incision and drainage. Patients receiving major tranquilizer therapy may experience unusual reactions when hypnotics or narcotics are prescribed by the dentist. The physician should be consulted before any additional drugs are suggested.

DENTAL HISTORY

Frequently the greatest problem causing failure to gain patient acceptance of a treatment plan is that the patient's wishes are not solicited. A new patient comes to the dental office and is examined by radiographs, study models, explorer, and periodontal probe. A careful diagnosis is made, and a treatment plan is formulated and presented. All this will have taken considerable time, and excellent judgment but may be rejected because of lack of pertinence to the patient's goals.

Many problems are averted by merely asking the patient simple questions, such as "What may I do for you?" or "What problems are you having with your teeth?" or "What would you like to accomplish with your dental treatment?" The last question indicates both your desire to hear about and respond to the patient's problem and your understanding that there should be an overall objective reached rather than a series of patchwork, piecemeal treatments given.

During the initial consultation, a number of other questions should be asked either verbally by the dentist or, as suggested by many experts in the field of practice management, by a patient questionnaire. Typical among these questions are "Do your gums bleed?" "Does food pack between your teeth?" "Does dental floss catch on your fillings?" These queries set the wheels in motion for stressing to the patient the importance of periodontal therapy, restorations of proper contour, and other sophisticated facets of dentistry, of which endodontics is an important branch.

After hearing the replies to these questions, the dentist should record in the patient's own words the answers given. When the case presentation is made, referral to these answers will show that the treatment plan is aimed at accomplishing the patient's objectives. If the current objectives are not appropriate to best dentistry, the patient must be given a thorough explanation that indicates the need for reappraisal and adjustment to reach a suitable goal of dental health. A patient's failure to respond positively to a realistic and progressive treatment plan usually indicates a lack of receptivity to modern dentistry and that the patient is a poor candidate for inclusion in an effective dental practice.

A patient seeks dental treatment for one of five purposes, as follows:

1. Relief of pain or discomfort—as with pulp exposure, fractured or mobile tooth, bleeding gingiva, acute abscess (either periapical or periodontal), TMJ pain, broken prosthesis, dislodged restoration, etc.
2. Correction of masticatory inefficiency or insufficiency—result of multiple missing teeth, severe malocclusion, prematurities, etc.
3. Improvement of cosmetics—unesthetic appearance due to large unsightly synthetic restorations, missing teeth, obvious metal restorations, large carious lesions, edematous gingiva, poorly matching or shaped jackets, diastemas, malocclusion, etc.
4. Examination for oral-systemic relationship—patient usually referred by a physician, when a disease state is suggestive of having originated in or spread to the oral cavity or when a disease is determined to be present but the rest of the body appears to be normal
5. Checkup—periodic with many people but also needed for women during pregnancy and for patients who are to have a surgical procedure (when the surgeon wants to be sure that the patient has no chronic dental problem that might interfere with healing)

It is important to ascertain which of these reasons has brought the patient to the dental office. Occasionally a patient indicates to the dentist a reason that is a cover-up for the true one. A typical example of this is the patient who fears that an oral ulcer is malignant yet states a completely different reason for seeking dental treatment.

Much of the dental history is recorded in the patient's dentition and must be related to the verbal information that is supplied. Multiple edentulous areas without replacement, heavy stain accumulation, obvious carious lesions, and minimal

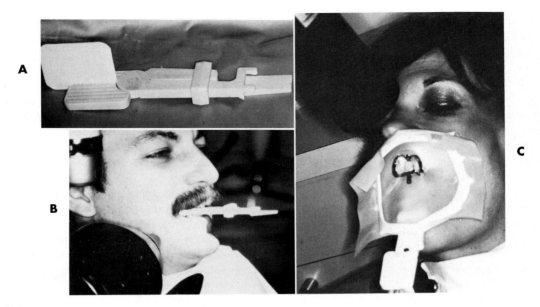

Fig. 2-3. **A,** Film holder, which is very useful in taking any intraoral radiograph. **B,** Patient is able to close on the holder while the film is being exposed, a much more comfortable position than having to keep the mouth open while film is finger held. With this technique the film has no opportunity to move between the time of placement and exposure. **C,** During treatment the film holder may be used for anterior teeth so that working length and master cone films can be acquired without the patient having to touch the film or holder and with the rubber dam still in place. Merely slip mounted film under rubber dam, and it will be held in place perfectly during exposure.

restorations indicate that the patient has a poor appreciation for dental treatment. Unless a strong motivation is supplied by the dentist or the patient's family and fully accepted by the patient, it is fruitless to attempt to formulate a treatment plan, including sophisticated procedures.

Multiple missing teeth replaced with poorly designed or fabricated bridges and partial dentures indicate that the patient has desired good dentistry but has been treated by practitioners incapable of supplying the best treatment. Usually this patient realizes that dental health is important but may be reluctant to undergo further extensive therapy for fear that the same result will occur. In this type of case, it must be indicated to the patient that a more progressive form of treatment will be followed. The use of periodontal and endodontic therapy must be emphasized so that the philosophy of extracting teeth is averted.

Patients with excellent restorative work rarely require introduction to sophisticated dentistry. They may have left their previous dentist because of a personality conflict but not from dissatisfaction with treatment. Taking time to explain some of the facets of therapy is frequently all that is required to gain control of the problem and restore a desirable dentist-patient relationship.

RADIOGRAPHS—THE MOST IMPORTANT DIAGNOSTIC AID

Use of the radiograph is mandatory in the diagnosis of any dental situation. In endodontics the radiograph is the most important single diagnostic aid, since it is the only reliable method for gaining needed information concerning the pulp canal space and periapical tissues, which are not observable to the naked eye. Any of the routine radiographic techniques described in textbooks or taught in dental schools can give the desired results necessary for adequate endodontic diagnosis. Either bisected-angle or long-cone techniques may be used, as long as careful planning precedes every exposure.

Film holder.   Use of a film holder is an excellent aid in obtaining reliable radiographs, particularly for posterior teeth. Film holders are commercially available or may be made from wooden blocks or impression compound (Fig. 2-3). They are mandatory for the long-cone technique.

Because of the angle of the hard palate, radio-

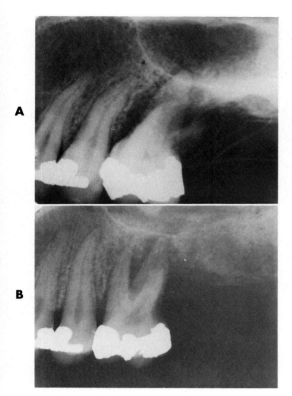

Fig. 2-4.   A, Radiograph of maxillary molar taken by having patient hold film with his thumb. Film was bent toward palate, distorting image, and was rotated. **B,** Same view taken with film holder. Note more normal relationship of root lengths and much better diagnostic quality of film.

graphs that are held by thumb or finger usually show the maxillary molars as having short buccal roots and a long palatal root. In actuality, the palatal root is rarely more than 2 mm longer than the buccal roots—a relationship that is correctly shown on films held by a film holder (Fig. 2-4).

For mandibular molars, film in a holder is exposed with the teeth closed rather than open as in finger-held views. Therefore the film has less chance to gouge the tissues on the floor of the mouth when a film holder is used, since the mylohyoid muscle is relaxed when the jaws are closed.

The film holder ensures that the film will be parallel to the occlusal surfaces of the teeth and aids in the positioning of the x-ray tube. It is easier to reproduce film angles for a series of the same area, and the film holder provides a method by which a particular tooth may be centered in the

film. Since many articles have been written in nonprofessional magazines concerning the dangers of radiation, patients are more comfortable when a device other than their own finger is used in holding the film.

For working films on anterior teeth, the opposite end of the film holder may be used so that the patient need not touch either the film holder or the film (Fig. 2-3, *C*). The mounted film is placed under the dam and positioned behind the tooth to be radiographed. The plastic rubber dam frame keeps the holder in position, and an excellent film is obtained.

Types of intraoral views to take for endodontic therapy.   In addition to the normal 18 to 22 views of a routine full-mouth radiographic survey, endodontic therapy requires supplementary films. Any tooth for which therapy is considered must have a minimum of two views, and posterior teeth may require three. One view should be the normal straight-on or direct exposure that shows the tooth to be treated well centered and allows for visualization of its mesiodistal dimensions. By altering the horizontal angulation of the cone, the dentist takes the additional films from a mesial and/or distal angle that retains the centering of the tooth in question but also gives some clues as to its buccolingual dimensions. Since much diagnostic information is available from a radiograph, examination with a magnifying glass or projector for enlargement is encouraged.

The direct view should give the following information concerning the tooth:

1. *Approximate overall length.* Depending on the vertical angulation required for the particular area, the measured length of the tooth image on the film may or may not correspond to the true tooth length. Views of mandibular molars and bicuspids taken at close to zero-degree angulation, with the film parallel to the teeth, result in a close correlation of tooth length to measured length of image. Maxillary anterior teeth, particularly cuspids, which require increased angulation, have a poorer correlation. However, if the film holder is used routinely and careful radiographic technique is followed, examination of the image gives significant clues as to relative tooth length so that sufficient warning is available before treatment when teeth are either much shorter or much longer than normal (Fig. 2-5).

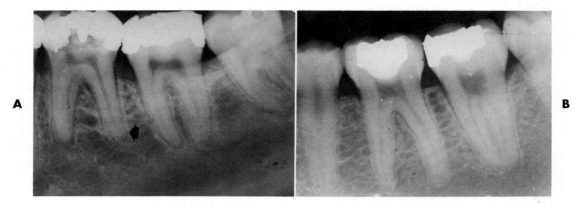

Fig. 2-5.   A, Mandibular first molar measured 17 mm on preoperative straight-on radiograph, shorter than average for that tooth. When the tooth was under treatment, the working lengths of the mesial canals were 17.5 mm. Also, note that this view shows distal canal curving off and exiting short of the apex. **B,** Another mandibular first molar measured 23.5 mm on the preoperative direct view, longer than average. The working lengths calculated during treatment were 23.5 mm for the mesial canals and 24 mm for the distal canal.

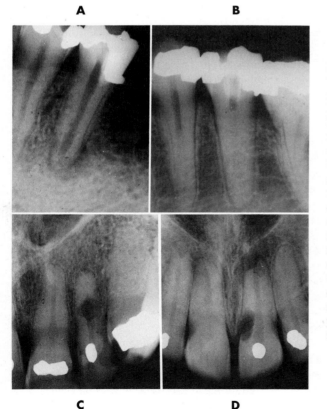

Fig. 2-6. Preoperative radiographs taken before treatment of mandibular second bicuspids of two patients, both 24 years of age. **A,** Very wide, irregular canal, at least size 70 or larger, before treatment. Heavy irrigation and rasping of walls with Hedstrom files (Chapter 7) are needed for proper debridement of this canal. **B,** Very narrow sclerotic canal, probably because of longstanding chronic pulpitis. Referring dentist's attempt to locate canal was unsuccessful. Careful exploration and enlargement with use of chelating agents and incremental instrumentation (Chapter 7) are needed to prepare this canal. **C,** An internal resorption defect alters shape of canal. As the canal is followed apically from coronal portion of tooth, there is obvious ballooning in middle third. (For completion of this case, see Fig. 14-3.) **D,** An external resorption defect, on the other hand, does not alter canal shape. This central incisor has a pulpoperiapical problem, but resorption from mesial is external only.

2. *Mesiodistal width of the pulp canal space.* Radiographs instantly reveal something about the width of the pulp canal space in general terms: that it is of normal width, is sclerotic, is very wide, or shows resorption. Such information is of obvious value during the course of therapy or in determining the method of therapy. Normal width may vary with the patient's age but is indicated by a definite radiolucent line from some position in the crown to the apical area. The sclerotic canal is vague on the film, is uneven in width or perhaps disappearing from view, and may only begin beneath the cervical line (Fig. 2-6, *B*). The very wide canal is one much wider than the patient's age would suggest and may or may not be associated with other entities, such as an open apex (Fig. 2-6, *A*).

Resorptive defects are also discernible on the radiograph and may cause an alteration in canal shape. An internal resorption defect alters the canal shape by causing a radiolucent bulge somewhere between the coronal and the apical portion of the canal (Fig. 2-6, *C*). Instituting endodontic therapy on these teeth almost always halts the resorption. Chapters 9 and 16 will discuss treatment methodology for these cases. An external resorption defect does not start within the pulp canal but rather begins adjacent to the periodontal ligament. Therefore external resorption does not cause any alteration in pulp canal shape (Fig. 2-6, *D*). Endodontic therapy may or may not halt the resorption. Unless there is a definite indication that a change from normalcy has occurred in the pulp or immediately periapical tissues, I do not recommend instituting endodontics for external resorption problems.

3. *Position of the orifice to other elements of the crown.* Since it is most important to find the canal, the radiograph shows some of the relationships to the other elements of the crown to aid in location of the orifice. These other features radiographically discernible in the crown are the enamel, caries, restorations, basis, pulpotomy dressings, cementoenamel junction, and dentinoenamel junction. The etiology for pulpal or periapical injury must be noted (Fig. 2-7).

4. *Mesial or distal curvature of the root.* It is rare to find a tooth whose root is perpendicu-

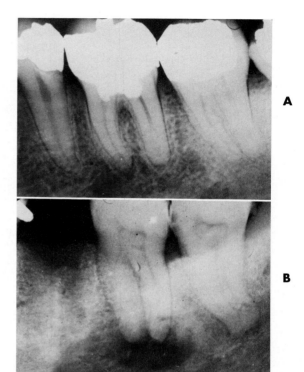

A

B

Fig. 2-7. **A,** Preoperative view of mandibular posterior area. Note following features, all indicative of probable need for endodontic treatment. Second bicuspid—deep restoration with base or pulp capping; some secondary dentin deposition on distal side of pulp canal, which is side toward restoration. First molar—pulpotomy dressing past cervical line; distal canal may divide in middle third; mesial canals not sclerosed. Second molar—possible pulpotomy or pulp cap; distal canal indistinct. **B,** Mandibular first molar has large periapical radiolucency, typical of the kind associated with necrotic pulp. However, etiology of pulpal death is not apparent, since no restoration or decay is present and there is no fracture. Pulp proved to be vital, and biopsy of lesion demonstrated eosinophilic granuloma. Had endodontic therapy been performed without consideration for cause of pulpal death, serious error would have delayed diagnosis and prevented correct treatment. (Courtesy Dr. William Shafer, Indianapolis.)

lar to the occlusal plane. The straight-on radiograph indicates the relative angulation of the root and discloses if a mesial or distal curvature is present. The film also indicates in general terms the type of dilaceration present, either gradual or sharp (Fig. 2-8).

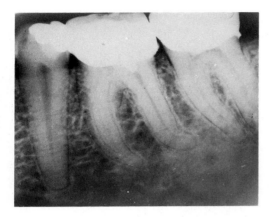

Fig. 2-8. Mandibular first molar with sharp distal dilaceration of canal in distal root.

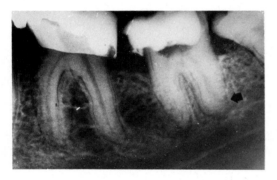

Fig. 2-9. Mandibular second molar with canal of distal root exiting short of apex *(arrow).*

5. *Some guides to the position of the apical foramen.* Factors such as root curvature, areas of occlusal stress, amount of cementum deposition, and tooth morphology determine the position of the apical foramen to the root. The direct radiograph indicates when the exit is definitely short of the radiographic apex if such emergence occurs on either the mesial or the distal surface of the root (Fig. 2-9). The film does not indicate if the exit occurs on the buccal or the lingual surface. However, if it appears that the pulp canal space abruptly halts at a point near the apex, this is usually indicative that the canal does exit short of the radiographic apex on either the buccal or the lingual aspect.

6. *Existence of apical radiolucencies resulting from pulpal damage and/or treatment.* The condition of the periapical tissues may be quite difficult to discern from radiographs. However, it is of prime importance in diagnosis, treatment planning, and therapy for endodontics to make such a determination. The difference between a normal periodontal ligament space and a widening of the space or between a widening of the space and a radiolucency must be determined. Magnification or, even better, projection with a slide projec-

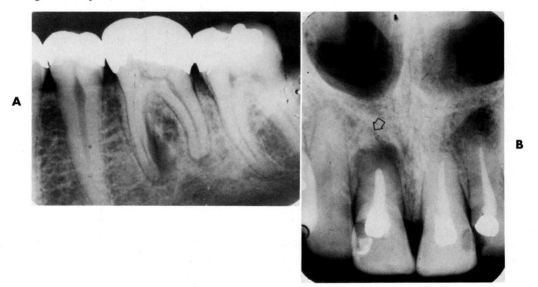

Fig. 2-10. Interesting radiolucencies. **A,** On distal border of mesial root of mandibular first molar. Note canal leaving root short of apex toward defect. **B,** Associated with endodontically treated right central incisor. Patient gave history of apical surgery to all three treated anterior teeth. The retained root *(arrow)* and an incomplete seal are probably responsible for lesion.

tor is particularly helpful in this area. The site of exiting of the canal (Fig. 2-10, *A*) is often disclosed by the position of the change in the periodontal ligament space. Evaluation of previously treated cases depends tremendously on the position and shape of radiolucencies present (Fig. 2-10, *B* to *F*). When evaluating radiolucencies, one must always remember that the true size of the lesion is much larger than the image seen on the radiograph.

7. *Radiolucencies not caused by pulpal damage and/or treatment.* The mere finding of a radiolucency in proximity to a tooth in itself does not indicate the need for endodontic treatment. In addition to those caused by pulpal damage and/or treatment, radiolucencies of the jaws may occur for many other reasons, totally unrelated to the pulpal condition or any local treatment. Because much of the total area of the maxilla and mandible is

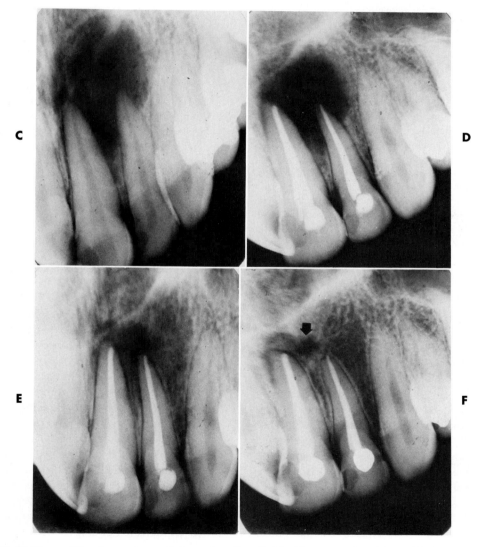

Fig. 2-10, cont'd.   Interesting radiolucencies. **C** to **F,** Maxillary central and lateral incisors treated surgically. **C** is preoperative; **D** was taken 3 months after surgery; **E** and **F** were made at yearly intervals. Without earlier radiographs for comparison, all postoperative films might be interpreted to indicate endodontic failure. Radiolucency shown in **F** *(arrow)* is fibrous tissue scar, does not indicate diseased tissue, and may never fill in with bone. The maxillary lateral incisor is the most common tooth to exhibit fibrous scar tissue after healing, particularly if periapical surgery was performed.

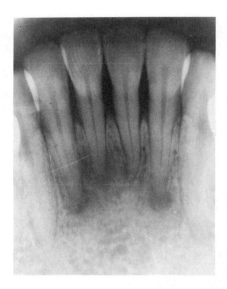

Fig. 2-11. Radiograph of mandibular incisors of a 35-year-old white female, indicating multiple periapical radiolucencies. Although the patient was referred for therapy for the four teeth, I would not treat them without confirming information. The patient was certain that the teeth had never been traumatized, and there was no visible damage to the crowns. All the teeth responded to electric pulp testing, indicating a diagnosis of multiple periapical fibrous dysplasia, formerly referred to as cementomas.

taken up with the roots of the teeth, any radiolucencies present for other reasons may appear in contact with, adjacent to, or superimposed on a root(s). A careless examination and evaluation may cause such teeth to be treated endodontically. There is no worse feeling than entering a pulp canal in a tooth with an apical radiolucency and then finding a normal, vital pulp present. Therefore incorrect treatment has been performed when the etiologic agent is misunderstood and does not result from pulpal damage or treatment. Care must always be exercised *before* starting treatment to verify that the pulp is involved and/or that the periapical tissues have been affected by the pulpal damage.

The most common periapical radiolucency that causes unneeded endodontic treatment is the so-called cementoma, also referred to as periapical fibroma, now called *periapical fibrous dysplasia* (Fig. 2-11).

Several other benign neoplasms may mimic periapical disease but are more serious and usually require some type of surgically related treatment, such as the ameloblastomas or the various developmental cysts. Avoiding errors in treatment for these entities requires the use of pulp testing (see later discussion) to rule out the cementoma. For the benign neoplasms, pulp testing coupled with knowledge of the radiographic appearance for these lesions (ameloblastomas often are multilobulated) and the anatomic position of developmental cysts (globulomaxillary cysts are found between the maxillary cuspid and lateral incisor; many cysts are in the third molar vicinity) is very helpful.

The most common anatomic condition that may be confused with periapical disease is the mental foramen because of its appearance on radiographs in proximity to the mandibular second bicuspid. The nasal cavity and sometimes even the maxillary sinus may appear to be a lesion involving a maxillary tooth. Pulp tests and angled radiographs (root tips move away from the anatomic radiolucencies) help to make a correct diagnosis. Fig. 2-12 demonstrates a lingual mandibular salivary gland depression, first reported by Stafne in 1942. It is a congenital defect and may be bilateral. One of the interesting aspects of the radiolucency shown in Fig. 2-12 is that 20 years later, the depression had smoothed out and was barely apparent radiographically.

Fig. 2-7, *B,* illustrates an eosinophilic granuloma mimicking periapical disease of a mandibular molar. This condition is often associated with sore or loose teeth. Therefore periodontists or endodontists may be called on to evaluate these symptoms. Together with Hand-Schüller-Christian disease and Letterer-Siwe disease, eosinophic granuloma forms the histiocytosis X group, each of which may mimic periapical disease. Histologic evaluation of biopsy specimens leads to the correct diagnosis.

Hormonal dysfunctions may also lead to radiolucent areas of the jaws. In hyperparathyroidism the first clinical sign or symptom may be a cyst of the jaws or a "ground-glass" appearance of bone. Sarco-

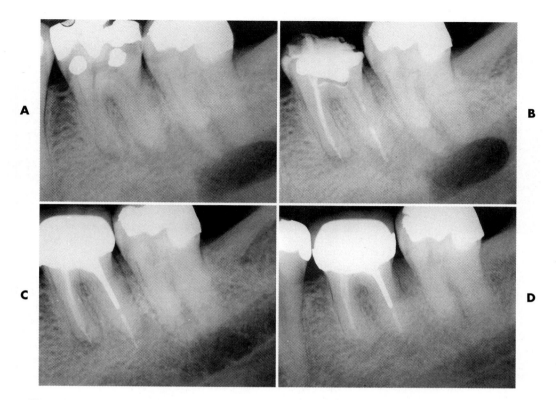

Fig. 2-12. Lingual mandibular salivary gland depression mimicking periapical disease. **A,** Preoperative radiograph of mandibular molar area indicating large radiolucency seemingly associated with the second molar and two smaller radiolucencies, each associated with a root of the first molar. Potential etiology for pulpal damage to the first molar is a large, distal carious lesion surrounding a large inlay. The second molar also has a large casting. Electric and temperature testing of the first molar gave no responses, but the second molar did respond. The first molar was slightly tender to percussion; the second molar reacted normally to percussion. **B,** It was decided to treat the first molar only and reevaluate the second molar later, considering the lesion to be a lingual mandibular salivary gland depression. Accordingly, the first molar was filled with laterally condensed gutta-percha and Wach's paste, with some sealer extruded past both apices. **C,** One year after treatment, periapical lesion on the distal root of the first molar is gone and that on the mesial root is decreased considerably. The radiolucency is still associated with the second molar, although slightly different in shape, and the tooth still responds to electric and pulp testing. **D,** Twenty years after original treatment, perfect healing is apparent on the first molar, with all excess sealer gone and tooth comfortable. The second molar still responds to electric and temperature testing, same casting is still present, and tooth is comfortable. Whereas the radiolucency is still present, it is much less radiolucent than in the first film. A study by Karmiol and Walsh indicated that salivary gland depression was present in the mandible in 18 of 4963 full-mouth radiographs investigated (0.4%) several times bilaterally. This patient did not exhibit the same radiographic finding on the opposite side.

mas of the jaws may exhibit a "sunburst" appearance on radiographs. Multiple myeloma also may cause radiolucent features in bones, including the maxilla or mandible. If the dentist cannot locate an etiologic agent for pulpal damage and pulp tests are negative

with these conditions, consultation with a physician is mandatory.

The traumatic bone cyst (not a true cyst) is an interesting condition that may be found in conjunction with a tooth requiring endodontic treatment. As suggested by its name, the

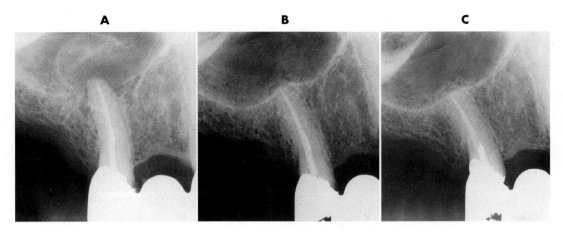

Fig. 2-13. Multiple lateral canals demonstrated after canal filling with laterally condensed modified chloropercha. **A,** Immediate postfilling film of maxillary second bicuspid indicating periapical and lateral lesions and chloropercha in many lateral canals. There is a disruption of the floor of the maxillary sinus. **B,** Film taken 2 years after treatment, indicating complete healing of the apical and lateral lesions and reconstitution of the floor of the sinus. **C,** Film taken 20 years after treatment, perfect healing of periapical, lateral, and sinus floor lesions still apparent. (Restorations by Dr. Sherwin Strauss, Chicago.)

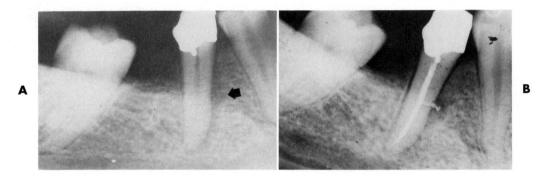

Fig. 2-14. A, Radiolucency on mesial surface of mandibular bicuspid *(arrow)* probably indicating a significant lateral canal with necrotic material, and only a minimal periapical lesion. **B,** Immediately after canal filling with laterally condensed gutta-percha and Wach's paste as sealer. The sealer is extruded toward the radiolucency.

lesion results from trauma, which may also have caused pulpal damage or death and resultant periapical extension. The surgical appearance after raising a flap is pathognomic. The cavity may be totally empty or contain a small amount of reddish exudate or clotted blood. Merely opening and lightly curetting this lesion lead to healing. If the root of an involved tooth is within the lesion, it should be treated before surgery.

In summary, many situations may give rise to radiolucencies of the jaws that may be confused with periapical disease. Some are

perfectly normal, some are mild, but some are quite serious. Before initiating endodontic treatment, the etiology should be clearly established. If an unanticipated condition is found on entry, further consideration should be rendered, including the possibility of consultation with other medical professionals.

8. *Existence of lateral radiolucencies and observations concerning lateral canals.* The lateral surfaces of roots should be carefully examined for areas of pathosis and exiting of canals. A definite lateral radiolucency often indicates the presence of a significant lateral canal that

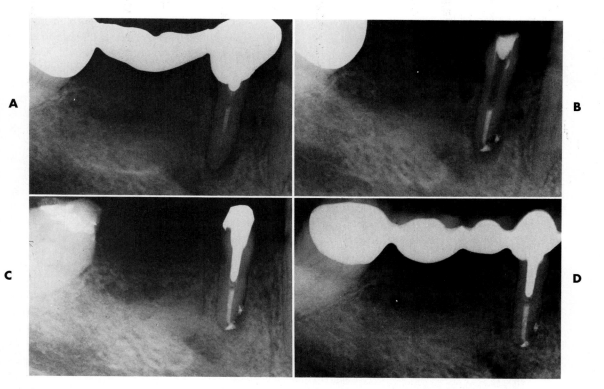

Fig. 2-15. **A,** Mandibular bicuspid with failing endodontics due to insufficient canal preparation and filling. Two radiolucencies are present, one apical and one lateral. **B,** Canal filling with laterally condensed gutta-percha and Wach's paste as sealer. Excess sealer has been expressed beyond apex and through the lateral canal. **C,** Three months after filling, a post has been placed and the radiolucency is beginning to heal. **D,** Eighteen months after canal filling, healing is quite advanced. (Restorations by Dr. Robert Salk, Chicago.)

is housing necrotic material. Some endodontists believe that the frequent display of filling materials demonstrating lateral canals in postoperative films indicates that the filling technique used is superior. I do not share this view because I have seen lateral canals demonstrated by sealer using every canal filling method. Fig. 2-13 indicates a maxillary bicuspid with a large periapical lesion, both apical and lateral, and a disruption of the floor of the maxillary sinus. The canal filling film indicates the presence of multiple lateral canals, perhaps eight or more. A postoperative film taken 20 years later indicates perfect healing and reestablishment of the floor of the sinus. The canal filling method was with modified chloropercha, not my favorite choice, and a method repudiated by some as ineffective. Several other modified chloropercha cases appear near the end of Chapter 9 and in Fig. 6-30 with lateral canals demonstrated.

I believe that the condition of the pulp of the tooth is a much better indicator for whether or not lateral canals will be demonstrated. Teeth with necrotic pulps have a much higher percentage of sealer in such canals than teeth with vital pulps. In a survey of patients treated by graduate students from Loyola University and myself, we found that when the pulp was necrotic, lateral canals were demonstrated 38% of the time, whereas if the pulp had been vital, the percentage of lateral canals decreased to only 3%

Many different types of lateral lesions are observable by radiographs. From a developmental standpoint, the first to discuss is the situation in which the lateral lesion is quite obvious, but there is no periapical lesion or only a minimal lesion at the apex (Fig. 2-14, *A*). Usually this is indicative of an apically progressing necrotic pulp that has allowed the exit of irritating materials through a significant lateral canal before the noxious elements reaching the apex. It is possible that there is true breakdown at the apex as well, but it is barely observable because of thicker overlying bone or insufficient apical breakdown of bone. Generally, at the time of filling, the sealer is extruded through the lateral canal to the site of the lateral radiolucency (Fig. 2-14, *B*).

If allowed to progress without endodontic intervention, this condition may next be seen as the second type, in which one or more lateral lesions exist plus a periapical lesion, but the lesions are separate and distinct (Fig. 2-15, *A*). Now, sufficient numbers of irritating

materials have emerged through both the lateral and the apical orifices in the root to allow for visualization of both sets of lesions.

If still allowed to progress without treatment, the periapical and lateral lesions coalesce into a single lesion. This type of lesion has been called a "wraparound" lesion, since it involves both the tip of the root and one or both of the mesial and/or distal lateral walls (Fig. 2-16). However, the etiology of the lesion remains as separate exit sites off the root.

Another type of periapical lesion closely resembles this "wraparound" type, but it may not involve etiology from the lateral canal. Fig. 2-17, *A*, demonstrates such a case in which the lesion expands down a side of the root rather than ballooning out apically, as is usually the situation. When the immediate postfilling film is viewed (Fig. 2-17, *B*), the clinician may be disappointed to observe no sealer exiting to the lateral lesion. However, subsequent films (Figs. 2-17, *C* to *E*) indicate that healing has taken place. Healing in this type of situation means either that no lateral canal was present to cause the lesion and that the source was solely from the apex, or that the lateral canal need not be demonstrated with sealer for healing to

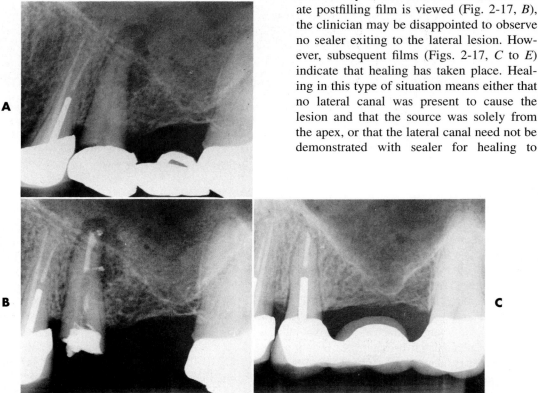

Fig. 2-16.   **A,** Preoperative mesial-angled view of maxillary second bicuspid with a "wraparound" periapical lesion, encompassing the apical area and a portion of the lateral distal surface of the root. **B,** Immediate postoperative view, after canal filling with laterally condensed gutta-percha and Kerr's Antiseptic Root Canal Sealer. That a lateral canal was involved in the pathogenesis of the lesion was verified by the sealer expressed through the root to the distal. **C,** Four years after treatment, straight view. The entire lesion has healed, with minimal amounts of sealer observable in the surrounding bone. The maxillary sinus, although adjacent to the lesion, was not involved, as it was in Fig. 2-13. (Restoration by Dr. Ascher Jacobs, formerly of Chicago.)

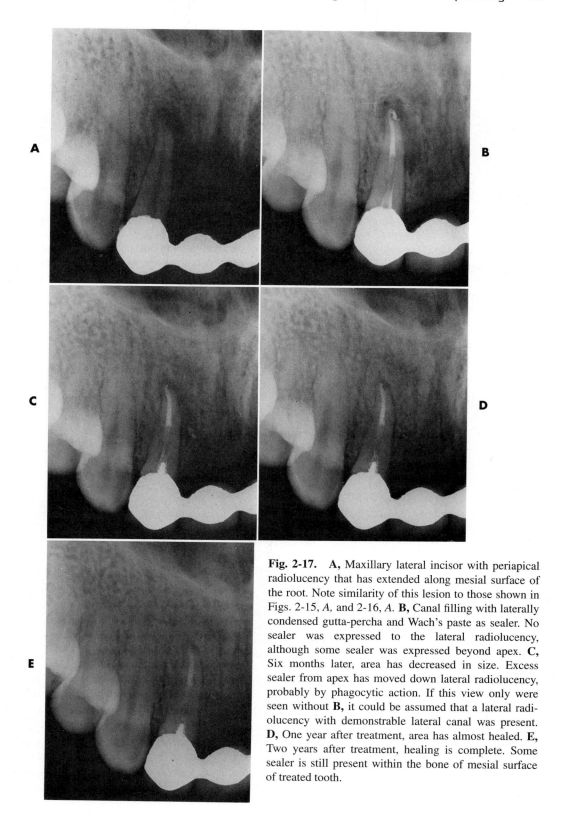

Fig. 2-17.   A, Maxillary lateral incisor with periapical radiolucency that has extended along mesial surface of the root. Note similarity of this lesion to those shown in Figs. 2-15, *A,* and 2-16, *A.* **B,** Canal filling with laterally condensed gutta-percha and Wach's paste as sealer. No sealer was expressed to the lateral radiolucency, although some sealer was expressed beyond apex. **C,** Six months later, area has decreased in size. Excess sealer from apex has moved down lateral radiolucency, probably by phagocytic action. If this view only were seen without **B,** it could be assumed that a lateral radiolucency with demonstrable lateral canal was present. **D,** One year after treatment, area has almost healed. **E,** Two years after treatment, healing is complete. Some sealer is still present within the bone of mesial surface of treated tooth.

A   **B**   **C**

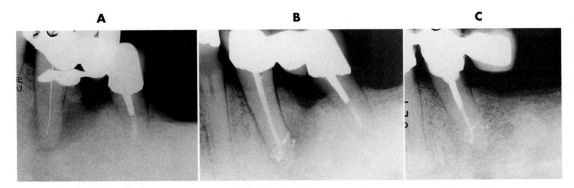

Fig. 2-18.   "Wraparound" lateral canal. **A,** Radiograph of file in place on mandibular second bicuspid, indicating canal exiting mesially. A sinus tract was present to the distal portion of the tooth, and the film indicates the lesion exiting distally. **B,** Immediate postfilling film after laterally condensed gutta-percha and Kerr's Antiseptic Root Canal Sealer. Several lateral canals are present, with the sealer wrapping around from the mesial to the distal either on the buccal or lingual portion of the root. **C,** Posterior abutment has been lost due to periodontal disease, but 11 years after treatment, the periapical lesion has healed perfectly while the path of sealer, although slightly resorbed, is still apparent. (Restorations by Dr. Maurice Slivnick, Skokie, Ill.)

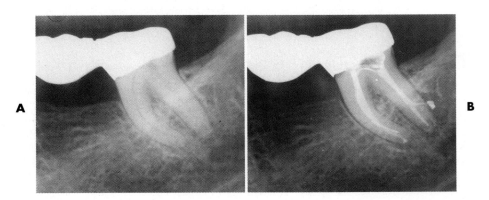

A   **B**

Fig. 2-19.   **A,** Preoperative film of mandibular second molar, with clinical symptoms of pulpitis thought to be caused by large restoration. No periapical or lateral lesions were seen in association with the tooth. An access cavity was prepared at an emergency appointment, the pulp extirpated, and all symptoms disappeared. The patient had been very pleasant and cooperative for several other endodontic cases, but for various reasons, it took almost 6 months to complete treatment for this tooth. **B,** Viewing this film after filling with laterally condensed gutta-percha and Kerr's Antiseptic Root Canal Sealer indicated two large lateral canals, both in association with lateral lesions, that were quite unexpected. The lateral lesions apparently had developed during the long period that it had taken to complete treatment. A possible cause for the pulpitis is now apparent as the caries on the mesial side.

transpire. In the latter case, perhaps dentin chips covered over the lateral canal, preventing necrotic tissue within it from feeding the lateral lesion but also stopping sealer from exiting to the periodontal ligament area.

Fig. 2-18 demonstrates another "wraparound" condition. A chronic draining sinus tract was present, extending to the distal area of the mandibular second bicuspid, but the file-in-place film (Fig. 2-18, *A*) indicated that the canal exited to the mesial. When the canal was filled (Fig. 2-18, *B*), the sealer exited from several sites and seemed to wrap around the buccal or lingual portion of the tooth from the mesial to the distal. Excellent healing was observed later.

In the cases demonstrated by Figs. 2-15, 2-16, and 2-18, demonstration of lateral

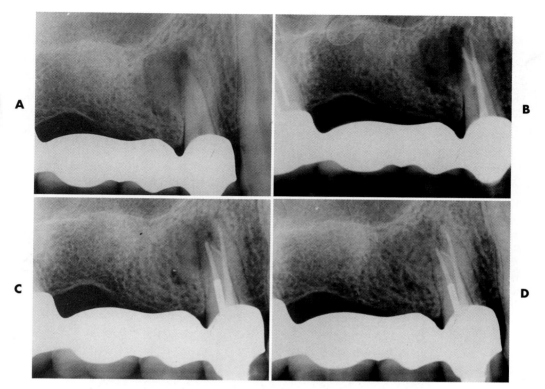

Fig. 2-20. **A,** Preoperative film of maxillary first bicuspid, indicating large periapical radiolucency with considerable distal extension of the lesion, a condition often seen with lateral canal lesions (see Figs. 2-16 and 2-21 as well). **B,** Although I did not anticipate a lateral canal for this case, when I filled the canals with laterally condensed gutta-percha and Kerr's Antiseptic Root Canal Sealer, a large lateral canal was demonstrated, branching off several millimeters from the tip of the palatal root (root to the right) to the buccal area. Post room was prepared in the buccal canal. **C,** Excellent healing 1 year after treatment. **D,** Perfect healing 5 years after treatment, with material in the lateral canal still visible. (Restoration by Dr. Morton Rosen, Chicago.)

canals was fully expected. In Fig. 2-17, it was anticipated but did not appear. Many times, however, lateral canals of considerable size are demonstrated without being expected. The case shown in Fig. 2-14 was one of my first to demonstrate a lateral canal. In retrospect, I could see that I should have anticipated it, but at that time I did not.

Fig. 2-19 is another instance in which I did not expect to see a lateral canal demonstrated. The patient had required that several teeth be treated endodontically and was always most cooperative. At the start of treatment (Fig. 2-19, *A*), the pulp was vital, with all the symptoms of a pulpitis present, and no lesions, lateral or apical, were seen. Treatment was started successfully and the pulpitis eliminated, but due to a variety of reasons,

completion was delayed for 6 months. When I finally filled the canals (Fig. 2-19, *B*), I was shocked to see several lateral canals, both exiting to lateral lesions that were not present before treatment. The cause for the pulpitis was also seen as the recurrent decay under the mesial portion of the bridge abutment. Some pulp, vital at the start of treatment, was present in these lateral canals. Because of the long time required for therapy, the tissue became necrotic but was removed, probably by the sodium hypochlorite irrigant, and allowed for passage of the sealer into the tissues surrounding the lateral canals.

Fig. 2-20 illustrates a tooth with a large periapical lesion with some lateral extension associated with a maxillary first bicuspid (Fig. 2-20, *A*), symptomatic before treatment.

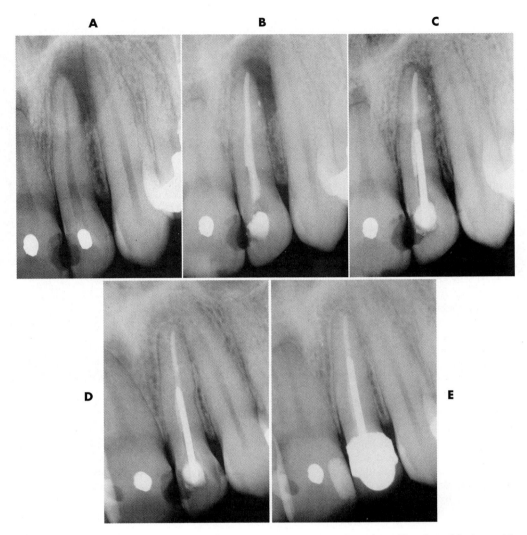

Fig. 2-21. Lateral lesion deflecting adjacent tooth. **A,** Preoperative film of maxillary lateral incisor, with lesion extending slightly apically but considerably distally, a sign often indicative of a lateral canal lesion. **B,** Immediately after filling with laterally condensed gutta-percha and Wach's paste, a lateral canal is demonstrated, coursing exactly to the distal portion of the lesion. **C,** After 1 year, lesion has decreased considerably, and it appears that the distance between the lateral and adjacent cuspid has decreased. Note that the contact areas on both the mesial and the distal are identical to those shown on film **A. D,** Two years after treatment, with complete healing. Lateral incisor and cuspid are very close to each other at their apices. **E,** Six years after treatment, perfect healing. (Restoration by Dr. Arnold Wax, Chicago.)

Again, although not anticipated, a lateral canal was filled with sealer, several millimeters from the apex of the palatal root (Fig. 2-20, *B*), pointing toward the major portion of the radiolucency. Excellent healing resulted from the treatment (Fig. 2-20, *C* and *D*).

Lateral lesions may cause pressures that deflect teeth. A large lesion, perhaps a "wraparound," associated with a maxillary

lateral incisor (Fig. 2-21, *A*) was treated, and the canal filling indicated a lateral canal extending to the lesion (Fig. 2-21, *B*). Subsequent films indicated excellent healing but also decreased distance between the lateral and the adjacent cuspid (Fig. 2-21, *C* to *E*).

Damage from a lateral canal lesion may be revealed subsequent to treatment. The maxillary cuspid shown in Fig. 2-22, *A,* required

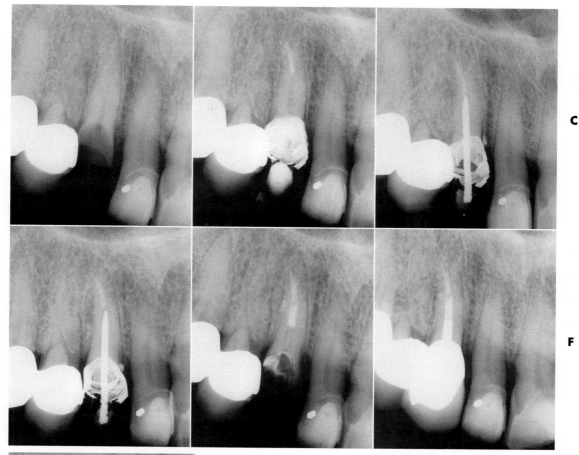

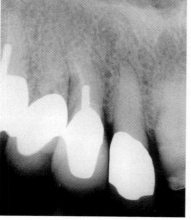

Fig. 2-22. Lateral canal lesion developing after canal filling and post room preparation. **A,** Preoperative film of maxillary cuspid. Considerable decay beneath the gingival margin is apparent. No periapical or lateral lesions are present, and the pulp was vital. **B,** Cooperative referring dentist constructed a temporary crown with a contoured metal band and acrylic, allowing me to treat the tooth with a well-adapted rubber dam to maintain asepsis. Canal filled with laterally condensed gutta-percha and Wach's paste, with post room prepared as long as possible due to necessarily considerable length of the anticipated clinical crown. **C,** Crown could not be completed because the patient became quite ill. This film, taken 6 months later, indicated possible development of a lateral lesion adjacent to the post space. **D,** Patient was forced to undergo cardiac surgery, further setting back restoration. This film was taken 1 year after completion of endodontic treatment, and now there is an obvious lateral lesion. The root is tender to palpation in the proximity of the lesion. **E,** Small portion of the canal filling apical to the post room was removed. The apical segment of the post room was reprepared and filled with laterally condensed gutta-percha and Kerr's Antiseptic Root Canal Sealer. This film was taken 3 months later, indicating healing of the lesion. The root is no longer tender to palpation. **F,** Eighteen months later, a post/core system and crown have been constructed, lesion has healed, and area looks excellent. **G,** Eleven years after original treatment, another post/core and crown were constructed, but area continues to look excellent. (Restoration by Dr. Steve Potashnick, Chicago.)

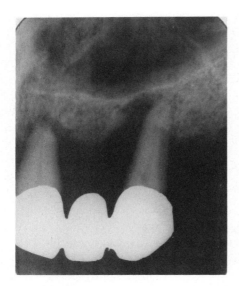

Fig. 2-23.   Insufficient alveolar support contraindicates endodontic treatment for the cuspid.

endodontic treatment. At treatment the pulp was vital, and no apical or lateral lesions were noticed. After filling and post room preparation (Fig. 2-22, *B*), the tooth was temporized (Fig. 2-22, *C*), but because the patient required cardiac surgery, final restoration was delayed. When the patient returned for evaluation, a lateral lesion was noted in the area of the post room. Re-treatment of this segment of the canal yielded a filling with sealer entering the lateral lesion (Fig. 2-22, *D*). Excellent healing followed (Fig. 2-22, *E* to *G*).

When a sinus tract is traced with a gutta-percha cone and the marker goes to a lateral surface of the root (Fig. 2-30, *A* and *B*), it probably indicates a lateral canal lesion, a root perforation, or a cracked tooth.

In summary, lateral canal lesions are interesting, may have several types of configurations, and can be indicated by a variety of filling techniques. In my opinion, they are much more likely to be demonstrated in teeth with necrotic pulps and, although occurring rarely, may cause problems after seemingly correct treatment.

9. *Periodontal defects.* Although the radiograph made before endodontic therapy is examined to aid in the treatment to be performed within the tooth, it should always be remembered that the alveolar bone holds the tooth. Because the pulp and the periodontal tissues have an intimate relationship and because sufficient support must be present before endodontic therapy is performed, the periodontal condition must always be evaluated (Fig. 2-23).

The finding of a periodontal pocket, even an extensive one, does not necessarily indicate that endodontic therapy will be fruitless on the tooth. It is not only important to examine the tooth to be considered for treatment, but also to evaluate the periodontal condition of the other teeth. Fig. 2-24 illustrates a case in which the mandibular molar, which had already received endodontic treatment, had a pocket in the furcation that could be probed from the labial direction. The patient was young, and no other areas of even moderate periodontal disease were present. Because the endodontic treatment did not appear adequate (Fig. 2-24, A to C), it was decided to attempt re-treatment. The subsequent radiographs (Fig. 2-24, F and H) indicate the desired result obtained.

Fig. 2-24.   **A,** Preoperative view, straight, and **B,** angled view of mandibular first molar. Tooth had received endodontic treatment, but periapical lesions were present on both roots. Even worse, a pocket could be probed into the furca, and some mobility was present. **C,** Crown and post were removed, and floor of the chamber was examined to see if any perforations or other causes for furcal involvement were present. There were none. Patient was otherwise free of periodontal problems. Accordingly, the existing canal fillings were removed. The distal canal could be instrumented to a desirable site, but not much length could be gained in the mesial canals. **D** and **E,** Straight and angled views after canal fillings with laterally condensed gutta-percha and Wach's paste as sealer. The furca was no longer probeable. **F** and **G,** Straight and angled views 2 years after treatment. The periapical areas healed, the pocket in the furca could not be probed, and the tooth was tight. **H,** Ten years after original treatment, furcation area remains normal, with periapical lesions healed. (Restoration by Dr. Doug Shindollar, Chicago.)

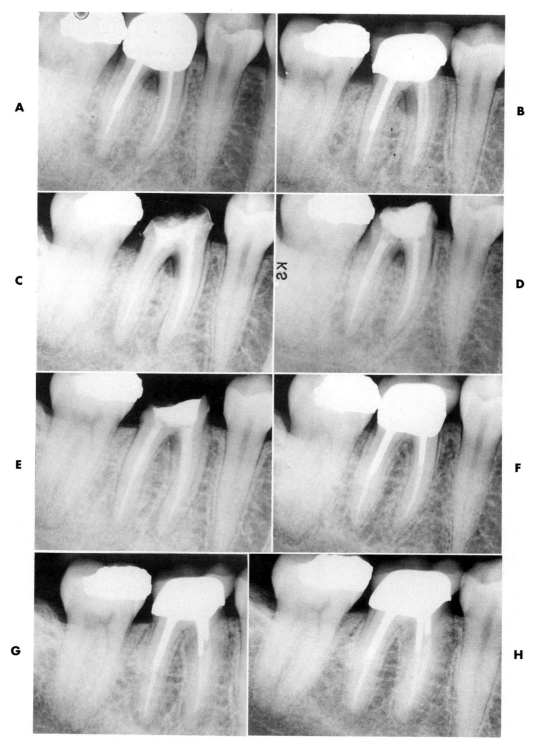

Fig. 2-24. For legend see opposite page.

Many cases in Chapter 13 illustrate seemingly hopeless periodontal conditions alleviated successfully by endodontic therapy alone or combined endodontic and periodontal therapy. This statement should not be misconstrued to suggest that teeth with advanced periodontal conditions should be treated endodontically on a routine basis. Surely the cuspid shown in Fig. 2-23 would not gain longevity if the canal were cleaned and filled. However, the suggestions for proper evaluation of periodontally involved teeth stated in Chapter 13 must be considered always.

The mesial and/or distal angulation view should add the following information:

1. *Number of roots present.* Although the straight-on view normally indicates the number of roots present in molars, the angle view is the one that discloses unanticipated root bifurcations. The additional roots are superimposed in the direct view and would lead to false information if no additional views were taken (Fig. 2-25).

2. *Number of canals present.* The presence of a single-rooted tooth does not necessarily indicate a single root canal. A bifurcated canal or separate canals may be present in any root. Such an occurrence is certainly not infrequent in single-rooted bicuspids (both mandibular and maxillary), distal roots of lower molars, and mesiobuccal roots of maxillary molars. They may be found in mandibular anterior teeth as well. Because of superimposition in the straight-on radiograph, the angle view is most important in this determination (Fig. 2-26).

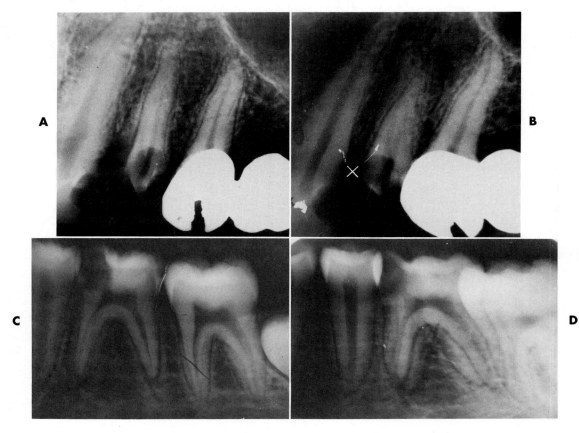

Fig. 2-25. Maxillary bicuspids have the greatest variation in root and canal configuration. Therefore radiographs from straight and angled positions are necessary to clarify the condition to be treated. **A,** Straight-on view gives information concerning the relative size and shape of the canal, but no information on the number of roots and canals present. **B,** View from distal toward mesial aspect (identified by the x placed on film) shows that two roots are present. Mandibular molars may have a number of variants, too. **C,** Direct view of mandibular first molar seems to indicate presence of two mesial canals but only one distal canal. **D,** View toward distal side shows two separate and distinct distal roots.

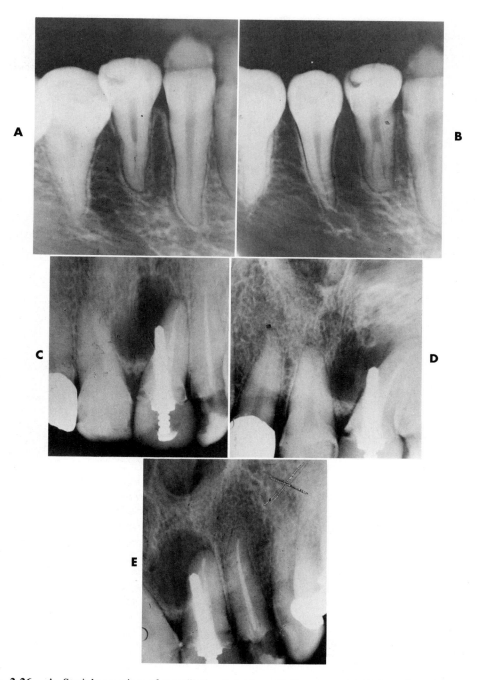

Fig. 2-26. A, Straight-on view of mandibular first bicuspid shows canal with large lateral canal or bifurcation in apical third. **B,** Angled view shows accurate configuration of bifurcation in middle third, leading to two separate and distinct canals. **C,** Routine direct view discloses mesial root perforation by post. As additional information for setting up treatment plan, it would be helpful to know whether perforation is toward labial or palatal surface. Therefore both mesial, **D,** and distal, **E,** views are taken. For identification in later viewing, an x is placed on the distal view film. By using the buccal object rule (Chapter 6), the dentist can determine that perforation is toward the palatal side.

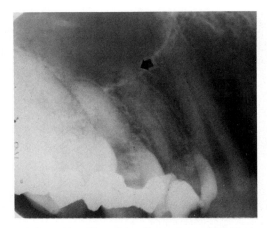

Fig. 2-27. First bicuspid radiograph, made with sharp angulation from mesial toward distal aspect, discloses that canal has a palatal curvature *(arrow)* not apparent in the direct view.

3. *Presence of buccal or lingual root or canal curvature.* These conditions may not be seen in the direct view, but indications are seen in the angle film (Fig. 2-27).

All the intraoral views should show the apices of the tooth and some degree of the surrounding periapical tissue. If a radiolucency is present, one of the views must reveal the complete limits of the defect. If the defect is too large to be completely seen in one view of periapical film size, supplementary films must be taken using occlusal, lateral jaw, or panoramic exposures (Fig. 2-28). Certain lesions of the jaws may appear to be typical of those due to pulpal pathosis, except for size or shape. Unless they are viewed in their entirety by one or more of the supplemental extraoral views, endodontic therapy might be instituted on a tooth unnecessarily. Worse yet, the true condition would not receive the needed treatment until the error was determined. Since some of these conditions are potentially dangerous, loss of time might be extremely serious.

Radiographs for tracing. The dentist should take supplemental radiographs whenever a chronic draining sinus (fistula) is found, to be certain as to the source of the tract. A gutta-percha cone of approximately size 40 is gently placed into the tract with cotton forceps until a solid stop is felt. This is usually performed without any need for anesthesia, but in some cases an injection is necessary. A radiograph is taken with the cone in place, and the tip of the gutta-percha points to where the drainage originates (Figs. 2-29 and 2-30). Ortho-

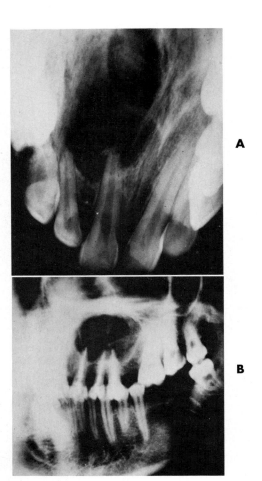

Fig. 2-28. **A,** Occlusal film gives complete view of large radiolucency that could not be completely visualized on any periapical film. **B,** Panoramic exposure gives excellent view of structures not usually seen on routine periapical films.

dontic wire has been suggested for tracing a chronic draining sinus, but gutta-percha appears to be far superior. The wire is sharp enough to perforate the wall of the tract and burrow into another site, which the softer and weaker gutta-percha is unable to do. The tract may take a very tortuous route through the soft tissue and bone. The wire will penetrate and go erratically, whereas the gutta-percha cone will probably remain within the confines of the tract (Fig. 2-30, *B*). This is most useful in determining whether the sinus is from a pulpal or a periodontal condition, which tooth is involved, or which root of a multirooted tooth is responsible. It is surprising how frequently the cause of the draining is found to differ from the apparent culprit.

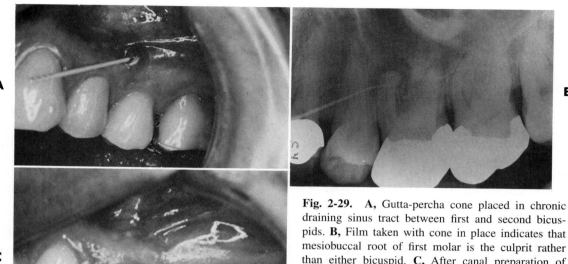

Fig. 2-29. **A,** Gutta-percha cone placed in chronic draining sinus tract between first and second bicuspids. **B,** Film taken with cone in place indicates that mesiobuccal root of first molar is the culprit rather than either bicuspid. **C,** After canal preparation of molar, the sinus tract heals within a few days. This is a constant finding when endodontic treatment is performed on teeth with sinus tracts.

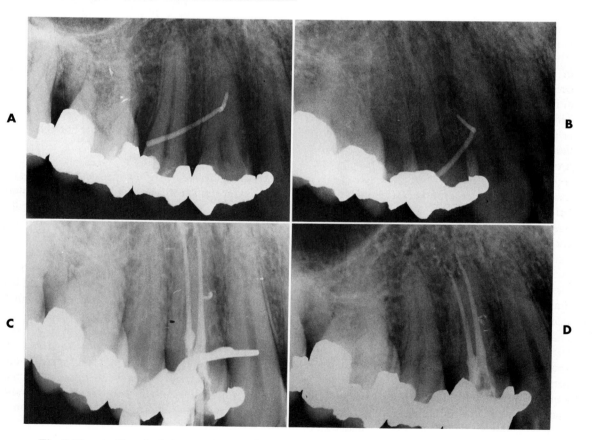

Fig. 2-30. **A,** Chronic draining sinus tract on the palate is traced with a gutta-percha cone to the lateral surface of a first bicuspid root, straight-on film. **B,** Angled view demonstrating tortuous route these tracts may take. **C,** Angled view taken during canal filling. Sealer is exiting exactly to site of traced sinus tract. **D,** Final film.

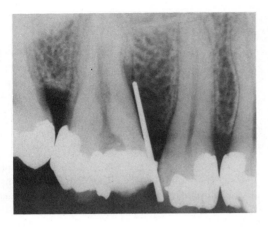

Fig. 2-31. Periodontal pocket is traced by radiograph of silver point placement along the mesial surface of maxillary molar. For tracing of periodontal defects, x-ray cone angulation is the same as that used for a bite-wing view; thus apex of tooth may not appear on the film.

Periodontal lesions may also be traced radiographically to determine their depth and extent. A silver point of approximately size 30 is placed into the tract until it is stopped by the sulcus depth or bone and is then radiographed. The relation of the pocket depth to the root or apex is now apparent. This method is useful in determining factors such as the depth of a pocket, the amount of supporting bone on a periodontally involved tooth, or which root of a multirooted tooth should be amputated (Fig. 2-31).

The size 30 silver point is stiff enough to place but small enough to trace a tortuous pocket and light enough to remain in place while a radiograph is taken. For diagnostic differentiation, when radiographs are reviewed or projected at a later date, it is always obvious where the radiopaque material was placed, since gutta-percha is used in chronic draining sinuses and silver points in pockets. Both materials are readily available in any office where endodontic therapy is performed.

Newer types of radiography. Over the past 20 years, many improvements and innovations have occurred in the field of radiology. There is no segment of dentistry in which radiographs are more important than in endodontics, so any improvement in this area will have a direct and positive effect during root canal therapy.

Several years ago, aspects for using xerography were applied to endodontics. Unfortunately, this was soon abandoned. Applications of video-type screens, with and without computers, have expanded interest in this area recently, and one of the areas of effort and promise has been radiovisiography (RVG).

RVG combines a conventional x-ray generator to a solid-state sensor with a scintillation screen to provide instant imaging. This created image may be enhanced for contrast and density, enlarged several times, and may focus on specific portions of the image, such as apices. Printing capabilities are also present, and storage in a computer system of charts is possible.

Calculation of working length or fitting of trial cones are obvious uses in addition to preoperative films. One of the major advantages of RVG is that approximately 80% less radiation is required for each exposure compared with current conventional machines.

With instant imaging, time is saved during treatment. Decreasing the hazards of radiation is certainly a valuable feature for the product. Being able to focus on a specific area, such as root tips, lateral lesions, or potential canal divisions, certainly would lead to better endodontic results.

Such interesting additions to our armamenteria for endodontics are always welcome, particularly when it may improve our results and decrease possible damage to our patients. I would hope that further improvements are also on the horizon.

OTHER DIAGNOSTIC AIDS

Although radiographs are the most important of the diagnostic aids for endodontics, they are by no means the only ones (Fig. 2-32). They should never be the sole source used for making a diagnosis; they should be evaluated with other tests and determinations before a final diagnosis is made. As will be illustrated in the section on differential diagnosis of periapical radiolucencies, reliance on the radiograph only will lead to erroneous diagnosis in many instances.

Among the other diagnostic aids are visual and digital examination of soft and hard tissues, thermal pulp testing, electric pulp testing, percussion, selective anesthesia, test cavity, and transillumination. In addition, certain laboratory tests may be required in diagnostic procedures.

Visual and digital examination of hard and soft tissues

The danger of too great reliance on radiographs is that the use of the eyes and fingers is over-

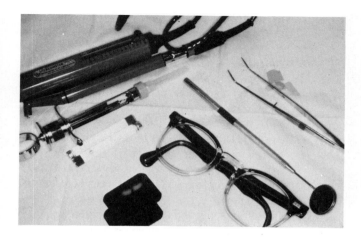

Fig. 2-32. Diagnostic tests useful in endodontic evaluation include *(upper left)* electric pulp tester and syringe with anesthetic Carpules for selective anesthesia; *(lower left to right)* radiographs, glasses representing eyes for visual examination of hard and soft tissues, mouth mirror for examination of teeth and butt end for percussion test, and cotton forceps with gutta-percha for hot test.

looked, although often they are of prime diagnostic value.

Severe discoloration of the crown of a tooth, particularly after a traumatic injury, usually indicates severed apical vessels leading to a nonvital pulp. In addition to aiding in the diagnosis, the existence of discoloration also suggests methods involved in treatment. In making the access cavity, the dentist should remove the discolored dentin with a large round bur or a prepared-tip fissure bur. Chlorinated soda used as canal irrigant should be allowed to remain within the crown during canal preparation to help in bleaching out the blood pigments.

Of course, severe carious lesions are usually obvious, and large lesions often cause pulpal involvement. Such lesions may occur through buccal or lingual areas and thus are difficult to ascertain from radiographs but are apparent to visual examination. Crown fractures are similarly rarely revealed by x-ray examination, particularly when they occur in a mesiodistal direction. Visual examination and probing with a sharp explorer clarify the condition.

Chronic draining sinus tracts (fistulas) are important aids in diagnosis. As stated previously, they must be traced with gutta-percha to identify the site of origination. The existence of a tract is also of importance during therapy, since it is some insurance that an exacerbation during treatment will not occur. Any buildup of pressures or exudates will simply "blow out" through the communication of apex and soft tissue.

The appearance of soft tissue may also be noted visually and may aid in diagnosis. If a patient is in pain, the pulp is the most obvious and frequent site of discomfort. However, an incipient lateral periodontal abscess or necrotizing gingivitis may be similarly painful and may thus be recognized. Before endodontic therapy on any tooth is started, the gingival sulcus must be probed with an endodontic explorer and/or a pocket probe to determine if a periodontal condition is present. This aids in determining the type of treatment plan to be used, the need for coordination with other areas of therapy, the possible etiology of the pulpal problem, and the prognosis (Chapter 13).

Palpation of the soft tissues overlying the buccal plate may induce pain in certain areas, indicative of a possible site of damage, or reveal hard or soft swelling. Complete examination of the tooth with this problem is warranted, including further radiographs and pulp and percussion testing. Existence of swelling in the apical area of a tooth requiring endodontic therapy may indicate that a destruction of the apical foramen is needed to gain successful drainage in the area, that apical surgery may be needed, or that an incipient alveolar abscess is present.

Thermal pulp testing

Thermal pulp testing may not be as sophisticated a procedure as electric pulp testing but is often a much more reliable and easily performed diagnostic procedure. The equipment required is inexpensive and easy to use, and the result is usually conclusive (Fig. 2-33).

One of the main reasons why thermal pulp testing is a valuable diagnostic tool is that certain painful conditions of the pulp may be brought on

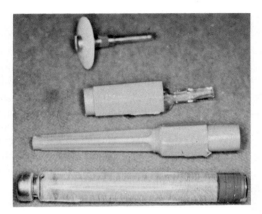

Fig. 2-33. For thermal testing, a rubber wheel *(top)* against a gold crown provides an excellent hot test. Disposable anesthetic needle holders *(middle)* or empty anesthetic Carpules *(bottom)* filled with water and placed in freezer compartment of refrigerator give sticks of ice, excellent for application to teeth for a cold test.

or relieved by sudden, severe temperature changes. Therefore the patient's reaction after application of heat or cold to specific teeth not only pinpoints the involved tooth, but also strongly suggests the condition present.

For teeth without crowns or deep restorations, baseplate gutta-percha is used to elicit a response to heat. As in all pulp testing, the teeth to be treated are dried and walled off with cotton rolls, and a saliva ejector is placed. A strip of the material (7 × 7 mm) is cut and, while being held in a cotton pliers, is heated to just short of smoking and applied to the cervical area of the tooth. A temperature greater than 65.5° C (150° F) is developed, sufficient to elicit a response from a normal or hyperemic pulp. To keep the patient unaware that a hot material is being applied, the heating must be done away from the patient's area of vision; otherwise, when the hot gutta-percha is brought to the tooth, the patient may recoil or react to what he or she thinks is going to happen rather than to what is felt.

Cast crowns are too thick to allow the heated gutta-percha to raise the temperature of the underlying tooth structure sufficiently to react. Therefore an alternative method of producing heat must be used if a hot test is needed on a tooth with full coverage. Sufficient heat is produced by using a rubber wheel mounted on a mandrel revolving at a polishing speed against the precious metal. Any-

one who has had a casting polished in the mouth or who has held an inlay during rubber wheeling will attest to the heat generated.

The rubber wheel is best used on a lingual area of the crown where the polishing will not materially affect the shape of the casting yet will be close enough to the more sensitive areas of the tooth.

Cold tests are easily performed with ice or ethyl chloride spray. The latter is useful if no refrigerator is in the office. The spray is directed at a cotton pellet held in pliers until a frosting is noted on the fibers. The pellet is then placed at the cervical area of the dried tooth and the response noted.

For testing with ice, cubes from an ice tray are unwieldy because of their bulk. As the ice melts from a large cube, cold water may drip on the gingival tissues, and the patient may react to that cold sensation rather than to an application against the tooth. Therefore a thin rod of ice is better for application. This may be obtained by filling with water the plastic containers that have held disposable needles and then placing them in the refrigerator's freezer compartment. When needed, the top of the container is removed, leaving a sharply pointed stick of ice that can be directly applied to the tooth to be tested.

Electric pulp testing

The electric pulp tester is an instrument that uses gradations of electric current to excite a response from susceptible elements of the pulpal tissues. The use of an electric tester for evaluation of the condition of the pulp is widespread and is valuable in many instances yet frequently misunderstood. It is important to emphasize that the results of electric pulp testing are always subject to the error of human interpretation and should be evaluated along with results from the other diagnostic aids before a final diagnosis is made.

Pulp testers are available with cords that plug into electric outlets for a power source and also as battery-operated portable instruments. Each type has possible electrical deficiencies. The pulp testers of the future may be operated by transistors, which would let them be smaller in size, able to deliver the expected current routinely, and able to supply many minutes more of use than battery-powered equipment. On the other hand, future instruments may be developed to determine the degree of blood supply rather than nerve supply to the pulp. Since the vascularity rather than the

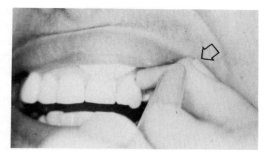

Fig. 2-34. Electric pulp test. Cotton roll has been placed, and the teeth have been air dried. Electrode is placed at gingival area of crown after electrolyte is applied. One finger *(arrow)* in contact with the patient completes the circuit.

innervation determines the vitality of pulp, such a test would be infinitely more descriptive of the pulp condition. It has been shown that a considerable loss of blood supply may occur before sufficient degeneration of nerve supply to alter an electrical response takes place.

Before the use of an electric pulp tester, the tooth or teeth to be evaluated should be surrounded by cotton rolls and air dried. Saliva present on the teeth may conduct to adjacent gingival tissue and yield a reaction from that source rather than from the underlying pulp. Removal of supragingival calculus may be needed, particularly in mandibular anterior teeth, to gain access to the cervical areas (see Fig. 2-34).

All pulp testers require an electrolyte to transmit the current from the machine to the hard structures of the tooth, and toothpaste is frequently used with good results. The jelly used for electrocardiograpy is superior for transmission, however, and its viscosity ensures that it will remain where placed. The tooth electrode is lightly dipped into a mound of jelly and placed as close to the cervical portion of the tooth as possible without contacting the gingiva.

The enamel covering the crown acts as a protective barrier and buffer to any of the influences attempting to reach the more susceptible dentin, including electric current. No reaction will take place until sufficient intensity is developed to reach the dentin. However, near the cementodentinal junction the enamel decreases in thickness,

making this the more desired area of testing. If sufficient soft tissue recession has taken place, the electrode may be applied to the cementum covering the root surface. This is an excellent site for gaining a true response, since only a very thin layer of cementum separates the electrode and the dentin.

For most pulp testers of the plug-in type, the circuit must be completed by having the operator keep one finger in contact with the patient while current is applied to the tooth. This procedure is not necessary in battery-operated machines.

With the electrode contacting the tooth, an electric charge is applied by pressing the rheostat button, a small charge being given initially and increased until a response is felt. The patient experiences a sense of heat or tingling in the tooth when the nerve tissue is excited. All testers have rheostats that indicate on a scale of 1 to 10 or 1 to 15 the relative amount of current applied. It is important to go slowly up the scale from a small amount of current. Going too rapidly may cause a painful feeling in the tooth being tested before the patient is able to indicate that a response has been felt.

If the vitality of a particular pulp is in question, the pulp tester should be used on adjacent teeth and on the contralateral tooth, when present, as controls. The amount of current indicated by the rheostat is used to make a comparison in determining normalcy. If the current required to gain a response from a test tooth is the same as that needed to excite the control, the pulp of the test tooth is considered normal. The pulp of a test tooth is considered degenerating when much more current is required to gain a response compared with the control. If much less current is required for a response on the tooth in question, it is considered hyperactive. Lack of response indicates pulpal necrosis.

A single test on any individual tooth is insufficient for comparison. Two readings should be taken for each tooth and an average recorded. If the two readings are far apart, a third test should be run, with the average of the two closest readings accepted. Using an electric test on any tooth more than four times may defeat the purpose, since some of the stimulation may become additive and the nerve tissue may react at a lower-than-true threshold according to the rheostat reading.

The response of multiple nonreactive teeth should be disregarded, particularly when some apparently normal teeth are involved, since individual patients may be stoic or have an extremely high pain threshold. By the same token, certain patients may be highly excitable and react quickly to minimal or subliminal stimulation. When testing a tooth that is expected to be highly reactive, as in a severely acute pulpitis, a more normal tooth should be tested first to give the patient a basis for judgment.

Potential deficiencies of pulp testers. Since both battery and plug-in pulp testers may have electrical deficiencies, the output of current on a given reading may vary from time to time, or even from tooth to tooth. Batteries may run down and not deliver the full current expected by the operating dial. On plug-in models the drain by other electricity-requiring appliances or equipment may alter the true current level.

Large restorations or bases may prevent the current from reaching dentinal tubules attached to processes extending to the pulp. This is particularly true for teeth restored with crowns or with pulpotomy dressings.

Molars may give readings not indicative of the true pulpal condition, since some combination of vital and nonvital canals may be present. If the canal in proximity to the tooth electrode is vital, a relatively normal reading will be recorded even if the other canals are necrotic.

As mentioned earlier, reactivity of the nerves to electrical stimulation is not synonymous with normalcy. The nerve tissue, being highly resistant to inflammation, might remain reactive long after the surrounding tissues have degenerated. However, Mullaney et al. examined histologically 48 dental pulps that gave a painful response when extirpated, although they had obtained nonvital responses with electric pulp testing. Only two pulps had normal-appearing nerve fibers.

One must remember, when making a comparison between a tooth in question and the contralateral tooth, that the pulp of the control tooth itself may not be normal or that a large restoration or a pulpotomy dressing may be present. The validity of comparing a test tooth with a control holds only when the control tooth gives every indication of normalcy.

Reports have stated that teeth involved in an acute alveolar abscess responded positively to electric pulp tests. Since the pulp must be necrotic for an acute alveolar abscess to occur, it must be assumed that the gaseous or liquefied elements within the pulp canal transmitted the electric charge to the periapical tissues. This would appear to be a relatively rare occurrence.

Teeth involved in splints or bridges may test positive to electric current by virtue of transferring the stimulus to adjacent vital abutments for a reaction. This may happen with hot or cold tests as well. If it becomes necessary to test the pulp of a tooth involved in a nonremovable appliance, temporary stopping may be placed around the pontics or abutments adjacent to the test tooth to prevent any transference. The results of the tests still may be inaccurate.

Teeth are usually nonresponsive to electric pulp testing shortly after eruption. At the other end of the spectrum, "older" teeth, despite the patient's age, may be similarly unresponsive. The term *older* is used here to mean teeth in which deep erosion or abrasion has produced heavy areas of sclerotic dentin. Also, teeth with many restorations on multiple areas of the tooth may be unresponsive or difficult to test with an electric tester, since no available sites exist where the current can be applied.

Ideal situations for electric pulp testing. In certain instances, electric pulp testing has a high degree of accuracy and gives excellent essential information. In general, such testing on anterior teeth has a high degree of reliability, since these teeth are single rooted, are easy to isolate, and have large restorations less frequently than do posterior teeth, and since good access is available to reach cervical, responsive areas.

Excellent evaluation of teeth involved in traumatic accidents is available with an electric pulp tester. Usually, anterior teeth are affected, frequently teeth with no prior restorations or pulpal damage. The cervical areas are easily accessible on these teeth, and the results of pulp testing are reliable. In the initial few days after an injury, a temporary paresthesia of the nerves may occur and make them unresponsive to testing. However, if the pulp retains its vitality, it will respond within normal limits after 30 to 60 days. Teeth adjacent to the direct site of trauma should also be tested. These teeth may respond normally at the initial examination but later require greater current for stimulation and eventually become nonresponsive due to the presence of a chronic pulpitis.

The electric pulp test may be an important aid in determining when a problem is caused by pulpal or by periodontal damage. The clinical symptoms of an acute alveolar and an acute periodontal abscess are similar. It is a mistake to assume that the frequency of the abscess due to pulpal death compared with that of a periodontal problem justifies opening the pulp chamber for relief. An evaluation of the pulp by either electric or thermal testing would suggest the origin of the swelling. Pulp evaluation is a necessary adjunct in periodontal diagnosis to determine the correct course of treatment for lesions possibly requiring endodontic therapy in addition to periodontics. However, one should remember that pulp vitality does not necessarily mean pulp normalcy (Chapter 13).

A periapical radiolucency does not necessarily indicate pulpal death. Anatomic landmarks, inflammatory lesions, and neoplasms may produce radiolucencies adjacent to teeth, suggestive of the typical periapical granuloma or cyst. Pulp testing should precede institution of endodontic therapy on teeth with periapical radiolucencies, particularly when any question exists as to the etiology of the pulpal death.

The death of a single pulp may produce a radiolucency that involves the apices of adjacent teeth and suggest endodontic therapy for multiple members of the arch. This is particularly true in the lower anterior area, where the apices are in proximity. Electric pulp testing can indicate which teeth are responsible for the lesion and prevent the treatment of those that are uninvolved. Even if the diseased tissue surrounds the apex of a tooth, vital blood and nerve vessels may penetrate the lesion and retain the tooth in a normal condition (Figs. 2-35 and 2-11).

Carbon dioxide snow. This method of pulp testing is used in Europe and is very popular with Australian dentists because of the efforts of Ehrmann. It is virtually unheard of in the United States, where ethyl chloride sprayed onto a cotton pellet and ice have been recommended as the preferred cold tests. The apparatus for using carbon dioxide (CO_2) is much more expensive than ethyl chloride or ice, but it does overcome some inherent problems found in the more routine cold tests.

The principle for use involves passing compressed liquid CO_2 through a small orifice in a holding cylinder onto a plexiglass tube to create a dry ice "pencil." Some CO_2 evaporates when it reaches an atmospheric pressure, accounting for its conversion to dry ice at a temperature of -78°C (-108°F). This is much colder and remains at a more reliable temperature than the other cold tests, according to Ehrmann.

A major advantage to this method is that it can be used on teeth with metal restorations and, supposedly, on individual teeth under splinted abutments. Possible disadvantages also have been stated. The intense cold of the CO_2 may cause cracks in the enamel, but Ehrmann has stated that if it does occur, it will not be of clinical significance. Cryosurgery involves using extreme cold to remove soft tissue, and some might be concerned that the dry ice stick will cause damage if it touches gingiva, the floor of the mouth, or other oral tissues. However, no damage seems to occur, since cryosurgery requires pressure for effectiveness in addition to the low temperatures.

Percussion

The use of percussion as a diagnostic aid gives valuable information, since it discloses the existence of an acute periapical inflammation. Because some of the diseases of the pulp and periapical tissues cause apical periodontitis, such a determination is important in making the correct diagnosis and leads to the plan of treatment.

The test is simple to perform, requiring only the butt end of a dental mirror handle used to tap gently the crown of the tooth. Some dentists claim that the type of noise or "thud" of a percussed tooth indicates the condition of the periapical tissues, but this has not been proved reliable.

Hard percussion of teeth known to be involved in a severely acute periapical condition is cruel. However, the test may be performed on adjacent teeth to rule out multiple etiologic agents when such a finding is determined.

It is important to mention that a normal tooth and one involved in a chronic periapical inflammation respond the same to percussion. Only when the condition becomes acute is the test reliable.

Test cavity

The use of a test cavity preparation is the final and unquestionably the most accurate of the pulp vitality tests. It involves the removal of dentin by a bur in a handpiece without the use of a local anesthetic to determine the vitality of an underlying pulp. Because it removes sound tooth structure, plus in most instances some portion of a restoration, this test should be performed only as a last resort. When thermal and electric tests have been inconclusive or impossible to perform and yet a determination of pulp vitality is mandatory, the test cavity will supply the answer.

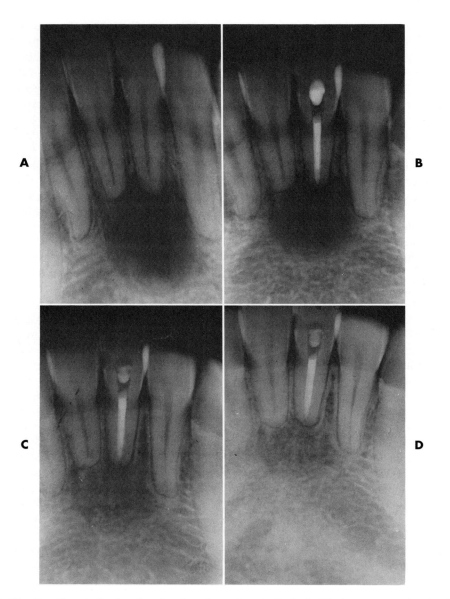

Fig. 2-35. Excellent indication for electric pulp testing. **A,** Periapical lesion seems to involve both mandibular central incisors. However, the central to the left on the film responded within normal limits to the electric pulp tester, whereas the central to the right gave no response. **B,** Accordingly, only the nonresponsive tooth was treated. **C,** Six months later, lesion is healing well. **D,** One year after treatment, verifying electric pulp tester results as accurate.

One example of this situation might be the finding of a radiolucency near the apex of an incisor restored with a porcelain jacket crown. Another example might be an acute swelling of the mandible where teeth in the area are splinted together with gold or bonded porcelain restorations.

For producing a test cavity, the preparation is placed in the lingual or palatal surface of an ante-rior tooth or the occlusal area of a posterior tooth. It is then relatively simple to restore the preparation without causing unesthetic damage to the tooth.

The cavity is best produced by using an airotor without water spray to give the most possible heat production to elicit a pulpal response. If a restoration is present, it may be penetrated with water spray until the underlying dentin is reached. Pain to the patient when undergoing the casting of a splint or bridge abutment is meaningless, since it might be reflected by the pulps of adjacent teeth.

When the dentin is drilled, the patient will know in no uncertain terms if the pulp is vital, even if he or she has a high enough threshold to have routine cavity preparation without anesthetic. Once a vital response is elicited, no further heat-producing work should be performed lest pulpal damage be caused that might require endodontic therapy.

After the response is noted, the cavity may be temporarily restored with ZOE before permanent restoration with foil, a casting, or amalgam. If the pulp is nonvital, the preparation may be enlarged to accommodate the normal access opening and the tooth then closed or left open according to the condition present.

Selective anesthesia

Selective anesthesia refers to administration of a local anesthetic to facilitate identification of the tooth causing a painful episode. Other diagnostic aids may be able to eliminate all but two teeth as possible etiologic agents but be unable to make the final choice. If one tooth is in each arch or if both are maxillary teeth and at least one tooth intervenes between them, selective anesthesia may be used to pinpoint the culprit.

If a maxillary tooth and a mandibular tooth are the possible causes, the correct local anesthetic injections (including a palatal injection) necessary to extirpate a vital pulp of the maxillary tooth are administered. If the pain vanishes, the maxillary tooth is identified as the causative agent. If pain has been brought on or intensified previously by thermal changes, the patient is instructed to rinse with water of the type that earlier produced the discomfort to test further that the correct tooth has been found.

If pain is not diminished by anesthesia of the maxillary tooth, the suspect mandibular tooth is indicated as the source of the problem and appropriate treatment administered to it. The maxillary tooth is selected for the initial injections because of the greater degree of deep anesthesia normally obtainable in the maxillary arch. The likelihood of missing a mandibular block injection is always present. If the mandibular injection was given first but did not take completely and pain persisted, the maxillary tooth might be wrongly treated.

If two maxillary posterior teeth are involved, the more anterior tooth is given the selective anesthetic and observation is made for change in degree of pain. Should the pain disappear, the anterior tooth is responsible; the posterior tooth is indicated for treatment if the pain remains. The more anterior tooth is tested first because innervation of the palatal root for posterior teeth is from the more posterior portion of the palate by way of the greater palatine foramen, adjacent to the second molar. If a palatal injection were given, an inflamed pulp in the palatal canal of any tooth anterior to the site would be anesthetized.

Transillumination

Emergence of the fiberoptic as a dental instrument has been a great aid in the use of transillumination for diagnosis. The test requires shining a bright light from the lingual or palatal surface of a tooth, with viewing in a darkened room.

In teeth with necrotic pulps the shadow of the pulp canal space appears darker than the rest of the tooth because of the breakdown of the blood cells. In teeth with vital pulps, no differentiation is noted. Periapical tissue may be similarly transilluminated if the plates of bone are close to each other, as in mandibular anterior teeth. Teeth with radiolucencies reveal a shadow around the apex, whereas normal teeth show no difference in the area.

Transillumination may be helpful in diagnosing the presence of a vertical fracture. With the fiberoptic shining at right angles to the fracture line, the segment of the tooth on the side of the crack illuminates, whereas the segment on the far side remains dark.

Vertical fractures of posterior teeth

JAMES A. DEWBERRY, JR.

One of the most puzzling and frustrating diagnostic problems encountered by the dental practitioner is the vertical fracture. Symptoms of this condition are often characterized by a sharp but brief pain during mastication. The conditions required to elicit this pain may be so unique that it can be extremely difficult for the patient or the dentist to reproduce and therefore to locate. The type and degree of pain can run a broad gamut. It may be sharp but only momentary so that the patient does not seek advice or treatment, since total relief comes by abstinence from mastication in the affected area. Usually that type of pain comes from a specific type of vertical fracture—a tiny crack extending into the dentin but not yet intersecting the pulp space. The sharp pain probably comes from exposing, stretching, and rupturing odontoblastic processes in the fracture plane. Eventually this type of fracture will progress farther apically, possibly intersecting the pulp space and infecting its contents.

A tiny crack that just intersects the pulp space or is a close tangent to it may cause a pulpal inflammation that can result in spontaneous pain referred throughout any or all of the areas served by the fifth cranial nerve. The source of pain may be impossible to locate because pulp tissue has no proprioceptive (location sense) capability. This can lead to bizarre medical treks by the patient from the otolaryngologist to the neurologist to the psychiatrist. These patients do not belong in psychiatric therapy, whereas those with seemingly similar (but occasionally bilateral) pain arising from spasm of musculature of the head and neck may benefit from such treatment. Once this subtle fracture progresses to the pulp space, resulting in pulp necrosis, the inflammation extends to the periodontal ligament and periapical bone. Both the ligament and the bone have proprioceptive fibers so that the resultant tenderness to percussion reveals the pain source. With the inflammation confined to the pulp tissue *before* extension periapically, localization is difficult unless the pain responds to thermal stimuli or the stick-bite test. The latter is virtually the only viable test for early cracks not involving the pulp. Often they can be seen on a visual examination, but many enamel cracks are of no clinical significance.

Radiographic evidence. Radiographic examination seldom reveals the fracture because it is usually parallel to the film. However, a vertical fracture is often suspected in the absence of an apparent cause for pulpal involvement (Fig. 2-36). For example, if symptoms, radiographs, and/or clinical tests show the presence of pulpal pathosis in a posterior tooth, and if the radiograph shows no caries or restoration near the pulp, this is virtually pathognomonic of a vertical fracture. Whereas horizontal root fractures or buccolingual crown fractures may occasionally be demonstrated radiographically, a mesiodistal vertical fracture is impossible to reveal, since the line of fracture is not in the plane of the radiograph even in a deep and separated split. When these teeth are extracted and radiographed in a *mesiodistal plane,* multiple fracture lines are frequently seen (Fig. 2-37). An advanced fracture may show what appears to be a periodontal pocket (Fig. 2-36, *B*). It is an area of bone loss caused by the necrosis of periodontal bone in the fracture line.

External evidence. The external clinical evidence of a cracked tooth is usually a fractured marginal ridge extending into a prominent fissure (Fig. 2-38) or a single, uniformly poor margin of a restoration. *Cracks and fractures of the enamel may have no clinical significance;* however, they may be suggestive of deeper dentin involvement. Frank separation or movement in the fracture line is proof of a fracture of the dentinal body of the tooth. If the tooth has a large, temporary restoration across the occlusal surface with a crack from mesial to distal, this is very often indicative of a similar crack in the tooth structure beneath.

To locate the tooth and cusp(s) involved, the dentist has the patient bite on an orangewood stick or a cotton-tipped applicator. Noting the cusps that occlude when the pain occurs aids in the location of the fracture site.

Once the tooth is located, a window in the dentin in the plane of fracture should reveal it. This window is usually in the form of a Class I cavity (Fig. 2-39). Caries does not seem to invade these fractures, although some are black, whereas others show no discoloration. Because the cracks often can barely be seen with the naked eye, a magnifying lens in the two-power range with a good direct light followed by transilluminating light in a darkened room are important diagnostic aids. Dyes such as methylene blue or washable ink are of little value. The floor of the preparation of the exploratory window should be smoothed as much as possible to avoid linear marks on the cavity floor that might be difficult to distinguish from a subtle crack.

In some cases it is tempting to remove dentin in the fracture line until it is no longer visible and place a restoration. This only creates a wedge into the fracture plane that *worsens* the problem rather than relieves it.

Occasionally, if a crack encircles a single cusp, that cusp may be relieved severely from occlusion,

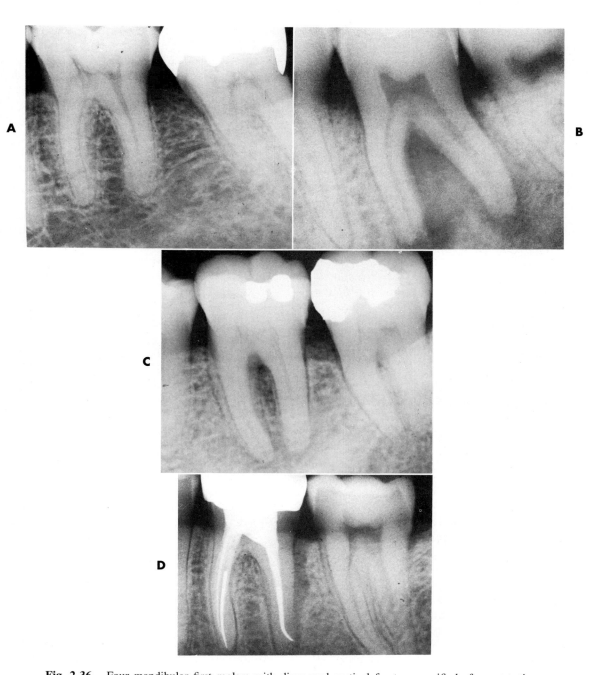

Fig. 2-36. Four mandibular first molars with diagnosed vertical fractures verified after extraction. Note that no restorations are present in **A** and **B,** and only two small occlusal amalgams are in **C.** Because the fractures are parallel to the film, no routine intraoral view will disclose the defect. **D,** If endodontic treatment is attempted on such teeth, failure will result. Seemingly excellent therapy was performed on this tooth 3 months earlier at the patient's insistence despite the fracture. Note the diffuse radiolucency extending the entire root length of the distal portion of the distal root, pathognomic of a vertical fracture.

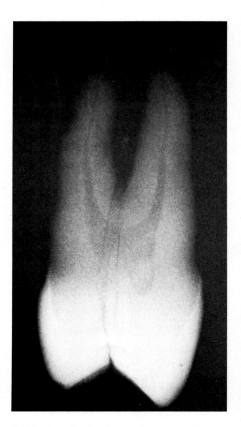

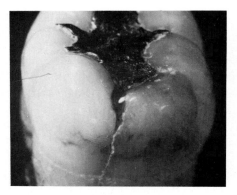

Fig. 2-38. Fractured marginal ridge was only external evidence of a crack on this mandibular second molar. No cavity was present, and no fracture line was discernible on a routine radiograph.

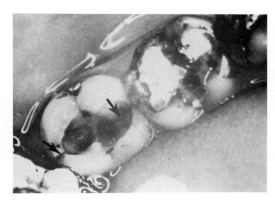

Fig. 2-37. Proximal view of extracted two-rooted maxillary first bicuspid demonstrating multiple mesiodistal fracture lines. Normal intraoral radiograph showed no crack.

Fig. 2-39. Occlusal amalgam was removed from mandibular first molar to trace down fracture line *(arrows)*.

relieving symptoms. If a coronal fracture's apical terminus traverses the epithelial attachment, it creates a defect in the attachment, the periodontal ligament, and the adjacent alveolar bone. This results in an infrabony pocket that will remain until the tooth is extracted (Fig. 2-40). These pockets may be tolerable for a time but are never reversible.

Fractures of anterior teeth. When an anterior tooth fractures, it generally occurs in a more horizontal plane, and the cause is accidental trauma of extraoral origin. Aspects of treatment are discussed in Chapters 10, 11, and 14. It should be noted here that many untreated *horizontal* fractures of the roots of anterior teeth heal uneventfully without stabilization or treatment, provided sufficient root length remains on the coronal segment.

Prognosis. There are many variables in the evaluation and prognosis of vertical fractures. Among them are the direction and depth of the fracture plane, separation or movement in the frac-

ture line, evidence of pulpal involvement, and the occlusal dimension or length of the fracture. One must remember that even after removing all restorations, *only the occlusal cross-sectional aspect of a vertical fracture can be seen* unless the pulp chamber is entered. Even then, placing the apical terminus of the fracture is guesswork, despite the use of a transilluminating light and a magnifying lens. However, with this limited information a predictive clinical judgment of the salvage prospects for the tooth must be made. Other factors that play a role in the decision are the strategic value of the tooth, the economics of treatment (the endodontic therapy must be followed by a *full*-coverage crown), and the patient's commitment or lack of it to attempt to retain the tooth.

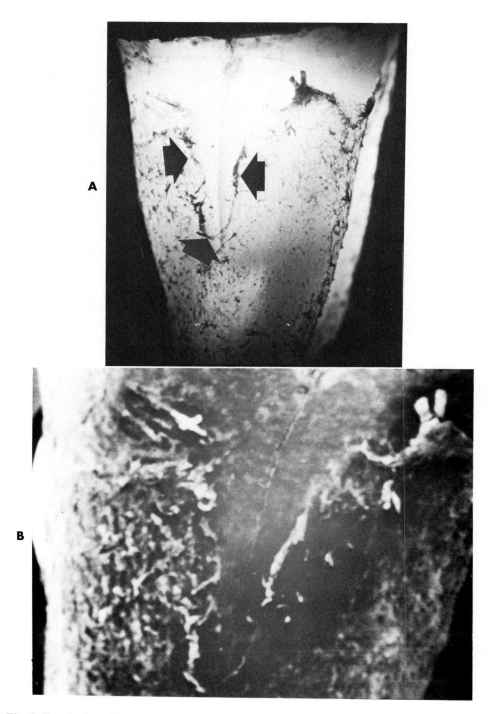

Fig. 2-40. **A,** As a fracture extends toward the apex, it creates a defect in the periodontal ligament space to cause an irreversible pocket. Note that the epithelial attachment divides as the fracture line progresses apically (*arrows*). **B** to **D,** Scanning electron microscope views of increasing magnifications, demonstrating the crack.   *Continued*

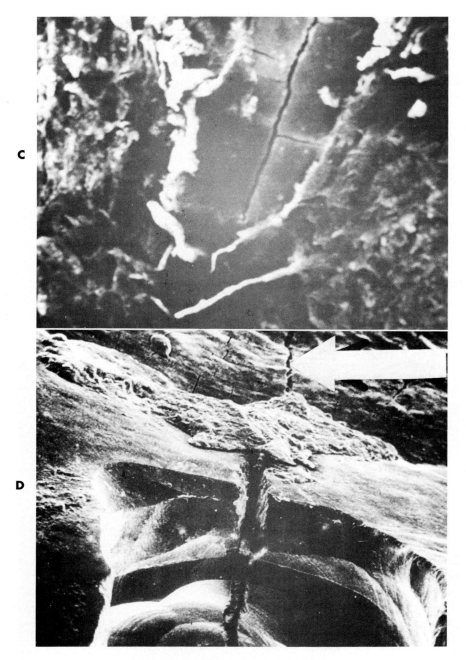

Fig. 2-40, cont'd.   For legend see p. 75.

Generally it can be said that a fracture traceable all the way from mesial to distal offers a very poor prognosis. If *any* movement is noted in this fracture line, the tooth should be condemned.

Causes and susceptibility of posterior fractures. The single most common cause of the vertical frac-

ture is the masticatory accident—an unexpected encounter with a hard object during confident, crushing mastication. The most common history of a remembered incident is an encounter with a piece of bone remaining in meat. Although many teeth are fractured from injudicious *voluntary* mastica-

Table 2-1. Distribution of cracked teeth

Location of teeth affected, in order of occurrence	Number of teeth cracked	Percentage (%) by location of 475 teeth
Mandibular first molar	146	30.7
Mandibular second molar	131	27.5
Maxillary first molar	99	20.8
Maxillary first bicuspid	34	7.1
Maxillary second bicuspid	29	6.0
Maxillary second molar	27	6.0
Mandibular second bicuspid	8	1.7
Mandibular first bicuspid	1	0.2
TOTALS	475	100.0

tion on objects such as ice, hard candy, or nuts, usually caution reigns in chewing these. The *unexpected* encounter of the masticatory accident seems to be the most destructive.

Patients with cracked teeth are most often healthy. It is unusual to see supporting bone in any condition but excellent in the patient with a cracked tooth. Even more unusual is a cracked tooth opposing a denture or even a bridge pontic. When this happens, or in any fracture with a large restoration, an iatrogenic cause may be considered, such as the overzealous effort to seat a poorly fitting casting or the injudicious use of a mechanical amalgam condenser. The plane of most compound restorations in posterior teeth (i.e., mesial to distal) coincides with the most common fracture plane, creating a metallic wedge through the enamel cap and a major portion of the dentinal body of the crown. Much of the remainder of the crown is pulp space almost to the furcation area, leaving little dentin available to protect against a split.

The use of molar teeth as crushers and grinders subjects them to incredible pressures. Anthropologists examining lead balls found bitten out of shape by prisoners during beatings at Fort Ticonderoga determined that 1600 pounds of pressure were required to reproduce the distortion in a similar ball. The morphology of posterior teeth, with their deep grooves, bifurcations, high cusps, and cuspal interrelationships, also creates susceptibility to fracture.

Table 2-1 lists the breakdown of 475 fractured teeth according to anatomic distribution. A strong majority (58%) were found in lower molars, with a slight preference for the first molar (31%) over the second (27%). This reflects not only the extremely heavy work of the molars but the potentially divisive force of a prominent palatal cusp of the maxillary molar driving far down into the central fossa of the opponent. This force tends to divide the lower molar vertically and laterally. If a masticatory accident is an additional mechanical component, the result is often a vertical fracture.

The maxillary molars follow far behind their mandibular opponents in incidence of fractures, with much greater occurrence in the first molar (21%) than in the second (6%). Maxillary first and second bicuspid features occurred with about equal frequency. Only one mandibular first premolar was diagnosed.

The mean age of the patients in this study was 50 years. The youngest patient was 23 years old. Perhaps the more pliable and cushiony periodontal ligament of young persons along with a more resilient and less mineralized dentin prevents fractures at earlier ages. Conversely, the senile or invalid patient has a selectively softer diet high in carbohydrate with little need for great masticatory effort. Further, elderly persons often have fewer opposed molars.

Little difference exists in sex distribution, with 52.3% males and 47.7% females. Most patients in the study showed high peaks and valleys of intercuspal arch relationships, but two or more teeth were found in four patients with severe occlusal abrasion exposing dentin on the entire occlusal surface. Contrary to many clinicians' opinions, bruxism was not noted as a contributory factor.

Treatment. Unrealistic or overambitious case selection leads to a high degree of failures. Efforts have been made to retain all the fractured segments with full coverage in a binding type of restoration. No statistical data are available concerning the success in treatment of fracture cases; however, a realistic pessimism will save the practitioner considerable embarrassment and the patient much time and economic penalty.

Many posterior teeth lost because of a fracture after endodontic therapy probably had the problem unrecognized before the treatment. A full crown is not a guarantee that fracture will not progress. Several lower molars have been noted to fracture years later even with full coverage. In the opening of any posterior tooth for endodontic therapy, *a careful look at the dentin floor* for evidence of a subtle fracture *before removal of the roof of the chamber* will minimize the chances of failure.

If the fracture does not intersect the pulp space and does not terminate beneath the epithelial attachment (i.e., a common fracture of the lingual cusp of an upper premolar) and no esthetic problem results, no treatment is necessarily indicated.

If the fracture intersects the pulp space and no movement is evident in the fracture line with a wedging test, an attempt to salvage the tooth would necessitate both endodontic therapy and full coverage. If treatment is elected, the occlusal surface should be reduced radically (as if to prepare for a full crown) at the time of the pulpectomy. This will, for a short time, limit occlusal forces that would tend to fracture the tooth further before a full crown can be placed.

Remember, *watching a vertical fracture is not appropriate.* It will only go one way—to worsen. It cannot heal. Further, there is no way to see the extent of a vertical fracture without extracting the tooth to examine it with extensive magnification. The rest is guesswork. Finally, do not be an optimist. If you see a fracture that has separated and you cannot remove a mobile piece without leaving a severe pocket, condemn the tooth. It is not my intent to show how to salvage cracked teeth, but rather how to avoid the expense, pain, poor public relations, and so forth in an often hopeless situation.

ENDODONTIC THERAPY IN TOTAL TREATMENT PLANNING

The need for endodontic therapy may occur in any one of three ways: (1) as a result of a painful or traumatic episode requiring emergency treatment, (2) as part of a total treatment plan to restore a patient's oral health, or (3) as a result of discovery of pulpal or periapical damage during a periodic checkup after completed treatment. If emergency therapy is involved or if only endodontic treatment is required, the needed work is performed as soon as practical. However, if endodontic therapy is part of a total treatment plan, the proper timing for the therapy is important.

Significance of a total treatment plan. The concept of total patient care has become the dominant approach in treatment planning. The advantages of this philosophy over the "one-tooth-at-a-time, let's-wait-and-see-what-happens" method need no further discussion. Total patient care includes evaluation of the patient's medical conditions, soft and hard tissues of the mouth, teeth and their supporting structures, and edentulous areas. By using the diagnostic aids discussed earlier, plus additional clinical and laboratory tests, the dentist makes a careful determination of what is wrong—the diagnosis of the patient's dental disease. Without knowing what is wrong, the dentist has no way to correct the problems present in a manner designed to prevent recurrence.

For some patients the total treatment plan may require only minor restorative treatment plus prophylaxis. For others all the specialized areas of dentistry will be needed to return the patient to oral health.

Total treatment plan for complex cases. Just as no complex apparatus can be built without a master plan, so there must be a specific plan of treatment to correct the dental disease present. Although no general agreement exists as to the correct order of treatment procedures, the following outline offers an effective pattern for treatment of most complex cases. Since I believe that periodontal health is the most important objective to be gained in caring for patients with complicated dental problems, this is emphasized in the treatment plan. Furthermore, since almost all adult patients have some degree of periodontal damage, it is assumed that periodontal treatment is required in most complex cases.

A. Diagnostic phase
   1. General oral examination—including use of diagnostic aids: intraoral and extraoral radiographs, study models, recordings of occlusal relationships, laboratory tests, etc.
   2. Periodontal evaluation—to identify the hopeless teeth, those with guarded prognosis, and those that are treatable, with the type of temporary splinting required, if necessary

3. Excavation of deep carious lesions—with pulpotomy if pulp is exposed, until endodontic therapy may be initiated, and with placement of sedative dressing if unexposed
4. Final establishment of treatment plan—recording of specific treatment needed for each tooth and/or area, time requirements for each phase, and coordination if the services of more than one dentist are to be utilized

B. Treatment phase
1. Surgical treatment—including extraction of hopeless or superfluous teeth and ridge preparation for prosthetic appliances, if necessary
2. Temporary splinting—to support weakened teeth during periodontal and/or endodontic therapy
3. Periodontal therapy—including all the needed ramifications, such as scaling, curettage, surgery, equilibration, and directions for home care
4. Endodontic therapy—if needed, performance possible at the same time as periodontal treatment; if different dentists are involved, coordination of work necessary for the timing of certain procedures, such as root amputation, periapical surgery, and periodontal surgery
5. Restorative and replacement procedures

In certain cases, additional areas of dental treatment, such as orthodontics, may be required.

C. Maintenance phase
1. Routine oral prophylaxis and supervision of correct home care
2. Radiographic examination—periapical films of all endodontically involved teeth plus any areas of possible problems, periodic bite-wing x-ray films every 4 to 6 months, and complete series every 1 to 3 years
3. Repair—needed treatment as required, should be only minor in nature for at least the first few years after return to oral health

The treatment plan is not infallible and must have some degree of flexibility. There must be some allowance for possible failure of response on the part of key teeth that are difficult to treat and for setbacks during phases of therapy.

Timing for endodontics in total patient care. Endodontic therapy must be initiated early in the treatment phase for two important reasons. If treatment is indicated but not started, the patient may have a painful experience from a deep carious lesion causing a pulp exposure, from a chronic pulpitis or periapical lesion becoming acute, or from an acute alveolar abscess. Also, there must be sufficient time to evaluate the results of treatment on any teeth in which the prognosis was questionable. Although most endodontic therapy is predictable, certain key teeth may be treated but the final result remain in doubt because of difficulties encountered during treatment or because of the preoperative condition of the tooth. When some time is available for observation before the tooth is restored or involved as an abutment, a better determination may be made concerning the result (Fig. 2-41). If the questionable tooth appears to be failing, the treatment plan must be altered.

Endodontic therapy is frequently performed concomitantly with periodontal measures. Since certain teeth may require treatment of both types, combined therapy is important. If one condition is treated while the other area is even temporarily neglected, the untreated condition may delay the normally expected healing of the treated phase.

Case presentation. Many patients have a completely erroneous idea of endodontic therapy. The thought of having a "nerve" removed or falsehoods heard from acquaintances are sufficient to create fear in even the most cooperative individuals. A brief and sincere explanation of the significant points of treatment is important in allaying suspicions and gaining the ultimate in patient cooperation. The type of case presentation varies with the personality of the practitioner and the attitude of the patient. A brief example of the presentations that I normally use in my practice will be described here. Modifications may be needed when used by others, but these samples should be an aid to dentists wanting to develop a case presentation suited to their individual practice.

A slight variation exists between the case presentation for a tooth with a definite periapical radiolucency and that for a tooth with no obvious radiographic damage. For a tooth with a relatively normal radiographic appearance in which the preoperative condition is acute or chronic pulpitis or necrosis, the following description of treatment is given the patient. "According to the information gained from the x-ray films that were taken and the tests that were performed, it is clear that the pulp, which is in the center of your tooth, has become inflamed (or has started to die or died, as the case may be). Some people refer to the pulp as the nerve because pain emanates from it; however, because much more is present than just nerve tissues— blood vessels and packing cells in particular—pulp is the correct term. Unfortunately, pulp tissue has a very poor ability to heal after injury, so you are

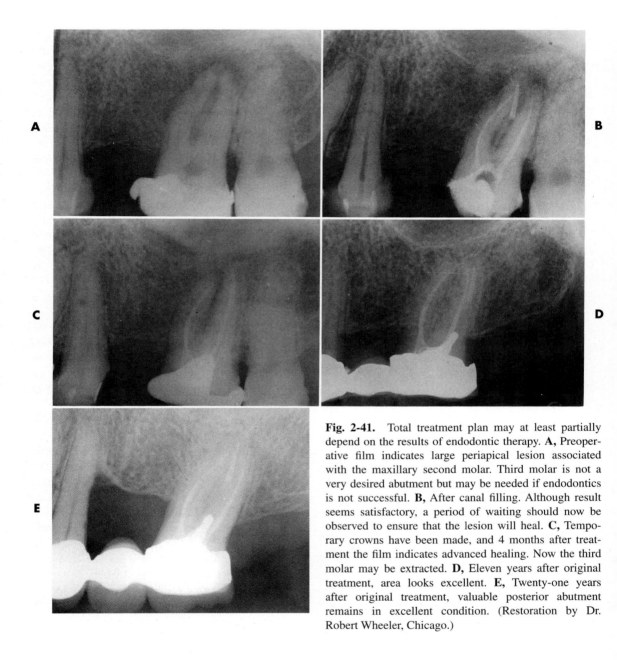

Fig. 2-41.   Total treatment plan may at least partially depend on the results of endodontic therapy. **A,** Preoperative film indicates large periapical lesion associated with the maxillary second molar. Third molar is not a very desired abutment but may be needed if endodontics is not successful. **B,** After canal filling. Although result seems satisfactory, a period of waiting should now be observed to ensure that the lesion will heal. **C,** Temporary crowns have been made, and 4 months after treatment the film indicates advanced healing. Now the third molar may be extracted. **D,** Eleven years after original treatment, area looks excellent. **E,** Twenty-one years after original treatment, valuable posterior abutment remains in excellent condition. (Restoration by Dr. Robert Wheeler, Chicago.)

faced with the choice of removing the tooth or removing the pulp and retaining the tooth."

For a tooth with an obvious periapical lesion, the start of the case presentation is slightly changed. The area on the x-ray film is shown and the following told to the patient. "According to the x-ray films taken and the tests performed, it is clear that you have an abscessed tooth. There are various types of abscesses and yours is a chronic abscess, one that is in a quiet state rather than causing a swelling. The abscess started because the pulp inside the tooth has died and has attracted bacteria, debris, or other irritating substances to the bone surrounding the tooth. Some people refer to the pulp as the nerve because pain may come from it; however, since blood vessels and packing cells are also present, pulp is the correct term. The abscess will heal if the tooth is removed, but it will also heal if the inside of the tooth is properly cleaned and sealed."

Both presentations are completed in the same way: "In order to retain the tooth, two to four relatively painless appointments will be required. First, the pulp tissue will be removed from its canal in the root, and then the interior of the tooth will be cleaned with instruments that act like small scrub brushes. Once all the debris, bacteria, and pulp are removed, the root is packed with an inert material that seals the tip and prevents any further damage.

"The tooth has been weakened by the irritants that damaged the pulp, and some tooth structure must be removed to perform the necessary treatment. Therefore, after this work is completed, a large filling or crown is placed to protect the tooth. The properly treated pulpless tooth may function as normally as any other tooth, hold a bridge or partial denture, and last for many years. In your case it is to your advantage to save the tooth in this way."

Visual aids may be included, such as radiographs, models, or pictures of successful cases or the parts of a tooth. Certain slight deviations may be made to include pertinent clinical symptoms present, such as sensitivity to temperature changes, chronic draining sinus, or swelling. When treating a tooth with a periapical radiolucency, the dentist should emphasize that no anesthetic will be required—a big plus with many patients who dislike injections.

The pamphlet produced by the ADA on endodontics may be given to the patient in addition to or instead of portions of the case presentation. Most of the possibilities for treatment are explained and illustrated in the booklet in a logical and clear manner.

Typical questions and simple answers. After a case presentation for endodontics, the patient may have questions about therapy. Questions typically asked and simple but direct answers follow:

"Will my tooth discolor?" Discoloration typically seen associated with "dead" teeth is due to hemorrhage of the blood vessels in the pulp after an injury or from a cement within the tooth that stains. If your tooth is not discolored now, it will probably not darken. If it is discolored, an improvement will occur during treatment or the tooth may be "capped" to give it a normal appearance.

"Why can't the work be finished in one long appointment rather than three or four shorter ones?" Time is necessary between appointments to allow medications placed within the tooth to kill bacteria and soothe the irritated tissue around the tooth. If a culture test is taken to see that the bacteria are destroyed, it takes a few days to observe the results.

"Is the treatment very painful?" Rarely is any pain felt during the appointments, except when the patient has severe pain at the outset. When needed, local anesthetic is used. Often the treated tooth is slightly tender to touch for 1 or 2 days after each appointment.

"What do you use to remove the pulp?" A small instrument that resembles a fishhook is used to engage the pulp tissue and remove it from the tooth.

"Is a pulp necessary in a tooth?" After the root of a tooth has reached full length and width, the pulp need not be present. In certain cases the root will continue to full growth even without the pulp.

"Why do you need to give me an injection, since you removed the nerve last appointment?" Some shreds of pulp tissue may remain that are sensitive. Even if the entire pulp has been removed, the tissues around the roots of the tooth have nerve tissue intact and may be irritable from the previous treatment.

"Could my other teeth that were extracted have been saved by endodontics?" Many excellent advances have been made in endodontics recently, making possible the retention of teeth that were formerly extracted. Even so, not all teeth are amenable to endodontic treatment, and treatment is not successful in every case.

"Why does the treatment cost so much more than ordinary fillings?" The work that is needed may be difficult and is time-consuming, since all the removal of irritants and cleaning of the tooth interior are performed with instruments by hand rather than with the drill. If the tooth is retained, the total fee for this endodontic therapy plus the filling (or crown) will be less than the fee for replacing the tooth with a fixed partial denture. In addition, and even more important, a tooth will be saved.

"Is this work surgery?" In most cases, endodontic treatment is performed through the tooth and is not considered surgery, as such. In some cases, if the abscess or area of irritation does not heal properly, surgery may be needed. Under a local anesthetic the tissues at the tip of the root are painlessly removed to retain the tooth.

REFERENCES
Textbooks on oral medicine and oral diagnosis

Burket LW: *Oral medicine: diagnosis and treatment,* ed 5, Philadelphia, 1965, Lippincott.

Cheraskin E, Langley LL: *Dynamics of oral diagnosis,* Chicago, 1956, Year Book.

Kerr DA, Ash MM, Millard HD: *Oral diagnosis,* ed 6, St Louis, 1983, Mosby.

Lynch MA, Brightman VJ, Greenberg MS, editors: *Burket's oral medicine,* ed 9, Philadelphia, 1993, Lippincott.

Mitchell DF, Standish SM, Fast TB: *Oral diagnosis: oral medicine,* ed 3, Philadelphia, 1978, Lea & Febiger.

Shafer WG, Hine MK, Levy BM: *A textbook of oral pathology,* ed 4, Philadelphia, 1983, Saunders.

Wood NK, Goaz PW: *Differential diagnosis of oral lesions,* ed 4, St Louis, 1991, Mosby.

Zegarelli EV, Kutscher AH, Hyman GA: *Diagnosis of diseases of the mouth and jaws,* ed 2, Philadelphia, 1978, Lea & Febiger.

Psychology in dental treatment planning

Berman CL, Berman LG: The psychological implications of tooth loss, *Dent Clin North Am* 13:961, 1969.

Borland LR, editor: Foreword to Symposium on Psychology in Dentistry, *Dent Clin North Am,* Nov 1962, p 579.

Brody HA, Nesbitt WR: Psychosomatic oral problems, *J Oral Med* 22:43, 1967.

Cinotti WR, Grieder A, Springob HK: *Applied psychology in dentistry,* ed 2, St Louis, 1972, Mosby.

DeLeon EL: Facial pain of non-odontegenic origin. *J Oral Med* 23:119, 1968.

Elfenbaum A: Causalgia in dentistry: an abandoned pain syndrome, *Oral Surg* 7:594, 1954.

English S: *Psychosomatic medicine,* ed 2, Philadelphia, 1949, Saunders.

Gier RE: Management of neurogenic and psychogenic problems, *Dent Clin North Am,* March 1968, p 177.

Harrigan WF: Psychiatric considerations in maxillofacial pain, *J Am Dent Assoc* 51:408, 1955.

Lang PJ: Experimental studies of fear reduction, *J Dent Res* 45:1618, 1966.

Lazarus RS: Some principles of psychological stress and their relation to dentistry, *J Dent Res* 45:1620, 1966.

Mackenzie RS: Psychodynamics of pain, *J Oral Med* 23:75, 1968.

Manhold JH: *Introductory psychosomatic dentistry,* New York, 1956, Appleton-Century-Crofts.

Morris AL, Little JW: Oral medicine in general practice. In Morris AL, Bohannan HM: *The dental specialties in general practice,* Philadelphia, 1969, Saunders.

Tobin DF, Behrens D: Understanding: an adjunct to periodontal therapy, *J Oral Med* 25:21, 1970.

Weckstein MS: Basic psychology and dental practice, *Dent Clin North Am* 14:379, 1970.

Weckstein MS: Practical applications of basic psychiatry to dentistry, *Dent Clin North Am* 14:397, 1970.

Vertical fractures of posterior teeth

Cameron CE: The cracked tooth syndrome, *J Am Dent Assoc* 68:405, 1964.

Cameron CE: The cracked tooth syndrome: additional findings, *J Am Dent Assoc* 93:971, 1976.

Hawks ML, Mullaney TP: A false diagnosis of a cracked tooth: report of a case, *J Am Dent Assoc* 114:478, 1987.

Luebke RG: Vertical crown-root fractures in posterior teeth, *Dent Clin North Am* 28:833, 1984.

Stanley HR: The cracked tooth syndrome, *J Am Acad Gold Foil Oper* 11:36, 1968.

Other references

Abbey LM: Screening for hypertension in the dental office, *J Am Dent Assoc* 88:563, 1974.

American Medical Association: Prevention of bacterial endocarditis, recommendations by the American Heart Association, *JAMA* 264:2929, 1990.

Bender IB, Seltzer S, Freedland J: The relationship of systemic diseases to endodontic failures and treatment procedures, *Oral Surg* 16:1102, 1963.

Bender IB, Seltzer S, Tashman S, Meloff G: Dental procedures in patients with rheumatic heart disease, *Oral Surg* 16:466, 1963.

Chamberlain FL: Management of medical-dental problems in patients with cardiovascular diseases, *Mod Conc Cardiovasc Dis* 30:697, 1916.

Chambers IG: The role and methods of pulp testing in oral diagnosis: a review, *Int Endod J* 15:1, 1982.

Drinnan AJ, Fischman SL: Medical-dental relationships, *Dent Clin North Am,* March 1968, p 31.

Ehrmann EH: Pulp testers and pulp testing with particular reference to the use of dry ice, *Aust Dent J* 22:272, 1977.

Elfenbaum A: In Levy S: *Dentist's handbook of office and hospital procedures,* Chicago, 1963, Year Book.

Frank AL: Extracanal invasive resorption—an update, *Compend Contin Educ Dent* 16:250, 1995.

Glick M, Garfunkel AA: HIV disease: pathogenesis and disease progression—an update, *Compend Contin Educ Dent* 13:80, 1992.

Knapp, DE: Therapeutic control of apprehension and pain in adult dental patients, *Dent Clin North Am,* March 1968, p 229.

Leddy BJ, Miles DA, Newton CW, Brown CE Jr: Interpretation of endodontic file lengths using radiovisiography, *J Endod* 20:542, 1994.

Little JW, Bartlett RC: Differentiation of common local and systemic disease in oral soft tissues, *Dent Clin North Am,* March 1968, p 141.

Little JW, Jakobsen J: Management of the hypertensive patient in dental practice, *J Oral Med* 29:13, 1974.

Miller DA, Wyrwa EB: Ear pain: a dental dilemma, *Compend Contin Educ Dent* 13:676, 1992.

Mitchell DF: Undesirable side reactions to drugs, *Dent Clin North Am,* March 1968, p 257.

Molinari JA: HIV, healthcare workers and patients: how to ensure safety in the dental office, *J Am Dent Assoc* 12:51, 1994.

Mullaney TP, Howell RM, Petrich JD: Resistance of nerve fibers to pulpal necrosis, *Oral Surg* 30:690, 1970.

Mulligan R: Late infections in patients with prostheses for total replacement of joints: implications for the dental practitioner, *J Am Dent Assoc* 101:44, 1980.

Rosenthal SL: Some clinical aspects of oral medicine, *J Oral Med* 25:112, 1970.

Shearer AC, Horner K, Wilson NHF: Radiovisiography for length estimation in root canal treatment: an in vitro comparison with conventional radiography, *Int Endod J* 24:233, 1991.

Uchin R: Management of problem endodontic patients. Paper presented before the E D Endodontic Study Club, Chicago, Feb 1968.

Wahl MJ: Myths of dental-induced endocarditis, *Compend Contin Educ Dent* 15:1100, 1994.

Weine FS: The enigma of the lateral canal, *Dent Clin North Am* 28:833, 1984.

Weine FS, Elfenbaum A: The legs as an aid in patient evaluation, *J Indianapolis Dist Dent Soc* 20:12, 1965.

Weine FS, Silverglade LB: Residual cysts masquerading as periapical lesions: three case reports, *J Am Dent Assoc* 106:833, 1983.

Weisman MI: American Heart Association revises the antibiotic regimen for the prevention of bacterial endocarditis, *J Endod* 12:34, 1986.

Marshall H. Smulson • Steven M. Sieraski

3 Histophysiology and diseases of the dental pulp

HISTOPHYSIOLOGY
Gross morphology of the dental pulp

An intact vital pulp may be removed from the root canal in one piece with a barbed broach; on examination, it is found to be a firm, cohesive, and resilient unit, maintaining its original shape. This is possible because the pulp is composed principally of a gelatin-like material called ground substance, which is reinforced throughout by irregularly arranged and interlaced collagen fibers and fiber bundles. Embedded in this stroma are the cells, blood vessels, and nerve fibers that make up the loose connective tissue frequently categorized as the *dental pulp organ.*

The term *vital pulp* is an arbitrary one, since varying degrees of inflammation, retrogressive changes, or necrosis may be present. *Semivital* pulps showing clear histologic evidence of tissue decomposition (proteolysis) have been extirpated from teeth that demonstrate normal ranges of response to vitality tests. With the occurrence of more and more proteolysis of ground substance, fibers, and cells, it becomes increasingly difficult to remove the pulp in one piece. This pulp is no longer capable of physiologic responses and is referred to as *necrotic* or *nonvital.*

Special environment of the dental pulp

Connective tissue elements of the dental pulp respond to changes in environment the same as any other loose connective tissue. However, the unique environment—unyielding walls of dentin surrounding a resistant and resilient fiber-reinforced ground substance—makes the dental pulp a special organ (Figs. 3-1 and 3-2).

The dental pulp has a rich circulatory force that, by virtue of the dynamics of fluid interchange between capillaries and tissue, establishes and maintains an extravascular hydrostatic (hydraulic)

pressure within this noncompliant chamber. The intrapulpal pressure, which has been measured to be about 10 mm Hg (Table 3-1), varies with each arterial pulse wave. An increase in intrapulpal pressure in an isolated region of the pulp may exceed the threshold limits of the peripheral sensory structures in the area and produce pain (Figs. 3-18 and 3-45).

Although multirooted teeth show a coronal anastomosis of blood vessels coming from each of the roots, and all teeth demonstrate accessory canals of various numbers, no consistent effective collateral circulation exists to overcome a severe irritant force, a phenomenon essential to the survival of any organ.

In summary, pulp injury is frequently irreversible and painful because of certain restrictions in its environment:

1. A low-compliance environment
2. Resilience of the connective tissue
3. An ineffective collateral circulation

For purposes of study the dental pulp may be subdivided into four zones (Figs. 3-2 and 3-3).

The first is the *central zone,* or pulp proper, a core of loose connective tissue (stroma) containing the larger nerves and blood vessels that begin to arborize toward the peripheral pulpal areas.

Outlining the central zone is an area richly populated with reserve (undifferentiated mesenchymal) cells and fibroblasts. This *cell-rich zone* serves as a reservoir for replacement of destroyed dentin-producing cells (dentinoblasts). Although most frequently observed in the coronal pulp, this zone can exist in the radicular pulp.

Peripheral to the cell-rich zone is the *subdentinoblastic zone* of the pulp, or *zone of Weil.* This area appears to be relatively free of cells and is often referred to as the *cell-free* or *cell-poor zone.* This zone may diminish in size or temporarily dis-

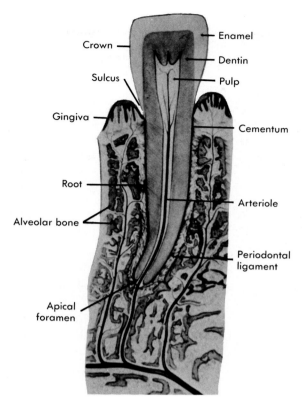

Crown

Sulcus

Gingiva

Root

Alveolar bone

Apical
foramen

Enamel

Dentin

Pulp

Cementum

Arteriole

Periodontal
ligament

Fig. 3-1. The tooth and its environment. The bone lining the tooth socket (alveolar bone proper) is known as cribriform because of its sievelike character. Note continuum of connective tissue from pulp to marrow spaces. (From Brescia N: *Applied dental anatomy,* St Louis, 1967, Mosby.)

appear when dentin formation is occurring at a rapid rate. When present, it has been measured to be approximately 40 µm wide.* The cell-free zone abounds in nerve fibers that have lost their outer wrappings (myelin sheaths). These terminal, naked, free fibers are dendrites of sensory nerves and are specific receptors for pain. Many enter the *dentinoblastic zone,* where they terminate as filaments, beads, or varicosities (Fig. 3-20, *A* and *B*). Many of the nerve fibers (10% to 20%) terminate in the tubules of the predentin and inner mature dentin (Figs. 3-6, 3-27, 3-29, and 3-30).

The combined dentinoblastic layer and subdentinoblastic free nerve network form a sensory complex *(peripheral sensory units)* that completely envelops or encapsulates the central pulp core.

*1 millimeter (mm) = 1000 microns (µm)
  1µm = 0.001 mm = 10,000 Angstrom units (Å)

Structural elements of the dental pulp

The components of the dental pulp, basically the same as in loose connective tissue anywhere else in the body, consist of *cells, intercellular substance,* and *intercellular fluid.*

The cells include fibroblasts, reserve cells, defense cells, and special cells.

The *fibroblast,* the principal cell distributed throughout the pulp, is especially abundant in the cell-rich zone (Fig. 3-16, *C*). It produces gelatinous intercellular matrix, in which all pulpal components are embedded, as well as collagen fibers that reinforce the matrix. Young fibroblasts may undergo mitosis and differentiate into replacement dentinoblasts. The shape of the fibroblasts varies from fusiform (cigar shaped) with long, slender, protoplasmic processes to stellate (star shaped) with shorter numerous branches. These processes appear to form a network with other fibroblasts. The health state of the fibroblasts reflects the age and vitality of the pulp and consequently the potential of the pulp to respond favorably to deleterious changes in its environment. As a result of the aging process, whether it occurs in a natural sequence or is accelerated by caries, abrasion, or pulp capping, there is a diminution in the size and number of these cells. (See discussion of retrogressive pulp changes, p. 158)

The *reserve cell,* found principally along capillaries and in the cell-rich zone, is a primitive undifferentiated cell that forms a reserve of pluripotential cells (Fig. 3-4). Such cells have the capacity to differentiate into various cell types as the need arises. They may become fibroblasts or change into dentin-producing (dentinoblastic) cells. During inflammation they may differentiate into macrophages or resorption cells (dentinoclasts).

The *histiocyte* (tissue macrophage) is another type of defense cell found in the connective tissue of the pulp. When activated, histiocytes migrate to the inflammatory site and become phagocytes (macrophages) that engulf bacteria, foreign bodies, and dead cells.

The *dentinoblast* (odontoblast) is a highly specialized connective tissue cell of the dental pulp, it is "special" because of the unique role it plays in both dentin and pulp function. We prefer the term dentinoblast rather than odontoblast because it more accurately describes the cell function and is more consistent with the accepted nomenclature of comparable cells. If a cementoblast produces

Table 3-1. Effect of pulp pathoses on intrapulpal pressure

Classification	Clinical considerations	Nature of pulp	Average intrapulpal pressure (mm Hg)
Normal pulp		Structures intact; tissue resilient; usually extirpation in one piece	10 (range, 8–15)
Reversible pulpitis (hyperalgesia)	Transitory pain, hyperreactive pulp; requires stimulus	Structually intact, but evidence of increased vacularity	13
Irreversible pulpitis (painful pulpitis)	Pain may be spontaneous and persist; persistent response to cold stimuli	Structurally intact; but engorged / Areas of necrosis or abscess formation	34.5
Nonvital pulp, exudative	Varies, but may be heat sensitive; prime finding in percussion sensitivity	Fluid filled	35.6
Nonvital pulp, dehydrated	No response to vitality tests; periapical radiolucency may be present	Dry granulated tissue ("mummy dust")	Unknown; capillary attraction of dentinal tubules and hygroscopic nature of canal contents may result in apparent negative pressure

Modified with permission of Dr. Henry Van Hassel (unpublished data).

cementum, an osteoblast produces bone, a chrondroblast produces cartilage, and an ameloblast secretes enamel matrix, the cell that produces dentin should be called a dentinoblast. In the words of Dr. Harry Sicher: "Odontoblast! A silly name, because they don't make teeth, only dentin. Odontoblasts make a little bit of dentin everyday. By extending its arm into the dentin, it also preserves and maintains the life and biochemical balance of the tissue."*

The dentinoblasts form a palisade arrangement at the pulp periphery. Although a single row of dentinoblasts may be present around the entire pulp periphery, a compound pseudostratified layer of as many as six to eight rows is sometimes observed, especially in the pulp horn regions. This is due mainly to the crowding of the cells in the continuously narrowing lumen; in addition, however, microscopic sections may vary in thickness and are frequently cut at an angle, so the adjacent cells appear as an additional row (Figs. 3-5 and 3-6). When cells are packed into multiple layers, their contours may be irregular. The variation in size and shape of these cells also depends on their location; they range from high columnar in the

pulp chamber, to low columnar and cuboidal in the cervical or midroot area, to flattened at the apex. The intercellular spaces between the dentinoblast may vary from 200 to 300 Å* (Fig. 3-7).

Columnar dentinoblasts have been described as being prismatic or polygonal in cross section and, having a "sweet potato" shape. Their lengths vary from 8 to 25 or more μm, with diameters ranging from 3 to 8 μm. The size depends on their functional activity, the more functional cells generally being taller. The dentinoblasts not only are in close physical contact with each other, but also communicate via numerous junctional complexes (p. 87), so that if one dentinoblast is injured, others are immediately affected. They do not undergo mitosis and may therefore be considered *postmitotic,* or *end, cells.* When dentinoblasts die, their matrix secretory function is carried out by neighboring dentinoblasts or by new dentinoblasts that arise from pluripotential cells from the underlying connective tissue. Although *reserve (undifferentiated mesenchymal) cells* are known *pluripotential cells,* some investigators consider *younger fibroblasts* to be endowed with the same capability. Electron micrographs show the cell body to contain a nucleus in the basal

*From Sicher H: Goteborgs Tandlak. Sallskaps, *Artikelserie*, no 250, Sept 1955.

* 1 millimeter (mm) = 1000 microns (μm)
1 μm = 0.001 mm = 10,000 Angstrom units (Å)

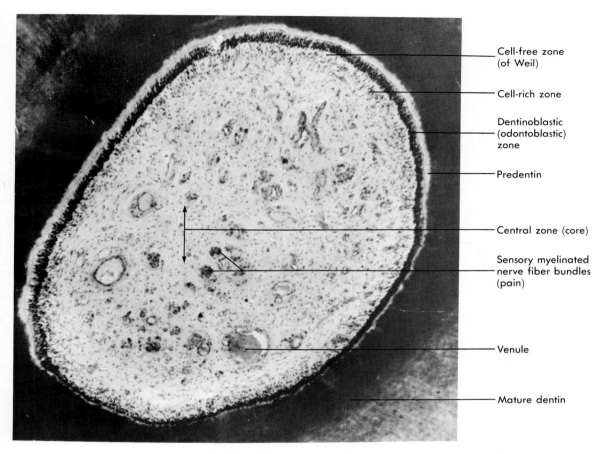

Cell-free zone (of Weil)

Cell-rich zone

Dentinoblastic (odontoblastic) zone

Predentin

Central zone (core)

Sensory myelinated nerve fiber bundles (pain)

Venule

Mature dentin

Fig. 3-2.   Cross section of a human tooth root showing elements of dental pulp. Structures in cell-free and dentinoblastic zones comprise peripheral sensory units (Courtesy Dr. Harold Grupe.)

portion, an extensive rough-surfaced endoplasmic reticulum, a large and well-developed centrally located Golgi complex, numerous mitochondria, and numerous granules and vesicles (Figs. 3-8 and 3-9).

By means of light microscopy, the dentinoblastic layer appears to be demarcated from the predentin by a heavily stained (hyperchromatic) line called the *pulpodentinal membrane*. Although not a membrane, it is an indication of the close contact of the dentinoblasts at their dentinal border. The dark dots or dense bars observed at these junctions were called *terminal bars* by earlier investigators who examined the structures under the light microscope. Disruption of this pulpodentinal (pseudo) membrane or the palisade arrangement of the dentinoblasts is microscopic evidence of pathologic change. No structure analogous to the pulpo-

dentinal membrane has been found by electron microscopy. According to Garant (personal communication), the pulpodentinal membrane corresponds to the point at which adjacent cells are tightly attached by a modified junctional complex and its associated fine cytoplasmic filaments called the *terminal web*. It is the terminal web that picks up the added stain. (See Fig. 3-8 and description.)

Observations with the electron microscope have indicated that these junctions (places of joining or meeting) between cells have multiple components forming a complex. Thus the term *junctional complex* more accurately describes the intercellular areas of contact. Junctional complexes have been observed in the pulp (Fig. 3-7), which Seltzer and Bender have classified as impermeable junctions, adhering junctions, and communicating junctions.

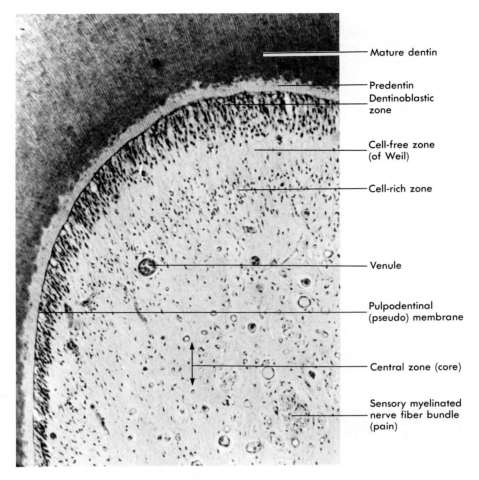

Mature dentin

Predentin
Dentinoblastic
zone

Cell-free zone
(of Weil)

Cell-rich zone

Venule

Pulpodentinal
(pseudo) membrane

Central zone (core)

Sensory myelinated
nerve fiber bundle
(pain)

Fig. 3-3. Periphery of dental pulp showing numerous fibroblasts and reserve cells in cell-rich zone. The cell-free zone contains a tangle (plexus) of free nerve fibers and capillaries. The myelinated nerve fiber bundles carry pain sensations to central nervous system.

1. Impermeable junctions. The tight junction, or zonula (little girdle) occludens, is so classified because of the fusion of adjacent plasma membranes. In the intestine, tight junctions serve as a barrier between luminal contents and underlying tissues. Corpron and Avery have reported tight junctions between dentinoblasts that probably maintain a positional relationship of the cell row as it moves uniformly away from the newly formed predentin. They have further postulated that tight junctions may be responsible for the aspiration of several or more dentinoblasts into one tubule when pressure is applied to the pulp during tooth extraction. It should be noted, however, that the zonula occludens in the dentinoblastic layer is not complete (Fig. 3-7) because substances pass easily

from blood vessels into the predentin (e.g., albumin from serum and molecular tracers).
2. *Adhering junctions.* Under light microscopy, adhering junctions were referred to as *intercellular bridges.* When viewed under the electron microscope, adhering junctions are characterized by small threads of tonofilaments that project from the cellular cytoplasm into and out of an electron-dense material called *plaques* or *patches* but do not cross over to neighboring cells (Fig. 3-7). The most frequently observed junctional, complex of this category are the *modified desmosomes,* or *intermediate junctions* (*zonula adherens*), where the membranes are separated by a space approximately 200 to 200 Å through which extracellular material (e.g., collagen, proteo-

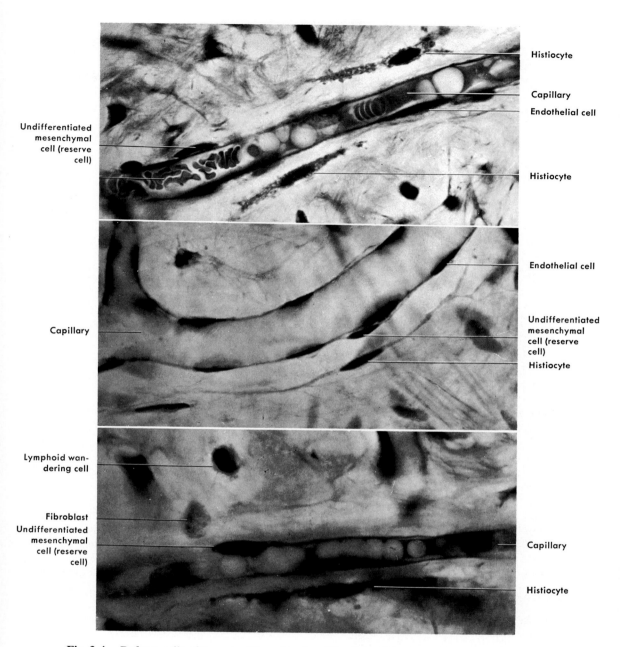

Fig. 3-4. Defense cells of the pulp. (From Bhaskar SN, editor: *Orban's oral histology and embryology,* ed 11, St Louis, 1991, Mosby.)

glycans) may diffuse. *Desmosomes* (*desmos,* band; *soma,* body), or *macula* (spot) *adherens,* do not appear to be characteristic of adhering junctions between dentinoblasts. However, Iguchi et al. observed numerous macula adherens between the dentinoblasts of rat incisors.

3. *Communicating junctions.* Communicating junctions, or *gap junctions* (*nexus-type junctions*), are sites of cell-to-cell communication between adjacent dentinoblasts and between dentinoblasts and fibroblasts of the subdentinoblastic layer (Figs. 3-7, 3-10, and 3-28, B). The intercellular space of the gap junction is

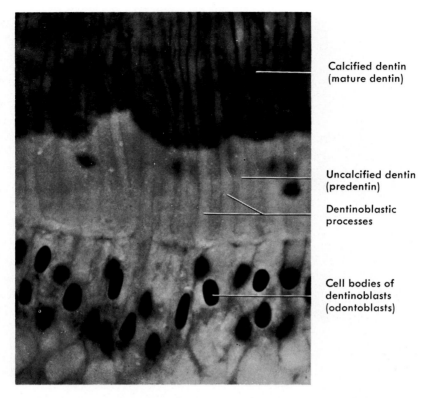

Fig. 3-5. Dentinoblasts (odontoblasts) and their processes. (From Bhaskar SN, editor: *Orban's oral histology and embryology,* ed 11, St Louis, 1991, Mosby.)

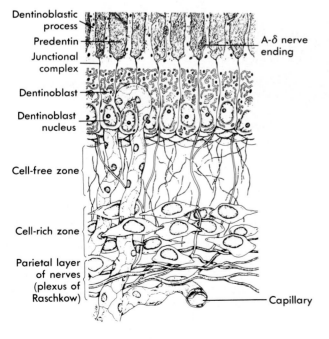

Fig. 3-6. Pulp periphery illustrating the dentinoblastic, cell-free, and cell-rich zones with capillaries and free nerve endings among the dentinoblasts. (From Bhaskar SN, editor: *Orban's oral histology and embryology,* ed 11, St Louis, 1991, Mosby. Courtesy Dr. James K. Avery, University of Michigan, Ann Arbor.)

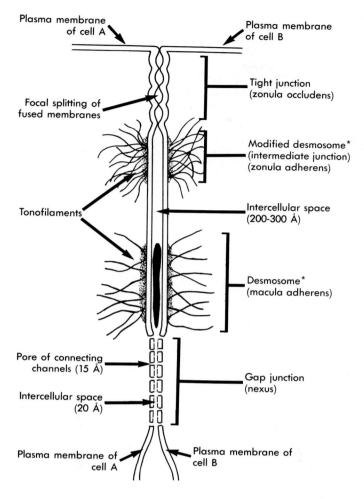

Plasma membrane
of cell A

Plasma membrane
of cell B

Tight junction
(zonula occludens)

Focal splitting of
fused membranes

Modified desmosome*
(intermediate junction)
(zonula adherens)

Tonofilaments

Intercellular space
(200-300 Å)

Desmosome*
(macula adherens)

Pore of connecting
channels (15 Å)

Gap junction
(nexus)

Intercellular space
(20 Å)

Plasma membrane of
cell A

Plasma membrane of
cell B

Fig. 3-7. Four types of junctions (junctional complex) observed at borders of neighboring cells (not to scale). Small filaments, believed to play a supportive role in cytoplasm, enter electron-dense plaque and loop back into cytoplasm. An electron-dense material is also seen in the intercellular space associated with the desmosome. The modified desmosome appears to be more characteristic of dentinoblastic junctional complexes than the desmosome.

narrowed but not obliterated (about 20 Å wide). At low magnification of the electron microscope, this type of junction may be mistaken for a tight junction; at higher magnification, however, an intercellular gap of 10 to 20 Å and a constant width throughout can be observed, and at no point do the opposing membranes appear to be fused. We do not know the exact nature of the signals that pass between the dentinoblasts at the gap junctions, but it can be postulated that they play an important role in the coordination of intercellular function.

Gap junctions differ from the other types because the juxtaposed plasma membranes contain special proteins called *connexons* that extend across the narrow intercellular space to connect the two cells.

The connexons contain channels (or pores) passing through the cell membrane and across the intercellular gap (Garant, personal communication).

The pores have a diameter of 15 Å and allow passage of low-molecular-weight materials between cells (metabolites, steroid hormones, vitamins, nucleotides) but not the higher-molecular-weight proteins and nucleic acids. Trowbridge suggests that the gap junctions provide a low-resistant pathway through which electrical excitation can pass from cell to cell, which may permit the dentinoblasts to function as a syncytium. Holland has observed that gap junctions often occur between dentinoblasts, dentinoblastic processes, and nerve fibers, as well as between dentinoblasts and fibroblasts (Fig. 3-10, *A*).

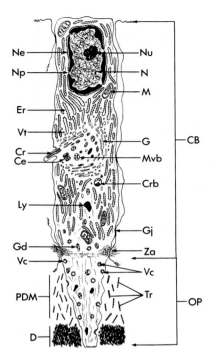

Fig. 3-8. Fully differentiated mouse dentinoblast. *CB,* Cell body; *Ce,* centriole; *Cr,* rudimentary cilia; *Crb,* crystalloid body; *D,* dentin; *Er,* endoplasmic reticulum; *G,* Golgi complex; *Gd,* dense granules; *Ly,* lysosome; *M,* mitochondria; *Mvb,* multivesicular body; *N,* nucleus; *Ne,* nuclear envelope; *Np,* nuclear pore; *Nu,* nucleolus; *OP,* dentinoblastic process; *PDM,* predentin matrix; *Gj,* gap junction; *Tr,* secreted tropocollagen (soluble collagen precursor, see p. 000); *Vc,* coated vesicle; *Vt,* transitional vesicle; *Za,* zonula adherens (terminal web, see p. 92). (From Garant PR, Szabo G, Nalbandian J: *Arch Oral Biol* 13:857, 1968.)

According to Holland and to Garant, the most prominent junctional complexes are those closest to the dentin and therefore at the junction between the dentinoblast cell body and its process. It takes the form of a *modified junctional complex* consisting of an incomplete zonula occludens, a partial zonula adherens (modified desmosome), and several gap junctions. The numerous fine cytoplasmic filaments that insert into the dense plaques (patches) of the zonula adherens are referred to as a terminal web (Fig. 3-8). This modified junctional complex does not completely encircle the cells. Small openings in the interdentinoblastic spaces occur to permit the passage of unmyelinated sensory nerves.

A cross-sectional view of dentin reveals 30,000 to 75,000 tubules per square millimeter. Dentinoblasts extend their cytoplasm and plasma membrane into these tubules as a dentinoblastic process (Tomes fiber) (Figs. 3-6 and 3-11). Under light microscopy the processes appear to reach the dentinoenamel and cementodentinal junctions, where they arborize (Fig. 3-27), but in transmission electron microscopic (TEM) studies the process appears to terminate in the pulpal half of the dentin. Recent scanning electron microscopic (SEM) studies and antibody techniques studies suggest the process may indeed extend to the dentinoenamel junction; however, the cellular nature of the structures observed in this area has not been confirmed. Thomas observed that the dentinoblastic process completely fills the dentinal tubule at the dentin-predentin junction, but farther into the dentin, the process separates from the tubule wall (Figs. 3-30 and 3-38). This peridentinoblastic space contains granular material and collagen fibrils.

Lateral branching and contact with neighboring processes may be seen at all levels. This communication permits the synchronization of cellular activity and pathways for the movement of nutrients and matrix constituents. A greater flow of tubular fluid is also permitted, thereby exposing a broader segment of the pulp to pressure changes. On the negative side, the lateral branching also may facilitate the lateral spread of acid in dental caries.

The processes are larger at the pulpal end than at the periphery (approximately 4:1). They are circular in cross section and, according to Sicher, have an average diameter of 2 μm and an average length of 2 mm (2000 μm). He concluded that at this length the cell process has four times the volume of the cell body, if all the processes extend to the dentinoenamel junction.

The dentinoblastic process is a direct extension of the cell body, and the plasma membranes are continuous. The cytoplasm, however, changes gradually as it extends through the predentin into the calcified dentin. The cytoplasm of the dentinoblastic process, unlike the cell body, is usually devoid of major cytoplasmic organelles, although fragments of isolated endoplasmic reticulum, mitochondria, and ribosome-like granules are frequently observed in the segment traversing the predentin. The predominant structures in the dentinoblastic process are microtubules (200 to 250 Å diameter),

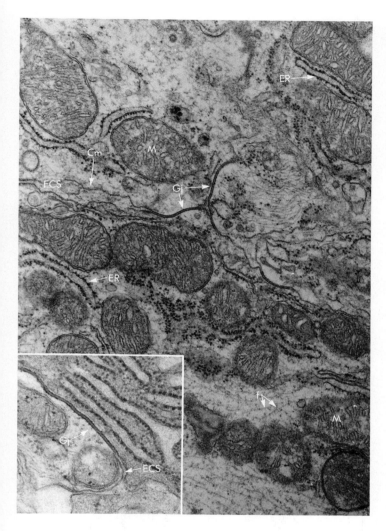

Fig. 3-9. Portions of several dentinoblasts showing regions of close apposition *(Gj)* of opposing cell membranes *(Cm)*. Note presence of fine filaments *(f)* within the cytoplasm. *ECS,* Extracellular space; *ER,* endoplasmic reticulum; *M,* mitochondria. (×35,400.) (*Inset,* Adjacent cell membranes of two dentinoblasts form a gap junction [G*J*]; × 48,000.) (From Garant PR, Szabo G, Nalbandian J: *Arch Oral Biol* 13:857, 1968.)

which serve as a transport system for peritubular dentin matrix, and filaments (50 to 75 Å diameter), thought to serve as a support mechanism for the process. The great number of vesicles present along the periphery of the process, which also originate in the process, contain the transported matrix that will ultimately be deposited on the tubule wall (Figs. 3-12 and 3-38). (See discussion of peritubular dentin, p. 129.)

The dentinoblastic processes are bathed by intercellular fluid from the dental pulp (dentinal lymph). The dentinal fluid is attracted into the tubules by capillary action. The dynamics of this capillary attraction is influenced by the intrapulpal pressure and whether or not the tubules at the outer surface are open or closed. Tanaka, using lanthanum tracers, confirmed that dentinal fluid emanates from terminal capillaries and diffuses to the dentinoenamel junction through peridentinoblastic spaces. The dentinoblasts are not nerve cells by origin or function, but their cell bodies and processes are in close contact with the nerve terminals (receptors for pain transmission). Thus, when injured or deformed, they may produce stimuli that are perceived by the free endings in contact with any part of the dentinoblast. One such stimulus may be the release of a neurotransmitter substance by the dentinoblast, which alters the permeability of the free nerve endings (producing an action potential). Another stimulus may also be in the form of a mechanical deformation of the dentinoblast (cell body or process), which acts as a

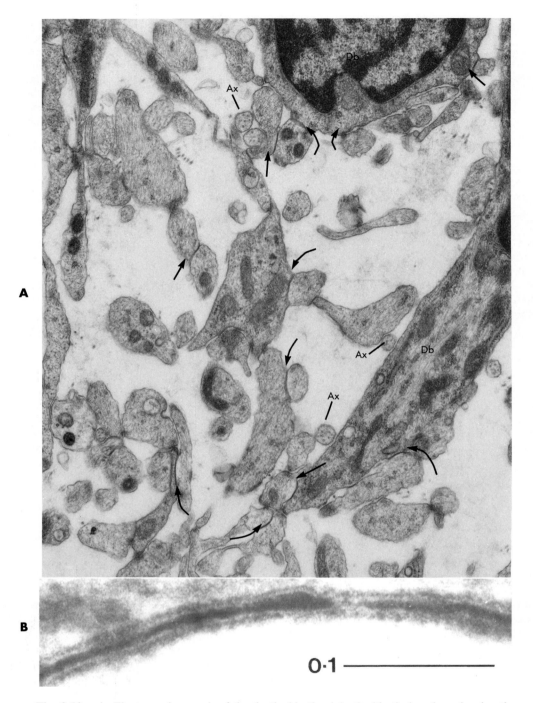

Fig. 3-10. A, Electron micrograph of the dentinoblasticsubdentinoblastic junction, showing the myriad of fine cell processes, which include axons *(Ax)* and dentinoblasts *(Db)*. Gap junctions *(arrows)* appear to be the dominant junctional complex in this region. (× 30,000.) (Courtesy Dr. G.R. Holland, University of Alberta, Edmonton, Canada.) **B,** Gap junction in dentinoblastic layer cut transversely and labeled with lanthanum hydroxide. Section has been stained with uranyl acetate and lead citrate to delineate inner leaflets of the apposed cell membranes. (×98 400,000; bar = 1.0 μm.) (From Holland GR: *Anat Rec* 186:121, 1976.)

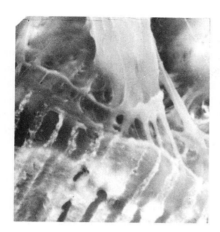

Fig. 3-11. Scanning electron micrograph of the dentinoblastic layer. Dentinoblasts are bunched together as a result of being torn from the dentin when tooth was cracked open. Dentinoblastic processes enter the dentinal tubules. (× 1800.) (From Seltzer S, Bender IB: *The dental pulp,* ed 3, Philadelphia, 1984, Lippincott.)

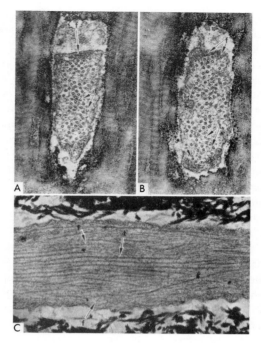

Fig. 3-12. A and **B,** Cross-sectioned dentinoblastic processes deeply situated within demineralized dentin. Closely packed microtubules *(t)* are major structural feature. Note dense aggregation of filaments in cortical regions of processes *(f)*. Asterisk denotes microtubules containing a central electron-dense dot. (× 60,000.) **C,** Longitudinal section of dentinoblastic process. Note parallel alignment of microtubules *(t)* and cytoplasmic filaments *(f)*. Microtubules appear equidistantly spaced over several microns, suggesting the presence of an intertubular stabilizing structure. (× 40,000.) (From Garant PR: *Arch Oral Biol* 17:1047, 1972.)

transducer mechanism converting mechanical energy into electrical energy. Thus dentinoblasts and A-delta (δ) nerve terminals function together as *intradental sensory units,* according to Trowbridge, and can be considered a *peripheral sensory capsule* because they completely envelop or encapsulate the central pulp core (Fig. 3-2).

As a columnar and specialized cell, the dentinoblast is more vulnerable to injury than the fibroblast. As the cell closest to the outer environment, it is also the first cell to be injured by environmental irritants. Therefore, in addition to the sensory role previously described, the dentinoblast initiates one or more of the following defense responses of the pulpodentinal complex: (1) tubular sclerosis, (2) irritation (reparative) dentin formation, and (3) inflammation. (See discussion of defense functions, p. 127.)

The intercellular components of the pulp are the collagen fibers, the amorphous ground substance matrix (both produced by the fibroblasts), and the intercellular tissue fluid (which comes from the capillaries). The collagen molecule, called tropocollagen, consists of three polypeptide chains. Differences in the amino acid composition and sequences provide the designation of alpha one (α1) and alpha two (α2). Four more collagen families or types have been recognized as a consequence of the different combinations of these

tropocollagen molecules. Types I, II, and III are referred to as *interstitial* collagen because they form the fibers in the intercellular spaces of various tissues. Type IV occurs in basement membranes. *Pulpal* collagen, produced by both dentinoblasts and fibroblasts, is a mixture of Types I and III at a ratio of 55:45. Since *dentin* collagen is principally Type I, it has been suggested that Type I is produced by the dentinoblast alone.

Several sizes of collagen fibers are found throughout the pulp. The smaller ones (reticular, argyrophilic, precollagenous) are dominant in developing and young pulps. They are very fine in diameter (100 to 120 Å) and do not show the typical collagen 640 Å wide cross-striations. With age, they increase in length and diameter to form mature collagen fibers. These larger collagen fibers are made up of bundles of several to a few dozen fibrils. The fibrils measure 400 to 700 Å or more in diameter and do demonstrate the 640 Å wide cross-striations. Once mature collagen is formed, it is less able to be destroyed and removed from the pulp. This is due to intrinsic chemical and structural changes related to the aging process. Thus, in an aging pulp, the mature collagen accumulates (accretion). As the pulp chamber becomes narrower with age, the collagen's inability to disintegrate to accommodate the smaller lumen results in *fibrosis,* a congestion that could be called a "crabgrass effect" (Fig. 3-52).

The amorphous component of intercellular material is the ground substance. The principal chemical components that give the form and properties to the ground substance are complex protein carbohydrate compounds called mucopolysaccharides, also referred to as glycosaminoglycans (GAGs) or proteoglycans. There are two types of mucopolysaccharides in the dental pulp: a nonsulfated type called *hyaluronic acid* (acid mucopolysaccharide), which is predominant in the dental pulp, and sulfated type, *chondroitin sulfuric acid.* Hyaluronic acid varies from a slightly viscid fluid that serves as a lubricant (synovial joint of the knee) to the soft gelatin-like material seen in the dental pulp. The chondroitin sulfuric acid components in the pulp are called chondroitin-4 sulfate (chondroitin A), dermatan-4 sulfate (chondroitin B), and chondroitin-6 sulfate (chondroitin C).

Since all pulpal components are embedded in this gelated matrix, it must be miscible with intercellular fluid. Water-soluble metabolites from the plasma (e.g., amino acids, salt, vitamins, hormones, oxygen) must pass through the selectively permeable arterial capillary walls to the cells. The dissolved waste products of cellular metabolism also must traverse the pulp tissue to enter the venous capillary flow and the lymphatic channels.

The ground substance is hydrophilic; i.e., it has the ability to hold a large amount of water (tissue fluid). The water is not free water, as observed in tissue fluid, but is bound in a colloidal or gel state (fluid colloidal system), which aids in the passage of the water-soluble metabolites and wastes through the medium. This binding to the ground substance is probably due to the long and featherlike framework of polysaccharide molecular chains, which have an extensive surface area within their meshes. These structures permit the molecule to hold varying amounts of water. Free water, however, is rapidly released wherever the ground substance is affected by injury and inflammation. The mucopolysaccharide molecules are highly polymerized (i.e., tightly bound together) thereby providing the viscid consistency and turgidity characteristic of the "gelated" pulpal ground substance. When the polymerization of these hydrophilic molecules increases, the viscosity (gelation) of the ground substance increases and the permeability decreases. When the degree of polymerization is less, the ground substance becomes more fluid (less gelated) and more permeable. The reinforcement by the collagen fiber bundles makes the ground substance even more rigid.

Any change in the nature or quality of the ground substance (i.e., the state of polymerization) directly influences the spread of inflammation and infection.

1. Van Hassel has demonstrated that local increases in fluid pressure are exactly that—local—confined to the site of injury or irritation by a resilient connective tissue. The viscosity of the gelated ground substance reinforced with collagen fibers does not permit fluids to move readily from one part of the pulp to another or the pressure to be transmitted throughout the tissue.

2. The gelated ground substance acts as a barrier against the spread of microorganisms and toxic products. However, organisms such as the hemolytic streptococcus can elaborate a spreading factor (the enzyme, hyaluronidase) that may dissolve the barrier and allow a faster invasion.

3. Although the turgidity of the ground substance resists the spread of inflammation, the process moves apically by increments from a particular site. Pressure from the increased tissue fluid collapses the thin-walled veins and venules, causing a vascular stasis and ischemia and resulting in local cellular death (Fig. 3-40).

4. Chemical mediators, (e.g., proteolytic enzymes, hyaluronidase), edema, and heat may also alter the quality of the ground substance (hydrolytic agents).

5. Chemotactic factors, chemicals liberated from injured cells, not only alter the viscosity but also exert chemotactic influence on polymorphonuclear leukocytes (neutrophils) and macrophages.

6. The viscosity can be further decreased by an excessive accumulation of inflammatory fluid (edema) and a localized temperature rise, both resulting from inflammation.
7. The temperature alters the state of ground substance in much the same way as in a reversible hydrocolloid, a sol-gel type of interplay. The heat of an inflamed pulp, by separating (depolymerizing) the molecules, diminishes the natural barrier of the gelated state.

Aging pulps (pulps undergoing retrogressive change) have less bound water, and the tissue therefore becomes increasingly dehydrated and *more viscous*. Oxygen and metabolites from the capillaries have more difficulty traversing the tissue. Cells that cannot obtain enough precursor materials are "sick" cells with a diminished ability to defend, heal, or repair themselves. They compete for available nutrition and for survival, with only a small number of cells capable of cell division (mitosis). The net result is fewer and smaller cells crowded in a sea of collagen accumulation. (See discussion of retrogressive pulp changes, p. 158.)

Functions of the dental pulp

The dental pulp carries out the four basic functions ascribed to all loose connective tissues: formative, nutritive, nervous, and defensive. It has a *formative* function because it forms dentin and continues to do so throughout the life of the tooth, which is also a defensive measure to minimize possible pulpal exposure through attrition (abrasion) or caries. The pulp has a *nutritive* function because its vascular tree nourishes all the vital elements of the pulpodentinal complex. It has a *nervous* function because of the critical roles that both sensory and motor nerves play in pain transmission and blood vessel (vasomotor) control. Finally, the pulp has a *defensive* function because of the protective roles played by the dentinoblasts (odontoblasts) and the underlying connective tissue components against harmful physical, chemical, and microbial irritants.

Formative function.

Dentin formation occurs throughout the life of the tooth at different rates of apposition and demonstrates different forms. The initial or primary dentin is tubular and regularly arranged because the dentinoblasts are not crowded and the tooth is under minimal functional strain. As more functional stresses are placed on the tooth, dentin

formation increases to such an extent that there is encroachment on the pulp cavity. As the dentinoblasts secrete the dentinal matrix and retreat toward the pulp center, they become crowded and their direction is altered. The dentin produced is wavier and contains fewer tubules per unit area. This type of dentin is appropriately called *functional*, or *secondary*, *dentin*.

Excessive environmental stimulation produces an atypical type of dentin. Operative procedures, caries, severe attritional stimulation (abrasion), and erosion produce initial episodes of rapid formation of dentin. This is a defense mechanism to compensate for regional dentin loss on the surface. Mjör considers it a specialized type of scar tissue formed in response to a local lesion (Fig. 3-34). The tubules are irregular or frequently are absent. This *tertiary* type of dentin is usually called *reparative, irregular,* or *defensive,* but more accurately has been termed *irritation dentin* by Langeland (Fig. 3-37). Irritation dentin is less sensitive to external stimuli because of the disruption in the continuity of the dentinoblastic process. (See discussion, p. 130.)

Severe trauma may activate the dentin-forming cells to such a degree that the canal lumen is almost entirely obliterated. The dentin produced under these circumstances may be referred to as *traumatic dentin* but is in reality an extensive form of irritation dentin. The term *osteodentin* has been applied to dentin when the matrix is laid down so rapidly that it entraps cells or tissue, giving it a bonelike appearance.

Dentin formation seems to follow essentially the same basic pattern as bone formation. The matrix-forming cells are either dentinoblasts or undifferentiated mesenchymal cells (reserve cells), which may differentiate into dentin-forming cells. Some investigators believe that less-differentiated, younger fibroblasts also have this capability. Seltzer outlines the steps in irritation (reparative) dentin formation as follows:

1. *Injury to the dentinoblasts*
2. *Inflammatory response* of the subjacent pulpal connective tissue
3. *Differentiation of new dentinoblasts* (matrix-forming cells)
   a. *Synthesis of cytoplasmic granules (collagen precursors).* Other granules within the cytoplasm of the dentin-forming cells contain both protein and GAGs, which assemble to form the proteoglycans.

The GAGs are composed of hyaluronic acid connected to core and link proteins that aggregate sulfated glycans. The granules also contain the enzyme *alkaline phosphatase,* which assists in making dentin matrix mineralizable (calcifiable).

   b. *Sulfation.* Although the precursors of the ground substance are within the dentinoblast, they are nonsulfated GAGs. Sulfation is initiated in the cytoplasm by attachment of negative sulfate ions (SO_4^{--}) to chondroitin. The sulfated GAGs serve to attract, bind, and neutralize positively charged calcium ions (Ca^{++}).

4. Secretion of the ground substance matrix and the soluble collagen precursors, tropocollagen (procollagen). "Soluble" refers to its solubility in an aqueous environment (e.g., water and saline).

5. Formation of the collagen fibrils. Dentinoblasts synthesize the soluble collagen precursors (tropocollagen) and secrete them into the ground substance matrix (Fig. 3-8). These simple chain molecules of tropocollagen mature by forming side chains with adjacent molecules to produce collagen fibrils. In other words, the collagen polypeptides become linked with adjacent polypeptides, mediated by a cell adhesion molecule (CAM), fibronectin. The new fibrils are still in a soluble state; however, the greater the side linkages and the larger the collagen fibrils, the more insoluble they become. The new fibrils now serve as a matrix for calcification.

6. Attraction of the mineral salts (calcification). The enzyme alkaline phosphatase removes phosphate ions from hexose phosphate (sugar present in predentin secretion) and phosphoproteins. The free phosphate binds with calcium ions (from the blood) to form calcium phosphate, $Ca_3(PO_4)_2$. The newly formed collagen molecules, linked by the CAM fibronectin, becomes coated with the sulfated GAGs (proteoglycans), which in turn absorb the calcium phosphates. The initial calcification of the predentin now serves as a nidus for hydroxyapatite crystal formation. An additional source of calcium also is provided from calcium-containing granules within the cytoplasm of the dentin-forming cells.

Tetracycline is incorporated into dentin during the mineralization process because of its high affinity for calcium (metallic ions). A tetracycline-calcium-orthophosphate complex is formed, resulting in clinically observable discoloration.

Nutritive function

The dental pulp must maintain the vitality of the dentin by providing oxygen and nutrients to the dentinoblasts and their processes, as well as providing a continuing source of dentinal fluid. Fulfillment of the nutritive function is made possible by the rich peripheral capillary network (terminal capillary network, or TCN) and its numerous projections into the dentinoblastic zone. Water-soluble metabolic substrates, components of plasma, filter across the capillary wall. This occurs when the pressure within the capillary from the pumping action of the heart (hydrostatic) is greater than the tissue pressure (osmotic) of the pulp. The tissue fluid reenters the capillaries at the venular end, where the osmotic pressure difference favoring reabsorption exceeds the hydrostatic pressure favoring filtration (Fig. 3-18).

The dental pulp chamber can vary from 2 to 5 mm in diameter at its widest portion. However, the extensive vascular arborization in the tissue that occupies this space emanates from only a few arterioles that enter foramina whose diameter may be as narrow as the tip of a size 10 file (0.1 mm). In addition to the arterioles, the foraminal space contains small venules, lymphatic vessels, and sensory nerves (Fig. 3-13). The arteries and veins are the dental branches of the superior and inferior alveolar vessels. They enter the apical foramina and begin to branch as they pass coronally. The branching occurs at all levels but is greater in the coronal pulp. Multirooted teeth have a rich anastomosis in the pulp chamber. However, no significant collateral circulation exists because of the relatively few communicating vessels from the accessory canals. The larger arterioles branch into smaller *terminal arterioles, precapillaries (metarterioles),* and ultimately *capillaries* as the arborization proceeds toward the pulp periphery (Fig. 3-14 and 3-17). Although capillaries are present in all areas of the pulp, there is a greater capillary concentration in the subdentinoblastic area to satisfy the functional demands of the large cellular population in the neighboring dentinoblastic and cell-rich zones (TCN) (Fig. 3-15). A striking feature of the blood vessels in the pulp is their small diameter and their thin, delicate walls (Fig. 3-16, *C*). The largest arterial vessels in the human pulp are 50 to 100 µm in diameter, which equals the size of arterioles found in most areas of the body.

The three characteristic layers of the arterioles reflect this delicateness: (1) an outer, scant connective tissue wrapping (the adventitia); (2) a thin, smooth muscle cell bed of several layers in the tunica media; and (3) the intima with its endothelial lining of flattened cells. The smaller terminal arterioles consist of endothelium, scattered smooth

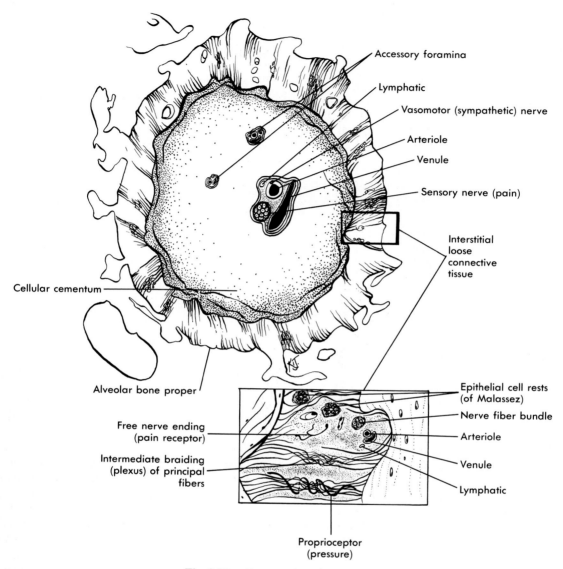

Fig. 3-13.   Cross section of root apex.

muscle cells spiraling around the endothelial tube forming the tunica media, and some supporting adventitia. One smooth muscle cell may wind around an arteriole several times so that contractions of the muscle cells control the diameter of the arteriole (Fig. 3-16, *A* and *B*). Inability of these muscle cells to contract results in vasodilation and increased blood volume (engorgement).

At rest, most capillaries are in a collapsed state and may carry as little as 5% of the circulating blood. In this state the blood may bypass the capil-laries, flowing from the arterioles to the venules (arteriovenous shunts) (Fig. 3-14). These arteriovenous anastomoses (AVAs) are present throughout the pulp but are more prevalent in the apical half. Kim has shown that as the intrapulpal pressure rises (which reduces blood flow) during an inflammatory response, these anastomosing vessels may open up in an effort to reduce the intrapulpal pressure and maintain the normal blood flow. Venous-to-venous anastomoses (VVAs) are also present.

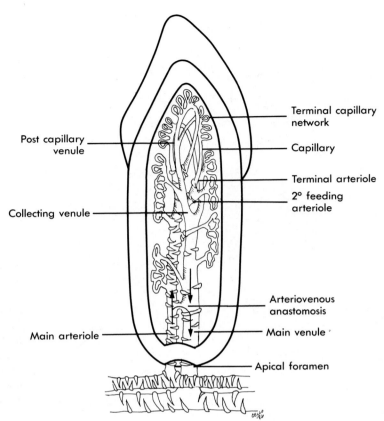

Fig. 3-14. Schema of pulp microcirculation.

Terminal capillary network

Capillary

Terminal arteriole

2° feeding arteriole

Post capillary venule

Collecting venule

Arteriovenous anastomosis

Main arteriole

Main venule

Apical foramen

There is no tunica media or adventitia in the capillary structure (Fig. 3-16, *D*). Capillaries are made up entirely of a single layer of flattened endothelial cells (endothelium) that is continuous with the endothelial lining of both arterioles and venules and is surrounded by a loose group of reticular and collagenous fibers. Two flat endothelial cells together can form a capillary tube approximately 8 to 10 μm in diameter. The capillary wall is therefore extremely thin and selectively permeable to electrolytes and particles of a small molecular size. The capillaries at the pulp periphery have pores or fenestrations between contiguous endothelial cells. Excessive dilation of these small vessels will injure the endothelial cells and diminish selective permeability. The intercellular fenestrations become larger, allowing the escape of larger (colloidal) blood protein particles into the tissue. The osmotic pressure difference across the capillary wall is now altered, and edema ensues (Fig. 3-18).

The capillaries are not innervated; their dilation after increased blood volume is passive and dependent on the diameter of the larger muscular vessels. Not all capillaries in a capillary bed function at the same time. Many remain collapsed until there is a sudden increase in blood volume, and many function only intermittently in the maintenance of tissue metabolism. Because of the nutritional requirements of the large number of cells there, the highest concentration of capillary loops is in the *peripheral plexus* (TCN) in the subdentinoblastic and cell-rich zones. During active dentinogenesis, capillaries are observed among the dentinoblasts and usually retreat pulpally as dentinogenesis slows down.

In the efferent venous system the capillaries coalesce into a sequence of venules (Figs. 3-14; 3-16, *E* and *F*; and 3-17) whose walls are even thinner and more delicate in structure than the arterial vessels. The larger lumina (50 μm or larger) are surrounded by a tunica intima, which consists of an endothelial lining, an extremely thin media, and an adventitia that is either scant or totally absent. The walls of the smaller venules are so delicate that fluid exchange occurs here as well as at the capillary level.

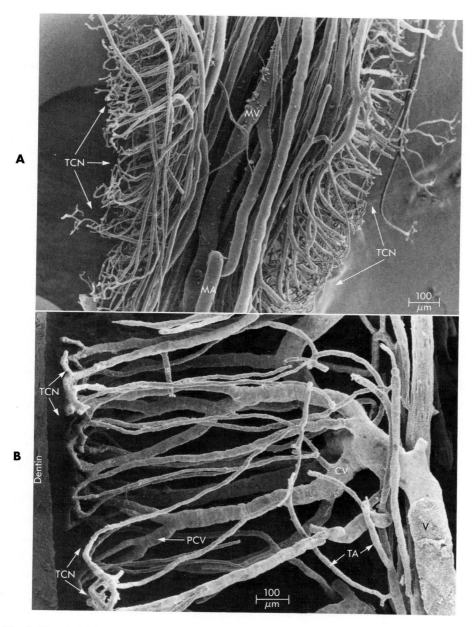

Fig. 3-15. **A,** Main arteriole of the dog dental pulp runs through central part of root canal, forming bundles. Branches are sent out either obliquely or perpendicularly toward dentinoblastic layer. Part of main arteriole forms a U-turn loop. From tip of loop, small branches run toward coronal pulp. *MA,* Main arteriole; *MV,* main venule; *TCN,* terminal capillary network beneath dentin. **B,** Terminal capillary network *(TCN)* is positioned almost perpendicular to the main trunk vessels, similar to teeth of a comb and its handle. Capillaries form continuous round connections between arterioles and draining venules. *a,* Arteriole; *CV,* collecting vein; *PCV,* postcapillary venule; *TA,* terminal arteriole; *V,* venule. (Bar = 100 μm.) (From Takahashi K, Kishi Y, Kim S: *J Endod* 8:132, 1982. © by American Association of Endodontists.)

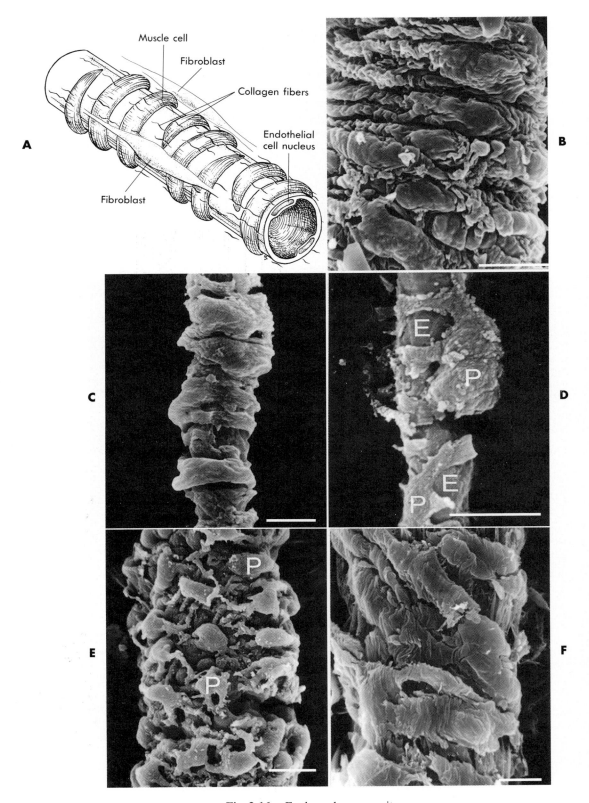

Fig. 3-16. For legend see opposite page.

Fig. 3-16.   A, Arteriole that conducts blood into precapillaries and capillaries. In essence it is a capillary surrounded by one layer of circular, smooth muscle fibers that form a simple tunica media. Connective tissue elements outside the muscular layer form the tunica externa (adventitia). **B,** Muscular arteriole (vessel runs vertically). Tunica media consists of two compact layers of spindle-shaped, circumferentially oriented smooth muscle cells. (Original magnification ×6000; bar = 5 μm.) **C,** Precapillary arteriole. Endothelium is dotted with scattered smooth muscle cells, which show no distinct evidence of constriction. (Original magnification ×4000; bar = 2 μm.) **D,** Capillary. Endothelium *(E)* is partially covered with pericytes *(P)*. (Original magnification ×8000; bar = 2 μm.) **E,** Postcapillary venule. Endothelium is covered with many pericytes *(P)*, which extrude several cytoplasmic processes. (Original magnification ×2500; bar = 2 μm.) **F,** Muscular venule. Flattened smooth muscle cells run obliquely or longitudinally to the vessel axis. (Original magnification ×2500; bar = 5 μm.) (**A** from Elias H: *Dent Dig* 56:489, 1950; **B** to **F** from Zhang J, Iijima T, Tanaka T: *J Endod* 19:55, 1993.)

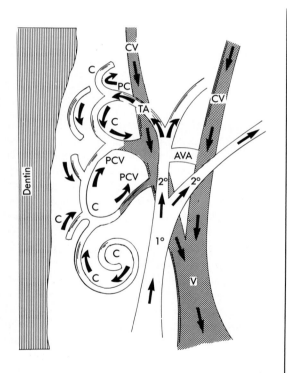

Vessel type	Diameter (μm)	Vm (mm/sec)
1° feeding arteriole	35-45	1.5
2° feeding arteriole	24-34	1.1
Terminal arteriole (TA)	16-23	0.6
Precapillary (PC)	12-15	0.5
Capillary (C)	>8	0.3
Postcap. venule (PCV)	12-23	0.2
Collecting venule (CV)	24-50	0.4
Venule (V)	>50	0.6

Vm = mean velocity

Fig. 3-17.   *Left,* Tracing from direct microscopic observation of a segment of the pulpal microvascular bed of the rat. *AVA,* Arteriovenous anastomosis; see figure table for other abbreviations. *Right,* Tabulation of hemodynamic parameters (diameter and velocity of flow). (From Kim S et al: *Microvasc Res* 27:28, 1984. © American Association of Endodontists.)

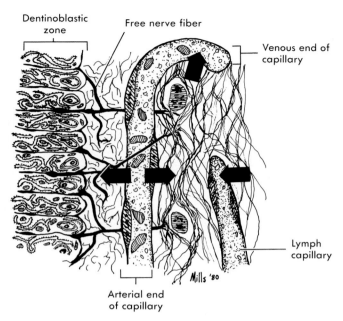

Dentinoblastic zone

Free nerve fiber

Venous end of capillary

Lymph capillary

Arterial end of capillary

Mills '80

Fig. 3-18. Fluid interchange among plasma, connective tissue, and lymphatics. Outward driving force is the capillary hydrostatic (heart) pressure. Inward pulling force is the protein osmotic pressure (due to higher concentration of large protein colloidal particles in the blood). At the arterial end, outward force is higher and fluid leaves vessels with metabolic nonosmotic particles (crystalloids). At the venous end, inward pulling force is higher and waste products enter venous and lymphatic circulation. Prolonged vasodilation, increased capillary permeability, and loss of plasma colloidal protein particles result in edema and increased intrapulpal pressure.

The presence of *lymph vessels* has been a subject of controversy. They are probably present, although they are not readily demonstrable. Dyes injected and/or perfused into the dental pulp have been isolated in the regional lymph nodes (submaxillary and submandibular) that drain the dental pulp. Using iron hematoxylin or periodic acid-Schiff hematoxylin to outline the blood and lymphatic vessels, Bernick studied the difference in lymph drainage among pulps of noncarious, carious, and restored teeth. He considered the lymphatic vessels of the human pulp in carious teeth to be a means of removing fluid, reducing pressure, and resolving incipient inflammation. The lymphatic vessels dilate and provide a drainage system for continuous removal of excess interstitial fluid, protein, cellular debris, and organisms. As a consequence, pulp pressure decreases; with the removal of the toxic stimulus, healing may occur in incipient inflammation where pulpal damage may not be severe (Fig. 3-18).

The existence of free interstitial fluid in pulps of normal teeth has been a controversial subject, but the presence of this fluid has been demonstrated and its effect measured by Beveridge and Brown and by Van Hassel. Taps inserted through the crowns and just up to the surface of the pulp tissue have registered the mean intrapulpal tissue pressure at an average 10 mm Hg. This is in the range of fluid pressures in other noncompliant areas such as the cerebrospinal fluid, with 5 to 14 mm Hg pressure. In a motion picture film, *Photographing the Microcirculation of the Dental Pulp* (Brown, Van Hassel, and Gadd), dentin was slowly and carefully shaved with a scalpel. The pulp could be observed, and clear fluid was seen rising from its surface pulsating with the heartbeat.

According to Van Hassel, a slight inflammatory response that raised the intrapulpal pressure to 13 mm Hg might be a reversible response (Table 3-1). However, a pressure of approximately 35 mm Hg in all probability indicates an irreversible state. Van Hassel further demonstrated that the nature of the resilient (turgid) fiber-reinforced gelated ground substance limits intrapulpal pressures to the site of irritation or injury.

Tönder and Kvinnsland were able to observe significant pressure differences at sites only 1 to 2 mm apart; therefore, when the structural integrity of pulp tissue is generally intact, an increase in intrapulpal pressure is not a generalized response that causes sudden strangulation of the pulp at the apex. It is, instead, a local phenomenon confined to the injury site by the turgidity of the pulpal tissue and followed by a progressive (circumferential) involvement of the pulp tissue as the inflammation and necrosis spread. The process moves apically by increments from the initial site. Pressure from the increased tissue fluid collapses the thin-walled veins and venules only in the area of the affected pulp tissue, causing a localized vascular stasis and ischemia. This results in local cellular death. This process repeats itself coronoapically (Fig. 3-41), as though the pulp were a series of compartments. The inflammation and resultant intrapulpal pressure changes proceed in a sequential manner from compartment to compartment. Strangulation can occur only if there is gross destruction of tissue.

Based on the work of Tönder, Heyeraas* outlined the mechanisms that prevent or limit the rise and spread of locally increased tissue pressure during pulpal inflammation (Fig. 3-40). These "edema-preventing mechanisms" explain why the pulp does not "strangulate itself" as a consequence of the "vicious cycle" of local inflammation. These events are:

1. A raised tissue pressure will, in itself, prevent further filtration.
2. Increased net filtration will automatically tend to lower the tissue fluid protein concentration and thus the colloid osmotic pressure.
3. Increased lymph flow will transport fluid and protein away from the inflamed area.
4. Net absorption into the capillaries in the adjacent normal pulp tissue will transport fluid out of the tooth.

Heyeraas further noted, as did Van Hassel, that in a case of a severe, persistent inflammation (where the structural integrity of the remaining pulp tissue is not intact), the increased tissue pressure could spread with a resultant compression of the blood vessels and total necrosis.

According to Van Hassel, intrapulpal pressure variations provide much of the pain phenomena associated with pulpitis. He suggests further that heat and cold are two distinctly different diagnostic tools because they represent two different phenomena:

1. Heat stimulation
    a. Heat causes vasodilation and subsequent increases in intrapulpal pressure. If the threshold of the sensory structures is reached, pain is produced.

*Presented at the International Workshop on the Biology of Dentin and Pulp, University of North Carolina, June 10–13, 1984.

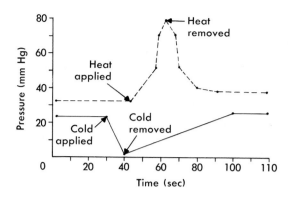

Fig. 3-19.   Effect of hot and cold on intrapulpal pressure based on the work of Beveridge and Brown. Eight seconds after the application of cold (ethyl chloride spray), the intrapulpal pressure had dropped to almost zero. Fifteen seconds after the application of heat (gutta-percha), the intrapulpal pressure doubled. Removal of the heat did not return the pressure to its original measurement. (Modified from Beveridge EE, Brown AC: *Oral Surg* 19:655, 1965.)

    b. Intrapulpal pressure rises directly and predictably as heat is applied to the tooth (Fig. 3-19). In an intact pulp a specific pulpal temperature must be reached before there is pain from heat. Therefore application of heat to normal teeth gives a delayed response. Table 3-4 reveals extremely different responses of low-threshold A-δ and high-threshold C fibers to rapid heat and slow, sustained heat stimulation.

    c. In a tooth with an inflamed pulp an increased intrapulpal pressure already exists; therefore one would expect an immediate painful response to gradual or sudden heat increase.

2. Cold stimulation
    a. The response to cold of a tooth with a normal or intact pulp is immediate. Since cold decreases intrapulpal pressure, pain from this source cannot be caused by increased pressure.
    b. Brännström attributes the pain from cold to a hydrodynamics mechanism (p. 119). The contraction of the fluid results in a rapid outward flow of fluid in the dentinal tubules and the subjacent pulpal tissue. Such a movement deforms intratubular and peripheral (A-δ) nerve membranes, which activates an action potential.
    c. In advanced acute pulpitis (advanced acute pulpalgia) when coronal necrosis is present in varying degrees, cold may not exacerbate the painful symptoms. If the peripheral coronal A-δ receptor units are not viable, they cannot be activated by fluid movement. Instead, cold relieves the pain

immediately because the vasoconstrictor effect reduces the blood volume. This in turn lowers the intrapulpal pressure to a subthreshold level for still viable C fibers (Table 3-4). Removal of the cold results in the return to pain within 30 to 60 seconds as the intrapulpal pressure returns to its former suprathreshold level.

Nervous function (neurogenic factor)

The dental pulp, as with any other connective tissue, requires a nerve supply to provide its primary but related functions: *vasomotor control* and *defense.*

Vasomotor innervation controls the movements of the muscular layer in the wall of the blood vessels, which results in expansion *(vasodilation)* or contraction *(vasoconstriction).* Such control regulates the blood volume and rate of blood flow of a particular arteriole. This in turn affects the fluid interchange between tissue and capillaries and influences the intensity of the intrapulpal pressure. A persistent flow of nerve impulses to the central nervous system (CNS) *(afferent)* and a return flow of impulses from the CNS *(efferent)* to the smooth muscle cells in the wall of arterial blood vessels (tunica media) may initiate the first phase of inflammation—transitory vasoconstriction followed by vasodilation.

Survival of any living organisms depends on its ability to recognize, respond, and adjust to harmful changes in the environment. This basic nervous and defense function is applicable to the dental pulp. A conscious recognition of irritants to the tooth gives the patient an opportunity to have the problem corrected before irreversible effects can occur. This recognition is possible because pain receptors in the pulpodentinal complex are linked to the CNS by an afferent pathway. Precise recognition, however, is not always a simple matter because it is subject to interpretation by the patient. Pain is multidimensional in scope, modified by cognitive, emotional, and motivational influences. In other words, the patient's personality, past experiences, and emotional state are major factors in localizing and interpreting the pain modality.

Afferent-efferent pathway. The precise mechanism for the transmission of pain, as well as the afferent-efferent pathway itself, is not completely known and is therefore subject to speculation and numerous hypotheses. Before reviewing a few of these theories, an overview of the basic components of this system are necessary.

Two types of nerve cells *(neurons)* are associated with the dental pulp:

1. The afferent (sensory) neuron (Fig. 3-20, *A*) is called a *pseudounipolar neuron* with two processes. The peripheral process *(dendrite)* originates in the dental pulp, and its terminals are the receptors at the pulp periphery. The cell body is located in the semilunar ganglion of the fifth cranial nerve *(trigeminal).* The second process *(axon)* proceeds to the CNS, where it terminates *(synapses)* in an island of gray matter *(nucleus)* called the *spinal nucleus of the fifth cranial nerve.* A second-order neuron decussates (crosses to the other side) and carries the impulse to the *thalamus,* synapsing with the third-order neuron (which terminates in the *postcentral gyrus of the cerebral cortex).*

2. The efferent system of nerve cells from the CNS (Fig. 3-20, *A*) to the dental pulp are *multipolar* neurons. They have many incoming shorter processes (dendrites) and one outgoing process (axon) of varying lengths. The figure shows their cell bodies to be located in the lateral horn of gray matter of the spinal cord's upper thoracic levels *(preganglionic)* and the superior cervical ganglion *(postganglionic).* The neuron contains the same organelles as any other cell: mitochondria, Golgi apparatus, endoplasmic reticulum, and lysosomes. In physiologic terms, *dendrite* implies a neuronal process carrying impulses toward the cell body; *axon* implies a neuronal process carrying impulses away from the cell body. However, since both pseudounipolar dendrites and axons of the afferent (sensory) system are the same morphologically, the term *axon* is frequently applied to both.

The nerve impulse depends on a change in the permeability of the neuronal membrane and one the *sodium-postassium pumps* of the cell. When the nerve fiber is at rest *(resting potential),* positively charged sodium ions (Na^+) are more concentrated in the extracellular tissue fluid than in the cytoplasm of the nerve itself. At the same time, positively charged potassium ions (K^+) are more concentrated in the cytoplasm than in the extracellular fluid. Because of this unequal concentration of ions, the nerve fiber membrane is polarized; i.e., the inside of the membrane is negative to the outside. Depolarization of the membrane is required

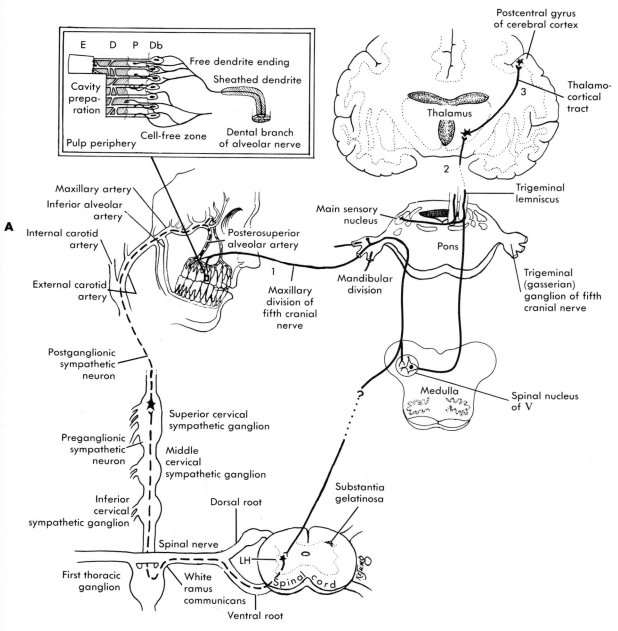

Fig. 3-20. A, Afferent-efferent pathway for sensory and vasomotor impulses. *E,* Enamel; *D,* dentin; *P,* predentin, *Db,* dentinoblast; *LH,* lateral horn (upper thoracic region); -----, efferent nerves; ——, afferent nerves; *1, 2, 3,* sensory neuron sequence.   *Continued*

for the propagation of the nerve impulse along the axon. Fig. 3-21 demonstrates the sequential mechanism of this phenomenon:

1. Stimulation increases the permeability of the axon membrane to Na$^+$, permitting their movement into the axon. As a result, a mo-

mentary depolarization occurs at the point of stimulation. The depolarized point on the membrane has become positive and acts as a stimulus to the next segment on the membrane.

2. As the impulse moves away, the membrane is recharged by the outward migration of K$^+$.

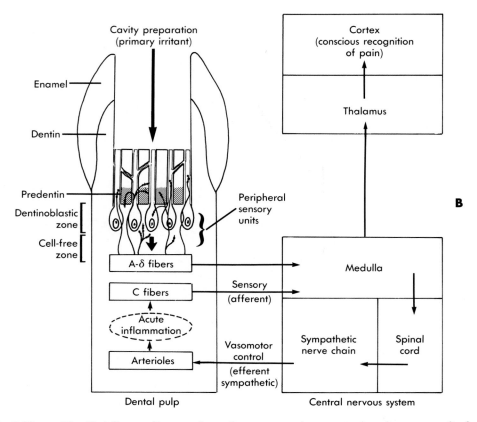

Fig. 3-20, cont'd.   B, Afferent-efferent pathway for sensory and vasomotor impulses as a result of severe dentinal stimulation.

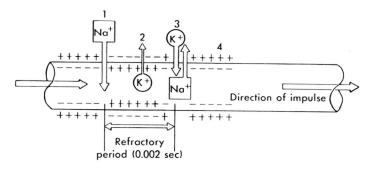

Fig. 3-21. Self-propagating waves of depolarization along a nerve fiber (action potential or nerve impulse). Note duration of refractory period (i.e., minimum time possible between impulses).

3. Subsequently the sodium pump expels Na^+ into the extracellular fluid while the potassium pump returns K^+ to the intracellular fluid.
4. The resting potential is now restored locally because the membrane is once again positive on the outside and negative on the inside of the axon membrane.

This cycle repeats itself down the length of the nerve as a self-propagating wave of depolarization *(action potential* or *action current)*. Each successive depolarized point on the conducting membrane soon becomes repolarized.

When the electrical impulse arrives at the *synaptic terminal, neurotransmitter molecules* are released from small *synaptic vesicles* in the terminal where they have been stored. The transmitter molecules (acetylcholine, norepinephrine, etc.) diffuse across a narrow synaptic cleft to generate (or inhibit) an electrical impulse in the receptors of the dendrites or on the cell bodies of other neurons. An *inhibitory synapse* alters membrane permeability, permitting an outward flow of K^+ but not an inward flow of Na^+. In effect, the inside of the membrane is more negative than it was during the resting state, thereby inhibiting the initiation of an action potential.

The *receptor* is a transducer, converting one form of energy (heat, mechanical, chemical) into electrical energy. Just as in hearing or sight, energy in the form of sound waves or light waves is converted into electrical energy. In the receptor, there is a much smaller amount of electrical activity (generator potential as opposed to action potential), measurable in millivolts. The generator potential must build up enough electrical activity until it finally reaches the nerve fiber's threshold. Then, suddenly, an action potential is set off in the neuron terminal *(all-or-none phenomenon)*. The exact mechanism for this is not completely understood. However, we can say that the stronger the stimulus, the more frequent will be the firing rate (number of impulses per second).

The dental pulp contains both sensory and motor nerves to fulfill its vasomotor and defense functions.

The larger sensory nerves are encased in a sheath of living cells *(Schwann cells)* whose plasma membrane consists of a lipoprotein material. The plasma membrane of the Schwann cell wraps itself around the nerve fiber in a "jelly roll" fashion (Figs. 3-23, *B,* and 3-24, *B*). This multilayered wrapping (sheath) is called *myelin* and is referred to as a *myelin sheath.* And action potential (impulse) in a myelinated nerve axon may be initiated at the nodes of Ranvier, where the myelin sheath is absent (Fig. 3-23, *B*). Unmyelinated fibers are also surrounded by Schwann cells, but the myelin spirals are absent. Schwann cells are indispensable for the life and function of peripheral nerve fibers. During the regeneration process, these cells create a pathway for the new axon to follow.

The sensory (afferent) nerves of the pulp are branches of the maxillary and mandibular divisions of the fifth cranial nerve (trigeminal). These small branches enter the foramina (Figs. 3-13 and 3-22) and arborize in the same manner as described for blood vessels. The larger nerves are found in the *central zone* (Fig. 3-23, *A*); as they proceed coronally and peripherally, they divide into smaller and smaller units. Subjacent to the cell-rich zone, the nerves branch extensively, forming the *parietal layer of nerves,* also known as the *plexus of Raschkow* (Fig. 3-24, *A*). This layer of nerves contains both myelinated A-δ fibers (2 to 5 μm in diameter) and the minute unmyelinated C fibers (0.3 to 1.2 μm). A subpopulation of these nerve fibers (mostly unmyelinated) contain neuropeptides, including substance P, calcitonin gene-related peptide (CGRP), and neurokinins. Johnsen has noted that the configuration of this plexus changes with increased dentin formation. The CGRP immunoreactive nerve fibers have been shown in animal studies (Khayat and others) to sprout extensively in the subdentinoblastic region and into dentin as a response to pulpodentinal injury. At about the level of the *cell-rich zone* (Fig. 3-6), myelinated fibers begin to lose their myelin sheath. In the *subdentinoblastic (cell-free) zone,* they form a rich network or tangle of naked (free) nerve fibers that are specific receptors for pain. Many of these fibers enter the dentinoblastic zone, where they pass between or wrap around the dentinoblasts; some penetrate into the predentin zone as well as the inner dentin, seen embedded along or around the dentinoblastic process (Figs. 3-20, *B,* and 3-31). Ochi and Matsumoto found the approximation of the nerve fibers and dentinoblastic processes to be about 20 nm, with no gap junctions or synapses present. Coated pits were found on the cellular membranes of the dentinoblastic processes adjacent to nerve fibers.

Nerve endings do not exist in every tubule. Intratubular nerves appear in 10% to 20% of the tubules in the coronal pulp horn region, compared with less than 1% at the level of the cementoenamel junction, and only occasional nerves are found in the radicular dentin (Fearnhead, and confirmed by Avery). The nerves may appear deeper in the inner dentin as a result of increasing dentin deposition rather than the growth of nerves peripherally. They are probably trapped in the tubules by dentin deposition. Avery et al. have shown that the neural tissue is one of the last to enter the highly vascular developing pulp. Although these nerves enter the pulp after dentin formation, they do not enter the peripheral region until the tooth is about to erupt. *Not until the tooth*

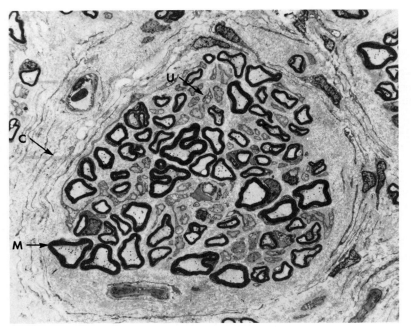

Fig. 3-22. Cross section of a sensory (afferent) nerve near the apical end of the pulp (human premolar). *C,* Connective tissue sheath: *M,* myelinated A fibers; *U,* unmyelinated C fibers. The difference in diameter between these two types of nerve fibers is readily apparent. (From Johnsen DC: *J Dent Res* 64:555, 1985.)

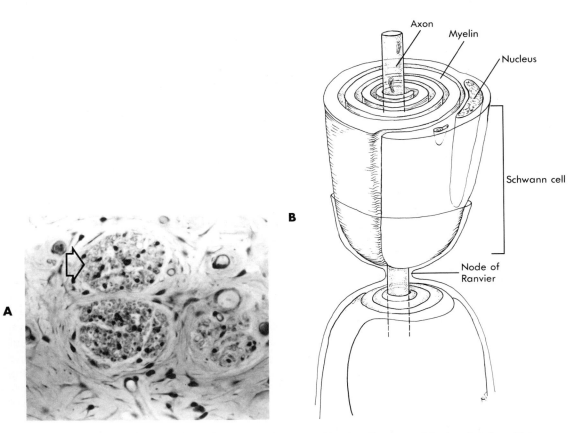

Fig. 3-23. **A,** Cross section of sensory (pain) nerve fiber bundles *(arrow)* in dental pulp, which carry impulses to the central nervous system. As A-delta nerve fibers leave their peripheral terminal positions, each becomes ensheathed by myelinated Schwann cells (see also Fig. 3-22). **B,** Structure of a myelinated sensory nerve fiber according to interpretation of electron microscopists (see also Fig. 3-24, **B**). (From Elias H, Pauly J: *Human microanatomy,* ed 2, Chicago, 1961, DaVinci.)

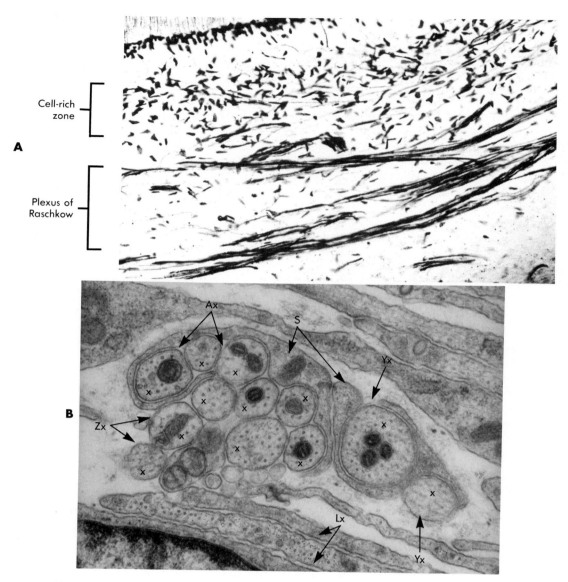

Fig. 3-24. A, Parietal layer of nerves (plexus of Raschkow). Although the larger-diameter myelinated nerves are readily apparent, minute unmyelinated C fibers are also present in this area. Cell-rich zone curves upward to the right. (× 1000.) **B,** Electron microscopic view (× 40,000) of the plexus of Raschkow, showing both cross sections *(X)* and longitudinal sections *(Lx)* of unmyelinated nerve fibers. Evident are characteristics that make these fibers particularly suited for pain reception: incomplete ensheathment by the Schwann cells *(S)* and multitudes of axon-to-axon contacts *(Ax). Yx,* Open Schwann cell sheath exposing axolemma (nerve membrane); *Zx,* several axons leaving the ensheathment of the Schwann cell. (**A** from Avery JK: In Bhaskar SN, editor: *Orban's oral histology and embryology,* ed 11, St Louis, 1991, Mosby; **B** from Holland GR: *Proc Finnish Dent Soc,* Nov 1986.)

nears functional occlusion can nerves be demonstrated among the dentinoblasts.

The motor nerves are supplied by the *sympathetic division* of the autonomic system. Sympathetic nerves *(postganglionic)* enter the foramina of the root in the outer wrapping of the arteries *(tunica adventitia)* (Fig. 3-13) and terminate as varicose fibrillar processes in the muscle cells of the middle muscular arterial wall *(tunica media).* The terms *vasomotor* and *vasomotor control* are appropriate names for these sympathetic fibers because by innervating the blood vessels and their musculature, they control the diameter of the vascular lumina and therefore the blood volume and blood flow, and ultimately the intrapulpal pressure. (See discussion on effect of the return impulse, p. 126.)

The speed with which a nerve impulse passes along a neuron varies directly with the diameter of the axon: *the larger the diameter, the faster the conduction* (Tables 3-2 and 3-3). Fibers having the largest diameter are classed as A fibers, those with the smallest diameter as C fibers, and those of the intermediate size as B fibers. The A fibers are myelinated and subdivided into the larger-diameter A-alpha (α) and A-beta (β), the intermediate A-gamma (γ), and the small A-delta (δ) fibers. The A-β and A-γ fibers carry touch, pressure, and proprioceptive impulses at a speed as high as 70 m/sec. The A-δ fibers carry pain (nociceptive) sensations at a speed ranging between 2 and 30 m/sec. The afferent sensory C fibers are unmyelinated and carry pain sensations at a slower speed (0.5 to 1.0 m/sec) because of their lack of myelin and smaller diameter. Unmyelinated C fibers average three to four times the number of myelinated A fibers (Johnsen). However, not all the C fibers are sensory; approximately 10% are sympathetic (Holland).

Neuropeptides are proteins that have been associated with central and peripheral nervous systems through immunohistochemistry and radioimmunoassay. Substance P, CGRP, and neurokinin A are sensory neuropeptides that have been demonstrated in the dental pulp. These sensory neuropeptides originate from the trigeminal ganglion and distribute in a population of unmyelinated C fibers. On excitation, these nerve fibers release the neuropeptides and produce an inflammatory response (vasodilation, hyperexcitation of nerve endings) called *neurogenic inflammation.* A sympathetic neuropeptide, neuropeptide Y (vasoconstrictor effects), and a parasympathetic neuropeptide, vasoactive intestinal polypeptide (vasodilator effects), have also been located in the dental pulp. The nonsensory neuropeptides are frequently associated with nerve fibers of blood vessels and are absent in the peripheral pulp (dentinoblastic layer).

It has been postulated that the A-δ fibers produce the initial momentary sharp pain response to external stimuli because of their peripheral location, low threshold of excitability, and greater conduction speed. On the other hand, continuous, constant, or throbbing pain is a result of sustained smaller C fiber activity; these C fibers have a

Table 3-2. Classification and function of fibers in peripheral nerves

Fiber	Diameter (µm)	Conduction velocity (speed of impulse, m/sec)	Function
A-alpha (α)	6-20	15-80 (myelinated)	Afferent fibers for touch, pressure, proprioception, vibration (mechanorecptors)
A-beta (β)	5-12	30-70	
A-gamma (γ)			
A-delta (δ)	1-5	2-30 (myelinated)	Afferent fibers for pain and temperature
B	1-3	3-15 (myelinated)	Visceral afferent fibers; preganglionic visceral efferent fibers
C	0.4-1.0	0.4-2 (unmyelinated)	Afferent fibers for pain and temperature; post ganglionic visceral efferent fibers

Table 3-3. Pain fibers in the pulp (nociceptive/algogenic)

	A-delta (δ) fibers	C fibers
Diameter (μm)	2-5 Measurement of parent fiber, which includes myelin sheath; smaller terminal processes (telodendrites) emerge from parent fiber	0.3-1.2 Fibers remain this diameter throughout their length.
Conduction velocity (m/sec): speed of electrical impulse or action potential traveling along nerve	5-30 As many as eight smaller terminals (telodendrites) feed into one larger myelinated parent fiber to produce greater velocity because of increased diameter.	0.4-2
Myelinated	Yes; parent axons located in cell-rich and central zones No; myelination lost by terminal branches of parent axon in dentinoblastic and subdentinoblastic zones	No; "Jelly roll" spirals of Schwann cell membranes absent Fibers enveloped by Schwann cells but not with myelin
Location of terminals	Superficial; terminals in dentin tubules in dentinoblastic and subdentinoblastic zones (pulp-dentin border zones)	Probably near blood vessels throughout pulp; small C fibers difficult to differentiate from other cell processes
Pain characteristics	Sharp, pricking, and unpleasant but bearable (fast and momentary)	Throbbing, aching, and less bearable; lingering and extremely unpleasant sensation
Stimulation threshold	Relatively low; does not take much to initiate (fire) an impulse; can be stimulated without injury to tissue	High threshold to stimulate these fibers; stimulus may have to be so intense that tissue is damaged; from pathologic standpoint, pain associated with inflammatory process (exudative lesion and tissue damage)

As suggested by Dr. Henry Trowbridge.
Dr. Trowbridge cautions that this is an interpretation of available but inconclusive data and is speculative to a certain degree.

much higher threshold of excitability. It should be noted that A-δ fibers can be stimulated without injuring the tissues (see discussion on hyperalgesia), whereas C fiber stimulation is associated with tissue damage and the inflammatory process. Tables 3-3 and 3-4 review the physiologic characteristics of both A-δ and C fibers and their reactivity to various stimuli. Note in Table 3-4 that only the A-δ fibers are activated by the frequently used electric and cold "vitality" tests. This may explain why these tests are not reliable on the immature teeth of young patients. These teeth contain significantly fewer A-δ fibers than mature teeth because myelinated nerves do not reach their maximal development and penetration into the pulp until the apex completes its development.

As previously mentioned, the precise mechanism for the transmission of pain and the afferent-efferent pathway itself are not completely understood and are therefore subject to postulation. Three of many theories attempting to explain the mechanism of pain transmission are the specificity theory, the pattern theory, and the gate control theory.

The specificity theory (advanced by von Frey in 1894) states that different sensory fibers mediate different sensory modalities such as pain, heat, cold, touch, and pressure. The receptors for pain are specific and are mostly unmyelinated free nerve endings. When stimulated, these fibers transmit impulses along specific pathways.

The pattern theory proposes that pain is generated by nonspecific receptors. It assumes that all

Table 3-4. Responses of pulpal A-δ and C nerve fibers to special stimuli

Stimulus	A-δ (low threshold)	C (high threshold)
Intrapulpal pressure changes		
Sudden nerve compression	Increased response	Increased response
Prolonged nerve compression	Decreased response (may block pain impulses)	Resistant to pressure increase (impulses will continue)
Vitality tests		
Electric	Positive (immediate)	Negative (except at high levels of stimulation)
Cold (ice)	Positive (immediate)	Negative (no apparent effect)
Rapid heat* (two-phase response) ⟶	Immediate: first response (sharp, localized) ⟶	Delayed: second response (dull, radiating)
Slow and sustained heat*	Negative	Positive (after 45° to 47° C [113° to 116.6° F])
Resistance to oxygen depletion		
Hypoxia/anoxia	Decreased fiber activity (short survival time in presence of pulp necrosis)	Fiber activity resistant to oxygen depletion (longer survival time in presence of pulp necrosis)

As suggested by Dr. Henry Trowbridge.
*Based on the experiments of Dr. M.V. Närhi (1985).

nerve fiber endings are alike and that the pattern for pain is produced by a more intense stimulation than for the other sensations. The summation of the pain impulses produce a pattern that the brain receives and recognizes.

The specific pain pathway and pattern theories have been challenged by evidence from Melzack and Wall, who introduced the *gate control theory* of pain transmission. The actual mechanism is a subject of controversy. The reader who may take exception to some aspects of our explanation must bear in mind that some of this area is still theoretic and still requires much research. Our attempt to relate this spinal cord phenomenon to the trigeminal complex and to the pulp itself is, at best, speculative.

According to the gate control theory, two of the factors that regulate pain transmission are as follows:

1. A gating mechanism located in a specific area of gray matter in the spinal cord is called the substantia gelatinosa. This gating mechanism receives painful (sensory or afferent) impulses from peripheral nerves and permits their passage to the brain by opening the gate, or prevents their passage by closing the gate. Whether the gate opens or closes depends on (a) the speed (velocity) of the impulse (the larger the fiber, the greater the velocity), (b) the interaction between noxious (nociceptive) pain stimuli transmitted along smaller-diameter fibers, and (c) those stimuli of touch and pressure (mechanoreceptors) that are transmitted along the larger-diameter fibers.

2. Descending central control from intrinsic brain mechanisms modulates the gating mechanism. This control arises from emotional, motivational, psychic, peripheral, and visual stimuli as well as from past learned experiences.

Basic anatomy of the gate control system. The gray matter of the spinal cord is organized into 10 laminae (layers or segments) referred to as *laminae of Rexed.* Layers I to VI are in the dorsal horn, layer X surrounds the central canal of the spinal cord, and layers VII to IX make up the remainder of the gray matter. Layer II (in the dorsal horn) is called the *substantia gelatinosa* (gelatinous substance), so named because of its gelatin-like physical appearance (Fig. 3-25, *B*).

Confined for the most part to the substantia gelatinosa are small neurons with short processes, referred to as *substantia gelatinosa cells* or SG cells. Located adjacent to the substantia gelatinosa in the spinal cord gray matter are the cell bodies of neurons, called *transmission cells* or T cells. These are larger than the SG cells and have short dendrites that enter the substantia gelatinosa to synapse with the SG cell bodies or cell processes (Fig. 3-25). The axon of the T cell is long and sends branches to the lateral area of white matter in the contralateral area of the spinal cord. It is joined by other T cell axons from different levels of the spinal cord. Collectively, these axons ascend by two routes: the *lateral spinothalamic* (fast and sharp pain) and the *spinoreticulothalamic* (slow and dull pain) pathways. These fibers then proceed to the subcortical areas of the brain, where they terminate in the *ventral posterior* and the *intralaminar thalamic nuclei,* respectively. A *nucleus* is a group of nerve cell bodies located within the brain and spinal cord. (A *ganglion* is a group of nerve cell bodies located outside of the brain and spinal cord.) In the thalamus the nerve fibers synapse with third-order neurons whose axons go to the postcentral gyrus of the cerebral cortex (Fig. 3-20, *A*).

How the gate works. Before proceeding, review Tables 3-2 and 3-3.

1. Axons of large-diameter afferent neurons (A-α, A-β, A-γ) enter the spinal cord through the dorsal root (Fig. 3-25). The principal branch of the large-diameter axon enters the dorsal horn, synapsing with T cells. A collateral (branch) of the same fiber enters the substantia gelatinosa and terminates on the SG cells. Another branch may ascend to the higher centers (see step 8).

2. Axons of small-diameter afferent neurons (C and A-δ) also enter the dorsal horn of the spinal cord to synapse with T cells. They also send a collateral to the substantia gelatinosa to terminate on the SG cells.

3. The SG cells send branches to synapse with incoming axon (afferent) fibers entering the T cell pool. Branches from the SG cells do not contact the T cells directly but rather the terminal area of the A and C axons (*presynaptic inhibition*). *The only activity that the SG cells can do is send inhibitory impulses to the T cells, preventing them from firing an impulse.*

4. Large-diameter fibers can only *excite* the SG cells, which in turn send out inhibitory impulses to the T cells (presynaptic inhibition). Since the T cells are unable to transmit an impulse, the *gate is closed* to pain.

5. Messages (impulses) from the branches of the smaller A-δ and C fibers can only *inhibit* the SG cells, stopping them from sending inhibitory impulses to the T cells. This action *opens the gate* to pain.

6. Since T cells are not receiving inhibitory impulses from the SG cells, they are free to send a painful response when activated by the smaller C or A-δ fibers.

7. Thus smaller fibers, A-δ and C, *open* the gate to pain by inhibiting SG cells; larger A-α, A-β, and A-γ fibers *close* the gate by exciting the SG cells. Stimuli such as touch, pressure, vibration, and rubbing send impulses via the large fibers, which *close* the gate when pain is present from small-fiber activity.

8. The large-diameter axons can also send an ascending collateral branch to *central control,* the higher centers of the brain. As a result, signals from the brain, by means of *descending tracts,* can influence (modulate) the gate control.

9. It is postulated that the gate control mechanism may be further modulated by intrinsic brain mechanisms (periaqueductal gray, reticular formation, thalamus) and through emotional, motivational, peripheral, psychic, and visual stimuli as well as by past learned experiences. Final response will depend on the balance or net result of the initial input from all three systems: large-diameter fibers, small-diameter fibers, and central control.

10. Accompanying the pain response are other neurologically related manifestations:
    Behavioral: crying, screaming, rage, stoicism
    Muscular: grimacing, withdrawal reflexes
    Visceral: syncope, respiratory increase, digestive reaction

Clinical applications of the gate control theory of pain.   Although the clinical applications of the gate control theory are speculative at best, the explanation of a number of clinical manifestations can be reasonably postulated.

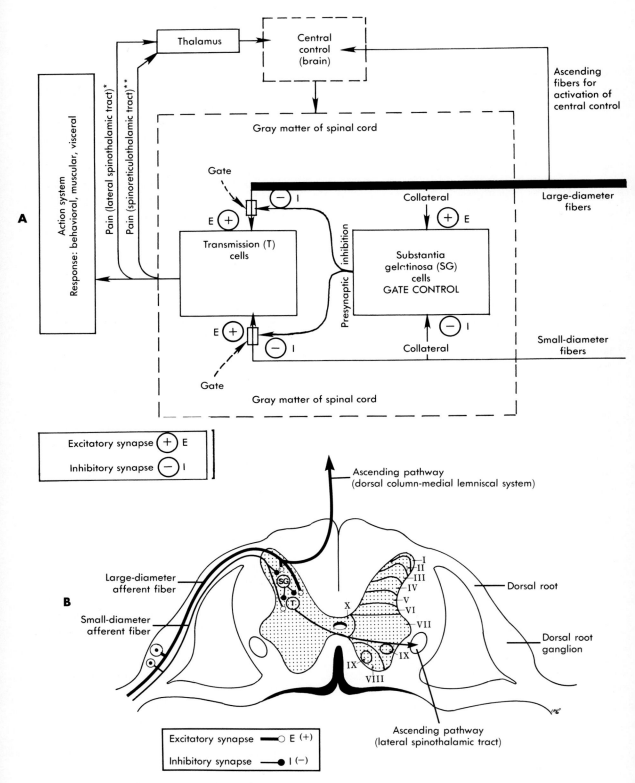

Fig. 3-25. **A,** Mechanism of gate control theory. (*), Fast, direct, sharp pain; (**), slow, indirect, dull pain. **B,** Components of gate control mechanism are transposed onto a sketch of spinal cord cross section. Roman numerals indicate the laminae of Rexed. *SG,* Substantia gelatinosa cells; *II,* substantia gelatinosa; *T,* transmission cells. (Courtesy Geraldine Gaik, Ph.D., Loyola University, School of Dentistry, Maywood, Ill.)

Higher-center modulation. Modulating influences of the higher centers may be visual, auditory, past experience, or temperament. Dentists regularly experience the distraught patient with a toothache. Such emotional stress may enhance the pain as a result of the influence of central control on the gate. The opposite effect may be demonstrated by an injured parent whose child is also injured. The parent, concerned over the safety of a loved one, might not be fully aware of his or her injuries. In this person the higher centers may be influencing the gating mechanism. The expression "mind over matter" could apply.

Spontaneous, intermittent, and continuous pain. Seltzer (personal communication) suggests that the A-β may be the larger fibers of the pulp, as A-α are the larger skin fibers. He further suggests that if the A-β fibers are not stimulated, pain is a result of C fiber and A-δ fiber activity. If a cavity preparation is cut, these smaller fibers produce the painful response because there are few A-β fibers at the periphery. If there is a pulpitis and A-β fibers deeper in the pulp are stimulated, they close the gate to pain from C fiber activity. Conversely, if A-β fibers are not activated by the inflammatory process, the C fiber summation can cause pain. Alternate A-β and C fiber stimulation as a result of pulp inflammation closes and opens the gate, thus explaining intermittent and spontaneous pain. The phenomenon of *summation* is the accumulation of the lesser impulses of smaller pain fibers at the points of synapse. This collective input will surpass the threshold where one or two impulses might not evoke a response. Liebman suggested that summation of lesser nerve fiber activity produces pain because the "mechanism for gate closure does not exist or is severely impaired." He states that this phenomenon may also explain the continuation of pulpal pain after such stimuli as cold and heat have been removed in cases of irreversible pulpitis.

Pulpal anoxia. Both Liebman and Närhi suggest that oxygen deficiency in a diseased pulp (anoxia, hypoxia) would adversely affect the larger fibers first (Table 3-4). As a consequence, the gate is allowed to remain open, and stimuli that were not noxious to a normal pulp, such as hot and cold fluids or slight increases in intrapulpal pressure, could trigger a more painful response because of the small-fiber activity.

Counterirritation, pressure, and massage. A common nondental example would be a bruised knee. The immediate pain is due to the C fiber stimulation, which opens the gate, producing intense pain. Rubbing diminishes the pain because the larger-diameter A fibers close some of the gate, and pain perception by the higher centers is diminished.

The use of poultices containing capsicum (cayenne pepper) is an old treatment that once played an important part in the clinical practice of dentistry. Such treatment is still available commercially as Poloris Pads (Block Drug Co., Jersey City, NJ). A small cloth pad containing the irritant is applied to the mucosa overlying the offending tooth. Mucosal hyperemia is produced, and most likely, A-α fiber stimulation causes the SG cells to close the gate. The same principle may be applied to massaging an area adjacent to an affected tooth or pressing firmly against the anterior border of the ramus just before inserting the anesthetic needle. Both actions modulate the final effect by stimulating large-fiber activity, which closes the gate.

Acupuncture. Continuous rotation of the acupuncture needle stimulates the peripheral nerves. The larger fibers such as the A-α are pressure nerves and transmit the impulse faster than the smaller fibers. They activate the SG cells, which send out inhibitory impulses to the T cells, closing the gate. Pain then is not perceived by the higher centers (central control).

Mechanism of referred pain. Referred pain originates at one site (e.g., mandibular first molar) and is experienced at another site (e.g., the ear). This phenomenon may be partially explained by the *convergence theory,* which states that the pain is referred because of several factors:

1. *Convergence of afferent nociceptive (algogenic) pain fibers from various regions of the head and neck into the subnucleus caudalis of the spinal nucleus V.* The multiple sources include the fifth, seventh, ninth, and tenth cranial nerves and cervical plexus nerves C2 and C3 (Fig. 3-26). This means that pain information from the face, teeth, temporomandibular joint (TMJ), ear, pharynx, larynx, scalp, and other assorted structures is converging into a pool of nociceptive (algogenic) neurons located at the brainstem level, namely, in the subnucleus caudalis of the spinal nucleus V (medulla). The proximity of these converging terminals from diverse sources suggests a complex synaptic communication in the subnucleus caudalis.

2. *Summation effect of persistent incoming stimuli on nociceptive neurons.* Neurotransmitter

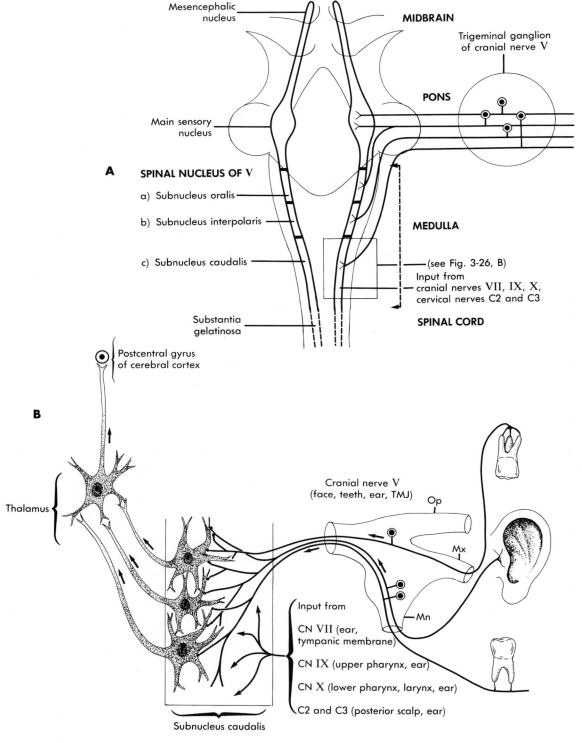

Fig. 3-26. Pattern for referred pain. **A,** Trigeminal nuclear complex showing the location of spinal nucleus V, the principal site for pain referral. The trigeminal nuclear complex consists of the mesencephalic nucleus (midbrain), main sensory nucleus (pons), and spinal nucleus V (medulla), which is continuous with the spinal cord substantia gelatinosa. The spinal nucleus V is further subdivided from rostral to caudal into a subnucleus oralis, interpolaris, and caudalis. (Courtesy Geraldine Gaik, Ph.D., Loyola University, School of Dentistry, Maywood, Ill.) **B,** Enlargement of the subnucleus caudalis of the spinal nucleus V, illustrating the pattern of convergence of incoming nociceptive fibers of cranial nerves *(CN)* and cervical nerves *(C)*. Ophthalmic *(Op)*, maxillary *(Mx)*, and mandibular *(Mn)* divisions of the trigeminal cranial nerve *(V)*. *TMJ,* Temporomandibular joint.

substance accumulates at the synaptic points of the converging fibers. When the threshold limits of the approximating terminals are surpassed, action potentials are initiated.

Theories of pulpodentinal pain fiber excitation. It is an established fact that, no matter what stimulus is applied to the tooth surface, only one conscious sensation is engendered—pain. However, no agreement exists on the exact mechanism that transmits the stimulus through the dentin to initiate a nerve impulse (pain).

Three theories or hypotheses of pain transmission have been proposed: (1) dentin innervation, (2) hydrodynamic mechanism, and (3) dentinoblastic deformation or injury (transduction).

Dentin innervation. The theory of dentin innervation states that there are nerve fibers within the dentinal tubules that, when injured, initiate the nerve impulse (action potential).

However, the extent of observable nerve fiber penetration has been limited to the predentin and inner dentinal zones. Penetration of the nerve fibers all the way to the dentinoenamel junction has not been observed with any certainty or consistency. One explanation given for this is as follows: in the predentinal zone the nerve fiber follows a straight course in a concavity or groove on the surface of the dentinoblastic process; peripheral to the inner dentin, however, the nerve fiber and the dentinoblastic process are intertwined in a corkscrew pattern and therefore extremely difficult to detect.

Gunji described four types of terminal configurations and ending sites. They include:

1. *Simple marginal pulpal fibers* that run from the subdentinoblastic plexus (of Raschkow) to the dentinoblastic layer, but *not to the predentin*
2. *Simple predentinal nerve fibers* that run a straight or spiral course through the tubule
3. *Complex predentinal nerve fibers* with terminal multiple branches and multiple ending-like enlargements on each branch. Although one terminal complex may cover an area in excess of 100,000 μm^2, *actual penetration into the dentin is limited to a few microns.*
4. *Nerve fibers that, without branching, run a direct course into the dentin* to a distance of 100 to 200 μm

Johnsen cited a number of investigators who have estimated that more than 40% of the dentinal tubules in the areas of the pulp horns have innervated tubules. This number diminishes rapidly

coronoapically: 4% to 8% (midcrown), 0.2% to 10% (cervical area), and 0.02% to 0.2% (midroot).

Experimental evidence by investigators (e.g., Närhi et al., Brännström and Åström, Anderson and Naylor) suggests that nerve fibers are not present in peripheral tubules. Such evidence includes:

1. Algogenic (pain-producing) substances such as KCI, bradykinin, acetylcholine, and histamine do not produce pain when applied to exposed peripheral dentin.
2. Hypertonic NaCl solution, capable of depolarizing nerve membranes in the deeper layers of dentin or the exposed pulp, will not initiate a nerve impulse when applied to peripheral dentin.

Yamada's electrophysiologic studies on dentin in dogs revealed that the dentinoenamel junction produced more action potentials than in the deeper cavity preparations. Yamada concluded that the reduced sensitivity may be the result of injury to the process. Others may argue that the dentinoenamel junctional area contains a multiplicity of terminal arborizations of the dentinal tubules and therefore a greater surface area to stimulate. Holland demonstrated a greater number of tubules in the predentin and inner 200 μm. The number diminished to about one third in the middle zone of calcified dentin, rising again in the periphery because of the terminal branching. These observations by both Yamada and Holland give credence to the common clinical observations of most dentists that dentin sensitivity is greatest at the periphery, decreases in the middle third, and increases again in the inner zones, closest to the pulp.

Hydrodynamic mechanism (fluid force effecting motion). The naked nerve (neuronal) endings in the subdentinoblastic and dentinoblastic zones and in the tubules of the inner dentin are exquisitely sensitive to sudden pressure changes, fluid movement, or mechanical deformation if the stimulation exceeds their threshold. It makes no difference whether the source of movement or pressure is from the pulp (intrapulpal) or is transmitted through the dentinal tubules (intratubular).

Brännström has proposed that dentinal pain is due to a hydrodynamic mechanism. The dentin contains more than 300,000 capillary tubes per square millimeter (Fig. 3-27) and constitutes about 10% of the dentin's volume. This percentage is higher near the pulp than peripherally. The fluid in these tubules, which comes from the intercellular fluid of the pulpal connective tissue, is clear as

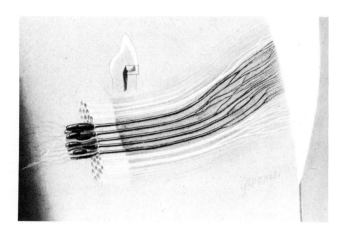

Fig. 3-27. Peripheral ramifications of dentinoblastic processes at dentinoenamel border. Capillary tube configuration of the dentin serves to attract pulpal tissue fluid into the lumina. (Courtesy Dr. John Bucher, University of Florida, Gainesville.)

water and has a composition similar to that of synovial or cerebrospinal fluid. The tubular fluid obeys the same laws of physics as do liquids in glass capillaries. Any displacement, no matter how slight, causes a flow of intratubular fluid. A rapid displacement in thousands of tubules at the same time produces a corresponding movement in the tubules as well as a significant movement in the contiguous pulpal tissue. This movement, either pulpward or outward, exerts a direct mechanical deformation on the low-threshold A-δ free nerve fibers within the tubules (Figs. 3-29 and 3-30) or in the subjacent pulp tissue (Fig. 3-28). The fluid movement may also cause a concomitant movement of dentinoblasts, which may in turn deform nerve fibers in contact with their process or cell body. The deformed nerve membrane increases its permeability to Na$^+$ ions. The rapid inward movement of the sodium depolarizes the A-δ fiber membrane, and an action potential (pain impulse) is initiated (Fig. 3-21).

Any stimulus that extracts tubular fluid from its outer surface causes an outward flow. The lost fluid is immediately replaced by pulpal tissue fluid responding to the capillary force within the dentinal tubules. Dry frictional heat caused by a bur during cavity preparation dehydrates the dentin (evaporation). To some degree the frictional stress may also mechanically press fluid out of the tubules. The pressures of chiseling or scraping the surface may have the same effect. In addition to the outward flow produced by these agents, dentinoblasts and nerve terminals may also be stretched or aspirated into the tubules, evoking a painful response (Fig. 3-39). This phenomenon occurs with much less frequency during cavity prepara-

tion when the field is kept moist with water spray. An air blast produces the same results (Fig. 3-31, *A*). However, Brännström found that if compressed air is applied to the dentin for a sufficiently long time, it becomes insensitive for at least 20 minutes because of the blockage to fluid flow by protein accumulation. Other stimuli that dehydrate causing outward movement are absorbent materials and hygroscopic pastes.

Candy bars and other sweets frequently trigger pain from a tooth with a defective restoration (e.g., open margins). Sugar and hypertonic solutions create an osmotic gradient, causing fluid movement from the deeper tubular areas of lesser concentration. The initial surge of dentinal tubular fluid results in firing of the low-threshold A-δ fibers and a resultant sharp pain. If a concomitant inflammation is present in the subjacent pulpal tissue, a dull persistent ache may follow as a consequence of activation of the higher-threshold C fibers.

The gap in a defective margin or loose filling contains salivary seepage between the filling and the tooth. Percussion or chewing on hard foods may cause pain if the loose filling material exerts a plunger action against the tubule orifices, driving the tubular fluid pulpward.

The pain associated with thermal stimulation may be due to the movement of fluid within the tubule, since fluids have a coefficient of expansion about 10 times greater than that of the tubule wall. Cold causes a contraction of the fluid and its *outward* flow, whether the tubule is open or closed at its outer surface (Fig. 3-31, *B*). Heat, on the other hand, causes expansion of the fluid and movement *toward* the pulp if the tubule is closed at the outer surface (i.e., covered by enamel or cementum). A

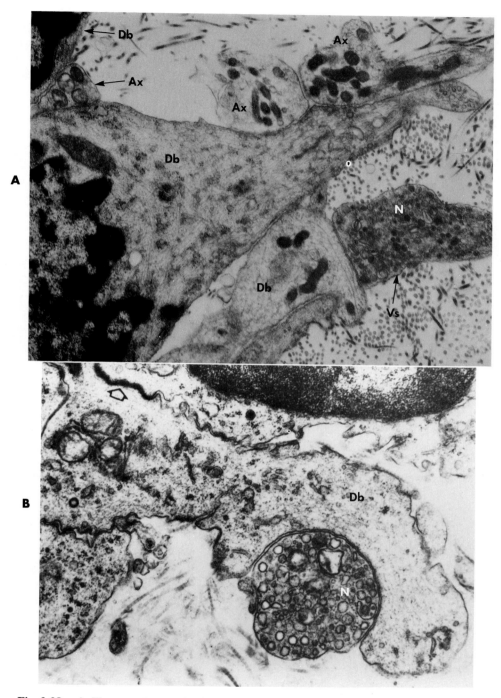

Fig. 3-28. **A,** Electron micrograph of the subdentinoblastic zone demonstrating close communication of nerve axons *(Ax)* with dentinoblasts *(Db)*. Nerve ending *(N)* in contact with a dentinoblast contain numerous dense-cored vesicles *(Vs)*. (×30,000.) **B,** Nerve ending *(N)*, containing numerous vesicles, indents, and part of dentinoblast *(Db)*. A 200 Å cleft appears between the nerve and the plasma membrane of the cell. Arrow at upper left denotes a gap junction. (**A** from Holland GR: *J Dent Res* 64:557, 1985; **B** from Avery JK: *Transactions of the Sixth International Conference on Endodontics,* New York, 1979, Masson.)

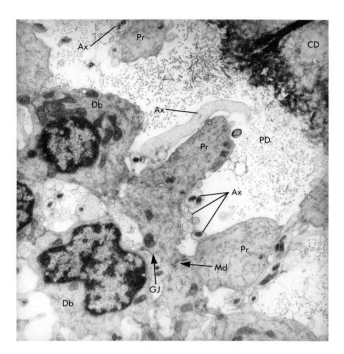

Fig. 3-29. Dentinoblastic-predentin junction. Dentinoblastic processes *(Pr)* and nerve axons *(Ax)* are seen entering the dentinal tubules in the predentin *(PD)*. Both gap junctions *(GJ)* and modified desmosome junctions *(Md)* are evident. *Db,* Dentinoblast cell bodies; *CD,* calcified dentin. (×15,000.) (Courtesy Dr. G.R. Holland, University of Alberta, Edmonton, Alberta, Canada.)

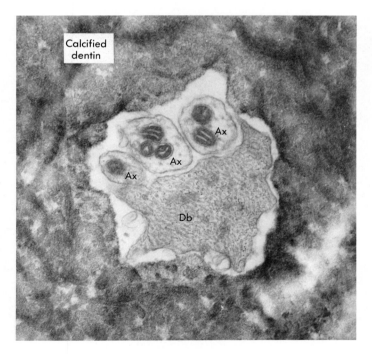

Fig. 3-30. Tubule in inner calcified dentin with the dentinoblastic process *(Db)* and accompanying axons *(Ax)*. (×80,000.) (Courtesy Dr. G.R. Holland, University of Alberta, Edmonton, Alberta, Canada.)

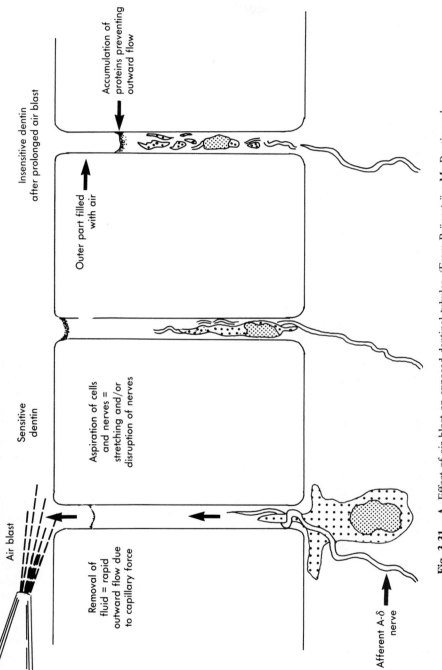

Fig. 3-31. A, Effect of air blast on exposed dentinal tubules. (From Brännström M: *Dentin and pulp in restorative dentistry,* London, 1982, Wolfe Medical.)

Continued

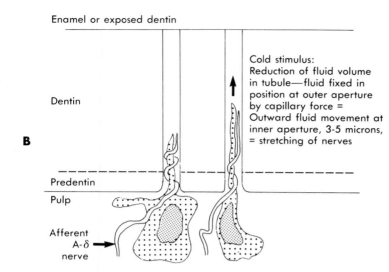

Enamel or exposed dentin

Dentin

B

Cold stimulus:
Reduction of fluid volume
in tubule—fluid fixed in
position at outer aperture
by capillary force =
Outward fluid movement at
inner aperture, 3-5 microns,
= stretching of nerves

Predentin

Pulp

Afferent
A-δ
nerve

Fig. 3-31, cont'd. B, Effect of cold on dentinal tubules. (From Brännström M: *Dentin and pulp in restorative dentistry,* London, 1982, Wolfe Medical.)

temperature increase of 20° F at the outer third of the tubule will result in an expansion of tubule contents and an immediate displacement of about 5 μm. If the tubule is open at the outer surface, the expansion from heat will cause the fluid to move away from the pulp and overflow its aperture. Dry heat also causes both movement and evaporation, resulting in the aspiration of dentinoblasts. A painful response to cold is faster than to heat because there is rapid outward movement of the tubule contents, whereas with heat a larger volume of the dentin must be affected before a sufficient pronounced dislocation of the tubule contents is produced. Heat in a normal (intact, not inflamed) pulp does not cause pain very often, but when it does, it is a duller sensation and of longer duration because of the vasodilatory effect (refer also to Van Hassel's hypothesis, p. 104). This phenomenon is probably due to the activation of the C fibers located deeper in the pulpal tissue (Table 3-3).

Johnson et al. measured in vitro the mean flow of fluid in fractured dentin (open tubules) by a hydrostatic pulpal pressure of 30 mm Hg. They found that a patent tubule can be emptied about 10 times a day. Histologic examination of 12 extracted teeth suggested that a reduction of the dentinoblastic layer occurred because of aspiration of the cells into dentinal tubules under exposed dentin, caries, or leaky fillings. This phenomenon, they concluded, was caused by a physiologic pressure gradient that caused an outward flow in the tubules.

Outward fluid flow may be minimized by precipitates from desensitizing tooth pastes that block the dentinal tubules at the surface. Such agents used are 5% potassium nitrate (Denquel), 10% strontium chloride (Sensodyne, Thermodent), dibasic sodium citrate (Protect), potassium nitrate plus sodium monofluorophosphate (Sensodyne F), and potassium oxalate (DDS-1, DDS-2). Greenhill and Pashley have shown that a 30% potassium oxalate solution applied to the open tubules results in the formation of calcium oxalate crystals. These crystals block the tubule apertures and reduce the hydraulic conduction of dentin about 98% (Fig. 3-32).

Dentinoblastic deformation or injury (transduction). Dentinoblasts can be injured by any stimulant applied to the dentin: thermal, mechanical, chemical, or osmotic.

The dentinoblast and its process may function as a transducer mechanism when the membrane stimulation is transformed into a chemical or electrical message. Dentinoblasts do not act as receptors of stimuli; when deformed or injured, however, they may produce stimuli that are received by the free nerve endings within the tubules (Figs. 3-30 and 3-33) or in contact with any part of the dentinoblast (Fig. 3-28). The stimulus produced by the dentinoblasts may be due to chemicals released by the injured cells, to changes in their electrical surface potential, or to movement associated with their deformation.

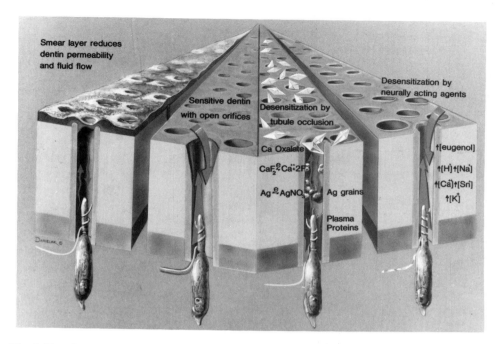

Smear layer reduces
dentin permeability
and fluid flow

Sensitive dentin
with open orifices

Desensitization by
tubule occlusion

Desensitization by
neurally acting agents

Ca Oxalate

$CaF_2 \overset{e}{\rightleftharpoons} Ca^+ 2F^-$

$Ag \overset{e}{\rightleftharpoons} AgNO_3$

Ag grains

Plasma
Proteins

↑[eugenol]

↑[H]↑[Na]

↑[Ca]↑[Sn]

↑[K]

Fig. 3-32. Summary of the mechanisms for desensitizing dentin. Patent dentinal tubules *(left center panel)* permit hydrodynamic forces (magnitude indicated by size of *arrow)* to stimulate mechanoreceptor nerves, thus causing pain. Desensitization by tubule occlusion *(right center panel)* can restrict fluid movement (magnitudes indicated by size of *arrows),* thereby decreasing pain. The creation of an authentic smear layer *(far left panel)* is very effective, as is an equivalent layer of crystalline precipitates. Desensitization by blocking nerve activity *(far right panel)* does not interfere with fluid flow but does reduce nerve response. Potassium salts and eugenol are but two examples of this type of desensitization. (From Pashley DH: *J Endod* 12:472, 1986.)

1. *Chemoactivation.* The injured dentinoblast may release polypeptides, called *neurotransmitter substances,* that cause the approximating naked nerve fibers to fire off an impulse. These chemicals apparently combine with unmyelinated pain fibers in the involved area, altering their permeability and causing the nerve to fire impulses (action potentials). The presence of "coated pits" on dentinoblastic processes in areas approximating nerve fibers suggests a stimulus transmission process through substance transfer.

2. *Electroactivation.* An injury to the dentinoblastic process changes the electric surface charges of the plasma membrane at the point of injury. These changes travel along the plasma membrane and stimulate pain receptors in contact with any portion of the dentinoblast. Because of the highly calcified peritubular matrix, the action potentials are confined to spread within the tubules, which prompted noted neurophysiologist Lord E.D. Adrian (1963) to refer to them as "built-in electrodes." Avery indicated that any movement of the cytoplasm of the dentinoblastic process will have the same effect. Sicher noted that

this hypothesis explains the sensitivity of the dentinoenamel junction, where the concentration and arborization of dentinoblastic processes are greatest. At this juncture the stimulus will effect a greater change in the electric charge on the body of the dentinoblast.

3. *Mechanoactivation.* The mere movement of the dentinoblasts may, in turn, move or jar the A-∂ terminal fibers, which have a low threshold of excitability. The deformation of the nerve plasma membranes increases their permeability to sodium ions. The resultant rapid inward movement of the sodium depolarizes the fiber membrane, and an action potential is initiated (Fig. 3-21). Hydrodynamics may not be responsible for the pain associated with light brushing of an explorer tip across exposed dentin because of insufficient tubular fluid displacement and flow. Another answer that does not conflict with the hydrodynamic theory is that the pain is due to direct stimulation of the dentinoblastic processes, which serve as transducers, transferring the stimulus to the nerve fibers. Ochi

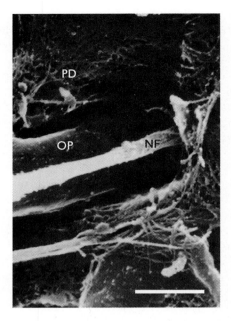

Fig. 3-33. Nerve fiber *(NF)* running along surface of the dentinoblastic process *(OP)* is seen using scanning electron microscopy. *PD,* Predentin. (Original magnification ×36,000; bar = 1 μm) (From Ochi K, Matsumoto K: *J Endod* 14:601, 1988.)

and Matsumoto theorize that when dentin is stimulated, a morphologic change (a momentary swelling or contraction) occurs in the dentinoblastic process. This then transmits the stimulation to the nerve fibers, resulting in pain.

Effect of the return impulse (efferent response). No matter which theory of pulpal pain fiber excitation is accepted, the fact remains that the afferent nerve impulse is activated by a stimulus applied to the dentin and that the net effect of the impulses on the dental pulp will depend on the *strength of the irritant,* the *duration of the irritant,* and the *prior health state of the dental pulp.*

The precise mechanism for activating the efferent response from the CNS is not clear. However, Kim, Edwall, Tönder, and other investigators have demonstrated by electric or chemical methods that *activation of the cervical sympathetic nerve causes pulpal vasoconstriction and a reduction of blood flow.* Anneroth and Norberg, as well as Polito and Antila, have observed that sympathetic innervation from the superior cervical ganglion forms plexuses around pulpal arterioles. A study by Avery et al.

noted a significant number of adrenergic endings in odontogenic areas (usually near the basal ends of dentinoblasts), endings that were both free and vascular related. Such findings suggest that these adrenergic nerve endings may play a role in regulating dentinogenesis as well as the blood flow.

The efferent sympathetic impulse returns from the CNS by way of postganglionic sympathetic neuron fibers located in the arterial adventitial layer. These fibers penetrate the muscle wall (tunica media) to the neuromuscular junctions of the arterioles. At the neuromuscular junctions, the transmitter substance *norepinephrine* is released, causing contraction of the smooth muscle cells. The resultant constriction of the arterial lumina occurs in the affected part of the pulp, thereby reducing its blood flow. Capillaries, which have no muscular wall, are not innervated. These small vessels can dilate or constrict passively, i.e., when the blood flow through the muscular vessels is increased or decreased.

The pulp is known to have *alpha-adrenergic receptors* in the walls of the arteriolar vessels. Their stimulation by the alpha-receptor agonist norepinephrine causes vasoconstriction and a decrease in blood flow. Studies by Kim have demonstrated that these pulpal vessels may also have *beta-adrenergic receptors,* which when activated will result in vasodilation and increased blood flow. However, Kim has reported that isoproterenol, a classic vasodilating agent, causes a *reduction* of blood flow *in the dental pulp.* To explain this paradox, he suggests that the *dilation of the arterioles by isoproterenol in the low-compliance environment of the dental pulp causes a compression of the venules that, in turn, reduces the blood flow.* Kim has stated further that beta receptors exist on all muscular vessels and may play a role in vascular permeability. Various humoral substances that can cause either vasoconstriction or vasodilation include catecholamines (epinephrine, norepinephrine, dopa), prostaglandins, substance P, and bradykinin. Separate studies by Edwall (personal communication) indicate that vasodilation may also be due to a *reflex phenomenon* following vasoconstriction and is mediated by tissue metabolites that exert a negative feedback.

Under normal homeostatic conditions, mild to moderate vasoconstrictor action of norepinephrine at neuromuscular junctions is inactivated or neutralized by accumulated catabolic products and their attendant lowering of the pH and diminished energy source (ADP $\leftrightarrows$ ATP*). These events cause the blood vessel smooth musculature to relax, permitting vasodilation and a concomitant increase in both rate and volume of blood flow,which in turn permits the removal of accumulated waste products (CO_2, H_2O) and the replenishment of oxygen and energy sources.

If a strong and/or sustained dentinal irritant results in an excessive number of efferent sympathetic impulses,this normal homeostatic reflex control mechanism is altered. The smooth muscle walls of the arterial vessels go into a state of prolonged contraction (spasm), resulting in an even greater accumulation of catabolic products, a greater lowering of the pH, and a depletion of energy source. The period of smooth muscle relaxation is now extended, and passive vasodilation ensues.

The dilated arterial vessels bring a greater blood volume into the pulp (hyperemia). Capillaries normally function on an intermittent basis, but an increased number brought into function now dilate passively because they have become engorged with blood. As a consequence, the flow of blood slows and a vascular congestion follows. This is the first step toward inflammation (pulpitis) and increased intrapulpal pressure. (See discussion of hyperemia, p. 140.) Stated simply:

1. Mild to moderate transitory pulpodentinal irritation
   $\downarrow$
   Transitory regional intrapulpal vasoconstriction
   $\downarrow$
   Transitory regional intrapulpal vasodilation
2. Strong and/or sustained pulpodentinal irritation
   $\downarrow$
   Prolonged regional intrapulpal vasoconstriction
   $\downarrow$
   Prolonged regional intrapulpal vasodilation → Hyperemia → Inflammation (Fig. 3-41)

Defense function

Because of their peripheral location and the extension of their cytoplasm into the dentinal tubules, the dentinoblasts are more vulnerable to injury than any other pulp cells. When irritated or injured, they contribute to one or more defense functions of the pulpodentinal complex (Fig. 3-34):
1. Dentinal pain
2. The smear layer
3. Tubular sclerosis
4. Irritation (reparative) dentin formation
5. Inflammation of the subjacent connective tissue

*ADP, Adenosine diphosphate; ATP, adenosine triphosphate.

If the injury is mild and of short duration, the response may be limited to the dentinal tubules and the dentinoblasts in the form of *sclerotic* and/or *irritation dentin*. As the severity of the irritant increases, the underlying pulp tissue responds with progressive inflammation, first in the sub-dentinoblastic zone and ultimately in the central zone.

Dentinal pain. Refer to theories of pulpodentinal pain fiber excitation (pp. 119 to 127).

The smear layer. Scaling, abrasion, attrition, caries, and cavity preparation (cutting, grinding) leave microcrystalline debris or a smear layer that extends slightly into the dentinal tubules (smear plugs), covers the dentinal surface, and is usually several microns in thickness (Fig. 3-35). This debris is mixed with saliva, water, and/or dentinal fluid. Such a closure of the dentin wound reduces both sensitivity and permeability. In a way this is a defense mechanism, even though it is not related to dentinoblastic function. Organic solid material and microorganisms may also contribute to the plugging of the outer tubule apertures (Fig. 3-36, *A* and *B*). According to Brännström, after several weeks and with the assistance of dentinal fluid and substances from the saliva, thin mineralized areas may be evident on the exposed dentin (Fig. 3-36, *C*). Brännström compares this mechanism with that of mineralization of enamel plaque, the remineralization of enamel caries, and the development of calculus. After a longer period, a thin mineralized "carpet" may cover the whole surface (Fig. 3-36, *D*). This phenomenon may not occur when there is too much acid food, defects in the composition of saliva, and overzealous brushing.

Pashley et al. considers the smear layer per se as an iatrogenically produced cavity liner that reduces permeability better than any of the varnishes. On the negative side, however, it (1) interferes with the apposition or adhesion of dental materials to dentin and (2) has the potential to provide a media for recurrent caries and bacterial irritation of the pulp.

Tubular sclerosis. Tubular sclerosis is produced by milder or moderately irritating agents such as slowly progressing caries, mild acute injury of cavity preparation, abrasion, erosion, attrition, and age changes (Fig. 3-37). It is the cumulative effect of several factors: continuing peritubular dentin formation by the dentinoblastic processes *(physiologic sclerosis)* and *intratubular calcification (pathologic sclerosis).* Sclerosis of the tubules

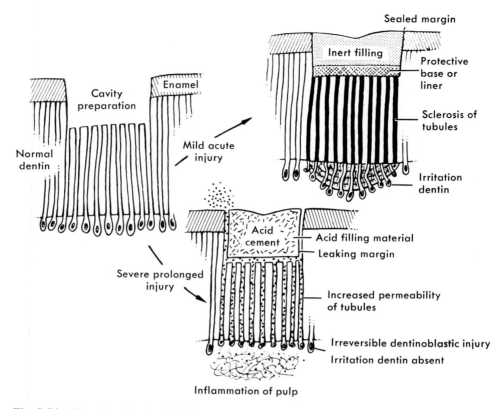

Fig. 3-34. Reaction of pulpodentinal complex to mild and severe injury. After cavity preparation and insertion of an inert filling, mild acute injury produces tubular sclerosis and irritation dentin. However, severe prolonged injury causes irreversible dentinoblastic injury, which in turn initiates pulpal inflammation. (From Massler M: *Dent Clin North Am,* March 1965.)

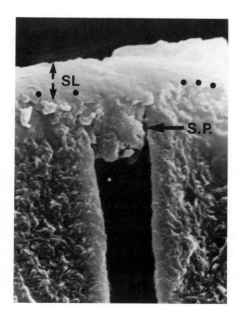

Fig. 3-35. Longitudinal section of dentinal tubule containing a smear plug *(SP)* beneath the smear layer *(SL)*. (Original magnification ×18000.) (From Pashley D: *J Endod* 16:70, 1990.)

will not occur if the dentinoblasts have been previously destroyed by such agents as strong chemicals applied to the open apertures, severe heat generated by high-speed cavity preparation (without coolant), or rapidly advancing caries. The resultant *dead tracts* may permit caries to spread faster and may even allow a more rapid egress of chemical agents into the pulp tissues (Fig. 3-34). Sclerotic dentin, on the other hand, may be considered a defense mechanism of the pulpodentinal complex because its formation alters the permeability of the tubules, blocking the access of irritants to the pulp.

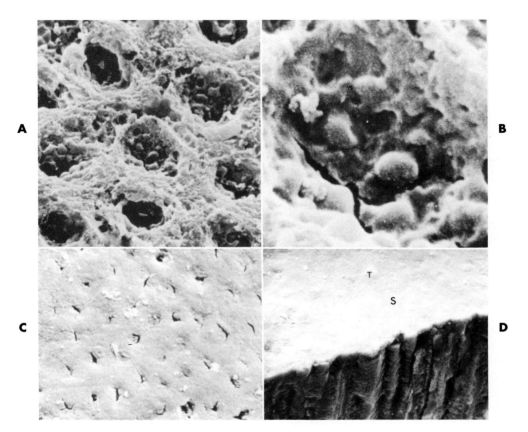

Fig. 3-36. Progression of surface mineralization of smear layer. **A,** Dentin on a buccal cusp was exposed by grinding 2 weeks before extraction and examined under scanning electron microscope. The pulp revealed slight inflammation, but sensitivity tests with probing and an air jet revealed an almost insensitive dentin surface. Microorganisms are plugging the tubule apertures and seem to have contributed to the organic material accumulating within the tubules nearest the surface. (×3800.) **B,** Detail of one tubule aperture seen in **A.** (×15,000.) **C,** Another tooth treated in the same way as the one seen in **A.** After 2 weeks this surface was almost insensitive. Bacteria are absent, and a small granulated structure, indicating mineralization, covers many tubule apertures. (×13000.) **D,** Dentin occlusal surface *(S)* produced by attrition, which had a glossy appearance in the clinic. A fracture perpendicular to the surface is seen below. At the attrited surface the positions of tubule apertures are seen as slight elevations *(T),* and the surface is covered with a thin mineralized layer. (×1300.) (See also description of surface mineralization, p. 127.) (From Brännström M: *Dentin and pulp in restorative dentistry,* London, 1982, Wolfe Medical.)

Peritubular dentin (physiologic sclerosis) is a calcified secretion of the dentinoblastic process. The numerous vesicles observed in the process are probably secretory products that are going to become the matrix of the peritubular dentin. These products, formed in the endoplasmic reticulum of the dentinoblast cell body, pass through the Golgi complex and now appear in the vesicles of the dentinoblastic process to be released as peritubular dentin matrix (Figs. 3-8, 3-12, and 3-38). The spar-

sity of organic matrix and the high concentration of calcium salts in the dentin environment permit the peritubular dentin to be more highly mineralized than the intertubular dentin. *As a result of both peritubular dentin formation and intratubular calcification, the tubules become narrower and may ultimately close completely (sclerosis).*

Intratubular calcification (pathologic sclerosis) is a physicochemical process caused by the precipitation of mineral salts within the dentinal tubules

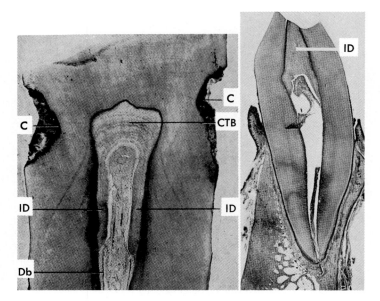

Fig. 3-37. Irritation dentin *(ID)* formed in response to abrasion and caries *(C)*. Rapid matrix formation and irregular mineralization pattern produce calciotraumatic lines or bands *(CTB)*. *Db,* Dentinoblastic layer. (From Coolidge ED, Kesel RG: *Endodontology,* ed 2 Philadelphia, 1956, Lea & Febiger.)

and is therefore fundamentally different from peritubular dentin. This type of calcification is found in the translucent zone of carious dentin and in the dentin of severe attrition, erosion, and abrasion. One of the sources of the calcium salts of pathologic sclerosis is recrystallized calcium and phosphate ions that previously had been dissolved during the demineralization phase of caries. Frank et al. identified the intratubular deposits as hydroxyapatite crystals (needle shaped) and Whitlockite crystals (rhomboidal). A hypothesis for another source of pathologic sclerosis is the precipitation of the calcium phosphate salts from the supersaturated dentinal fluid, which may obliterate the dentinal tubules by being deposited in or around degenerating dentinoblastic processes.

Irritation dentin formation. The formation of irritation (reparative) dentin has already been described. It may be referred to as defensive dentin because it is the second line of pulpodentinal defense. The tubular structure of this rapid-forming dentin can be erratic. The tubules are frequently twisted and less numerous than in regular dentin and at times are completely absent.

The formation of irritation dentin is an attempt to compensate for the dentin loss; just as importantly, however, it provides a barrier that has a higher degree of calcification than does regular dentin and is less sensitive because of lack of continuity of the dentinoblastic processes. Dentinoblas-

tic cells that die as a result of injury may be replaced by cells from the cell-rich zone, which move up to the dentinoblastic zone and secrete dentin matrix. They may not assume the columnar-polygonal shape of the dentinoblast but rather a cuboidal or flattened appearance. The resultant newly formed dentin has a lost continuity of the dentinal tubules. This dentinal barrier helps block irritants from the exterior but also prevents reinnervation of injured dentin by sprouting pulpal nerve fibers. Adjacent surviving dentin with intact dentinal tubules may become heavily innervated (CGRP immunoreactive fibers) in the repair process.

As a result of the injury to the dentinoblasts and the subsequent matrix formation by many atypical dentinoblastic cells, irregularities in the mineralization pattern occur and are evident by the presence of alternating light and dark concentric rings or bands, which appear like growth rings on a tree. These are called *calciotraumatic lines* or *bands* (Fig. 3-37).

Inflammation. Mild and moderate injury to the dentinoblastic processes may produce tubular sclerosis and irritation dentin, but prolonged and/or severe irritation can irreversibly affect the plasma membrane and the nucleus of the dentinoblasts, thus initiating the first step toward an inflammatory response (pulpitis) (Fig. 3-34). For example, the irritation of deep cavity preparations less than 2 mm from the pulp may be intensified by:

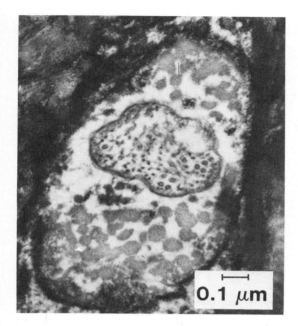

Fig. 3-38. Tubule at the edge of the inner third of dentin with uncalcified matrix apparently filling in the lumen around the process. (From Holland R: *J Dent Res* 64:508, 1985.)

1. Inadequate water coolants
2. Acid cements
3. Inadequate insulation of metal fillings
4. Microleakage of restorations

Five facets of inflammation will be considered:
1. Nature of the inflammatory response
2. Role of the dentinoblast
3. Primary factors that initiate the inflammatory response
4. Types of inflammation
5. Immunologic considerations

Nature of the inflammatory response. Inflammation is the reaction of living tissue to any type of injury. Direct action against deleterious agents requires the mobilization and coordination of vascular, neurologic, cellular, and humoral responses. The objectives of the inflammatory process are (1) to destroy the irritant at the site of the injury, (2) to at least neutralize it temporarily by dilution or containment while additional defense forces are brought into action, and (3) to set the stage for repair of the damaged tissue. Achieving the first two objectives may evoke clinically evident symptoms sometimes referred to as the cardinal signs of acute inflammation: heat (calor), redness (rubor), swelling (tumor), pain (dolor), and loss of function (function laesa).

Inflammation and repair are interdependent phenomena. They should not be considered as separate processes but as *exudative (acute) and proliferative (chronic) phases of the same process— inflammation.* No difference exists between the dynamics of pulpal inflammation and that of periapical inflammation; only the environment is different.

The *exudative (acute) response* is the initial immediate response of the pulpal or periapical tissue to any irritant—mechanical, chemical, thermal, or microbial. This emergency action to overcome and neutralize the injurious agent is characterized by an influx of fluid exudate (inflammatory edema) to dilute and detoxify and by the infiltration of white cells to ingest and immobilize. The dominant cells in this phase are the polymorphonuclear leukocytes (neutrophils) (Table 3-5).

The *proliferative (chronic) response* is a secondary or delayed action. Its presence depends on the ability of the exudative (acute) forces to decrease the toxicity of the irritant. It is an attempt of the connective tissue components of the pulp and periapex to form new cells (fibroblasts), blood vessels (angioblasts), and fibers. Pulpal and periapical nerve fibers (CGRP immunoreactive fibers) proliferate in response to acute pulpal injury. Sprouting of these nerve fibers occurs in pulpal areas subjacent to the injury site but also in corresponding periapical tissues before apical progression of pathosis. These elements constitute *granulation tissue,* whose function is to repair and replace the damaged tissue. The granulation tissue is called *granulomatous* when lymphocytes, plasma cells, and macrophages are present in great numbers. Granulomatous tissue is therefore not only a healing tissue, but a defense tissue as well, where organisms are destroyed, not nurtured.

Both exudative (acute) and proliferative (chronic) responses may coexist in the pulp or periapex undergoing inflammation (see Table 3-6), although the latter lags behind and is peripheral to the former. Ultimately, according to Fish and MacLean, a spectrum of zones develops in both pulpal and periapical disease (Fig. 3-48; see also Figs. 4-7 and 4-8). The characteristics and capacity of one zone's hyperactivity to dominate over another depend on (1) the zone's distance from the toxic agent (Table 4-2), (2) the strength and duration of the toxic agent, and (3) the health of the host and the affected tissue.

Table 3-5. Differences between acute and chronic inflammation

Inflammation	Stimuli	Types of reaction	Principal cells	Pain	Chemical mediators*
Acute	Transient	Exudative	Polymorphonuclear leukocytes (PMNs)	(+)	Vasoactive amines Kinins Complement
			Macrophages		Arachidonic acid derivatives (prostaglandins, leukotrienes, etc.)
Chronic	Persistent	Proliferative	Macrophages Lymphocytes	(−) (+), if subacute	Antibodies Lysosomal enzymes
			Plasma cells		Lymphokines

Modified with permission of Dr. Mahmoud Torabinejad.
*See Chapter 4.

Role of the dentinoblast. The following sequence of changes can be observed as the dentinoblastic injury increases progressively:

1. *Increased permeability of the dentinal tubule* (Fig. 3-34) because of the destructive effect of the injury to the dentinoblast and its process. Microorganisms and chemical irritants now have easier access to the pulp.
2. *Disturbance of the pulpodentinal membrane.* This is not a true membrane but a three-dimensional illusion caused by the junctional complexes (pp. 88 to 91). The disturbance is a reflection of the aggregate breakdown of the dentinoblasts.
3. *Disruption of the palisaded dentinoblastic layer.* The continuous uninterrupted contact between dentinoblasts results in a field effect response in which many dentinoblasts are affected by a single stimulus (Fig. 3-43, *B*).
4. *Aspiration of many of the dentinoblastic nuclei* into the dentinal tubules (also referred to as *displacement* or *migration*). This phenomenon may be due to the outward flow of tubular fluid (Brännström) (Fig. 3-39) as a result of dry frictional heat, air blast (Fig. 3-31), etc. (See p. 119.)
5. *Irreversible dentinoblastic injury,* which results in the release of the *tissue injury fac-*

tors (Fig. 3-42). When the dentinoblasts are severely injured or die, they liberate a variety of chemical substances that affect neighboring dentinoblasts and underlying connective tissue. Some of these substances are enzymes that dissolve or hydrolyze the cell (autolysis), as well as intracellular substances. The sprouting of CGRP immunoreactive nerve fibers and the initiation of irritation dentin formation are possible reparative responses at this stage of dentinoblastic injury.

6. *Inflammatory changes* in the dentinoblastic zone. These include dilation of capillaries and the resultant stasis of their blood flow. Autolysis can also occur if oxygen and metabolites are denied because of congestion of nearby blood vessels (within 2 to 4 minutes). The subsequent effect of such severe injuries is the further disruption of the palisade arrangement of the cells and the accumulation of edematous fluid within the tissue gaps created *(vacuolization)* (Fig. 3-43).
7. *Subdentinoblastic inflammatory changes* (vasodilation, leukocytic infiltration, edema). In addition to effecting a neurologic response, some of the chemical mediators released (tissue injury factors) cause local dilation of the blood vessels as well as an

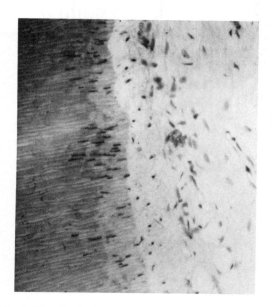

Fig. 3-39. Aspiration (displacement) of dentinoblasts into dentinal tubules after cavity preparation on a dry surface. Dry frictional heat from the bur causes outward fluid movement in tubules (away from the pulp), sucking in dentinoblasts and their nuclei. This phenomenon occurs less frequently when the field is moist. Note absence of inflammatory changes. (Courtesy Dr. Samuel Seltzer, Temple University, Philadelphia) (Refer also to discussion of hydrodynamic mechanism, p. 119.)

increase in the permeability of the capillaries (Figs. 3-40 and 3-42). Dilation of the capillaries from increased arterial pressure and blood volume stretches the wall, causing the pores (fenestrations, gaps, interendothelial junctions) between adjacent endothelial cells to enlarge. Coupled with endothelial swelling, this results in the escape not only of excessive amounts of plasma fluid, but of larger blood protein particles as well. The walls of pulpal arteries are made up of a single layer of endothelial cells and possess the property of selective permeability; i.e., smaller particles such as glucose and amino acids are able to pass through the wall but not the larger colloidal plasma protein particles.

If these blood proteins (colloids) are depleted and the tissue osmotic pressure is increased, the osmotic pressure of the capillary is insufficient to attract enough tissue fluid back into the return (venous) flow (Starling's hypothesis). The resultant accumula-

tion in the tissues is called *edema.* Excessive loss of plasma fluid results in hemoconcentration and a slowing or even cessation of the blood flow *(stagnation* or *stasis).*

The reduced current also allows the leukocytes to leave their position in the central (axial) stream and line up along the blood vessel wall *(margination).* By ameboid motion they pass through the wall *(diapedesis)* and surrounding (perivascular) tissue (Fig. 3-40, *D* and *E*). Substances called chemotactic agents cause leukocytes to migrate to the site of injury. This directional reaction of mobile cells is appropriately called *chemotaxis. Inflammation,* the third mechanism of pulpal defense, is now well established. The reversibility of the pulpal inflammation depends on the elimination of the pulpal irritants (caries excavation) and the repair potential of the pulp itself. Khayat and others have shown in animal studies that teeth with limited pulpal inflammation often have fibrous pulp tissue intervening between the inflamed area and sprouting nerves in the uninflamed pulpal boundary tissues. Fig. 3-43, *C,* shows the marked cellular infiltration and approaching abscess formation. In addition, the dentinoblast layer has been destroyed and predentin is absent.

8. *Central zone inflammation* reflects the circumferential and apical progression of irreversible total pulpitis, as outlined by Van Hassel (Fig. 3-41).

Primary factors that initiate the acute inflammatory response. The two primary factors responsible for pulpal and periapical inflammation are the nerve factor (neurologic response) and the tissue injury factor (cellular response). Both vascular and humoral responses are mediated by these two phenomena (Fig. 3-42).

The *nerve factor* is the activation of neurologic responses by environmental irritants (mechanical, chemical, microbial) that injure the dentinoblasts. Such primary irritants may cause the following:

1. *Immediate and transitory (primary) pain perception* as a result of pulpal intratubular pain fiber excitation (due to A-δ fiber activity). (Refer to the theories of pulpal pain fiber excitation, p. 119.)

2. *Vasodilation* that persists (prolonged) if the injury is severe enough, leading to increased capillary (and small venule) permeability,

Table 3-6. Summary of inflammatory activity in pulpal and periapical connective tissue

Histopathologic activity

I. Preinflammatory phase
  A. Prolonged vasodilation
  B. Capillary bed engorgement
  C. Incipient fluid exudation and cellular infiltration

II. Inflammation
  A. Exudative stage—*acute response*
    1. Early exudative phase
      a. Fluid exudation (edema)
        (1) Serum (dilutes irritant)
        (2) Complement
        (3) Fibrinogen (becomes a mechanical barrier of fibrin)
        (4) Kininogen (converted to kinins)
      b. Released from damaged tissue
        (1) Kininogen converted to
          (a) Bradykinin
          (b) Lysylbradykinin (kallidin)
        (2) Arachidonic acid derivatives (prostaglandins, leukotrienes, etc.)
          (a) Unstable intermediates (PGG_2, PGH_2, HETE, etc.)
          (b) Stable end products (PGE, PGF, etc.)
      c. Cellular exudation
        (1) From blood
          (a) Neutrophils (PMNs)
          (b) Monocytes (become macrophages)
        (2) From connective tissue
          (a) Histiocytes (macrophages)
          (b) Reserve cells (become macrophages)
      d. Suppurative response—formed when there is a sufficient number of injured and dead cells and neutrophils present
    2. Late exudative phase (incipient chronic response)
      a. Fluid exudation
        (1) Components seen in acute inflammation
        (2) Antibodies
          (a) Opsonins (enhance phagocytosis)
          (b) Agglutinins ("clump" bacteria)
          (c) Precipitins (precipitate soluble foreign substances)
          (d) Antitoxin (neutralize toxins)
      b. Cellular exudation
        (1) Cells seen in acute inflammation
        (2) Sensitized lymphocytes
          (a) Plasma cells (produce antibodies—humoral immune response)
          (b) Sensitized T cells (produce lymphokines—cell-mediated immune response)
      c. Advanced suppurative response (occurs when early suppuration does not resolve)
  B. Proliferative phase: initiation of repair and healing—*chronic response*
    1. Granulomatous tissue: granulation tissue plus chronic inflammatory cells
      a. Macrophages from monocytes, histiocytes, and reserve cells (phagocytosis)
      b. Sensitized lymphocytes (plasma cells and sensitized T cells)
      c. Fibroblasts (produce new fibers)
      d. Angioblasts (form new capillaries)
    2. Encapsulation: orientation of peripheral collagenous fibers (productive fibrosis)

Histopathologic classification

Pulp		Periapex

Hyperemia
(hyperalgesia),
(reversible pulpitis),
(hyperactive pulpalgia)

Incipient
apical
periodontitis

↓

Acute
pulpitis

↓

Acute
apical
periodontitis

Exudative (acute) hyperactivity

Acute
periapical
abscess

Subacute

↓

Subacute

↓

Chronic
pulpitis

Proliferative (chronic) hyperactivity

Chronic
apical
periodontitis
(abscess,
granuloma,
cyst)

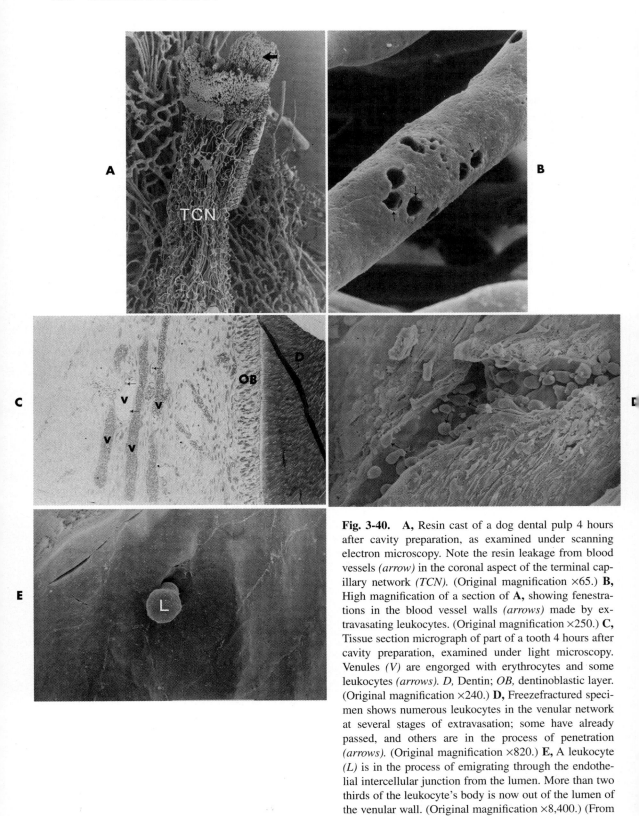

Fig. 3-40. **A,** Resin cast of a dog dental pulp 4 hours after cavity preparation, as examined under scanning electron microscopy. Note the resin leakage from blood vessels *(arrow)* in the coronal aspect of the terminal capillary network *(TCN)*. (Original magnification ×65.) **B,** High magnification of a section of **A,** showing fenestrations in the blood vessel walls *(arrows)* made by extravasating leukocytes. (Original magnification ×250.) **C,** Tissue section micrograph of part of a tooth 4 hours after cavity preparation, examined under light microscopy. Venules *(V)* are engorged with erythrocytes and some leukocytes *(arrows)*. *D,* Dentin; *OB,* dentinoblastic layer. (Original magnification ×240.) **D,** Freezefractured specimen shows numerous leukocytes in the venular network at several stages of extravasation; some have already passed, and others are in the process of penetration *(arrows)*. (Original magnification ×820.) **E,** A leukocyte *(L)* is in the process of emigrating through the endothelial intercellular junction from the lumen. More than two thirds of the leukocyte's body is now out of the lumen of the venular wall. (Original magnification ×8,400.) (From Kogushi M et al: *J Endod* 14:476, 1988.)

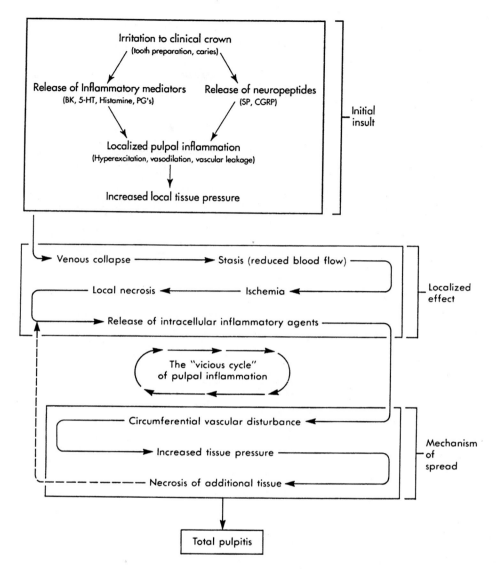

Fig. 3-41. Profile of pulpal pathophysiology. The "vicious cycle" of pulpal inflammation is the progression from localized coronal inflammation to irreversible total pulpitis and is consistent with data from intrapulpal pressure recordings (see also Fig. 3-42 and Table 3-1). (Modified from Van Hassel HJ: *Oral Surg* 32:126, 1971.)

ity). (Refer to the theories of pulpal pain fiber excitation, p. 119.)

2. *Vasodilation* that persists (prolonged) if the injury is severe enough, leading to increased capillary (and small venule) permeability, fluid exudation (edema), and leukocyte infiltration. This reaction marks the beginning of the exudative (acute) phase of inflammation.

3. *Increased intrapulpal pressure* in the affected pulpal region as a result of the increased blood volume *(hyperemia)* and tissue exudate.

4. *Secondary (spontaneous) pain response* if the intrapulpal pressure from the exudative (acute) response surpasses the threshold limits of the C nerve fibers in the affected area. The presence of necrotic tissue *(secondary irritant)* maintains the exudative response and allows the pain to persist. The pain may now

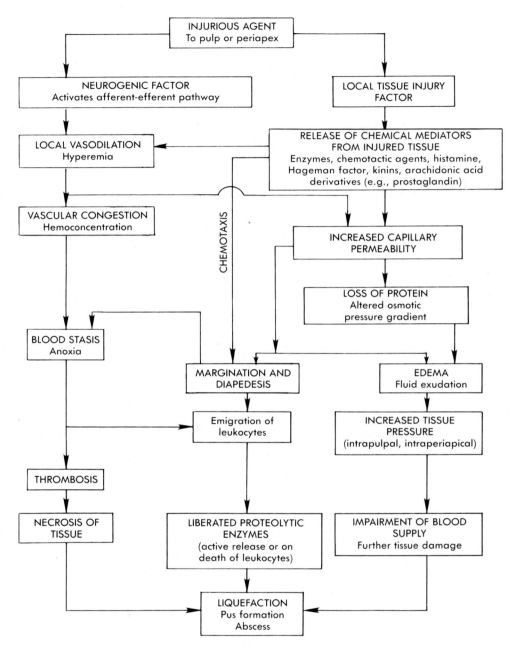

Fig. 3-42.   Mechanism of pulp and periapical exudative (acute) inflammatory response. Sequential outline of the pulp and periapical vascular changes at site of injury due to cellular (tissue injury factor) and neurogenic (nerve factor) responses. (Modified from Anderson WAD, Scotti TM: *Synopsis of pathology,* ed 10, St Louis, 1980, Mosby.)

The *tissue injury factor* is due to the release of mediators by the injured dentinoblasts, the chemical substances (described earlier), which set into motion the process of inflammation *locally* (Fig. 3-42). These mediators produce the same local effects described for the nerve factor: (1) prolonged local vasodilation if the injury is severe enough, leading to fluid exudation and infiltration of leukocytes; (2) increases of regional intrapulpal volume and pressure; and (3) pain perceived by the patient to be of a spontaneous and/or continuous nature. The role of mediators in initiating a painful response has not been clearly defined.

Types of inflammation. Inflammation may be classified according to the nature of the exudate (serious, fibrinous, purulent, sanguinous, etc.) or according to the causative agent (tuberculous, syphilitic, staphylococcal, etc.). For our purpose the classification used is related to *duration* and *severity* (acute, chronic, or subacute) as well as to the presence or absence of pain (Table 3-5).

The term *acute* implies hyperactivity of the exudative inflammatory forces (Table 3-6), which are closest to the source of the injury or infection *(exudative zone)* even though peripheral chronic activity may be evident. If the *primary irritant* force intensifies, so will the exudative response in an attempt to overcome and neutralize the invader. As the intrapulpal (or intraperiapical) pressure increases beyond the threshold limits of the sensory receptors, varying degrees of pain will be felt. The terms *painful pulpitis* and *painful periapical pathosis* are applicable. The absence of pain does not mean that an acute inflammatory response is absent. It means that the intrapulpal pressure is below the threshold of excitability of the pain fibers. Langeland, Seltzer, and others have demonstrated histologically the presence of an acute inflammatory response when the clinical diagnosis was *nonpainful pulpitis*. The predominant cell in the acute response is the polymorphonuclear leukocyte (PMN, neutrophil). Tissue macrophages, which are less motile and survive longer than PMNs, make their appearance later.

Chronic inflammation signifies the emergence of the *proliferative phase* of the inflammatory cycle. In the areas peripheral to the exudative (acute) activity (Table 3-6; see also Table 4-2), there occurs a proliferation of tiny, fragile blood vessels (angioblastic activity) as well as marked fibroblastic proliferation of new collagen. These two components constitute *granulation tissue,*

essential to the healing process. When the cell population includes lymphocytes, plasma cells, and mononuclear phagocytes (tissue macrophages), *granulomatous* must replace the term *granulation* because the tissue is now both defensive as well as healing in its function. Justification for the use of the controversial term *granulomatous* when referring to dental lesions appears on p. 173. This response may arise on the heels of an acute inflammation or may develop from the onset, when a low-grade irritation to the pulp or periapex is neutralized by effective tissue resistance. The term *chronic* implies a tissue pressure below the threshold limits of pain receptors. The products of the exudative zone are draining onto a surface, being absorbed into the venous or lymphatic flow, moving (pointing, spreading) into adjacent connective tissues, or utilizing any combination of these outlets for pressure release. Since the pressure against sensory units is subthreshold, pain is absent and the term *nonpainful pulpitis* or *nonpainful periapical pathosis* is applicable. When the strength of the irritant has been significantly reduced by the exudative defense, the granulomatous tissue (granulation tissue plus chronic inflammatory cells) becomes hyperactive and dominates the inflammatory complex in its attempt to heal and repair. Complete repair, however, cannot occur as long as the toxic agents are still present in the pulp chamber or root canal. Although the predominant cells in chronic inflammation are lymphocytes, plasma cells, and macrophages, a limited number of PMNs are usually present.

The term *subacute* implies a seesaw of hyperactivity between the exudative (acute) and proliferative (chronic) inflammatory components and is applicable to pulpitis as well as advanced forms of apical periodontitis. Clinically it is characterized by periods of mild to moderate symptoms caused by a mild to moderate exacerbation of a chronic (nonpainful) lesion. The painful symptoms occur when the exudative zone becomes hyperactive to a slight or moderate degree and the regional tissue pressure increases. (See the descriptions of chronic pulpalgia and subacute periapical abscess, pp. 149 and 169.)

Immunologic considerations. The field of immunology has in recent years developed into one of the most interesting, exciting, and challenging areas of the medical and dental professions. Its multitudinous aspects in relation to the body's defense are only now beginning to be unraveled. Because of the potential importance of immunology in the diagnosis and treatment of oral infection as well as an understanding of the pathogenesis of these diseases, a basic knowledge of this field is vital. For these reasons, an overview or synthesis of the immunologic mechanisms involved in pulpal and periapical diseases is presented in a separate section of Chapter 4.

DISEASES OF THE DENTAL PULP

1. Inflammatory diseases of the dental pulp
   a. *Hyperalgesia** (reversible pulpitis, hyperreactive pulpalgia, hypersensitivity)
      (1) Hypersensitive dentin
      (2) Hyperemia
   b. *Painful pulpitis*
      (1) Acute pulpalgia[†] (acute pulpitis)
      (2) Chronic pulpalgia (subacute pulpitis)
   c. *Nonpainful pulpitis*
      (1) Chronic ulcerative pulpitis (due to caries)
      (2) Chronic pulpitis (carious lesion absent)
      (3) Chronic hyperplastic pulpitis (pulp polyp)
2. Additional pulp changes
   a. *Necrosis* (sequela to inflammatory or retrogressive changes)
   b. *Retrogressive changes* (degeneration, pulposis)
      (1) Atrophy and fibrosis
      (2) Dystrophic calcification (calcific degeneration, calcific pulposis)
   c. *Internal resorption,* which may be sequela to persistent chronic inflammation
3. Refer to Table 3-7.

Inflammatory diseases of the pulp

Hyperalgesia (reversible pulpitis, hyperreactive pulpalgia, hypersensitivity). This is a general category that histologically may represent a spectrum of responses ranging from *dentin hypersensitivity,* without a concomitant inflammatory response of the underlying pulpal connective tissue, to an *early (incipient) mild phase of inflammation.* It is an indication of peripheral A-δ fiber stimulation (Table 3-3).

The point at which reversibility of hyperalgesia ends and irreversibility begins is entirely specula-

*Algesia: a state of increased sensitivity to pain; provoked by stimuli not normally painful.
†Algia (Greek *algos,* pain): suffix meaning pain or painful condition.

tive. Determination of reversibility is a clinical judgment influenced by an evaluation of the patient's history and clinical symptoms (Table 3-8). A history of recent dental procedures (root planing, cavity preparation, etc.) or the presence of periodontal disease, a faulty restoration, or cervical erosion may influence that judgment. A painful episode of short duration requiring an external stimulus (touch, cold, heat) also influences that judgment because the *spontaneous* and *continuous* pain of *irreversible pulpitis* is an indication of the presence of dead and dying tissue *(secondary irritant).* Necrotic tissue presence activates and maintains the inflammatory response and the resultant increase in intrapulpal pressure (Table 3-1).

Hypersensitive dentin. Hypersensitive dentin may be due to two factors:

1. Transmission of pain-producing stimuli as a result of opened apertures of dentin tubules. (See Brännström's hydrodynamics theory, p. 119.) Vasodilation or inflammation need not be present in the underlying pulp tissue. Hypersensitive dentin may be associated with exposed dentinal tubules as a result of abrasion, erosion, or following root planing. The symptoms may be minimized or controlled through the use of commercial desensitizing toothpastes. (See p. 124.)
2. Lowered pain threshold of peripheral receptors as a result of underlying prolonged vasodilation (hyperemia) or local incipient inflammation (classic or neurogenic).

Hyperemia. Pulpal hyperemia is a capillary bed engorgement with a predisposition to edema (Fig. 3-40, *C*). This predisposition is a result of prolonged vasodilation and its sequelae: elevated capillary pressure and increased vascular permeability. Electron microscopy has demonstrated that venules (20 to 30 μm diameter) also contribute substantially to the fluid exudate. An increased blood volume in the confined environment of the dental pulp increases intrapulpal pressure in the affected area.

The hyperemic response in a localized part of the pulp may also be accompanied by an incipient inflammatory response of mild to moderate severity (Fig. 3-43, *A* and *B*). The cell-free zone may be obscured by inflammatory cells subjacent to the affected dentinal tubules, and small hemorrhages may be present. The dentinoblastic layer may be partially disrupted because many of the dentinoblasts have been displaced (aspirated) into the tubules. The predentin may be reduced in width if

Table 3-7. Comparative terminology and classifications of pulpal pathoses

	Classification used at Loyola University	Ingle's classification	Seltzer and Bender (histologic classification)
	I. Inflammatory changes		

Painful pulpitis	1. Hyperalgesia (reversible pulpitis)
	   a. Hypersensitive dentin
	   b. Hyperemia
		1. Hyperreactive pulpalgia
		   a. Hypersensitivity
		   b. Hyperemia
			1. Intact pulp with scattered chronic inflammatory cells (transitional stage) (incipient form of chronic pulpitis)

	2. Acute pulpalgia (acute pulpitis); most frequently, severely painful exacerbation of existing chronic inflammation	2. Acute pulpalgia Incipient (may be reversible) Moderate (may be referred) Advanced (may be relieved by cold)	2. Acute pulpitis
	3. Chronic pulpalgia (subacute pulpitis); Mildly painful phase of chronic pulpitis ("smouldering pulpitis")	3. Chronic pulpalgia	3. Chronic partial pulpitis with partial necrosis
Nonpainful pulpitis	4. Chronic pulpitis (nonpainful phase)	4. Chronic pulpalgia	*or* 4. Chronic total pulpitis with partial liquefaction necrosis
	5. Chronic hyperplastic pulpitis	5. Hyperplastic pulpitis	5. Chronic partial pulpitis (hyperplastic form)
	6. Pulp necrosis	6. Pulp necrosis	6. Pulp necrosis
	II. Retrogressive (degenerative) changes		
	1. Atrophy 2. Dystrophic calcification	1. Atrophic pulposis 2. Calcific pulposis	1. Atrophic pulp 2. Dystrophic mineralization

there has been prolonged interference with predentin formation.

Hyperemia is an initial and potentially reversible pulpal response that sets the stage for the inflammatory cycle. The capability for resolution (reversability) depends on the strength and duration of the irritant, the extent of pulp tissue affected, and the prior health status of the pulp itself.

Etiology. Pulpal reaction to external stimuli (caries, restorative procedures) is largely related to the permeability of the dentin. The tubular structure of dentin is an integral part of the hydrodynamic theory of dentinal pain and also provides a permeable intermediary between the pulp and the enamel and cementum. Under normal circumstances the enamel and cementum act as a relatively impermeable barrier to block the patency of the dentinal tubules at the dentinoenamel or dentinocemental junction. When caries or cutting procedures interrupt this natural barrier, the dentinal tubules become bidirectionally patent; the dentinal fluid flows outward as a result of the intrapulpal pressure (10 mm Hg), and external substances (bacteria, bacterial products, restorative material solutes) diffuse inward toward the pulp.

The movement of substances (potential pulpal irritants) through dentin is related to dentin permeability. Permeability of dentin is directly related to the number of dentinal tubules, providing a continuity between the external surface of the tooth and the pulp. An increase in the number of these

Table 3-8. Differential diagnosis of potentially reversible affected pulps*

	Potentially reversible	Probably irreversible
Pain	Momentary—dissipates readily after stimulus is removed (e.g., cold) (A-δ fiber stimulation)	*Continuous*—persists for minutes to hours after stimulus is removed; presence of internal (secondary) irritant (C fiber stimulation) *Throbbing*—may be present; due to arterial pulsation in area of increased intrapulpal pressure (C fiber stimulation)
Stimulus	Requires external stimulus (e.g., cold, heat, sugar)	*Spontaneous*—does not require external (primary) stimulus; dead or injured pulp tissue present in chamber or canal (internal or secondary irritant)† *Intermittent*—spontaneous pain of short duration
History	Patient may have undergone recent dental procedures (e.g., root planing, cavity preparation); cervical erosion or abrasion may be present	Patient may have had extensive restoration, pulp capping, deep caries, trauma, etc.
Electric pulp test	May be premature response	May be premature, delayed, or mixed
Percussion	Negative response unless problem related to occlusal stress	May respond in advanced stage of pulpitis when concomitant acute apical periodontitis is present
Referred	Negative because of minimally affected pulp tissue and short duration of pain	Common finding (Table 3-10, Fig. 3-26, p. 151)
Lying down	Negative because of minimally affected pulp tissue	Common finding because increase in cephalic blood pressure increases already excessive intrapulpal pressure
Color	Negative	May be present as result of tissue lysis and intrapulpal hemorrhage
Radiograph	Probable cause (e.g., restoration and/or caries), periodontal pocket, cupping of alveolar crest	Probable cause as for reversible
	Periapex, negative	Periapex, may be slight widening of apical periodontal space

*Diagnosis should not be made on the basis of the results of any one test but on the supportive confirmations of at least three (e.g., percussion, vitality [thermal and/or electric], radiographic). Refer also to Chapter 2.
†Secondary irritant perpetuates the inflammatory response, which increases regional intrapulpal pressure.

"open" dentinal tubules increases the dentin permeability. The permeability of an individual dentinal tubule relates to the fourth power of its tubular radius. For example, if the opening of a dentinal tubule is reduced to one-fourth its original size, then the permeability of that tubule is reduced to one-sixteenth its original value. The length of the dentinal tubules or thickness of dentin is related to its resistance to permeation. The greater the length of a dentinal tubule, the greater is its resistance to permeation (Table 3-9).

Microbial agents. Microorganisms must be present in sufficient numbers and/or virulence to initiate a hyperemic response. Low concentrations are immediately destroyed and phagocytosed by the local defense cells. This relationship may be expressed by this basic formula:

Pulpal disease state =

$$\frac{\text{Number of microorganisms} \times \text{Virulence}}{\text{Tissue resistance}}$$

Microorganisms may invade through carious or traumatic exposures or through the dentinal tubules when the protective enamel is lost as a result of fracture, abrasion, erosion, caries, or anomalies such as dens in dente. Microorganism

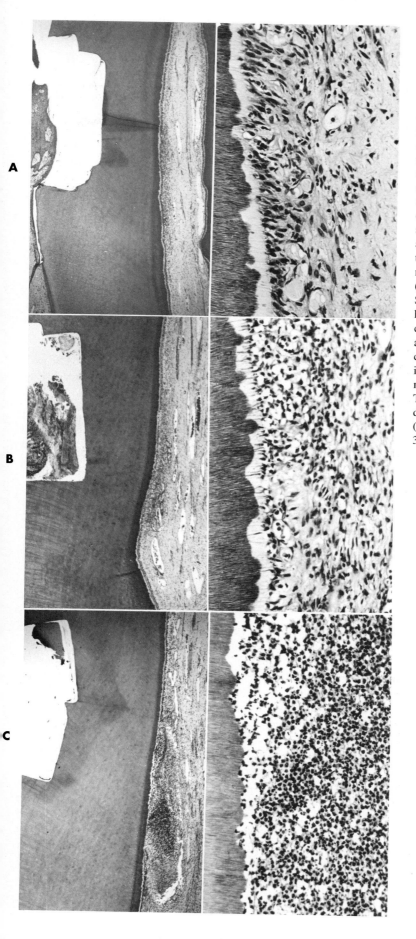

Fig. 3-43. Pulp reactions to experimental traumatic manipulation of monkey dentin. **A,** Slight pulp reaction after cavity preparation and temporary gutta-percha dressing for 8 days. Higher magnification (×300) of subjacent pulp tissue shows increased cellularity obscuring the cell-free zone. More capillaries can be seen than are normally found in the dentinoblastic and subdentinoblastic regions. **B,** Moderate pulp reaction after cavity had been left open for 8 days. Higher magnification (×300) shows localized increased cellularity and vascularity as well as disruption of the dentinoblastic layer. Some dentinoblastic nuclei have been displaced (aspiration) into the dentin tubules. **C,** Severe pulp reaction after soft carious human dentin has been placed in the cavity, which was then filled with amalgam for 8 days. Higher magnification (×300) shows marked cellular infiltration, approaching abscess formation, of the subjacent pulp tissue. The dentinoblastic layer has been destroyed, and predentin is absent. (From Mjör I, Tronstad L: *Oral Surg* 34:102, 1972.)

Table 3-9. Area of surface of dentin available for diffusion at various distances from the pulp

Distance from pulp (mm)	Average number of tubules (1000/mm^2)	Average diameter of dentin tubules (μm)	Average dentin surface available (%)*
Pulp	45	2.5	22.1
0.1–0.5	43	1.9	12.2
0.6–1.0	38	1.6	7.6
1.1–1.5	35	1.2	4.0
1.6–2.0	30	1.1	2.9
2.1–2.5	23	0.9	1.5
2.6–3.0	20	0.8	1.1
3.1–3.5	19	0.8	1.0

Modified from Garberoglio R, Brännström M: *Arch Oral Biol* 21:355, 1976.
*From Pashley D: *Oper Dent Suppl* 3:13, 1984.

invasion of the pulp may be induced by dental procedures related to pressure, especially in deep cavities. Cementing and condensing of restorative materials, impression taking for indirect techniques, and the use of rotary instruments are all operative procedures that exert pressure against the dentin. They are capable of driving organisms through the tubules and into the dental pulp. If the resistance of the pulp is low and the virulence and/or concentration of the dentinal microorganisms are high, a hyperemia may result. If the pulp is already hyperemic or inflamed, a more severe inflammatory state (exacerbation) will follow.

Dentinal caries has been classically described by Sarnat and Massler as existing as either an active or arrested lesion. An active carious lesion is dynamic in its advance toward the pulp, whereas the arrested carious lesion is static, having developed a sclerotic zone in the dentin (a natural defense barrier to permeation). Dentin involved with caries can be subdivided into *infected dentin*, which is invaded by bacteria, and *affected dentin*, which is only exposed to the permeating bacterial products. Reeves and Stanley examined teeth with carious lesions and only found significant pulpal pathosis in those where bacteria had invaded reparative dentin or penetrated closer than 1.11 mm of the pulp. Bergenholtz has demonstrated in animal studies that bacterial byproducts alone can produce pulpal inflammation when sealed in dentinal cavities. Pashley et al. summarized the following as important variables that affect the pulpal diffusion of microbial products through permeable dentin:

1. The thickness of the remaining dentin. (The thicker the dentin, the lower is the concentration of microbial products.)

2. The surface area of the exposed, permeable dentin. (A thin, crescent-shaped area of exposed cervical dentin permits much less permeation than a leaking full-crown preparation.)
3. The presence or absence of a smear layer. (The more plugged dentinal tubule apertures, the less is the permeation of microbial products.)
4. The "potency" of the microbial products.
5. The rate of pulpal blood flow. (The greater the pulpal blood flow, the better is the removal of accumulated pulpal irritants; interference in blood flow could result in accumulation of pulpal irritants, resulting in an exacerbation of the inflammatory condition.)

When a concomitant generalized systemic bacteremia is present, previously inflamed or partially necrotic pulps are susceptible to bacterial invasion. Microorganisms may escape into the affected pulp tissue through the injured and leaky blood vessels. This attraction or fixation of microorganisms in areas of inflammation is referred to as *anachoresis*. Pulpal contamination or infection can also extend from lateral, apical, or furcal canals that communicate with periodontal pockets.

Physical agents. The amount of pulpal vasodilation as a result of physical irritation depends on the strength and duration of the irritant as well as the *ability of the pulpal microvasculature to remove any accumulation of inflammatory mediators.* Cutting procedures can produce varying magnitudes of pulpal damage, depending on applied pressure, speed, bur size, temperature, cavity depth, and postoperative insulation protection.

Stanley has shown that speeds of 50,000 rpm and greater were biologically acceptable to the pulp when the operator controlled (1) *temperature* with adequate coolants, (2) *force* (pressure) by using smaller cutting tools, (3) *remaining dentin thickness* with proper cavity depth, and (4) *postoperative protection of deep cavities* with sedative cements such as zinc oxide–eugenol (ZOE).

The most critical factor in determining the degree of pulpal response is the *remaining dentin thickness,* which is measured from the floor of the cavity to the pulp tissue. Given a constant cutting speed and technique, the intensity of the pulpal response increases as the remaining dentin decreases. Minimal effects are transmitted to the pulp if the remaining dentin thickness is 2 mm or more. Stanley found that burn lesions will not result at any cavity depth as long as adequate water coolant accompanies the procedure. Adequate coolant will allow the floor of low-speed preparations or high-speed preparations (greater than 200,000 rpm) to be brought to within 0.3 mm of the pulp with minimal danger of severe inflammatory response. Speeds between 3000 and 30,000 rpm appear to be the most harmful to the pulp even though a water coolant is used. The traumatic capacity of cutting techniques can be minimized by the production of irritation dentin, which is produced sooner and in greater amounts with the low-speed technique than with high-speed techniques despite remaining dentin thickness. However, it must be kept in mind that the greater the irritant force and the deeper the cavity preparation, the greater is the damage to the dentinoblasts, thereby requiring a longer recovery period for the dentinoblastic zone.

Cutting procedures can affect the permeability of the remaining dentin after cavity preparation. As cavity preparation into sound permeable dentin progresses toward the pulp, the exposed dentinal tubules increase in number per unit area and increase in tubular diameter. Approximately a 20-fold increase in potential dentin permeability can result from extending a cavity preparation that is 3 mm from the pulp to within 0.5 mm of the pulp (Table 3-9). Similarly, an acid etchant applied to dentin in a cavity preparation has the potential to increase dentin permeability four- or fivefold as a result of enlargement of the dentinal tubule apertures. Pashley et al. demonstrated with an in vivo animal study that shortly after dentinal cavity preparation, there is an appreciable decrease in dentin permeability. They attribute this to a precipitation of intratubular protein (i.e., fibrinogen) after dentin is exposed during cavity preparation.

Kim cautions against the use of periodontal ligament injection anesthesia for restorative procedures on teeth with vital pulps. Local anesthesia by this technique requires the use of a vasoconstrictor-containing solution that has the side effect of completely stopping or greatly reducing pulpal blood flow. Under these conditions, normally well-tolerated cutting procedures have the potential to allow accumulation of inflammatory mediators, resulting in pulpal damage (e.g., pulpal hemorrhage).

Other physical irritants are:

1. Loss of coronal enamel or cervical cementum through erosion, abrasion, or fractures that expose the dentin to repeated insults and a possible hyperalgesic response
2. Cementation and impression procedures that exert a pressure against the tubular dentin floor, causing dentinoblastic displacement
3. High fillings, tooth drift, injudicious use of the mechanical separator, or too rapid orthodontic movement, which may produce a secondary pulpal response as a result of periapical or periradicular compression

Thermal agents. The degree of friction heat generated by cutting instruments depends on the size and type of cutting tool, the speed of rotation, the cavity depth, and the effectiveness of the coolant. Larger burs affect more dentin surface than do small ones, and grinding instruments require more pressure than do cutting ones. However, instruments used in cavity preparation are not the only source of *thermal irritation.* Metal fillings without the proper insulation of liners and bases transmit environmental thermal change immediately to a pulp already irritated by the cavity preparation. The same is true for the heat generated by setting cement or the polishing of a restoration. Polishing of metallic restorations with powders and Burlew wheels after cementation with an acid cement is a frequent cause of hyperemia.

Chemical agents. Many chemical agents and restorative materials have been cited as irritating to the pulpodentinal complex.

1. *"Sterilizing" or disinfecting chemical applied to the exposed dentin surface* may be highly irritating and produce severe dentino blastic injury. These include phenol, alcohol, chloroform, hydrogen peroxide, and silver nitrate. To be effective, phenol requires prolonged contact with the dentin. Seltzer has shown that few pulp changes are evident when the remaining dentin thickness was 3 mm, but in deep cavities in which only 0.6 mm of dentin remained, there was severe pulp damage.

Alcohol and chloroform not only produce a thermal irritation through evaporation, but also dehydrate the tubules, allowing the acid from zinc phosphate cement to penetrate to a greater depth. Pohto and Scheinin, in their film *Microcinematography of the Dental Pulp,* demonstrated that hydrogen perioxide may travel through the dentinal tubules of deep cavity preparations and into the pulp, producing emboli and thus altering and perhaps even arresting pulpal circulation. Silver nitrate is not as self-limiting as was once thought. In deep cavities it can penetrate readily into the pulp, even though sclerosed and irritation dentin barriers are present.

2. *Dentin-conditioning and dentin-bonding agents.* Classic acid etchants (e.g., 37% phosphoric acid) used on dentinal surfaces have the potential of demineralizing peritubular dentin. The resultant widening of dentinal tubule apertures results in a potential increased dentin permeability and pulpal irritation. To minimize pulpal responses, dentin-conditioning procedures should employ weaker acids, passively applied to the dentin surface (without rubbing and scrubbing) for short periods (5 to 15 seconds). These techniques are used to remove the superficial smear layer but leave the smear plugs in the dentinal tubule apertures (blocking permeability). At the same time the passive application is used so as not to disrupt the remaining collagen framework at the dentin surface. The collagen framework later interacts with the hydrophilic priming agents and forms a hybrid layer that improves the penetrability of adhesive resins and thus the micromechanical interlocking or bonding.

3. *Acid-liquid components of cements.* Initial acidity of zinc phosphate cements, once frequently used silicate cements, and to a lesser extent zinc polycarboxylate cements, have been associated with pulpal irritation for many years. Recently, glass ionomer cements have attained popularity, but instances of postcementation sensitivity have been reported. Glass ionomer cements mixed to a luting (cementing) consistency have been found to retain a longer period of acidity (below pH 3) than zinc phosphate or zinc polycarboxylate cements. This, in conjunction with the cytotoxicity of other ingredients

(e.g., fluoride), may lead to hyperalgesia. It is generally accepted that fewer adverse pulp responses have been experienced when glass ionomer cements are used with a higher powder/lower liquid ratio for restorations per se.

4. *Acrylic monomer,* used in the catalyst system of composite resins and in conjunction with self-curing resins, can be harmful. In addition to the shrinkage potential of these filling materials, their inability to seal effectively leads to yet further pulpal irritation as a result of marginal leakage.

5. *Eugenol* released from ZOE has the potential to diffuse through dentin and produce either beneficial or irritating effects on pulpal tissue. The therapeutic properties ascribed to eugenol include (1) antiinflammatory activity through the inibition of prostaglandin synthesis, (2) antibacterial effects of inhibitory properties, and (3) anodyne effects through desensitization and blockage of pain impulse transmission. Eugenol applied for prolonged periods or in high concentration can be cytotoxic or neurolytic or can produce vasodilation, protein denaturation, cellular edema, or necrosis.

Restorative materials. Brännström attributes minimal pulpal irritation directly to today's accepted restorative materials but believes bacterial contamination results from microleakage of restorative materials as a primary pulpal irritant. A restoration placed in a cavity preparation can develop a "contraction gap" between the restoration and the tooth surface. The contraction gap then fills with fluid from the outflow of dentinal tubules or saliva from the external surface. An environment is created for bacterial growth and failure of the restoration. Bergenholtz et al. studied bacterial leakage and associated pulpal response under restorations of composite, amalgam, silicate, gutta-percha, and ZOE in monkeys. The amount of bacterial leakage under restorations correlated directly with the degree of inflammatory response in the pulp. *ZOE was found to be the most effective sealing agent against bacterial leakage.* Intermediate levels of bacterial leakage occurred with gutta-percha, composite, and amalgam, whereas silicate evidence the highest degree of bacterial leakage.

The possible routes for microleakage increase with interfaces between dentin, smear layer, cavity varnish or cement, and restorative material (Fig. 3-44). Brännström contends that the smear layer produced in prepared dentinal cavities is nonpermanent and has the potential to foster bacteria for recurrent caries and irritation of the pulp. He advises the use of an antibacterial detergent for the removal of the infected superficial smear layer. The reduced dentin permeability created by the production of a smear layer should then be retained by the residual smear plugs in the dentinal tubule apertures. To counteract the development of the contraction gap, Brännström recommends desiccation of the disinfected cavity followed by the use a hydrophilic liner under the restoration. A hydrophilic liner would expand to fill any space that would otherwise produce a contraction gap. An antibacterial liner would also be in ideal position to affect any residual bacteria left in the dentinal tubule apertures.

Histopathology and clinical symptoms. The increased blood volume associated with hyperemia also increases the intrapulpal pressure in the involved area, which may be limited to a segment of the pulp chamber.

The viscosity of the gelated ground substance (reinforced by collagen fiber bundles) plays a major role in the containment of these local pockets of intrapulpal pressure. A prolonged vasodilation may result in capillary injury with an initial loss of plasma fluid (edema), a minimal amount of white cell infiltration, and possibly some erythrocyte extravasation (incipient stage of pulpitis). The pressure exerted against the dentinoblasts and the A-δ nerve fibers in the affected peripheral area is subliminal, i.e., not great enough to initiate a pain impulse. Their threshold, however, *is lowered* so

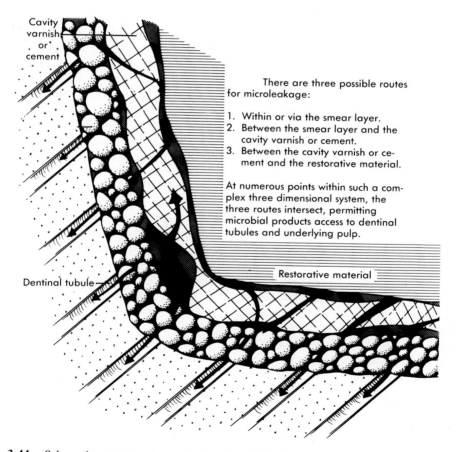

Cavity varnish or cement

Dentinal tubule

Restorative material

There are three possible routes for microleakage:

1. Within or via the smear layer.
2. Between the smear layer and the cavity varnish or cement.
3. Between the cavity varnish or cement and the restorative material.

At numerous points within such a complex three dimensional system, the three routes intersect, permitting microbial products access to dentinal tubules and underlying pulp.

Fig. 3-44.   Schematic representation of the interface of dentin and restorative material in a typical cavity. The granular constituents of the smear layer have been exaggerated out of their normal proportion for emphasis. Three theoretic routes for microleakage are indicated by arrows. (From Pashley DH: *Oper Dent Suppl* 3:13, 1984.)

that the dentin is in a hypersensitive state and therefore more sensitive to external (primary) stimuli such as cold. The role of mediators in lowering this threshold has not been clearly defined. These mediators *(endogenous algogenic agents)* initiate pain either by direct excitation of the nerve terminals or by lowering their threshold of excitability to such stimuli as heat, cold, or mechanical forces Serotonin (5-hydroxytryptamine, 5-HT), a vasoconstrictor liberated by injured platelets, may also have an algogenic effect. Olgart introduced 5-HT experimentally into the pulp and noted the increased excitability of the A-δ fibers. Neuropeptides released from unmyelinated C nerve fibers mediate neurogenic inflammation, which can result in hyperexcitability of nerve endings.

External (primary) mild irritants (heat, cold, sweet, sour) applied to these hypersensitive structures activate a nerve impulse, which results in an exaggerated painful response. Trowbridge refers to this phenomenon of hypersensitivity as *hyperalgesia* and compares it with sunburned skin. Although affected sunburned areas feel warm, there is no pain unless touched. If the primary external irritant is removed, the pain stops immediately. *Although hyperemia may be accompanied by hypersensitive dentin, the presence of hypersensitive dentin does not necessarily mean that hyperemia or incipient inflammation is also present.* It may signify only the absence of the protective enamel or cervical cementum with the resultant exposure of dentinal tubules to the environment.

Another condition of hypersensitivity is the *dentinal crack syndrome.* This frequently occurs in extensively restored teeth without cuspal protection in which an occlusal crack into dentin has developed. The most frequent complaint is a sharp, momentary pain during mastication that is poorly localized to one quadrant. In this situation, forces against cuspal inclines bordering the crack result in its separation. The opened crack now fills with fluid from dentinal tubules or saliva. When the cuspal force is released, the crack reopposes (closes), resulting in a pulpward hydrodynamic stimulus. The subsequent sharp, momentary pain is caused by the movement of dentinal tubule fluid and stimulation of A-δ fibers. A complaint by the patient of this type of pain can be diagnosed by selective closure against a cotton applicator tip placed between cusps of the suspect tooth and its antagonist. A positive diagnosis can be made when a visual crack is identified and a reproducible

sharp, momentary pain occurs as the pressure on the cotton applicator tip is released *(rebound tenderness).* A similar mechanism exists for a patient experiencing episodes of sharp, momentary pain as a result of a loose restoration. Movement of the loose restoration in the presence of salivary leakage exerts a plunger action against the dentinal surface, causing a hydrodynamic stimulus for pain. Further complications may occur in the form of *hyperalgesia* when *bacterial products diffuse to the pulp through exposed dentinal tubules contiguous with the leaky margin or crack,* initiating an inflammatory response (Brännström, 1986).

Diagnosis

Pain. The pain associated with hyperalgesia (reversible pulpitis) does not occur spontaneously. This condition is therefore asymptomatic, requiring an external stimulus *(primary irritant)* to evoke a painful response. The pain is sharp and of brief duration, ceasing when the irritant is removed. It has been described as a shock sensation (Table 3-8).

Visual examination and history. While examining for caries, restorations, fractures, or traumatic occlusion, the dentist may be able to elicit from the patient a timetable regarding the restoration and past treatment as well as a history of the subjective symptoms.

Radiography. Periodontal ligament space and lamina dura are normal Radiographs may show the depth of the caries or cavity preparation.

Percussion. Usually the response is negative to percussion. There may be a mild response if pulpal vasodilation has been prolonged, especially after cavity preparation. A reverse hyperemia also may develop as a result of occlusal stress against the periapex. The only treatment then is relief of the occlusal disharmony.

Vitality tests. With thermal testing, the hyperalgesic pulp responds more readily to cold stimulation than normal teeth. In such affected teeth, cold also evokes a more rapid response than heat because hot and cold represent two different diagnostic phenomena. (See discussion on hot and cold stimulation, p. 105.) With *electric testing* the hyperalgesic pulp can be expected to require minimal current to initiate a positive response. Such responses are a reflection of increased excitability of A-δ nerve fibers (Table 3-3).

Treatment. What is the best treatment for hyperalgesia? The answer is to be found in a review of the etiologic factors—*prevention.* Control of operative procedures and an awareness of the causative agents are essential. If the cavity preparation is extensive, placement of the permanent restoration should be avoided for several weeks or more. Multiple irritants should be avoided. A tooth with extensive caries, subjected to the pressure and frictional heat of cavity preparation, followed by an alcohol or ether swabbing, acid cements, and then continued thermal shocks through a metallic restoration, is vulnerable to the prolonged vasodilation of hyperemia and incipient pulpitis. A sedative base always should be used in deep cavities and may also serve as an insulator. (See discussions on zinc oxide and eugenol (p. 146), densitizing toothpastes (p. 124), and the smear layer (p. 127).)

Painful pulpitis

Definition. Painful pulpitis is a clinically detectable inflammatory response of the pulpal connective tissue to an irritant. *The exudative (acute) forces are hyperactive, and the painful symptoms are indicative of an intrapulpal pressure increase that has surpassed the threshold limits of pain fibers.*

Classification. Experience has shown that it is impossible to determine with any degree of certainty whether a tooth with painful pulpitis is in a serous stage, a suppurative stage, or a combination of these phases in different sections of the pulp. Speculation plays a key role. From a clinical standpoint, however, it is important to determine whether the patient has a reversible or irreversible pathologic process of the pulp, requiring either palliative treatment or root canal therapy. Applying a knowledge of the fundamentals of the inflammatory cycle to the closed, unyielding (noncompliant) environment of the pulp chamber and canal and to the special environment of the periapex can be important in determining the presence of pathosis, thereby removing some of the empiricism employed in patient treatment. The only valid *clinical* term is *painful* pulpitis. *A painful pulpitis examined histologically may show a chronic character of its tissue; however, increased exudative (acute) activity in the regions closest to the irritant may increase the regional intrapulpal pressure beyond the threshold of excitability of the sensory structures and produce pain.* Thus the histopathologic term *acute* may be used synonymously with *painful.* Painful pulpitis includes the following:

Acute pulpalgia (acute pulpitis). This is a severely painful and irreversible acute inflammatory response characterized by exudative hyperactivity. The histopath-

ologic features include vasodilation, fluid exudation (inflammatory edema, leukocyte infiltration, and ultimately a pulpal abscess (Table 3-6).

Chronic pulpalgia (subacute pulpitis). This is a mild exacerbation of a chronic pulpitis. The exudative (acute) response becomes hyperactive to a slight or moderate degree. It is characterized by intermittent episodes of mild to moderate pain induced by transient pressures emanating from the exudative zone. The term *subacute pulpitis* is used for cases that cannot clearly be classified as either acute or chronic pulpitis. It has sometimes been described as a "smouldering" inflammatory response. Ingle uses the word "grumble" when describing the discomfort from chronic pulpalgia.

Etiology. Since painful pulpitis is preceded by vasodilation (hyperemia), its etiologic factors are the same. However, painful pulpitis may also develop as an acute exacerbation of a previously existing, nonpainful, chronically inflamed pulp in which the exudative (acute) zones becomes hyperactive, as in the following situations:

1. Food impactions in a carious cavity with an exposed pulp may either block the drainage from the exudative zones subjacent to the caries or force carious contaminants deeper into mobilized granulomatous tissue. The resultant pulpal pressure buildup will produce painful symptoms. *Indiscriminate excavation of caries may have the same effect.*

2. A tooth that has become chronically inflamed either initially or as a sequela of acute inflammation may remain in an nonpainful state for months or years. The stimulus of additional operative procedures may activate or intensify the exudative (acute or subacute) response. The intrapulpal pressure increases and pain results.

Histopathology and clinical symptoms. Prolonged dilation and engorgement of pulpal blood vessels during regional hyperemia (subjacent to the affected tubules) result in increased vascular permeability and capillary pressure and loss of plasma proteins. The fluid exudation (inflammatory edema), leukocyte infiltration and subsequent localized abscess formation that follow add to the intrapulpal pressure, raising it beyond the threshold limit of pain receptors (Fig. 3-45 and Table 3-3). Early on, the rise in intrapulpal pressure will cause a spontaneous throbbing pain due to the pulsation of the intrapulpal pressure and only the peaks of the pulses reaching suprathreshold levels (Fig. 3-46). As the intrapulpal pressure increases, the entire intrapulpal pressure pulse becomes suprathreshold, and the pain is felt as a spontaneous constant pain. Evident in this *severe* reaction is the disruption or destruction or the dentinoblastic layer, and the predentin may be reduced in width or absent (Fig. 3-43, *C*). *The resultant pain is interpreted by the patient as spontaneous* (not evoked by any external primary stimulus). *If a primary (external) stimulus does trigger this response, the pain continues when the irritant is removed. The inflammatory response now is maintained and increased by a secondary (internal) irritant, the injured and dead cells, and later the products of proteolysis; thus the seeming spontaneity of the pain.*

As the blood flow slows, congestion and stasis result. The regional tissue cells, deprived of their oxygen (anoxia) and nutrition, die, producing small zones of necrosis (Fig. 3-41). Neutrophilic leukocytes by ameboid movement pass through the endothelial gaps (pores) of the capillary walls to the area of injury and engulf bacteria and tissue fragments (Fig. 3-45, *C*). This neutrophilic function (chemotaxis) is guided by chemicals (chemotactic agents) released from the injured and dead cells (Fig. 3-42 and Table 3-6).

Although a variety of leukocytes may be observed in any given histologic section, the PMN (neutrophil) is the characteristic principal cell. As the acute inflammation persists, blood-borne and tissue-borne macrophages make their appearance. The disintegration of the leukocytes releases proteolytic ferments (proteases) that liquefy (digest) the injured cells and tissue, resulting in pus formation. Many of the injured cells release their own proteases and undergo self-digestion (autolysis), which adds to the suppurative accumulation. As the suppurative core or pulp abscess is formed, the first two zones of the acute-chronic inflammatory spectrum are now evident (see Table 4-2). The suppurative core (zone I) may be referred to as the *zone of necrosis* or *infection* (Fig. 3-47). When microorganisms are present in sufficient numbers of virulence, the term *zone of infection* may be used. It contains the dead and dying cells as well as intermediate and end products of tissue proteolysis. Zone II is the inflamed connective tissue surrounding the suppurative core.

The irritant force has its greatest effect in this area, and the term *zone of contamination* is used to describe it. As a result of the exudative activity (vasodilation, fluid exudation, cellular infiltration)

in zone II, the term *exudative* (or *acute*) *inflammatory zone* is also applicable. As the inflammation persists, the toxic elements are diluted at the sites peripheral to the exudative (acute) zones. Here the proliferative (granulomatous, fibrous, chronic) activity of zone III initiates its appearance. (See discussion on histopathology of chronic pulpitis, p. 154.)

Intrapulpal pressure (and therefore pain) continues to increase as pus forms and hemorrhage occurs from ruptured blood vessels. The pressure may be so great that the patient feels a throbbing sensation produced by pulse wave stimulation of the C fibers.

Diagnosis

Pain. The severity of the clinical symptoms of *acute pulpalgia (acute pulpitis)* will vary as the inflammatory response increases. The degree of intensity of pain depends on the intensity of the intrapulpal pressure and the viability of peripheral sensory units. It will vary from a mild and readily tolerated discomfort to a severe, even excruciating, throbbing. The pain is *continuous or has periods of cessation (intermittent).* It is *spontaneous* because of the presence of necrotic tissue (the internal or secondary irritant), which further provokes and serves as a nidus for inflammation and the resultant "suprathreshold" intrapulpal pressure increase. Thus, unlike the pain of *reversible pulpitis (hyperalgesia),* this pain lingers after the *primary (external) irritant* has been removed. Painful pulpitis is generally diffuse and not readily localized by the patient until there is a concomitant positive response to percussion. The patient may be able to locate the general area of discomfort but usually will not be able to pinpoint the specific tooth until certain diagnostic tests are employed. Lying down or bending over may intensify the pain of acute pulpalgia because the overall increase in cephalic blood pressure is relayed to the confined pulp tissue.

The pain of *chronic pulpalgia (subacute pulpitis)* has clinical manifestations similar to acute pulpalgia. It also is diffuse, frequently referred, and difficult to localize. However, the pain is more moderate. Patients frequently tolerate the discomfort for months because the painful episodes are intermittent and readily controlled by aspirin. Diagnosis is very difficult because the tooth may not show any demonstrable periapical change on the radiograph or demonstrate a clearly defined tenderness to percussion. A common expression is: "Well … it feels

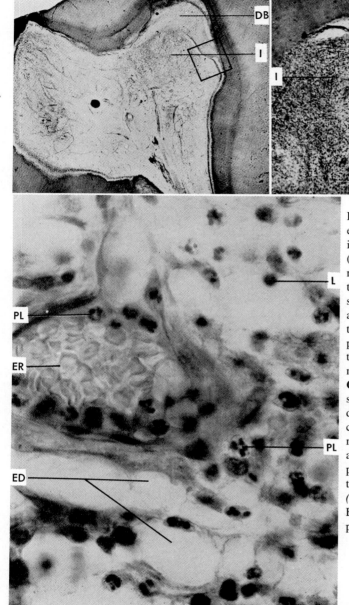

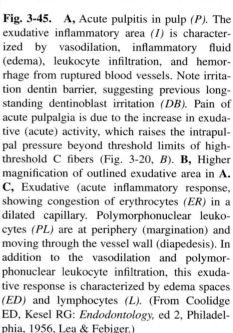

Fig. 3-45. **A,** Acute pulpitis in pulp *(P).* The exudative inflammatory area *(I)* is characterized by vasodilation, inflammatory fluid (edema), leukocyte infiltration, and hemorrhage from ruptured blood vessels. Note irritation dentin barrier, suggesting previous longstanding dentinoblast irritation *(DB).* Pain of acute pulpalgia is due to the increase in exudative (acute) activity, which raises the intrapulpal pressure beyond threshold limits of high-threshold C fibers (Fig. 3-20, *B*). **B,** Higher magnification of outlined exudative area in **A.** **C,** Exudative (acute inflammatory response, showing congestion of erythrocytes *(ER)* in a dilated capillary. Polymorphonuclear leukocytes *(PL)* are at periphery (margination) and moving through the vessel wall (diapedesis). In addition to the vasodilation and polymorphonuclear leukocyte infiltration, this exudative response is characterized by edema spaces *(ED)* and lymphocytes *(L).* (From Coolidge ED, Kesel RG: *Endodontology,* ed 2, Philadelphia, 1956, Lea & Febiger.)

different when you tap it, but I'm not sure it hurts." Chronic pulpalgia is frequently associated with caries, particularly recurrent caries not readily discernible under an existing restoration. This is one reason why diagnosis is so difficult. Partial necrosis of the pulp, a frequent postoperative finding,

accounts for (1) the milder symptoms, (2) the mixed and frequently inconclusive responses to vitality tests, and (3) the intermittence of the painful episodes over many weeks or months.

Pain referral. Localization by the patient of both acute and chronic pulpalgia is difficult

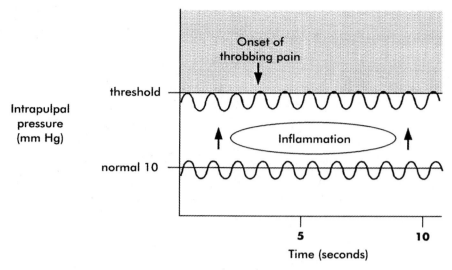

Fig. 3-46. Graphic interpretation of intrapulpal pressure and its relationship to throbbing pain from C nerve fibers. Normal intrapulpal pressure pulses at approximately a 10 mm Hg level. As inflammatory events cause intrapulpal pressure to rise and the peaks of the intrapulpal pressure pulse become suprathreshold, throbbing pain results.

because only pain receptors are found in the pulp. Localization is facilitated by the extension of the inflammatory response into the periapex, which contains both pain and pressure receptors. The pressure receptors of the periodontal ligament are also referred to as position sensors or proprioceptors (Fig. 3-13). Painful pulpitis may be referred to other areas of the same and opposing arches as well as to structures remote from the involved tooth. Glick has charted pain from mandibular premolars that was referred to maxillary molars, mandibular molars, or even to the mental and midramal areas. Pain from maxillary and mandibular molars may be referred into the body and angle of the mandible and to the ear (Fig. 3-26, *B*).

Examination of Table 3-10 reveals that (1) pain is referred to the opposite arch on the same side by posterior teeth only; (2) referral from incisor to posterior teeth, and vice versa, is not recorded; in their textbook *The Dental Pulp,* Seltzer and Bender observe that such referral seldom occurs with any of the anterior teeth; and (3) referral of pain across the midline is not recorded.

Experimental findings by Van Hassel and Harrington of electric pulp testing of 32 volunteers whose general and oral health was within normal limited demonstrated the following results:

1. Stimulation discrimination between the opposing arches was 95% accurate.

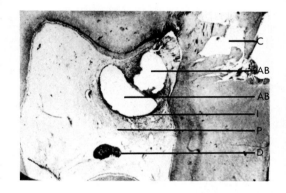

Fig. 3-47. Acute pulpitis (clinically, acute pulpalgia). Abscess *(AB)* in the zone of necrosis resulting from a carious exposure *(C)* is surrounded by the zone of contamination *(I)*. This exudative zone is characterized by vasodilation, fluid exudation (edema), and leukocyte infiltration. Proliferative (granulomatous) activity *(P)* has been initiated by diluted irritant in this area. Note denticle *(D)*. (From Coolidge ED, Kesel RG: *Endodontology,* ed 2, Philadelphia, 1956, Lea & Febiger.)

2. When the stimulus-localization choice was between two teeth in the same quadrant, teeth were correctly identified in 794 of 1014 tests (78%).

3. The ability to discriminate increases as the distance between the teeth increases.

Table 3-10. Referred pulpal pain

Site of pain referral	Tooth pulp initiating pain
Frontal (forehead) region	Maxillary incisors
Nasolabial area	Maxillary canines
	Maxillary premolars
Maxillary region above maxillary molars	Maxillary second premolars
	Maxillary first molars
Temporal region	Maxillary second premolars
Mandibular area below mandibular molars	Maxillary second and third molars
Ear	Mandibular molars
	Maxillary second and third molars (occasionally)
Mental region of mandible	Mandibular incisors, canines, and premolars
Angle of mandible	Mandibular first and second molars
Midramal region	Mandibular second premolars
Superior laryngeal area	Mandibular third molars
Maxillary premolars	Maxillary canines
Maxillary molars	Maxillary canines
	Mandibular premolars
Mandibular premolars	Maxillary canines
	Maxillary premolars
Mandibular first premolar	Mandibular first and second molars

Modified from Glick DH: *Oral Surg* 15:613, 1962.

4. Within the quadrant, posterior teeth in the mandible appear to have the greatest potential for erroneous identification.
5. Clinicians searching for the tooth responsible for poorly localized pain may rely with some confidence on the patient's choice as to quadrant.

(See discussion on mechanism of referred pain, p. 117, and Fig. 3-26).

Visual examination and history. Examination and review of the involved tooth may reveal previous symptoms or a traumatic experience.

Radiography and percussion. Radiographs may show the depth and extent of caries and restorations. The periapex usually has a normal configuration; however, a slight widening may be evident in the advanced stages of painful pulpitis as the periapical connective tissue begins to undergo the identical inflammatory changes demonstrated by the pulp during the incipient stage of pulpitis. Tenderness to percussion implies an *increased intraperiapical pressure as a result of hyperactive*

exudative (acute) inflammatory tissue. The term *acute pulpalgia* (or *acute pulpitis*) *with acute apical periodontitis* is applicable in this situation. Widening of the periodontal ligament space *without percussion tenderness* implies a nonpainful (chronic) state, and the term *acute pulpalgia* (or *acute pulpitis*) *with chronic apical periodontitis* may be used.

Vitality tests

THERMAL TEST. Irreversible pulpitis may respond in the same manner to thermal stimulation as reversible pulpitis (hyperalgesia), but the pain may persist after the stimulus is removed (Table 3-8). As pulpal inflammation progresses, heat will intensify the response because it has an expansive effect on the blood vessels, tissues, and gaseous products of proteolysis. Conversely, cold will tend to relieve the pain in advanced stages of pulpitis when coronal necrosis exists because it has a contractile effect on the remaining central or apical functional vascular bed, reducing the intrapulpal pressure below the threshold limits of excitability of still viable, more centrally located pain receptors (C fibers). Occasionally a patient will come to the office with a piece of ice in the mouth to relieve the pain, but as soon as the ice is removed, the pain intensifies as the increased intrapulpal pressure returns. Cold does not initiate pain in advanced pulpitis because the peripheral A-δ fibers in the inner dentin and in the dentinoblastic and subdentinoblastic zones are no longer viable and therefore are incapable of transmitting action potentials. Postoperative evaluation of this tissue usually demonstrates partial necrosis of varying degrees.

ELECTRIC TEST. A response to less current may be expected in the early stages because of the low threshold of the peripheral A-δ pain fibers. As the tissue becomes more necrotic, more current is required. Table 3-4 reveals that the electric pulp tester will activate only the A-δ fibers. This test may not be diagnostic in advanced cases of acute pulpalgia because of erratic mixed responses, particularly multirooted teeth.

Treatment. See Chapter 5.

Nonpainful pulpitis

Definition. Nonpainful pulpitis is an inflammatory response of pulpal connective tissue to an irritant. Here the *proliferative (chronic)* forces are hyperactive and play a dominant role. *Pain is absent because of diminished exudative inflammatory activity and a corresponding decrease in the intrapulpal pressure to a point below the threshold limits of pain receptors.*

Classification. Chronic inflammation signifies prolonged exudative changes and the appearance of granulation or granulomatous tissue peripheral to the exudative (acute) zones. This response immediately follows an acute inflammation or may develop from the onset when a low-grade irritation to the pulp is neutralized by effective tissue resistance. The term *chronic* implies a subthreshold intrapulpal pressure because the products of the exudative zone are (1) draining into the carious lesion, (2) being absorbed into the venous or lymphatic circulation, (3) moving (spreading, pointing) into an adjacent connective tissue area, or (4) utilizing any combination of these outlets for pressure release. Pressure against the pain receptors is below their threshold limits, and pain is absent. The term *nonpainful pulpitis* is applicable in this situation. When the strength of the irritant force is significantly reduced, the granulomatous tissue

response (proliferative) becomes hyperactive and dominates the scene in its attempt to heal and repair, even though exudative (acute) zones may still be present. Complete repair, however, cannot occur as long as the toxic agents are present. The predominant inflammatory cells are lymphocytes, plasma cells, and macrophages; however, PMNs may also be present.

Chronic pulpitis (ulcerative or open form). This is a chronic inflammation of the cariously exposed pulp characterized by the formation of an abscess at the point of exposure *(ulcer)*. The abscess is surrounded by granulomatous tissue (granulation tissue plus chronic inflammatory cells), and the terms *pulpal chronic abscess* or *pulpal granuloma* are also applicable to this inflammatory complex. The chronic inflammation may be *partial* or *total* depending on the extent of pulp tissue involvement (Fig. 3-48).

Chronic pulpitis (hyperplastic form). This chronic inflammation of the cariously exposed pulp is characterized by an overgrowth *(hyperplasia)* of granulomatous tissue into the carious cavity. The resultant *polyp* is usually lined by the stratified squamous epithelium of the oral mucosa (Figs. 3-49 and 3-50).

Chronic pulpitis (closed form: carious lesion absent). This may occur from operative procedures, trauma, or periodontal lesions extending apically to the foramina of lateral canals). *Excessive orthodontic movement* may affect the vascular supply to the pulp, producing localized areas of necrosis. Depending on the strength and duration of the inciting irritant, pulpitis may be chronic from the onset or become chronic after the exudative (acute) responses have subsided. (See discussion on etiologic factors of hyperemia, p. 141.) If pulpal damage is minimal, resolution of incipient chronic pulpitis may occur; however, the pulpitis may persist over long periods. Exacerbation is likely to occur if the teeth are subjected to additional operative procedures. Seeming resolution may leave a "scar" of denticles, diffuse calcifications, and increased irritation dentin, all of which diminish and obstruct the lumen of the pulp chamber and canal.

Etiology. The etiologic factors of nonpainful, chronic pulpitis are essentially the same as those for painful pulpitis. The nature of the pulpal response will depend on the strength and duration of the irritant, the previous health of the pulp, and the extent of tissue affected.

Histopathology and clinical symptoms

Chronic pulpitis (ulcerative). As the caries advances toward the pulp, both sclerotic dentin and irritation dentin are produced in an attempt to

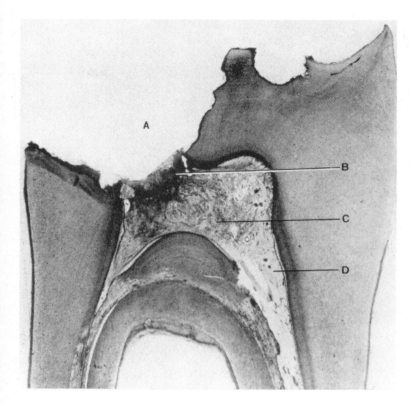

Fig. 3-48. Chronic ulcerative pulpitis (nonpainful pulpitis). This well-established chronic response shows the following: infected zone of necrosis at exposed pulpal surface *(A)*; exudative zone of contamination with dense PMN and lymphocytic infiltration *(B)*, which masks the edema and vasodilation; granulomatous zone of irritation *(C)*; and intact, noninflamed pulp tissue *(D)*. (From Coolidge ED, Kesel RG: *Endodontology,* ed 2, Philadelphia, 1956, Lea & Febiger.)

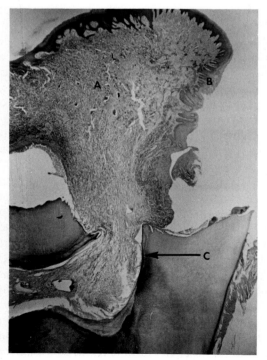

Fig. 3-49. Chronic pulpitis, hyperplastic form. Granulomatous tissue *(A)* has proliferated from pulp into carious cavity. Implanted epithelial cells from oral mucosa have established a stratified squamous covering *(B)* and an epithelial attachment to the pulp chamber wall *(C)*.

prevent exposure. When the slow-moving caries begins to destroy the defensive dentinal barrier, the irritation to the subjacent pulp tissue is mild, and a minimal amount of vasodilation and chronic mononuclear leukocyte infiltration (lymphocytes and machrophages) occurs. When the pulp is finally exposed, this regional vasodilation increases, followed by the exudative (acute) response. Cellular infiltration of neutrophils (PMNs) and inflammatory edema precede the ultimate abscess formation at the point of exposure (ulcer). Zone 1, the *zone of necrosis* (or *infection*), is now established. The inflamed tissue surrounding this ulcer contains the *exudative* (or *acute*) *inflammatory components* of zone II, the *zone of*

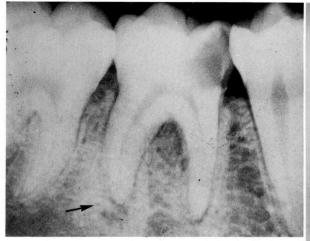
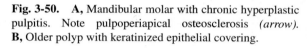

A

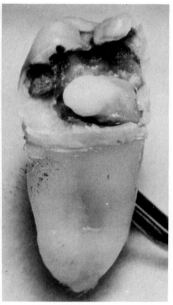

B

Fig. 3-50. **A,** Mandibular molar with chronic hyperplastic pulpitis. Note pulpoperiapical osteosclerosis *(arrow).* **B,** Older polyp with keratinized epithelial covering.

contamination (Fig. 3-48). As a result of the dilution of the toxic material and the antibacterial agents in zone II (see Table 4-2), the invading irritant has been downgraded. The stage is now set for the formation (proliferation) of the repair and healing tissue of zone III, the *zone of irritation.* Consequently, young fibroblasts and new capillaries develop and form granulation tissue in an attempt to replace the exudate in zone II and fill in any tissue gaps. This highly vascularized, new connective tissue represents the chronic or proliferative aspect of inflammation. It is a defense tissue as well as a healing and repair tissue. By itself, it is highly resistant to infection; a number of chronic mononuclear leukocytes are present, however, adding to the effectiveness of the defense response. These include lymphocytes and plasma cells (antibody source) and reserve cells and histiocytes (macrophage source). Because of the defense elements present, the term *granulomatous tissue* is substituted for *granulation tissue.* This pulpal "granuloma" then is mobilized to destroy the advance of microorganisms infiltrating from zones I and II. (See discussion of Kronfeld's "mountain pass concept," p. 179.) The total chronic response may be limited to the pulp

chamber only *(partial pulpitis),* with no evidence of affected tissue in the canal except for some vasodilation.

Pain is absent because the exudative (acute) forces of defense are not hyperactive and proliferative granulomatous (chronic) forces of repair dominate. The contaminant is under control. Since there is adequate drainage and absorption of the exudate, no buildup of intrapulpal pressure occurs. Painful symptoms develop if there is interference with the drainage by food packs or a sudden inoculation of the granulomatous tissue with contaminants. The resultant painful pulpitis is of the acute or subacute form.

Chronic pulpitis (hyperplastic). In an attempt to carry out its primary function of healing and repair, the granulomatous tissue of a young pulp with chronic ulcerative pulpitis may proliferate through a large carious exposure. Chronic hyperplastic pulpitis is usually found in teeth of children and adolescents, in which the pulp tissue has a high resistance, and large carious lesions permit free proliferation of the hyperplastic tissue. The polyp in the incipient stage is basically granulation tissue and appears as a pinkish red globule of tissue protruding from the pulp chamber. It varies in size and frequently fills the entire carious cavity. Few nerve fibers are present so it is relatively nonpainful to touch. The surface, however, is "raw" and bleeds easily when probed (Figs. 3-49 and 3-50, *B*).

Still-viable desquamated (exfoliated) epithelial cells from the oral mucosa may become implanted and grow on the rich granulation surface. As this polyp surface becomes covered with stratified squamous epithelium, the granulomatous tissue beneath may become less vascular, simulating the appearance of oral mucosa. In many cases an epithelial attachment to the pulp chamber or canal wall is evident. Theoretically, healing of the inflamed pulp is occurring; however, the carious destruction and inability to restore the tooth, with the polyp present, make endodontic treatment necessary.

Diagnosis.   Pain is absent except under the conditions previously described. Radiographic periapical evidence is lacking except when extensive or longstanding pulpal involvement may reveal an *incipient chronic apical periodontitis.* Frequently in young patients the low-grade longstanding irritation stimulates periapical bone deposition *(pulpoperiapical osteosclerosis; condensing osteitis).* Areas of dense bone develop around the apices of the involved teeth, usually mandibular molars with large carious lesions (Fig. 3-50, *A*; see also Fig. 4-5). (See discussion on pulpoperiapical osteoclerosis, p. 172.) Thermal and electric vitality tests may elicit normal responses. If the chronic response is extensive, greater stimulation than for the control tooth may be required. Visual examinations will reveal the caries or pulp polyp if present.

Treatment.   In cases of chronic hyperplastic pulpitis the polyp is first removed with a sharp curette before therapy is initiated on the remaining vital pulp tissue (Chapter 5).

Additional pulp changes

Pulp necrosis

Definition.   Necrosis or death of pulp tissue is a sequela of acute and chronic inflammation of the pulp or an immediate arrest of circulation by traumatic injury (Fig. 3-51). It may be partial or total depending on the extent of pulp tissue involvement.

Histopathology and clinical symptoms.   Two types of pulp necrosis may be observed: a flow of pus from an access cavity indicates *liquefaction necrosis,* which is associated with a good blood

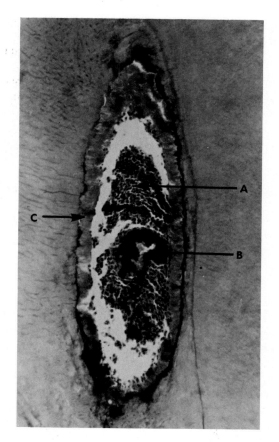

Fig. 3-51.   Tangential section showing canal with pulp necrosis. Masses of polymorphonuclear leukocytes *(A)* are seen, as well as a plaque of bacteria *(B).* Peripheral necrotic predentin *(C)* must be removed during canal preparation.

supply and inflammatory exudate (proteolytic enzymes have softened and liquefied the tissues); *coagulation necrosis* is associated with the diminishing or cutting off of the blood supply to an area *(ischemia).* The tissue can have the appearance of a soft solid mass, occasionally of a cheesy consistency (caseation), composed principally of coagulated protein, fats, and water. The products of necrosis are toxic to the periapical tissues and can initiate an inflammatory response and subsequent abscess formation without the presence of microorganisms.

Decomposition of proteins by anaerobic bacteria is termed *putrefaction.* Some of the poisonous intermediate and end products found in this decomposed (necrotic) and infected protein are as follows:

1. Intermediate proteolytic products, which emit a foul odor
   a. *Indole* and *skatole,* produced by deamination of tryptophan (i.e., loss of amine molecules from an amino acid)
   b. *Putrescine* and *cadaverine* (also referred to as *ptomaines*), from tryptophan decarboxylation (loss of carboxyl molecules of an amino acid)
   c. *Indican,* derived from indole (potassium indoxyl sulfate)
2. End products, such as hydrogen sulfide, ammonia, water, carbon dioxide, and fatty acids
3. Exotoxins that are secretions of bacteria
4. Endotoxins that are released when microorganisms are destroyed
5. Foreign bacterial protein

Diagnosis. Pain is absent in a tooth with total necrosis. Any pain associated with such a tooth emanates from the periapical tissues. Swelling, mobility, and response to percussion and palpation are negative unless associated with concomitant periapical inflammation. Radiographic findings are normal unless there is a concomitant apical periodontitis or pulpoperiapical osteoclerosis. There is no response to vitality tests. Sometimes a positive electric response is related to liquefaction necrosis, acting as an electrolytic transmitter to the periapex or to the presence of some residual viable pulpal nerve fibers (Tables 3-3 and 3-4). Multirooted teeth may present a mixed response because only one canal may contain totally necrotic tissue. There may be a definite color change because of altered coronal translucency. Discoloration may be caused by hemolysis of red blood cells or decomposition of pulp tissue. The history may reveal past trauma or past episodes of pain.

Treatment. See Chapter 5.

Retrogressive pulp changes. Attrition and abrasion, trauma, operative procedures, caries, pulp capping, and reversible pulpitis all induce changes in the pulp tissue that cannot be classified as inflammatory. Various terms such as *retrogressive, degenerative, aging, dystrophic, catabolic,* and *pulposis* have been applied. These altered pulp conditions are (1) atrophy and fibrosis and (2) dystrophic calcification (calcific metamorphosis).

Atrophy and fibrosis. Wasting away or decrease in size of an organ is usually attributable to faulty nutrition. Atrophic changes may occur slowly as the tooth grows older. Normal age changes in pulp tissue are characterized by a gradual shift in the ratio and quality of the tissue elements. Mature collagen fibers per unit area increase, and the size and number of pulp cells decrease (Fig. 3-52)

An increase in mature collagen fibers is called *fibrosis.* It occurs in aging connective tissue anywhere in the body, whether in the skin or in the spinal column. The fibrosis in the atrophied dental pulp may be so severe that the cells appear as shrunken solid particles in a sea of dense fibers. The fibroblasts have lost their processes and are rounded, with pyknotic (shrunken) nuclei. Even the dentinoblasts appear to be reduced in length, presenting a cuboidal and sometimes flattened appearance.

The speeding of the aging process is referred to as *induced aging* and may result from the hyperactive stimuli listed at the beginning of this section. Severe attrition (abrasion), for example, increases the production of irritation dentin and *decreases the size of the canal lumen.* At the same time, the apical canal and foramina may be diminished by the formation of periapical cementum, a compensatory mechanism for the occlusal wear. The net result is an altered blood flow to the pulp tissue (see Fig. 4-1).

As a result of diminished vascularity, the ground substance in aging pulps becomes increasingly dehydrated and viscous. Fewer new collagen fibers are being formed, but more of the older collagen fibers are present because they do not die off. Instead they accumulate *(accretion)* and crowd the environment, resembling crabgrass *(fibrosis).* The fibers seem to orient themselves and become bound together in larger bundles. The cells, unable to obtain enough nutrition and oxygen, are struggling for survival and unable to defend, heal, or repair effectively.

As a result of caries, a young person may already have a tooth with an aging and sick pulp. Operative procedures followed by pulp capping may now induce or speed up the aging process, with an increasing amount of irritation dentin (decreasing the size of the pulp chamber), fibrosis, and calcification. The patient's chronologic age therefore is not always an indication of the health or physiologic age of the pulp.

A study by Bernick and Nedelman demonstrated that in the aging process the following occurred:

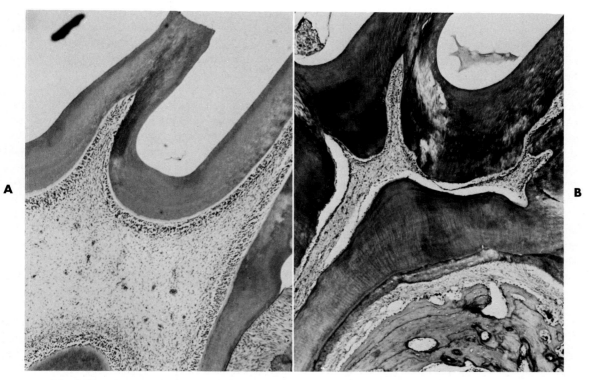

Fig. 3-52.   **A,** Normal pulpal connective tissue of a young rat molar (30 days). **B,** A 300-day-old rat molar showing reduced chamber and canal lumen, marked fibrosis, and diminution in cell size and number. (Courtesy Dr. Patrick Toto, Loyola University, School of Dentistry, Maywood, Ill.)

1. Progressive reduction in the size of the pulp chamber
2. Progressive deposition of calcium masses that originate in the root pulp and progress into the coronal pulp
3. Decrease in the nerves and blood vessels of the coronal pulp because of the calcification in these structures
4. Persistence of the connective tissue sheaths of the affected blood vessels and nerves, giving the pulp a fibrotic appearance

Calcifications. These are found in both healthy and aging pulps, although their incidence increases with age. Willman found calcifications in 87% of 164 teeth selected at random. Many of the calcifications (15%) were not discernible on a radiograph. Hill reported calcifications in 66% of all teeth in individuals between 10 and 20 years of age and 90% between 50 and 70 years of age. *Dystrophic calcification* is a deposition of calcium salts in dead or degenerating tissue. It may be due to local alkalinity of the destroyed tissue that attracts the salts. This mineralization thus may occur in minute areas of young pulp tissue affected by minor circulatory disturbance or in blood clots, or even in and around single degenerating cells.

Calcifications that begin in the connective tissue walls of blood vessels and nerves (Fig. 3-16, *C*) follow the course of these structures. When the deposits fuse, they become long, thin, and fibrillar. *Diffuse calcifications* are generally observed in the root canal but may also be seen in the pulp chamber. The larger, well-outlined denticles or stones develop more frequently in the pulp chamber. Pulp denticles are classified according to location (free, embedded, or attached) and according to structure (true or false). *Free denticles,* lying free in the chamber, may become attached or embedded as more dentin is laid down around them. *True denticles* are not dystrophic structures, since they are composed of dentin and formed by detached dentinoblasts or fragments of Hertwig's sheath, which may stimulate undifferentiated cells to assume dentinoblastic activity. *False denticles* are formed when a degenerating tissue structure serves as a nidus for deposition of concentric layers of calcified tissue. Calcifications usually are readily removed from the pulp chamber, but they may be a problem when present in the pulp canal. The use of chelating agents has greatly facilitated this procedure. Although not proved, it is improbable that pulpal pain results from the presence of the calcifications. Pain associated with affected teeth probably arises from the pulpal conditions responsible for the calcification.

Internal resorption. The term *idiopathic resorption* is used synonymously with internal resorption because the precise etiology is unknown. It is, however, generally believed that trauma or persistent chronic pulpitis is responsible for the formation of dentinoclasts by activating undifferentiated reserve connective tissue cells of the pulp. These cells fuse to form the multinucleated clastic cells, the same type that is observed during bone and cementum removal (osteoclasts and cementoclasts). Trauma may produce intrapulpal hemorrhage that can organize and be replaced by granulation (repair) tissue. Dentinoclasts differentiate when the growing granulation tissue compresses the wall of the pulp chamber or canal. The same process may occur after pulp capping or partial pulpectomy of a tooth with chronic pulpitis. Microscopic examination shows a scalloped dentinal wall in the affected area (Fig. 3-53). Multinucleated dentinoclastic cells are seen in these little bays (Howship's lacunae), and the entire region is filled with granulomatous (chronic) tissue. In addition, there may be several areas of repair of

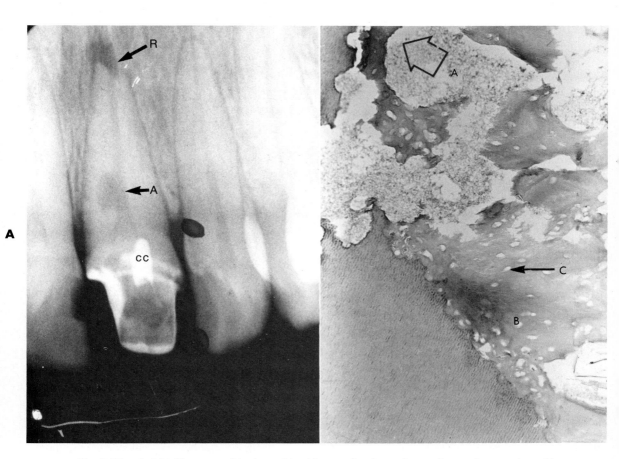

Fig. 3-53. **A,** Maxillary central incisor with a history of caries, pulp capping, and restoration with a jacket crown. Attempt was made to locate canal through a calcified chamber *(cc)*. Persistent chronic pulpal inflammation has produced internal resorption *(A)*. Note apical resorption *(R)*. **B,** Photomicrograph of internal resorption showing resorptive defects *(A)* and an attempt at repair by a tissue resembling bone *(B)* and containing numerous lacunae *(C)*.

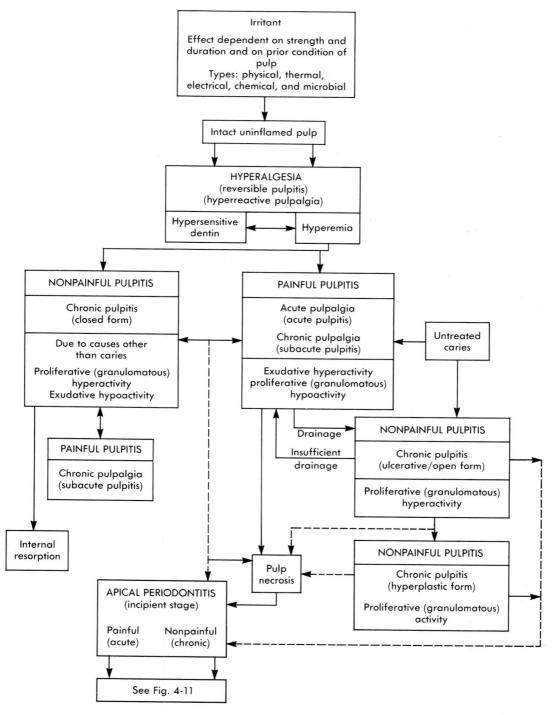

Fig. 3-54. Sequence of pulp pathosis related to inflammation. Refer also to Fig. 4-11 (sequence of pulpoperiapical pathoses related to inflammation).

the resorbed areas with an atypical dentin or bonelike tissue. These zones of resorption and repair are consistent with the patterns established in granulomatous and fibrous zones of irritation and stimulation (see Table 4-2).

When the resorption occurs in the pulp chamber, the red capillary granulations may be seen through the enamel (pink spots). Internal resorption in the root canal may perforate into the periodontal ligament. Diagnosis then is more difficult because of the possibility that the condition was initially external resorption that perforated the pulp canal.

Treatment of these teeth must be carried out immediately. To "wait and see" may mean the loss of the tooth or possible surgical intervention to retain it. During the inflammatory transition toward total necrosis of the pulp, episodes of internal resorption frequently occur (Fig. 3-54). *Once the pulp tissue dies, all internal resorption ceases.*

REFERENCES

Ahlberg KF: Influence of local noxious heat stimulation on sensory nerve activity in feline dental pulp, *Acta Physiol Scand* 103:71, 1978.

Anderson DJ: Chemical and osmotic excitants of pain in human dentine. In Anderson DJ, editor: Sensory mechanism in dentine, Oxford, 1963, Pergamon.

Anderson DJ, Naylor MN: Chemical excitations of pain in human dentin and pulp, *Arch Oral Biol* 7:413, 1962.

Andrews S, Van Hassel HJ, Brown A: Correlation between intrapulpal pressure and sensory response in pulpal pathoses (abstract), 49th General Session, International Association for Dental Research, March 1971.

Anneroth G, Nordberg KA: Adrenergic vasoconstrictors innervation in the human dental pulp, *Acta Odontol Scand* 26:83, 1968.

Aubin JE: New immunological approaches to studying the odontoblast, *J Dent Res* 64:515, April 1985.

Avery JK: Mechanism of reparative dentin formation and pain. In Grossman LI, editor: *Transactions of the Sixth International Conference on Endodontics,* Philadelphia, 1978, New York, 1979, Masson.

Avery JK: Repair potential of the pulp, *J Endod* 7:205, 1981.

Avery JK: The dental pulp. In Bhaskar SN, editor: *Orban's oral histology and embryology,* ed 3, St Louis, 1986, Mosby.

Avery JK, Cox CF, Chiego DJ: Presence and location of adrenergic nerve endings in the dental pulp of mouse molars, *Anat Rec* 198:59, 1980.

Baume LJ: The biology of pulp and dentine, *Monogr Oral Sci 8,* Basel, 1980, S Karger AG.

Bender IB: Pulp biology conference: a discussion, *J Endod* 4:37, 1978.

Bergenholtz G: Effect of bacterial products on inflammatory reactions in the dental pulp, *Scand J Dent Res* 85:122, 1977.

Bergenholtz G, Cox CF, Loesch WJ, Syed SA: Bacterial leakage around dental restorations: its effect on the dental pulp, *J Oral Pathol* 11:439, 1982.

Bernick S: Vascular supply to developing teeth of rats, *Anat Rec* 137:141, 1960.

Bernick S: Differences in nerve distribution between erupted and non-erupted human teeth, *J Dent Res* 43:406, 1964.

Bernick S: Age changes to the blood supply of human teeth, *J Dent Res* 46:544, 1967.

Bernick S: Morphologic changes to lymphatic vessels in pulpal inflammation, *J Dent Res* 56:841, 1977.

Bernick S, Nedelman C: Effect of aging on the human pulp, *J Endod* 1:88, 1975.

Beveridge EE, Brown AC: The measurement of human dental intrapulpal pressure and its response to clinical variables, *Oral Surg* 19:655, 1965.

Bhaskar SN, editor: *Orban's oral histology and embryology,* ed 10, St Louis, 1985, Mosby.

Brännström, M: The transmission and control of dentinal pain. In Grossman LI, editor: *Transactions of the Sixth International Conference on Endodontics,* Philadelphia, 1978, New York, 1979, Masson.

Brännström M: Dentin and pulp in restorative dentistry, London, 1982, Wolfe Medical.

Brännström, M: Communication between the oral cavity and the dental pulp associated with restorative treatment, *Oper Dent* 9:57, 1984.

Brännström M: Smear layer: pathological and treatment considerations, *Oper Dent Suppl* 3:35, 1984.

Brännström M: The cause of postrestorative sensitivity and its prevention, *J Endod* 12:475, 1986.

Brännström M: The hydrodynamic theory of dentinal pain: sensation in preparations, caries, and the dentinal crack syndrome. *J Endod* 12:453, 1986.

Brännström M, Åström A: The hydrodynamics of the dentin: its possible relationship to dentinal pain, *Int Dent J* 22:219, 1972.

Brännström M, Garberoglio R: The dentinal tubules and the odontoblastic processes, *Acta Odontol Scand* 30:291, 1972.

Brännström M, Johnsson G: Movement of the dentin and pulp liquids on application of thermal stimuli, *Acta Odontol Scand* 28:59, 1970.

Brännström M, Johnsson G: The sensory mechanism in human dentin as revealed by evaporation and mechanical removal of dentin, *J Dent Res* 57:49, 1978.

Chien S: Hemodynamics of the dental pulp, *J Dent Res* 64:602, 1985.

Copron RE, Avery JK: Ultrastructure of odontoblasts in dentinal tubules, *J Dent Res* 50:511, 1971.

Dewhirst FE, Goodson JM: Prostaglandin synthetase inhibition by eugenol, guaiacol and other dental medicaments (abstract 199), *J Dent Res* 53(spec iss):104, 1974.

Edwall LG: Pulpal blood flow. Paper presented at the Pulp Biology Conference, Philadelphia, March 1977.

Fearnhead RW: The neurohistology of human dentine, *Proc R Soc Med* 54:877, 1961.

Fearnhead RW: The histological demonstration of nerve fibers in human dentine. In Anderson DJ, editor: *Sensory mechanisms in dentine,* New York, 1963, MacMillan.

Fish WE: *Surgical pathology of the mouth,* Philadelphia, 1951, Lippincott.

Fox LT, Senia ES, Zeagler J: Another look at the odontoblast process, *J Endod* 10:538, 1984.

Frank RM: Attachment sites between the odontoblast process and the intradentinal nerve fibers, *Arch Oral Biol* 13:833, 1968.

Frank RM, Wolfe F, Gutmann B: Microscopie electronique de la carie au niveau de la dentine humaine, *Arch Oral Biol* 9:163, 1964.

Garant PR: The organization of microtubules within rat odontoblast processes revealed by perfusion fixation with glutaraldehyde, *Arch Oral Biol* 17:1047, 1972.

Garant PR, Cho MI: Ultrastructure of the odontoblast. In Butler WT, editor: *The chemistry and biology of mineralized tissues*, Birmingham, 1985, EBSCO Media.

Garant P, Szab G, Nalbandian J: The fine structure of the mouse odontoblast, *Arch Oral Biol* 13:857, 1968.

Garberoglio R, Brännström M: Scanning electron microscopic investigations of human dentinal tubules, *Arch Oral Biol* 21:355, 1976.

Glick DH: Locating referred pulpal pains, *Oral Surg* 15:613, 1962.

Greenhill JD, Pashley DH: The effects of desensitizing agents on the hydraulic conduction of human dentin in vitro, *J Dent Res* 60:686, 1981.

Grossman L: *Endodontic practice,* ed 10, Philadelphia, 1981, Lea & Febiger.

Gunji T: Morphological research on the sensitivity of dentin, *Arch Histol Jap* 45:45, 1982.

Gunji T, Kobayashi S: Distribution and organization of odontoblast processes in human dentin, *Arch Histol Jap* 46:213, 1983.

Heyeraas KJ: Pulpal, microvascular and tissue pressure, *J Dent Res* 64:585, 1985.

Hill T: *Oral pathology,* ed 4, Philadelphia, 1949, Lea & Febiger.

Hirvonen TJ, Närhi M, Hakumäki M: The excitability of dog pulp nerves in relation to the condition of dentin surface, *J Endod* 10:294, 1984.

Holland GR: Membrane junctions on cat odontoblasts, *Arch Oral Biol* 20:551, 1975.

Holland GR: Lanthanum hydroxide labelling of gap junctions in the odontoblast layer, *Anat Rec* 186:121, 1976.

Holland GR: Non-myelin nerve fibers and their terminals in the subodontoblastic plexus of feline dental pulp, *J Anat* 130:457, 1980.

Holland GR: Nerves in dentine. In Lisney SJ, Mathews B, editors: *Current topics in oral biology,* Bristol, Great Britain, 1985, University of Bristol Press.

Holland GR: The odontoblast process: form and function, *J Dent Res* 64:499, 1985.

Holland GR: Odontoblasts and nerves: just friends. In *Proceedings of the Finnish Dental Society,* Helsinki, Nov 1986.

Hume WR: An analysis of the release and the diffusion through dentin of eugenol from zinc oxide–eugenol mixtures, *J Dent Res* 63:881, 1984.

Iguchi Y et al: Intercellular junctions in odontoblasts of the rat incisor studied with freeze-fracture, *Arch Oral Biol* 29:487, 1984.

Ingle JI: Differential diagnosis and treatment of oral and perioral pain. In Ingle JI, editor: *Endodontics,* ed 3, Philadelphia, 1985, Lea & Febiger.

Inoki R, Kudo T, Olgart L: Dynamic aspects of dental pulp—molecular biology, pharmacology and pathophysiology, New York, 1990, Chapman and Hall.

Johnsen DC: Innervation of teeth: qualitative, quantitative and developmental assessment, *J Dent Res* 64:555, 1985.

Johnsen DC, Harshbarger J, Rymer HD: Quantitative assessment of neural development in human premolars, *Anat Rec* 205:421, 1983.

Johnson G, Olgart L, Brännström M: Outward fluid flow in dentin under a physiologic pressure gradient: experiments in vitro, *Oral Surg* 35:238, 1973.

Khayat BG et al: Responses of nerve fibers to pulpal inflammation and periapical lesions in rat molars demonstrated by calcitonin gene-related peptide immunocytochemistry, *J Endod* 14:577, 1988.

Kim S: Regulation of pulpal blood flow, *J Dent Res* 64:590, 1985.

Kim S: Microcirculation of the dental pulp in health and disease, *J Endod* 11:465, 1985.

Kim S: Neurovascular interactions in the dental pulp in health and disease, *J Endod* 16:48, 1990.

Kim S: Pulpal blood flow. Paper presented at the Pulp Biology Conference, Philadelphia, March 1977.

Kim S, Lipowsky HH, Usami S, Chien S: Arteriovenous distribution of hemodynamic parameters in the rat dental pulp, *Microvasc Res* 27:28, 1984.

Kogushi M et al: A study of leukocyte extravasation in early inflammatory changes in the pulp, *J Endod* 14:475, 1988.

Kramer IRH: Vascular architecture of the human dental pulp, *Arch Oral Biol* 2:177, 1960.

Langeland K: The histopathologic basis in endodontic treatment, *Dent Clin North Am,* Nov 1967, p 491.

Liebman F: Pain and pressure in the human pulp, *Oral Surg* 33:122, 1972.

Lilja J: Innervation of different parts of the predentin and dentin in young human premolars, *Acta Odontol Scand* 37:339, 1979.

Lilja J, Nordenvall K, Brännström M: Dentin sensitivity: odontoblasts and nerves under desiccated or infected experimental cavities, *Swed Dent J* 6:93, 1982.

Linde A: The extracellular matrix of the dental pulp and dentin, *J Dent Res* 64:523, 1985.

Lowenstein WR: Cellular communication through membrane junctions, *Arch Intern Med* 129:299, 1972.

Lundy T, Stanley HR: Correlation of pulpal histopathology and clinical symptoms in human teeth subjected to experimental irritation, *Oral Surg* 27:187, 1969.

Melzack R, Wall PD: Pain mechanism: a new theory, *Science* 150:971, 1965.

Menke R, Weine F, Ulinski P, Smulson M: An autoradiographic demonstration of trigeminal nerve terminations in a rat's tooth, *J Endod* 3:128, 1977.

Michelich VJ, Schuster GS, Pashley DH: Bacterial penetration of human dentin in vitro, *J Dent Res* 59:1398, 1980.

Mjör, IA: Reaction patterns in human teeth, Boca Raton, Fla, 1983, CRC Press.

Mjör IA: Dentin-predentin complex and its permeability: pathology and treatment overview, *J Dent Res* 64:621, 1985.

Mumford JM: *Orofacial pain,* ed 3, New York, 1982 Churchill Livingstone.

Mumford JM: The role of restorative treatment in the genesis of hypersensitive teeth. In Rowe NH, editor: *Proceedings of Symposium on Hypersensitive Dentin: Origin and Management,* Ann Arbor, Nov 1985, University of Michigan.

Närhi MV: The characteristics of intradental sensory units and their responses to stimulation, *J Dent Res* 64:564, 1985.

Närhi MV: Evaluations of the methods used to test the sensitivity of teeth. In Rowe NH, editor: *Proceeding of symposium on Hypersensitive Dentin: Origin and Management,* Ann Arbor, Nov 1985, University of Michigan.

Närhi MV et al: Activation of heat sensitive nerve fibers in the dental pulp of the cat, *Pain* 14:317, 1982.

Ochi K, Matsumoto K: A morphological study of dentinal nerve endings, *J Endod* 12:601, 1988.

Olgart LM: Excitation of intradental sensory units by pharmacological agents, *Acta Physiol Scand* 92:48, 1974.

Olgart LM: The role of local factors in dentin and pulp in intradental pain mechanisms, *J Dent Res* 64:572, 1985.

Pashley DH: Smear layer: physiological considerations, *Oper Dent Suppl* 3:13, 1984.

Pashley DH: Dentin permeability, dentin sensitivity, and treatment through tubule occlusion, *J Endod* 12:465, 1986.

Pashley D: Clinical considerations of microleakage, *J Endod* 16:70, 1990.

Pashley DH, Kepler EE, Williams EL, Okabe A: Progressive decrease in dentine permeability following cavity preparation, *Arch Oral Biol* 28:853, 1983.

Pohto M, Scheinin A: Microscopic observations on living dental pulp, *Acta Odontol Scand* 16:303, 1958.

Polito P, Antila R: Innervation of blood vessels in the dental pulp, *Int Dent J* 22:228, 1972.

Provenza D: *Oral histology: inheritance and development,* ed 2, Philadelphia, 1986, Lippincott.

Rapp R, Avery JD, Strachan DS: The distribution of nerves in human primary teeth, *Anat Rec* 159:89, 1967.

Reeves R, Stanley HR: The relationship of bacterial penetration and pulpal pathosis in carious teeth, *Oral Surg* 22:59, 1966.

Ruch JV: Odontoblast differentiation and the formation of the odontoblast layer, *J Dent Res* 64:489, 1985.

Rugh TV: Visceral sensation and referred pain. In Fulton JF, editor: *Howell's textbook of physiology,* Philadelphia, 1947, Saunders.

Salzberg BM: New approaches to the neurophysiology of the dental pulp, *J Dent Res* 64:597, 1985.

Sarnat H, Massler M: Microstructure of active and arrested dentinal caries, *J Dent Res* 44:1389, 1965.

Scott D: Physiologic considerations in the arousal of pain in teeth. Paper presented at the Workshop on Mechanisms of Pain and Sensitivity in the Teeth and Supporting Tissues, Nov 1973, Fairleigh Dickinson University, Hackensack, NJ.

Seltzer S: Reparative dentinogenesis, *Oral Surg* 12:595, 1959.

Seltzer S: Hypothetic mechanisms for dentin sensitivity, *Oral Surg* 31:387, 1971.

Seltzer S, Bender IB: *The dental pulp,* ed 3, Philadelphia, 1984, Lippincott.

Seltzer S, Bender IB, Ziontz M: The dynamics of pulp inflammation: correlations between diagnostic data and actual histologic findings in the pulp, *Oral Surg* 16:846, 969, 1963.

Sessle BJ: Recent developments in pain research: central mechanisms of orofacial pain and its control, *J Endod* 12:435, 1986.

Sicher H: The odontoblast, *Bur* 54:2, 1953.

Sigal MJ, Aubin JC, Ten Cate AR, Pitaru S: The odontoblast process extends to the dentinoenamel junction: an immunocytochemical study of rat dentine, *J Histochem Cytochem* 32:872, 1984.

Smith DC, Reese ND: Acidity of glass ionomer cements during setting and its relation to pulp sensitivity, *J Am Dent Assoc* 112:654, 1986.

Stanley HR: Reaction of the human pulp to cavity preparation: results produced by eight different operative grinding technics, *J Am Dent Assoc* 58:49, 1959.

Stanley HR: Biologic effects of various cutting methods in cavity preparation: the part pressure plays in pulpal response, *J Am Dent Assoc* 61:450, 1960.

Stanley HR: Design for a human pulp study, *Oral Surg* 25:633, 756, 1968.

Stanley HR: Pulpal responses: In Cohen S, Burns R, editors: *Pathways of the pulp,* ed 3, St Louis, 1984, Mosby.

Stanley HR: Pulpal responses to conditioning and bonding agents, *J Esthetic Dent* 5:208, 1993.

Stanley H, Broom CA, Spiegel EH, Schultz MS: Detecting dentural sclerosis in decalcified sections with the Pollak triderome connective tissue stain, *J Oral Pathol* 9:359, 1980.

Stanley HR et al: The detection and prevalence of reactive and physiologic dentin, sclerotic dentin, reparative dentin and dead tracts beneath various types of dental lesions according to tooth surface and age, *J Pathol* 12:257, 1983.

Takahashi K: Vascular architecture of dog pulp using corrosion resin casts examined under a scanning electron microscope, *J Dent Res* 64:579, 1985.

Takahashi K: Changes in the pulpal vasculature during inflammation, *J Endod* 16:92, 1990.

Takahashi K, Kishi Y, Kim S: A scanning electron microscopic study of the blood vessels of dog pulp using corrosion resin casts, *J Endod* 8:131, 1982.

Tanaka T: The origin and localization of dentinal fluid in developing rat molar teeth studied with lanthanum as a tracer, *Arch Oral Biol* 25:153, 1980.

Thomas HF: The extent of the odontoblast process in human dentin, *J Dent Res* 58:2207, 1979.

Thomas HF: The dentin-predentin complex and its permeability: anatomical overview, *J Dent Res* 64:607, 1985.

Tönder KJH: Vascular reactions in the dental pulp during inflammation, *Acta Odontol Scand* 41:247, 1983.

Tönder KJH, Kvinnsland I: Micropuncture measurements of interstitial fluid pressure in normal and inflamed dental pulp in cats, *J Endod* 9:105, 1983.

Tönder KJH, Naess G: Microvascular pressure in the dental pulp and gingiva in cats, *Acta Odontol Scand* 37:161, 1979.

Trowbridge HO: Pathogenesis of pulpitis resulting from dental caries, *J Endod* 7:52, 1981.

Trowbridge HO: Pulp histology and physiology. In Cohen S, Burns R, editors: *Pathways of the pulp,* ed 3, St Louis, 1984, The C. V. Mosby Co.

Trowbridge H: Mechanisms of pain induction in hypersensitive teeth. In Towe NH, editor: *Proceedings of Symposium on Hypersensitive Dentin: Origin and Management,* Nov 1985, Ann Arbor, University of Michigan.

Trowbridge HO: Intradental sensory units: physiological and clinical aspects, *J Endod* 11:489, 1985.

Trowbridge HO, Edwall L, Panopoulos P: Effect of zinc oxide–eugenol and calcium hydroxide on intradental nerve activity, *J Endod* 8:403, 1982.

Trowbridge H, Emling C: *Inflammation, a review of the process,* ed 2, Bristol, Pa, 1983, Comsource/Distribution Systems.

Van Hassel HJ: Physiology of the human dental pulp, *Oral Surg* 32:126, 1971.

Van Hassel HJ, Ervin M: Correlation of sensory response with intrapulpal temperature and pressure, *IADR abstract no* 342, 1973.

Van Hassel HJ, Harrington GW: Localization of pulpal sensation, *Oral Surg* 28:753, 1969.

Wakasaki S: Neuropeptides in the dental pulp: distribution, origins, and correlation, *J Endod* 16:67, 1990.

Weber DF: Human dentinal sclerosis: a micrographic survey, *Arch Oral Biol* 19:163, 1974.

White RK et al: A study of the odontoblast process with transmission electron microscopy, *Oral Surg* 62:569, 1986.

Willman W: Calcifications of the pulp, *Bur* 34:73, 1934.

Yamada M: Electrophysiological studies of excitation of dentin evoked by chemical means. In Anderson DF, editor: *Sensory mechanisms in dentine,* Oxford, 1963, Pergamon.

Yamada M: Recording of nerve potential, *Int Dent J* 19:239, 1969.

Zhang J, Iijima T, Tanaka T: Scanning electron microscopic observation of the vascular wall cells in human dental pulp, *J Endod* 19:55, 1993.

Marshall H. Smulson • James C. Hagen • Susan J. Ellenz

4 Pulpoperiapical pathology and immunologic considerations

HISTOPHYSIOLOGY OF THE PERIAPEX

The apical periodontium consists of root cementum, periodontal ligament, and the bone of the alveolar process—all interdependent tissues.

Cementum

Along the coronal two thirds of the root, the cementum is thin and lamellated; as a result of greater functional stresses, cementum in the apical third is wider, irregularly lamellated, and at times quite cellular (Fig. 4-1). Although its basic function is to attach the principal fibers of the periodontal ligament to the tooth, cementum has a number of other functions that can and do affect endodontic diagnosis and treatment:

1. The continuous deposition of cellular cementum around the apical third of the root (passive eruption) compensates for coronal attrition. This deposition results in increased tooth length and multiple constricted apical canals. Excessive constriction of the apical canals can affect the blood flow into the pulp and induce retrogressive or age changes. (See discussion on retrogressive pulp changes, p. 158.) Even though the root length is increased, the working length may decrease proportionately if the cementodentinal junction is the criterion for measurement. Continuous deposition of apical cementum after filling of the root canal will, in time, increase the distance between that junction and the apex of the root (Fig. 4-1).

2. The terminal area for intracanal preparation is the cementodentinal junction, which is usually estimated to be 1 mm from the apical foramen and more than 1 mm in older teeth. Cementum lines the canal in this area and may even overlap into the dentinal portion of the canal; thus the cementodentinal junction is the narrowest (minor) diameter of the canal and may also be referred to as the *histologic foramen* because it represents the junction

of pulpal connective tissue with the interstitial loose connective tissue of the periodontal ligament. This *minor diameter* may aid in locating the terminal canal position for intracanal instrumentation. For obliteration procedures, it provides a bottleneck area where an *apical dentin matrix* may be established to prevent overextension of the filling materials. (See discussion of apical anatomy and its effect on canal preparation, Chapter 7.)

3. Cementum repairs root resorption, which is pathologically produced by a granuloma or physiologically induced by the drifting movement of teeth (migration). As a result of the resorption followed by cementum replacement in migrating teeth, the apical foramen may be changed to a more lateral position.

4. The loss of cementum from the cervical position of the tooth may render the tooth hypersensitive to thermal change because of the exposed dentinal tubules. This may complicate identification of an approximating tooth requiring endodontic treatment.

5. Michanowicz et al. and Andreason and Hjörting-Hansen have shown evidence to support the cementogenic theory of root repair. Continuous deposition of cementum can occur at the fractured ends of two segments of a horizontal root fracture, joining them and effecting root repair.

6. Torneck et al., Heithersay, and others have shown that cementum contributes significantly to the hard tissue barrier formed at the root end as a result of apexification procedures (Chapter 16).

Periodontal ligament

The periodontal ligament consists of two different tissues, each with separate and distinct functions: (1) a suspensory ligament and (2) a periosteum. The suspensory ligament is made up of regularly arranged, dense connective tissue colla-

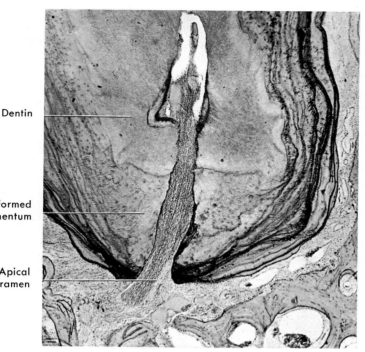

Dentin

Apex formed
by cementum

Apical
foramen

Fig. 4-1. Increase in root length and constriction of the apical canal due to increased cementum deposition around root apex. Note cementodentinal junction and coalescence of pulpal and periapical connective tissues. (From Bhaskar SN: *Orban's oral histology and embryology,* ed 11, St Louis, 1991, Mosby.)

gen fibers (principal fibers) that pass from cementum to bone (see Fig. 3-13). The spaces (interstices) between the principal fiber bundles are occupied by irregular loose connective tissue. This interstitial loose connective tissue performs the multiple functions of periosteum: formative, nutritive, nervous, and defense. The histologic makeup of these tissues provides several endodontic considerations.

Nervous function. Pressure receptors terminate in and around the bundles of principal fibers; thus the ligament portion provides a sensory function of proprioception or position localization. The interstitial loose connective tissue contains the free nerve endings that are the specific receptors for pain. Identifying a tooth with acute pulpalgia is difficult because only pain receptors are evident in the pulp. Localization of the pain is facilitated by the extension of the inflammatory response into the periapex (acute apical periodontitis), which activates both pain and proprioceptive responses.

Mobility. According to Sicher, individual *principal fibers* do not run a continuous uninterrupted course from bone to cementum but become disoriented midway to form an intermingling, splicing, or braiding relationship. He called this arrangement an "intermediate plexus." Although subsequent studies provide no support for the existence of a definitive plexus, there is no other explanation for tooth mobility (not related to bone loss) except the lack of fiber continuity from bone to cementum.

Certainly, as Sicher points out, "such movement cannot be due to the separation of Sharpey's fibers from their insertion sites." Even an avulsed tooth will not perform this feat. According to Melcher, the fibers run from one bundle to another and are probably spliced with or incorporated into their new neighbors.

Pressure from pulpoperiapical inflammation exerted against the tooth is, in turn, transmitted to the periodontal ligament. The upward pull in the intertwining fibers may cause an unwinding (disassociation) that results in tooth mobility, even though there may be ample bony support. Stability of the tooth may return within hours after the periapical pressure has been relieved.

Pulpoperiodontal junction. Pulp tissue response to an irritant does not necessarily end at a "magical" point of demarcation called the apical foramen. The connective tissue of the pulp forms a continuum (coalescence) with interstitial loose connective tissue of the periodontal ligament at the juncture of root canal foramina and continues into the marrow spaces. An inflamed vital pulp therefore may be accompanied by tenderness to percussion with or without radiographic evidence of periapical change.

Periapical cyst formation. Remnants of Hertwig's epithelial root sheath remain in the interstitial loose connective tissue as clusters of cells called *rests of Malassez*. These cells remain dormant until activated by periapical inflammation to play a principal role in cyst formation. (See discussion on periapical cyst, p. 175.)

Alveolar bone

The alveolar process consists of the *alveolar bone proper* and the *supporting bone*. The alveolar bone proper is the thin layer of compact bone that lines the socket. It appears as a radiopaque line on the radiograph and is referred to as the *lamina dura* (hard layer). The intensity of this radiopacity will vary with the angle of the x rays and the diameter of the root (Fig. 4-2). The alveolar bone proper is made up of lamellated bone. The lamellae are arranged parallel with the surface of the periodontal ligament space, as well as in small haversian systems. Sicher used the term *bundle bone* to describe alveolar bone containing the attachment of the principal fiber bundles (Sharpey's fibers).

The term *cribriform plate* has been used to describe the alveolar bone proper because a surface view shows a sievelike appearance (see Fig. 3-1). The many openings are due to perforations by interalveolar nerves and blood vessels as well as the coalescence of the interstitial loose connective tissue of the periodontal ligament with the loose connective tissue of the marrow spaces. Since the cribriform nature makes the periodontal ligament space less confining than the noncompli-

ant environment of the pulp chamber and root canal, the pain from inflammatory pressure may be less intense than pulpal pain. In addition, during stress periods, osteoclastic cells are found to increase this space. Persistent periapical inflammation will result in resorption of the periapical lamina dura. Radiographic detection of disruption in the continuity of this compact bone is an effective diagnostic aid. However, the absence of a break in the lamina dura does not rule out the presence of an early periradicular inflammatory lesion. In addition, radiographic evidence lags behind the actual degree of tissue destruction. It is estimated that at least a 30% to 50% loss of minerals from bone is needed to make the lesions become visible on the radiograph.

The supporting bone that surrounds and gives support to the alveolar bone proper of the tooth socket consists of the facial and lingual cortical plates of compact bone and the intervening spongy or trabecular bone. In their study of experimental bone lesions, Bender and Seltzer demonstrated the following:

1. If a lesion does not encroach on the junction between the cortical bone and the cancellous bone, it will not be visible on the radiograph. A lesion around the mesial root of a lower first molar would become more readily visible on a radiograph than would a distal root because it is usually closer to the cortical plate.
2. The angulation of the x rays will determine the accuracy of interpretation of the healing or breakdown of clinical lesions.

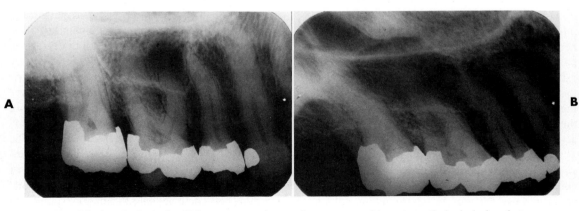

Fig. 4-2. A, Periapical radiolucency superimposed over root end is not a pathologic lesion, but a buccal extension of the maxillary sinus. **B,** Intact periodontal ligament space and lamina dura evident in angled radiograph confirm the diagnosis.

The trabecular (cancellous) bone has a septal or labyrinthine arrangement of bone lamellae, with its marrow forming a continuum with the interstitial loose connective tissue of the periodontal ligament. Since specific receptors for pain are not present in the trabecular spaces, the feeling associated with extension of the inflammatory response into the marrow spaces is one of fullness or continuing pressure. Pain receptors present in the blood vessel sheaths or pressure on nerves passing through the area may give referred sensation.

Pain receptors, however, are numerous in the periosteum that covers the cortical plates and in the specialized periosteum of the periodontal ligament, which is the *interstitial loose connective tissue.* Pressure in these areas produces pain of varying intensities. A patient with an acute periapical abscess may tolerate this more readily than pulpal pain because the environment is less confining, which permits inflammatory pressures to be dispersed more readily. However, sudden increases in periapical (or periradicular) pressure from percussion and mastication will result in episodes of sharp and jolting pain.

Pulpoperiapical disease (periapical pathoses of pulpal origin)

Review Table 3-6, Fig. 3-54, and discussion on types of inflammation, p. 139.
1. Painful pulpoperiapical pathoses
    a. Incipient acute apical periodontitis
    b. Advanced acute apical periodontitis
       (1) Acute periapical abscess
       (2) Recrudescent abscess (acute exacerbation of advanced chronic apical periodontitis)
       (3) Subacute periapical abscess: painful phase of the chronic periapical abscess cycle
2. Nonpainful pulpoperiapical pathoses
    a. Pulpoperiapical osteosclerosis (condensing osteitis, sclerosing osteitis)
    b. Incipient chronic apical periodontitis
    c. Advanced chronic apical periodontitis
       (1) Periapical granuloma*
       (2) Chronic periapical abscess (nonpainful phase)
       (3) Periapical cyst*
3. Refer to Table 4-1 and Fig. 4-11.

*Not identifiable clinically; therefore the term *advanced chronic apical periodontitis* should be used until there is confirmation from biopsy findings.

Painful pulpoperiapical pathoses

Painful pulpoperiapical pathoses are inflammatory responses of the periapical connective tissue to pulpal irritants in which the exudative (acute) forces become hyperactive and play a dominant role. The painful symptoms are caused by a great increase in intraperiapical pressure as well as algogenic mediators released by the injured cells.

Acute apical periodontitis. This is the incipient (initial) exudative and mildly symptomatic inflammatory reaction of the periapical connective tissues. It is caused by contaminants from the pulp canal, which produce vasodilation, fluid exudation, and white cell infiltration in the periapex (Fig. 4-3).

Acute periapical abscess. The acute periapical abscess is an advanced exudative and severely symptomatic inflammatory response of the periapical connective tissues (Fig. 4-4). It is caused by contaminants from the pulp canal that produce a steadily increasing amount of inflammatory exudate (edema), leukocyte infiltration, and suppuration. (Refer to definition of exudative [acute], p. 139.)

Recrudescent abscess (phoenix abscess). An acute periapical exacerbation that *arises from a previously existing chronic (granulomatous) lesion* develops as the granulomatous zone becomes contaminated or infected by elements from the root canal (zone of necrosis). Diagnosis is based on the acute symptoms plus radiographic examination, which reveals a large periapical radiolucency. (Refer to Kronfeld's mountain pass concept, p. 179.)

Subacute periapical abscess. This is the painful phase of a *chronic periapical abscess cycle.* During the nonpainful phase of the chronic periapical abscess, the pain and swelling readily regress because there is drainage through the stoma (mouth) of the *sinus tract.* When the sinus tract becomes blocked with coagulum and/or proliferation of mucosal epithelium over the stoma, drainage ceases, periapical pressure increases, and the tooth becomes mildly tender to percussion. The inflammation may now spread to the soft tissue adjacent to the sinus tract stoma. The pressure causes the tissue to balloon outward. A *parulis* (gumboil) develops on the mucosa, and the gingiva may develop a circumscribed red swelling. The exudative changes of acute inflammation are present, as are the proliferative changes characteristic of chronic inflammation. There is a delicate interplay for the dominance of one phase over the other. Symptoms, when present, are generally mild and of low intensity.

Table 4-1. Comparative terminology and classification of pulpoperiapical pathoses

Classification used at Loyola University	Ingle's classification
Painful pulpoperiapical pathoses	
1. *Incipient* acute apical periodontitis (describes the beginning stage only)	1. Acute apical periodontitis
2. Advanced acute apical periodontitis (describes the advanced, more symptomatic stages only)	2. *Terms listed below describe advanced stages of acute apical periodontitis:*
a. Acute periapical abscess	a. Acute apical abscess
b. Recrudescent abscess (acute exacerbation of prior existing advanced chronic apical periodontitis)	b. Phoenix abscess (acute exacerbation of prior existing chronic lesion)
c. Subacute periapical abscess (*painful* phase of the chronic periapical abscess cycle)	c. Suppurative apical periodontitis (chronic apical abscess) (terms used to describe both painful and nonpainful phases of the chronic apical abscess cycle)
Nonpainful pulpoperiapical pathoses	
1. Pulpoperiapical osteosclerosis	1. Condensing osteitis
2. *Incipient* chronic apical periodontitis (describes the beginning stage only)	2. Chronic apical periodontitis (describes both incipient and advanced stages)
3. Advanced chronic apical periodontitis (describes the more extensive stages)	3. Chronic apical periodontitis (describes both incipient and advanced stages)
a. Periapical granuloma	a. Periapical granuloma
b. Periapical cyst	b. Apical cyst
c. Chronic periapical abscess (nonpainful phase of the chronic periapical abscess cycle)	c. Suppurative apical periodontitis (chronic apical abscess) (terms used to describe both painful and nonpainful phases of the chronic abscess cycle)

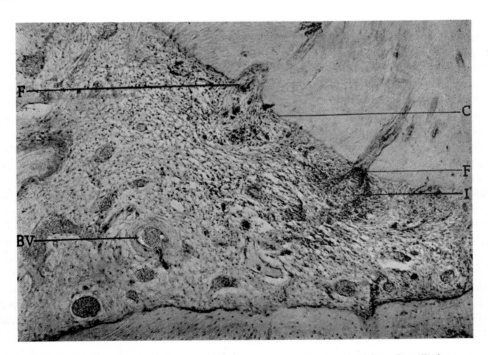

Fig. 4-3. Mild exudative (acute) response *(I)* surrounding multiple apical foramina *(F)* due to root canal irritants. Leukocyte infiltration (PMNs and lymphocytes), edema space, and vasodilation may be seen. *C,* Cementum; *BV,* blood vessels. (From Coolidge ED, Kesel RG: *Endodontology,* ed 2, Philadelphia, 1956, Lea & Febiger.)

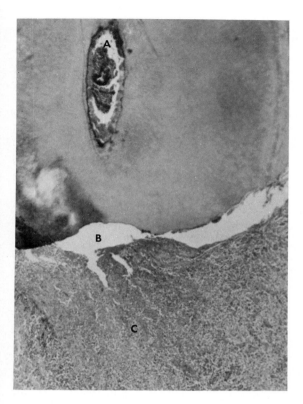

Fig. 4-4. Tangential section showing acute periapical abscess caused by necrotic debris *(A)* in the root canal. Pus core *(B)* is surrounded by dilated and congested blood vessels and a heavy infiltration of inflammatory cells *(C)*, which includes PMNs and lymphocytes. A higher magnification of the root canal can be seen in Fig. 3-51.

Etiology. When the inflammatory process or the toxic components of pulpal necrosis approach the connective tissue of the pulpoperiapical junction, an apical periodontitis ensues. However, persistent periapical tissue compression from traumatic occlusion may also produce an apical inflammatory response; and if the occlusal disharmony is not corrected, there may be secondary pulpal involvement as well.

Etiologic factors related to root canal procedures. Several complications can arise from improper endodontic technique:

1. *It is impossible to extirpate a pulp without initiating an inflammatory response because a wound is created.* Pulp extirpation may tear the tissue at the apical region of coalescence with the interstitial loose connective tissue of the periodontal ligament, or beyond, because the operator has no control as to where the pulp tissue stump will eventually be. A second sequential irritant is provided by the subsequent manipulation with intracanal instruments, which crush residual tissue within the canal. In addition, contaminated filings may be pushed up into the injured tissue and act as a foreign body, providing a nidus for the resultant periapical inflammation. *Routinely filling these canals during the same appointment as the cleanse-and-shape procedure will most certainly increase the possibility of postoperative exacerbation.* Leaving teeth with vital pulps open after an emergency appointment has been shown by Weine et al. to be a source of postoperative complications, thereby increasing the treatment time (Chapter 5). New and large numbers of microorganisms are introduced into what might have been a sterile environment to feed and grow on the rich substrate provided in the accessory canals and dentinal tubules, as well as in the main canal.

2. *Using strong or excessive amounts of interappointment intracanal chemicals may induce periapical inflammation.* **Medicaments used to sterilize the root canal are of secondary importance and should be used only to augment the cleansing and shaping operation.** Even the strongest antimicrobial agents are ineffective if the canal contains pus and debris and its walls are irregular. Cleansing and shaping of the canals in the presence of sodium hypochlorite and intermittent debridement is the most effective way to achieve canal sanitation.

3. *Improper manipulation of instruments within the root canal or overextension as a result of inaccurate measurement of canal length will force dentinal debris, irrigating solutions, and toxic components of necrotic tissue into the periapex.* If microorganisms are present, not only will the periapical connective tissue be inoculated, but a transient bacteremia may develop as well. The physical injury caused by the instrument itself will add to the intensity of the ensuing inflammatory response.

Histopathology and clinical symptoms. Following is an account of the development of a periapical abscess:

Acute apical periodontitis is the initial exudative (acute) response of the periapex. The sequence of events described for incipient pulpitis is identical to that for events occurring in the interstitial loose connective tissue of the apical periodontium. The clinical symptoms differ only because the environment is different. Periapical hyperemia must first take place; and if the irritant persists, the prolonged vasodilation in the narrow apical periodontal space is followed by inflammatory exudate and leukocyte infiltration. The increased pressure may elevate the tooth slightly, stretching the ligament fibers. The nerve endings in the area are subliminally stimulated, so even a slight pressure against the tooth will cause mild pain. The constant increase in pressure will activate osteoclast formation to resorb the bone and increase the periodontal ligament space. The process will continue as long as the pulpal contaminants persist in irritating the periapex.

The tooth becomes increasingly tender as the process advances toward the next stage—*acute periapical abscess.* Vascular congestion results in regional anoxia and cell breakdown (autolysis). Neutrophils increase in number, releasing their proteolytic ferments to form the pus core. Acute exudative zones of inflammation develop that are identical with those described for pulpal inflammation (p. 150).

The intensity of the pain increases as pus formation adds to the periapical pressure and the pus seeks a pathway of least resistance through the trabecular spaces. The pain becomes more intense and steady with an additional feeling of fullness in the area. Unless drainage can be established, the exudative inflammatory response may spread diffusely, creating peripheral areas of cellulitis. Periapical inflammation of incisors may produce soft tissue swelling of the lip; periapical response of maxillary canines may affect the area of the ala of the nose; and an acute periapical abscess of the maxillary premolars may produce swelling of the eyelid. The soft vestibular tissues overlying the root end may become inflamed and painful to palpation even though there may be little radiographic evidence of periapical bone resorption. At this point the patient may be febrile.

The most intense pain occurs as the pus penetrates the outer plate of bone and begins to raise the periosteum. Once the periosteum and mucosa are ruptured (whether by the pressure of the suppurative material or by the operator's scalpel), the pain subsides and will not return unless the drainage is blocked. Since the acute or exudative aspect of the inflammation no longer plays an aggressive role and the irritant force has been downgraded through drainage, the chronic or proliferative (repair) phase of the inflammatory cycle becomes increasingly active as granulation and granulomatous tissue formation increases. Both the clinical and the histopathologic pictures are now characteristic of a *nonpainful chronic pathosis.*

Diagnosis

Pain. Painful pulpoperiapical pathosis will range from the slight tenderness of the earlier stage of *acute apical periodontitis* to the frequently intense and continuous throbbing of the *acute periapical abscess.* Often a localized sense of fullness accompanies the pain. At all stages the pain is readily localized as the tooth becomes increasingly tender to percussion. In the late stages of abscess formation the patient usually can tolerate the discomfort if the tooth is not touched.

Swelling and palpation. In the early stages swelling is usually not present, but a *firm pressure against the mucosa over the root end may incite a positive painful response.* As the abscess extends towards the surface, swelling increases. It may be preceded by edema and cellulitis. Resorption of the overlying cortical bone and localization of the suppurative mass beneath the mucosa produce *a palpable fluctuant swelling.*

Vitality tests. When the periapical pathosis is a sequela of pulpal necrosis, no response is to be expected to either electrical or thermal tests. In the early stage of painful pulpoperiapical pathosis, a positive response to a vitality test may be recorded because of residual viable type C nerve fibers that are resistant to the hypoxia of necrotic tissue (see Table 3-4); the same may occur in multirooted teeth when the tissue in one canal may be less affected than the tissue in another.

Radiography. Some periapical change is usually evident. It ranges from a slight widening of the apical periodontal ligament space to the large periapical radiolucency of a *recrudescent (phoenix) abscess.*

Treatment. Refer to Chapter 5.

Nonpainful pulpoperiapical pathoses

Nonpainful pulpoperiapical pathoses are inflammatory defense responses of periapical connective tissue to a pulpal irritant. In them the proliferative (chronic or granulomatous) components are hyperactive and play a dominant role. Pain is absent because of diminished (subthreshold) intraperiapical pressure. (See definition of chronic [proliferative], p. 139.)

Pulpoperiapical osteoclerosis (condensing osteitis, sclerosing osteitis). This productive response of periapical bone to a low-grade longstanding pulpal irritation is manifested as an increase in the density of the periapical bone, not because of a greater concentration of minerals (hypercalcification), but because of osteoblastic hyperactivity. The bony trabeculae increase in thickness to such a degree that the marrow spaces are eliminated or reduced to small tags of fibrous tissue; i.e., there is more bone tissue in a given space. This response is typically found in young persons around the apices of mandibular teeth with large carious lesions and chronically inflamed pulps. A return to the normal trabecular pattern may occur after root canal therapy (see Figs. 3-50, *A,* and 4-5). Pulpoperiapical osteoporosis (bone resorption), on the other hand, is caused by osteoclastic activity resulting from extension of pulpal disease into the periapex.

Incipient chronic apical periodontitis. This initially chronic periapical connective tissue response to pulpal irritants is characterized by a slightly widened apical periodontal space containing dilated blood vessels, a mild inflammatory exudate, and a dense accumulation of chronic inflammatory cells (plasma cells and lymphocytes). If the pulpal contaminants are not removed, the response will intensify to one of the advanced chronic or acute forms.

Periapical granuloma. This more advanced form of chronic apical periodontitis is characterized by the growth of granulation tissue and the presence of chronic inflammatory cells (granulomatous tissue) in response to continued pulpal irritation. A peripheral collagenous fiber capsule is usually present (Figs. 4-6 to 4-8). A massive invasion of this tissue by pulpal contaminants will result in the formation of an acute abscess (*recrudescent* or *phoenix abscess*).

If equated with the classical terminology used in pathology, *dental granuloma* is a misnomer. This is not a tumor, as the suffix intimates, nor does it resemble clinically or microscopically the *infectious* or *tuberculoid* granuloma. The term is in common usage, however, and until an alternate and more appropriate term is found, we will use it in the context just defined. The granulomatous lesions of tuberculosis, syphilis, and leprosy are forms of chronic inflammation and contain lymphocytes and occasionally plasma cells, but they also contain large fibroblasts and histiocytes (macrophages) that have been transformed into epithelium-like cells called *epithelioid cells.* They may also develop a peripheral collagenous capsule, but unlike dental granulomas, some of these lesions have large numbers of multinucleated giant

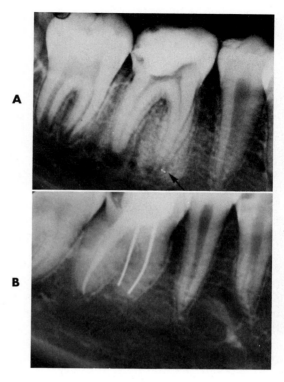

Fig. 4-5. **A,** Pulpoperiapical osteosclerosis related to nonpainful (chronic) pulpitis and later to pulp necrosis. Osteoblastic activity around mesial root *(arrow)* of the mandibular first molar in this 13-year-old patient was stimulated by longstanding low-grade irritant. Note pulpoperiapical *osteoporosis* at apex of distal root. **B,** Resolution of both osteoporosis and osteosclerosis 8 months after completion of endodontic therapy.

cells and may develop a central area of caseation necrosis.

Chronic periapical abscess (suppurative apical periodontitis). This longstanding low-grade inflammatory reaction of the periapical connective tissue to pulpal irritants is characterized by the formation of a *parulis* and active pus formation draining through the *stoma* (mouth) of a sinus tract. The chronic periapical abscess usually develops from a chronic apical periodontitis but may also result from an acute periapical abscess that has found a pathway and subsequent drainage through the oral mucosa. Mild painful symptoms occur when the sinus tract stoma is blocked with coagulum and/or proliferation of mucosal epithelium over the stoma. During this symptomatic phase the term *subacute periapical abscess* is appropriate (Figs. 4-9 and 4-10).

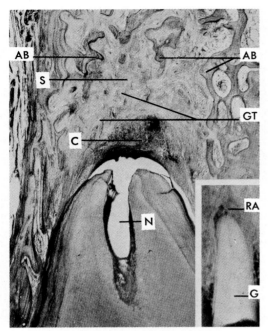

Fig. 4-6.   Maxillary central incisor with Type I pulpoperiapical lesion: periapical granuloma (see Hirsch classification, p. 183). Zonal responses evident include zone of necrosis *(N)*, zone of contamination *(C)*, granulomatous tissue *(GT)* in the zone of irritation, and fibrous activity in the zone of stimulation *(S)*. *AB,* Alveolar bone. Inset shows radiolucency *(RA)* and inadequate root canal filling *(G)* as they appear on a radiograph. (From Coolidge ED, Kesel RG: *Endodontology,* ed 2, Philadelphia, 1956, Lea & Febiger.)

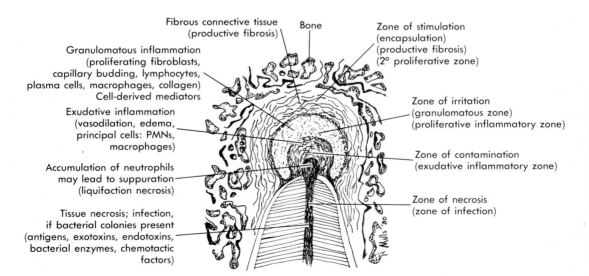

Fig. 4-7.   Zones of a well-established granuloma as described by Dr. W. E. Fish (Type I pulpoperiapical lesion (see Hirsch classification, p. 183). See also Figs. 4-6 and 4-8. (Illustration as suggested by Dr. Henry Trowbridge, University of Pennsylvania, Philadelphia.)

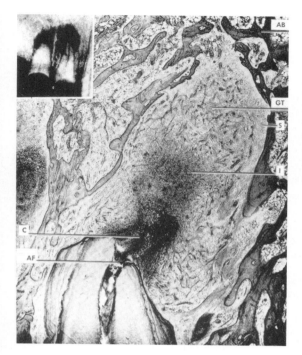

Fig. 4-8. Mesiodistal section through apex of a maxillary first premolar with a periapical granuloma (Type I pulpoperapical lesion; see Hirsch classification, p. 183). The radiograph shows large area of bone resorption. Necrotic tissue at apical foramen *(AF)* feeds zone of contamination *(C)*, which results in an exudative (acute) response. Toxicity and leukocyte infiltration diminish as distance from the canal foramen increases *(I)*. Granulomatous tissue *(GT)* and peripheral encapsulation *(S)* are evident. *AB,* Alveolar bone. (From Boyle P: *Kronfeld's histopathology of the teeth,* ed 4, Philadelphia, 1955, Lea & Febiger.)

Periapical cyst. A periapical cyst is a chronic inflammatory response of the periapex that develops from chronic lesions with preexisting granulomatous tissue. It is characterized by a central fluid-filled epithelium-lined cavity surrounded by granulomatous tissue and peripheral fibrous encapsulation (Fig. 4-14).

Etiology. The etiologic factors for *nonpainful pulpoperiapical pathoses* are the same as those listed for *acute apical periodontitis.* If the irritant is of low enough intensity, the chronic periapical response may develop from the onset, or it may develop from an acute apical periodontitis whose acute features have dissipated. *Incipient chronic apical periodontitis* is the first stage of nonpainful, chronic periapical pathosis, which, if allowed to continue, will develop into a *periapical granuloma* or *cyst* (Fig. 4-11). The formation of the periapical cyst depends on a previously existing granulomatous form. The *chronic periapical abscess* may also develop from the *apical periodontitis* but frequently is a sequela of an *acute periapical abscess* after drainage has been established.

The appearance of a periapical pathosis in the presence of a vital pulp requires an explanation other than that usually given for multirooted teeth, i.e., vital tissue in one canal and necrotic tissue in the other. Langeland et al. explain, in terms of inflammation and immunology, the "seemingly illogical" presence of intact pulp tissue between two areas of severe inflammation. The toxic bacterial and proteolytic products travel from the affected region through the lymph vessels to the periapical tissue, where they accumulate and effect an inflammatory response.

Histopathology and clinical symptoms. The following describes the development of the incipient and advanced forms of chronic apical periodontitis.

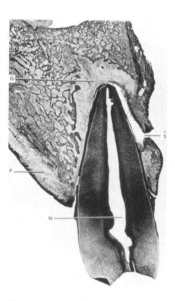

Fig. 4-9. Chronic periapical abscess (suppurative apical periodontitis) with formation of a sinus tract. Labiolingual section through a maxillary central incisor with a necrotic pulp *(N)*. Granulomatous tissue *(G)* surrounds apex. Stoma (mouth) of the sinus tract *(S)* opens into labial vestibule. *P,* Mucoperiosteal tissue of palate. (From Boyle P: *Kronfeld's histopathology of the teeth,* ed 4, Philadelphia, 1955, Lea & Febiger.)

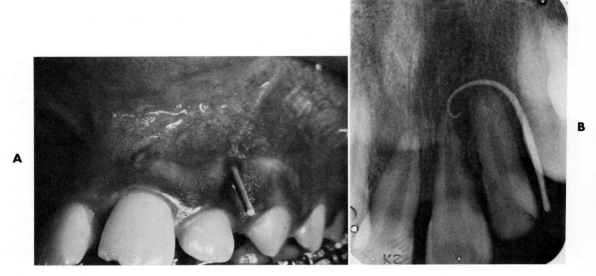

Fig. 4-10. **A,** Pliable gutta-percha cone placed in stoma of a sinus tract located distal to the maxillary lateral incisor. **B,** Cone bypasses lateral incisor to reveal the central incisor as the source of the sinus tract. Care should be taken to ensure that the cone is pliable and not dry and brittle.

The presence of necrotic pulp tissue in the root canal (zone of necrosis/infection) results in diffusion of the toxic material into and slightly beyond the area of coalescence of pulpal and periodontal connective tissue. Without any radiographic evidence, centers of cellular infiltration will appear around each foraminal opening. Capillary dilation occurs, and leukocytes are attracted to the area. Closest to the *zone of necrosis* (zone I) are the neutrophilic leukocytes (PMNs). These are surrounded by large masses of lymphocytes and plasma cells. The initial mild chronic response *(incipient chronic apical periodontitis)* increases as more of the necrotic products and microorganisms, if present, diffuse from the pulp canal into the periapex. The toxicity of the root canal irritant is reduced by the fluid and cellular exudative activity in the *zone of contamination* (zone II). This reduction in toxicity stimulates undifferentiated cells to join together to form multinucleated osteoclasts, which resorb the contaminated periapical bone. Radiographic evidence of a widened apical periodontal space now becomes evident. The gap that is opened in the bone surrounding the lesion will ultimately be filled with granulomatous tissue to form zone III, the *zone of irritation* (Table 4-2). Granulomatous tissue has a repair and

healing function because it contains granulation tissue formed by the new capillaries and young fibroblasts. It also has a defense function because its resistance to infection is augmented by the presence of lymphocytes and plasma cells as well as undifferentiated cells and histiocytes that have become scavengers (macrophages). *When plasma cells are observed, active antibody synthesis is most likely occurring.* Enlarged mature or degenerating plasma cells that contain large inclusions, thought to be immunoglobulin, are called *Russell bodies.* They have a homogeneous (hyaline or glassy) appearance and are acidophilic (pink color) when stained with hematoxylin and eosin (Fig. 4-13, *B*). Some of the macrophages observed are called *foam cells* because they have ingested fatty material found in many of the degenerating cells in the area (fatty degeneration). Ultimately the lipid material is released by the foam cells, and needles or crystals of cholesterol are found. Many granulomas also may contain strands or islands of epithelium (see cyst description, p. 179). It is important to note that in this zone of irritation viable microorganisms are absent.

The periapical granuloma may be compared to the pulpal granuloma (see discussion of chronic ulcerative pulpitis, p. 154); unlike the chronic

Table 4-2.   Mobilization of a well-established periapical granuloma (Type I pulpoperiapical lesion)

Zone	Description
I **Zone of necrosis** *(zone of infection)*	**I** ***Necrotic or infected root canal contents*** 1. Pus fluid contains dead cells, destructive components released from phagocytes, intermediate and end products of protein decomposition (proteolysis) 2. Polymorphonuclear leukocytes (neutrophils) present 3. Microorganisms present or absent; if present: exotoxins, endotoxins, antigens, bacterial enzymes, chemotactic factors

II
Zone of contamination *(exudative inflammatory zone)*
	II
	Immediate response to toxic elements coming out of root canal
	1. Principal *exudative* (acute) defense response (vasodilation, fluid exudation, cellular infiltration); dilution of toxic elements plus antibacterial action of inflammatory fluid (see Table 3-6)
	2. Principal defense cells
	  a. Polymorphonuclear leukocytes (PMNs) (early)
	  b. Macrophages: blood-derived mononuclear cells and tissue-derived histiocytes (appear later because they are less motile and survive longer than PMNs)

The left two rows are bracketed as **Exudative (acute) zones.**

Transitional area

Zone	Description

III
Zone of irritation *(granulomatous zone, proliferative inflammatory zone)*
	III
	Toxicity diminishing as distance from canal foramina increases
	1. Function: defense, healing, repair
	2. Principal proliferative (chronic) response: granulation tissue (capillary proliferation and fibroblastic activity).
	3. Granulomatous: granulation tissue plus chronic defense cells
	4. Principal chronic defense cells: lymphocytes, plasma cells, blood-derived macrophages, tissue macrophages that develop from histiocytes, and reserve cells (undifferentiated mesenchymal cells).
	5. Cell-derived mediators of inflammation: antibodies from plasma cells, lymphokines from sensitized T cells (T-type lymphocytes), histamine and serotonin (5-hydroxytryptamine) from basophils
	6. Russell bodies: enlarged plasma cells with numerous antibody inclusions (Fig. 4-13, *B*)
	7. Eosinophils (later): attracted by mast cell *eosinophil chemotactic factor* (ECF-A) and lymphokine ECF-A eosinophils modulate inflammation and allergy by destroying certain vasoactive substances:
	    Platelet activating factor (PAF)
	    Slow-reacting substance of anaphylaxis (SRS-A)
	8. Foam cells: macrophages after ingesting cells with fatty degeneration
	9. Favorable environment for osteoclasts
	10. Occasional cholesterol crystals
	11. Epithelial clusters and strands

IV
Zone of stimulation *(zone of encapsulation, zone of productive fibrosis)*
	IV
	Toxicity reduced to a mild stimulant
	1. Peripheral orientation of collagen (fibroblastic activity)
	2. Favorable environment for osteoblastic activity
	  a. Bone apposition and reversal lines evident during recessive and rest periods
	  b. Occasional *reactive hyperostosis* when lesion encroaches on the cortical plate

The left two rows (III and IV) are bracketed as **Proliferative (chronic) zones.**

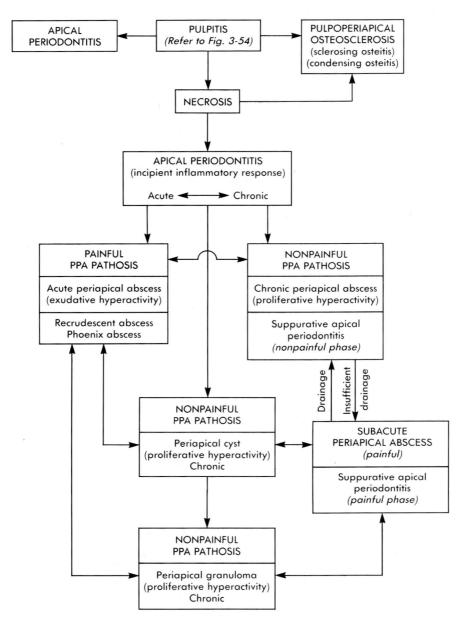

Fig. 4-11. Sequence of pulpoperiapical *(PPA)* pathoses related to inflammation. Refer also to Fig. 3-54 (sequence of pulpal pathoses related to inflammation).

response of the pulpal connective tissue, however, a fourth zone *(zone of stimulation)* becomes well developed. At the periphery of the granulomatous zone the toxicity of the root canal irritants becomes so diluted and diminished that the irritants act as a stimulus to fibroblasts and osteoblasts in the area. A wall of collagen fibers is laid down by the fibroblasts in an attempt to *encapsulate* the entire

inflammatory complex, separating the granulomatous tissue from the bone. Osteoblasts function best in this zone, and during periods of regression, they lay down additional bone matrix over the surface of the older resorbed bone. *Root-end resorptive defects of varying degree are usually a sequela of longstanding granulomatous lesions. When the defect is irregular or cup shaped, a readjustment of the working length must be made to obtain a solid apical dentin matrix* (see Fig. 8-14).

Kronfeld's mountain pass concept.   A study by Langeland et al. of 35 biopsy specimens revealed bacterial cells in the periapical granulomatous tissue in only one case.

A half century earlier, Kronfeld had pointed out that the granuloma is not an environment in which bacteria live but one in which they are destroyed. He compared the bacteria in the root canal (zone I) with an army entrenched "behind high and inaccessible mountains," the foramina serving as mountain passes. The exudative and granulomatous (proliferative) tissue of the granuloma represents a mobilized army defending the plains (periapex) from the invaders. If only a few invaders enter the plain through the mountain pass, they are destroyed by the defenders (leukocytes). A mass attack of invaders results in a major battle, analogous to acute inflammation (acute or exudative forces of zone II). Only complete elimination of the invaders from their mountainous entrenchment will eliminate the need for a defense force in the "plains." Once this is accomplished, the defending army of leukocytes withdraws, the local destruction created by the battle is repaired (granulation tissue of zone III), and the environment returns to its normal pattern.

The objective, therefore, in nonsurgical root canal therapy of teeth with periapical pathoses is elimination of the irritant from the canal and keeping it out by a "three-dimensional" filling of the canal. If the contents of zone (i.e., necrosis and infection) are eliminated, the granuloma can complete its function of healing and repair.

Chronic periapical abscess (suppurative apical periodontitis).   The chronic periapical abscess has been described as a sequela to an acute abscess after free drainage of the pus has been established. It may also form when there is a steady increase of canal irritants into a previously existing incipient chronic apical periodontitis or periapical granuloma. The zones established are comparable to those of a periapical granuloma except for the amount of pus formation around the apex. Great masses of neutrophilic leukocytes are evident in the exudative zone. The sinus tract carrying the discharge is usually lined with granulomatous tissue but may be lined with stratified squamous epithelium characteristic of the mucosal surface surrounding the stoma (Fig. 4-9). (Refer also to p. 182.)

Periapical cyst.   The periapical cyst has been defined as a periapical granuloma with a central, fluid-filled epithelium-lined cavity (Fig. 4-14). Where do these epithelial cells come from? How does this central cavity form? The source of the epithelial cells may be traced to Hertwig's epithelial root sheath, a double-layered tissue of epithelial cells (inner and outer enamel epithelium) that proliferates apically from the enamel organ. Root formation will not occur without its organizing influence. As dentin is deposited against this sheath, the continuity of the epithelial cells is broken up by invading connective tissue from the dental sac. Cementoblasts are formed in the connective tissue, and cementum is deposited on the surface of the newly formed dentin. Some of the epithelial cells degenerate, but many persist as small clusters called epithelial rests of Malassez (see Fig. 3-13). These clusters remain dormant until activated by the irritation present in a granulomatous response. The epithelial cells undergo mitosis and proliferate in all directions simultaneously; thus a ball of epithelial cells is formed. Shear compares it to the morula stage in the early embryo. The epithelium does not have its own blood supply but depends on its nutrition and oxygen diffusing from the surrounding granulomatous tissue. The nutrition source is enhanced by the projection of the chronically inflamed connective tissue into the ball of cells from all directions. This same principle is seen in the lamina propria of the oral mucosa. When such a tissue is sectioned, the epithelium appears to form arcades (arches or columns) and rings surrounding cores of vascular connective tissue as a "spongework" of epithelium (Figs. 4-12 and 4-13).

If the chronically inflamed connective tissue invaginations are inadequate to supply nutrition to the central cells of the epithelial ball, they degenerate and die. Intercellular fluid (edema) appears, giving the epithelial cells a spongelike characteristic *(spongiosis).* The spaces between the cells increase, and soon complete separation of the central epithelial cells occurs. A definite central cavity develops containing fluid and a number of cells in different stages of degeneration. Fluid from the surrounding granulomatous tissue is attracted to the center of the mass because the cyst wall acts as a semipermeable membrane and the protein of the dead cells has increased the osmotic pressure. The cyst grows by attracting tissue fluid into the cystic lumen as more and more epithelial cells die and

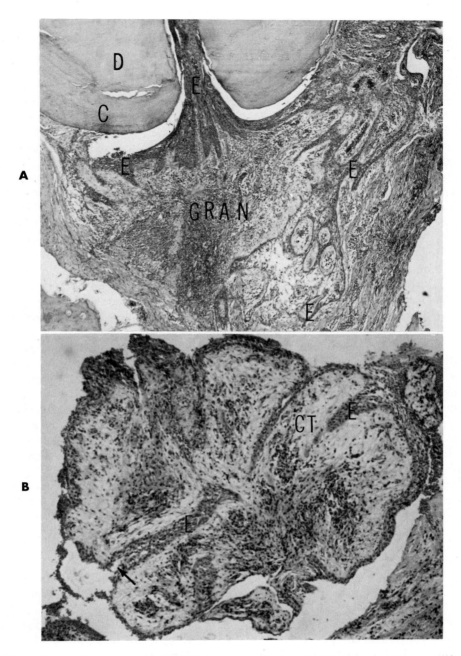

Fig. 4-12. **A,** Granulomatous *(GRAN)* is present periapically. Epithelium *(E)* has proliferated within the granuloma. *D,* Dentin; *C,* cementum. (×32.5.) **B,** Arcading of epithelium consistent with Type II pulpoperiapical lesion: *epithelial granuloma* (see Hirsch classification, p. 183). Epithelial trabeculae *(E)* surround cores of connective tissue *(CT).* (×58.5.) (**A** from Seltzer S, Soltanoff W, Bender IB: *Oral Surg* 27:111, 1969; **B** and **C** from Seltzer S: *Endodontology: biologic considerations in endodontic procedures,* ed 2, New York, 1988, McGraw-Hill.)

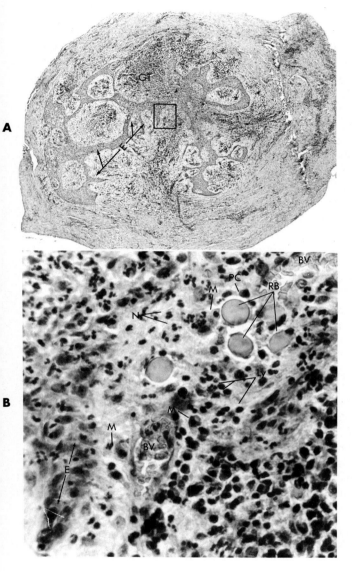

A

B

Fig. 4-13. **A,** Granuloma with proliferating stratified squamous epithelium (Type II pulpoperiapical lesion: *epithelial granuloma* (see Hirsch classification, p. 183). Note arcading effect on the underlying tissue. Arcades and rings of epithelial cells *(E)* surround cores of connective tissue and granulation tissue *(GT)* that have penetrated into epithelium. **B,** Higher magnification outlined by rectangle in **A.** Note inflammatory cells and structures. *M,* Macrophages; *PC,* plasma cells,; *Ly,* lymphocytes; *N,* neutrophils (polymorphonuclear leukocytes); *BV,* dilated capillaries; *E,* proliferating stratified squamous epithelium with intercellular edema and moderate neutrophilic infiltration; *RB,* Russell bodies.

contribute to the continued increase in the osmotic pressure of the cystic cavity. The cystic growth causes pressure on the capillaries in the surrounding connective tissue, producing an ischemia. This in turn causes more epithelial cells to die from the lack of oxygen and nourishment, and the cycle is repeated.

The cyst cavity contains a fluid that varies from clear amber to viscous yellow. In about a third of the cases in his study, Shear found cholesterol present, which is a product of cellular fatty degeneration and is deposited in the cyst wall in the form of crystals. *Cholesterol clefts* or *slits* appear in histo-

logic sections as clear areas because the crystals are dissolved during the preparation.

Diagnosis

Pain.   Pain is associated with nonpainful periapical pathoses only in terms of a history of acute or subacute episodes. Epithelium may close the sinus tract opening (stoma). Pressure buildup by the continuous formation of pus will produce subacute symptoms and a ballooning out of the epithelium (parulis, or gumboil). The symptoms will subside when the epithelium ruptures.

Pressures exerted during operative procedures on a tooth with a periapical granuloma may create negative pressures in the apical periodontium. As a result, necrotic pulp debris may be sucked into the highly mobilized periapex. The resultant acute exacerbation *(recrudescent* or *phoenix abscess)* is described in the discussion on painful pulpoperiapical pathoses.

Swelling and palpation. A chronic periapical abscess may show evidence of a slight swelling in the area around the sinus tract stoma, particularly during episodes of subacute exacerbation. Occasionally the sinus tract will open onto the surface of the face, floor of the nose, or other portions of the head and neck in proximity to the periapical area of the involved tooth. In these cases the patient may have a history of treatment by a physician for a skin lesion. Elimination of the necrotic contents of the canal will effect a cure.

Zone IV of a periapical granuloma is characterized by osteoblastic and fibroblastic activity. When the granuloma approaches the outer cortical bone of the alveolar process, periosteal cells are activated and a hard tissue bulge may appear *(reactive hyperostosis).* When the contaminants of zone I are removed, the bony configuration can be expected to return to normal (remodeling).

Percussion and mobility. Both percussion and mobility tests are negative. However, increased mobility, when present, may be related to excessive periradicular bone loss, whereas mobility in acute periapical pathosis is generally due to exudative pressure exerted against the root end, which is transmitted laterally to the principal fibers of the periodontal ligament. (Refer to discussion of mobility, p. 167.)

Color. Frequently there is a definite color change because of the loss of translucency. *Transillumination with a fiberoptic unit* is an effective diagnostic aid. Considerable discoloration may be caused by hemolysis of erythrocytes or decomposition of pulp tissue.

Vitality tests. All vitality tests will be negative because the nerve fibers are not viable. Sometimes a positive electric response is related to liquefaction necrosis acting as an electrolytic transmitter to the periapex, or it may be related to the presence of still viable apical nerve fibers (see Table 3-4). Positive responses may occur with multirooted teeth where viable nerve tissue remains in one of the canals.

Radiography. An accessory pliable (not brittle) gutta-percha cone can be inserted into the stoma of the sinus tract of a chronic periapical abscess to obtain radiographic confirmation of the involved tooth or root (Fig. 4-10). The chronic periapical abscess may show a diffuse area of bone rarefaction, whereas the granuloma and cyst tend to be well defined, highlighted by an opaque hyperostotic border. The inflammation and destruction are always greater than the radiography shows. *It is impossible to diagnose periapical lesions with any degree of accuracy unless a biopsy is taken and the tissue is examined under the microscope, even though the incidence of cysts is greater for larger lesions.* The terms *advanced chronic apical periodontitis* or *pulpoperiapical osteoporosis* may be used until the nature of the lesion is confirmed.

Treatment of nonpainful pulpoperiapical pathoses. Successful treatment depends on effective removal of the root canal contents (zone of necrosis), followed by adequate apical seal so healing and repair can take place.

The prognosis for successful healing without surgical intervention is very favorable. Resolution of a *chronic periapical abscess* usually occurs without any special treatment of the sinus tract. If closure is not apparent before the obliteration, judicious curettage of the tract and the lesion (via the tract) with a small endodontic excavator may be considered. This procedure will break up any organized epithelium (if present), facilitate drainage, create hemorrhage, and initiate an acute tissue response. If this action fails to bring results, surgical intervention using a full surgical flap will be necessary.

Many clinicians believe that when the lesion is large, healing is facilitated only by surgery. However, if the dominant periapical tissue is granulomatous, surgical intervention removes a tissue already mobilized for healing and repair. Large lesions as well as small ones have the capacity and potential for healing (see Figs. 1-10 and 11-2). The indications for surgical intervention are presented in Chapter 11.

Do pulpoperiapical cysts have the potential for healing without surgical intervention? Correlating histopathologic and clinical evidence with deductive reasoning implies that this potential does exist.

Histopathologic evidence. Nonodontogenic (fissural) and follicular odontogenic cysts differ from pulpoperiapical cysts both etiologically and histologically.

The fissural (developmental) cysts (e.g., the globulomaxillary) arise along the lines of fusion of embryonic bony processes (Table 4-3). Follicular

Table 4-3. Classification and etiology of cysts

Type of cyst	Etiology
Odontogenic	

Follicular
  Primordial
  Dentigerous
  Multilocular
	Epithelial cells of dental organ (follicle)

Pulpoperiapical (radicular)	Activation of dormant epithelial rests in periodontal ligament
Residual	Residual epithelial cells or rests after tooth extraction
Nonodontogenic	

Fissural
  Globulomaxillary
  Midpalatine (median palatal)
  Nasoalveolar
  Median mandibular
	Epithelial cells entrapped between embryonic facial processes of bones at lines of fusion

Incisive canal (nasopalatine)	Epithelial remnants of nasopalatine duct

odontogenic cysts (e.g., the dentigerous) arise from the enamel organ or follicle. Chronic inflammatory cells (lymphocytes and plasma cells) admixed with neutrophils in the subepithelial connective tissue may be present in varying degrees.

The pulpoperiapical cysts, on the other hand, are inflammatory cysts. They are part of an inflammatory complex and usually contain two components not found in the fissural and follicular cysts:

1. A causative factor (zone I) that can be removed without surgical intervention
2. A granulomatous zone that has the potential for repair and healing by the proliferation of its fibrous and vascular components (granulation tissue), once the causative factor has been removed (Fig. 4-14)

It is speculated that pulpoperiapical cysts having the least potential for healing without surgical intervention are older longstanding cysts that show very little evidence of granulomatous tissue (Type V lesion; see classification, p. 183). The epithelium in these cases is surrounded by a dense fibrotic stroma with few chronic inflammatory cells (Fig. 4-15).

Hirsch et al. (1979) classified surgically excised pulpoperiapical lesions as follows:

I. Periapical granuloma. Consists of a delicate (collagenous) fibrillar network, rich in blood vessels and chronic inflammatory cells (granulomatous tissue). The endothelial cells appear swollen, and large numbers of macrophages and foam cells are present. Cholesterol crystals and associated foreign body giant cells may also be observed. The periphery of the lesion may demonstrate a fibrous capsule (Figs. 4-7 and 4-8).

II. Epithelial granuloma. Similar to the periapical granuloma except for the presence of proliferating solid strands of epithelium (arcading effect) (Figs. 4-12 and 4-13).

III. Radicular cysts with modern (chronic inflammation. A continued development of an epithelial granuloma. Central necrosis has already occurred, resulting in a cavity surrounded by epithelium (usually stratified squamous). There is evidence of strong proliferative activity. Cholesterol crystals and foreign body giant cells are common in the connective tissue of the richly vascularized cyst wall. A peripheral dense fibrous capsule is usually present (Fig. 4-14).

IV. Radicular cyst with strong (acute or subacute) inflammation and epithelial necrosis. Such inflammation is present in the wall of the cyst, resulting in widespread necrosis and loss of the cyst epithelium. Histologic sections show a cystic lumen covered by partly necrotic epithelium, surrounded by granulomatous tissue. The peripheral capsule is often missing, and bone fragments may have an osteolytic appearance.

V. Radicular cyst without inflammation (chronic or acute). The epithelium is well developed and surrounded by a dense fibrous capsule, and inflammatory cells are absent (Fig. 4-15).

Clinical evidence. Table 4-4 reveals that of the nine biopsy studies listed, six were based on 200 or more cases. Note that the incidence of cysts ranged from 14% to 47%. Surgical intervention, however, is not required 14% to 47% of the time for the successful treatment of all cases with periapical lesions. *We must therefore conclude by deductive reasoning that some pulpoperiapical cysts have the potential to heal following the adequate removal of root canal contaminants and the obliteration of the root canal space.*

Morse et al. have devised a test for determining the nature of a pulpoperiapical lesion (granuloma or cyst) before endodontic treatment. An endodontic instrument is used to penetrate into the periapical lesion to induce fluid flow into the root canal. Fluid is then withdrawn from the canal and subjected to differential diagnosis by *polyacrylamide*

A

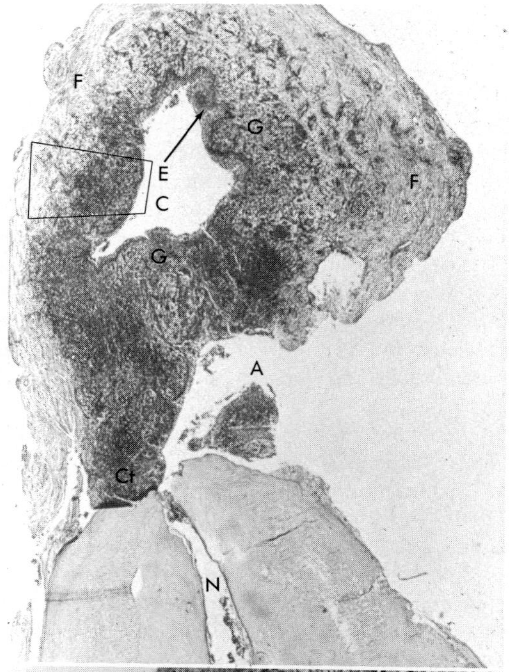

B

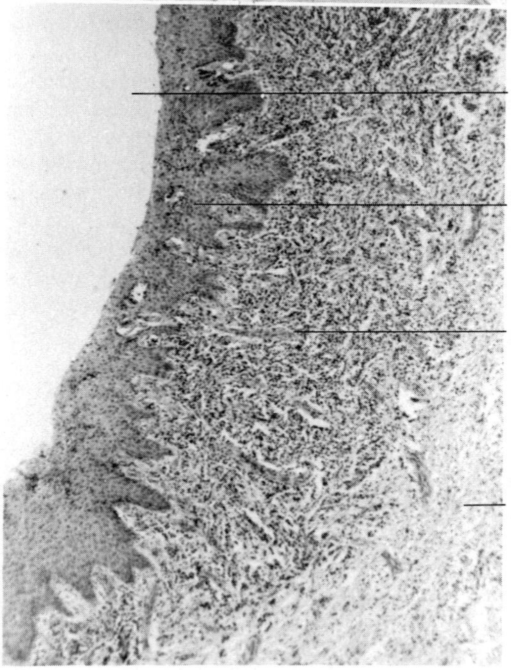

Cyst cavity

Stratified
squamous
epithelium

Granulomatous
tissue

Fibrous
capsule

Fig. 4-14. A, Type III pulpoperiapical lesion: *periapical cyst with moderate chronic inflammation* (see Hirsch classification, p. 183). Stratified squamous epithelium *(E)* lines fluid-filled cavity *(C)* and is surrounded by granulomatous tissue *(G)* and fibrous encapsulation *(F)*. Artifact *(A)* was caused by tissue separation during the slide preparation. Zone of necrosis *(N)* in root canal communicates with zone of contamination *(Ct)*. **B,** High-power magnification comparable to the area outlined in **A.** (A from Shafer WG, Hine MK, Levy BM: *Textbook of oral pathology,* ed 4, Philadelphia, 1983, Saunders.)

gel electrophoresis, a process that causes proteins to migrate in an electrical field according to their charge and molecular weight. In this test an electrophoretic pattern is formed by the albumin and globulin proteins present in the aspirated fluid. The cystic pattern differs from the one formed by a granuloma. In this way, diagnosis is possible without histologic examination. The semipermeable nature of the epithelial lining of a cyst allows plasma proteins to pass into the cyst lumen. The resulting increase in osmotic pressure yields an inward movement of fluid containing protein, gen-

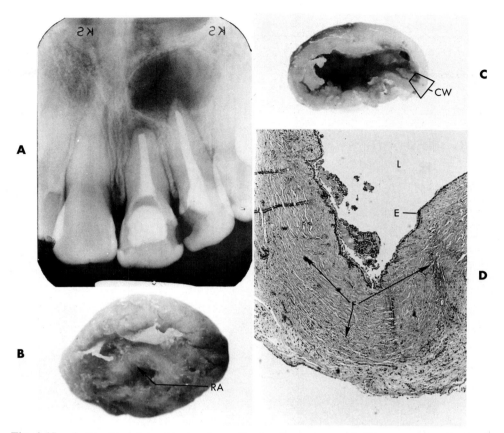

Fig. 4-15. **A.** Maxillary lateral incisor immediately after a root canal filling procedure. **B,** Small opening in center of completely enucleated lesion marks position previously occupied by the root apex *(RA)*. **C,** Hemisection of fibrous specimen revealed large cavity with an irregular but smooth lining surface. **D,** Microscopic examination of the wall *(CW)* showed a Type V pulpoperiapical lesion: *radicular cyst without inflammation* (see Hirsch classification, p. 183). Stratified squamous epithelium *(E)* lining the cystic cavity *(L).* Very few, scattered inflammatory cells are present, as well as a defense fibrotic stroma *(F).* This type of cyst has the least potential for healing without surgical intervention because of the absence of granulomatous tissue.

erally albumin and gamma globulins. With gel electrophoresis the presence of a higher percentage of protein can be confirmed in cyst fluid, whereas a lower percentage indicates a granuloma (Fig. 4-16). The accuracy of the electrophoretic method to differentiate a radicular cyst from a periapical granuloma was corroborated in a research study by Barlocco and Poladian.

Healing mechanism of pulpoperiapical cysts. Although there is no histologic evidence that proves conclusively the mechanism of inflammatory cyst repair, a number of theories have been advanced.

1. Seltzer et al. (1969) observed, in a series of 1-year studies, the entrapment and degeneration of epithelium by newly formed collagen fibers during the repair process. They concluded that pulpoperiapical cysts have the potential for healing without surgical intervention.

2. Bhaskar, as a result of his study, hypothesized that at least two mechanisms lead to destruction of the epithelial lining: (a) a transitory acute inflammation attracting PMNs, which liberate lysosomal enzymes to disrupt or destroy the epithelium, and (b) subepithelial

Table 4-4.   Reported percentages of periapical lesions

Investigator (yr)	Granuloma (%)	Cyst (%)	Other lesions (%)	Total no. of cases
Periapical lesion biopsies (200 or more cases)				
Grossman and Esther (1963)	63	17	20	503
Patterson, Shafer, and Healey (1964)	84	14	2	510
Bhaskar (1966)	48	42	10	2308
Lalonde and Luebke (1968)	45	44	11	800
Mortensen, Winther, and Birn (1970)	59	41	0	396
Ross and Birch (1976)	51	47	2	206
Electrophoretic differentiation of radicular cysts and granulomas				
Morse, Patnik, and Schacterle (1973)	77.5	22.5	0	40
Morse, Schacterle, and Wolfson (1976)	76.7	23.3	0	43
Barlocco and Poladian (1979)	82.5	17.5	0	40

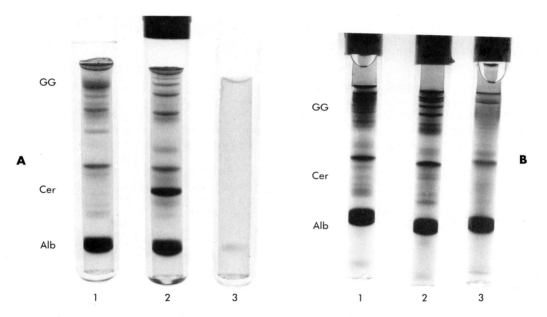

Fig. 4-16.   Polyacrylamide gel electrophoretic patterns for a periapical granuloma (**A**) and a periapical cyst (**B**). *1*, Fingertip plasma. *2*, Periapical plasma. *3*, Root canal fluid. *Alb*, Albumin: *Cer*, ceruloplasmin region; *GG*, gamma globulin region. (From Morse D, Patnik J, Schacterle G: *Oral Surg* 35:249, 1973.)

hemorrhage and subsequent ulceration of the epithelium. He suggested that, no matter how careful the operator, the pericystic inflammatory response and/or hemorrhage into the cystic cavity occurs when the canals are instrumented. This is especially true if the instrumentation goes beyond the foramen. Bhaskar further noted that, *whenever apical lesions become recrudescent, conservative endodontic therapy, when performed after drainage has been established and acute symptoms disappear, is almost always successful.*

Bender's response to Bhaskar's hypothesis reiterated certain biologic principles with respect to repair:

1. *Drainage* is one of the basic principles in repair because excess cellular fluid, pus, and extravasated blood must be eliminated before fibroplasia can occur.

2. *Unless pressure is removed* by either drainage or absorption of the fluid, cell migration will not occur.

3. *The repair process occurs from the periphery toward the center.* Healing never starts from the center, as can be evidenced radiographically. Bender indicated that direct penetration of instruments to the center of the cyst to establish drainage and reduce pressure has more merit than does artificial creation of a mild acute response (as suggested by Bhaskar).

IMMUNOLOGIC CONSIDERATIONS

In our brief description of immunologic mechanisms involved in pulpal and periapical diseases, it would be impossible to give an in-depth understanding or knowledge of the theoretic aspects of immunology. Rather, this overview is for the purpose of defining the components of the immunologic system and to give a working knowledge of their interrelationship with the inflammatory process, with special attention to the pulp. Mechanisms involved will be given as general concepts, with a description of specific reactions in the pulpal and periapical tissues where this information is available.

It has been well established that antigens placed in the pulp are able to sensitize the host. Walton and Langeland placed zinc oxide and eugenol–based materials on pulp stumps after removal of the coronal pulp. These materials were seen at various time intervals in blood vessels, lymphatics, and other lymph nodes. Barnes and Langeland found that bovine serum albumin placed in powder form into the pulp chamber resulted in high blood antibody titers, whereas introduction of packed sheep erythrocytes resulted in a somewhat lower titer. In another study (Torabinejad and Kiger) cats were injected with keyhole limpet hemocyamin (KLH). After time for sensitization, the KLH was injected into pulp tissue. Radiographic and histologic evidence demonstrated the formation of antigen-antibody complexes at the apex of the teeth. Antigen placed in the pulp of nonsensitized animals resulted in no radiographic or histologic changes. Other data confirm the pulp as a route by which antigen may be introduced, thereby sensitizing the host to antigenic stimulus (DeDeus and Han, Feiglin and Reade, Page et al., Rosengren).

Induction of the immune response

Processes that initiate the early exudative phase of inflammation may result in the introduction of foreign substances such as microbes, microbial products (e.g., endotoxin), or altered cellular components into pulpal or periapical tissues (Fig. 4-17). Granulocytic phagocytes are the initial cells called to the area and are most effective at halting the invasion. If foreign material persists, macrophages begin to appear at the site of response. Although a primary function of all phagocytes is to destroy and rid the body of foreign material by enzymatic and nonenzymatic means (Fig. 4-18), the blood-derived and tissue-derived macrophages have another extremely important role. Along with other antigen presenting cells (APCs), they are responsible for triggering the immune response. If the irritation continues or if phagocytes are unable to cope with foreign or damaged tissue, the body will mount a more massive, highly efficient response that is capable of specificity as well as memory—*the immune response.*

Induction of the immune system to an optimal level requires interaction between an APC, the foreign substance (antigen), and cells of the lymphoid system. This interaction may take place at the site of response, although it more often occurs in lymphoid tissues such as the spleen, thymus, or lymph nodes draining the peripheral site. Once this interaction is initiated, startling transformations occur in the two major lymphoid cell populations.

Components of the immune system

The lymphoid system consists mainly of two basic cell types: *B cells,* gaining their identity from the human equivalent of the avian bursa of Fabricius, and *T cells,* which gain their identity from the thymus.

In birds it is well known that lymphocytes differentiate in the bursa of Fabricius (B cells). In human beings, however, it appears that B lymphocytes arise directly from hemopoietic cells in fetal liver or in fetal and adult bone marrow. They then

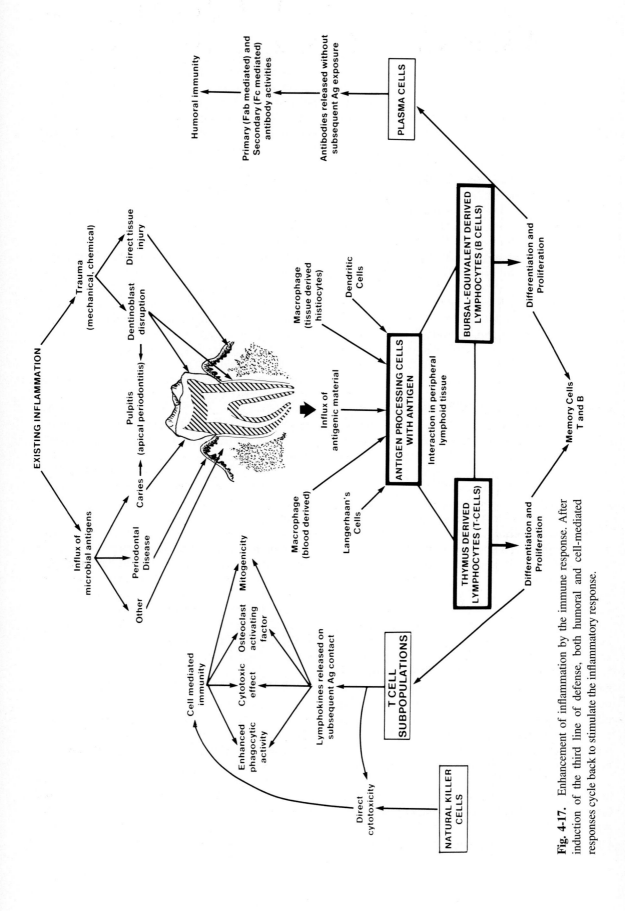

Fig. 4-17. Enhancement of inflammation by the immune response. After induction of the third line of defense, both humoral and cell-mediated responses cycle back to stimulate the inflammatory response.

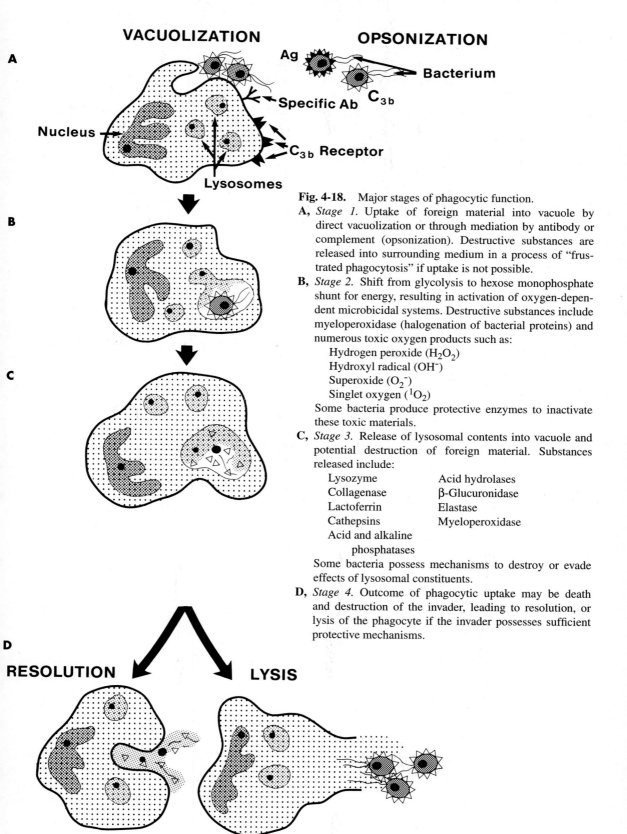

Fig. 4-18. Major stages of phagocytic function.

A, *Stage 1.* Uptake of foreign material into vacuole by direct vacuolization or through mediation by antibody or complement (opsonization). Destructive substances are released into surrounding medium in a process of "frustrated phagocytosis" if uptake is not possible.

B, *Stage 2.* Shift from glycolysis to hexose monophosphate shunt for energy, resulting in activation of oxygen-dependent microbicidal systems. Destructive substances include myeloperoxidase (halogenation of bacterial proteins) and numerous toxic oxygen products such as:

  Hydrogen peroxide (H_2O_2)
  Hydroxyl radical (OH^-)
  Superoxide (O_2^-)
  Singlet oxygen ($^1O_2$)

Some bacteria produce protective enzymes to inactivate these toxic materials.

C, *Stage 3.* Release of lysosomal contents into vacuole and potential destruction of foreign material. Substances released include:

Lysozyme	Acid hydrolases
Collagenase	β-Glucuronidase
Lactoferrin	Elastase
Cathepsins	Myeloperoxidase
Acid and alkaline	
phosphatases	

Some bacteria possess mechanisms to destroy or evade effects of lysosomal constituents.

D, *Stage 4.* Outcome of phagocytic uptake may be death and destruction of the invader, leading to resolution, or lysis of the phagocyte if the invader possesses sufficient protective mechanisms.

are distributed throughout the lymphoid tissues of the body. When stimulated by an appropriate APC-antigen complex, with the assistance of "helper" T cells, they are capable of producing mediators of the *humoral response,* the *antibody.*

Five classes (isotypes) of antibodies may be secreted by stimulated B cells (plasma cells): IgG, IgM, IgA, IgE, and IgD. Because of their basic structure, antibodies are able to cross-link antigens on cells together, causing the cells to clump *(agglutinate).* This process also occurs with smaller soluble antigens such as protein and is called *precipitation.* IgM and IgG (Fig. 4-19) are called circulatory antibodies because of their predominance in blood (80% to 85% of human serum immunoglobulin) and are the most important serum antibodies in the immune armamentarium. IgM, also called macroglobulin, is a large pentameric form with five basic antibody structures held together by the proteinaceous J chain; it is the first antibody to be produced when host is stimulated by antigen. Plasma cells then shift to an IgG production (IgM-IgG shift). IgM and IgG have the ability to bind to macrophages through specific receptor sites. When involved in this process, the antibodies are called opsonins and the process is termed *opsonization.* In combination with complement, they enhance the inflammatory process, thereby mediating destruction and clearance of the antigens that induced their production. IgG is the one class of antibody able to cross the placenta, providing temporary immunity to a newborn child.

IgA (Fig. 4-19) is the major antibody found in secretions such as saliva, colostrum, tears, and secretions of the respiratory and gastrointestinal (GI) mucosa. It is thought to help maintain a stable relationship between host and normal flora as well as to serve a major protective function at those sites. As with IgM, IgA has multimeric forms held together by J chains. The dimeric form (secretory IgA) is secreted through the mucous membranes and is relatively stable to acidic conditions and proteolytic enzymes. These properties are due to attachment of another protein, the *secretory component* (SC or T protein). By binding to the bacteria, secretory IgA can inhibit adherence of these organisms to mucosal and tooth surfaces. Torres et al. showed a significant correlation between canals open to oral flora and higher concentration of secretory IgA. The authors theorize that leaving canals open to the oral cavity may result in periapical cysts as a result of activation of rests of Malassez by epithelial growth factor present in saliva.

IgE, in conjunction with eosinophils, serves a function of protecting against parasitic infections. However, it is most often associated with host tissue damage in allergic immediate hypersensitivity reactions. The function of IgD has not yet been clarified. However, it is a surface receptor on B lymphocytes and may play a role in antigen-triggered lymphocyte differentiation.

T lymphocytes, as with B lymphocytes, originate as pluripotential stem cells in the bone marrow. They become committed to a specific type of stimulation as they pass through the thymus and are then distributed throughout the lymphoid tissues. Four basic functional subpopulations of T cells have been identified: (1) suppressor T cells (T_S) and (2) cytotoxic T cells (T_C), defined by the presence of the T4/Leu2a surface maker; and (3) helper T cells (T_H) and (4) T cells primarily involved with lymphokine production and macrophage activation (T_D) defined by the T4/Leu3a marker. When contacted by the appropriate antigen (antigen alone, or after processing by APCs), they become sensitized and mediate the *cell-mediated immune response* (CMI). When APCs are involved, additional recognition between T cells and certain major histocompatability complex (MHC) markers is required. T_H and T_S cells are primarily involved in modulation of the immune response, and T_H/T_S ratio defines, in part, level of immune responsiveness against certain antigens. They may be triggered by antigen-bearing APCs to produce response-mediating factors. These factors might then prevent or enhance B and T cell responsiveness.

T_C cells, along with other non–antigen-sensitized cells such as killer (K) or natural killer (NK) cells, act to lyse target cells to which they are sufficiently closely bound. Recognition of antigen by helper and cytotoxic T cells appears to require interaction with antigen-bearing APCs possessing appropriate tissue markers (MHC markers) on their membranes. On production of interleukin-1 from the APC and interleukin-2 (IL-2) from the T cell, antigenactivated cells are driven into proliferation.

T_D cells exert their effect mainly by production of lymphokines. They recognize free antigen and

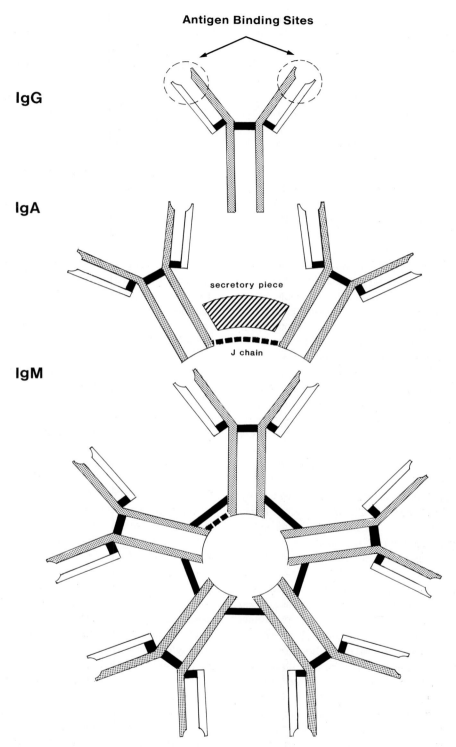

Fig. 4-19.   Basic structure of IgG, IgM, and secretory IgA. Multimeric forms are pictured along with the J chain thought to assist in polymerization. The secretory piece seen on secretory IgA is essential to the secretion process and in the protection of this immunoglobulin from destruction by proteolytic enzymes.

become sensitized T cells, although lymphokines are not produced until these cells are presented with antigen borne by an APC such as the macrophage.

The *lymphokines,* primarily exerting their effects on the macrophage population, are a large heterogeneous group of proteinaceous substances that either directly affect foreign substances or alter existing inflammatory reactions. A few examples of lymphokines are *lymphotoxin, macrophage activating factor* (MAF), *migration-inhibiting factor* (MIF), *osteoclast-activating factor* (OAF), and *eosinophil chemotactic factor of anaphylaxis* (ECF-A). Lymphotoxin has a direct lethal effect on cellular invaders. MAF alters macrophages to a more active state, whereas MIF holds these cells in the area of response. ECF-A exhibits a modulating suppressive effect on inflammation by calling eosinophils to the area. Eosinophils have the capability of destroying certain vasoactive substances such as histamine and serotonin (5-hydroxytryptamine). OAF is one lymphokine mediator shown to be extremely important in bone resorption (Horton et al., Raisz et al.). The stimulation of osteoclasts to resorb bone is a significant finding in many chronic inflammatory disorders, including periodontal disease. Horton et al. noted the importance of biologically active effector molecules released at local sites by infiltrating leukocytes and later demonstrated the release of OAF from lymphocytes of patients with periodontal disease. Its mechanism of activation has been critically investigated by Yoneda and Mundy and Bockman and Repo. These investigators and others have defined the necessity of certain prostaglandin (PGE) series, as produced by adherent monocytes, in lymphokine-mediated bone resorption.

Torabinejad and Luben implicated the potential importance of OAF in periapical bone destruction by demonstrating OAF in human periapical lesions. Interleukin-1β (IL-1β), a cytokine responsible for approximately 60% of bone-resorbing activity in inflammatory supernatants, has been identified as a major component of OAF. Lim et al. demonstrated a trend toward higher levels of IL-1β in symptomatic as opposed to asymptomatic periradicular lesions. Tumor necrosis factor α (TNFα), tumor necrosis factor β (TNFβ), and interleukin-1α (IL-1α) as well as synergistic interaction between these cytokines have been reported to be responsible for the remainder of OAF activity. Wang and Stashenko have demonstrated that the most resorptive activity in human periapical lesions is mediated by IL-1β and TNFβ. The levels of IL-1β were determined by Matsuo et al. to be almost double those of IL-1α in periapical exudates of infected root canals. The levels of IL-1β were found to decrease and the levels of IL-1α increase during the course of root canal therapy, possibly suggesting different roles for IL-1α and IL-1β during the healing process.

Memory cells (memory B or memory T cells) are also produced during initial exposure to an antigenic stimulus and are most important in the development of immunity. If memory cells subsequently meet the same antigen that originally induced them, they undergo a rapid transformation to plasma cells and sensitized T cells without the time-consuming induction period observed in the initial response. This secondary (or anamnestic) response occurs to a much smaller antigen dose, in a much shorter time after introduction of antigen, and results in more massive and longer-lived antibody levels.

It should be noted that, in some cases, sensitized T cells and plasma cells are observed relatively early in an inflammatory response. This indicates that memory cells are recognizing antigens that had been seen previously and are begin stimulated in an anamnestic response.

Chemical mediators of the inflammatory and immune responses

Although a wide variety of mediators and cell components are involved in the immune response and inflammation (Table 4-5), four of the most important substances or systems—histamine, complement, kinins, and arachidonic acid derivatives such as prostaglandins—will be described for a more complete understanding of inflammatory mechanisms. It should be realized that, unlike many other inflammatory mediators, kinins and prostaglandins may be normally involved in a variety of homeostatic mechanisms in the body.

On damage to normal tissue by infection or nonmicrobial trauma, several chemical mediators are released to initiate the inflammatory response (Fig. 4-20). These include mast cell products such as histamine and the arachidonic acid derivatives.

Mast cells have been shown to exist in connective tissues throughout the body (Selye), although some investigators (Anneroth and Brännström,

Table 4-5.   Major chemical mediators of inflammation

Origin	Group	Mediators
Plasma	Kinin system	Bradykinin
		Lysylbradykinin
	Complement system	C_{3a}, C_{5a}, $C_{5,6,7}$
	Clotting system	Hageman factor
		Fibrinopeptides
	Fibrinolytic system	Plasmin
Tissue	Vasoactive amines	Histamine
		5-Hydroxytryptamine (5-HT)
	Arachidonic acid derivatives	PGE, PGF
		Leukotrienes
		Others
	Acidic lipids	Slow-reacting substance of anaphylaxis (SRS-A)
	Lysosome (lysosomal granule) components	Fig. 4-18
	Lymphocyte products	Antibodies
		Lymphokines (Fig. 4-17)
	Others	Substance P
		Neurotensin

Eda and Langeland) have questioned their existence in human periapical lesions (Perrini and Fonzi) and inflamed dental pulp (Möller). Triggering of mast cell degranulation by tissue injury, drugs, and immune mechanisms causes many clinical effects associated with inflammation and allergic phenomena (Fig. 4-21). More recently, Farnoush demonstrated mast cells in both inflamed and non-inflamed human pulp. Mast cells in inflamed pulp gave histologic evidence of having degranulated. The role of mast cells in release of histamine and proteolytic enzymes elsewhere in the body (Dvorak and Dvorak, Selye, Uvnas) has been clearly shown. Histamine has been demonstrated to be the most important of the vasoactive amines (Owen and Woodward) and potentially plays a major role in early vasodilation of the pulp.

Complement is actually a series of at least nine major serum proteins in the blood. This system (Fig. 4-22) may be set in motion in a *cascading effect* nonenzymatically by bacteria, bacterial by-products, or lysosomal enzymes (alternate pathway) or by immune activation via antigen-bound IgG or IgM (classic pathway). Not only can complement activation cause lysis of cellular antigens and destroy nearby tissue cells in a bystander lysis phenomenon, it also results in release of certain breakdown products that mediate other proinflammatory processes. C_{3b} that is bound to antibody-antigen complexes can adhere to leukocytes, platelets, or erythrocytes, causing an agglutination in the process of *immune adherence.* C_{3a} and C_{5a} act in the chemotaxis of PMNs and macrophages and as anaphylatoxins, causing release of vasoactive substances from mast cells and basophils such as histamine, slow reacting substance of anaphylaxis (SRS-A), and prostaglandins. $C_{5,6,7}$ is also chemotactic and can cause bystander lysis. Although little data are available as to complement levels in inflamed pulpal tissue, elevated C_{3a} levels in periapical lesions have been reported by several investigators (Kettering and Torabinejad, Kuntz et al., Pulver et al.).

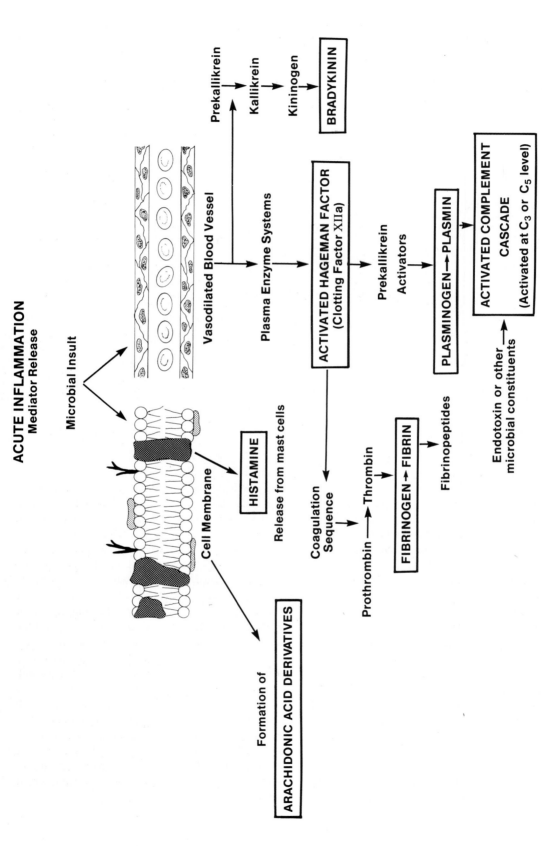

Fig. 4-20. Major mediators released during the inflammatory response.

MAST CELL ACTIVATION

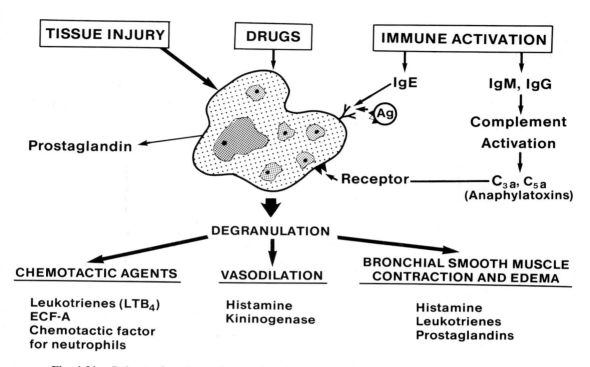

Fig. 4-21. Release of mediators from activated mast cells and the role of these mediators in the inflammatory process.

The *kinins* (Fig. 4-20) are vasoactive polypeptide molecules, including bradykinin and lysylbradykinin, that are capable of attracting leukocytes, causing vasodilation and smooth muscle contraction, as well as producing high levels of pain. Kinins and other vasoactive substances, including histamine, serotonin, and SRS-A, are capable of altering vascular permeability, increasing vasodilation, and enhancing the inflammatory reaction.

Kallikrein, the enzyme responsible for causing formation of kinins, is released from damaged tissue, or plasma kallikrein is indirectly activated by *Hageman factor* (Factor XII of the clotting system). Factor XII is itself activated by tissue damage or bacterial products such as endotoxin. The kallikrein then converts kininogen (circulating globulin) to kinin.

The arachidonic acid derivatives (Fig. 4-23) are involved in complex interrelationships in inflammation, as well as in homeostatic mechanisms. They appear to be major regulatory components

and have been called the *hormones of inflammation*. Many substances involved in the inflammatory state are derived from arachidonic acid, which is released from cell membrane lipids by the enzymatic action of cyclooxygenase and lipooxygenase. They are released from damaged tissue or actively secreted from phagocytes in contact with immune complexes or opsonized particles. On appropriate stimulation, the arachidonic acid derivatives produced include prostaglandins and thromboxanes (derived by use of the enzyme cyclooxygenase), and the leukotrienes, hydroperoxyeicosanoic and hydroxyeicosanoic acids (derived using the enzyme lipooxygenase). Prostaglandins E and F (PGE, PGF) seem to be involved in potentiating bradykinin-induced and histamine-induced pain as well as causing fever, edema, vasodilation, chemotaxis, platelet aggregation, and various other reactions correlated with inflammation, although no one prostaglandin can be said to account for all reactions observed in inflammation. Rather, these reactions may result from an imbalance of prosta-

COMPLEMENT ACTIVATION

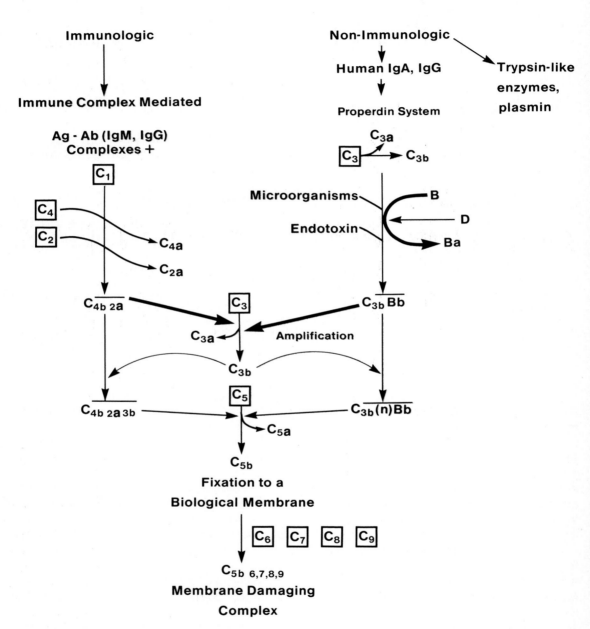

Fig. 4-22. Overview of the complement cascade. Activation by both classical and alternate pathways is shown.

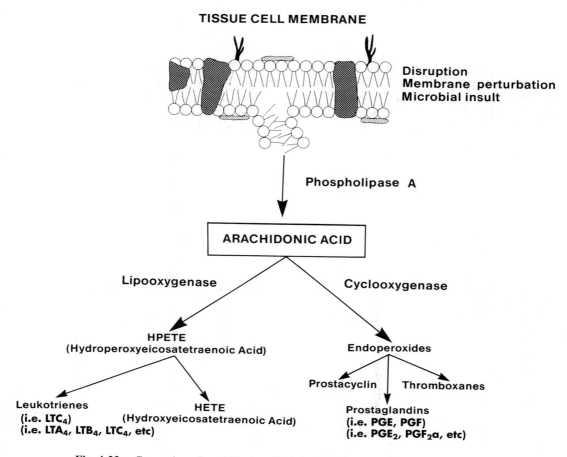

Fig. 4-23. Generation of arachidonic acid derivatives through membrane perturbation.

glandin types. Since certain prostaglandins exert their action by altering levels of secondary compounds within cells (the cyclic nucleotides), a so-called second messenger system for controlling inflammation has been suggested. Although these interactions are obviously very complex, it is easy to see the elegant types of control that must exist. Along with their roles in homeostasis, regulation of blood flow and pressure, and hormonal regulation, prostaglandins play a central role in inflammation and mediation of pain. Olm et al. and El Attar and Lin demonstrated levels of prostaglandins, thromboxanes, and leukotrienes in gingival tissues, whereas Lessard et al. demonstrated that levels of all three were elevated in inflamed dental pulp of dogs. Increased biosynthesis was usually also demonstrated. Cohen et al. specifically defined elevated levels of PGE_2 and PGF_2 in painful human pulp compared with nonpainful pulps.

Arachidonic acid metabolites have also been implicated in the pathogenesis of human periapical lesions. Torabinejad et al. found a positive correlation among high concentrations of leukotriene B_4 (LTB_4), the presence of high numbers of PMNs, and symptomatic periapical lesions. Leukotriene is a lipooxygenase metabolite of arachidonic acid. McNicholas et al. showed that PGE_2 is present in significantly higher levels in the periapical tissues of patients with symptoms of acute apical periodontitis compared with patients with chronic apical periodontitis or normal controls. Oguntebi et al. confirmed the involvement of prostaglandins in bone resorption via an experimental rat model. Periapical granulomas induced in rats that had been injected with indomethacin, a potent inhibitor of prostaglandin synthesis, showed a significantly lower degree of periapical bone resorption and much lower level of inflammation than the control group.

It is important to note that the mediators just mentioned do not, as a rule, exert prolonged activity. Rather, some are extremely unstable (e.g., certain complement components and arachidonic acid derivatives) or natural inhibitors exist to destroy their activity (e.g., C_{3b} inhibitor, anaphylatoxin inhibitor for complement; α-antitrypsin, α-macroglobulin, C_1-esterase inhibitor for kinin-forming systems; components of a certain fraction of human serum, the Cohn fraction IV-α globulin for prostaglandin-forming systems). These substances are important in fine control of the inflammatory and immune responses.

Role of the immune system in the inflammatory process

Induction of the immune response does not imply that other more acute inflammatory processes cease to function. Rather, besides exhibiting protective mechanisms of its own, the immune system augments and enhances the acute aspects of inflammation. These types of complex interactions of the immune system within the inflammatory process are difficult to describe in this short overview. However, knowledge of inflammation, inflammatory mediators, immune cells, and lymphocyte products must be integrated if the body's protective mechanisms are to be understood.

Immunoglobulin and immunoglobulin-bearing cells have been identified in periapical lesions (Morton et al., Naidorf, Pulver et al., Stern et al., Torabinejad et al.), including immunoglobulins of several isotypes. On the basis of electron microscopy (Farber) and cell dispersion (Stern et al.), T lymphocytes have also been identified within periapical lesions. Cymerman et al. tested the existence and subpopulation identify of T cells using monoclonal antibody techniques. Both T cytotoxic/suppressor lymphocytes and T helper/ inducer lymphocytes were identified. Quantitation was not attempted. Torabinejad and Kettering reported that in sections examined from periapical lesion specimens, T cells outnumbered B cells. Lukic et al. studied the prevalence of B and T cells in periapical lesions. T cells were found to be more prevalent than B cells in the same specimen. B cells were more dominant in focal infiltrates, whereas T cells of suppressor/cytotoxic phenotype dominated in granulomas with proliferating epithelium and initial cyst formation. The authors concluded that the presence and ratios of different immunocompetent cell subsets may reflect the pathogenesis of granuloma and transformation to cyst.

The humoral response provides many functions that enhance inflammation (Fig. 4-17). Antibodies function mainly to specifically bind and agglutinate or precipitate antigens that induced their production. Phagocytic cells can then more easily take up and destroy foreign substances. IgG and IgM enhance phagocytosis by the process of opsonization described previously. By the interaction of complement with antigen-antibody complexes, complement components cause release of vasoactive substances and call more phagocytes to the area of response. The inflammatory process then becomes self-perpetuating, since the presence of more phagocytes causes increased tissue damage and more antigen processing by macrophages. An enhancement spiral of inflammation and the immune system may then occur.

The cell-mediated response also assists in greatly stimulating inflammation (Fig. 4-17). First, certain sensitized T cells (helper T cells) assist in the B cell response, causing higher levels of antibody. Second, lymphokines obviously have a major effect on inflammation. Due to the nonspecific nature of certain lymphokines, these effectors are not released from sensitized T cells until the cells meet the appropriate antigen (contrast this to the constant release of antibody from plasma cells after primary sensitization). Lymphotoxin will nonspecifically lyse human cells as well as invaders. This further tissue damage enhances inflammation. MAF and MIF increase the number of phagocytes in the area of response.

Human periapical lesions develop as a result of the immune response to continuous stimuli from infected root canals. Matsuo et al. identified a correlation between the presence of immunoglobulin-containing cells and CD4+ (helper/inducer T cells) cell-rich lesions. These cells appeared to be acting in concert against antigenic stimuli from root canals, thereby surrounding the site of invasion to defend the host. The proportion of macrophages (CD11+ cells) were found to be greater in symptomatic teeth. Therefore it appears all cell types contribute to the pathogenesis of human periapical lesions.

Damaging effects of the immune response

Although it goes without saying that the immune system is a potent defense mechanism of the body, certain situations exist in which it can become self-destructive (Fig. 4-24). These harmful reactions associated with antigen are called allergies or hypersensitivities. Two general types of

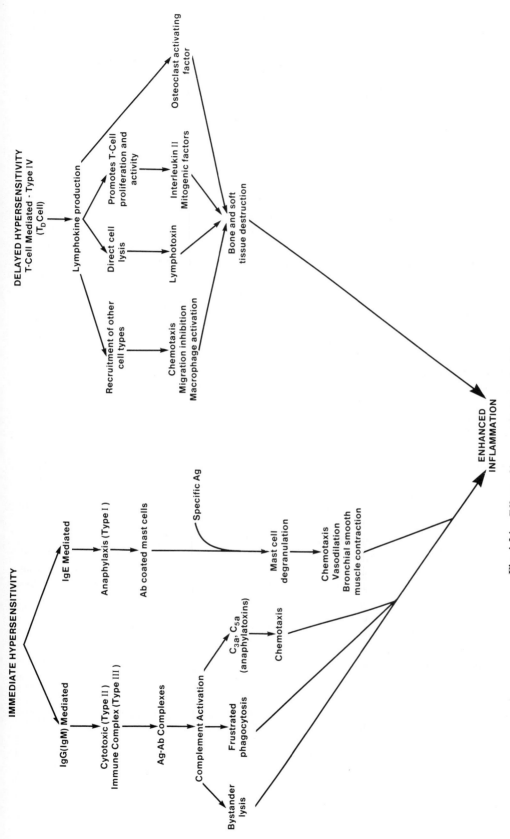

Fig. 4-24. Effects of hypersensitivity on the inflammatory process.

allergic reactions exist: *immediate,* which usually occurs within seconds or minutes and is caused by interaction with specific antibodies (humoral immunity), and *delayed,* which may take days to occur and is caused by the CMI. Previous sensitization by the provoking antigen, or an antigen similar in structure, is necessary.

Immediate hypersensitivity can be of three basic types. The most common type is mediated by IgE and is termed *anaphylactic.* Under certain conditions, antigen-IgE complexes cause degranulation of mast cells and basophils, with resultant release of severely damaging vasoactive substances and platelet-activating factor (PAF, inducing platelet aggregation and secretion of further vasoactive substances by platelets). Individuals who have a tendency to form IgE rather than the other antibody classes are called *atopic* and often have a variety of allergies. The other two types are IgG and/or IgM mediated and involve activation of complement, and eventual production of complement cleavage products C_{3a} and C_{5a} (mentioned previously), and eventual lysis of host cells. Inflammation and tissue damage may result.

Delayed hypersensitivity involves the CMI. Bacterial infection of dental pulp stimulates the activation of host protective mechanisms to eliminate this same bacteria from the infected root canals. Macrophages are called in great numbers to the site of response, and reactions occur that appear to be due to an overstimulation of CMI. Large quantities of lymphokines are released, normal inflammation is enhanced, further tissue damage occurs, and immune self-enhancement continues. Periapical lesions are local accumulations of immune inflammatory cells. Wang and Stashenko have discussed the resultant apical bone destruction as a host protective mechanism that creates space for this influx of cells. This helps to localize bacteria to the root canal and permit bone to retreat from the sites of infection and possibly the development of osteomyelitis. When the bacterial stimulus is removed, the lesion can be repaired by new bone.

It is extremely important to realize that an acute inflammatory response in the pulp and periapex has the potential of progressing through the chronic phase of inflammation and into a subacute response without the presence of clinical symptoms. This type of chronic lesion (or granuloma) contains antigens, phagocytes, necrotic material, and components of the immune system, both humoral (plasma cells, antibodies) and cellular (other lymphocytes, lymphokines). Therefore it contains materials necessary to trigger most, if not all, of the reactions mentioned in this description of immunology. Trowbridge suggested that T cells and macrophages played a key role in chronic inflammation. Activated T cells were instrumental in producing lymphokines capable of modifying the behavior of other cells, thus possibly facilitating or suppressing the immune response. Irreversible destruction of parenchymal tissue was replaced with fibrous connective tissue. Cytokines, produced by T cells and macrophages, enhanced the proliferation of fibroblasts, collagen production, and neovascularization. Such a lesion may exist for a prolonged time (even years) in a smoldering state. If the balanced state of the granuloma is altered by trauma or endodontic therapy, resulting in introduction of large quantities of antigen and immune cells into the surrounding area, the entire array of inflammatory reactions could be set in motion within a very short time. In this case, immune reactions would be superimposed on acute aspects of inflammation (flare-up), making it difficult to distinguish between the characteristics of each, since both would probably be present even if only one aspect were dominating.

REFERENCES

Andreason JO, Hjörting-Hansen E: Intraalveolar root fractures: radiographic and histologic study of 50 cases, *J Oral Surg* 25:414, 1967.

Anneroth G, Brännström M: Autofluorescent granular cells and mast cells in the human gingiva and dental pulp, *Odontol Rev* 15:10, 1964.

Bailey JM: Prostacyclins, thromboxanes and cardiovascular disease, *Trends Biochem Sci,* March 1979, p 68.

Barlocco JC, Poladian AJ: Una tecnica diagnostica de quistes y granuloma periapicales, *Odontol Bonaerense.* April 1979, p 22.

Barnes GW, Langeland K: Antibody formation in primates following introduction of antigens into the root canal, *J Dent Res* 45:111, 1966.

Bartels HA, Naidorf IJ, Blechman H: A study of some factors associated with endodontic "flare-ups," *Oral Surg* 22:225, 1968.

Baumgartner JC, Picket AB, Muller JT: Microscopic examination of oral sinus tracts and their associated perapical lesions, *J Endod* 10:146, 1984.

Bender IB: A commentary on General Bhaskar's hypothesis, *Oral Surg* 34:469, 1972.

Bender IB, Seltzer S: Roentgenographic and direct observation of experimental lesions in bone. I and II, *J Am Dent Assoc* 62:152, 708, 1961.

Bhaskar SN: Periapical lesions—types, incidence, and clinical features, *Oral Surg* 21:657, 1966.

Bhaskar SN: Nonsurgical resolution of radicular cysts, *Oral Surg* 34:458, 1972.

Bhaskar SN, editor: *Orban's oral histology and embryology,* ed 11, St Louis, 1991, Mosby.

Bockman RS, Repo MA: Lymphokine-mediated bone resorption requires endogenous prostaglandin synthesis, *J Exp Med* 81:154, 1981.

Bonta IL, Parnham MJ: Prostaglandins and chronic inflammation, *Biochem Pharmacol* 27:1611, 1978.

Cohen JS et al: A radioimmunoassay determination of the concentrations of prostaglandins E2 and F2 in painful and asymptomatic human dental pulps, *J Endod* 11:330,1985.

Cymerman JJ, Cymerman DH, Walters J, Nevins AJ: Human T lymphocyte subpopulations in chronic periapical lesions, *J Endod* 10:9, 1984.

DeDeus QD, Han SS: The fate of H3-cortisone applied on the exposed dental pulp, *Oral Surg* 24:404, 1967.

Donlon WC: Immunology in dentistry, *J Am Dent Soc* 100:220, 1980.

Dvorak H, Dvorak A: Basophilic leucocytes: structures, function and role in disease, *Clin Hematol* 4:651, 1975.

Eda S, Langeland K: The alteration of mast cell staining due to various fixatives and demineralizing agents, *Scand J Dent Res* 78:217, 1970.

El Attar T, Lin H: Prostaglandins in gingiva of patients with periodontal disease, *J Periodontol* 52:16, 1981.

Farber PA: Scanning electron microscopy of cells from periapical lesions, *J Endod* 1:291, 1975.

Farnoush A: Mast cells in human dental pulp, *J Endod* 10:250, 1984.

Feiglin B, Reade PC: The distribution of 14C leucine and 85Sr labeled microspheres from rat incisor root canals, *Oral Surg* 47:277, 1979.

Fish WE: *Surgical pathology of the mouth,* Philadelphia, 1951, Lippincott.

Frank MM: The complement system in host defense and inflammation, *Rev Infect Dis* 1:483, 1979.

Fujii S, Moriya H, Suzuki T: *Kinins II,* New York, 1979, Plenum.

Green DB, editor: Conference on inflammation, *J Endod* 6, 1977.

Grossman L: *Endodontic practice,* ed 10, Philadelphia, 1981, Lea & Febiger.

Grossman LI, Esther S: Estudic comparativo clínico e histologiopatológico de reaçotes periapicales crónicas, *Rev Brasil Odontol* 22:226, 1963.

Harrison JW, Larson WJ: The epithelized oral sinus tract, *Oral Surg* 42:511, 1976.

Heithersay GS: Stimulation of root formation in incompletely developed pulpless teeth, *Oral Surg* 29:620, 1970.

Hirsch J et al: Periapical surgery, *Int J Oral Surg* 8:173, 1979.

Horton JE, Oppenheim JJ, Mergenhagen SE, Raisz LG: Macrophage-lymphocyte synergy in the production of osteoclast activating factor, *J Immunol* 113:1278, 1974.

Horton JE, et al.: Bone resorbing activity in supernatant fluid from cultured human peripheral bone leukocytes, *Science* 177:793, 1972.

Horton JE, et al.: Partial purification of a bone resorbing factor elaborated from human allogenic cultures, *Cell Immunol* 43:1, 1979.

Kettering JD, Torabinejad M: Concentrations of immune complexes, IgG, IgM, IgE, and C3 in patients with acute apical abscesses, *J Endod* 10:417, 1984.

Kuntz DD, Genco RJ, Guttuso J, Natiella JR: Localization of immunoglobulins and the third component of complement in dental periapical lesions, *J Endod* 3:68, 1977.

Lalonde ER, Luebke RG: The frequency and distribution of periapical cysts and granulomas, *Oral Surg* 25:861, 1968.

Langeland K, Block R, Grossman L: A histopathologic study of 35 periapical endodontic surgical specimens, *Oral Surg* 3:8, 1977.

Lehner T: Cell mediated immune response in oral disease, *J Oral Pathol* 1:39, 1972.

Lessard GM, Torabinejad M, Swope D: Arachidonic acid metabolism in canine tooth pulps and the effects of non-steroidal anti-inflammatory drugs, *J Endod* 12:146, 1986.

Lim G et al: Interleukin 1B in symptomatic and asymptomatic human periapical lesions, *J Endod* 20:225, 1994.

Lukic, Arsenijevic N, Vujanic G, Ramic Z: Quantitative analysis of the immunocompetent cells in periapical granuloma: correlation with the histological characteristics of the lesions, *J Endod* 16:119, 1990.

Matsuo et al: Quantitative analysis of immunocompetent cells in human periapical lesions: correlations with clinical findings of the involved teeth, *J Endod* 18:497, 1992.

Matsuo et al: Interleukin-la and interleukin-1B in periapical exudates of infected root canals: correlations with the clinical findings of the involved teeth, *J Endod* 20:432, 1994.

McNicholas S, Torabinejad M, Blankenship J, Bakland L: The concentration of prostaglandin E2 in human periradicular lesions, *J Endod* 17:97, 1991.

Melcher AH: Repair of wounds in the periodontium of the rat: influence of periodontal ligament on osteogenesis, *Arch Oral Biol* 15:1183, 1970.

Melcher AH, Correia MA: Remodeling of periodontal ligaments in erupting molars of mature rats, *J Periodontol Res* 6:118, 1971.

Michanowicz A, Michanowicz J, Abou-Rass M: Cementogenic repair of root fractures, *J Am Dent Assoc* 82:569, 1971.

Möller E, editor: Role of macrophages in the immune response, *Immunol Rev* 40:1, 1978.

Morse D, Patnik J, Schacterle G: Electrophoretic differentiation of radicular cysts and granulomas, *Oral Surg* 35:249, 1973.

Morse D, Schacterle G, Wolfson E: A rapid chairside differentiation of radicular cysts and granulomas, *J Endod* 2:17, 1976.

Morse D, Wolfson E, Schacterle G: Non-surgical repair of electrophoretically diagnosed radicular cysts, *J Endod* 1:158, 1975.

Morse R: Immunologic aspects of pulpal-periapical diseases, *Oral Surg* 43:436, 1977.

Mortensen H, Winther JE, Birn H: Periapical granulomas and cysts: an investigation of 1,600 cases, *Scand J Dent Res* 78:241, 1970.

Morton TH, Clagett JA, Yavorsky DJ: Role of immune complexes in human periapical periodontitis, *J Endod* 3:261, 1977.

Movat HZ, editor: *Inflammation, immunity and hypersensitivity,* New York, 1979, Harper & Row.

Naidorf I: Immunoglobulins in the periapical granulomas: a preliminary report, *J Endod* 1:15, 1975.

Naidorf IJ: Correlation of the inflammatory response with immunological and clinical events, *J Endod* 3:223, 1977.

Oguntebi BR, Barker BF, Anderson DM, Sakumura J: The effect of indomethacin on experimental dental periapical lesions in rats, *J Endod* 15:117, 1989.

Olm K, Alberts HK, Lisboa BP: Measurement of eight prostaglandins in human gingival and periodontal disease using high pressure liquid chromatography and radioimmunoassay. *J Periodontal Res* 19:501, 1984.

Owen DDA, Woodward DF: Histamine and histamine H1- and H2-receptor antagonists in acute inflammation, *Biochem Soc Trans* 8:150, 1980.

Page DO, Trump GN, Schaeffer LD: Pulpal studies. Part I. Passage of 3H tetracycline into the circulatory system through rat molar pulps, *Oral Surg* 35:555, 1973.

Patterson S, Shafer W, Healey H: Periapical lesions associated with endodontically treated teeth, *J Am Dent Assoc* 68:191, 1964.

Perrini N, Fonzi L: Mast cells in human periapical lesions: ultrastructural aspects and their possible physiopathological implications, *J Endod* 11:197, 1985.

Pulver WH, Taubman MA, Smith DJ: Immune components in human dental periapical lesions, *Arch Oral Biol* 23:435, 1978.

Raisz LG, Trummel CL, Mundy GR, Luben RA: Immunologic factors influencing bone resorption: role of osteoclast activating factor from human lymphocytes and complement mediated prostaglandin synthesis. In Talmage RV, Owen M, Parsons JA, editors: *Calcium-regulating hormones,* Amsterdam, 1975, Excerpta Medica.

Reed WP: The immunologic substrate: role of local and systemic immunity in the head and neck, *Otolaryngol Clin North Am* 9:581, 1976.

Roitt IM, Lehner T: *Immunology of oral disease,* Oxford, 1980, Blackwell.

Rosengren L: Inoculation of *Streptococcus mutans* and other bacteria into dental pulps of rats, *Isr J Dent Med* 19:1, 1970.

Ross PN, Birch BS: A clinical histopathologic study of conservative endodontic failures, *J Dent Res* 55 (special issue B), abstract 271, 1976.

Sela M: Antigenicity—some molecular aspects, *Science* 166:1365, 1969.

Seltzer S: *Endodontology: biologic considerations in endodontic procedures,* ed 2, New York, 1988, McGraw-Hill.

Seltzer S, Bender IB, Ziontz M: The dynamics of pulp inflammation: correlations between diagnostic data and actual histologic findings in the pulp. *Oral Surg* 16:846, 1963.

Seltzer S, Soltanoff W, Bender IB: Epithelial proliferation of periapical lesions, *Oral Surg* 27:111, 1969.

Seltzer S et al: Biologic aspects of endodontics. III. Periapical tissue reactions to root canal instrumentation, *Oral Surg* 26:694, 1968.

Selye H: *The mast cells,* Washington, DC, 1965, Butterworth.

Shear M: The histogenesis of the dental cyst, *Dent Pract* 13:238, 1963.

Sinai I et al: Biologic aspects of endodontics. II. Periapical tissue reactions to pulp extirpation, *Oral Surg* 23:664, 1967.

Spector WG, Willoughby WG: The inflammatory response, *Bacteriol Rev* 27:117, 1963.

Stashenko P, Yu S, Wang C: Kinetics of immune cell and bone resorptive responses to endodontic infections, *J Endod* 18:422, 1992.

Stern MH, et al: Quantitative analysis of cellular composition of human periapical granuloma, *J Endod* 7:117, 1981.

Stern MH, Preizen S, Mackler BF, Levy BM: Isolation of characterization of inflammatory cells from human periapical granuloma, *J Dent Res* 61:1408, 1982.

Taubman MA, Smith DJ: Oral immunology. In Shaw HJ et al, editors: *Textbook of oral biology,* Philadelphia, 1978, Saunders.

Toller PA: Protein substances in odontogenic fluids, *Br Dent J* 128:317, 1970.

Tomasi TB, Bienenstock J: Secretory immunoglobulin. In Tomasi TB, editor: *The immune system of secretions,* Englewood Cliffs, NJ, 1976, Prentice-Hall.

Torabinejad M, Bakland LK: Immunopathogenesis of chronic periapical lesions, *Oral Surg* 46:685, 1979.

Torabinejad M, Bakland LK: Prostaglandins: their role in the pathogenesis of pulpal and periapical disease. Part I, *J Endod* 6:733, 1980.

Torabinejad M, Bakland LK: Prostaglandins: their role in the pathogenesis of pulpal and periapical diseases. Part 2, *J Endod* 6:769, 1980.

Torabinejad M, Clagett J, Engel D: A cat model for the evaluation of mechanisms of bone resorption: induction of bone loss by simulated immune complexes and inhibition by indomethacin, *Calcif Tissue Int* 29:207, 1979.

Torabinejad M, Cotti E, Jung T: Concentrations of leukotriene B4 in symptomatic and asymptomatic periapical lesions, *J Endod* 18:205, 1992.

Torabinejad M, Eby WC, Naidorf I: Inflammatory and immunological aspects of the pathogenesis of human periapical lesions, *J Endod* 11:479, 1985.

Torabinejad M, Kettering JD: Identification and relative concentration of B and T lymphocytes in human chronic periapical lesions, *J Endod* 11:122, 1985.

Torabinejad M, Kettering JD, Bakland LK: Localization of IgE immunoglobulin in human dental periapical lesions by the peroxidase-antiperoxidase method, *Arch Oral Biol* 26:677, 1981.

Torabinejad M, Kiger RD: Experimentally induced alterations of periapical tissues of the cat, *J Dent Res* 59:87, 1980.

Torabinejad M, Luben RA: Presence of osteoclast activating factor in human periapical lesions (abstract), *J Endod* 11:145, 1985.

Torneck C, Smith J, Grindell P: Biologic effects of endodontic procedures on developing incisor teeth, *Oral Surg* 35:378, 1973.

Torres J, Torabinejad M, Matiz R, Mantilla E: Presence of secretory IgA in human periapical lesions, *J Endod* 20:87, 1994.

Trowbridge H: Immunological aspects of chronic inflammation and repair, *J Endod* 16, 54, 1990.

Trowbridge HO, Emling RC: *Inflammation: a review of the process,* ed 2, Bristol, Pa, 1983, Distribution Systems.

Uvnas B: Release processes in mast cells and their activation by injury, *Ann NY Acad Sci* 116:880, 1964.

Walton RE, Langeland K: Migration of materials in the dental pulp of monkeys, *J Endod* 4:167, 1978.

Wang C, Stashenko P: Characterization of bone resorbing activity in human periapical lesions, *J Endod* 19:107, 1993.

Wasserman MA: Prostaglandins: birth of a new therapeutic era, *Am Pharm* 19:15, 1979.

Weine F, Healey H, Theiss E: Endodontic emergency dilemma: leave tooth open or keep tooth closed, *Oral Surg* 40:531, 1975.

Wood NK, Goaz PW: *Differential diagnosis of oral lesions,* ed 4, St. Louis, 1991, Mosby.

Yoneda T, Mundy GR: Prostaglandins are necessary for osteoclast-activating factor production by activated peripheral blood leukocytes, *J Exp Med* 149:279, 1979.

5 Endodontic emergency treatment

Approximately 90% of patients requesting treatment for the relief of pain to a dental office have pulpal and/or periapical disease and thus are candidates for endodontic therapy. This fact was originally reported by Mitchell and Tarplee and then reaffirmed by Hasler and Mitchell in an exhaustive study of 1628 patients with toothaches. Not all these people will receive endodontic treatment. Some of the involved teeth may not be treatable or restorable, whereas some of the patients may not be interested in saving the affected tooth or be able to afford the required treatment. However, 90% of those calling the office for relief may be potential endodontic patients.

Despite this impressive information, if one examines dental publications or programs for dental society meetings, articles or presentations on endodontic emergency treatment are conspicuous by their absence. At the time of the writing of this edition, infection control, esthetics, implants, and practice management seem to have a huge segment of the postdoctoral information market. However, knowing how to treat successfully and adequately 90% of those requiring pain relief represents a huge segment of problems to be solved in any dental office.

In addition to the pain experienced by the patient, the need for endodontic emergency treatment usually has some upsetting effect on the practitioner. Time must be taken from another scheduled patient to dispense the needed relief. Being conscientious, the dentist wishes to spend any necessary time that is required to get the patient out of pain yet wishes to disrupt the normal schedule only minimally.

This chapter will discuss the methods essential in making a rapid yet accurate diagnosis of pulpal and periapical pain, the kinds of emergency treatment needed to relieve pain, and the correct procedures to follow to gain a successful endodontic result.

EFFECTS OF EMERGENCY TREATMENT

Flare-ups even with the best therapy. There is often some embarrassment felt by dentists when one of their patients requires emergency treatment. They may believe that the painful episode could have been prevented or that it was caused by their past dental work. This feeling should be dispelled, since a flare-up may occur sometimes with the best therapy and a particular exacerbation may not be directly associated with recent treatment.

An excellent example of this situation is a patient requiring replacement of an old and inadequate restoration for a tooth with a chronic pulpitis. Because the pulp had been in a quiet state, the operator was unaware of the true condition. As a result of cavity preparation, impressions, temporarization, and restoration placement, the chronic pulpitis was converted to an acute situation and pain developed. However, the tooth has received a better restoration as a result of treatment. Although the major source of pulpal irritation may have occurred many years earlier when the previous work was performed, the present treatment might be erroneously blamed as the major source of the problem.

It is impractical to remove every deep restoration to examine the underlying tooth structure, particularly when there is no clinical or radiographic evidence of damage. Teeth with fillings or bases in proximity to the pulp may be difficult to evaluate with available diagnostic aids. Also, the response to pulp injury varies with individuals. The pulps of some patients may have an excellent recovery after extensive operative procedures, whereas in others pulp tissue will remain in a permanently damaged state after less complex treatment, even if all the normally used pulpal protective agents and devices are utilized.

Emergencies in cases under construction. During the course of tooth preparation, pulp exposure or irreversible damage may occur without the operator's realizing the situation. In excavating the last vestiges of decay or preparing abutments for parallelism, a wafer-thin wall of dentin may remain that is sufficient to protect the pulp to withstand the procedures that follow. A pulp exposure may occur in a tooth with chronic pulpitis or pulp necrosis, and thus no bleeding occurs to alert the dentist. Within a day or two of such an occurrence, the patient probably suffers a serious toothache, and an endodontic emergency has developed. This type of pain is much more severe than the sensitivity to thermal changes normally associated with many operative procedures.

Method for reaching new patients. As stated earlier, programs on practice management are very popular at present. Intensive courses are given on how to attract and then retain new patients into a dental practice. Such programs are often given by various combinations of psychologists, time and money management experts, and marketing analysts.

In my opinion, efficient and effective endodontic treatment is one of the best ways to attract and retain new patients into a specific practice. A patient coming into a dental office for the first time, in pain and in jeopardy of losing a tooth, is in a very vulnerable position.

If applicable, at the time of the emergency appointment the dentist should suggest that endodontic therapy might be employed to retain the involved tooth. If the necessary treatment is administered and the pain is relieved, patients are impressed with the dentist's interest in their oral health, as shown by preventing an extraction and by the effectiveness of the treatment. In these circumstances it would not be unusual for the patient, prompted by the excellence of the emergency treatment, to make further appointments for evaluation of dental problems and needed therapy.

Sometimes the need for endodontic emergency treatment may be considered to be beneficial for both the patient and the dentist. Some potential patients avoid dental treatment for various reasons, most often fear, but are forced to seek relief due to pain. If treated by a caring person, with skill and effectiveness, such a patient can be won over, proper treatment can be gained for any and all dental problems present, and the patient can be on the way to dental health.

Demonstration of continued interest in past patients. In addition to reaching new patients,

effective emergency treatment reassures the patient already within the practice that the dentist is maintaining a continued interest. If an emergency befalls a patient during the interim period between checkup appointments, the necessary treatment must be promptly provided. The patient's feelings about the need for an emergency appointment may not coincide with a true emergency as far as the dentist is concerned. However, if patients are not obliged in what they consider their time of need, they have every right to be upset. Recurrence of procrastination in these circumstances may lead to the loss of patients so handled.

Self-satisfaction. In addition to the relief that the patient feels after successful emergency treatment, the dentist feels a definite amount of self-satisfaction. The patient came in with a serious problem, consisting of pain and the threat of tooth loss. By correct endodontic emergency treatment the pain is relieved, yet the endangered tooth is to be retained. The hero of this drama is the dispenser of this excellent treatment, and the dentist has every right to feel proud of the work.

INITIAL THERAPY FOR "HOT" TEETH

Initial therapy for "hot" teeth refers to what needs to be done to give relief from pain at the first appointment for a tooth with pulpal or periapical involvement. Further portions of this chapter will discuss the needed emergency treatment for a tooth for which endodontic therapy had already been started and for traumatic injuries.

Two types of emergency treatment will be described and are listed in Table 5-1; choosing one or the other depends on the time available for administering therapy. If little time is available and the emergency treatment must be dispensed while seeing the patient in pain between normally scheduled patients, a specific regimen will be presented. However, if a full appointment is available without time constraints, a longer treatment session will be described. In all circumstances the suggested therapy is designed to get the patient out of pain and retain the relief of pain for a reasonable amount of time—until the patient can be fit into the regular schedule again. Getting the patient out of pain for a short while, only to be seen again in pain very soon, is counterproductive.

Need for making diagnosis. Before any endodontic treatment is performed, of either routine or emergency nature, an accurate diagnosis must be made to determine what is wrong. A classification of

Table 5-1. Emergency treatment for "hot" teeth

Diagnostic tests		Condition of periapical tissues according to radiograph	Clinical condition	Treatment, minimal or considerable amount of time available	Medicament	Open/close
Pulp vitality	Percussion					
+	0	Normal	Acute pulpitis	Minimal amount of time:		
				Single-rooted tooth—pulpectomy	None	Close
				Multirooted tooth—pulpotomy	Formocresol	Close
				Considerable amount of time:		
				Single-rooted tooth—pulpectomy and canal preparation	None	Close
				Multirooted tooth—pulpectomy	None	Close
+	+	Normal to slight thickening to small radiolucency	Acute pulpitis with acute apical periodontitis	Minimal amount of time:		
				Nonmolar—pulpectomy	None	**Close!**
				Molar—pulpotomy of largest canal	CMCP	**Close!**
				Considerable amount of time:		
				Nonmolar—pulpectomy and canal preparation	None	**Close!**
				Molar—pulpectomy	None	**Close!**
0	0	Radiolucency	Pulp necrosis	Canal debridement	None	Close
0	+	Small to large radiolucency, may be diffuse	Acute periapical abscess	Minimal amount of time:		
				Incision and drainage, preferably through tooth; otherwise through tissue	Often systemic antibiotics	Open
				Second appointment, canal debridement	None	Open
				Third appointment, irrigate and dry, **do not file**	None or sulfa point	Close
				Considerable amount of time: Open through tooth and let drain until exudation stops; mild preparation	None	Close

pulpal and periapical disease is made, since each major category of clinical condition requires slightly different treatment. If an indifferent attempt is made in diagnosis and the wrong condition is thought to be present, an incorrect method of therapy will be initiated. This is particularly serious in emergency treatment, since a minimal amount of time is available because of the press of other patients, and the patient in pain may have an increase in symptoms if the wrong treatment is provided.

Fortunately the conditions that require emergency endodontic treatment may be divided into four major categories, each requiring different handling for relief of pain but all based on making only two clinical determinations. The four conditions are acute pulpitis, acute pulpitis with apical periodontitis, pulp necrosis, and acute periapical abscess. Any acute condition may have been converted from a chronic inflammation or may be the initial inflammatory lesion. The exact pathogenicity is really not too important at the time of the emergency treatment, since the major objective is to relieve the pain rather than decide what conditions preceded it.

Table 5-1 summarizes the emergency treatment required for initial endodontic therapy for patients in pain. After a diagnosis is made, on the basis of response to pulp testing and percussion, the needed treatment, medication, and closing of the access preparation are listed.

Types of diagnostic aids needed. According to Table 5-1, three clinical determinations are required before instituting endodontic emergency treatment: (1) determine the presence or absence of pulp vitality, (2) analyze the reaction of the offending tooth to percussion, and (3) evaluate the radiograph.

As discussed in Chapter 2, the thermal tests for reaction to heat and cold and the electric pulp tester are the most reliable diagnostic aids for determining pulp vitality. The test cavity may be employed if question still exists. For cold, using either ice sticks or ethyl chloride spray is best. Either hot gutta-percha or rubber wheeling on metal restorations is used for heat.

In some cases no diagnostic aid is needed to establish that the pulp is vital, but merely questioning of the patient is sufficient. If the patient supplies the facts that changes in temperature either increase or decrease pain, the pulp is considered to have vitality.

Percussion is an important test because it determines whether inflammation has extended to the periapical tissues. The test is best performed by lightly tapping the teeth with the butt end of a mirror handle.

Radiographs are critically important in all stages of endodontic therapy, particularly in deciding on the correct emergency treatment when minimal time is available to gain pain relief. The presence or absence of a periapical lesion, or even a thickening of the periodontal ligament, may dictate different therapy. As discussed in Chapter 2, and as seen in Figs. 5-1, 5-3, 5-9, and 5-10, each of these conditions require individual analysis as related to other clinical symptomatology to arrive at the correct form of treatment.

Acute pulpitis

For a diagnosis of acute pulpitis to be made, the pain must be coming from a vital pulp in a tooth without tenderness to percussion. These two determinations establish that the inflammation has not yet reached the apical portions of the root canal and probably is confined to the coronal pulp. Radiographically there is no change from normal in the periapical tissues, since the inflammation has not reached that area. However, some cause of coronal pulp inflammation, such as deep caries, extensive restoration, trauma, or pulp capping, must be shown (Fig. 5-1).

Accordingly, when minimal time is available, in a posterior tooth the correct emergency treatment is a pulpotomy. Local anesthetic is administered and the correct access cavity prepared (Chapter 6). By means of spoon excavator and large round bur, the coronal portion of the pulp is removed, leaving

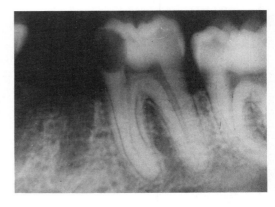

Fig. 5-1. Radiograph reveals large carious lesion with probable pulp exposure but no deviation from normal in periapical tissues.

vital tissue inside the pulp canals (Fig. 5-2, *A*). A cotton pellet is moistened with formocresol and placed over the canal orifices for 1 minute. This pellet is discarded; a new pellet very lightly dampened with formocresol is placed in the chamber (Fig. 5-2, *B*), and the access cavity is closed with zinc oxide–eugenol (ZOE), accelerated with zinc acetate crystals (Fig. 5-2, *C*). The patient is then given another appointment for completion of the endodontic treatment.

Only a pulpotomy need be performed at the emergency appointment for acute pulpitis because the pulp in the roots probably has remained in a relatively normal condition. After removal of the tissue in the chamber, the site of inflammation precipitating a painful response is gone. The action of the formocresol is to fix the noninflamed tissue left in the root until subsequent treatment thoroughly debrides the canal contents. Because formocresol is caustic, its action must be kept within the pulp canals. As long as vital tissue remains between the drug and the periapical tissues, there is little chance of periapical damage. Therefore neither of the cotton pellets used within the chamber is to be saturated with formocresol; if a complete pulpectomy is performed at the emergency appointment, an alternative medication should be used.

In single-rooted teeth it is just as easy to remove the pulp totally as to perform a pulpotomy at the emergency treatment for acute pulpitis. Accordingly, this procedure is followed if sufficient time and canal width allow for complete pulpectomy. With the entire pulp removed, a cotton pellet with no drug is sealed in as before with ZOE.

After the temporary seal is placed, occlusion should be checked with marking paper to ascertain that no high spots exist (Fig. 5-2, *D*). Supraocclusion might cause a pericementitis. This would complicate the next phases of endodontic therapy, since the healing of periapical tissue is the objective of

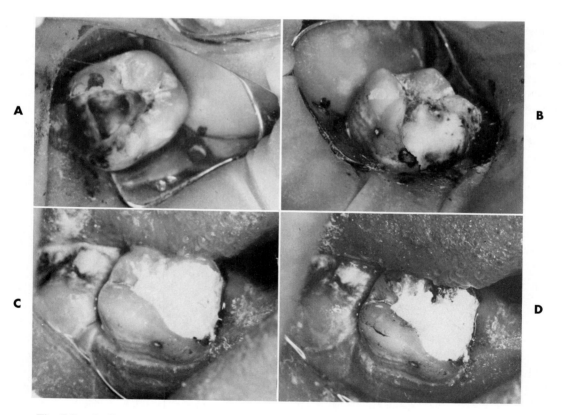

Fig. 5-2. **A,** Coronal pulp is removed, leaving vital tissue within canals. **B,** Cotton pellet dampened with formocresol is placed over canal orifices. **C,** Preparation is closed with zinc oxide–eugenol (ZOE). **D,** Marking paper indicates that no high spots exist on temporary restoration, which might cause dislodgement. The patient may now be released.

any endodontic treatment. Also, if the temporary seal is too high, portions of the ZOE might break out, opening the access preparation to the contaminants of saliva. Since one of the important factors in treating an acute pulpitis is to keep the tooth sealed between appointments, loss of the temporary filling would be undesirable.

When considerable time is available at the emergency visit, more treatment may be afforded. In multirooted teeth a complete pulpectomy may be performed rather than merely a pulpotomy. The removal of the entire pulp will ensure that the pain that brought the patient to the dental office will be eliminated. With the entire pulp removed, no medicament is necessary, and the access is closed with a dry, sterile cotton pellet and ZOE.

For single-rooted teeth with more time available, the pulpectomy is performed and then the working length is calculated (Chapter 8), followed by initiation of canal preparation. Again, no medicament is needed, and the access is closed as with multirooted teeth.

Acute pulpitis with apical periodontitis

The most difficult emergency condition to treat is acute pulpitis with apical periodontitis. This is particularly true in mandibular molars, where an insufficiency in depth of anesthesia is not an uncommon problem. Considerable time is usually required for the emergency treatment of this condition because the inflamed tissue that must be

removed is in the apical portion of the root canal.

The diagnosis of acute pulpitis with apical periodontitis is usually simple to make. The patient is aware of the tooth's tenderness to percussion and may request that the dentist not tap that particular member of the arch during the oral examination. In the most typical classic situation, heat causes the intense pain whereas cold relieves. Some patients may actually come to the dental office with a glass of ice water that they have been taking periodically to keep the pain to a minimal level of intensity. Sensitivity to *both* heat and cold is not unusual. Therefore the determinations of tooth vitality and tenderness to percussion are obvious.

A radiograph of a tooth with acute apical periodontitis may show a small periapical radiolucency, exhibit a thickening of the periodontal ligament space, or appear normal (Fig. 5-3). In a multirooted tooth, one root may show one radiographic condition, whereas another root may demonstrate a different situation.

Heavy dosage of local anesthetic is administered, with two Carpules being required for most posterior teeth. The correct access cavity is prepared. In some cases when the pulp has been severely inflamed for a considerable time, the patient may complain of sensitivity to access preparation, even after good signs of paresthesia have been obtained, increasing in intensity as the pulp is approached. When this occurs, the proper approach is to be sympathetic about the patient's

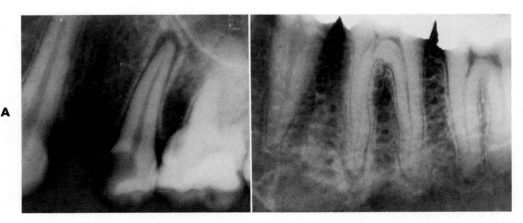

Fig. 5-3. **A,** Radiograph reveals small radiolucency around apex of maxillary second bicuspid. **B,** Radiograph shows thickening of periodontal ligament space on mesial root, but no apparent change adjacent to distal root of the mandibular first molar. Radiopacity around both roots indicates presence of pulpoperiapical osteosclerosis. Both teeth were tender to percussion and had vital pulp tissue. Diagnosis of acute pulpitis with apical periodontitis was made for each.

pain, explain that the severe inflammation has prevented the anesthetic from attaining full effectiveness, and request the patient to endure a few more minutes of discomfort until anesthetic can be applied directly to the irritated tissue. When water spray is used to complete the access preparation, its cooling effect may make approach to the pulp more endurable.

Once the roof of the chamber has been removed, anesthetic is applied directly to the vital pulp (Fig. 5-4), and generally no further pain will be experienced.

Best therapy for the condition is a complete pulpectomy, and this should be performed in non-molar teeth in all cases and in molar teeth when sufficient time is available. The inflamed tissue in an acute pulpitis with acute apical periodontitis is found in the apical portion of the canal(s). If only a pulpotomy is performed, the patient probably will not gain relief from pain. It is the pulp near the apex that must be removed.

Although complete pulpectomy is feasible in nonmolar teeth in minimal time, this is rarely possible if a molar is causing the problem. Therefore it is permissible in this condition for a complete pulpectomy to be performed on the largest canal only in the molar tooth, that is, the palatal canal of a maxillary molar or the distal canal of a mandibular molar (Fig. 5-5). This will involve the taking of a radiograph and removal of bulk tissue, but this procedure still requires much less time than a complete pulpectomy and usually is effective.

Generally the single-canal pulpectomy for molar teeth works well to gain relief, since it is the largest canal that usually houses the tissue carrying the pain in an acute pulpitis with acute apical periodontitis. However, in a low percentage of cases the inflamed tissue causing the pain will be in the undebrided smaller canals. In that instance, not only will pain relief not be obtained, but the pain might intensify. The patient should be called the next day after the emergency treatment to verify that the condition has been alleviated. If not, another appointment must be scheduled quickly, and then all the remaining pulp is removed.

If sufficient time exists, the complete pulpectomy is preferable for molar teeth with this condition. Care must be exercised to ensure that all canals have been located and debrided. This means that radiographs with files in place (Fig. 5-6) must be taken and evaluated. The second distal canal of a mandibular molar or a second canal in a maxillary second bicuspid may house sufficient pulp tissue to cause a continued painful condition if undiscovered and hence uncleaned. The access cavity is closed with a sterile cotton pellet and ZOE, accelerated with zinc acetate crystals, and the occlusion is checked. For some erroneous reason, many practitioners believe that any tooth that is tender to percussion before treatment should be left open at an emergency appointment to gain pain relief. Nothing could be further from the truth. Although it is true that leaving open a tooth that has a condition of acute pulpitis with apical

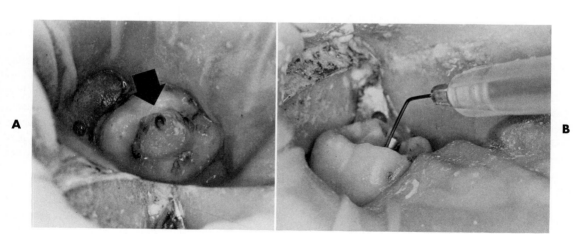

Fig. 5-4. Direct injection into pulp. **A,** Small hole is drilled through roof of chamber *(arrow).* Entire roof must not be removed because the intrapulpal injection will not be effective. **B,** Injection solution is forcibly inserted into pulp through the small hole in roof of chamber.

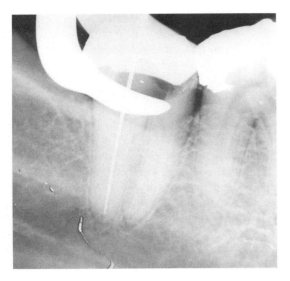

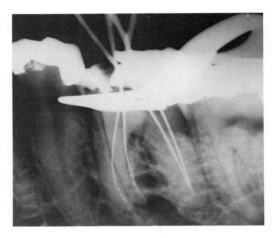

Fig. 5-6. The best emergency treatment for a tooth with acute pulpitis and acute apical periodontitis is to have the entire pulp removed. In mandibular molars the possibility of tissue remaining in a second distal canal must be managed.

Fig. 5-5. Mandibular second molar with preoperative symptoms of tenderness to percussion, severe pain, and a vital pulp, indicating an acute pulpitis with acute apical periodontitis. Because minimal time was available for the emergency appointment, a pulpotomy was performed, the pulp from the distal canal was removed, and that canal was enlarged. The patient was free of pain that evening. Had more time been available, a complete pulpectomy would have been the treatment of choice.

periodontitis will diminish the pain response initially, such relief will be merely transitory. Unless the apical tissue is removed, pain must return, and after the tooth has been open, the inflamed tissues will be further irritated by the ingress of contaminants from the oral fluids.

Even though some relief may have been gained, the later treatment will have been greatly complicated. In one study, Weine et al. investigated the total number of appointments needed to complete treatment after teeth with vital pulps had been left open at the emergency appointment. When such teeth were left open, 5.11 appointments were needed to complete therapy and 25 out of 81 cases exacerbated during treatment. However, in teeth kept closed, 3.31 appointments were needed to complete therapy and only 11 of 144 cases exacerbated during the course of treatment (Fig. 5-7). Therefore, in the condition of acute pulpitis with apical periodontitis, all the pulp tissue within the canals must be removed and the access cavity sealed to gain best results.

Pulp necrosis

Pulp necrosis rarely causes an emergency procedure. Usually the condition is first discovered through periapical films during radiographic examination or through the findings of a swelling or distention of periapical tissue during digital examination. However, the patient may notice a swelling and request emergency treatment. Even though a true emergency does not exist, a patient with this problem must not be kept waiting more than a day or two. The area might become acute and a severe condition result. The patient may worry excessively about the situation and attempt to incise the area or use local phlogistic agents (Fig. 5-8).

The radiograph usually reveals a radiolucency ranging from a definite thickening of the periodontal ligament space to a large periapical lesion (Fig. 5-9). If the apex of the root is close to the buccal plate or protrudes through it, no periapical change may be evident. The tooth is not sensitive to percussion, or is only mildly sensitive, and does not respond to pulp vitality tests.

The proper treatment for pulp necrosis is canal debridement. No anesthetic is necessary in most instances, although some patients may insist that one be administered despite explanations by the dentist that the pulpal nerve tissues are no longer responsive. In some cases there are still enough pain receptors to cause discomfort during the pro-

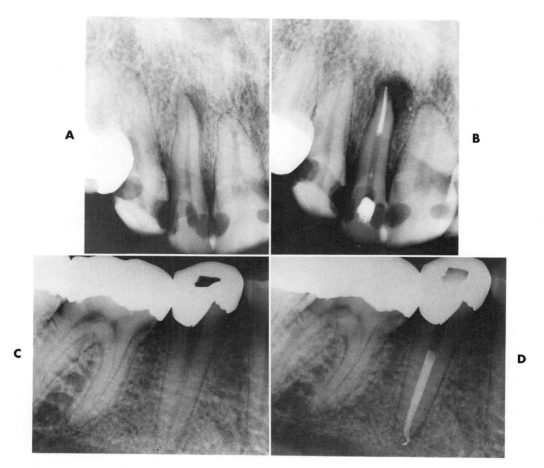

Fig. 5-7. **A,** Maxillary lateral incisor was referred for treatment after having been left open at the emergency treatment appointment. Referring dentist reported that pulp had been vital; but since some periapical damage was seen on radiograph and the tooth had been tender to percussion, it was decided to keep the access open. **B,** After six appointments and two intratreatment exacerbations, periapical surgery was performed. **C,** Mandibular second bicuspid referred for treatment after being left open at an emergency appointment. Tooth had been tender to percussion, but pulp was vital. **D,** Seven appointments were required to complete the case, and the tooth exacerbated twice. Both these teeth would have been much easier to treat if the access cavities had been kept closed.

cedure, and anesthetic may be required. The correct access cavity is prepared and the tooth length determined. Sufficient canal enlargement with heavy irrigation (Chapter 7) is performed to permit removal of the necrotic pulp tissue, a pellet of cotton is placed in the chamber, and the access is sealed with ZOE.

Acute periapical abscess

The diagnosis of acute periapical abscess is obvious. The patient has a large diffuse swelling; the responsible tooth is tender to percussion, is mobile, and lacks vitality. Generalized pain may be absent despite the discomfort of the swelling. In many patients, pain is present before the swelling occurs as the toxic products build up pressure. Once the bone is perforated and there is room for the exudate to expand through the soft tissues, pain may be relieved and certainly is lessened.

Radiographs for acute periapical abscess range from no periapical change, when the inflammation is rapid, to definite radiolucency (Fig. 5-10, *A*). In the latter case the acute abscess may develop from a chronic lesion, whereas in the former the abscess is

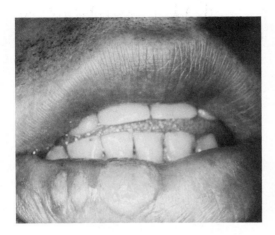

Fig. 5-8. Aspirin burn. Patient placed a tablet on a chronic draining sinus tract in mandibular areas and held it in place with his lip.

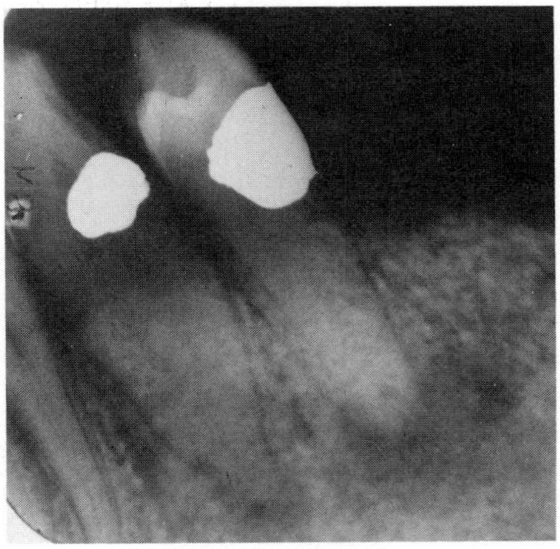

Fig. 5-9. Pulp necrosis of mandibular cuspid with small periapical radiolucency and first bicuspid with a larger lesion.

acute before it has had a chance to destroy sufficient periapical tissue for radiographic visualization.

Whenever possible, the acute periapical abscess should be incised and drained through the root canal space, even if this requires damage to an existing restoration (Fig. 5-10). The indications for an incision and drainage (I and D) through the tissue are few but are discussed in this chapter. The correct access cavity is prepared, always using the highest-speed handpiece available to minimize the vibrations that are so painful in this condition. If the patient still experiences painful vibrations, stick impression compound may be softened by hot tap water and tightly placed across the labial surfaces of the abscessed tooth and the teeth adjacent. Cool water makes the compound solidify and acts as a splint to lessen the vibrations.

Local infiltration anesthetic should not be administered in the distended area because of the pain caused by injection, the chance for dissemination of virulent organisms, and the ineffectiveness of such anesthesia. Block anesthesia usually is effective, however, and may be administered when the patient remains uncomfortable during the initial phases of the emergency treatment.

In many cases, drainage will occur immediately on removing the pulp chamber roof, with a bloody and/or purulent exudate discharging through the access opening (Fig. 5-10, B).

Aspiration using any mild suction device will further aid in establishing drainage through the canal. A wide-gauge needle placed in the saliva

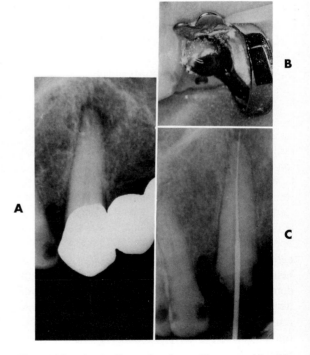

Fig. 5-10. **A,** Radiograph of maxillary cuspid with small periapical lesion and clinical symptoms of an acute periapical abscess. **B,** After removal of bridge, canal is opened to allow bloody exudate to discharge. **C,** If drainage does not occur, apex is enlarged with a size 20 or 25 file.

ejector will give sufficient negative pressure to establish and maintain exudation in many cases. Other teeth may appear to be dry within the canal, and one might suspect that a noncausative tooth has been erroneously opened or that all the exudate had been discharged through the tissue. This is not correct. What has happened is that the apical constriction is preventing the inflammatory products from draining through the tooth.

To relieve this problem, the apical constriction is purposely violated and enlarged to a minimum of a size 20 or 25 instrument, to allow for exudate drainage through the tooth (Fig. 5-10, *C*). Such a procedure usually results in gaining the desired drainage. Again, negative pressure aids in continuing the exudation. If drainage does not occur after the use of a size 20 or 25 file through the apex, it is permissible to attempt further to gain drainage with a size 30 file, followed by negative pressure. If drainage does not result with the size 30 file, do *not* continue attempting to widen the apex further. If drainage does not result with the size 30, going to sizes as big as 70 or 80 will be equally ineffective.

When sufficient drainage has resulted and if the patient is afebrile, no antibiotic coverage is needed. If the patient is febrile and minimal drainage has occurred, an antibiotic should be prescribed (Chapter 20). When the patient is febrile and drainage has been gained or when minimal drainage has resulted with an afebrile patient, an individualized evaluation must be made to decide whether an antibiotic is needed. It may be well to remain in contact with the patient for the next 24 hours; then only if the symptoms persist should an antibiotic be prescribed.

For many years, after establishment of drainage, the patient was dismissed with the access cavity left open. In most patients the swelling continued to subside and the symptoms decreased acceptably. The patient was reappointed for further therapy, as will be discussed later, and although some exacerbations did occur, the treatment generally came to a successful conclusion even though four to six total appointments were required.

Recently there has been an alteration in the most desirable method for treating an acute periapical abscess with drainage. This regimen allowed for drainage, but the emergency appointment ended with the access cavity closed. To accomplish this, it was necessary for the dentist to have an extra chair available, since the patient had to be allowed to sit with the tooth draining for as long as an hour or even more. Also, the dentist had to have sufficient time available to check on the patient to observe the stages of draining and then be able to do some canal preparation before closing the tooth. For best therapy, it was necessary for a dental assistant to remain with the draining emergency patient while the doctor was in another operatory treating a different patient.

The drainage follows a very predictable pattern, starting with pus of a yellowish, whitish, or greenish color mixed with blood. Gradually the pus decreases, and primarily blood drains. Finally the blood flow decreases, and only a clear serum exudation emerges. The sight of the serous fluid indicates that the forceful exudation has dissipated, and this may take from 15 minutes to well over an hour to occur.

At this point a film with files in place is taken and the correct working length calculated. The canal is enlarged several sizes and then may be closed with a sterile cotton pellet and ZOE. The patient is reappointed from 2 to 5 days later and therapy continued. In some cases the patient may have further problems and must be seen the next day. Usually I attempt to allow for more drainage and then reclose one more time. If flare-ups persist, the canal probably is best left open with adjunctive antibiotic treatment.

There are several advantages for this type of therapy. With the tooth kept closed, no new type of microorganism systems are introduced into the infected periapical tissues than were present at the initial opening. This is very significant in teeth with multicanaled systems where ribbon-shaped anastomoses exist going from canal to canal. There is no problem attempting to reclose a tooth left open, and the total number of appointments decreases (Fig. 5-11). Neither food nor debris are packed into an open canal. The single major disadvantage is that a very long and sometimes inconvenient initial appointment is needed to start the program.

If it is not possible to allow the time for closing such a tooth, the long-used method of drainage through the canal and access left open may be utilized. Once the drainage has been gained, there is no attempt to close the tooth, thus allowing any further exudation to exit in the interim between appointments; the patient is rescheduled 3 to 7 days later. At that time the canals are enlarged to approximately one size smaller than the estimated final width. Again each canal is left open. The patient is next seen 2 to 7 days later. After the rubber dam is

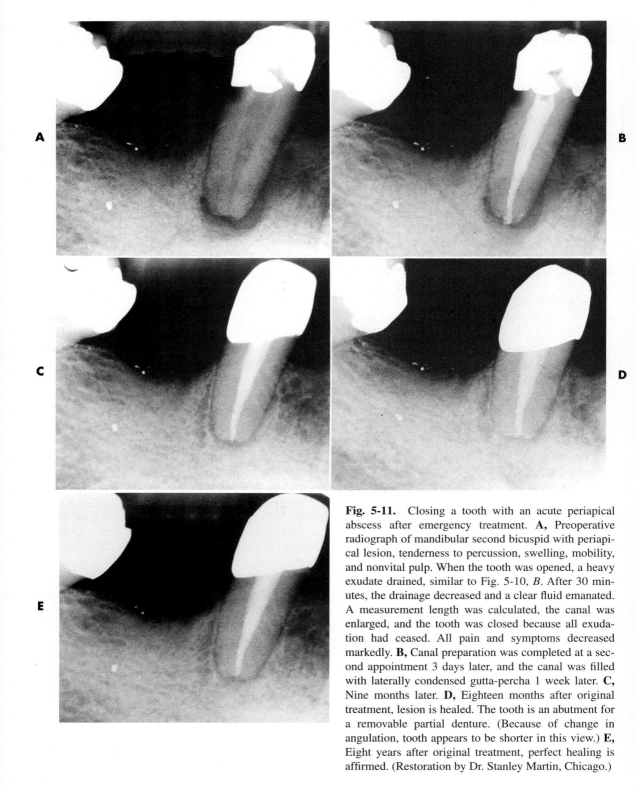

Fig. 5-11. Closing a tooth with an acute periapical abscess after emergency treatment. **A,** Preoperative radiograph of mandibular second bicuspid with periapical lesion, tenderness to percussion, swelling, mobility, and nonvital pulp. When the tooth was opened, a heavy exudate drained, similar to Fig. 5-10, *B*. After 30 minutes, the drainage decreased and a clear fluid emanated. A measurement length was calculated, the canal was enlarged, and the tooth was closed because all exudation had ceased. All pain and symptoms decreased markedly. **B,** Canal preparation was completed at a second appointment 3 days later, and the canal was filled with laterally condensed gutta-percha 1 week later. **C,** Nine months later. **D,** Eighteen months after original treatment, lesion is healed. The tooth is an abutment for a removable partial denture. (Because of change in angulation, tooth appears to be shorter in this view.) **E,** Eight years after original treatment, perfect healing is affirmed. (Restoration by Dr. Stanley Martin, Chicago.)

applied, the canals are heavily irrigated, aspirated, and dried with absorbent points. Broaches may be used to remove any debris that has lodged within the tooth, but no files or reamers may be employed.

As suggested by Frank et al., paper points with a sulfonamide powder may be used for intracanal medicament. Sulfanilamide or sulfathiazole powder is obtainable in any pharmacy. A sterile paper point is dampened by dipping into sterile distilled water. The sulfonamide is fluffed in its container by shaking, and the point is inserted. The powder adheres to the dampened point, and one point is placed in each dried root canal. A dry sterile pellet of cotton is placed in the chamber and the access sealed with ZOE. If the patient's medical history indicates an allergy to sulfonamides, that medication is not sealed but a sterile pellet of cotton is substituted.

The timing for sealing of the access cavity after treatment of an acute periapical abscess requires further discussion. As may be noted in Table 5-1, this condition is the only one that involves leaving the tooth open as part of the emergency treatment. Clinical experience has shown that when a tooth has been left open, if the access is sealed for the first time at the same appointment in which canal enlargement is performed, a high percentage of exacerbations will occur. To avoid this, the following rules are made governing closure *in cases that have been left open for drainage:*

> *If you file, don't close.*
> *If you close, don't file.*

This statement has been misquoted by many dentists and taken out of context for the last few years. Leaving teeth open after filing is done for teeth that have already been left open to discharge an active exudate. If a tooth is closed, it should be kept closed throughout treatment if possible. Leave teeth open only when that is the only choice.

During canal enlargement of an opened tooth, mass contaminants from the microorganisms and debris within the canal are inoculated into the periapical areas, even when the instruments are confined to the interior of the canal. Closing at the same appointment does not allow for the venting of the elements and products of inflammation, thereby causing a high percentage of flare-ups. When the tooth is closed after only the irrigating and drying of the canals, few irritants are pushed through into the irritable periapical tissues, and the medication placed aids the body in producing a healthy reaction.

Culturing the exudate. Whether or not one utilizes culturing in one's endodontic technique, taking a culture of the exudate during an acute periapical abscess or a recrudescent abscess is a wise idea. It takes only a few minutes to perform, and its information when an antibiotic is needed to control a recalcitrant case is invaluable. The culture should not be taken of the initial portion of the exudate when considerable purulence discharges because the majority of the microorganisms at that time are dead and thus incapable of reproduction. However, when the exudate starts to change from yellowish to a reddish hue, the culture sample may be taken with a sterile paper point or sterile cotton swab. At that time, viable microorganisms will be picked up to produce a positive growth.

If the patient has few or no problems after the emergency appointment, the culture may be discarded. However, if the symptoms remain, become worse, or recur, the culture should be sent to a laboratory for antibiotic sensitivity testing (Chapter 15).

Irrigants used in treating acute abscesses. The constituents and uses for the intracanal irrigants are listed in Chapter 7. When an acute abscess is being treated, it is suggested that the irrigants normally used during canal preparation be altered somewhat to provide important functions not usually required.

At the emergency appointment the preferred irrigant in the initial stages of inducing drainage should be warm sterile water or saline. The sodium hypochlorite normally used has a tendency to clump the exudate, which might cause plugging of the apical constriction and halt the drainage. When patency through the apex is maintained, sodium hypochlorite may be used if further canal preparation is to be performed at the emergency appointment.

When the patient returns after having a tooth left open for the appointment when the access will be closed without filing, another adjustment is recommended. The preferred irrigants are the alternating use of sodium hypochlorite and hydrogen peroxide. These two solutions cause foaming when used together and will aid in the bubbling out of any debris that might be packed in the canal. This reduces the need for files or reamers to clean an open canal when it is necessary to close a case without canal preparation. To prevent buildup of nascent oxygen, the sodium hypochlorite must always be the final irrigant used, until all foaming has stopped. This must be done before sealing of the access cavity.

Drainage through the tissue and bone. The presence of a post and core crown, sectioned silver point, or heavily calcified canal prevents obtaining intracanal drainage after an acute periapical abscess. Therefore the drainage must be accomplished through the apical tissue and frequently apical bone by a process of *trephination* (defined as cutting a hole in the bone) or artificial fistulation (artifistulation for short). When it is possible to obtain drainage through the canal, trephination should not be used, even if it would take less time. With the nidus of infection remaining undisturbed within the canal, the relief will be short-lived and the tissue in the area of incision unnecessarily damaged.

Artifistulation or trephination should not be performed until the swelling is sufficiently localized to permit adequate drainage following incision. If the swelling is diffuse, antibiotic cover is prescribed along with hot mouth rinses. Once the area is fluctuant and localized, incision and drainage procedures may be instituted.

For artifistulation a stab incision is made just below the most dependent point of the swelling with a no. 11 scalpel. Usually a heavy purulent exudate is obtained immediately. The apical bone is probed with an endodontic explorer to locate a perforation, which may be enlarged with a spoon excavator or endodontic file to ensure venting of the apical area.

The incision is not closed but is purposely left open to allow for any further drainage. To accomplish this, a strip of rubber dam material (20 by 20 mm) is cut to resemble the letter H or rolled into a tube and disinfected by dipping into a suitable chemical solution. One half of the dam drain is placed underneath the flap, with the wings allowed to extend underneath the tissue. A suture is placed to attach the isthmus to the unretracted edge of the flap. An antibiotic is prescribed, and the patient is then scheduled for another appointment 4 to 7 days later.

Only if artifistulation fails to give sufficient drainage and pressure remains within the periapical bone should trephination be utilized. The flap should be increased in size to allow for visualization of the apical bone. By using a fissure bur in the airotor with water spray, the periapical bone is removed until the tip of the root is uncovered and the necessary drainage obtained. The H or tube drain is placed, an antibiotic prescribed, and the patient rescheduled for 4 to 7 days later (Fig. 5-12).

At the subsequent appointment the drain is removed and an apicoectomy performed (Chapter 11). During this operation the tissue along the lines of incision is removed so more normal areas are in contact when the site is sutured after apical surgery.

EMERGENCY TREATMENT OF TRAUMATIC INJURIES—FRACTURES

Emergency endodontic treatment may be required as a result of traumatic injury: a crown fracture, root fracture, luxation, or avulsion. As a result of sports or horseplay, the anterior teeth of young boys, ages 7 through 14 years, are the most frequently involved. However, impact injuries to the dentition as a result of an automobile accident, household mishaps, assault, or other traumatic event may result in an endodontic emergency for patients of any sex or age on any tooth.

Emergency treatment may be complicated by local edema, bleeding, or other consequences of the accident. Frequently the patients involved have had few or no previous dental problems, having enjoyed excellent dental health until the mishap, but may now be faced with a serious situation. In most impact injuries a temporary paresthesia of the nerves to the pulp occurs as a result of the trauma. Therefore there may be no way to evaluate the condition of the injured pulp accurately by using diagnostic aids. As has been stressed in the discussion of diagnosis and treatment planning, an accurate assessment of what is wrong should be made before any treatment is performed.

Still, the patient with a traumatic injury requires emergency treatment to guard against discomfort that might develop and to enhance the chances for the success of any therapy that may be required in the future.

Crown fracture without pulp exposure. A patient may be brought in for emergency treatment of a fractured tooth that has no direct pulp exposure. The injury may have produced a fracture deep into the dentin or may have merely chipped a small portion of enamel. In the latter case smoothing the jagged edge with a sandpaper disk and rubber wheel will prevent irritation to the tongue and lips.

However, exposure of dentin requires more definitive treatment. A thin mixture of ZOE is placed over the exposed dentin. Then a celluloid

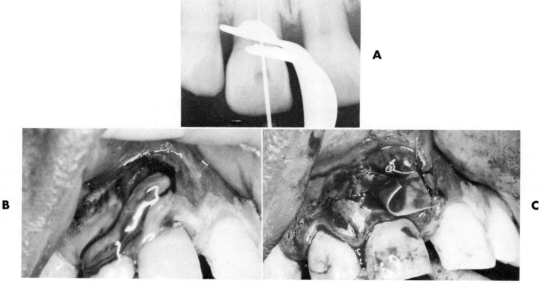

Fig. 5-12. Incision and drainage through the tissue. The patient was referred for treatment of the right central incisor, which had been left open by the referring dentist for the previous 5 days. Now swelling has worsened, raising the lip. **A,** Size 30 file was passed through the apex attempting to reinstitute drainage through the tooth, but no discharge could be obtained. **B,** With no. 11 scalpel blade, a stab incision was made into the dependent area of swelling, resulting in a heavy purulent discharge. **C,** A rubber dam segment was rolled into a tube and sutured to place to prevent premature closure of tissue. The lingual access was closed 2 days later and the drain removed 5 days after the incision. No further problem was encountered in treatment.

crown is festooned, filled with a thick mix of ZOE accelerated with zinc acetate crystals, and cemented into place. These celluloid crowns often become dislodged, and a more permanent type of covering may be needed after a relatively short time. If the initial dressing stays in place for merely a few weeks, the sedative effect may greatly aid in the recuperation of the pulp and its function will be served.

The fractured tooth should be checked with radiographs and pulp testing before any extensive permanent restoration is placed. Adjacent teeth should be similarly examined, since it is not unusual for the pulp of a fractured tooth to recover while the pulp of a neighboring tooth that was seemingly unaffected by the injury becomes necrotic. The reason for such occurrences is that the fracture dissipates the force of a blow while the effect of the blow to the adjacent whole tooth is received at the periapical area and may sever or seriously damage the apical nerve and blood vessels.

Crown fracture with vital pulp exposure. The presence or absence of apical closure must be determined by radiograph, since emergency therapy differs for these two entities. If closure has taken place, the emergency treatment is identical to that previously listed in Table 5-1 as treatment for acute pulpitis, which is the condition present. The canal is broached and the pulp removed in anterior teeth and a pulpotomy performed on posterior teeth, suitable medication is placed, and the access is closed. For a fractured anterior tooth with pulp exposure a lingual opening is unnecessary, but the exposure through the incisal is widened with a tapered fissure bur and direct access to the apex is available. The patient is given another appointment for the completion of endodontic therapy.

If apical closure has not yet taken place, a formocresol pulpotomy is performed to keep the apical pulp tissue unimpeded in its function of completing apexogenesis (Chapter 16). Pulpotomy is preferred to pulp capping even if the exposure is of minimal size. In fractured teeth it is always a problem to retain the temporary crowns or dressings. If a pulp capping is to be performed and the temporary seal is lost or dislodged, the underlying pulp will become contaminated and require redressing. Worse yet, the pulp may become necrotic because of the invasion of microorganisms, and the apex may cease developing. The pulpotomy dressing is placed deeply enough into the canal so that it will be unaffected if the crown covering becomes loosened.

At periodic intervals, 3 to 6 months, radiographs are taken to evaluate the degree of apical development. Once apical development has been completed, routine endodontic treatment may be instituted. (Chapter 16).

Crown fracture with necrotic pulp exposure. After crown fracture into the pulp chamber, it may be determined that the pulp tissue is nonvital. This condition may occur as a result of an earlier accident, caries, or deep restoration or by a severing of the pulpal blood vessels in the most recent traumatic incident. It is interesting that certain children are highly accident prone and may suffer repeated injuries to teeth and jaws (see later discussion).

Emergency treatment follows the pattern shown in Table 5-1. The condition present is diagnosed as either an acute periapical abscess or pulp necrosis, as determined by the clinical symptoms and the response to vitality and percussion tests. The presence or absence of apical closure does not have any effect on the emergency treatment but will have important bearing on the therapy that will follow. If apical closure has taken place, routine endodontic treatment will be performed. If the apex has not developed, apexification procedures will be instituted after cessation of acute symptoms (Chapter 16).

Horizontal root fracture. Horizontal root fracture does not always mean that endodontic therapy will be necessary. Although the dentin and cementum have been cleaved, the pulp tissue may have been stretched by the injury but still may retain its integrity in a recoverable state. If little or no mobility is present, no emergency therapy is indicated. The area should be reevaluated periodically by radiographs and pulp vitality testing. When definite mobility is present, some type of stabilization is required. This is needed to reappose the fractured segments in the hope that the pulp has retained vitality and that any fractured alveolar

bone will heal to retain the loosened tooth (Fig. 5-13). Stabilization may be afforded by orthodontic wire, arch bars, acrylic and wire combination, or any other satisfactory method. The method for treating horizontal root fractures will be discussed in Chapters 10 and 11.

EMERGENCY TREATMENT OF TRAUMATIC INJURIES—AVULSED TEETH

The replacement of a tooth that has been removed from the alveolar socket, either intentionally or by accident, is called *replantation*. As an emergency procedure to replace a traumatically avulsed tooth, it is spectacular but unfortunately has a rather low long-range success ratio compared with routine endodontic therapy. However, one must consider that the avulsed tooth represents a foreign body when it is replaced and is therefore subjected to all the fuctions of the body that may be employed to counteract such intruders. Replantation success should not be compared with other types of endodontic therapy in which the treated tooth remains in its alveolar housing and is benefited by the periodontal attachment. Rather, it should be viewed as a last-ditch heroic attempt to retain alveolar bone and tooth-to-tooth relationships for a period of time. The resorption that so frequently follows the procedure takes some time to cause tooth mobility (Fig. 5-14). Once this occurs, a temporary removable prosthesis, followed by a fixed partial denture, may be constructed at the convenience of the dentist and the patient. Shortly after the accident, it might have been difficult to prepare adjacent teeth as fixed partial denture abutments because of the large size of the pulp commonly found in youngsters. In the period while the replant was in place, even though in a resorbing condition, precious time has been gained to allow for diminution of the pulp canal size of abutments. Construction of such appliances immediately following the traumatic injury is considerably more complex.

Newer philosophies of replantation. For many years, endodontists were advised to enlarge and fill the root canal of an avulsed tooth before replantation. This procedure has been replaced in the last ten years by the method suggested by Andreasen, based on clinical and experimental research. An extensive bibliography for the subject of replantation appears at the end of this chapter.

It had been observed that a relatively good success rate was achieved when patients, or someone else present, replanted the avulsed tooth

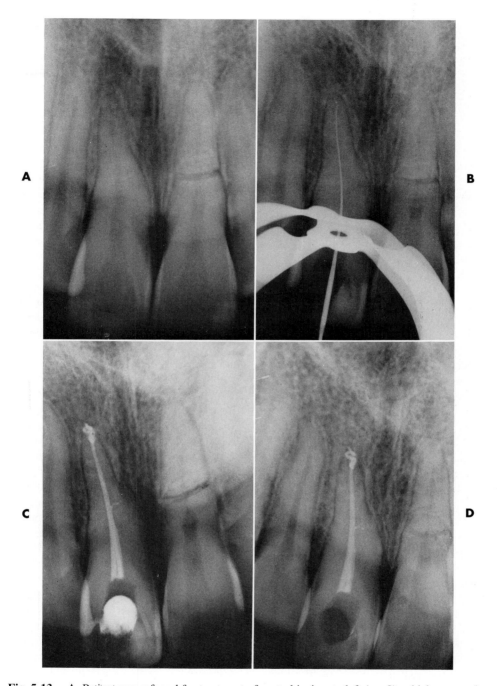

Fig. 5-13.   A, Patient was referred for treatment of central incisor to left (no. 8), which was tender to percussion and sensitive to hot and cold. Central incisor to right (no. 9) was not mobile and was symptom free. Both teeth had vital pulps. Patient was involved in an automobile accident 3 months earlier. **B,** File in place for no. 8. **C,** Canal filling for no. 8. Symptoms all subsided after canal preparation. Note lateral canal exiting to site at the same level as fracture of no. 9. Still no symptoms on 9. **D,** Eighteen months later, no. 9 still remains vital and symptom free.

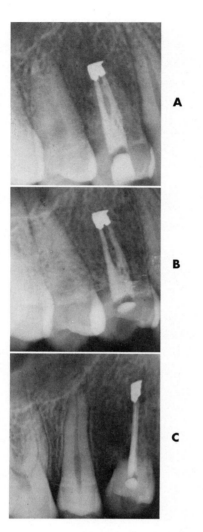

Fig. 5-14.   **A,** Tooth replanted with apical amalgam plug and gutta-percha canal fillings. **B** and **C,** Five years postoperatively, root has resorbed almost completely, leaving only canal fillings in place. Crown of tooth is still tight.

immediately after the trauma compared with replantation by a dentist, despite the absence of canal filling, sterility, or stabilization. Practitioners and researchers began to realize that when the time out of the mouth was minimized, the outlook for the avulsed tooth improved dramatically. Studies by Andreasen and others verified that the longer the period between the traumatic extraction and the reinsertion, the greater is the chance for failure. Therefore the technique for replantation that follows assumes that the avulsed tooth is located quickly after the incident and may be replanted at the site of injury or that the

tooth will be taken quickly to the dental office, where a dentist is able to replant it.

It has been reported that immature teeth that are rapidly replanted without pulp extirpation may require no further endodontic treatment, other than stabilization. The open apex allows for a replacement and/or repair of the severed pulpal vessels, and root resorption is diminished.

A study by Sherman indicated that the presence of the original periodontal ligament on the root surface of replanted teeth improved the prospect for secondary cementum deposition and root resorption repair. When the original periodontal ligament was scraped and the tooth replanted with absorbable surgical sponge, root resorption was more extensive and progressive and a greater degree of ankylosis took place compared with the nonscraped replants.

Technique.   Much research on this subject was done by Andreasen and his coworkers. Other Scandinavians also reported on studies with avulsions and replantations, and their investigations have been valuable in designing the most ideal combination of treatment modalities. At present, some controversy still surrounds the best method for treatment, and alternative techniques are being suggested and investigated constantly. Five specific areas of treatment must be considered, and various combinations of therapy are available.

The method of treatment suggested here follows closely the recommendations by Andreasen. Because of the many studies that he performed over long periods, evaluating treatment modalities where only a single variable was altered, I believe that his theories are the most reliable. However, even then I have made slight modifications in a few areas. In these cases, I have included the treatment methods of Andreasen as well, whenever they differ from mine.

The reader should be warned that although the treatment schedule suggested here has been used successfully in many cases, it is still subject to further research and evaluation, which may lead to future changes.

Suggested treatment of the avulsed tooth

Part I: Emergency treatment at the site of injury

1. Best results occur if the tooth is replanted as soon as possible after the avulsion. The parent, playground supervisor, gym teacher, or responsible adult present who can replace the tooth as quickly as possible will be doing a great favor to the patient. If someone calls

you and states that a tooth has been knocked out, try to have a responsible adult replace the tooth in its socket. Even if the tooth has been badly contaminated by being found in mud or animal fecal matter, it should be replanted *without* sterilization or scrubbing with soap or detergent. The tooth may be rinsed under running tap water until it appears that foreign matter has been washed away, but no tissue clinging to the root surface should be scraped.

2. After rinsing, if necessary, the tooth should be firmly and directly reinserted into the socket, handling the crown only. The family dentist, or nearest practitioner, should be telephoned and the child taken to the dentist's office as soon as possible. A small towel may be placed in contact with the biting edges (incisal edges) of the replanted and the adjacent teeth, and firm pressure applied to keep the tooth in its socket on the trip to the dental office.

3. If it is impossible to reinsert the tooth, the tooth should be placed in a suitable transport medium (see following discussion) and brought to the dental office.

Part II: Emergency treatment at the dental office

1. When the patient arrives at your office, put the tooth in a glass of saline (a pinch of salt in a glass of water produces 0.7% salinity). Take a health history, examine the area, and take radiographs as thoroughly but as *quickly* as possible. If the tooth has been replaced, and seems in an acceptable position, splint as described in step 3 below.

2. If the tooth has not been replanted, do not curette or attempt to sterilize either the root surface or the socket. Handle the tooth at all times with a sponge soaked in saline, grasping the crown only. Wipe away gross debris *gently* from the root surface with the wet sponge. Irrigate the socket with saline. Do not make an access cavity, do not cut off any of the root tip, and do not perform an apical fenestration. *Measure the tooth length and record it on the patient's chart.*

3. As soon as possible, implant the tooth firmly into the socket with the sponge. Radiograph to check the position (Fig. 5-15, *A*). Splint with a soft arch wire (Figs. 5-15, *B*, and 5-16) and acid-etch or similar system. A soft diet is advised (no apples, ribs, sandwiches,

chewy or hard candy). Dairy products, soft ice cream or ice milk, and well-done hamburgers are acceptable foods.

Part III: Completion of endodontic treatment

1. One week after replantation, prepare the access cavity, perform canal debridement and preparation using the previously recorded tooth length, and place a ZOE temporary filling in the access. Teeth with undeveloped apices may be watched without pulp extirpation because some of these pulps may revitalize sufficiently for continued apical development. If pulp necrosis develops later, canal debridement and apexification procedures may be undertaken (Chapter 16). To prevent ankylosis, remove the splint at the conclusion of this appointment. The soft diet must be continued.

2. Two weeks after replantation (1 week after canal preparation), place calcium hydroxide paste in the canal to inhibit and reduce external resorption (Fig. 5-15, *C*). If the paste is placed too soon, before the periodontal ligament is regenerated, it may cause increased resorption. Recall monthly (Fig. 5-15, *D*, *E*, and *F*).

3. After the periodontal ligament and the apex have reformed radiographically, which takes 3 to 6 months, reopen the tooth. Refresh the canal walls with mild preparation and fill with gutta-percha and sealer (Fig. 5-15, *G*) (see Chapter 8). Recall initially at 1 month, then at 3-month intervals. External resorption usually occurs in the first year or not at all (Fig. 5-15, *H*, *I*, and *J*).

Use of transport medium. As mentioned in part I, step 3, if the avulsed tooth cannot be replanted at the time and site of the accident, it becomes incumbent to transport the tooth to the dentist in a manner that will be conducive to a successful reattachment. To accomplish this, a suitable transport medium must be selected.

For many years it was common for an avulsed tooth to be brought to the dental office wrapped in a tissue paper. This led to a drying out of the tooth and any remaining periodontal ligament, decreasing chances for success. Information was made available to the public that this choice was poor, and for a while, the preferred transporting method was to wrap the tooth in a wet tea bag. This was better; the tooth was kept moistened, but water was not the best liquid for transport.

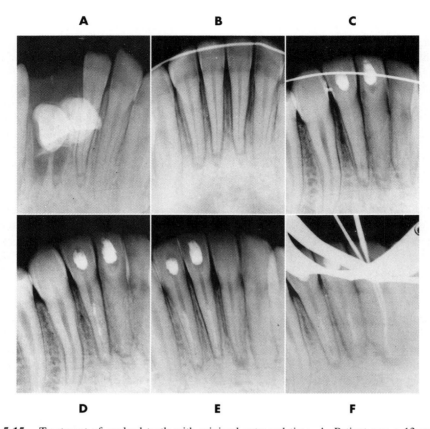

Fig. 5-15. Treatment of avulsed teeth with minimal extraoral time. **A,** Patient was a 13-year-old girl injured by a swing that had backed up prematurely when she was not looking, knocking the crowns of the mandibular right central and lateral incisors totally to the lingual, forcing the apices out of their sockets to a position where the root tips were completely visualized pushing the lower lip forward. Several other areas of trauma were apparent, including bruises on both lips, fractured root tips on three mandibular incisors, and multiple sites of bleeding in the mouth. The mother brought her to my office within 60 minutes of the accident, where this film was taken. **B,** I was able to realign the teeth and replace them in their sockets. Even though the vessels to the apices were completely severed and the pulps devitalized, no attempt was made to handle, clean, or initiate endodontic treatment on the teeth. An acid-etch soft arch wire splint was placed (Fig. 5-16). One week later, access cavities were prepared in the replanted incisors, the pulps extirpated, and canal preparation performed. Both teeth had figure-eight types of canal shape and were enlarged as Type II canals (Chapter 6). The splint was removed, but the teeth seemed to be very mobile. Therefore, I put the splint on again, using an acid-etch attachment system. **C,** An additional week later, 2 weeks after replantation, the accesses were reopened, mild preparation was performed, and calcium hydroxide paste was placed. The splint was removed and left off for the rest of therapy. **D,** The lateral incisor had a brief period of soreness, so the tooth was opened, mildly enlarged with heavy irrigation, and reclosed with calcium hydroxide paste. **E,** After 4 months, the two treated teeth were firm and were prepared for completion of treatment. This film revealed a lesion at the apex of the left central incisor. Electric and temperature tests gave no response. **F,** The pulp was totally necrotic on opening. As expected, this tooth had a similar canal configuration (Type II) to the others. **G,** The teeth were filled with laterally condensed gutta-percha with Wach's paste as sealer. **H** and **I,** Films taken 2 years after treatment indicated total periapical healing and no signs of lateral resorption. For the left central incisor, the lingual portion of the canal did not fill totally, but the canal appears to be sealed both apically and coronally to that site. **J,** Three years after treatment, excellent healing still.

G   **H**

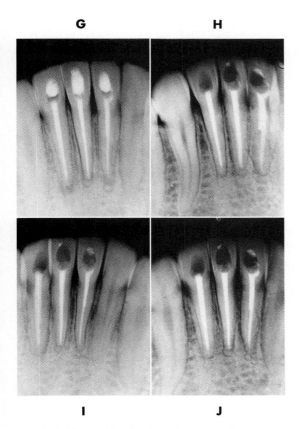

I   **J**

Fig. 5-15, cont'd.   For legend see opposite page.

Hank's Balanced Salt Solution (HBSS).   Best information at this time seems to indicate that HBSS is a very favorable transport medium for the avulsed tooth. A retrospective study reported by Krasner and Person (Krasner is the originator for the use of this product in endodontics) indicated that the solution was highly successful when used in 85.3% of replantation cases. HBSS contains sodium chloride, glucose, potassium chloride, sodium bicarbonate, sodium phosphate, calcium chloride, magnesium chloride, and magnesium sulfate. It has been used in the past as a tissue culture support for mammalian tissues and has demonstrated the ability to preserve and reconstitute the cells of the periodontal ligament.

Krasner has developed an avulsed tooth storage system, named the Emergency Tooth Preserving System* (ETPS), which contains HBSS, a net for holding the tooth atraumatically, and a container for bringing the submerged tooth to the dentist.

*Biological Rescue Products, Inc., Conshohocken, PA 19428.

This system is available to schools, gymnasiums, park district fieldhouses, and other sites where tooth trauma may occur.

Unquestionably, HBSS and the transporting system are valuable in treating avulsion cases. Still, I have some reservations concerning its use. Present information strongly indicates that the best chance for success is by immediate replantation at the site of trauma. The transporting system should be used *only* when such a procedure is not possible.

In the suggestions for use of the ETPS, soaking of the tooth in HBSS before reinsertion is suggested in certain cases. I believe that this is acceptable if the tooth has been allowed to dry out, but if the tooth has been handled properly and is moist, it is better to keep the extraoral time to a minimum and replant as soon as possible without soaking.

Saliva.   In my opinion the patient's own saliva is the best transport medium for an avulsed tooth. Favorable reports on using it have been published, and the logic for its use and its availability are obvious. After trauma to the face and jaws, youngsters generally drool saliva and blood constantly. Often a child comes to the dental office after any trauma to the mouth with a dish or hand towel around his or her neck to absorb this constant flow. There is no problem collecting several inches of saliva, tinged with blood, in a cup or small juice glass and then dropping the tooth into this very biologic liquid.

Also, it has been suggested that when the tooth cannot be replanted at the site of injury and acceptable transport media are not present, it be placed in the patient's mouth or under the tongue. This method has received favorable reports. In such cases the transport medium being used successfully is saliva. For such a method for transporting to be considered, the patient must be an older child or adult. If the child is young, is unreliable, or has a severe gag reflex, there is too great a chance for swallowing the tooth on the trip to the dentist's office.

Milk.   Andreasen favors milk over saliva as a transport medium. Many accidents that cause an avulsion occur related to athletics: on a baseball field, football field, playground, or gym. Except for when an accident happens in the home, milk is not readily available, whereas saliva is always present. Also, milk may contain many antigens that could act negatively from an immunologic standpoint on the reattachment process.

Water.   If no other acceptable transport medium is present, water is the liquid of last resort, as opposed to allowing the tooth to dry out. It is readily available, even at athletic fields, where drinking fountains are always present, and decreases the speed with which periodontal ligament tissue will die.

Stabilization. Stabilization is mandatory to retain the replanted tooth in the desired relationship until a new periodontal attachment is initiated. Many methods of splinting have been utilized, but most have had definite disadvantages because of bulkiness, possibility of loss, irritation of gingival tissues, prevention of normal oral hygiene, and interference with subsequent endodontic procedures.

Adhesive cements have been introduced, which bind directly to enamel and have been widely used in orthodontics. Heiman et al. discuss a procedure for using an adhesive system designed expressly for stabilizing avulsed teeth. The method is rapid and effective, and it circumvents all the problems mentioned that were encountered with other splinting techniques. The teeth to be incorporated in the splint—normally at least two or three teeth, both mesial and distal to the replant—are cleansed by pumicing with a fluoride prophylaxis paste. The teeth are rinsed, dried by air spray, and kept dry with cotton roll placement. A cotton pellet dampened with two drops of the surface-treating agent is applied to the labial enamel surface of each tooth in the splint and kept in contact for 1 minute; it is then rinsed off and the teeth dried. A strip of heavy-guage rectangular orthodontic wire (0.0215 by 0.028 inch) is measured, cut, heat treated, and contoured to approximate contact with the teeth in the area that has been surface treated. the ends of the wire are bent around the most distal teeth in the splint and held with carding wax.

The powder and liquid components are mixed according to the manufacturer's recommendations until a smooth mass is obtained. The cement is applied to the teeth and wire, but because of the rapid set, only two or three teeth may be involved with a single mix. The carding wax is removed after the cement has set, and the wire ends and excess cement are trimmed and smoothed with sandpaper disks and rubber wheels to prevent irritation to the gingiva and inner surfaces of the lips (Fig. 5-16).

After sufficient stability of the replant has been gained by reattachment, the splint is easily removed by cutting through the cement with a bur to free the wire and flicking off the adhesive with a scaler.

Andreasen suggests that the splint be removed 1 week after replantation. (Formerly it was suggested

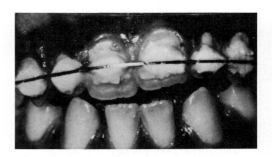

Fig. 5-16. Stabilization afforded a replanted central incisor by adhesive system. Note absence of impingement on gingival tissues. (Courtesy Dr. Gerald Heiman, Glenview, Ill.)

that the splint remain for 4 to 8 weeks.) He believes that keeping the splint in place too long leads to ankylosis or inflammatory resorption, since the periodontal ligament is not kept in function. It is difficult to remove the splint this early, with the tooth still exhibiting a degree of mobility, and not experience mental reservations about this course of therapy. However, Andreasen has followed cases for long periods and maintains the advisability of early splint removal.

Postoperative instructions and systemic treatment. In addition to advice concerning the soft diet, several other instructions must be given after the replantation procedure. In most of my cases I did not prescribe antibiotics. However, Andreasen has reported that systemic antibiotics strongly contribute to replantation success. When one considers the potential contamination that might befall the root during the avulsion, it does seem logical to prescribe antimicrobial agents for the initial few days after the replantation. Currently I do prescribe antibiotics adjunctively unless I am certain that the avulsion and extraoral period were such that no serious contamination could occur.

The patient's physician should be consulted very soon after the replantation concerning the need for an antitetanus booster. Differing views concerning the frequency of these inoculations exist, so it is important to have the medical records reviewed to make the correct decision.

Mild postoperative swelling is normal, and severe pain rarely results from the dental treatment. Mild analgesics should be prescribed for 1 to 4 days. When the adhesive system splint is used, normal oral hygiene may be followed.

Replantation after an extended extraoral period. There is no question that rapid reinsertion of the avulsed tooth enhances success of the procedure. In some cases, however, it becomes very difficult to replace the tooth quickly. Sometimes the tooth is not found until several hours to several days later. It may be that the accident occurs in an area far from a convenient dental office. The trauma may be so extensive that the tooth avulsion was a relatively minor injury compared with other damage (Fig. 5-17). When these events do occur, if at all possible, even though the treatment was delayed, considering the benefits that might result from therapy, replantation should be attempted.

Some have suggested that when the tooth has not been replaced within several hours, it is acceptable to perform endodontic treatment before replantation. I do not agree. The sooner that the tooth is returned to its environment, with the least extraoral manipulation, the better it will be. The pulp tissue may be removed several days later and treatment continued as described earlier in part III.

If the tooth has been allowed to dry out during the extraoral period, according to Mattson et al., soaking in a pH-balanced solution, such as HBSS, will wash off undesirable adhesions to the root surface and may reconstitute depleted cellular metabolites. A soaking of 30 minutes is suggested and would seem to be a logical procedure to follow. Treatment is continued as suggested.

Typical posttreatment sequelae. After completion of routine endodontic therapy, the patient should be seen at regular 6-month intervals, at which time radiographs are taken. It is hoped the treated tooth or teeth will be doing well (Fig. 5-15, H, I, and J), but one of two undesirable conditions may occur to replanted teeth: root resorption (Figs. 5-14 and 5-17) or ankylosis.

Resorption is initially seen radiographically on the lateral surfaces of the root, in irregular bays. As it becomes more extensive, most of the root structure may be replaced by bone, and only the canal filling material remains behind to indicate the earlier treatment. Even though extensive root resorption occurs, the crown may remain relatively tight (Fig. 5-14).

Ankylosis is certainly preferable to resorption. Although the tooth fails to undergo passive eruption with this condition and therefore appears shorter than the adjacent teeth, a jacket crown can be fabricated to alleviate undesirable esthetics.

The periodontal ligament space is absent on the radiograph, and periapical bone appears to attach directly to root surface. Probably some root resorption took place before the area filling in with bone.

Some teeth will exhibit both resorption and ankylosis. However, it is only the progressive resorption that will ultimately dictate loss of the replant and replacement by prosthetic means. As long as the tooth remains relatively firm, it will do its part and be worth the effort to retain it.

At the 6-month recall appointments, it is wise to take radiographs of the teeth adjacent to the treated teeth (Fig. 5-15, E) and the matching teeth in the opposite arch (Fig. 5-18). Often when trauma occurs and an acute phase is noticed and treated, some residual chronic response shows in these members of the arch. If these problems are not discovered and treated promptly, changes may occur that resist endodontic treatment: dystrophic calcification, which may make canal location very difficult, or resorption, either external or internal.

Ultimate long-term prognosis for replanted teeth. There is no area of endodontics, or perhaps in all of dentistry, where more anecdotal information is available than on the subject of replantation. This fact is verified at dental society lectures when the subject is replantation and a member of the audience rises to describe a case treated many years ago, in total defiance of the present suggestions for treatment—and sometimes without any treatment at all, other than reinsertion of the tooth—and yet the tooth is perfect in every way. Articles are published in the more local journals describing similar situations.

I do not want to disparage the authenticity of these reports, but the observers of events should realize that such results are a very small fraction of the total attempts to treat in these ways. The huge majority of such treatment regimens have been abysmal failures, and teeth were extracted early in the game. The reason that these successful cases are still brought up is because of their rarity rather than their frequency.

The long-term prognosis for replantation is still poor, although the recent efforts by Andreasen, his colleagues, and others has undoubtedly caused a significant increase in the success rate. The clinician should be aware that these teeth sometimes do well for long periods, and then, for no apparent reason, problems arise. I have had many cases where I replaced the calcium hydroxide paste several times

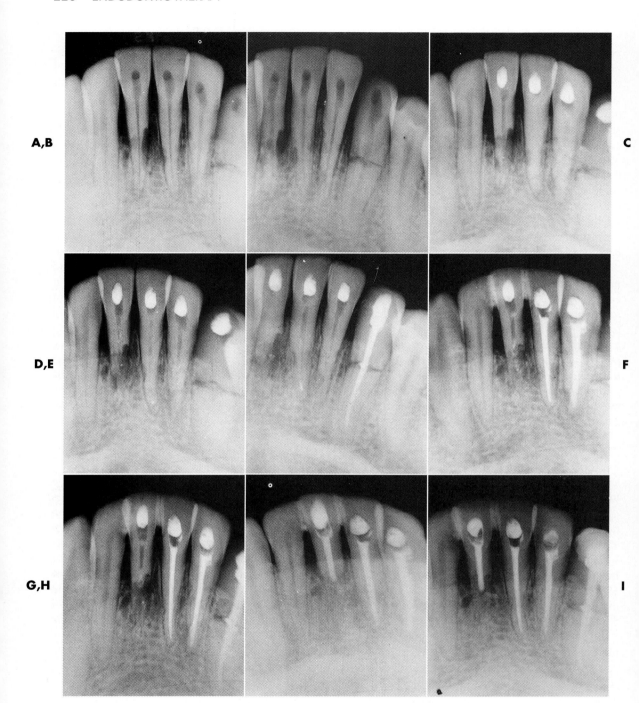

A,B

C

D,E

F

G,H

I

Fig. 5-17.   For legend see opposite page.

J   K   L

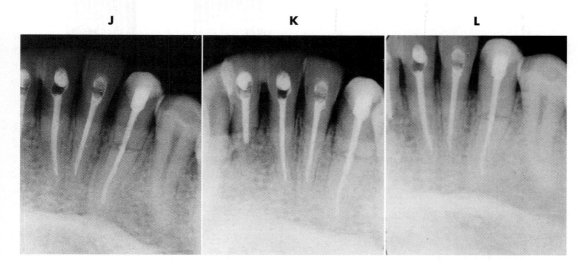

Fig. 5-17, cont'd.   The patient was an 18-year-old male involved in a serious accident when a car with a drunken driver drove off an overpass and fell on top of his car. The young male was unconscious and injured so seriously that it was anticipated that he would expire. Three mandibular teeth were knocked out and located on the floor of his vehicle, but nothing was done to replace them because of the grave outlook. Three days later, he was making a miraculous recovery and had awakened. An oral surgeon from the hospital staff was called in to replace the teeth and perform other intraoral procedures caused by the accident. The patient continued to recover and left the hospital after several weeks. After 8 weeks he went to the oral surgeon, who referred him to me for continuation of treatment. **A** and **B,** My preoperative radiographs of the anterior mandibular teeth, taken several weeks later, 3 months after the accident. The mandibular left cuspid (no. 22) had a midroot fracture, and the oral surgeon had extirpated the pulp from the coronal portion after preparing access. The mandibular left lateral (no. 23) and central (no. 24) incisors and the right central incisor (no. 25) had access cavities prepared and the pulp extirpated. All four teeth had been left open for almost 3 months. Tooth no. 25 and the crown of no. 22 were mobile, but no. 23 and no. 24 were fairly tight. Much debris was in the pulp canals, and the tissue around the teeth was still inflamed and tender to the touch. Severe sites of resorption were associated with no. 25 and the fracture line of no. 22. Several sites of resorption were noted on no. 23 and no. 24, but none were as severe as seen on no. 25. **C,** Radiograph taken 3 months later, 6 months after the replantations. The remaining pulp had been removed from no. 22, the entire canal prepared, and calcium hydroxide paste placed past the fracture line. Teeth no. 23, no. 24, and no. 25 were all treated identically, with canal preparation accompanied by heavy irrigation and placement of calcium hydroxide paste. All access cavities were closed with a cotton pellet and ZOE. On this film it can be seen that the bays of resorption on no. 25 at the gingival line have increased considerably. **D,** Three months later, 9 months after replantation, no. 25 looks much worse and has increased mobility, and the resorption seems to have cut through the root, with the root tip still visible apical to the activity. The other three teeth are now tight. I had changed the calcium hydroxide paste twice on no. 25 but had not needed to do so on the others. **E,** Three months later, 12 months after replantation. Tooth no. 22 has been filled with laterally condensed gutta-percha and Sealapex as sealer. It is firm and comfortable. The bays of resorption on no. 23 and no. 24 seem to be reversing, and these teeth are also firm and comfortable. Tooth no. 25, however, continues to resorb and is mobile and sore despite several more canal cleanings and plaement of paste. **F,** Three months later, 15 months after replantation. Teeth no. 23 and no. 24 have been filled with laterally condensed gutta-percha and Wach's paste as sealer and are firm and comfortable. Continued resorption is apparent on no. 25, and the root tip is now seen separated from the remainder of the tooth. Because of continued mobility of this tooth, bonding has been used to splint it to the adjacent teeth. **G,** Three months later, 18 months after replantation. It was now possible to probe the apex of no. 25 from the gingivolingual, although the tooth was acceptably tight from the bonded splint. I feared that the tooth would start to decay within the canal, so I recleaned the canal and filled it with laterally condensed gutta-percha and Wach's paste. I knew that the tooth would not last much longer but believed that it was now functioning as a pontic and might be able to stay this way for a little longer. **H,** Radiograph taken after canal filling, indicating the gutta-percha at approximately the radiographic tip of the root. **I** and **J,** Radiographs taken 24 months after replantation. Teeth no. 22, no. 23, and no. 24 are comfortable and firm with resorptive bays reformed. Tooth no. 25 appears to be getting longer! One cannot tell if the firmness is due to the splinting or slightly increased root length. **K** and **L,** Radiographs taken 36 months after replantation. Continued healthy appearance of no. 22, no. 23, and no. 24, with no new resorption visible. Tooth no. 25 continues to be getting longer, with root surface visible approximately 3 mm from the gutta-percha. Obviously, further observation will be needed.

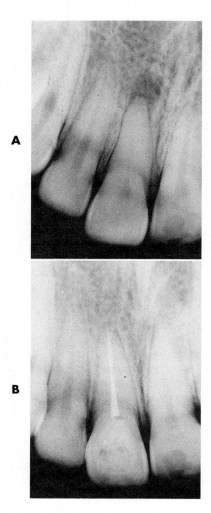

Fig. 5-18. A, Radiograph of maxillary central incisor of patient shown in Fig. 5-15, who had an accident causing avulsion of two mandibular anterior teeth and the need for endodontic treatment on an adjacent tooth. One year after initiating treatment of those teeth, the patient had returned for a recall appointment. Not only were the treated teeth evaluated, but also those teeth adjacent and occluding were examined and radiographed. This film indicates a periapical lesion associated with the right central incisor and considerable decrease in width of the root canal space. No symptoms were present. **B,** Canal had been located, prepared and at a second appointment filled with laterally condensed gutta-percha and Wach's paste, with some excess sealer being pushed past the apex. This film was taken 2 years later, demonstrating perfect healing of the lesion and a small strand of sealer still present. Had the lesion not been noted in the radiograph, the canal probably would have continued to become more narrow, making location at a later time more difficult. This might have led to a perforation or the need for surgical treatment. It was so much easier to treat at the time that the lesion was first discovered.

with changeable success, and yet, in the same mouth, other teeth responded well with a single application (Fig. 5-17). In some instances, teeth assumed to be responding properly were filled with gutta-percha, but after several years the resorptive defects were noted and further treatment was required.

When treating avulsions, the patients must be kept on perpetual recall, requiring a radiograph every 6 months. If an insurance coverage or legal event is involved, the patient or parents of the patient should be encouraged to wait until the long-term outlook is clearly understood, which is often impossible to assess. Insurance companies realize that these cases can be in therapy for many years with extended costs and therefore are anxious to settle the claims quickly. If one calculates the initial charges, perhaps several changes of paste, filling with gutta-percha, observation periods, perhaps loss of the tooth in 5 to 15 years, subsequent replacement by a fixed bridge, and then, depending on the patient's age, replacement with fixed bridges in the future, it is easy to see why the insurance companies are anxious to settle quickly.

When treating an avulsed tooth, the best advice that I can give to the operator is to be prepared for any event or eventuality and expect the unexpected.

Intentional replantation. Perhaps this subject should be listed in Chapter 11 since it is really a surgical rather than an emergency endodontic procedure. However, because the sequelae, splinting, and other procedures are often similar to those employed during a replantation that follows traumatic injury, intentional replantation will now be described.

Intentional replantation implies that a tooth requiring endodontic treatment is purposely removed from its alveolar housing, some type of canal or apical preparation and/or filling is performed, and the tooth is returned to its original socket. Two extensive studies, by Grossman and by Deeb, have been reported with rather good results.

Deeb intentionally replanted 274 teeth and stated that only 26% showed resorption after 5 years. However, at the Fourth International Conference on Endodontics, he disclosed some variances from his original report. He stated that among anterior teeth in which the periodontal ligament was curetted, 26% were lost after 5 years in those patients who returned for recheck examination. No estimate was made of retention ratio of all patients treated.

Having ascertained that curetting of the periodontal ligament was harmful, Deeb then did a further study concerning canal filling materials and methods while the ligament was allowed to remain. In a group of posterior teeth filled by apical preparation and amalgam filling, 54% displayed resorption. In anterior and posterior teeth when canals were filled with gutta-percha, the resorption rate was 60%.

Grossman's study reported on 45 replants, averaging 5.6 years, with an 82% success rate. However, files on some patients with replants were lost, and the sampling included only those who returned to the University of Pennsylvania for further dental treatment. It was possible that results would differ if all those treated by intentional replantation were surveyed.

Since the success ratio for intentional replantation is far below that for routine or surgical endodontic therapy, it was concluded by the Fourth International Conference that the procedure should be attempted only when every other possible technique had failed or was impractical. Only when extraction was the only alternative could intentional replantation be considered the treatment of choice.

Therefore the indications for intentional replantation would include situations described as follows:

1. When routine endodontic treatment of teeth is impractical or impossible, as in patients who are unable to keep their mouths open for the necessary length of time
2. When an obstruction of a canal is present, such as a broken instrument or a calcification, or a periapical radiolucency is present, yet routine surgery is impractical, as in a lower molar with the mandibular canal in proximity
3. When perforating internal or external resorption is present, yet surgery is impractical
4. When a foreign body, such as molten metal, is in the periodontal ligament or periapical tissue but surgery is impractical
5. When previous treatment has failed but nonsurgical retreatment or surgery is impractical

If a choice exists between periapical surgery and intentional replantation, the former should be selected, since it has by far the better prognosis. As listed in the indications, lower molars, in which periapical surgery may be complicated, provide the highest percentage of potential cases (Fig. 5-19).

Before the surgical procedure the root canals should be filled, preferably with gutta-percha, as far as possible in a partially obstructed canal and to the apical foramen in those completely negotiable. The anesthetic required for periapical curettage is administered. With maximum care used to prevent fracture of the tooth, which would make the entire procedure a failure, the tooth is extracted. There can never be too much time spent in performing the extraction, with slow buccolingual movement necessary and no attempt made to remove the tooth until it is very loose. Because the central portion of the tooth is weakened from the previous therapy, no squeezing of the forceps should be exerted, which might cause fracture.

When the tooth is finally luxated, it is immediately placed in a solution of sterile saline while the socket is packed with sterile gauze. If the canals have not been filled to the apex, the tooth is held in a saline-saturated gauze (2 by 2 inches) while the apices are trimmed with a fissure bur. A small Class I cavity preparation is made with an inverted cone bur, and the canals are sealed with amalgam. If the canals have been filled, any excess filling material is removed with the fissure bur. The tooth is then replaced in the sterile saline until it is time for replantation.

The gauze is removed from the socket and any necessary curettage performed. The tooth is replaced into the socket and stabilized by any of the acceptable methods. Biven et al. suggest a method for fabricating an acrylic splint for use with an intentional replantation procedure. At a prior appointment, alginate impressions are taken and stone models poured. Heavy-gauge stainless steel wire (0.03 inch) is adapted to the model around the most posterior tooth in the arch and surrounded by quick-cure acrylic. No plastic covers the posterior segment, allowing for a spring action to the splint. Holes are drilled interproximally so that ligature wire may be used to further support the tooth after replantation.

It is strongly suggested that two operators be involved in an intentional replantation case. All the studies seem to agree that time out of the mouth is critical in the prognosis for such treatment. Having two people present and able to perform the procedures allows for a minimal time for the tooth to be out of the mouth. One operator may extract the tooth, hand it in a sterile moist gauze pad to his colleague, and curette the area or otherwise prepare the socket. Meanwhile the other operator will be trimming the apices and probably placing reverse fillings or cutting back to previously placed gutta-percha.

Postoperative instructions are the same as those used for a replantation procedure.

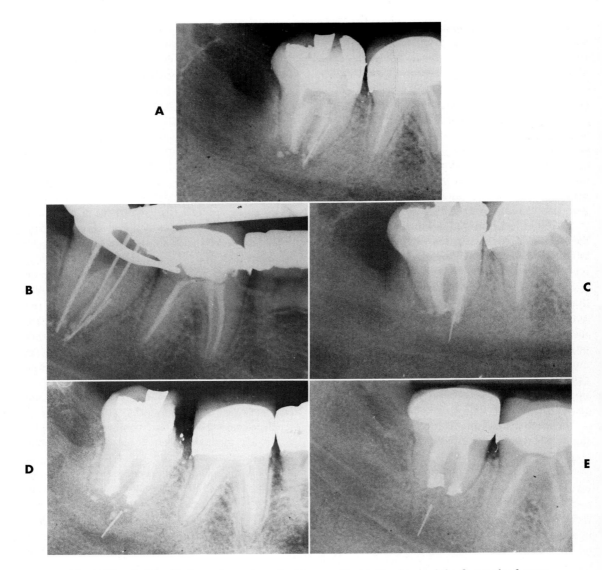

Fig. 5-19. **A,** Mandibular molar region of a 15-year-old girl. I had treated the first molar 3 years earlier, but the parents chose someone else to treat the second molar. Canals were filled with a paste material, and two separated files were present in the mesial canals. Tooth was tender to percussion. **B,** An attempt was made to remove the separated instruments. One was retrieved, but the other was pushed further out the apex. **C,** Canals were refilled with laterally condensed gutta-percha and Wach's paste. It was decided to perform an intentional replantation procedure because tooth remained tender to percussion. **D,** Tooth was extracted, and apices were trimmed and reverse filled. However, the file had slipped from the tooth and could not be located through the socket. To keep the tooth out of the mouth as short a time as possible, we replanted it with the file still in the mandible. **E,** Forty months after replantation, area has healed well and symptoms are completely absent. (Surgery by Dr. Charles Neach, Chicago, and myself.)

Prognosis for intentional replantation. The outlook for an intentionally replanted tooth is superior to that for a traumatically avulsed replanted tooth. The time during which the tooth is out of the mouth, which is certainly critical, is greatly reduced and the replant is kept moist during the needed manipulation. Venting is provided by the trimming of the root end or curettage of the periapical area. No curettage of the periodontal ligament attached to the tooth is performed. Therefore all the criteria for successful replantation are adhered to, which is not always the case after trauma.

EMERGENCY THERAPY FOR INTRATREATMENT PAIN

In the course of routine endodontic therapy, emergency treatment may be required to relieve pain, whether or not the originating need for the endodontic care involved emergency appointment. Based on the same general diagnoses listed in Table 5-1, the correct emergency treatment is now described.

Even though flare-ups can and do occur even with best therapy, carefully considered treatment will decrease these annoying occurrences. Attempting to treat flare-ups causes considerable inconvenience, as well as often initiating mental anguish to both the patient and the dentist. Therefore, when endodontic therapy is performed, considerable thought should be given each step to verify the efficacy of that treatment. Also, sufficient time should be allowed to reach a satisfactory stopping spot, as suggested by the tables in Chapter 19. It has been my experience that many flare-ups occur when improper treatment is rendered or when insufficient time is allowed for specific modalities in therapy.

Apical periodontitis secondary to treatment. It is upsetting to both the patient and the dentist when the tooth involved in endodontic therapy becomes sensitive to percussion during the course of treatment. This is particularly true when the symptom was not present before treatment. Secondary apical periodontitis may be extremely uncomfortable and cause a throbbing, gnawing, and/or pounding pain. The preoperative condition of the pulp usually is either chronic or acute pulpitis. If the access cavity is opened, no productive exudate or escape of gas is noted and culture tests may be negative, since no infection is present.

The cause of secondary apical periodontitis is most fequently overinstrumentation, but the condition may occur as a result of overmedication (too caustic or too much intracanal medicament) or of forcing debris into the periapical tissues. A simple test is available to confirm whether the apical tissues have been overinstrumented. With the rubber dam in place and the access cavity opened, a sterile paper point is selected that is thin enough in width to reach the apical portion of the preparation. The point is grasped with cotton pliers at a point approximately 2 mm more than the total working length of the tooth and inserted into the canal. If the apex is overinstrumented, the point will extend easily past the working length without obstruction. On withdrawal, the tip of the point will disclose a reddish or brownish color, indicating inflamed tissue in the periapical region and absence of a stop in the apical preparation (Fig. 5-20).

To give symptomatic relief in this condition, a corticosteroid-antibiotic medication is used. A paper point that will reach the periapical tissue is dipped into the mediament, which has a salvelike consistency (Fig. 5-21). The point is placed in the

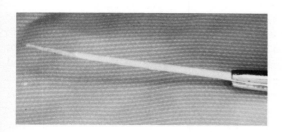

Fig. 5-20. Paper point passed into periapical tissue of an overinstrumented tooth. Reddish brown color is seen on point when it is withdrawn.

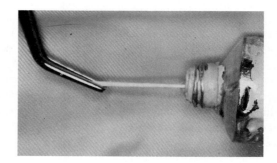

Fig. 5-21. Corticosteriod-antibiotic medication is applied to paper point and will be placed in periapical area to relieve symptoms of overinstrumentation.

canal with a pumping action, injecting the inflamed periapical tissues with the anti-inflammatory agent. The antibiotic is present to prevent any possible ovegrowth of microorganisms that might proliferate when the inflammatory response is lessened. The access is sealed with ZOE.

In a report by Van Cura and Remeikis, pain and hypersensitivity disappeared within an hour in 86% of patients treated with a cream composed of triamcinolone, nystatin, neomycin, and gramicidin. Ehrmann, Schneider, and Schroeder also separately reported excellent results with particularly rapid relief of pain when using similar combinations.

After this emergency treatment, routine endodontic therapy may be continued within 2 to 5 days. If the operator thought that the apex had not been violated but the telltale signs of overinstrumentation are verified, further adjustment of the canal working length should be made. Radiographs taken at various angles with a file in place may disclose that the apical foramen is exiting from the root surface at an unexpectedly high position.

Incomplete removal of pulp tissue. When treatment during the initial appointment for endodontic therapy has consisted of pulpotomy or partial pulpectomy after a diagnosis of acute or chronic pulpitis, the patient may experience pain due to incomplete removal of inflamed pulp tissue. When an acute pulpitis is present without apical periodontitis, usually the inflammation is confined to the coronal pulp, which is removed during the pulpotomy. However, in a chronic pulpitis and in some cases of acute pulpitis, the inflammation may have already extended into the radicular pulp. Although initially a pulpotomy might relieve such pain, discomfort frequently returns. The symptoms of such pain may be sensitivity to hot and/or cold or pain to percussion.

This condition is confirmed when the access is reopened after local anesthetic administration and rubber dam application. A sterile paper point is placed in the canal, definitely short of the apical foramen. When withdrawn, the point will display the brownish discoloration indicative of inflamed seeping tissues. Radiographs are taken to determine canal length, and the remaining pulp tissue is removed. A sterile cotton pellet is placed, and the access is sealed with ZOE.

If any chance of overinstrumentation has occurred and the tooth was tender to percussion, a corticosteroid-antibiotic combination should be used as previously described.

Recrudescence of a chronic apical periodontitis. Most teeth with necrotic pulps and apical lesions are asymptomatic, and the periapical condition is referred to as chronic apical periodontitis. They are usually noticed when routine full-mouth radiographs are taken, at which time endodontic therapy is often advised. Although most teeth with this condition are successfully treated uneventfully, a low percentage of the chronic lesions become acute after the first endodontic appointment. This condition is then referred to as a recrudescence (defined as breaking out anew) or a phoenix (rebirth) abscess.

The exact reason for the condition is merely an object of speculation. Some point out that facultative anaerobic organisms, multiplying slowly in the low-oxygen environment of the periapical tissues, suddenly receive air when the canal is opened by endodontic therapy. With the improved conditions present, the bacteria supposedly fulminate violently and produce an acute reaction. This particular theory, however, has a few holes. In some cases, culturing of the tooth reveals no bacterial growth. In other cases the bacteria recovered by culture do not grow as facultative anerobes.

However, the change in the environment within the root canal probably does have something to do with a recrudescense. Multiple strains may be harbored in a particular lesion. After initial canal instrumentation, some strains are severely reduced, whereas another may be relatively unaffected. Since there are fewer organisms with which to compete, a virulent strain may then begin rapid multiplication. Those cases of recrudescence without organisms being recovered may be due to faulty culture technique, to the acute reaction being caused by overinstrumentation, or to necrotic debris being forced through the apex with an area of low resistance present.

The symptoms of a recrudescense are identical to those of an acute periapical abscess: mobility, tenderness to percussion, and swelling. The same emergency treatments in Table 5-1 for an acute abscess, incision and drainage through the root canal, may be used (Fig. 5-22). If there is time and a chair is free, the tooth may be left open with a rubber dam in place and then reclosed when all the exudation has ceased. The initial exudation may be encouraged by irrigation with warm sterile saline or water. Generally the patient gains relief, and no further complication occurs. The tooth is completed one or two appointments later.

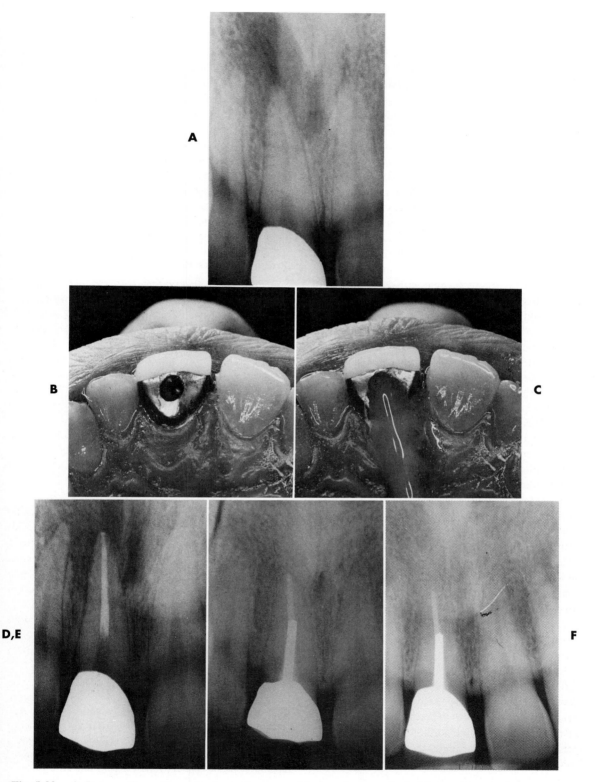

Fig. 5-22. **A,** Preoperative radiograph of maxillary central incisor. Large periapical lesion, history of trauma. Completely asymptomatic. **B,** Tooth was opened, canal prepared, and a temporary placed at the first appointment. Next day the patient experienced severe pain followed by a large swelling. The temporary was removed. **C,** An aspirator was applied to lingual access and a large purulent exudate discharged. The tooth was left open and reclosed a few days later. **D,** After several appointments, tooth is symptom free. A canal filling has been placed. **E,** Eleven years after original treatment, lesion exhibits perfect healing. **F,** Twenty-two years after original treatment, perfect healing demonstrated. (Restoration by Dr. Emory Bryant, Jr., Ft. Wayne, Ind.)

If the drainage refuses to stop or if there is not time or space to allow for drainage, the tooth may be left open and the patient dismissed. The tooth may be reclosed, without filing, when all the symptoms have disappeared 2 to 5 days later. Such cases may be closed with no medicament or with powdered sulfonamide on a paper point, plus ZOE.

To accomplish this, the rubber dam is applied and the access opened (Fig. 5-23), A). Generally a heavy exudate will drain. A sample is taken to culture for possible antibiotic sensitivity testing when the exudate changes to a bloody discharge. The canal is irrigated with warm sterile water or saline solution and gently enlarged, without forceful exertion of the instrument against the canal wall. The canal should be left open with the dam still in place for at least 15 minutes, until the exudation has ceased or a slight clear serum drains. The canal is irrigated with sodium hypochlorite, dried with sterile paper points, and a dry cotton pellet placed in the chamber. A thick mix of ZOE closes the access (Fig. 5-23, B).

The patient should be contacted within the next 24 hours to ensure that the tooth has remained quiet. A short appointment is scheduled within a week for a dressing change and slight additional canal enlargement. If symptoms remain absent, the canal is filled according to the normal schedule.

Recurrent periapical abscess. This condition refers to a tooth with an acute periapical abscess, relieved by emergency treatment, after which the acute symptoms return. Even with the access left open, packing of food debris or foreign objects such as segments of a toothpick, toothbrush, or chewing gum may prematurely stop the drainage. When an open tooth is both filed and closed at the same appointment, the abscess frequently recurs. In still other cases the symptoms of an abscess return a few days after the access is closed, without any intervening treatment.

The emergency and follow-up treatments are also the same as those used to treat the acute periapical abscess. In some cases the abscess may recur more than once. This is usually due to microorganisms of high virulence or to poor host resistance. When a particular tooth has two exacerbations, it may be best treated with periapical surgery. However, if the indications for surgery are poor, as with lower molars or a debilitated patient, nonsurgical treatment must still be pursued.

As will be discussed in Chapter 15, cultures and antibiotic-sensitivity tests should be taken from the exudate of a recrudescence or a recurrent periapical abscess. It will normally take 48 to 72 hours to receive a bacteriologic report disclosing the antibiotics to which the microorganisms found are particularly sensitive. If an abscess recurs a second time, the patient should receive premedication with the effective antibiotic, with four doses taken before the access is closed, commencing the drug 20 hours before the appointment and continuing for 3 additional days. This gives the body defenses additional help in attempting to keep the evidently virulent bacteria under control and may prevent the need for surgery.

Preventing flare-ups during treatment

Patients can accept that pain may continue or linger to a lesser extent when they come to the dental office for emergency treatment of a toothache. Following the often-used quotation, "Rome

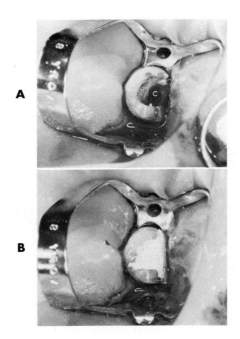

Fig. 5-23. Reclosing a recrudescent abscess. **A,** Mandibular second bicuspid had been asymptomatic before treatment, but a large periapical radiolucency was present. Canal had been enlarged to a size 40 at previous appointment, but patient returned next day with severe swelling and pain. Rubber dam was placed, and a heavy bloody exudate discharged. **B,** After allowing drainage to subside, I irrigated the canal, dried it, and reclosed at same appointment. Therapy was completed without further problems.

was not built in a day," the patient is able to understand that just as it took several days for the toothache to build up, so may it take several days to dissipate. Interestingly, if Table 5-1 is followed with great care and accuracy, a huge percentage of toothaches are gone completely within several hours of the emergency treatment.

What is difficult for patients to comprehend is when they enter the office virtually pain free but experience a sustained increase in pain after treatment or, even worse, when they have little or no pain before therapy but then encounter an explosive flare-up after the dental appointment.

As stated earlier, pain may follow even the best treatment and should not cause any patient/dentist problems if a good relationship exists before the flare-up, especially when the patient has been warned that such a change for the worse may occur. However, we must try our best to prevent flare-ups from occurring, and several steps can be taken to reduce these disturbing and perplexing problems.

Preventing postoperative percussion sensitivity—secondary apical periodontitis. Patients may come in for treatment with teeth tender to percussion or without such sensitivity (Table 5-1). A secondary apical periodontitis is the term applied to severe tenderness to percussion immediately *after* treatment was initiated, regardless of the condition before therapy. The initial appointment may have been to treat emergency pain or merely the normally scheduled first appointment of therapy.

The cause for this tenderness to tapping, eating, chewing, or striking the offending tooth is always the same—overinstrumentation of the apical foramen. Many dentists tend to file too close to the radiographic apex to ensure that all residual pulp tissue or any necrotic debris is removed. All the studies on apical anatomy endorse the concept that any filing within 0.5 mm of the radiographic apex is too long, and in more unusual cases, filing even several millimeters from that site may be too long. The desire to remove unwanted tissue from the canal is most commendable, but if carried to any extreme, it may lead to the undesirable acute secondary apical periodontitis.

The occurrence of this condition will be minimized if accurate radiographs are taken from several angles before any treatment and if the sites of canal exiting are located before any instrumentation. Then, when the measurement films are taken with files in place, several similarly angled views should be taken and analyzed with increased

magnification (Chapters 7 and 8). If a concerted effort is made to file canals to the apical constriction or, as described by Kuttler (Chapter 8) to the minor diameter, this problem becomes minimal.

Most importantly, if the operator determines that the apex has been severely violated by overinstrumentation, it is mandatory to take remedial steps immediately at that appointment rather than waiting for the patient to call with pain. The use of the corticosteroid-antibiotic combination paste is used at the appointment when the overinstrumentation occurs (Fig. 5-21), and the need for a separate emergency appointment with the attendant painful episode is avoided.

Preventing flare-ups when treating a tooth with a necrotic pulp. Prevention of a flare-up while treating a tooth with a necrotic pulp is much more difficult than when treating a tooth with a vital pulp. Generally the former already has some periapical breakdown, and thus the multiple immunologic and inflammatory factors are in place that might elicit the undesirable response (Chapter 4). Even so, some logical choices in treating such cases will decrease the number of flare-ups that do result.

It is unwise to use medicaments with immunologic potential, such as the phenolic derivatives. Debridement is much preferable to medication in order to remove gross tissue and substrate. Recent microbiologic studies have implicated anaerobes as important causative agents in pulpal necrosis and periapical breakdown (Chapter 15). Efforts to reduce the anaerobic population seem logical, including alternating the irrigants hydrogen peroxide and sodium hypochlorite. Also, short appointments with minimal exposure of the anaerobes to the irrigants should be converted to longer periods when the canal is bathed in these solutions.

In fact, I prefer to *lengthen* the time that I expose anaerobes to intracanal irrigants when first opening the tooth with a periapical lesion. After the canal has been measured carefully and initial enlargement, including flaring, performed (Chapter 7), rather than closing the tooth with the appropriate temporary, I increase the time that the irrigants remain in the canal.

With the rubber dam still in place, obviously, I place some sodium hypochlorite and peroxide (either hydrogen or carbamide) and allow them to react, with oxygen foaming resulting. Minimal manipulation of a small file, absolutely short of the apex, further enhances the foaming and gives wider distribution of the oxygen.

If I am quite busy, I may have my next patient seated, give an anesthetic, check a recall appointment, or perform a postoperative treatment. If I leave the treatment room of the patient with the endodontic case still open, I have a reliable dental assistant remain with the patient for assurance and to inform me if anything untoward occurs (rubber dam flies off, patient becomes ill, etc.). I explain to the patient that I am "soaking the canal," just as they might soak a finger, foot, blister, or sore site on another portion of their body. I rarely, if ever, have had any negative reaction to this, and I believe that this added time of exposure to anti-anearobic treatment has been valuable.

Extra time in ensuring well-debrided and cleaned canals to prevent flare-ups is much preferable to the need for extra appointments with patients in pain.

Use of antibiotic and other agents to prevent flare-ups. Some reports have been published recently that recommend the use of antibiotics, antihistamines, anti-inflammatories, and other agents to prevent endodontic flare-ups. I believe that most of these substances are vastly overused, unnecessary, and potentially dangerous. I agree that patients with certain systemic conditions (diabetes, connective tissue disorders, tendency to retain water, history of flare-ups after endodontic treatment, etc.) are best covered by antibiotics. Some of the nonsteroidal anti-inflammatory drugs (NSAIDs) (Chapter 20) have been shown to be valuable when taken before an endodontic appointment to prevent postoperative pain.

However, in the vast majority of endodontic cases, postoperative pain serious enough to require an additional unanticipated appointment or prescriptions for relief of severe pain occur infrequently. This is particularly true when canal debridement has been carried out sufficiently that the inflamed tissues within the pulp canal space have been removed adequately and that minimal or no instrumentation beyond the cementodentinal junction has occurred.

In a wide ranging study (946 patient visits), considering multiple types of cases, Walton and Fouad (from the University of Iowa, a dental school relying on adequate instrumentation as opposed to pharmacotherapeutics) reported the incidence of postoperative pain to be 3.17%. In this illuminating study the highest number of flare-ups occurred after treatment of an acute periapical abscess, where types of closure (Table 5-1) and

other factors of recrudescence may result. In cases of chronic apical periodontitis, for which many investigators recommend the use of antibiotics or antiinflammatories, the flare-up problem occurred in only 3.4% of patients. Considering the problem of possible antibiotic allergies, the difficulty in selecting the correct antimicrobial agent, and the strong information that the flare-up will be extremely infrequent, it would seem that the use of these agents is without efficacy.

Again, I wish to state emphatically, *there are a few cases when an antibiotic should be used when opening up an asymptomatic tooth with a periapical lesion*, but I *do not* believe that this should be a constant treatment modality.

In a recent report, Selden has stated that informing the patient about the possibility of a flare-up is an important part of postappointment instructions after initiation of endodontic therapy. I strongly agree with this. Rather than prescribing in advance for a condition that in all probability will not occur, it is better to maintain contact with the patient (e.g., after initial treatment of an acute periapical abscess or, if one wishes, after treatment of an asymptomatic tooth with a periapical lesion) and then prescribing when warranted.

Significance of a chronic draining sinus

The presence of a chronic draining sinus tract (often erroneously referred to as a fistula) is a favorable sign at the start of endodontic therapy. It is of considerable diagnostic aid and may be the indication that forces a patient to seek much-needed dental treatment. The closure of the tract after the debridement appointment is an excellent indication that there is an initiation of healing: this sign is equally obvious and impressive to the patient as well.

However, to the dentist the tract ensures that emergency therapy for intratreatment pain will not be needed, except when the apex is severely overinstrumented. Should any inflammatory products or microorganisms start to build up, they simply "blow out" through the sinus tract and prevent an exacerbation.

REFERENCES

Endodontic emergencies, general topics

August DS: Managing the abscessed open tooth: instrument and close. Part 2, J Endod 8:364, 1982.

Auslander WP: The acute apical abscess, *NY State Dent J* 36:623, 1970.

Balaban FS, Skidmore AE, Griffin JA: Acute exacerbations following initial treatment of necrotic pulps, *J Endod* 10:78, 1984.

Barnett F, Tronstad L: The incidence of flare-ups following endodontic treatment, *J Dent Res* 68:1253, 1989.

Bence R: Trephination technique, *J Endod* 6:657, 1980.

Brian JD Jr, Ranly DM, Fulton RS, Madden RM: Reaction of rat connective tissue to unfixed and formaldehyde-fixed autogenous implants enclosed in tubes. *J Endod* 6:628, 1980.

Chestner SB, Selman AJ, Friedman J, Heyman RA: Apical fenestration: solution to recalcitrant pain in root canal therapy, *J Am Dent Assoc* 77:846, 1968.

Dorn SD, Moodnick RM, Feldman MJ, Borden BG: Treatment of the endodontic emergency: a report based on a questionnaire. Parts 1 and 2, *J Endod* 3:94, 3:153, 1977.

Ehrmann GH: The effect of triamcinolone with tetracycline on the dental pulp and apical periodontium, *J Prosthet Dent* 15:149, 1965.

Forrest JO: Attitudes in endodontics, *J Br Endod Soc* 4:57, 1970.

Frank AL, Glick DH, Weichman JA, Harvey H: The intracanal use of sulfathiazole in endodontics to reduce pain, *J Am Dent Assoc* 77:102, 1968.

Genet JM, Hart AAM, Wesselink PR, Thoden Van Velsen SK: Preoperative and operative factors associated with pain after the first endodontic visit, *Int Endod J* 20:53, 1987.

Goldman M, Rankin C, Mehlman R, Santa C: The immunologic implications and clinical management of the endodontic flare-up, *Compend Contin Educ Dent* 10:126, 1987.

Harrison JW, Bellizzi R, Osetek EM: The clinical toxicity of endodontic medicaments, *J Endod* 5:42, 1979.

Harrison JW, Baumgartner JC, Svec TA: Incidence of pain associated with clinical factors during and after root canal therapy. Part I. Interappointment pain, *J Endod* 9:384, 1983.

Hasler JF, Mitchell DF: Analysis of 1628 cases of odontalgia: a corroborative study, *J Indianapolis Dist Dent Soc* 17:23, 1963.

Kleier DJ, Mullaney TP: Effects of formocresol on posttreatment pain of endodontic origin in vital molars, *J Endod* 6:566, 1980.

Luks S: Observed effects of traumatic injuries upon anterior teeth, *NY State Dent J* 28:65, 1962.

Marshall JG, Liesinger AW: Factors associated with endodontic posttreatment pain, *J Endod* 19:573, 1993.

Mata E, Koren LZ, Morse DR, Sinai IH: Prophylactic use of penicillin V in teeth with necrotic pulps and asymptomatic periapical radiolucencies, *Oral Surg Oral Med Oral Pathol* 60:201, 1985.

Mitchell DF, Tarplee RE: Painful pulpitis: a clinical and microscopic study, *Oral Surg* 13:1360, 1960.

Morse D et al: Infectious flare-ups and serious sequelae following endodontic treatment: a prospective randomized trial efficacy of antibiotic prophylaxis in cases of asymptomatic pulpal-periapical lesions, *Oral Surg Oral Med Oral Pathol* 64:96, 1987.

Naidorf IJ: Endodontic flare-ups: bacteriological and immunological mechanisms, *J Endod* 11:462, 1985.

Negm MM: Management of endodontic pain with nonsteroidal antiinflammatory agents: a double-blind, placebo-controlled study, *Oral Surg Oral Med Oral Pathol* 67:88,1989.

Nevins A, Verhelle R, Feldman MJ, Berman D: Local prophylactic Benadryl injections in an attempt to reduce post-instrumental pain, *J Endod* 20:296, 1994.

Nobuhara WK, Carnes DL, Gilles JA: Antiinflammatory effects of dexamethasone on periapical tissues following endodontic overinstrumentation, *J Endod* 19:501, 1993.

Schneider DW: Triamcinolone acetonide-demethylchlortetracycline HCl treatment in endodontic practice, *J Oral Med* 23:51, 1968.

Schroeder, A: Corticosteroids in endodontics, *J Oral Ther Pharm* 2:171, 1965.

Selden HS: Pain empowerment—a strategy for pain management in endodontics, *J Endod* 19:521, 1993.

Selden HS, Paris L: Management of endodontic emergencies, *J Dent Child* 37:260, 1970.

Seltzer S, Naidorf IJ: Flare-ups in endodontics. Etiological factors, *J Endod* 11:472, 1985.

Seltzer S, Naidorf IJ: Flare-ups in endodontics. II. Therapeutic measures, *J Endod* 11:559, 1985.

Smith RG, Patterson SS, El-Kafrawy AH: Histologic study of the effects of hydrocortisone on the apical periodontium of dogs, *J Endod* 2:376, 1976.

Torabinejad M et al: Factors associated with endodontic interappointment emergencies of teeth with necrotic pulps, *J Endod* 14:261, 1988.

Van Cura JE, Remeikis NA: Corticosteroid-antibiotic combination in the treatment of acute secondary apical periodontitis, *Ill Dent J* 39:307, 1970.

Walton R, Fouad A: Endodontic interappointment flare-ups: a prospective study of incidence and related factors, *J Endod* 18:172, 1992.

Weine FS, Healey HJ, Theiss EP: Endodontic emergency dilemma: leave tooth open or keep closed. *Oral Surg* 40:531, 1975.

Replantation

American Association of Endodontists: *Treatment of the avulsed permanent tooth: recommended guidelines of the American Association of Endodontists*, 1994, Chicago.

Anderson AW, Sharav Y, Massler M: Periodontal reattachment after tooth replantation, *Periodontics* 6:161, 1968.

Andreasen JO: The effect of splinting upon periodontal healing after replantation of permanent incisors in monkeys, *Acta Odontol Scand* 33:313, 1975.

Andreasen JO: Root fractures, luxation and avulsion injuries—diagnosis and management. In Gutmann LJ, Harrison JW, editors: *Proceedings of the International Conference on Oral Trauma*, American Association of Endodontists Endowment & Memorial Foundation, Chicago, November 1986.

Andreasen JO, Hjorting-Hansen E: Replantation of teeth. Radiographic and clinical study of 110 human teeth replanted after accidental loss, *Acta Odontol Scand* 24:263, 1966.

Biven GM, Ritchie GM, Gerstein H: Acrylic splint for intentional replantation, *Oral Surg* 30:537, 1970.

Camp J: Diagnosis and management of sports-related injuries to the teeth, *Dent Clin North Am* 35:733, 1991.

Coccia CT: A clinical investigation of root resorption rates in reimplanted young permanent incisors: a five-year study, *J Endod* 6:413, 1980.

Cvek M: Prognosis of luxated non-vital permanent incisors treated with calcium hydroxide and filled with gutta-percha.

A retrospective clinical study, *Endod Dent Traumatol* 45:8, 1992.

Deeb E: Intentional replantation of teeth in humans. Presented at the Fourth International Conference on Endodontics, Philadelphia, April 1968.

Deeb E, Prietto PP, McKenna RC: Reimplantation of luxated teeth in humans, *J South Calif Dent Assoc* 33:194, 1965.

Grewe J, Felts W: Autoradiographic investigation of tritiated thymidine incorporated into replanted and transplanted mouse mandibular incisors, *J Dent Res* 47:108, 1968.

Grossman LI: Intentional replantation of teeth, *J Am Dent Assoc* 72:1111, 1966.

Grossman LI, Chacker FM: Clinical evaluation and histologic study of intentionally implanted teeth. Presented at the Fourth International Conference on Endodontics, Philadelphia, April 1968.

Healey HJ: Replantation: a brief review and report of a case sequel, *Oral Surg* 6:775, 1953.

Heiman GR, Biven GM, Kahn H, Smulson M: Temporary splinting utilizing an adhesive system, *Oral Surg* 31:652, 1971.

Heimdahl A, Von Konow L, Lundquist G: Replantation of avulsed teeth after long extra-alveolar periods, *Int J Oral Surg* 12:413, 1983.

Kaplan RB, Ward HL: Some of the periodontal ramifications of replantation of avulsed teeth, *J Oral Med* 26:40, 1971.

Kemp WB, Grossman LI, Phillips J: Evaluation of 71 replanted teeth, *J Endod* 3:30, 1977.

Knight MK, Gans BJ, Calandra JC: The effect of root canal therapy on replanted teeth of dogs, *Oral Surg* 18:227, 1964.

Krasner P, Person P: Preserving avulsed teeth for replantation, *J Amer Dent Assoc* 123:80, 1992.

Krasner P, Rankow H, Ehrenreich A: Apparatus for storing and transporting traumatically avulsed teeth, *Compend Contin Educ Dent* 10:232, 1989.

Mattson L, Andreasen J, Cvek M, Granath LE: Ankylosis of experimentally reimplanted teeth related to extra-alveolar period and storage environment, *Pediatr Dent* 4:327, 1982.

Natiella JR, Armitage JE, Green GW: The replantation and transplantation of teeth, *Oral Surg* 29:397, 1970.

Oswald RJ, Harrington GW, Van Hassel HJ: Replantation. 1. The role of the socket, *J Endod* 6:479, 1980.

Oswald RJ, Harrington GW, Van Hassel HJ: A postreplantation evaluation of air-dried and saliva-stored avulsed teeth, *J Endod* 6:546, 1980

Rothschild DL, Goodman AA, Blakey KR: A histologic study of replanted and transplanted endodontically and nonendodontically treated teeth in dogs, *Oral Surg* 28:871, 1969.

Sherman P: Intentional replantation of teeth in dogs and monkeys, *J Dent Res* 44:1066, 1968.

Van Hassel HJ, Oswald RJ, Harrington FW: Replantation. 2. The role of the periodontal ligament. *J Endod* 6:506, 1980.

Weine FS: The case against replantation, *J Am Dent Assoc* 100:664, 1980.

6 Access cavity preparation and initiating treatment

After the establishment of a diagnosis and treatment plan, the first part of treatment directly applied to the tooth is the access cavity preparation, also known as the *endodontic entry*. It has already been emphasized that canal preparation is the most important segment of endodontic therapy. Canal preparation may be divided into two phases: the coronal portion and the intraradicular (within the root) portion. The coronal phase, which is the access cavity, must give direct access to the root canals and the apical foramina so that these areas may be properly cleaned and shaped by the intraradicular phase. Therefore all the treatment that follows hinges on the accuracy and correctness of the entry. If the access is improperly prepared as to position, depth, or extent, it will be difficult to reach an optimal result.

RULES FOR PROPER ACCESS PREPARATION

To ensure that the most efficient access cavity is prepared, the following rules should be observed.

1. *The objective of entry is to give direct access to the apical foramina, not merely to the canal orifices.* Since it is the apical foramen of each canal that must be sealed, the access cavity must allow for removal of any tooth structure that might impede the preparation and filling of that area. For that reason, the access cavity preparations suggested in this chapter may deviate slightly from those recommended by some other writers, whose main considerations were directed at the opening of the orifices.

2. *Access cavity preparations are different from typical operative occlusal preparations.* The typical occlusal cavity preparations used in operative dentistry are based on the topography of occlusal grooves, pits, and fissures and on the avoidance of underlying pulp. The access cavity preparations for endodontic therapy are designed for efficiently uncovering the roof of the pulp chamber and providing direct access to the apical foramina by way of the pulp canals. Since the two types of preparations must satisfy different criteria, it is only natural that they have differing configurations. By the same token, any attempt to use an operative cavity preparation as an endodontic access without considerable modification will greatly complicate the treatment.

The appropriate access cavity preparations suggested later in this chapter should be reviewed before endodontic therapy on any tooth is begun, until they become familiar to the operator.

3. *The likely interior anatomy of the tooth under treatment must be determined.* Each tooth has a typical length, number, and configuration of roots and canals, as listed in Tables 6-1 to 6-3. Before starting the access, radiographs taken from at least two different angles must be studied. Knowing what combinations of interior anatomy are possible and having the information given by the radiographs, the operator will be able to ascertain with great accuracy the canal system present in the tooth to be treated and the possible alternative configurations. This information gained before initiation of preparation will greatly facilitate the entry as well as further treatment.

4. *When canals are difficult to find, the rubber dam should not be placed until correct location has been confirmed.* It is often difficult to prepare access in a malposed tooth or one that is part of a bridge or splint. The occlusal anatomy, which ordinarily gives excellent clues to the position of the underlying canals, may be considerably altered. Teeth with large and/or deep restorations causing heavy dentinal sclerosis also may cause problems. Therefore it is best to make the initial portion of the access preparation before the placement of the rubber dam so that the shape and inclination of the

Table 6-1.   Typical tooth lengths, number of roots, and canal configuration for anterior teeth*

Tooth	Total length	Crown length	Root length	Number of roots	Types of canals
Maxillary central incisor	A = 23.0	10.5	12.5	One	I
	L = 28.0	12.0	16.0		
	S = 18.0	8.0	8.0		
Maxillary lateral incisor	A = 22.5	9.0	16.5	One	I
	L = 27.0	10.5	16.5		
	S = 17.0	8.0	8.0		
Maxillary cuspid	A = 27.0	9.5	16.5	One	I
	L = 32.0	12.0	20.5		
	S = 20.0	8.0	11.0		
Mandibular incisors	A = 21.0	9.0	12.0	One	I most frequent
	L = 25.0	10.5	14.5		II less frequent
	S = 16.0	7.0	9.0		III least frequent
Mandibular cuspid	A = 24.0	10.0	15.0	One; two, buccal and	I most frequent
	L = 30.5	12.0	20.5	lingual, rare	II less frequent
	S = 20.0	8.5	11.5		III least frequent

*Tables 6-1 to 6-3 present data from more than 9000 cases from my private practice. Working lengths for each tooth with a normal or restored crown were compiled. The average length *(A)* was the measurement from the cusp tip to apex of the median tooth; the long length *(L)* was the measurement of the tooth at the 95th percentile; the short length *(S)* was the measurement of the tooth at the fifth percentile. The lengths of the root and crown were derived from Black's *Descriptive Anatomy of the Human Teeth.*

Table 6-2.   Typical tooth lengths, number of roots, and canal configuration for bicuspids*

Tooth	Total length	Crown length	Root length	Number of roots	Types of canals
Maxillary first bicuspid	A = 21.0	8.5	12.5	Two most frequent	
	L = 24.0	10.0	14.5	(60%), buccal and	
	S = 17.5	7.0	10.0	palatal	Each I
				One (40%)	III most frequent
					II less frequent
					I rare
				Three rare	Each I
Maxillary second bicuspid	A = 21.0	8.5	12.5	One (85%)	I most frequent
	L = 25.0	10.5	15.0		II less frequent
	S = 17.0	7.0	9.5		III least frequent may have Type IV at apex
				Two (15%), buccal and palatal	Each I
Mandibular first bicuspid	A = 21.5	7.5	14.0		
	L = 25.0	9.0	17.0	One	See Table 6-4.
	S = 17.0	6.5	11.5		
				Two, buccal and lingual, rare	Each I
Mandibular second bicuspid	A = 22.0	8.0	14.0	One	I most frequent
	L = 25.0	10.0	17.0		II or III rare
	S = 17.0	6.0	11.5		IV very rare
				Two, buccal and lingual, very rare	Each I
				Three, two buccals and one lingual, extremely rare	

*See Table 6-1 for explanation of terms.

Table 6-3.   Typical tooth lengths, number of roots, and canal configuration for molars*

Tooth	Total length	Crown length	Root length	Number of roots	Types of canals
Maxillary first molar	A = 20.5	7.5	13.0	Three, two buccal and one palatal	Distobuccal and palatal: each I
	L = 24.5	9.0	16.0		Mesiobuccal: see Table 6-5.
	S = 17.0	7.0	10.0		
Maxillary second molar	A = 20.0	7.0	13.0	Three, two buccal and one palatal (90%)	Distobuccal and palatal: each I
	L = 24.0	8.5	15.5		Mesiobuccal: see Table 6-6.
	S = 17.0	7.0	10.0	Two, one buccal and one palatal (10%)	Each I most frequent; buccal root may have II or III infrequently
Mandibular first molar	A = 21.0	7.5	13.5	Two most common, mesial and distal	Mesial: III most frequent
	L = 24.5	10.0	15.0		II less frequent
	S = 18.0	6.0	11.5		Distal: I most frequent
					II less frequent
					III least frequent
				Three, one mesial and two distal	Mesial: same as above
					Distal: each I, distolingual very curved
Mandibular second molar	A = 20.0	7.0	13.0	Two most common, mesial and distal	See Table 6-7.
	L = 24.0	8.5	15.5		Distal: I most frequent
	S = 17.0	6.0	12.0		II or III rare
				One	II most frequent
					I less frequent
					III least frequent

*See Table 6-1 for explanation of terms.

adjacent teeth, the gingival tissues, and the hard structures covering the roots are of aid in determining the position of the canals. In addition, if the tooth to be treated is part of a bridge or splint, water spray may be used to keep the adjacent abutments from overheating until the gold is penetrated.

Once the roof of the chamber is penetrated and the correct access is verified, the rubber dam may be applied. Since the canals will be enlarged considerably with heavy irrigation, the effect of any microorganism contamination before dam placement is minimal. Under no circumstance should a file, reamer, or broach be used until the dam is securely in place.

If for some reason it is mandatory to use the rubber dam for every phase of treatment, the access cavity for complex cases should be prepared with multiple-tooth rather than single-tooth isolation. This will allow for visualization of adjacent teeth while the dam is in place (Fig. 6-1).

5. *Endodontic entries are prepared through the occlusal or lingual surface—never through the proximal or gingival surface.* In an attempt to be conservative, the dentist may elect to perform endodontic therapy through an already existing proximal or gingival restoration or carious lesion. When this is done, the canal-enlarging instruments must be bent at severe angles to pass through the access and still perform their function. Inadequate canal preparation and/or broken instruments may result.

When proximal or gingival tooth destruction occurs, affected areas should be excavated and restored, with either a temporary seal or a permanent filling material. Then the normal access cavity is prepared through the occlusal or lingual surface, as described later in this chapter.

6. *As part of the access preparation, the unsupported cusps of posterior teeth must be reduced.* Endodontic therapy requires the removal of much of the central portion of the treated tooth, greatly reducing resistance to stress. Although this problem is solved by the placement of a proper restoration after treatment, the tooth is severely weakened until that time.

Therefore, as part of access preparation, all unsupported cusps must be reduced by trimming with a tapered fissure carbide or diamond stone until a definite clearance in occlusal and lateral movement is obtained. This decreases the chance for cuspal fracture beneath the gingival or bony attachment, which is so difficult to repair, or vertical fracture of the root, which is hopeless!

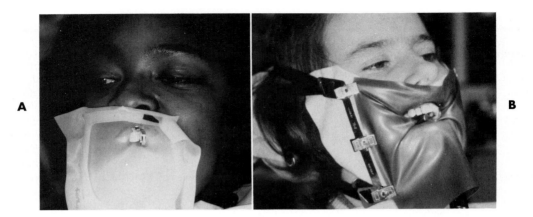

Fig. 6-1. Types of rubber dam applications. **A,** Single-tooth isolation for maxillary central incisor, using an Ostby frame. **B,** Multiple-tooth isolation from maxillary first bicuspid to opposite first bicuspid, using a Woodbury frame.

COMMON CANAL CONFIGURATIONS

Although the apical foramen must be sealed by endodontic therapy, the root canal is what provides the pathway to the apex. Therefore it is important for the dentist to be familiar with the various paths that the route takes in getting to the apex. These are the typical configurations of the root canals.

Canal configuration studies. For many years the standard works of referral for this subject had been the canal morphology studies published in the first third of the twentieth century. Hess, in particular, published several reports demonstrating huge numbers of pulpal vessels with intricate curvatures, anastomoses, and junctions, which were rarely recapitulated by canal fillings of that period. Wheeler published several textbooks dealing with this subject.

It is obvious that canal anatomy in human teeth has not changed for hundreds, if not thousands, of years. However, for some inexplicable reason, many of these early studies proved to be inaccurate. Then, in 1965, Rankine-Wilson and Henry, with their study club in Perth, Australia, published an illuminating report on the canal anatomy of mandibular anterior teeth. Many dentists were shocked at the frequency of two canals in mandibular incisors according to that study, and few really placed credence in the findings. However, because the mandibular anterior teeth were not often endodontically involved, the information did not have much impact clinically.

The Rankine-Wilson and Henry paper did serve to stimulate further research into the canal ana-

tomy of the more frequently treated teeth, particularly in those instances where a lesser degree of success than anticipated was obtained. Rankine-Wilson, a restorative dentist who learned to do his own endodontic treatment for his rehabilitation cases because of the absence of endodontic specialists in Perth, came to the United States in 1967 to teach at Northwestern University Dental School for 1 year in the Crown and Bridge Department. Weine, a young endodontist recently out of his master's program and also teaching at Northwestern, and Rankine-Wilson became fast friends and discussed possible future studies on canal configuration. Both agreed that the mesiobuccal root of the maxillary first molar had many more failures than could be anticipated, particularly in cases where postoperative inspection of the radiographs indicated reasonably well-treated cases.

The result of these discussions was the paper by Weine et al. in 1969, indicating that four canals were present in that tooth more often than three canals (51.5% versus 48.5%). Many teachers and clinicians ridiculed that study and claimed that the results were contrived and inaccurate. However, since 1969, a number of investigators have studied that root by various methods, essentially substantiating the results of the Weine study (Table 6-4), with several claiming an even greater occurrence for four canals in that tooth.

Once that study, as surprising as it was, had been verified, the dam was broken and many other teeth or roots were investigated, with new and

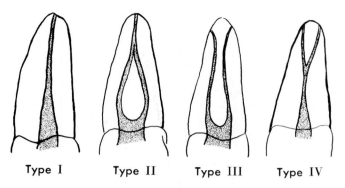

Type I   Type II   Type III   Type IV

Fig. 6-2. Four types of canal configuration present in one root are shown: *Type I*—single canal from pulp chamber to apex; *Type II*—two canals leaving the chamber and merging to form a single canal short of the apex; *Type III*—two separate and distinct canals from chamber to apex; *Type IV*—one canal leaving the chamber and dividing into two separate and distinct canals.

significant information reported. Such teeth as the mandibular first bicuspid (Table 6-5), the mandibular first and second molars (Table 6-6), and the maxillary second bicuspid and molar (Table 6-7) were the objects of illuminating studies. The net results of these reports were that many, many more teeth were treated successfully than had been previously, and when treatment was not successful, an intelligent assessment of failure and possible retreatment could be reached.

Types of configurations. Despite the many combinations of canals that are present in the roots of the 32 permanent teeth, it is possible to categorize the canal systems in any one root into four different types (Fig. 6-2). These four types can be described briefly.

Type I—single canal from the pulp chamber to the apex
Type II—two separate canals leaving the chamber but merging short of the apex to form only one canal
Type III—two separate canals leaving the chamber and exiting the root in separate apical foramina
Type IV—one canal leaving the pulp chamber but dividing short of the apex into two separate and distinct canals with separate apical foramina

Canal preparation of Type I and Type III canal systems is relatively straightforward, since each of the canals in these configurations is separate and distinct between orifice and apex. The only difference between the two is that the Type III system has two canals, whereas the Type I has only one.

However, Type II and Type IV systems are different because there are some areas in the root where the two canals share space and others where

the canals are separate. This requires individualized procedures in each of these conditions to obtain the most desirable results. Methods for preparing, as well as filling, Type II and Type IV systems are discussed in Chapter 7.

Vertucci has written extensively about canal anatomy and established a somewhat different classification, with seven major types rather than four. Some of his types are merely variants of those just listed, such as a single canal that divides in midroot but then remerges into one canal (considered to be Type I in this classification) or two canals leaving the floor of the chamber separately, merging in midroot and then separating into two canals as they exit the tooth (considered to be Type III in this classification).

Periodically a configuration is seen that is not specifically described in the classification used in this textbook, but this is a very rare occurrence (Fig. 6-3). I doubt that those types that fail to be described accurately with my classification occur any more frequently than 0.1%, if that often. Learning a larger number of configurations for such a minuscule number of cases seems unwarranted.

Vertucci did his studies by collecting minimally decayed and restored extracted teeth, decalcifying the hard tissues, removing the pulpal contents, and injecting dye into those spaces. These transparent specimens were designed to be viewed by students and dentists interested in pulpal anatomy. My classification is based on endodontic therapy, specifically as recorded on radiographs taken during and after endodontic treatment. Both systems are

Table 6-4. Canal configuration studies for the mesiobuccal root of the maxillary first molar

Author(s)	No. of teeth	Method of study	Type I (%)	Type II (%)	Type III (%)	Type IV (%)
Weine et al.	208	Vertical sectioning	48.5	37.5	14.0	0
Pineda and Kuttler	262	Radiographic	39.3	12.2	35.7	12.8
Green*	100	Vertical sectioning	64.0	22.0	14.0	
Seidberg et al.	100	Horizontal sectioning	38.0	37.0	25.0	
		Clinical cases	66.7	← 33.3 →		0
Pomeranz and Fishelberg	71	Decalcified and dyed	71.8	16.9	11.3	0
	100	Clinical cases	69.0	16.0	15.0	0
Vertucci	100	Decalcified and dyed	45.0	37.0	18.0	
Evenot	170, 208	Radiographic, several microscopic	28.8	23.5	38.8	8.8
Hartwell and Bellizzi	538	Clinical cases	81.4	← 18.6 →		0
Weller and Hartwell	835	Clinical cases	61.0	← 39.0 →		0

*Mesiobuccal root studied in both maxillary first and second molars.

Table 6-5. Canal configuration studies for mandibular first bicuspids

Author(s)	No. of teeth	Method of study	Type I (%)	Type II (%)	Type III (%)	Type IV (%)	Three canals
Pineda and Kuttler	202	Radiographic	69.3	4.9	1.5	23.4	0.9
Green	50	Vertical sectioning	86.0	4.0	← 10.0 →		Not reported
Vertucci	400	Decalcified and dyed	70.0	4.0	1.5	24.0	0.5
Baisden et al.	106	Transverse sectioning	76.4	0	0	23.6	0

Table 6-6. Canal configuration studies for mesial root of mandibular second molar

Author(s)	No. of teeth	Method of study	Type I (%)	Type II (%)	Type III (%)	Type IV (%)
Green	100	Vertical sectioning	13.0	49.0	38.0	0
Pineda and Kuttler	300	Radiographic	58.0	20.6	13.8	7.6
Vertucci	100	Decalcified and dyed	27.0	38.0	26.0	9.0
Weine et al.	72	Radiographic with files in place	4.0	52.0	40.0	0

Table 6-7. Canal configuration studies for mesiobuccal root of maxillary second molar

Author(s)	No. of teeth	Method of study	Type I (%)	Type II (%)	Type III (%)	Type IV (%)
Nosonowitz and Brenner	161	Clinical cases	68.9	25.5	5.6	0
Pomeranz and Fishelberg	29	Clinical cases	62.1	13.8	24.1	0
Pineda and Kuttler	294	Radiographic	64.6	8.2	12.8	14.4
Vertucci	100	Decalcified and dyed	71.0	17.0	12.0	0
Kulild and Peters	32	Access and bur penetration	21.8	← 78.2 →		0
	32	Sectioning and microscopic	6.3	← 93.7 →		0
Eskoz and Weine	67	Radiographic with files in place	59.7	20.9	16.4	3.0

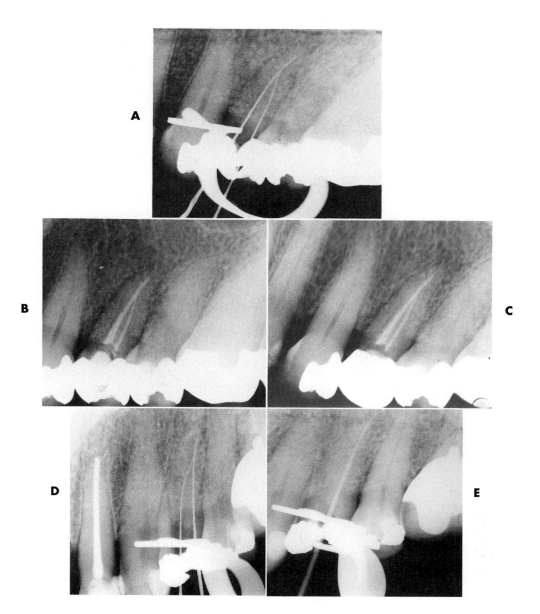

Fig. 6-3. Types of canal configurations that appear the same at the start but prove to be different. **A,** Radiograph of files in place for determination of canal configuration and working length calculation for a maxillary first bicuspid. This angled view from the mesial indicates that the palatal canal (*left*) is the master canal, with the buccal canal merging into it—clearly a Type II canal system. As also can be seen in this view, the orifices are quite far apart leaving the chamber but still merge short of the apex. **B,** Canals filled with laterally condensed gutta-percha and Wach's paste. **C,** One year later, after restoration, normal periapical tissue. (Restorations by Dr. Irving Fishman, Chicago.) **D,** Radiograph of files in place for determination of canal, configuration and working length calculation of another first bicuspid, also angled view from the mesial. The canal to the right (the buccal) is the master canal, according to this film, with the palatal canal merging into it—clearly another Type II canal system, very similar to that shown in view **A,** except having different master canals. **E,** Preparation was completed as a Type II configuration, with one master gutta-percha canal placed as master canal in the buccal canal. **F,** Immediate postfilling film, canals filled with laterally condensed gutta-percha and Wach's paste, post room prepared in buccal canal. It is obvious now that the canal configuration was of two canals exiting the floor of the chamber, merging into a single canal, and then redividing into two separate canals to exit at the apex. This type of configuration is quite unusual but does occur occasionally. It is neither Type II nor Type IV and, in fact, is not covered in the classification given. **G,** One year after treatment. **H,** Two years after treatment, periapical areas remain normal. (Restorations by Dr. Charles Greene, Skokie, Ill.) *Continued*

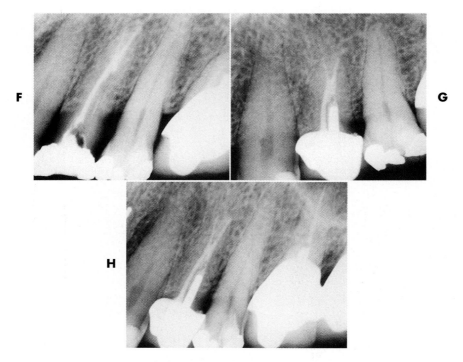

Fig. 6-3, cont'd. For legend see p. 245.

important and deserve attention, but my choice is to use a simple and clinically oriented classification system.

This classification does not consider the possible position of large auxiliary canals or the position at which the apical foramina exit the root. Any combination of these factors could be present in any of the canals without regard to any specific configuration.

In Tables 6-1 to 6-3 this classification is used to describe the canal configurations present in each root. Extremely unusual root and canal configurations were not considered in the compilation of data for these tables. The figures listed are those that are applicable to needed treatment in the greatest number of cases. Although no exact percentages are given for the possible combinations, the following terms have been used to indicate the frequency of occurrence:

Most frequent—present in more than 55% of cases
Less frequent—present in less than 45% but more than 25% of cases
Least frequent—present in less than 25% but more than 2% of cases

Rare—occurring in less than 2% of cases but still present occasionally

ARMAMENTARIUM FOR ACCESS PREPARATIONS

The tray setup for access preparations is shown in Fig. 6-4. Instruments to be included are as follows:

Front surface mirror—for best visibility
Endodontic explorer—one end comes to a point to aid in locating orifices while the other has a slight hook to check shelves at edges of the preparation (Fig. 6-5)
Endodontic excavator—to remove decay and pulp tags
Plastic instrument
Amalgam plugger
Spatula
Cotton pliers
Broaches
Glass slab
Cotton pellets—to hold medication and absorb blood
Burs—long shank, no. 701 or 558, no. 4, no. 2, and a specially prepared no. 701 or 558 with a rounded or safe-tipped end to prevent gouging (Fig. 6-6);

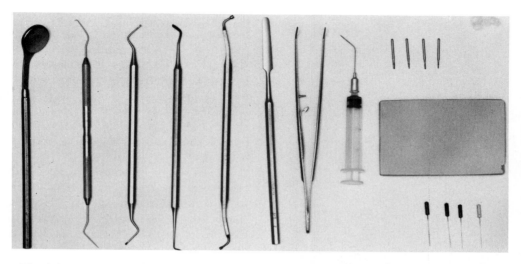

Fig. 6-4. Tray setup for access cavity preparation and canal preparation. *From left,* Front surface mirror, endodontic explorer, excavator, plastic instrument, amalgam plugger, spatula, cotton pliers, irrigating syringe. *At right, from top,* Cotton pellets, long shank burs, mixing slab, broaches.

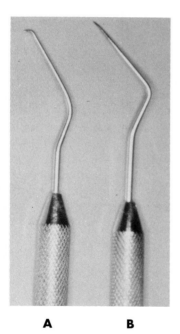

A   B

Fig. 6-5. Two ends of endodontic explorer. **A,** Hook end, used to check for shelves that might harbor microorganisms or cause crown discoloration. **B,** Sharp tip for locating canal orifices.

safe-tipped burs *only* to be used on floor of the pulp chamber after penetration of roof

Rubber dam materials also must be available for this appointment, including sheets of rubber dam, punch, frame, clamp holder, and clamps. Clamps needed are as follows:

Nos. 26* and 27*—wingless clamps for molars or
Nos. 12A† and 12B†—winged clamps for molars
No. 209*—for bicuspids and bulky anterior teeth
No. 211* or 9†—for small anterior and broken down teeth, or a similar assortment

In addition, temporary filling materials and intracanal medicaments must be available. (See Chapter 7.)

PULP CANAL ANATOMY AND ACCESS PREPARATIONS

Maxillary central incisor. The maxillary central incisor always has one root and Type I canal configuration. The root is bulky, with a slight distal axial inclination but rarely has a dilaceration. The typical length measurements are given in Table 6-1.

*S.S. White–Pennwalt Dental Products International, Philadelphia, PA 19102.
†Columbus Dental Manufacturing Co., Columbus, OH 43206.

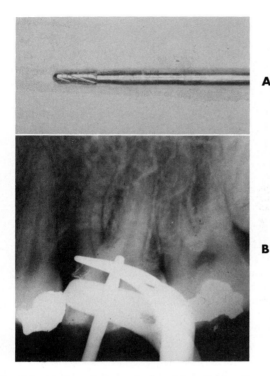

Fig. 6-6. **A,** Rounded or safe-tipped bur. Cutting flutes are present on sides but not tip of bur. Any fissure bur may be altered to become safe tipped by trimming flutes from end with a heatless stone. **B,** After canal orifices of posterior teeth have been located, safe-tipped bur is passed along floor of chamber. Cutting flutes on sides trim any overhanging dentin to give direct access to canals. Once roof of chamber has been penetrated, use of this bur prevents gouging or perforation of the floor.

A labiolingual section of the tooth shows that the pulp cavity comes to a point near the incisal edge, becomes wider as it approaches the cervical line, then narrows to the apex. The apical foramen frequently exits short of the apex, to the labial direction. A mesiodistal section discloses that the pulp cavity is wider toward the incisal area and then tapers to the apex.

The access cavity preparation is begun by using a tapered fissure bur in the exact center of the lingual surface. The bur should be directed parallel to the long axis of the crown rather than at a right angle, as has been suggested. If the access is begun at a right angle to the long axis, there is a possibility for penetration too far labially, or for completely missing the pulp canal on a tooth with considerable dentinal sclerosis. On the other hand, penetration along the long axis in the center of the tooth must eventually reach the canal (Fig. 6-7). The philosophy of right-angle penetration is a holdover from the era preceding the use of high-speed instruments, when it was difficult to penetrate enamel with slow speed using steel burs. With an airotor and carbide burs, direct penetration offers no problem. Access for each anterior tooth should be prepared in this newer manner.

A cross section of the tooth in the cervical area shows that the canal has a slightly triangular shape, with the apex toward the lingual surface and the base to the labial. For that reason the entry has a round but slightly triangular shape to give direct access to the entire canal (Fig. 6-8).

Once the canal is found, a safe-tipped tapered fissure bur is used to remove any dentin overhangs that would trap debris, sealer, or other materials, which might cause crown discoloration or prevent direct access to the apex. This procedure is followed in all anterior teeth, both maxillary and mandibular.

The maxillary central and lateral incisor and canine roots, and therefore canals as well, all have a distal axial inclination. This means that in penetrating along the long axis of the tooth, the bur must be slightly angled toward the distal surface (Fig. 6-9). Failure to provide for this situation may lead to penetration of the mesial portion of the root.

Maxillary lateral incisor. The maxillary lateral incisor always has one root and a Type I canal configuration. The root is more slender than in the maxillary central incisor and frequently has a distal and/or lingual curvature or dilaceration. The typical length measurements, given in Table 6-1, are slightly shorter than for the adjacent central incisor.

The general shape of the pulp canal, both in mesiodistal and in labiolingual section, is the same as shown by the central incisor. However, a cross section through the cervical area shows that the canal has an oval shape, and therefore the access preparation also has that shape (Fig. 6-10).

Maxillary cuspid. The maxillary cuspid always has one root and a Type I canal configuration. The root may appear to be slender from the labial view, as seen on a typical intraoral radiograph, but is bulky as viewed proximally, with an irregular outline (Fig. 6-11, *B*). The typical length measurements, given in Table 6-1, disclose that the tooth is the longest in the arch.

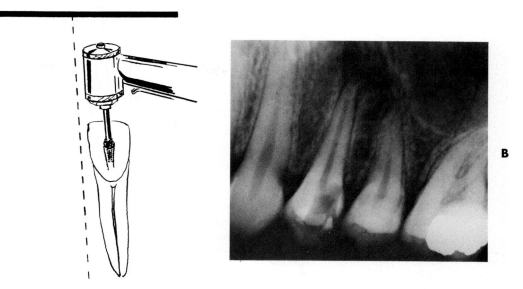

A

B

Fig. 6-7. **A,** All burs used in access cavity preparation must be angled along the long axis of tooth being entered. As long as bur remains in center of tooth parallel to long axis, the pulp, even if diminished by dentinal sclerosis, will be reached. Note that line parallel to long axis *(dotted line)* of this mandibular anterior tooth is not perpendicular to occlusal plane *(heavy line)*. This is true on most teeth; therefore, to determine true root angulation, the dentist must obtain radiographs and perform the clinical examination before beginning the access. **B,** Failure to direct bur along the long axis of tooth has led to a perforation of distal portion of first bicuspid into periodontal ligament space. Endodontic procedures to follow will be impeded by probable ingress of microorganisms and debris unless the perforation is sealed. Even then, restoration after treatment will be much more complicated than it would have been with a proper entry.

A labiolingual section shows that the pulp canal comes to a point near the incisal area but is wide through the cervical and middle root until it reaches the apical third of the root, where it narrows. Frequently the canal exits short of the root tip to the labial direction. A mesiodistal section shows that the pulp canal is much narrower than the labiolingual section, with a relatively regular shape all the way to the apex. In cross section through the cervical area, the canal has an oval outline, which is the correct shape for the endodontic entry (Fig. 6-11).

Mandibular central and lateral incisors. Central and lateral incisors in the mandible are so similar in shape, configuration, and dimension that one description will hold true for both. The endodontic implications of the mandibular incisor roots and canals were extensively studied and reported by Rankine-Wilson and Henry. Much of the information concerning these teeth had never been presented in such detail before this important study.

For that reason the configurations and access suggested here for these teeth differ from those recommended by earlier writers.

The mandibular incisors have only one root, which is narrow mesiodistally but relatively wide labiolingually, and may have a distal and/or lingual curvature. The canal configuration may be of Type I, II, or III, in that order of frequency. Of the 111 teeth examined by Rankine-Wilson and Henry, 60% had Type I, 35% showed Type II, and 5% were classified as Type III. Furthermore, noting a correlation between crown shape and canal configuration, they stated that short squatty crowns had blunted roots, usually with a divided or split canal.

When two canals were present, the labial canal was the straighter. The point of division for divided canals was in the cervical third of the root.

A labiolingual section reveals the great width of the pulp canal, never visualized by the routine intraoral radiograph, which allows room for two

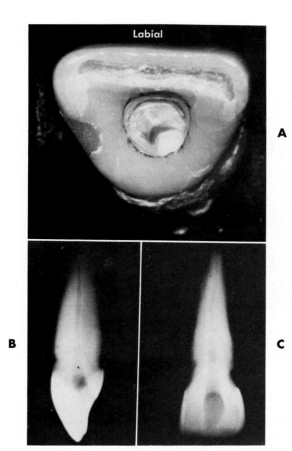

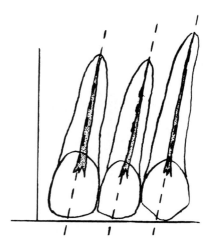

Fig. 6-9. Long axis of each maxillary anterior tooth angles distally in patients with normal occlusion. Attempting to enter these teeth on a path perpendicular to occlusal plane will lead to perforation. Because many variations in angulation do occur, it is necessary to consult radiographs, examine topography of bone over roots, and be aware of typical anatomic conditions before picking up handpiece to start the entry.

Fig. 6-8. **A,** Access cavity for maxillary central incisor is generally round, but extensions toward incisal region to allow for cleansing of pulp horns impart a slightly triangular shape. Triangle's base is toward incisal edge, whereas rounded apex is incisal to cingulum. Preparation shown is much closer to incisal edge than is usually depicted. However, this position gives direct access to apex, as seen in labial and proximal radiographs, **B** and **C.**

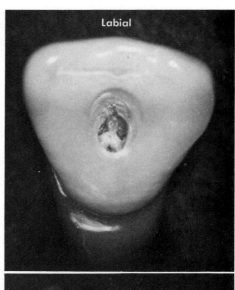

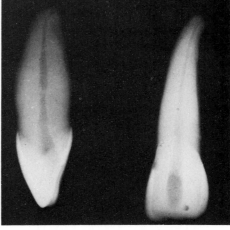

Fig. 6-10. **A,** Access preparation for maxillary lateral incisor is oval with greatest width incisogingivally. As in central incisor, the incisal extent is placed close to incisal edge for direct access to apex. Note common finding of a distal curve and exiting of canal seen in labial view, **C,** as would be visualized in typical intraoral radiograph. However, canal exits to palatal side in proximal view, **B,** which would ordinarily be missed in a clinical case. Exiting short of tip of apex is a common occurrence in lateral incisors.

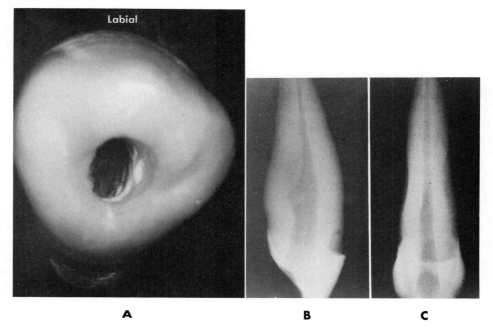

Fig. 6-11. **A,** Access preparation for maxillary cuspid is oval with widest diameter incisogingivally to give direct access to apex. Proximal view, **B,** shows great width of canal in middle third of tooth, which tapers down to a rather small diameter near apex. This taper is much more gradual as viewed labially, **C.**

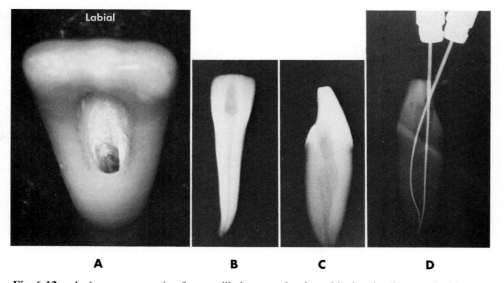

Fig. 6-12. **A,** Access preparation for mandibular central or lateral incisor is a long oval with greatest width incisogingivally and incisal extent close to incisal edge. Even though canal appears extremely narrow in typical intraoral radiograph as seen from the labial aspect, **B,** proximal radiograph, **C,** shows wide canal that demands a wide access preparation from incisal to gingival areas to gain proper intraradicular preparation. **D,** Width of tooth as viewed proximally allows for divided canal configuration that is present in a surprisingly high percentage of these teeth.

separate canals or one wide canal with an island of dentin in the middle (Fig. 6-12, *C* and *D*). A mesiodistal section shows that the pulp canal is quite narrow and is particularly constricted in the root portion of the tooth, with both the root and the canal taking a gradual distal curve (Fig. 6-12, *B*). Because of this narrow mesiodistal dimension, the access preparation must be extremely precise to avoid root perforation. Developmental depressions are found on both the mesial and the distal surfaces of the root, decreasing the mesiodistal dimension in the middle of the root. Therefore canal enlargement past size 70 or 80 may lead to lateral perforation in thin incisors.

A cross section in the cervical area demonstrates that the canal is a long, thin oval, very constricted mesiodistally. Because of the implications of canal configuration, the access preparation suggested is oval but is wide labiolingually to allow for proper instrumentation (Fig. 6-12). Rankine-Wilson and Henry demonstrated that the routine entry ordinarily used allows for the instrumentation of the labial canal only in divided-canal teeth or the labial wall of a single-canaled tooth.

The uninformed dentist may believe that mandibular incisors are relatively simple teeth on which to perform endodontic therapy. Nothing could be further from the truth. These teeth come right behind the molars and the multicanaled mandibular bicuspids in degree of difficulty. The major reason for this is the narrow mesiodistal dimension compared with buccolingual width, which makes it almost impossible to enlarge the canal or canals evenly in every direction. Also, the 40% of teeth with two canals reported by Rankine-Wilson and Henry is almost never reached by practitioners during clinical situations.

To add to the problems, because of their proximity, it is virtually impossible to radiograph these teeth from a sufficient angle to know in advance that two canals are present (Fig. 6-13). Interestingly, I have had a low percentage of two filled canals in mandibular incisors. However, in teeth in which the crowns have been badly decayed or in trauma cases when much of the crown is missing, I have cut the teeth down to slightly above the gingival margin and then have had a high percentage of two canals, even greater than the reported percentages.

Therefore, if I encounter difficulty with a case involving a mandibular incisor, I will decoronalize the tooth. Invariably, I discover a second canal (Fig.

6-13, *B*), and generally the problems desist after canal preparation. Follow-up films on these cases have been extremely satisfying (Fig. 6-13, *D*).

The reason why these teeth do not cause us as many problems as they might is that a high percentage of the two-canal cases rejoin near the apex (Fig. 6-14). In these teeth, if one of the canals is well prepared and the apex well-filled (Fig. 6-14, *C*) the result will be satisfactory (Fig. 6-14, *D*). These teeth should never be filled with a silver point, since the apical portion of the canal is broadly elliptic and must be sealed with a semisolid compactible material.

Mandibular cuspid. Mandibular cuspids usually have only one root but in rare cases may have two separate roots. Teeth with one root may have Type I, II, or III configuration, as do the mandibular incisors. These teeth are usually the longest of the mandibular teeth but have greater length variation than do maxillary cuspids, as indicated in Table 6-1.

The root canal is thin mesiodistally but wide labiolingually. The cervical cross section is oval, as is the suggested entry (Fig. 6-15). This tooth usually has a slightly labial axial inclination of the crown. Therefore the access is directed toward the lingual surface.

A bifurcated canal is possible in this tooth, and generally there will be at least a hint in the preoperative or file-in-place radiograph (Fig. 6-16, *A* and *F*). If this is the case, an access preparation buccolingually wider than usual should be used. Should only one canal be present, it will be quite wide buccolingually in any case (Fig. 6-15, *B*), so that the extra width, even when unnecessary, will not be a problem. However, if two canals are present, only the extra buccolingual width of the access will permit proper location, preparation, and filling (Fig. 6-16).

Maxillary first bicuspid. Maxillary first bicuspids have a number of variations in root and canal configuration. Approximately 60% have two roots, one buccal and the other palatal, each with a single canal. The two roots may be completely separate or merely twin projections rising from the middle third of the root to the apex, with the latter slightly more common. The two roots are usually equal in length from apex to cusp.

In approximately 38% of maxillary first bicuspids, only one root is present, usually with two separate canals (Type III). Type II canal configuration is present less frequently. Type I is very rare.

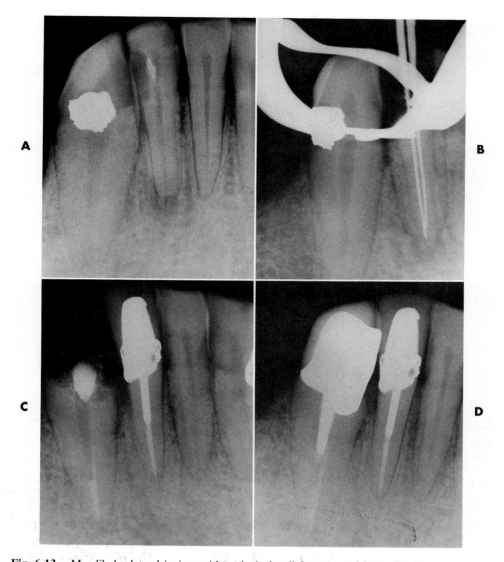

Fig. 6-13. Mandibular lateral incisor with periapical radiolucency and large distal carious lesion. **A,** Chronic draining sinus tract was present. **B,** Routine lingual access was prepared so one canal could be located and enlarged. The sinus tract persisted. Tooth was decoronalized and a second canal located. Note files in both canals. It was virtually impossible to angle film sufficiently to see that the canals were separate and distinct; but both went to their lengths independently, which does not happen in Type II canal configuration. **C,** Two canals were filled with laterally condensed gutta-percha. This film, taken 6 years later, indicates perfect apical healing. **D,** Nine years after treatment. (Restorations by Dr. Morton Schreiber, Highland Park, Ill.)

All the root and canal configurations of this tooth are present also in maxillary second bicuspids, but the frequency of occurrence changes considerably. The most common configuration in one is the least common in the other, and vice versa (Table 6-2).

The preoperative angled view is very helpful in determining the type of configuration present.

A cross section at the cervical line shows a ribbon-shaped canal or one shaped like a figure eight, with the widest dimension buccolingually.

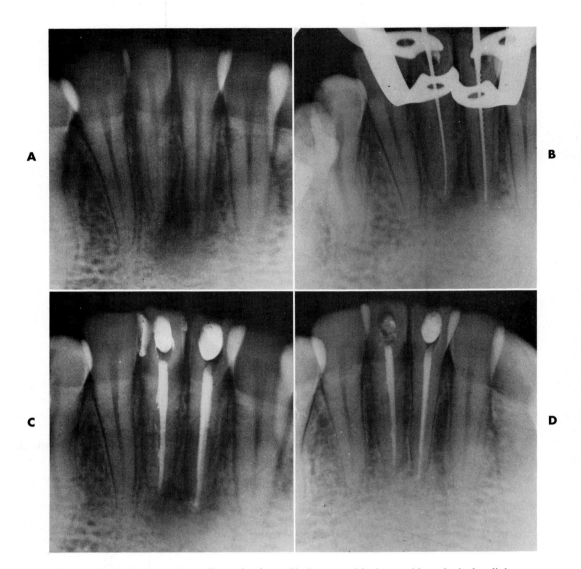

Fig. 6-14. A, Preoperative radiograph of mandibular central incisors with periapical radiolucencies. Pulps were nonresponsive to pulp testing. There was a history of trauma. **B,** Files in place give a hint of two canals. **C,** Despite making a large labiolingual extension of the access, I could not locate the second canal in either tooth. However, at the time of filling, I could see that Type II canal configurations were present. Canals were filled with laterally condensed gutta-percha and Wach's paste. **D,** Excellent healing 2 years later.

Therefore the access cavity preparation is a thin oval, with the greatest width in the same direction, exactly the opposite of the occlusal cavity preparation for maxillary bicuspids.

For all bicuspids, initial access preparation is begun by using a tapered fissure bur in the middle of the central groove. Buccal and lingual movement of the bur develops the oval shape needed for most bicuspids. Once the roof of the pulp chamber is penetrated, a safe-tipped fissure bur is used to uncover the orifices to give direct access to the apices. The buccal canal lies beneath the buccal cusp, whereas the palatal canal lies beneath the palatal cusp (Fig. 6-17).

In teeth with sclerotic canals, it is usually best to locate the canal that is farthest from the deep portion of decay or existing restoration and thus is the least calcified. Careful examination of the floor

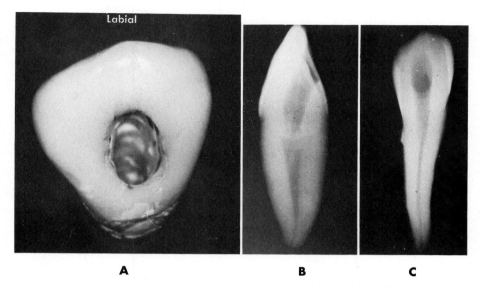

Fig. 6-15.   **A,** Entry for mandibular cuspid is oval with greatest width incisogingivally. Labial and proximal radiographs, **B** and **C,** demonstrate direct access to apex afforded by such a preparation.

of the chamber, aided by fiberoptic illumination, will show the ribbon-shaped outline of the presclerotic pulp canal. Further exploration at the end opposite the already discovered canal will soon reveal the missing channel.

Vertucci has stated that when two canals are present in one root, the distance between the orifices is a strong indicator of their ultimate relationship to each other. In other words, if the orifices are close to each other, the canals will merge short of the apex, and if they are far apart, they will remain separate and distinct. I have not found this to be consistently correct, particularly in maxillary bicuspids. Fig. 6-3 illustrates a case where the orifices of the two canals were quite far apart, each under their respective cusps (as can be seen in the angled radiograph with files in place, Fig. 6-3, *A*), and yet merged short of the apex into a single site of exiting. Similarly, I have treated bicuspids where the orifices were more centered, away from the buccal and palatal extents of their teeth, and yet these canals remained separate and distinct all the way to their apical exiting sites.

Vertucci's comments referred to molar teeth as well as bicuspids. In the mesial root of mandibular molars, his views are accurate. If the mesial canals in these roots are close together, the chances of them being merged are much higher than if they are far apart. The reason for this is that develop-

mentally in many cases, the mesial canal had a single, large, figure-eight shape. As the isthmus in the middle closed down, the large, single canal became two canals, many of which still joined at the apex in these cases.

However, in other molar roots and in some single-rooted molars, canals may have orifices close, but they remain separate and distinct to the apex (Fig. 6-18).

In treating bicuspids that have large restorations under bridges or splints, the dentist may have difficulty telling which of the two canals has been uncovered. If the wrong assumption is made as to which canal was located, preparation at the opposite end of the chamber will lead to a perforation. To avoid this, the *buccal object rule,* so important in the radiography of multicanaled teeth, is extremely useful. This rule states that the root or canal farther from the film (the buccal) moves a greater distance on an x-ray projection taken with the cone angled in the horizontal plane than does the root or canal closer to the film. To solve the problem of which canal has been found, a file is placed in the canal and a radiograph is taken. If the cone is pointed toward the distal direction, the buccal root will move more and therefore be more distal on the film, whereas the palatial canal will appear more to the mesial area (Fig. 6-19).

The buccal object rule is used in the determination of working lengths for posterior teeth (Chapter 7).

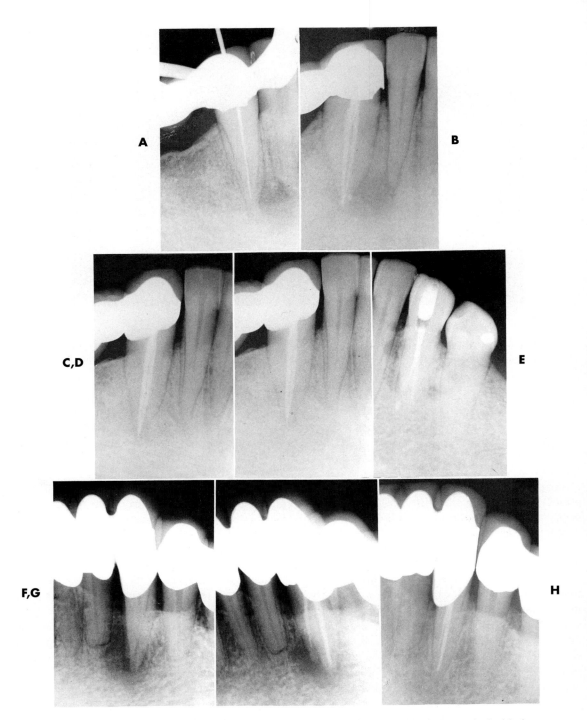

Fig. 6-16. **A,** Radiograph of mandibular cuspid with initial file in place indicates periapical lesion to the mesial and short placement of file. There is also an extreme fluting of the root on both the mesial and the distal, indicating the possibility for an additional canal. Accordingly the access was widened buccolingually. **B,** A second canal was located through this wider-access preparation. Both canals were prepared and filled with laterally condensed gutta-percha and Wach's paste. On this angled radiograph it appears that the canals merge at the apex. However, each canal was prepared separately, and there probably was a small distance between the two, but not wide enough to be seen at this angulation. **C,** One year later. **D,** Three years later, excellent healing. **E,** Another two-canaled mandibular cuspid, with site of separation much further apically. Canals were filled with chloropercha technique. **F,** Preoperative radiograph of mandibular cuspid with two roots and a large periapical lesion. **G,** Canals filled with laterally condensed gutta-percha and Wach's paste. **H,** Seven years later, perfect healing. (Restorations by Dr. Robert Wheeler, Chicago.)

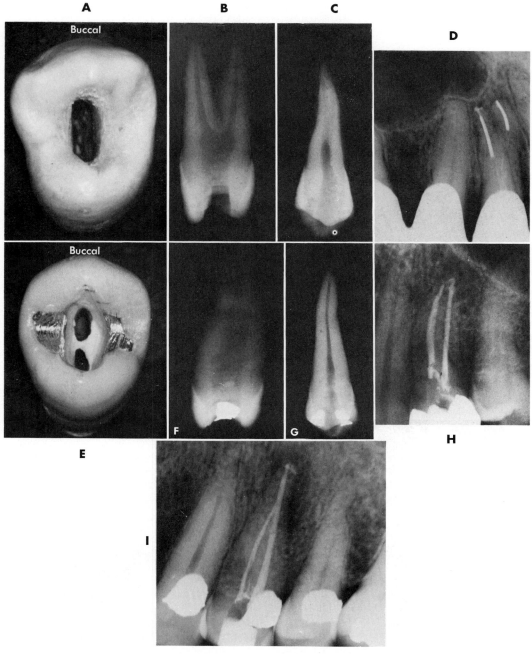

Fig. 6-17.   Access preparations for three typical types of maxillary bicuspids. **A,** Entry for tooth with two separate roots is oval with greatest width in buccolingual direction. Preparation must reach height of cusps because buccal canal lies beneath buccal cusp and palatal canal lies beneath palatal cusp, as seen in proximal radiograph. **B,** Attempting to narrow preparation by not extending to cusps will prevent direct access to apices. **C,** Preparation need not be very wide mesiodistally. **D,** Immediate postfilling radiograph of typical tooth with this configuration. **E,** Entry for single-rooted maxillary bicuspid with two canals leaving floor of chamber. Orifices are closer together than in birooted tooth, and extension to cusp height is not required for direct access to apices. **F** and **G,** Immediate postfilling radiographs show two types of teeth in which this access was used: two canals all the way to apex, **H,** or canals merging to form a single apical foramen, **I.** Access for single-canaled maxillary bicuspid.

Continued

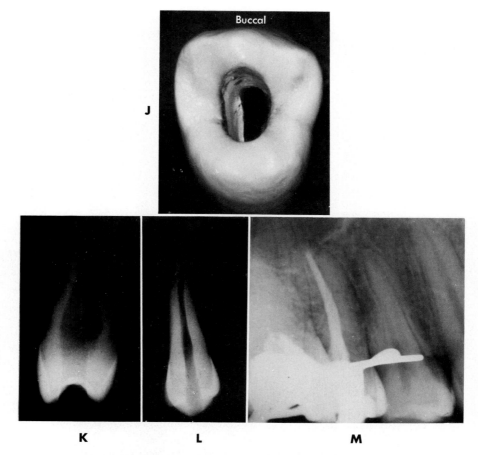

Fig. 6-17, cont'd. J, Same buccolingual extension as in **E** but slightly wider than other maxillary bicuspid entries in mesiodistal direction, as verified in labial view, **L.** As seen from proximal view, **K,** the canal is wide buccolingually. **M,** Angled view during canal filling shows typical single-canaled bicuspid, typically found in second bicuspids but very rare in first bicuspids.

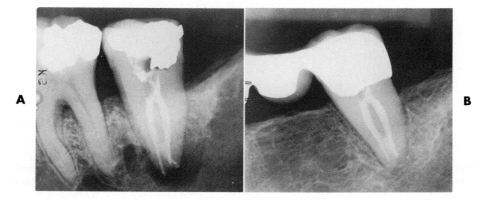

Fig. 6-18. A, Mandibular second molar with two canals close to each other at floor of the chamber, remaining separate and distinct to the apex. Film taken after canal filling. Note large periapical lesion. **B,** Area 18 years after treatment, indicating perfect healing. The first molar had been extracted several years earlier for periodontal reasons.

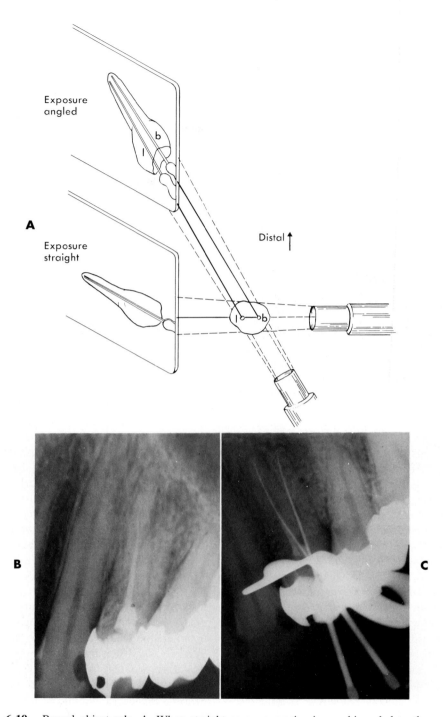

Fig. 6-19. Buccal object rule. **A,** When straight-on exposure is given a bicanaled tooth, canals become superimposed on film and no individual visualization is possible. If cone is turned to give an angled exposure, film will separate the roots. According to the buccal object rule, the root or canal farther from the film will move a greater distance on the radiograph than will the root or canal closer to the film. Therefore, when the cone is aimed to the distal, the buccal canal, *b,* moves more and appears distal to the lingual or palatal canal, *l.* This rule is used in radiographic evaluation and determination of canal length for maxillary bicuspids, bicanaled mandibular bicuspids, and mandibular molars. **B,** Typical case involving use of buccal object rule during access cavity preparation. Entry into a maxillary first bicuspid indicated a gutta-percha filling approximately in center of chamber floor, but no exact indication as to which of the two canals had been filled. Rather than chance a perforation by searching incorrectly, I consulted the angled preoperative radiograph. Film was taken with cone pointing to distal. Since buccal root moves more than palatal, it appears as distal on the film and is the unfilled canal. **C,** With this information, location of the other canal and establishment of working lengths became a simple matter.

Even though it is the best and most scientific method for distinguishing between canals on a radiograph, some dentists fail to understand the concept and substitute other methods for identification. Among these are the placement of file in one canal and a reamer in the other, or two files used but one much larger than the other to differentiate the canals on an x-ray film. However, since the buccal object rule is so helpful during endodontic therapy and is really not complicated, its mastery will greatly facilitate treatment of multicanaled teeth.

A rare combination of roots that occurs in less than 2% of maxillary first bicuspids and even less frequently in second bicuspids is the trirooted tooth, each root with one canal. Two buccal roots and one palatal root are present in these cases and closely resemble the configuration of a small maxillary second molar. There are two types of trirooted bicuspids, one where three separate orifices are present (Fig. 6-20), and the other where the two buccal canals come off a single orifice, whereas the palatal canal has its own orifice (Fig. 6-21). The latter is more difficult to treat.

Preoperative diagnosis is very important because once the condition is recognized, then further treatment is facilitated. The roots are not always easily recognizable, and the angled views in particular (Figs. 6-20, A, and 6-21, A) seem to give a confusing perspective of the tooth. The three orifices present reveal the underlying condition when that configuration exists and the operator is observant. Another hint of three roots occurs when the canals are entered and a moderate-sized file (no. 15, 20, or 25) fits in the palatal canal, whereas it is difficult to gain proper depth in the buccal even with a size 10 instrument.

When treating trirooted bicuspids with only a single buccal orifice, it is important to consider the buccal root to be a Type IV canal system. Both buccal canals must be widened mesiodistally so that separate sites for instrument and filling cone placement are developed. Remember that the buccal segment with this configuration is much wider mesiodistally when two roots are present than when only a single root is present, and plenty of room for this widening is available.

Maxillary second bicuspid. As stated in Table 6-2, the most common root configuration in maxillary second bicuspids is a single root, occurring approximately 85% of the time. Type I canal configuration is most common, but Type II, III, or IV may be present, with decreasing frequency.

Approximately 15% of the time, two separate roots are present, each with a single canal. An extremely rare variant has three separate roots (Fig. 6-22).

There is variation in the cervical cross section of maxillary second bicuspids, depending on the canal configuration. If only one canal is present, the canal shape is slightly oval. If two canals are present, the canal shape resembles a ribbon or figure eight, as in the first bicuspid. The access preparation is exactly the same as that for maxillary first bicuspids.

When only one canal is present, it is usually found rather easily in the center of the access preparation. If only one canal is found, but it is not in the center of the tooth, it is probable that another canal is present; one should be searched for on the opposite side. Radiographs from various angles, some with a file in place, may be helpful.

The finding of a Type IV canal in maxillary second bicuspids went virtually unnoticed until papers by Pineda and Kuttler and by Vertucci et al. reported that it did occur in a small percentage of teeth. I have found it as frequently as 10% of the time, which is a much higher percentage than in either of those reports. Type IV canals are the most difficult to prepare and fill. It becomes almost impossible to cleanse both apical segments adequately (Chapter 7). Although it is possible to express sealer into the segment that does not receive the direct placement of the master cone, a true sealing of the canal is problematic.

In many cases the finding of a Type IV is discovered when the canal filling is completed (Fig. 6-23, B), and for many years I thought that this was merely a large apical auxiliary canal. As with many other instances when problems occur during treatment of teeth, consider the possibility of a Type IV canal when a maxillary second bicuspid is not responding to seemingly correct therapy (Fig. 6-24, A to C). When the extra apical canal is located, prepared, and filled, the problems suddenly cease (Fig. 6-24, C to E).

When re-treating failing cases on this tooth, consider the possibility of a Type IV canal. Take an angled view from the distal similar to the projection used for a maxillary molar (Fig. 6-37, C), and the Type IV canal may become apparent (Fig. 6-25, A). The further treatment plan for the tooth becomes obvious (Fig. 6-25, B).

When a preoperative film (Fig. 6-26, A) indicates the possibility of the Type IV system and this

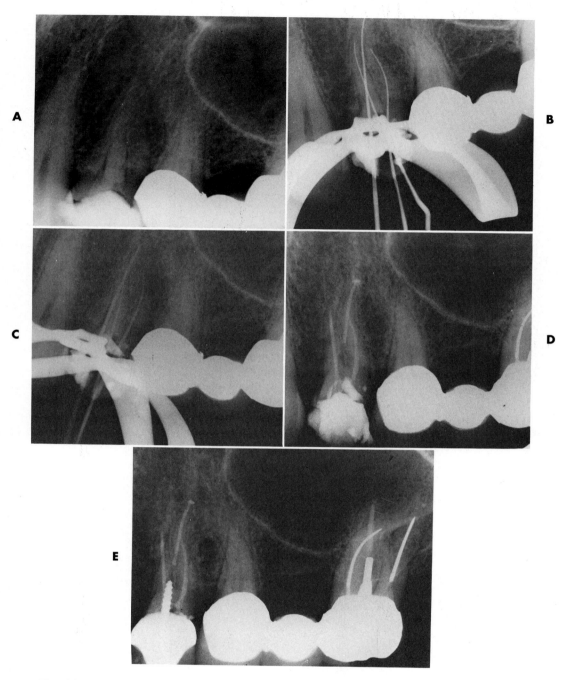

Fig. 6-20.   Trirooted first bicuspid with three separate orifices. **A,** Angled radiograph of maxillary first bicuspid gives strange perspective of the tooth. **B,** Problem is that it is a trirooted bicuspid. Files in place indicate two buccal and one palatal root. Note that files in buccal roots cross. **C,** Master cones in place. Due to canal preparation, the buccal cones no longer cross. **D,** Final canal filling with laterally condensed gutta-percha and Wach's paste, indicating separate orifices for the buccal canals. **E,** One year later, area looks excellent. I had treated second molar 11 years earlier. (Restorations by Dr. Gary Meyers, Highland Park, Ill.)

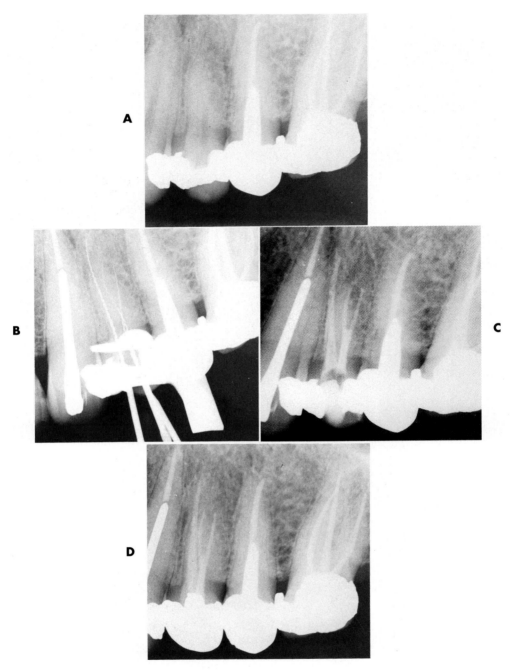

Fig. 6-21. Three canals in a maxillary first bicuspid, with both buccal canals coming off the same orifice. This type of configuration is much more difficult to diagnose and treat than that demonstrated in Fig. 6-20, where three separate orifices are present. **A,** Preoperative film angled view with appearance similar to Fig. 6-20, *A.* The adjacent cuspid also needs treatment. **B,** Angled view from the mesial, indicating that a size 15 Hedstrom file in the distobuccal canal and a size 10 K file in the mesiobuccal canal are coming through the same orifice. Note the difference between this film and the files in place in Fig. 6-20, *B.* **C,** Immediate postfilling film, canals filled with laterally condensed gutta-percha and Wach's paste. Note that the orifice portion of the buccal root has been widened significantly to the point of division of the two buccal canals. **D,** Radiograph 1 year later. (Restorations by Dr. George Morfas, Munster, Ind.)

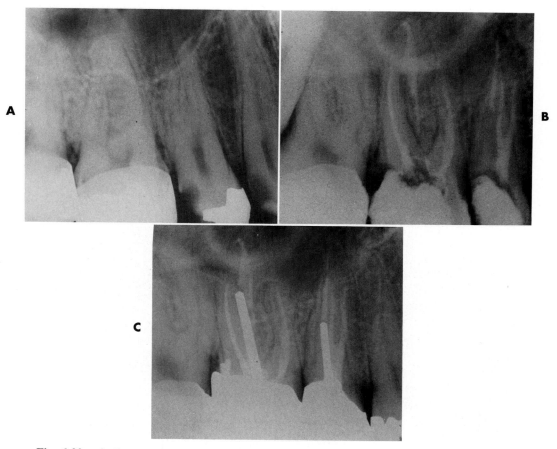

Fig. 6-22. **A,** Preoperative radiograph of maxillary second bicuspid with three roots. **B,** After canal filling with laterally condensed gutta-percha and Kerr's antiseptic sealer. **C,** Twelve years later. (Restorations by Dr. Herman Gornstein, Chicago Heights, Ill.)

important fact is verified at initial exploration (Fig. 6-26, *B* and *C*), a very desirable result can be obtained (Fig. 6-26, *D* to *F*).

Mandibular first bicuspid. The mandibular first bicuspid may cause great problems during treatment because of the relatively frequent existence of a bifurcated canal dividing in the middle or apical third (Type IV) into a buccal and a lingual branch. Although these teeth usually have one root and one canal, Types II and IV configurations may be present. The condition of two separate roots, each with one canal, is rarely present.

For many years this tooth was considered to have only one root with a single canal. However, there is no question that a single root that divides apically or a Type IV canal system is present in a very significant number of cases, ranging between 15% and 25%. Table 6-5 lists the studies discussing the various canal configurations typically found in this tooth.

The crown is bulky when compared with that of anterior teeth, giving the appearance of a very large total tooth. However, the root or roots are slender by comparison, being only slightly larger in circumference and generally shorter than the root of the adjacent cuspid. The narrower root should be kept in mind when the dentist is attempting to locate a canal that is difficult to find. It also may cause a problem when a post is required. If the canal or canals are widened too greatly, too close to the tip of the root, a strip perforation may result.

The pulp canal size and shape of the tooth with

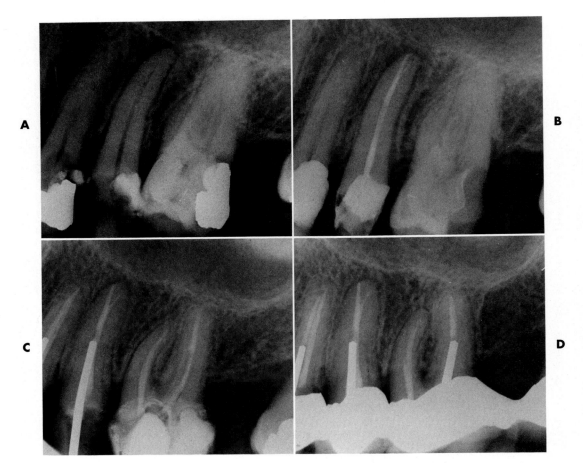

Fig. 6-23. **A,** Preoperative radiograph of maxillary left side. Second bicuspid has periapical lesion and requires endodontic therapy, as do first bicuspid and first molar. **B,** Canal filling in the second bicuspid completed with laterally condensed gutta-percha and Kerr's antiseptic sealer. It appeared that a lateral canal was picked up to the distal portion of the root. **C,** Six months later, healing underway. **D,** Two years later, areas well healed. Although I thought at the time that the second bicuspid had a lateral canal, I realize now that it was a Type IV canal. (Restorations by Dr. Ascher Jacobs, formerly of Chicago.)

a single canal is similar to the mandibular cuspid and mandibular second bicuspid as visualized in buccolingual and mesiodistal section. In cervical cross section the canal is slightly oval and thus the access preparation has the same shape (Fig. 6-27). When divided canals are present, the entry must be widened buccolingually (Fig. 6-28).

This Type IV canal is difficult to treat. In many cases the lingual canal cannot even be located and only the buccal is prepared and filled, a situation prone to failures. The buccal canal must be approached from the lingual direction and, conversely, the lingual canal from the buccal (Fig. 6-29, *B*). These canals have an original curvature that is usually straightened by the time the prepa-

ration is completed. This leads to some overextended canal fillings (Fig. 6-29, *C*). Because the canals are still small at the apex, there is an excellent chance for success (Fig. 6-29, *D*).

Because of the difficulties involved in preparing and filling this system, some cases require alternatives to the most routine therapy. In several instances I have used minimal canal enlargement at the apex and then canal filling with chloropercha (Chapter 9) in order to treat Type IV mandibular bicuspids with narrow, curved canals (Fig. 6-30). Attempting to widen these canals to sizes needed for routine lateral condensation leads to severe alteration of canal shape and resultant problems.

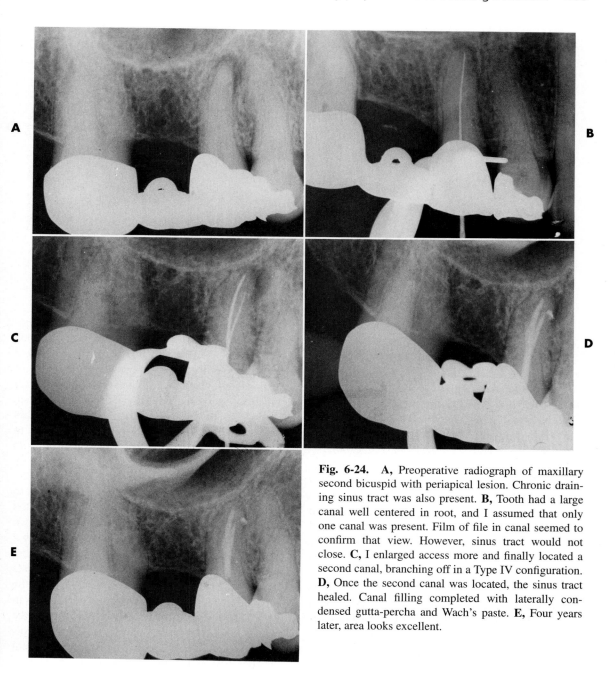

Fig. 6-24. **A,** Preoperative radiograph of maxillary second bicuspid with periapical lesion. Chronic draining sinus tract was also present. **B,** Tooth had a large canal well centered in root, and I assumed that only one canal was present. Film of file in canal seemed to confirm that view. However, sinus tract would not close. **C,** I enlarged access more and finally located a second canal, branching off in a Type IV configuration. **D,** Once the second canal was located, the sinus tract healed. Canal filling completed with laterally condensed gutta-percha and Wach's paste. **E,** Four years later, area looks excellent.

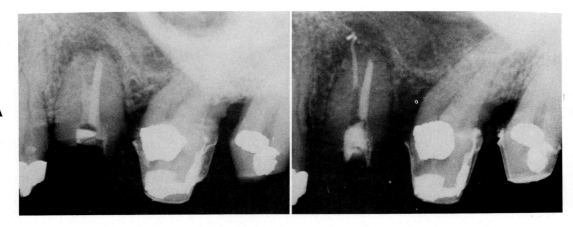

Fig. 6-25.   A, Sharply angled preoperative view from distal shows Type IV canal on second bicuspid. **B,** On basis of this information, location, enlargement, and filling of second canal are performed.

Mandibular second bicuspid.   The mandibular second bicuspid has far fewer variations than the first bicuspid, usually having one root and one well-centered canal. Rarely are Type II, III, or IV canal configurations present. (See Table 6-2.) The access preparation is generally round but may be slightly oval (Fig. 6-31). When two canals are present (Fig. 6-32), the entry is the same as for the bicanaled mandibular first bicuspid (Fig. 6-28).

A low percentage of mandibular second bicuspids, still less than 1%, are tricanaled, with two buccal canals and one lingual. This configuration is extremely difficult to treat and requires great skill plus some good fortune. Because of the small tortuous canals that are difficult to enlarge, filling with a chloropercha technique is recommended (Fig. 6-33).

Maxillary first molar.   The maxillary first molar always has three separate roots, two buccal and one palatal. The distobuccal and palatal roots always have one canal each, but the mesiobuccal may have a configuration of Type I, II, or III. The mesiobuccal root is similar in shape and canal configuration to single-rooted maxillary bicuspids, although slightly smaller. Evenot did an exhaustive study concerning the mesiobuccal root and stated not only that it was the most difficult root to treat endodontically, but also that some of the anatomic variations seen in this root defied any successful treatment.

A mesiodistal section through the buccal roots shows that the buccal canals are thin and well centered in their respective roots but with both orifices

on the mesial three fifths of the crown. Buccolingual section shows the palatal canal to be much wider than either buccal canal, with a buccal curve occurring near the apex in most teeth. The orifice of the palatal root is more prominent than either buccal orifice and is located beneath the mesiopalatal cusp. The orifice of the mesiobuccal canal is located beneath the mesiobuccal cusp, but the orifice to the distobuccal canal has no direct relation to its cusp. The distobuccal orifice is usually located by means of its relation to the mesiobuccal orifice, with the former found approximately 2 to 3 mm to the distal and slightly to the palatal aspect of the mesiobuccal orifice. The distance between the two buccal orifices will be greater when considerable dentinal sclerosis has occurred. Since the buccal roots diverge as they leave the crown, the canals form a V shape and approach each other near the floor of the chamber. As reparative dentin fills in the chamber and decreases canal diameter, the orifices are found farther up their respective roots and thus are farther apart. This is an important consideration when the dentist is attempting to locate these canals in patients with heavy dentinal sclerosis.

A cross section through the cervical area shows that the pulp chamber floor has the shape of a quadrilateral, with four unequal sides. Most writers describe access cavity preparation for molars, both maxillary and mandibular, as triangular in outline form. However, since the floor of the maxillary first molar is quadrilateral, the access cavity must have a similar shape. The large palatal canal

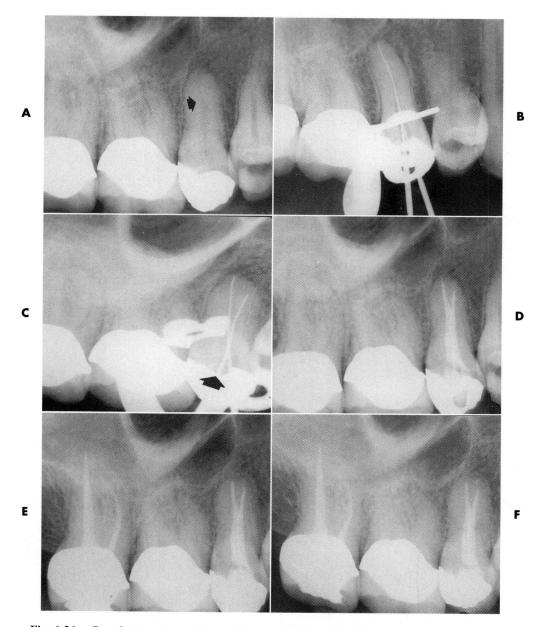

Fig. 6-26. Complete treatment of a maxillary second bicuspid with a Type IV canal system. **A,** Preoperative radiograph of maxillary bicuspid and molar area. Both second bicuspid and second molar reveal periapical lesions, large restorations, and the need for endodontic treatment. A wide canal in the center of second bicuspid root seems to divide into two apical canals *(arrow),* a Type IV configuration being possible. **B,** Size 20 Hedstrom file is in the palatal canal extension, but I was not able to locate the buccal extension in this straight view. **C,** View from the distal, indicating files in both apical extensions of the Type IV system. By going farther from the palatal *(arrow),* my file was able to enter into the buccal portion. **D,** Canal filling with laterally condensed gutta-percha and Wach's paste. **E,** One year later, treatment was completed on the second molar as well, and lesions on both teeth have healed. **F,** Nine years after treatment, healing still perfect on both teeth. (Restorations by Dr. Gary Meyers, Highland Park, Ill.)

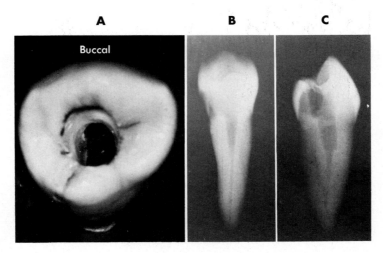

Fig. 6-27. Access preparations for typical mandibular first bicuspids. **A,** Entry for single-canaled tooth is slightly oval with buccolingual dimension only slightly wider than mesiodistal width. **B** and **C,** Buccal and proximal views show that canal is well centered. Direct access to apex is obtained with such an entry.

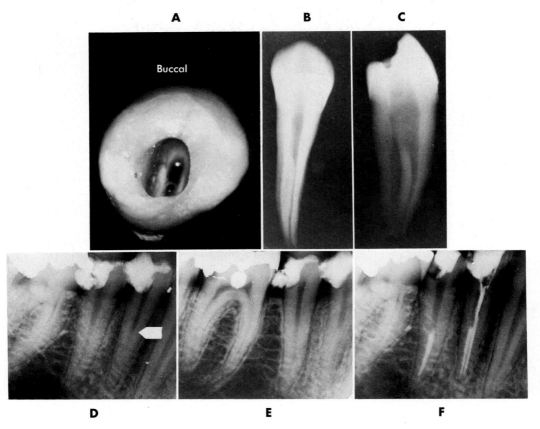

Fig. 6-28. Access preparation and canal configuration for mandibular first bicuspid with two canals. **A,** When two canals are present, oval preparation normally used for mandibular first bicuspids is widened buccolingually to afford access to both canals. Contrast this with access shown in Fig. 6-27, *A.* **B** and **C,** Lingual canal is usually smaller than buccal canal. When two canals are present, chamber is wide, a factor unnoticed in usual periapical film taken from a normal projection. **D,** In straight-on preoperative radiograph the canal in first bicuspid seems to disappear in midroot *(arrow).* This is an important indication that two canals are present. **E,** In angled view the divided canals are more clearly seen. **F,** Postoperative film shows the two canals filled and post room prepared.

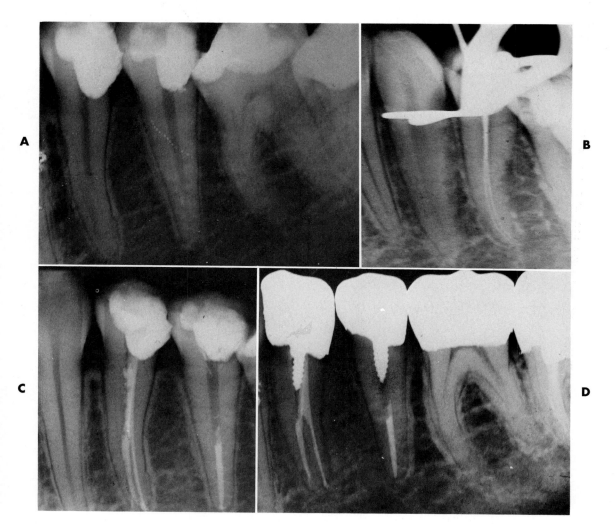

Fig. 6-29. **A,** Preoperative view angled from mesial of mandibular bicuspid area indicates knobby curved roots of first bicuspid with the canal image fading out in midroot, indicative of a Type IV system. **B,** Files in place. Note that file in lingual canal *(left)* is sharply curved. **C,** Canals filled with vertically condensed gutta-percha and Kerr's antiseptic sealer, and post room prepared. Some sealer has escaped past the apex. **D,** Three years later. (Restorations by Dr. Sherwin Strauss, Chicago.)

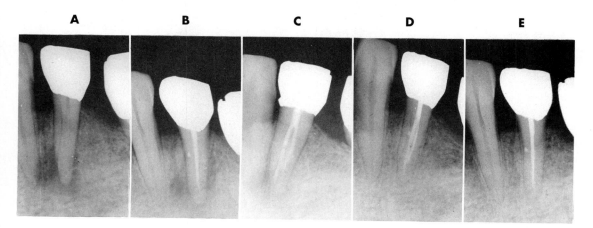

Fig. 6-30. **A,** Preoperative radiograph of mandibular first bicuspid, with two canals present and large periapical lesion wrapping around both mesial and distal sides of the tooth. **B,** It was difficult to insert my files close to the radiographic apex, and the two canals were very curved. I reached the minimal acceptable apical width, widened the orifice portions, and filled the canals by the chloropercha technique. Straight view is shown. **C,** Angled view. Multiple lateral canals are demonstrated in the postfilling radiographs. **D,** One year later. **E,** Two years later, lesions have healed perfectly.

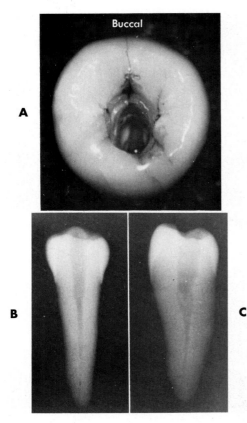

Buccal

A

B

C

Fig. 6-31. A, Access for mandibular second bicuspid is round, but it may be slightly oval if hint of two canals is present. **B** and **C,** Because canal is well centered in both buccolingual and mesiodistal dimensions, this tooth is one of easiest to treat endodontically.

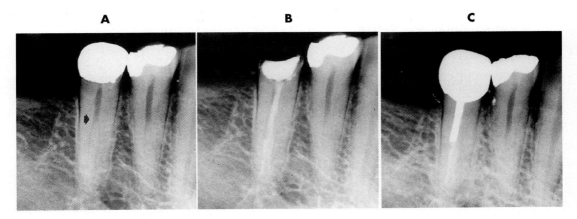

A   B   C

Fig. 6-32. Bicanaled mandibular second bicuspid. **A,** Preoperative radiograph. Because the tooth has rotated slightly, the point of division of the canals is easily seen *(arrow)*. Because this site is fairly close to the occlusal portion of the tooth, the treatment is not as complicated as if the division site were farther apically. **B,** Canals filled with laterally condensed gutta-percha and Wach's paste, and post room prepared. **C,** Four years later, periapical area remains normal. (Restorations by Dr. Irving Fishman, Chicago.)

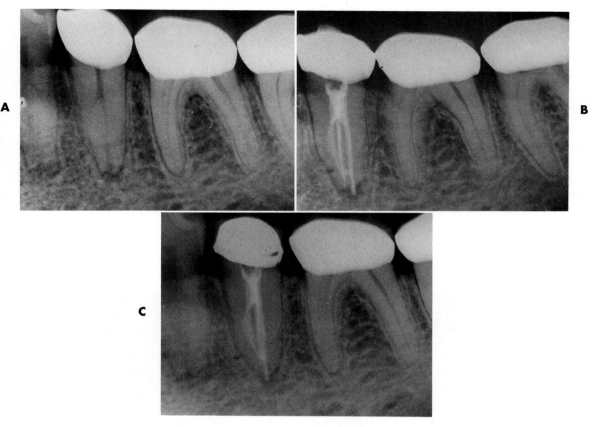

Fig. 6-33. **A,** Preoperative radiograph of tricanaled mandibular second bicuspid. Tooth is tender to percussion and sensitive to heat. Root canal configuration seems difficult to evaluate, but at least two canals must be present. **B,** Slightly angled view of canal filling indicates three canals, two buccal and one lingual. Canals were filled by chloropercha technique. **C,** One year after treatment. (Restorations by Dr. E. Beall, Tarrytown, N.Y.)

will not receive sufficient debridement of the canal walls if prepared through the confines of the apex of the triangle; it needs the greater width afforded by a more flattened side (Fig. 6-34, *A*). Therefore, for maxillary molar access preparations, a quadrilateral with rounded corners is recommended. The shortest side is the palatal, parallel to the central groove. The next shorter side is the buccal and has a slope toward the distopalatal aspect because the position of the distobuccal orifice is farther toward the palatal than the mesiobuccal orifice. The longest side is the mesial, with the opposite side toward the distal slightly shorter. Because of the quadrilateral rather than triangular shape, the mesial side does not make as sharp an angle toward the palatal, and more room is available for location of the frequently found second mesiobuc-

cal canal. Since all the orifices of this tooth lie on the mesial three fifths of the crown, there is no need to violate the oblique ridge in preparing the access cavity (Fig. 6-34, *B* to *D*).

To begin the preparation, a tapered fissure carbide bur is used to penetrate the enamel in the center of the central groove, and the access is increased in depth toward the mesiopalatal cusp. It is best to locate the palatal canal first, since this is the largest and easiest to find. Once the roof of the chamber has been penetrated, a safe-tipped bur is used to complete the palatal extension of the access near the mesiopalatal cusp. The endodontic explorer is used in this area to locate the orifice of the palatal canal. Once found, its position will aid in the uncovering of the smaller and more difficult to locate buccal canals.

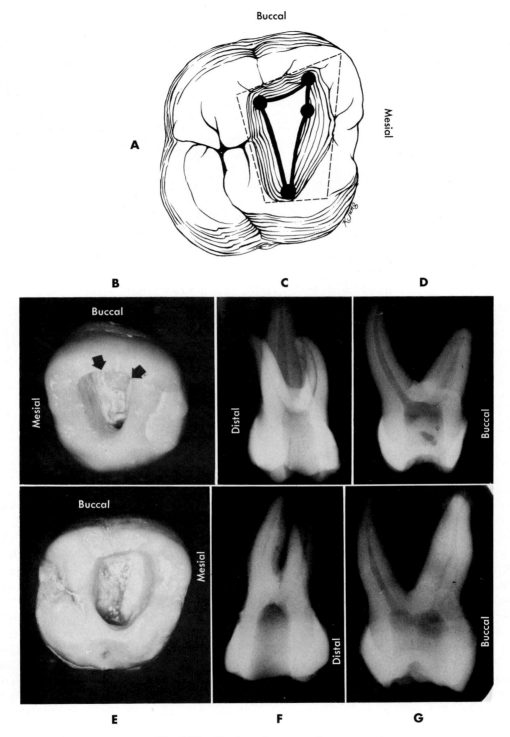

Fig. 6-34. For legend see opposite page.

Fig. 6-34.   Access cavity preparations for maxillary molars. **A,** General outline is quadrilateral with rounded corners rather than a triangle. Large palatal canal requires flat side for its proper preparation rather than apex of a triangle. Distobuccal canal is located 2 to 3 mm distally and slightly toward palatal canal from mesiobuccal canal. Second mesiobuccal canal is located 2 to 5 mm toward palatal canal from larger mesiobuccal canal. Entire preparation is on mesial three fifths of the crown. **B,** Occlusal view of access preparation for maxillary first molar. Note large palatal orifice and considerable distance between two buccal canals *(arrows)*. **C,** Buccal view shows entire entry on mesial three fifths of the tooth and verifies the distance of 2 to 3 mm between the buccal canals. Despite access being to the mesial, the opening is seen as well centered over root stock. **D,** Proximal view displays considerable width of palatal canal compared with buccal canals. Note gradual buccal curve of palatal canal, typically found in maxillary molars. **E,** Occlusal view of access preparation for a maxillary second molar. Note that buccal canal orifices are closer together than in first molar, whereas palatal canal is still quite large. **F,** Buccal view shows entire entry on mesial three fifths of tooth and proximity of two buccal roots and canals. **G,** Proximal view shows palatal canal to be widest, with a frequently present gradual buccal curve.

The safe-tipped bur is kept in contact with the floor of the pulp chamber and moved buccally to uncover the entire chamber. Once the mesiobuccal orifice is located beneath its cusp, the distobuccal canal will be uncovered by moving the safe-tipped bur distally and slightly toward the palatal surface. The second mesiobuccal canal either occurs as a separate canal or merges with the main canal in approximately 50% of all maxillary first molars and, with some frequency, in the maxillary second molar as well. To uncover this fourth canal, the safe-tipped bur is moved from the mesiobuccal orifice toward the palatal canal a distance of 2 to 5 mm. If present, the additional canal's orifice will be located in that area.

As with most molar roots, the buccal roots of the maxillary first molar are curved, although the mesiobuccal root is generally more curved. When viewed from the buccal, the mesiobuccal canal curves first to the mesial as it leaves the floor of the chamber and then to the distal, often quite abruptly. This is an important reason why this canal generally is so difficult to treat. The degree and abruptness of curvation cause frequent problems during canal preparation for loss of curvature, straightening of the canal, decrease in working length, and/or strip perforation.

From the mesial, the mesiobuccal canal curves initially to the buccal and then to the palatal. The buccolingual curvature is generally less than the mesiodistal curvature. The distobuccal canal is curved less frequently and is generally straighter than the mesiobuccal canal. Although the distobuccal canal usually will curve toward the mesial, giving a cowhorn appearance to the buccal roots (Fig. 6-35), it may curve to the distal. Because of the curviness of these buccal roots, the original working length determined by the first files in place to the apex (Fig. 6-35, *A*) may be diminished during the course of canal preparation (Fig. 6-35, *B* and *C*). This loss of working length (Chapter 7) is seen in many curved canals, but it occurs frequently in this tooth.

Despite the excellent overall success ratio for endodontic cases, the mesiobuccal root of the maxillary first molar has always been implicated with an excessively high failure rate. This has been due to the frequent occurrence of a second separate canal in this root, yet the rarity with which it is located and filled (Table 6-4). The canal configuration of maxillary bicuspids usually is determined before therapy by careful examination of angled radiographs. However, the proximity of the two canals in the mesiobuccal root plus the radiopaque structures in the area of the first molar often prevent preoperative forecast by x-ray examination.

Therefore it is suggested that some attempt be made to locate the orifice of the fourth canal whenever maxillary first molars are treated. If the radiograph seems to indicate that a second canal is present in the mesiobuccal root and the tooth appears to be shorter than average, this attempt should be pursued with some vigor until the canal is located or it appears that further preparation may cause perforation (Fig. 6-36). If the radiograph seems to indicate that only a single mesiobuccal canal is present and the tooth is longer than average, excessive time should not be spent attempting to locate the additional canal.

If only a single mesiobuccal canal is located, it

A   **B**   **C**

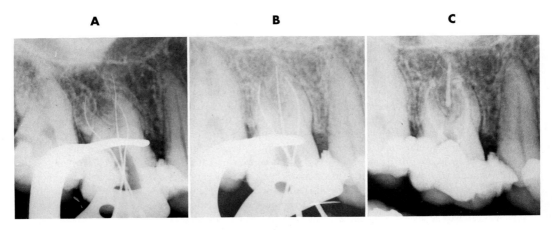

Fig. 6-35. **A,** Initial determination of working length in maxillary first molar in which both buccal canals were measured at 19.5 mm and the palatal canal at 20 mm. **B,** As canals were enlarged to size 30, the buccal canals were measured at 18 mm and the palatal canal at 19.5 mm. **C,** Postfilling radiograph indicates that even these shortened measurements were too long; a considerable amount of excess sealer has been expressed through apices of buccal roots.

should be prepared and filled in a routine manner. If any preoperative symptoms such as a chronic draining sinus, sensitivity to temperatures, or apical soreness over that root persist, further efforts to locate the additional canal should be made. If, after therapy that consisted of treating three canals, these symptoms return or a periapical radiolucency develops in association with that root, it should be assumed that an undiscovered second canal is responsible.

If nonsurgical re-treatment is performed, further efforts must be made to locate the missing canal. If surgery is to be performed, the techniques used to accommodate the sealing of an additional canal by the figure-eight reverse filling preparation must be utilized (Chapter 11).

It is not possible to locate the second mesiobuccal canal in every case even when it is present. The percentages listed in Table 6-4 indicate that results in clinical cases treated are always fewer than four canaled first molars investigated in pure laboratory in vitro studies. Attempting to locate the fourth canal at all costs will lead to perforations and/or weakening of the tooth. Therefore it is better to avoid serious procedural problems and stop short of disasters when the second mesiobuccal canal evades serious attempts at location. One must hope that the second canal, if present, merges with the canal already located. Performing excellent treatment on that canal will result in many such cases being successful. Remember that most studies on the mesiobuccal root indicate that merging canals

(Type II) are more frequently present than separate and distinct canals (Type III).

If periapical surgery is performed on the root, another problem may arise. In addition to the many teeth with two separate canals, many more cases will display two canals from the floor of the chamber merging to form a single apical foramen. If the root is cut down for an apicoectomy and reverse fill, it is possible that the second canal will be opened to the periapical tissue half the time. If this canal is unfilled, a postsurgical failure can develop. Therefore careful examination of the beveled root must be made and the figure-eight reverse filling preparation used if there is any chance for the presence of the additional canal (Chapter 11).

The routine periapical view of this tooth gives no additional information concerning the possibility of an additional mesiobuccal canal (Fig. 6-37, *A* and *B*). However, angled radiographs are helpful in anticipating the fourth canal before starting treatment. In most posterior teeth, angled views taken from the mesial toward the distal are the most helpful. On the contrary, for the maxillary first molar, greater information is gained by taking the film with the cone pointed from the distal to the mesial direction (Fig. 6-37, *C*). This projection gives a profile type of view of the mesiobuccal root and allows for visualization of the presence of the extra canal (Fig. 6-37, *D*). The same projection from the distal to the mesial direction is used when taking radiographs for the determination of working

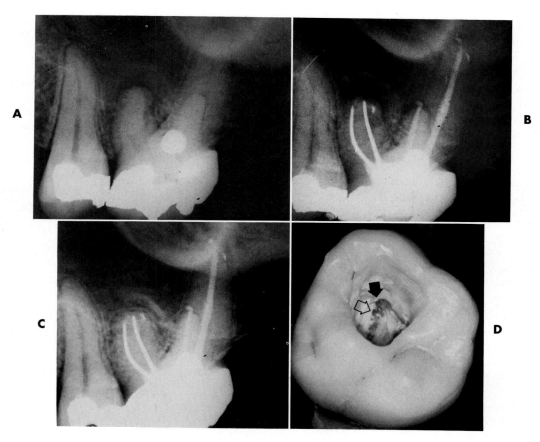

Fig. 6-36.   Second mesiobuccal canal of maxillary first molar. **A,** One canal was located and prepared in each of three roots, but a chronic draining sinus tract present before treatment failed to close. This view, angled mesially, projected mesiobuccal root away from any structures that might mask its appearance. Note double image of the root, suggesting a second root or canal. **B,** By next appointment, after second mesiobuccal canal had been located and enlarged, the draining sinus had closed. Immediate postfilling film shows two separate canals in mesiobuccal root filled with silver points. **C,** Excellent healing 1 year later. **D,** View into the mesiobuccal portion of the access preparation in a maxillary first molar. The larger canal *(solid arrow)* is located 2 to 5 mm buccally from the smaller canal *(open arrow).* (**A** to **C,** Restorations by Dr. Neal Baigh, LaGrange, Ill.)

length. The view is correct when the files in the distobuccal and palatal canals are approximately superimposed, or when the file in the distobuccal canal is slightly mesial to that in the palatal canal (Fig. 6-37, *E*). If the view is taken too far from the distal direction, the mesiobuccal root is projected over the second bicuspid, and visualization of the additional canal is difficult.

Because of the proximity of the two mesiobuccal canals, even this projection may not allow for complete visualization of two separate canals, even when there is strong indication that two are present (Fig. 6-38, *A*). The best method for verifying that two canals are present is to place files in both canals. If the canals do in fact merge to form

a Type II configuration, when a file is inserted to the full working length in one canal, the file in the other canal will be stopped short (Fig. 6-37, *E*). However, if both files go the full working length, a Type III configuration is verified, even if the film seems to indicate that the canals merge (Fig. 6-38, *B*). This might be further established by the final film (Fig. 6-38, *C*).

The Type II configuration is common in the mesiobuccal root. When this occurs, the final radiograph angled from the distal direction demonstrates the site of merging of the canals as a more radiopaque portion of the canal filling because of the superimposed effect of the sealer and cones on the film (Fig. 6-39).

There is a higher percentage of Type II configurations compared with Type III in the maxillary first and second molars. In some cases, therefore, the operator makes an exhaustive search for the mesiolingual canal, only to find that it merges with the mesiobuccal canal far into the body of the root. The tendency then is to assume that much time has been wasted in finding this additional canal because, since it joined the already-found canal, success would have resulted with only three canals filled.

This belief should be avoided. It is always favorable to locate, prepare, and fill the additional canal in any root, even if it does join another canal already being treated. I have had several cases where a chronic sinus tract did not heal in associa-

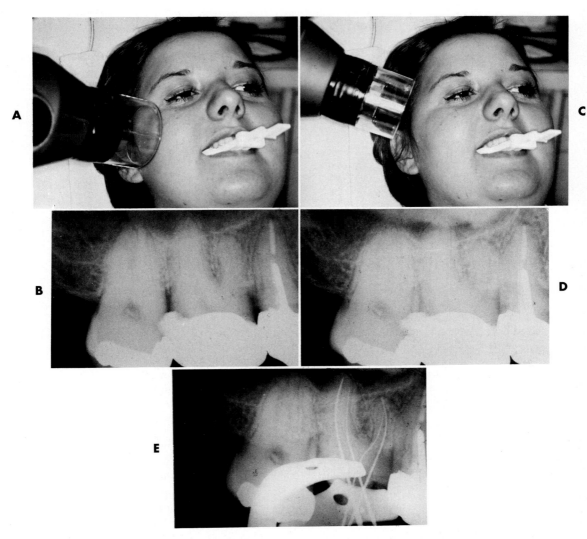

Fig. 6-37. Taking radiographs when treating maxillary first molars. **A,** Routine cone and film placement. **B,** Typical radiograph from this arrangement. Mesiobuccal root may seem to be in profile, but contrast this with **D. C,** Angled view is taken with film placed in routine position, but cone is placed distal to maxillary second molar and pointed to mesial. **D,** Typical radiograph as a result of such cone placement. Now mesiobuccal root is in profile, and the considerable width, capable of accommodating an additional canal, is more clearly seen. **E,** Radiograph for determining working length. Cone placement is the same as in **C.** File in distobuccal canal is slightly mesial to file in palatal canal. Second canal is present in mesiobuccal root and appears to merge with larger canal short of apex.

tion with a mesiobuccal root until the mesiolingual canal was located and prepared, even when a Type II condition was present (Fig. 6-40). The undiscovered canal contained sufficient irritants to perpetuate the lesion. Conceivably, it could hinder obtaining the most desirable filling of the mesiobuccal canal if left untreated.

There might be four separate roots in the maxillary first molar, with two roots at the mesiobuccal, each with a single canal. The radiograph angled from the distal direction will give a hint of this type of configuration (Fig. 6-41, *A*), which subsequently will be determined and confirmed during the course of treatment (Fig. 6-41, *B* to *D*).

Names of canals in mesiobuccal root. When the early studies on the configuration of the mesiobuccal canal were first reported, the newly discovered canal was often referred to as "the second

mesiobuccal," because no one expected more than one canal in this root. However, soon it was called, and properly so, "the mesiolingual" or occasionally "the mesiopalatal."

Recently it has become fashionable for some to refer to this canal as "MB-2." MB-2 is a poor and inappropriate name. It has no parallel in endodontic terminology and is, as will be clearly described soon, patently incorrect.

In the mandibular first or second molars (the situation closest to the maxillary molars), the canals are referred to as the mesiobuccal and the mesiolingual, not "MB-1" and "MB-2" or even "M-1" and "M-2." This canal is not an upstart that must be described in terms of the well-known father or older brother.

Anatomically the names of the canals typically describe the path of entrance to be opposite.

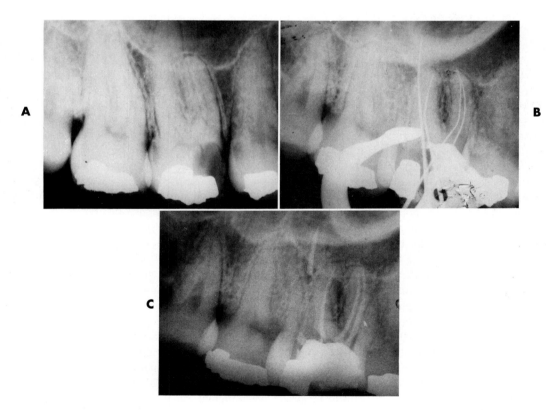

Fig. 6-38. **A,** Radiograph taken with cone placement as illustrated in Fig. 6-37, *C.* Mesiobuccal root is wide and probably will accommodate two canals. **B,** Angled view from distal to determine working length. Mesiobuccal root is in profile, and it appears that files in mesiobuccal root do merge. However, both files independently went to 20 mm. **C,** After canal filling with laterally condensed gutta-percha, radiograph was taken from slightly more distal direction. The two separate mesiobuccal canals are clearly seen.

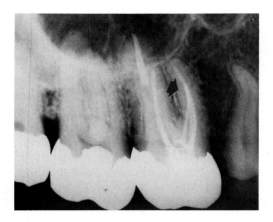

Fig. 6-39. Angled view of maxillary first molar after canal filling. Type II configuration was present in mesiobuccal root, and the site of merging *(arrow)* is more radiopaque than the rest of the fill.

Therefore, in the bicanaled mandibular first bicuspid, the buccal canal is reached from the lingual and the lingual canal from the buccal. In the maxillary molar the palatal canal is entered from the buccal, the distobuccal from the mesiolingual, and the mesiobuccal from the distolingual. Since the mesiolingual canal should be approached from the distobuccal, this verifies its proper name.

Mistakes are made in entering this canal by those who approach it from the distolingual, as one would to enter the mesiobuccal canal. The correct path of entry is from the distobuccal, and the name of the canal is the *mesiolingual.*

Maxillary second molar. The maxillary second molar usually has similar canal configuration combinations to the first molar: two buccal roots and one palatal root. The distobuccal and palatal roots each have one canal, but the mesiobuccal may have two canals (Fig. 6-42), with either canals merging short of the apex (Type II) or remaining separate and distinct (Type III). Until recently the exact percentages for the configurations present in the mesiobuccal root of the maxillary second molar were only the object of speculation. However, recent studies have published some interesting percentages, listed in Table 6-7. Even though the second canal is known to be present in many instances, it may be very difficult to locate and prepare it because the tooth is so far posterior in the mouth. Therefore the total number of maxillary second molars with four canals filled is certainly far below the total number with four canals present, even in the most conservative estimate.

In their in vitro study, Kulild and Peters found that in this tooth, 78.2% of the mesiobuccal roots had two canals (Type II plus Type III), as uncovered by access and bur penetration, rising to 93.7% when uncovered using a microscope and sectioning. These numbers can never be reached clinically with the presently available equipment.

The access cavity is prepared in the same manner and shape as for the first molar, except that the buccal side of the quadrilateral is not as long, since the buccal canals are usually found closer together (Fig. 6-34, *E* to *G*). In second molars with sclerotic canals or those that have crowns compressed mesiodistally, the distobuccal orifice may be located toward the center of the access rather than near the mesiobuccal orifice. If the distobuccal canal is not found near the mesiobuccal canal in teeth with these conditions, exploration in the center will usually yield the missing canal.

A differing type of root configuration may also be present in the maxillary second molar that contains only two roots, one buccal and the other palatal (Fig. 6-43). In still another modification these two roots merge near the apex (Fig. 6-44). The total frequency of the two-rooted maxillary second molar among all such teeth is approximately 10%, with the separate root condition much more common.

Mandibular first molar. The mandibular first molar generally has two separate and distinct roots, one mesial and the other distal. The mesial root always has two distinct canals leaving the floor of the pulp chamber, which exit as separate apical foramina in approximately 85% of cases (Type III canal configuration) but merge to form one apical foramen (Type II) in the remainder.

As the mesial root leaves the crown, initially it curves to the mesial but then it makes a gradual turn to the distal and generally has a distal curve in its apical third. From a buccal view this root has a crescent shape. The two mesial canals have the same directional curvatures when viewed from the buccal—first to the mesial and then to the distal.

From the mesial view the canals differ strongly. The mesiobuccal canal curves first to the buccal and then to the lingual. The coronal portion of the mesiolingual canal is straighter and then in the middle third begins a more gradual buccal curve. Therefore, from this view, the canals diverge coronally but then converge apically.

The distal root is slightly narrower buccolingually than the mesial root, but they are equal in mesiodis-

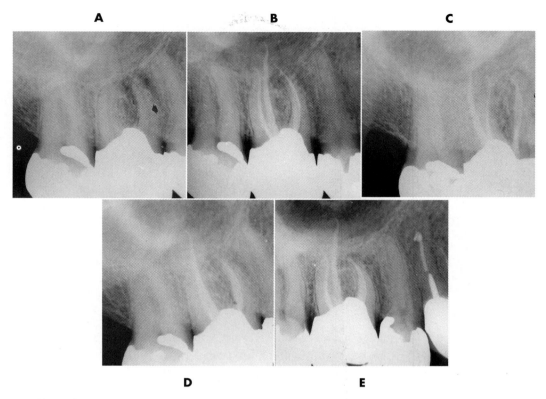

Fig. 6-40.   Type II canal in mesiobuccal root, but area would not heal until both canals were cleaned. **A,** Preoperative film of maxillary first molar, distal view, indicating a probable Type II canal system in the mesiobuccal root. The site of merging *(arrow)* can be seen in midroot. Before treatment, a chronic draining sinus tract was present, and the patient had apical tenderness at the apex of the mesiobuccal root. At the first appointment I was able to locate and enlarge the three major canals only and did not enter the mesiolingual canal. At the second appointment the tract was still draining and apical tenderness was still present. I located the mesiolingual canal, enlarged it to size 25 apically, flared to size 35, and did moderate enlargement of the previously located canals. At the next appointment the tract had closed and no tenderness was present, so I was able to fill the tooth. **B** and **C,** Straight view and angled view from the distal after filling tooth with laterally condensed gutta-percha and Wach's paste. Site of merging actually was much more toward the apex than it appeared in **A. D,** Two years after treatment. **E,** Five years after treatment, indicating perfect healing. (Restorations by Dr. Kerry Voit, Chicago.)

tal width. The distal root often has a mesial curvature. Usually only one distal canal is present, with a large, kidney-shaped orifice (Fig. 6-45), but Type II or III configurations are present occasionally.

The distal portion of the mandibular first molar has a tremendous number of variations, including types of canals, curvatures, shapes, and inclinations. To gain additional information, the straight-on projection normally taken (Fig. 6-46, *A* and *B*) must be supplemented by at least one angled view, with the cone placed at the mesial and pointing toward the distal direction giving the most infor-

mation (Fig. 6-46, *C* to *O*). During the course of treatment, these angled views taken from the mesial direction will aid greatly in correctly categorizing the configuration present (Fig. 6-47).

When two separate canals are present, they are much thinner than single distal canals. Therefore, when a distal canal will not accommodate a size 25 file at initial entrance, it is a good indication that the root has a Type II or III configuration. The presence of two separate distal roots is rare but does occur. The distolingual root is smaller than the distobuccal root and usually very curved (Fig. 6-47).

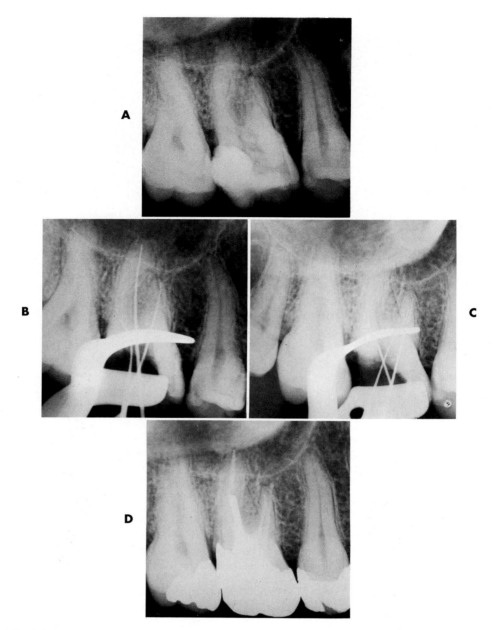

Fig. 6-41. Four-rooted maxillary first molar (a four-bagger). **A,** Preoperative angled film from distal aspect, giving hint of two separate mesiobuccal roots. **B,** Initial film for determination of working length shows that file in mesiobuccal root is not well centered. **C,** Further exploration yielded orifice to fourth root. **D,** Six months after treatment, film shows separate mesiobuccal roots. (Restorations by Dr. Edward LeMire, Chicago.)

The mandibular first molar is the most frequently exposed tooth and as such requires endodontic treatment frequently. However, many dentists are reluctant to perform the needed therapy because they believe such treatment is complex.

Although some mandibular first molars are taxing, often the tooth is treated without complications. Since the tooth usually has one large and two small canals, therapy should be thought of as treatment of a maxillary bicuspid (conforming to

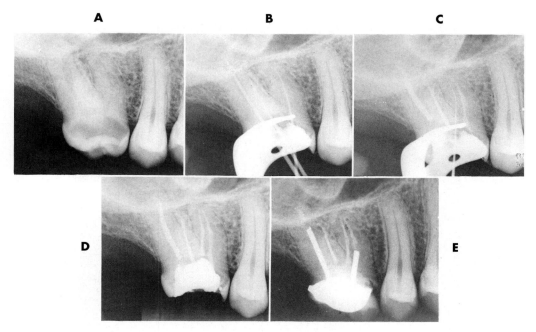

Fig. 6-42. **A,** Preoperative radiograph of maxillary second molar requiring endodontic therapy. The first molar had been extracted several years earlier, and the second molar had rotated somewhat to the mesial to close the space. **B,** Radiograph of three master cones in place before filling the canals. It appears that the master cone in the mesiobuccal root is well centered, indicating only a single canal in that root. **C,** After canal filling with laterally condensed gutta-percha and Wach's paste, I noticed an additional orifice palatal to the mesiobuccal canal and placed a file easily to this length. **D,** That canal was enlarged and filled similarly. **E,** Two years later, everything appears normal.

the distal canal) and two maxillary lateral incisors (the two mesial canals). Psychologically, treating the tooth under this assumption may be more supportive.

A mesiodistal section through the tooth reveals that the orifices of both the mesial and the distal canals lie in the mesial two thirds of the crown and that the canals are well centered in their roots (Fig. 6-45, *D*). A buccolingual section shows that the pulp chamber is in the center of the crown and that the distal canal is wide and ribbon shaped, whereas the mesial canals are thin. The cervical cross section shows that the chamber floor is trapezoidal. This means that the access cavity for this tooth is also trapezoidal, not triangular.

Access preparations for both first and second mandibular molars are essentially identical. The general outline is trapezoidal with rounded corners. The shortest side is to the distal aspect, and the mesial side is slightly longer. The buccal and lingual sides are of approximately the same length and taper toward each other distally. The mesiolingual canal lies beneath the mesiolingual cusp. The

mesiobuccal canal is the most difficult to locate, but it is usually found on a straight line to the buccal from the mesiolingual orifice and is tucked deeply beneath the mesiobuccal cusp. The orifices may be connected by a corridor extending part or all the way to the apex. When difficulty is encountered in locating the mesiobuccal canal, the operator should have no qualms about cutting down the mesiobuccal portion of the tooth, even as far as the height of the gingiva, to aid in visualization. If the canal is not properly found and debrided, the case would be a failure and conservation of tooth structure would be useless. If endodontic therapy is successful, the reduced cusp is easily built up with a casting.

Many authors have suggested the triangular-shaped entry for this tooth. However, the distal canal is kidney shaped in most cases, with the greatest width buccolingually. Also, two canals exiting the floor of the chamber are found in the distal root approximately 30% of the time, one on the buccal aspect and the other toward the distal and lingual aspects. Attempting to enlarge the single large canal or to locate the possibly present

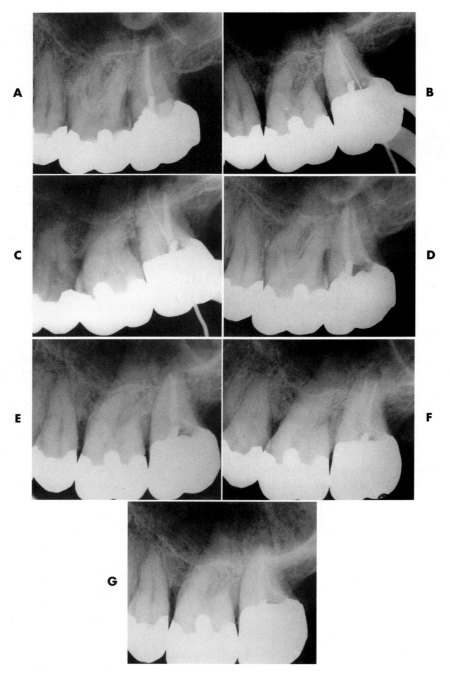

Fig. 6-43. Maxillary second molar with two roots and two canals. **A,** In preoperative film it appears that two roots are present, but only one canal has been filled. A periapical lesion is present, and the tooth is tender to percussion. When the access was opened, it was seen that the filled canal was to the palatal. A canal was located to the buccal and a file placed. **B** and **C,** Straight view and angled view from the distal were taken to verify that the file was within the canal and not a perforation. **D,** Tenderness to percussion stopped after location and preparation of the buccal canal, which was filled with laterally condensed gutta-percha and Wach's paste, as demonstrated by this immediate postfilling film, angled from the mesial. **E** and **F,** Straight and angled from the distal views 4 years after treatment, periapical lesion healed and no further problems. **G,** Nine years after original treatment.

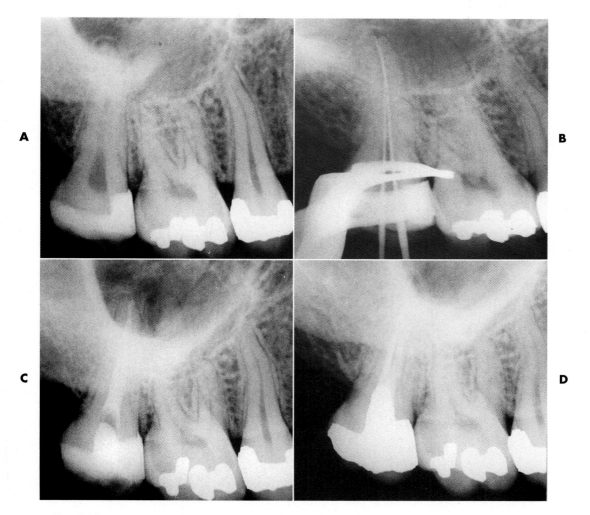

Fig. 6-44. Maxillary second molar with two roots merging near the apex. **A,** Preoperative radiograph of maxillary molar area shows temporary restoration in the second molar in proximity to the pulp. The tooth had been exposed by the referring dentist attempting to prepare the tooth for an onlay. Note the difference in the exterior shape of the second molar to the adjacent first molar. **B,** Two files in place, one in each canal, indicating site of merging several millimeters from the apex. Other angled views also indicated a site of merger for the two canals. **C,** Immediate postfilling film, two canals filled with laterally condensed gutta-percha and Wach's paste. **D,** Two years later, normal appearance.

second canal requires a much wider access than that afforded at the apex of a triangle. However, by widening this area buccolingually to produce a trapezoidal opening, sufficient space is made available for examination of the chamber floor, and a desirable canal preparation can be achieved (Fig. 6-45).

The distal canal is the largest and easiest to find. Therefore it should be located first, lying slightly distal to the buccal groove, closer to the buccal than the lingual wall.

A tapered fissure bur is used in the central pit and the preparation increased in depth by moving the bur mesially and distally from the central pit to the mesial pit. Once the roof of the pulp chamber is penetrated, the safe-tipped bur is used to remove the remaining overhanging tooth structure. The orifice of the distal canal is located with the endodontic

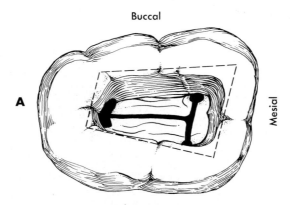

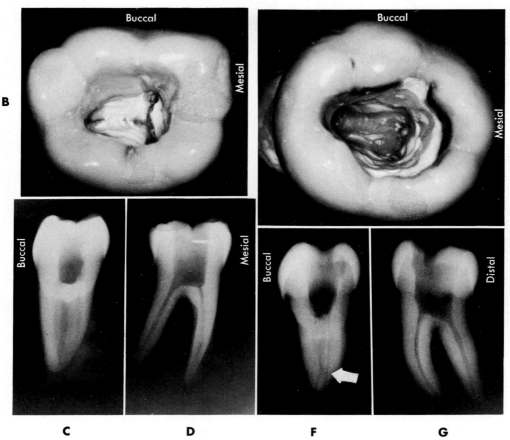

Fig. 6-45. Access canal preparations and canal configurations in mandibular molars. **A,** General outline advised for mandibular molars is a trapezoid with rounded corners rather than a triangle. Distal canal is usually kidney shaped, or two separate canals may be present. Working through apex of a triangular section does not give sufficient access for proper canal location and preparation. **B,** Occlusal view of access preparation for three-canaled mandibular first and second molars. Distal canal has a kidney-shaped orifice, widest buccolingually, whereas mesial canals are located beneath their cusps and are quite far apart with a line on the floor of the chamber connecting them. **C,** Proximal view shows entry funneled to afford access to apices, well centered in buccolingual dimension of the tooth. Note mesial canals far apart at their orifices but curving toward each other as they approach their apices. **D,** Buccal view shows distal canal to be straight while mesial canals have a gradual curve toward distal aspect. Entire access is within mesial two thirds of crown. **E,** Occlusal view of access preparation for mandibular first and second molars in which two mesial canals merge short of apex (Type II configuration). Mesial orifices are much closer together than in **B,** but the trapezoidal configuration is still required for large distal canal. **F,** Proximal view shows point of merging of two mesial canals short of root tip *(arrow).* Canal appearing to buccal side of merged canal is the distal one, since rays traveled through the tooth from the mesial aspect to the distal to give this film. **G,** Buccal view showing straight distal canal and curved mesial canals.

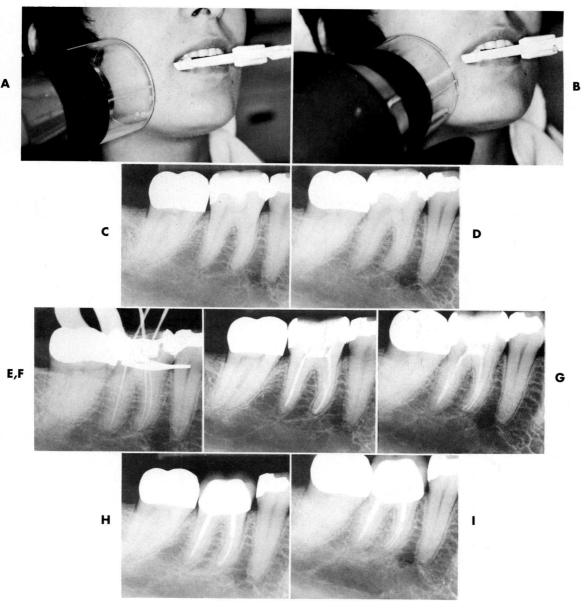

Fig. 6-46. Two most common configurations for the mandibular first molar and the radiographs needed for their evaluation. **A,** Routine cone and film placement. **B,** Angled view is obtained with film holder in the same position, cone tip in the same position, but cone head pointed to the distal at an angle of 20 to 30 degrees. **C** to **I,** Three canals present. **C,** Film taken as shown in **A. D,** Film taken as shown in **B. E,** Angled view of files in place. **F,** Immediate postfilling straight view, canals filled with laterally condensed gutta-percha and Wach's paste. **G,** Postfilling angled view. **H** and **I,** Three years after treatment, straight and angled views. (Restorations by Dr. Carle Kibbitt, Chicago.)

Continued

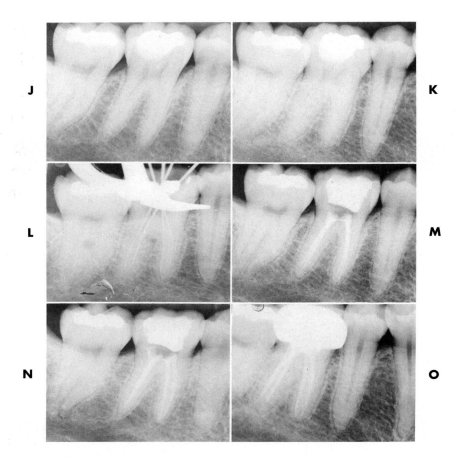

Fig. 6-46, cont'd. J to **O,** Four canals present. **J,** Film taken as shown in **A. K,** Film taken as shown in **B. L,** Angled view of files in place, indicating two separate and distinct distal canals. Compare with **E** and note that when only one distal canal is present, it is well centered in that root. This view is taken from the distal to separate the distal canals, since the distobuccal canal is often slightly mesial to the distolingual canal. A slight angle from the mesial will often superimpose the two distal canals (see **N**). **M,** Immediate postfilling straight view, four canals filled with laterally condensed gutta-percha and Wach's paste. **N,** In the angled view the distal canals seem to be only one because they have been superimposed. **O,** Angled view from the distal 3 years later. (Restorations by Dr. Wilbur Pettit, Chicago.)

explorer. The safe-tipped bur is placed in this area and moved mesially and slightly to the lingual side to uncover the mesiolingual canal. After the latter is located, the safe-tipped bur is moved buccally to expose the mesiobuccal orifice. The entire preparation is confined to the mesial two thirds of the crown (Fig. 6-45).

There is a rare variant of the typical two mesial plus one or two distal canals that is seen in some mandibular first molars. This type has one mesial root with two canals close to each other that almost file into one canal plus two separate and distinct distal roots (Fig. 6-48). In my experience,

most of these cases have occurred in Asian patients.

The roots in this situation are very short but quite curved. Both distal roots are crescent shaped; that is, the distolingual curves first to the distolingual and then to the mesiobuccal, whereas the distobuccal curves first to the distobuccal and then to the mesiolingual.

Mandibular second molar. This tooth has more variants than any of the molar teeth, even though the most common configuration is the same as that of the mandibular first molar—one distal canal and two mesial canals. In general the access cavity

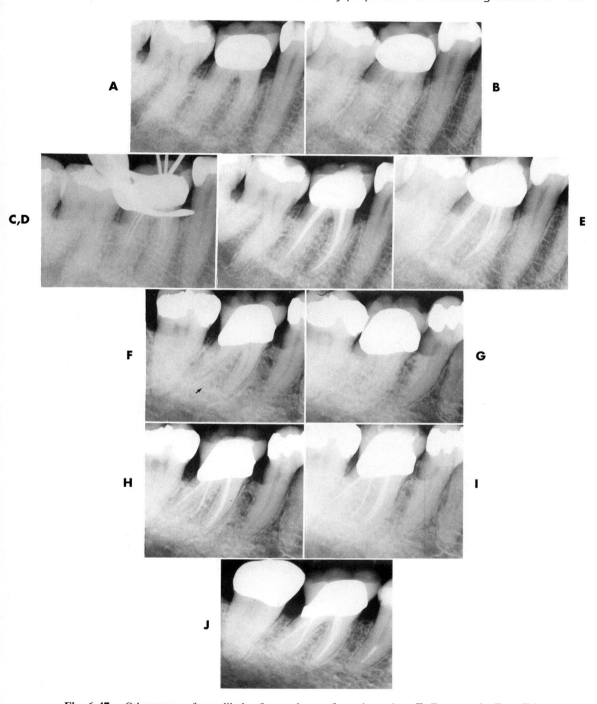

Fig. 6-47.   Other types of mandibular first molar configurations. **A** to **E,** Four canals, Type II in both roots. **A,** Straight view as shown in Fig. 6-46, *A.* **B,** Angled view as shown in Fig. 6-46, *B.* **C,** Angled view of files in place, indicating Type II canal systems in both mesial and distal roots. **D** and **E,** Immediate postfilling straight and angled views, canals filled with laterally condensed gutta-percha and Kerr's antiseptic sealer. **F** to **I,** Four separate roots. **F,** Straight view as shown in Fig. 6-46, *A,* where second distal root can be seen *(arrow).* **G,** Angled view as shown in Fig. 6-46, *B,* in which all four roots can be seen. **H** and **I,** Straight and angled views taken after canal filling with laterally condensed gutta-percha and Wach's paste. **J,** Twelve years after treatment, periapical tissues remain normal. (Restorations by Dr. Sherwin Strauss, Chicago.)   *Continued*

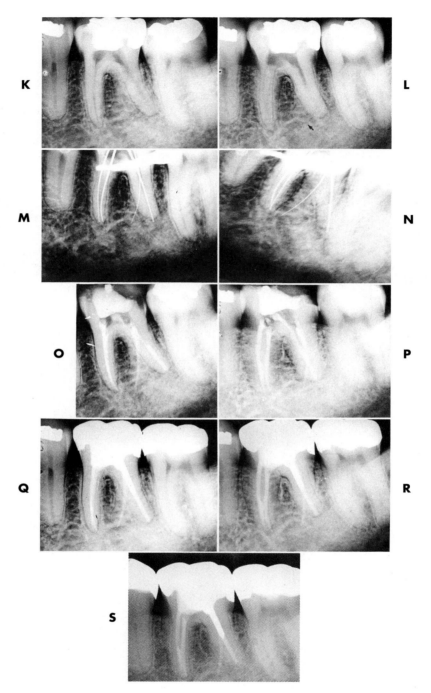

Fig. 6-47, cont'd. **K** to **S,** Four canals, three roots, with distobuccal root very curved. **K,** Straight view as shown in Fig. 6-46, *A.* **L,** Angled view as shown in Fig. 6-46, *B,* with very curved distolingual root *(arrow).* In cases with separate distolingual roots the canal is smaller than the distobuccal canal. Initially the distolingual canal curves to the distolingual and then turns to curve back to the mesiobuccal. **M** and **N,** Views of files in place, straight and angled from the distal. Note extreme curvature of the distolingual canal. **O** and **P,** Straight and angled views after canal filling with laterally condensed gutta-percha and Wach's paste. **Q** and **R,** Four years after treatment, area remains normal. **S,** Twenty years after original treatment, area still looks excellent. (Restorations by Dr. Arnold Wax, Chicago.)

preparation is the same for the adjacent first molar (Fig. 6-45, *A*). Although only one mesial canal is never present in the mandibular first molar, it does occur in the second molar. This bicanaled tooth has a slightly different access preparation, with the trapezoid narrowed to the mesial to be more rectangular (Fig. 6-49, *A*). The operator must be very certain on the basis of viewing radiographs (both straight and angled) and exploration before settling for treating only one mesial canal. Usually when only one canal is present, it is located in the middle of the mesial half of the chamber and will accept a size 20 or larger instrument at initial attempt. Routine treatment of only one mesial canal will lead to a high percentage of failures (Fig. 6-50). Some studies have reported that the percentage of one mesial canal in this tooth is greater than 50%. I disagree, and in the report of Weine, Pasiewicz, and Rice, only 4.0% were found to have a single mesial canal (Table 6-6).

When two mesial canals are present, a Type II system is more common than a Type III, which is much different than the relationship found in the mandibular first molar (Fig. 6-51).

The mandibular second molar may have only a single root with several variants: one single, large canal; two canals that merge (Fig. 6-52) or remain separate (Fig. 6-53); or the so-called C-shaped tooth (Fig. 6-54), first described by Cooke and Cox. The tooth looks like a routine second molar when viewed on the preoperative radiographs (Fig. 6-54, *A*). When the access cavity preparation is made, from the occlusal it appears that the orifices of the canals are not individually distinct but that there is a C-shaped trough on the floor of the chamber. If one file is placed in the mesial canal and one in the distal, the radiograph may reveal that both files are in the same canal (Fig. 6-54, *B*).

The C-shaped configuration refers to a continuous slit between all the canals so that a horizontal section through the root yields a space in the shape of the letter C. The closed area of the C may be to either the buccal or the lingual. If it is to the buccal, the canal is continuous from the mesiobuccal to the mesiolingual around the lingual to the distolingual to the distobuccal. If the area of closure is to the lingual, the slit goes from the mesiolingual to the mesiobuccal along the buccal to the distobuccal to the distolingual. When the canals are filled (Fig. 6-54, *D*), no individual canal really appears well condensed despite deep penetration of spreaders and a high number of auxiliary cones.

This is because the canals are really not wide in any dimension and the filling material must take up considerable space.

Two roots being present is the most common condition for the mandibular second molar (96% in the study by Weine, Paslewicz, and Rice). In the mesial root, Type I, II, or III configurations may be present. In the distal root a Type I canal is very dominant, but Types II and III systems also are possible, although rare. Three separate roots may be found (Fig. 6-55), but only rarely.

GENERAL SHAPE OF WALLS IN ACCESS PREPARATIONS

Each tooth requires its own individual lingual or occlusal shape for access preparation—quadrilateral, oval, or round. However, it is equally important to have the correct shape or taper of the walls of the preparation to give maximal access to the apical area of the canal and to retain the intertreatment dressing.

Removal of obstructions to the apex. Many of the errors in access cavity preparation are due to the dentist's desire to limit the removal of tooth structure. Believing that conservation of enamel and dentin will aid in the stability of the tooth during treatment and better retain the future restoration, the dentist prepares an access of minimal size. Unfortunately the result of such a philosophy is to restrict the direct access to the apex, causing incomplete removal of debris, insufficient preparation of dentin walls, failure to discover additional canals, and inability to produce maximal condensation of the canal filling (Fig. 6-56).

Most teeth require extensive restoration after endodontic therapy. The dentist should never hesitate to remove tooth structure if doing so will aid in producing a more nearly optimal endodontic result. Even if a satisfactory restoration is present before treatment but access and visibility are limited as long as that restoration is present, it must be understood that retaining the tooth is the priority. Such a restoration must be removed.

Typical of this situation is a mandibular molar in which there is a full gold crown and the mesiobuccal canal is not located through ordinary preparation because of dentinal sclerosis. If the crown is removed, the underlying dental structures are most easily viewed; then such landmarks as dentin rings, root shape, and the other canal orifices will generally lead to the missing canal. Teeth with unusual root size and shape under large restorations similarly can

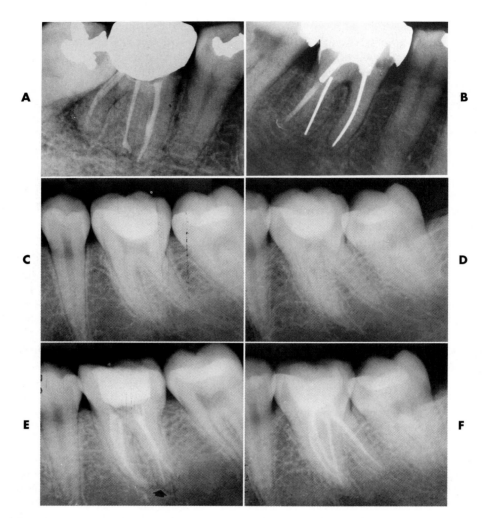

Fig. 6-48. Unusual mandibular first molars. **A,** Immediate postfilling film, two mesial canals close together and two separate and distinct distal roots. **B,** Ten years postoperative film of a mandibular first molar with a similar configuration. Most of the patients in whom I have treated such teeth have been Asians. **C** and **D,** Straight view and angled view from the distal of preoperative film of mandibular first molar with four separate roots, the two mesial roots being very close together but the distal roots far apart. **E** and **F,** Straight view and angled view from the distal, immediate postfilling films, four canals filled with laterally condensed gutta-percha and Wach's paste. The distolingual root *(arrow)* is the most curved, although it seems relatively straight on the film. That is because the root curves first to the lingual and then sharply to the buccal, both in the plane of the x-ray cone. This patient was Caucasian, so this combination is not limited to Asians.

be better treated when there is nothing to hamper direct visualization (Fig. 6-57).

Even in teeth with small or no restorations, direct access to the apex may be restricted by ledges of tooth structure that are left when direct preparation along the long axis is not followed. Levin has described the presence of incisal and

lingual triangles that keep the enlarging instruments from performing their tasks properly on anterior teeth. Such obstructions may be easily removed with the safe-tipped bur or with tapered diamond stones (Fig. 6-58).

Need for divergent walls. In the desire to provide a good temporary seal between appoint-

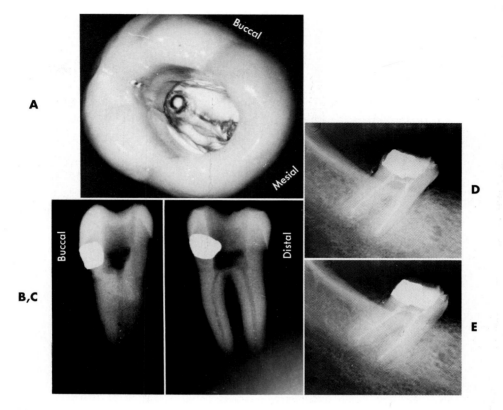

Fig. 6-49.   Access cavity preparations and canal configuration in bicanaled mandibular second molar. This is a rare configuration and, according to the study by Weine et al., occurs as infrequently as 4% of the time. **A,** Outline form is still trapezoidal, as in all mandibular molars, to allow for large distal canal and for careful examination of mesial portion to verify that only one canal is present. **B,** Proximal view displays large occlusal opening to allow examination for a second mesial canal, if present. In this view the two canals are superimposed. **C,** Buccal view, showing straight distal canal and mesial canal curving from the floor of the chamber first to the mesial and then to the distal. **D** and **E,** Immediate postfilling films after canal filling with laterally condensed gutta-percha and Wach's paste. To be certain that only one canal is present in the mesial root, two radiographs, angled differently from each other by at least 45 degrees, must be taken of both the initial file in place and the final filling. Film **D** was taken straight on, and film **E** was taken from the mesial at a horizontal angulation of 50 degrees. In both films the canal filling is well centered in the root. If another canal were present, in one of these two films the canal would be eccentric in the mesial root, as seen in Fig. 6-50, *B* and *C*.

ments, the dentist may shape the access preparation to be wider toward the floor of the pulp chamber than to the occlusal (or lingual) surface. With the philosophy that such a preparation will better retain silicate and resin restorations, the dentist utilizes this incorrect taper.

The difference is that in endodontic treatment there is no solid base for the temporary filling to butt against, but merely a pellet of cotton and an empty chamber. As forces of mastication are

applied to the temporary seal, there is no resistance to inward dislodgment, and exposure of the canals to contamination results. However, if the walls of the entry are prepared to diverge toward the occlusal (or incisal) aspect, the forces will tend further to seat the temporary filling. Even if some of the material at the periphery is lost, the seal is retained and contamination prevented (Fig. 6-59).

Access for badly worn or fractured anterior teeth.   When an attempt is made to prepare an

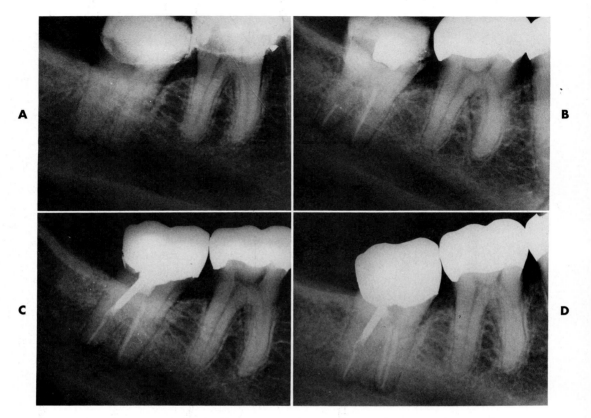

Fig. 6-50.   A, Preoperative radiograph of mandibular second molar. **B,** The operator assumed that there was only one mesial and one distal canal. **C,** Eighteen months after treatment, a radiolucency had developed around mesial root, and the tooth was tender to percussion. **D,** I located the additional canal, the mesiolingual, and the symptoms vanished.

entry on patients with badly eroded anterior teeth, some alteration in routine shaping is necessary. Because heavy dentinal sclerosis usually accompanies incisal wear, as a result of old age and/or bruxism, the most direct possible access is needed. This is accomplished by making the preparation directly through the incisal edge rather than through the lingual edge, thus allowing the preparation to follow the path of recession of the pulp chamber, which is easily visualized by its difference in color and texture from the surrounding dentin.

Fractured anterior teeth are similarly entered through the incisal edge. The trauma has reduced crown height, and restoration by a post-and-core type of crown becomes mandatory. The fractured crown is trimmed to be parallel with the occlusal plane, and any sharp edges are rounded to prevent irritation to the lips or tongue. Then, rather than angle in from the lingual area, the entry is placed

on the incisal edge to gain direct access to the apex (Fig. 6-60).

PREPARATION OF AREA FOR TREATMENT

Before an entry may be begun, certain preparation of the site of treatment must be made to reach a successful result from both the dentist's and the patient's viewpoint. To ensure patient comfort, the tooth must be correctly anesthetized. Also, the tooth to be treated must be able to accommodate a rubber dam.

Need for local anesthesia during endodontic therapy.   Correct use and administration of local anesthetics provide the best assurance of patient cooperation. When patients complain of pain during endodontic treatment, they are usually correct. The cause of the pain may be that the anesthesia is not sufficiently profound, that the injection technique did not deliver solution to the correct sites,

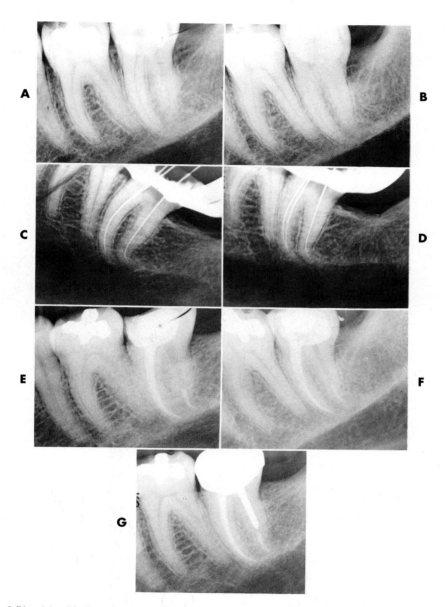

Fig. 6-51.   Mandibular second molar with Type II canal system in mesial root. **A,** Preoperative straight view. **B,** Preoperative angled view. These films were taken similarly to those shown in Fig. 6-46, *A* and *B,* except that the film and cone tip were slightly more to the distal. In these views only one mesial canal can be identified. However, when the correct access was prepared, similar to that shown in Fig. 6-45, *B,* three canal orifices were located. **C** and **D,** Straight and angled view with files in place. On the straight views the files are superimposed, but the site of convergence is seen on the angled view. **E** and **F,** Straight and angled views after canal filling with laterally condensed gutta-percha and Wach's paste. **G,** Straight view, 2 years later, area looks excellent.

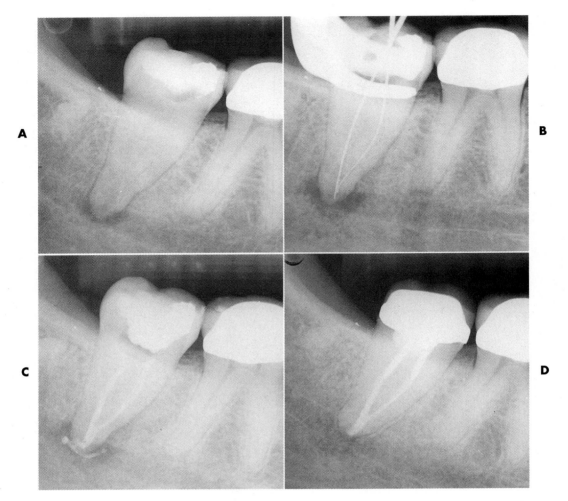

Fig. 6-52. **A,** Preoperative radiograph of mandibular second molar with a large, single root and periapical lesion. **B,** Two canals are present, merging into a single apical site of exiting. **C,** Canal filling with laterally condensed gutta-percha and Wach's paste. Some excess sealer was pushed out of the apex due to the relatively wide apical exit. **D,** Excellent healing 2 years after treatment, all excess sealer and periapical lesion are gone without periapical surgery. (Restorations by Dr. Neal Baigh, LaGrange, Ill.)

or that not all the needed injections were given.

Deeply profound anesthesia is a must for endodontic procedures such as pulp extirpation, canal enlargement when normal periapical tissue is present, and some instances of canal filling.

For some fearful patients, anesthesia may be needed for any phase of treatment and should be used if the patient is insistent, even if a large periapical radiolucency is present.

Types of anesthetic solutions used in endodontics. For profound anesthesia, two types of anesthesia solutions are widely used in endodontics:

lidocaine (Xylocaine) and mepivacaine (Carbocaine). Although both drugs are more toxic than procaine (Novocain), the old standby for dentistry, they have a more rapid onset, have much greater depth, and last longer than procaine. The potential problem of toxicity rarely arises, since smaller quantities of either preferred anesthetic are needed compared with procaine. Also, the qualities of onset and depth are important in endodontic treatment. For maxillary teeth and mandibular anterior teeth, usually one to two Carpules (1.8 ml per Carpule) are sufficient to gain deep anesthesia. For

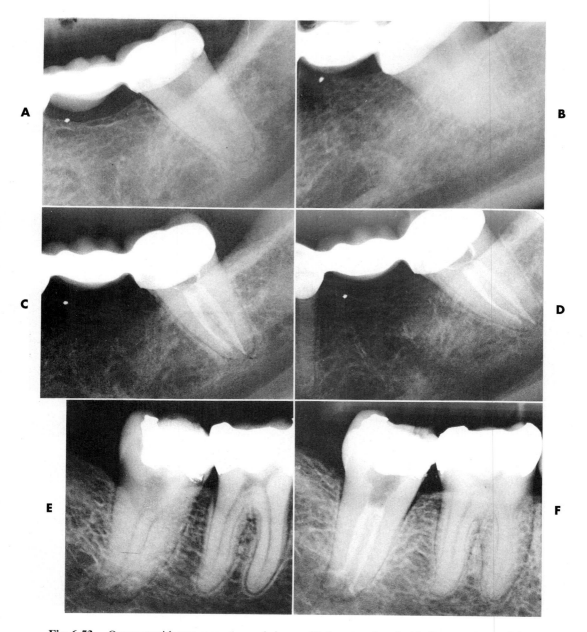

Fig. 6-53.   One root with two separate canals in mandibular second molar. **A,** Preoperative straight view, indicating a single root, but individual canal shape difficult to identify. It might have a single canal, two merging canals, or two separate canals. **B,** Preoperative angled view gives no additional information. **C** and **D,** Postoperative views, two separate canals, each filled with laterally condensed gutta-percha and Wach's paste. (Restorations by Dr. Sue Klyber, Chicago.) **E,** Preoperative view. **F,** Immediate postfilling film, canals filled with laterally condensed gutta-percha and Wach's paste. Both these teeth are similar to the C-shaped mandibular second molar (Fig. 6-54), only the canals have remained separate instead of merging.

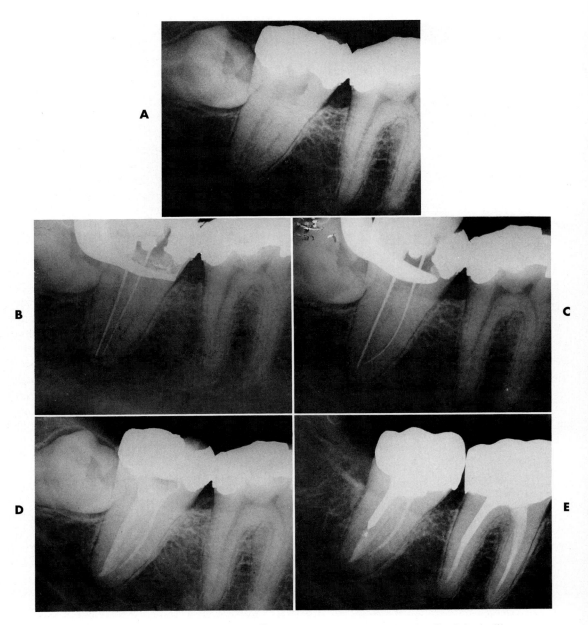

Fig. 6-54. **A,** Preoperative radiograph of C-shaped mandibular second molar. Tooth looks like any routine mandibular second molar. **B,** One file was placed in distal and one in mesiobuccal area. However, when film was developed, both files were in distal area. It was further feared that the file closer to the mesial might have resulted in a perforation. **C,** Additional efforts left one file in distal and one in mesial areas. **D,** Immediate postoperative film indicates fillings of only moderate density despite heavy lateral condensation and many auxiliary cones. **E,** Three years later, area looks excellent. (Restorations by Dr. Robert Lauren, Chicago.)

those mandibular posterior teeth requiring nerve block anesthesia, two Carpules, and often more, are necessary.

In those cases for which profound anesthesia is unnecessary, as for nonvital pulp removal or prevention of pain due to rubber dam clamp impingement, half a Carpule is sufficient.

Injections needed for removal of vital pulp tissue. Root and bone anatomy, condition of the pulp tissues, and patient pain tolerance all have a bearing on the types of injections that will be needed to remove vital pulp tissue. In most cases the routine injections listed in Table 6-8 should be given. If pain is still experienced, the supplementary injections are usually sufficient to gain patient comfort. In some cases, particularly mandibular molars with considerable pulpal inflammation, only intrapulpal injections are effective.

In maxillary anterior teeth, only labial infiltration of one Carpule is necessary, deposited directly over the apex. Some lateral incisors may have considerable thick bone over the apex and require an additional Carpule. Deposition beneath the periosteum usually ensures better anesthesia from all infiltrations. Supplementary anesthesia is rarely needed, but if necessary, a palatal infiltration to anesthetize the branches from the incisive canal is given.

For maxillary posterior teeth, local buccal infiltration and palatal infiltration to block the branches of the anterior palatine nerve are needed. One Carpule is sufficient for bicuspids, whereas two Carpules, one for each buccal root, are needed for molars. Only a few drops are required on the palate. Once the palatal canal has been thoroughly debrided, palatal infiltration is rarely needed for succeeding appointments. Supplementary anesthesia is available only by intrapulpal injection.

Mandibular incisors are anesthetized with one Carpule given by labial infiltration. The central incisor may have thicker bony covering and require slightly more. Supplementary injection is given by lingual infiltration.

For the mandibular cuspid and first bicuspid, the mental block injection gives extremely rapid and deep results. Lingual infiltration may be needed, particularly if two separate roots are present. The cuspid may require local infiltration as well if nerves from the opposite side cross over and anastomose.

The mandibular second bicuspid and molars must have a mandibular block. Whereas local infiltration may be useful for supplementary anesthesia, it alone is insufficient to remove vital pulp tissue. For supplementary anesthesia the second bicuspid may require lingual infiltration, directly beneath the tooth. Molars may need local infiltration and injections into the alveolar crest of the furcation and septum between the adjacent teeth.

For mandibular molars, ligamental anesthesia is optional but may be quite helpful, particularly when a tooth with a severe pulpitis is being treated. It is certainly much better than giving a long buccal injection, which anesthetizes the soft tissues but has no effect on the pulp.

When the patient complains of pain during access, despite the indications of good anesthesia and after the suggested injections, intrapulpal injection is needed. It should be explained to the patient that the anesthetic has not taken effect completely because of the degree of inflammation, but that more solution will soon be given and will

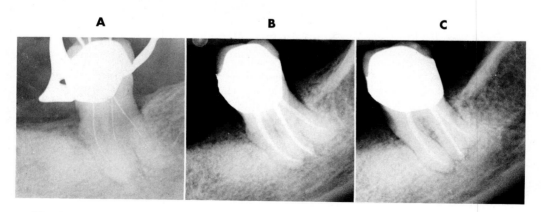

Fig. 6-55. Three separate roots in mandibular second molar. **A,** Files in place, indicating three separate roots, each quite curved. **B** and **C,** Immediate postfilling films, canals filled with laterally condensed gutta-percha and Wach's paste.

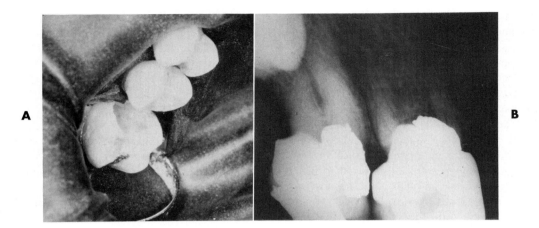

Fig. 6-56. A, Maxillary first molar with pulp exposures to mesiobuccal and palatal canals after caries excavation. Attempting to conserve tooth structure by using this mesial entry as access will severely hamper all procedures to follow. **B,** Large, multiple restorations on all surfaces of this maxillary first molar with considerable dentinal sclerosis will make canal location difficult. Rather than be conservative about tooth structure and risk root perforation while searching for the canals, it is better to cut down the crown of the tooth to slightly above gingival line, if necessary. This will give best visualization for finding the canals and for preparations that will follow.

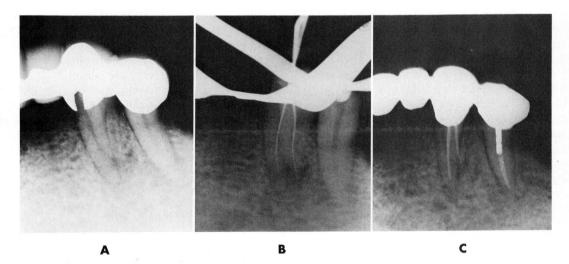

Fig. 6-57. Mandibular cuspid with two canals requiring endodontic treatment, as did the adjacent first bicuspid. **A,** Attempting to locate and enlarge two separate canals through a large restoration is extremely difficult. Understanding the situation, the cooperative referring dentist removed the crowns, even though it was part of the precision case. It was more important to ensure that the endodontics could be done in the best environment than to retain the crowns and risk perforation or inadequate therapy. **B,** Crown is sacrificed, but the canals are located and direct access to the apices is obtained. **C,** Two years after treatment, the periapical lesions have healed, and a new splint is in place. (Restorations by Dr. Joe Morros, Chicago.)

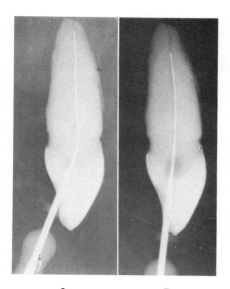

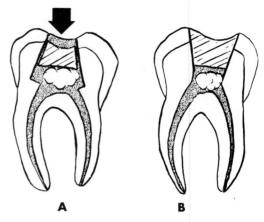

<table>
<tr><td>**A**</td><td>**B**</td></tr>
</table>

Fig. 6-58. **A,** Access to this central incisor seems correct, but proximal radiographic view discloses that incisal triangle was not removed and therefore the file does not have direct access to the apex. Note that bend forces file against labial portion of canal, thus not allowing for even preparation of walls. **B,** With access enlarged labially, the file had direct access to the apex.

Fig. 6-59. **A,** Incorrect access is prepared with greatest width toward floor of chamber, according to philosophy that such a preparation will give greater retention to intertreatment seal. However, without a solid floor to butt against, vertical force *(arrow)* pushes cement into preparation and results in contamination of canals. **B,** Correctly tapering preparation is widest at occlusal edge. Vertical forces will only serve to further seat the temporary seal.

Table 6-8.   Local anesthetic for treating teeth with vital pulp tissue

Tooth	Injections needed for	
	Routine anesthesia	Supplementary anesthesia
Maxillary central and lateral incisors and cuspid	Labial infiltration	Palatal infiltration
Maxillary bicuspids and molars	Labial infiltration Palatal infiltration	Intrapulpal injection
Mandibular incisors	Labial infiltration	Lingual infiltration
Mandibular cuspid and first bicuspid	Mental block	Lingual infiltration
Mandibular second bicuspid	Mandibular block	Buccal infiltration Lingual infiltration
Mandibular molars	Mandibular block Intraligamentary injections*	Intraseptal injection Intrapulpal injection

*Optional.

be effective. The patient will usually cooperate for the few minutes that are required to penetrate the roof of the chamber.

For effectiveness, intrapulpal injections require a bulk of vital tissue to transport the anesthetic throughout the canals. Therefore, when it appears that intrapulpal anesthetic may be needed for any tooth, it should be administered after a small hole in the roof of the pulp chamber has been made and before any tissue is extirpated. In molars the solution is deposited in the largest canal—palatal canal for maxillary molars and distal canal for mandibular molars—and will traverse the entire canal system in a few minutes.

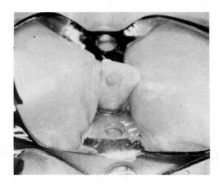

Fig. 6-60. Entries for badly abraded anterior teeth or those with fractured crowns should be made through incisal edge rather than with routine lingual access. Such a preparation gives more direct access to the apex.

Many textbooks advise the use of such exotic and usually painful methods of anesthesia as pressure anesthesia or intraosseous injection. I have never found these to be necessary. Rarely do maxillary or mandibular anterior teeth cause any problem, although for certain patients, additional solution may be required.

Special comments about mandibular block injections. Being able to extirpate a pulp from a mandibular first molar tender to percussion and sensitive to hot in a painless manner is the most demanding anesthetic test in dentistry. The depth of anesthesia required for this procedure transcends any other dental procedure for this tooth, including preparation for a crown, periodontal surgery, or even extraction.

A precisely placed mandibular block injection, more correctly referred to as an *inferior alveolar nerve (IAN) block,* is required for this procedure. The patient should experience lip paresthesia after injection within 90 seconds for the dentist to feel relatively safe in attempting to start the access preparation and expect to complete the extirpation totally and painlessly. When the patient requires 10, 15, or more minutes to gain numbness in the lip, usually more injections (intraligamentary and intrapulpal) are needed.

Methods are available to increase an operator's ability to gain a high percentage of lip paresthesia from IAN injections within this 90-second window. Generally it is accepted that if a dentist can obtain paresthesia in 90 seconds in 85% or more of IAN blocks administered, the technique being

used is excellent and cannot be improved. However, many dentists do not reach this 85% level, and the following remarks should be helpful in attaining this degree of effectiveness.

Administer correct amount of solution. Malamed has stated that the IAN injection may require as much as 1.5 to 3.0 ml of solution to be effective. Assuming that 1.8 ml is available in each injection and that some solution will be deposited during penetration to the site of the nerve, one can easily see that injection of one Carpule of local anesthetic may not be enough solution to attain acceptable pulpal anesthesia. Therefore, for these complicated cases, two Carpules of anesthetic should be injected for best results. If the patient has cardiovascular problems and two Carpules may contribute a greater amount of vasoconstrictor than desired, it is a simple matter to give one Carpule with a low amount of vasoconstrictor and a second Carpule of the same or another anesthetic agent without any vasoconstrictor.

Use of the short needle. The long needle has been recommended for dental injections for many years. The basic reason for its use originally was that in cases where the needle broke during the injection, more metal was available to grasp for removal. Also, since the most vulnerable site for needle breakage was at the hub, the longer needles would have less chance of being placed into the tissue to the hub and thus less chance of being broken. These are good and logical reasons, and to this day, most dentists use a long needle (28.9 to 41.5 mm in length, averaging about 36.0 mm) to deliver the IAN block.

However, when this view became prevalent, dental needles were much different than they are now, both in manufacture and use. The former needles were cut from a long tube and were more susceptible to breakage than the rolled metal needles of today. Forty years ago it was common practice to reuse needles dozens of times, with boiling the usual method for sterilization. Today, and for many years now, needles are disposable and are reused only at the same appointment for the same patient. Sterilization usually is by gas. Needle breakage in the last few years has been minuscule. Choice of needle length should be based on more significant conditions.

Many dentists think that the use of the long needle is predicated on the distance between the pterygomandibular raphe and the lingula being longer than a short needle (19.9 to 25.5 mm, averaging about 22 mm). Menke and Gowgiel, using cadaver material rather than dried specimens, measured this distance. Although previous literature had suggested that the penetration distance was as short as 12 mm to as long as 38 mm, they found the range to be 12 to 19 mm, with an average of 16 mm, all well within the length of 22 mm, the most popular length of the short needle.

Having the maximal penetration distance only a few millimeters from the total length of the needle allows for the anesthetist to visualize that distance easily when using a short needle, which would be nearly impossible when using a long needle, where the exposed metal would be approximately 20+ mm. Furthermore, the long needle has much more "drift," or needle deviation, to its tip. This fact and because many more anatomically important sites are found past the site of injection than before it make a miss being too long an undesirable error in administering the IAN block. The shorter miss, although still being an anesthetic failure, probably will not cause an untoward reaction or enter an undesirable position.

Use care when giving an IAN block with a short needle.   Malamed still discourages the use of the short needle because he believes that it is more apt to break than a long needle. He has stated that the weak point, the hub, may be reached with a short but is unreachable with a long needle. The answer to this problem is to always use a needle of 19 mm or longer. Furthermore, with virtually every short needle, if you approach within 1 or 2 mm of the hub, the needle has gone too far already. Remove it carefully and reinject. *Never go to the hub with any needle, regardless of length!*

If, however, one still insists on using a long needle but understands the advantage of knowing when penetration of 16 mm has been reached, I advise placing a sterile endodontic stop (Fig. 7-16) on the long needle at 16 mm. Then, as the IAN block is being given, the operator knows when the ideal penetration site has been reached.

Intraligamentary anesthesia.   Intraligamentary injections (ILIs) are neither new nor intraligamentary. They were used in the early 1920s, reintroduced in Italy by Colombo in 1972, and have gained popularity in the last few years since specialized syringes were manufactured. Even though early users and manufacturers claim that anesthesia is gained by the solution filtering down through the periodontal ligament to the apical vessels,

there can be no question that the injection is effective by being intraosseous.

Many other misconceptions and incorrect applications surround the so-called ILI. The injection works best with an anesthetic solution containing epinephrine, because the vasoconstriction evidently has effect on the apical vessels. According to Pashley, this effect goes farther systemically than merely the local site of the injection, so I prefer an epinephrine level no greater than 1:100,000. Because of the local ischemia produced in the pulp by such an injection, ILI is well used when endodontic procedures or extractions are performed, but, according to Kim, should not be used for operative dentistry when the pulp is to be conserved.

Because the injection is intraosseous rather than intraligamentary, the bevel of the needle must be pointed *away* from, not toward, the tooth being anesthetized. The injection is given into the interproximal space to the mesial and distal of the tooth; buccal or lingual injections do not seem to have any effect on the pulp. The injector must feel that pressure is needed to obtain the desired anesthesia, and only a few drops need to be expressed. If a large amount of solution enters the tissues easily, the injection will probably have little effect because it is not being forced into the bone. Specialized injection syringes need not be used, but a standard injection syringe is perfectly acceptable, as long as pressure can be built up. The ordinary syringe should have a plastic, metal, or glass sleeve to protect the Carpule of anesthetic solution, since in some cases the pressure built up can break the glass, thus causing an explosion of flying glass and solution that might cause injury to the patient or the dentist. I have found that 30-gauge and ultrashort (quarter-inch) needles seem to work best.

Dye distribution studies by Walton have demonstrated that the solutions pass into the teeth adjacent to the one being injected. Therefore the ILI cannot inject single teeth to isolate an individual tooth as the cause of pain. Erroneous results may occur if an attempt is made to affect only a single tooth and keep an adjacent tooth unanesthetized.

The patient will experience some pain in the area after the injection but probably very little more than in any other site of needle insertion. The injection should be used with great care in patients with periodontal disease, unless the tooth is to be extracted at that visit. The forceful injection into a diseased, septic area may cause a periodontal abscess to fulminate.

Not all clinicians are in agreement concerning the effectiveness of this injection, even though Kim reported as high as 88% full anesthesia on inflamed mandibular molars. My own experience is that ILIs provide an effective supplementary anesthetic choice when performing pulp extirpations on inflamed mandibular molars. They generally allow the dentist to gain access into the pulp itself relatively painlessly. Then an intrapulpal injection allows for the comfortable completion of the extirpation.

An ILI will not give pulpal anesthesia in mandibular molars for any extended time and may be useful for only 8 minutes or less. In a typical scenario a dentist may attempt a mandibular block for a painful mandibular molar, but the patient does not feel symptoms of paresthesia quickly. After 10 to 15 minutes, lip paresthesia seems adequate and the dentist starts access preparation. After some painless preparation, the patient starts to become uncomfortable, indicating lack of full effect from the block.

At this point the dentist administers the ILIs. Since it took over 10 minutes for the block to start to work, the dentist decides to allow that much time for the ILIs to work. This is a serious mistake. By that time, even if they were effective initially, the ILIs will have lost their anesthetic quality and the patient will again be in pain.

If ILIs are administered, the operator should wait only a minute or two and then continue preparation. Hopefully the hard tissue to the pulp will be uncovered relatively painlessly, and then the intrapulpal injection can be given to ensure total anesthesia for the extirpation.

Application of rubber dam for severely broken-down teeth. Some teeth with severe loss of tooth structure may present problems for the application of a rubber dam. Since the use of the dam is mandatory, certain procedures performed before access preparation is begun will aid in holding the clamp.

If sufficient tooth structure is present above the alveolar bone, an alveoloplasty procedure is required to expose sufficient portions of the root face. This may be accomplished with tapered diamond stones and water spray to remove the bone covering the root. After the endodontic appointment, a large amount of zinc oxide–eugenol (ZOE) may be used to cover the entire root face rather than merely the access cavity and to act as a pack, since ZOE is a major constituent of most periodontal dressings. This will prevent pain and keep the exposed bone covered until sufficient new soft tissue develops.

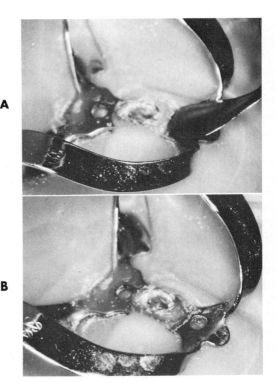

Fig. 6-61. **A,** Mandibular incisor has broken beneath gingiva but requires rubber dam application. Clamp is placed on tissue, and a periodontal knife is used to trim pinched tissue easily and bloodlessly. **B,** Root face is now completely exposed for performance of necessary endodontic treatment and to simplify the post, core, and crown preparation that will follow.

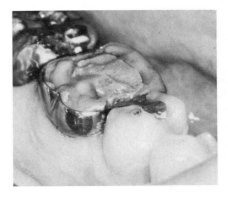

Fig. 6-62. Preformed band placed on mandibular first molar that was so badly broken down on buccal aspect that no rubber dam clamp could hold satisfactorily. Metal band will impinge minimally on gingiva, is relatively simple to place compared with a festooned copper band, and will support direct clamp placement.

If only soft tissue covers the tooth to be treated, gingivoplasty procedures will be needed. These may be rapidly and bloodlessly accomplished by the use of an electrosurgery unit. Gingivoplasty may be performed also by applying a sharp rubber dam clamp on the gingiva at the position of gingivectomy depth. The clamp pinches off the tissue, and the latter is easily trimmed and removed with a scalpel or surgical knife (Fig. 6-61). The oversized temporary-pack dressing is also used.

Use of bands. If a badly broken-down tooth requires endodontic therapy and sufficient crown length is present, a cemented preformed band may be useful to allow for rubber dam application and to retain the intertreatment dressing.

Several companies have these preformed bands (Fig. 6-62) available in many widths to accommodate every possible size and shape. They are contoured to resemble the gingival shape, thereby lessening the chance for soft tissue damage and aiding in retention of the band. Some authors suggest the use of a copper band. However, these bands take much longer to festoon and apply, are not precontoured to lessen gingival inflammation, and are not as sturdy.

Access when deep gingival decay is present. When deep gingival decay is present, using a preformed band may not seal off the area, and contamination of the canal would result. The correct procedure is to prepare the normal access through the occlusal (or lingual) surface. Contents of the canal are removed past the decay, and the cavity is excavated to sound dentin with sufficient retention to hold a temporary seal. A file or silver point is placed through the access, well past the gingival preparation. Silver amalgam is the material of choice to seal the preparation, particularly if the area must hold a rubber dam clamp at a succeeding appointment. ZOE, thickly mixed, is also acceptable but may tend to crumble under the pressure of clamp placement. Once the temporary seal has attained initial set, the file or point that was used to keep material from being pushed into the canal is removed, and patency of the canal is verified (Fig. 6-63).

Aid for a leaky rubber dam. In some instances the rubber dam fails to control seepage of saliva, resulting in constant contamination of the chamber of the tooth being treated. This condition may arise during treatment of splint or bridge abutments, where the series of castings prevents the dam from being tucked into the interproximal spaces around the treated tooth, or

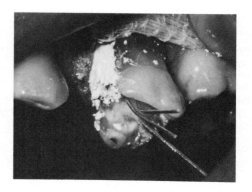

Fig. 6-63. Maxillary molar was severely decayed on mesial aspect. Normal access was prepared, canals enlarged, and caries excavated. A lubricated silver point was placed in each canal to keep the distance to the apex patent, and the preparation was packed with ZOE. After cement sets, points will be removed and a routine temporary seal placed. At next appointment, outer seal will be removed, but gingivally packed ZOE will remain in place to prevent contamination.

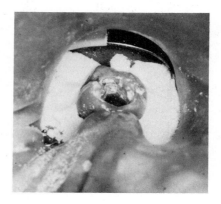

Fig. 6-64. Rubber dam seal was incomplete, and saliva continued to seep during appointment. A thick mixture of Ward's Tempak is placed around clamp to seal off area.

when the normal shape of the crown is lacking because of caries, loss of restoration, or abnormal axial inclination.

To avoid fighting saliva all during the appointment, the practitioner may use Ward's Tempak or other similar temporary cement to halt the seepage. A medium mix is prepared and packed around the rubber dam clamp. Because ZOE cements normally set faster when in contact with moisture, in a few minutes the leakage will be halted and treatment may continue normally (Fig. 6-64).

REFERENCES

Canal configuration

Amos ER: Incidence of bifurcated canals in mandibular cuspids, *J Am Dent Assoc* 50:70, 1955.

Baisden MK, Kulild JC, Weller RN: Root canal configuration of the mandibular first premolar, *J Endod* 18:505, 1992.

Carns EJ, Skidmore AE: Configurations and deviations of root canals of maxillary first premolars, *Oral Surg* 36:880, 1973.

Cooke HG, Cox FL: C-shaped canal configurations in mandibular molars. *J Am Dent Assoc* 99:836, 1979.

Eskoz N, Weine FS: Canal configuration of the mesiobuccal root of the maxillary second molar, *J Endod* 21:38, 1995.

Evenot M: Contribution a la connaissance des systemes endodontiques complexes la racine mesio vestibulaire de la premiere molaire maxillaire, approche, instrumentale, clinique et pedagogique, doctor's thesis, Academie de Paris, Universite Rene Descartes (Paris V), 1980.

Green D: Double canals in single roots, *Oral Surg* 35:689, 1973.

Hartwell G, Bellizzi R: Clinical investigation of in vivo endodontically treated mandibular and maxillary molars, *J Endod* 8:555, 1982.

Kulild JC, Peters DD: Incidence and configuration of canal systems in the mesiobuccal root of the maxillary first and second molars, *J Endod* 16:311, 1990.

Leven HJ: Access cavities, *Dent Clin North Am,* Nov 1967, p 801.

Neaverth EJ, Kotler LM, Kaltenbach RF: Clinical investigation (in vivo) of endodontically treated maxillary first molars, *J Endod* 13:506, 1987.

Nosonowitz DM, Brenner MR: The major canals of the mesiobuccal root of the maxillary 1st and 2nd molars. *NY J Dent* 43:12, 1973.

Pineda F: Roentgenographic investigation of the mesiobuccal root of the maxillary first molar, *Oral Surg* 36:253, 1973.

Pomeranz HH, Fishelberg G: The second mesiobuccal canal of the maxillary molars, *J Am Dent Assoc* 88:119, 1974.

Rankine-Wilson RW, Henry P: The bifurcated root canal in lower anterior teeth, *J Am Dent Assoc* 70:1162, 1965.

Seidberg BH, Altman M, Guttuso J, Suson M: Frequency of two root canals in maxillary permanent first molars, *J Am Dent Assoc* 87:852, 1973.

Skidmore AE, Bjorndal AM: Root canal morphology of the human mandibular first molar, *Oral Surg* 32:778, 1971.

Sykaras SN, Economou PN: Root canal morphology of the mesiobuccal root of the maxillary first molar, *Odontostomat Prodos* 24:99, 1970.

VandeVorde HE, Odendahl D, Davis J: Molar 4th canals: frequent cause of endodontic failure? *Ill Dent J* 44:779, 1975.

Vertucci FJ: Root canal anatomy of the mandibular anterior teeth, *J Am Dent Assoc* 89:369, 1974.

Vertucci FJ: Root canal morphology of mandibular premolars, *J Am Dent Assoc* 97:47, 1978.

Vertucci FJ: Root canal anatomy of the human permanent teeth, *Oral Surg* 58:589, 1984.

Vertucci FJ, Gegauff A: Root canal morphology of the maxillary first premolar, *J Am Dent Assoc* 99:194, 1979.

Vertucci FJ, Williams RG: Root canal anatomy of the mandibular first molar, *J NJ Dent Assoc* 45:27, 1974.

Vertucci FJ, Seelig A, Gillis R: Root canal morphology of the human maxillary second premolar, *Oral Surg* 38:456, 1974.

Weine FS: Initiating endodontic therapy in posterior teeth. Part I. General considerations and starting treatment of bicuspids, *Compend Contin Educ Dent* 3:377, 1982.

Weine FS: Initiating endodontic therapy in posterior teeth. Part II. Maxillary molars, *Compend Contin Educ Dent* 3:455, 1982.

Weine FS: Initiating endodontic therapy in posterior teeth. Part III. Mandibular molars, *Compend Contin Educ Dent* 4:153, 1983.

Weine FS, Healey HJ, Gerstein H, Evanson L: Canal configuration in the mesiobuccal root of the maxillary first molar and its endodontic significance. *Oral Surg* 28:419, 1969.

Weine FS, Pasiewicz R, Rice RT: Canal configuration of the mandibular second molar using a clinically oriented in vitro method, *J Endod* 14:207, 1988.

Weller RN, Hartwell G: The impact of improved access and searching techniques on detection of the mesiolingual canal in maxillary molars, *J Endod* 15:82, 1989.

Zillich R, Dawson J: Root canal morphology of the mandibular first and second premolars, *Oral Surg* 36:738, 1973.

Local anesthesia

Farsakian LR, Weine FS: The significance of needle gauge in dental injections, *Compend Contin Educ Dent* 12:262, 1991.

Kim S: Ligamental injection: a physiological explanation of its efficacy, *J Endod* 12:486, 1986.

Malamed SF: *Handbook of local anesthesia,* ed 3, St Louis, 1991, Mosby.

Menke RA, Gowgiel JM: Short-needle block anesthesia at the mandibular foramen, *J Am Dent Assoc* 99:27, 1979.

Pashley DH: Systemic effects of intraligamentary injections, *J Endod* 12:501, 1986.

Walton RE, Abbott BJ: Periodontal ligament injection: a clinical evaluation, *J Am Dent Assoc* 103:571, 1981.

Walton RE: Distribution of solutions with the periodontal ligament injection: clinical, anatomical, and histological evidence, *J Endod* 12:492, 1986.

White JJ, Reader A, Beck M, Meyers WJ: The periodontal ligament injection: a comparison of the efficacy in human maxillary and mandibular teeth, *J Endod* 14:508, 1988.

Wittrock JW, Fischer WE: The aspiration of blood through small-gauge needles, *J Am Dent Assoc* 76:79, 1986.

7 Intracanal treatment procedures, basic and advanced topics

The major objective of the intracanal treatment procedures is to remove the contents of the canal and adjacent tissues in such a way that the filling procedures that follow will be facilitated. This means not only that the pulp tissue, necrotic debris, microorganisms, and affected dentin must be removed from the treated tooth, but also that the canal walls must be prepared to receive a filling material that will seal the apical foramen.

To describe this aspect of treatment lucidly, Schilder has dubbed these procedures *cleansing and shaping* in emphasis of the need for debridement and development of a specific receptacle for the filling material. I prefer the term *canal preparation* but certainly acknowledge that cleansing and shaping must be performed to reach the desired goal. "Canal enlargement" should not be used; merely widening the diameter of the canal may not produce the correct shape that must be developed, neither does it always remove undesired contents from the canal.

The importance of canal preparation cannot be overemphasized. It is these intracanal procedures that allow for the initiation of healing by removing the irritants to periapical tissue that have been harbored within the canal. When for some reason a longer than routine period of time has elapsed between the start and the completion of therapy, it is not unusual to note radiographic evidence of healing of a periapical lesion on an x-ray film before canal filling (Fig. 7-1).

This chapter will discuss the instruments necessary to accomplish the desired objective, the procedures designed to produce results effectively and rapidly, and the adjuncts needed to retain the tooth in a desirable condition until the canals are filled. The treatment of teeth with complex problems will also be described.

The discussion on calculation of working length has been included in this chapter for the previous four editions of this textbook. However, for this edition, I have given this subject a chapter of its own, Chapter 8. Working length calculation may be an object of controversy, and I wanted to give sufficient space to each of the several techniques. Popularity of several types of apex locators also has increased recently. The bulk of material was great enough that it would have expanded this chapter—the most important phase of endodontic treatment—to more than 15% of the entire book.

Because aspects of working length are necessarily involved in canal preparation, it is my hope that this change does not become disorienting to the reader, who notes references to working length while reading Chapter 7, but has not yet read the basis for its calculation. Perhaps this should be treated as are some aspects of intricate spy novels, where characters and events are referred to but have not yet been introduced fully in the prose.

BASIC INTRACANAL INSTRUMENTS

The basic endodontic instruments used within the root canal are broaches, files (K-type and Hedstrom), and reamers.

Broaches. Broaches are available in two types: smooth and barbed. The smooth broach is used by some practitioners as an initial instrument to explore the patency and the walls of the canal. I do not follow this procedure, preferring to remove tissue bulk before the placement of any instrument near the apex to avoid forcing any inflamed or necrotic tissue through the apex.

The barbed broach has been used for many years in endodontics and was originally used in canal preparation. However, because of its ease of breakage, it is confined to removal of soft tissue

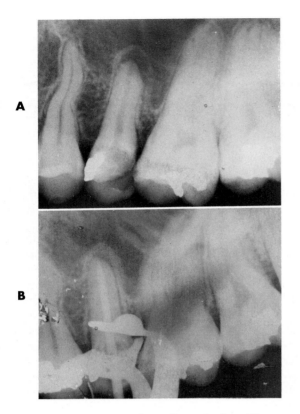

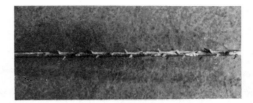

Fig. 7-2. Broach has small barbs protruding from shaft, highly susceptible to breakage when locked in canal.

Fig. 7-1. A, Preoperative radiograph of maxillary second bicuspid with large periapical radiolucency. Patient was a college student, home only for school vacations. Canal was debrided during Thanksgiving holiday, and second and third appointments were scheduled for Christmas recess. **B,** Five weeks later, when radiograph was taken for verification of fit for master cone, radiolucency had already healed. Poor fixing and scratches on this film have occurred because it is an intratreatment film developed ultrafast and is generally discarded at the conclusion of the fill appointment. The significance of this radiograph was not realized until later that day.

only. It is a tapered instrument of soft steel that is notched by a shredder to produce sharp barbs extending outward from the shaft (Fig. 7-2).

This design is responsible for the frequency of breakage, since the notching weakens the shaft by providing a place for fracture if stress or torque is applied. In addition, misuse within the canal may lead to disastrous results. If the operator attempts to force apically a barbed broach within a tightly fitting canal, the barbs will be bent toward the shaft, allowing for deeper insertion. However, when the instrument is withdrawn, the barbs will engage the adjacent dentin. As more force is

exerted in removal, the barbs will dig deeper and further fatigue may result in snapping of the instruments. *Therefore, once the hard surface of the dentin walls is felt, the barbed broach must not be inserted any farther.*

Correct use of the instrument involves its careful insertion through the access cavity until the dentin walls are felt or the approximate length of the canal is reached. The broach is slightly withdrawn, then rotated a few revolutions, and removed. Vital or necrotic pulp tissue and debris become ensnared on the barbs and removed so that much of the bulky content of the canal is debrided before files are placed toward the apical foramen.

The barbed broach is similarly used to remove the paper points or cotton pellets of intertreatment dressings, which may defy removal by excavator or explorer.

The smallest-sized broach available has approximately the width of a size 20 instrument. Since broaches should not be used until the canal is wide enough for comfortable accommodation, they are not used initially in narrow buccal canals of maxillary molars and mesial canals of mandibular molars. Once these have been enlarged to size 20 or larger, broaches should be used to remove the bulky tissue that has been packed into the apical portion of the preparation.

Methods for using reamers and files. Some confusion exists as to the actions for using enlarging instruments and the instruments themselves. Both reamers and files may be used with either a reaming or a filing motion.

Reaming. Reaming involves placement of the instrument toward the apex until some binding is felt and then turning the handle more than a full revolution. Clockwise turning will remove material from the canal by way of the flutes' revolution, whereas counterclockwise turning will force material apically. The major effectiveness of hard tissue removal by reaming is in the insertion of the instrument by shaving the dentin walls.

Filing.   Filing involves placement of the instrument toward the apex until some binding is felt and then removing the instrument by scraping against a side of the dentin wall with little or no revolution of the handle. This dragging against the side of the wall is also referred to as *rasping* action. The major effectiveness of hard tissue removal by filing is in the outstroke or withdrawal of the instrument by dragging the flutes on the dentin walls.

Considerable difference exists between using filing action and pistoning the canal. *Pistoning* involves going up and down forcefully. This push/pull motion tends to pack dentinal filings at the apex and alter canal shape in small, curved canals to create ledges and short fills. Filing involves a passive placement of the instrument to its working length and a drag motion against the canal wall.

Circumferential filing.   Circumferential filing is a method of filing whereby the instrument is moved first toward the buccal (or the labial) side of the canal, then reinserted, and removed slightly mesially. This continues around the preparation to the lingual aspect and then to the distal until all the dentin walls have received planing (Fig. 7-3). This technique enhances preparation when a flaring method is used by widening the orifice of the canal considerably, whereas the apical portion is kept relatively small.

Most roots are oval in cross section and are wider buccolingually than mesiodistally (the sole exception being the palatal root of the maxillary molar). If such a root contains only one canal, which many but not all do, it will be wider buccolingually as well. In these cases the circumferential filing is emphasized in the buccolingual direction. The oval canal is made into a wider and larger oval. This permits easier placement of precurved instruments, gutta-percha cones, and finger spreaders. Such a preparation is developed solely and specifically for gutta-percha canal filling rather than silver points.

Circumferential filing is modified by anticurvature filing (Fig. 7-12, *E*) when flaring the mesial canals of maxillary and mandibular molars and some other curved canals. This alteration will be addressed later in this chapter in response to avoiding strip perforations.

Studies have shown that the action of using the instrument, rather than the instrument used, determines the general shape of the canal preparation.

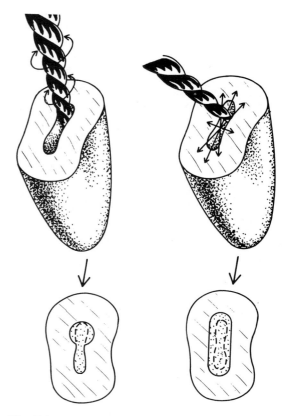

Fig. 7-3. Most roots are oval in cross section, and many have a single oval canal. If the dentist attempts to prepare such a canal with reaming action *(top left)*, the result will be a canal with a keyhole shape *(bottom left)*. This canal is overprepared in one segment and hardly prepared at the opposite side—an undesirable situation. However, circumferential filing *(top right)* involves placement of the file and dragging it out against peripheral walls, emphasizing buccolingual directions. The result *(bottom right)* is a wider oval that is enlarged in all dimensions and may be filled with compressible materials. This method also enhances making the orifice portion as wide as possible without gutting the crown. Circumferential filing is modified in some canals with anticurvature filing (Fig. 7-12, *E*).

Therefore reaming action produces a canal that is relatively round in shape. The use of filing action develops a preparation that is irregular, usually increasing any eccentricities in the original canal shape.

Reamers.   Reamers were the original intracanal instruments, used since the nineteenth century for removal of the contents of the pulp canal and for widening and smoothing the canal walls.

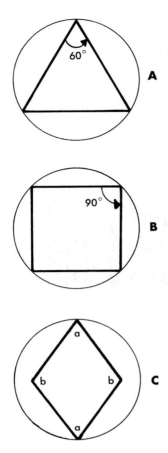

Fig. 7-4. Shapes of blanks for basic instrument systems. Each are twisted to give a different type of instrument. **A,** Triangular blank, as classically used for the reamer but now used in some files, has three angles of 60 degrees each to provide cutting efficiency and a moderate cross-sectional diameter for flexibility. **B,** Square blank, as classically used for the file, has four angles of 90 degrees each, not as sharp as those of the triangular blank, with a wide cross-sectional diameter that decreases flexibility. **C,** Diamond blank, as used for the K-Flex file, has opposite angles equal. Angle *a* is less than 90 degrees, sharper than those of the square blank, but these are the only two cutting angles. The cross-sectional diameter (line connecting the two angle *b*'s) is narrower than the square blanks of the same size, so this instrument has greater flexibility. Angle *a* plus angle *b* always equals 180 degrees.

They are manufactured by twisting triangular blanks (Fig. 7-4, *A*) to produce cutting edges. Because each angle of the blank is approximately 60 degrees, a sharp knifelike edge is available to shave and reduce canal walls. The cross-sectional

area of the blank is not excessively wide, so the instrument has a high degree of flexibility.

Reamers are used during canal preparation to shave dentin. When used with a rasping action, they are less efficient than a file. They remove intracanal debris with clockwise reaming action and are used in this manner to remove old gutta-percha canal fillings that have been softened with chloroform or xylene. By turning reamers counter-clockwise, the dentist can place materials such as root canal sealer and creamy medicaments in the apical portion of the canal.

Files. Files are useful instruments in endodontics for the removal of hard tissue during canal enlargement.

Whereas the reamer was the original endodontic instrument, the file was developed by changing some of the principles of design in an effort to make a more efficient instrument, one that would remove tooth structure faster. The triangular blank was replaced with a square blank (Fig. 7-4, *B*) and was twisted more to give greater numbers of cutting edges. Because the Kerr Manufacturing Company was the first to adopt this method, these files were called K-type for many years. The square blank had angles of 90 degrees, which did not cut as well as the 60-degree angle of the reamer. However, reamers had a half to one flute per millimeter, whereas files were given one and a half to two and a half flutes per millimeter (Fig. 7-5, *A*) and thus had many more cutting edges. The cross-sectional area of the file (from angle to opposite angle in the blank) was greater than that of the reamer, making it less susceptible to breakage, which was considered a very valuable property in the days of the weaker carbon steel instruments. However, the tighter wind of the file and its greater cross-sectional diameter decreased its flexibility.

The action of the file is to scrape the flutes against the canal walls to gouge a portion of the dentin and pull it from the canal. This action requires periodic cleaning of the instrument by the operator so the dentin shavings do not clog the flutes.

Files are efficient removers of tooth structure in any one of three techniques because of the multiplicity of cutting edges. They may be used with rasping or pure filing action only, in which they are placed in the apical portion of the canal carefully and dragged against one wall of the canal during removal. They may be used with quarter-turn filing, in which the instrument is carefully placed, rotated 90 degrees, and dragged out at the

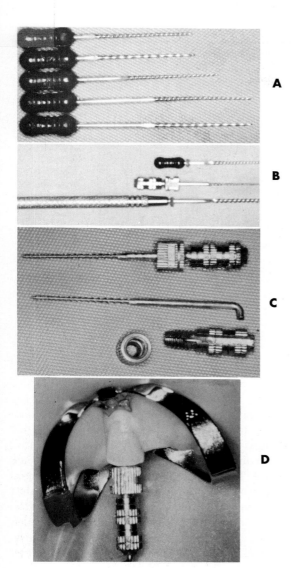

Fig. 7-5. **A,** Instruments are manufactured in different lengths as well as widths. *From top,* File, 21 mm; reamer, 21 mm; two files, 25 and 31 mm; and reamer, 31 mm. **B,** Different types of handles are available. *From top,* Short plastic handle, measurement control (or test) handle, long metal handle. **C,** Measurement control handle *(top)* is adjustable to allow for varying canal working lengths. Assembly consists of a file shaft *(middle)* placed in a handle and bolt *(bottom).* **D,** Once correct working length is set, bulky handle prevents overinstrumentation of apex by being physically stopped by incisal edge of tooth.

same time. They also may be used with pure reaming action and turned as they enter the canal.

Files alone may be adequately used in canal preparation. Some techniques suggest the use of reamers first and then files of the same size before going to the next greater width. The rationale for such a method is that the reamer used clockwise removes debris remaining within the canal and that, since reamers are slightly smaller than files, enlargement is facilitated. I have not found this necessary. Heavy and frequent canal irrigation followed by aspiration of excess lavage fluid will satisfactorily remove canal debris and dentin filings. Also, some companies manufacture reamers larger than files, or this difference may occur because of inaccurate quality control of instrument width.

There were virtually no innovations in instrument design since Kerr began making files early in the 1900s. Then, suddenly, in a year's time, several startling changes occurred in instrument manufacturing that tremendously widened the choices available. This is an extremely advantageous situation and verifies the important position that endodontics has gained with the general public and the dental community.

Need for flexible files. From the start of this century until the 1970s, molar teeth and teeth with sharply curved canals were rarely treated. When they were, a high percentage of failures resulted. In fact, Grossman wrote in his textbooks as late as 1967 that teeth with canal curvatures of 45 degrees and greater could not be treated successfully without surgery. Although this was not known at that time, the reason was that most endodontic files used then were rather inflexible.

As mentioned in the discussion of files, increasing cross-sectional diameter decreases instrument flexibility. Since the triangular blank, used for the reamer (Fig. 7-4, *A*), has a narrower cross-sectional diameter than the square blank, used for the file (Fig. 7-4, *B*), the reamer has greater flexibility than the file in similar sizes. However, files became the dominant instrument for canal preparation, and as such, a total decrease in flexibility of intracanal instruments resulted. Smaller files, such as sizes 10, 15, and 20, have narrow diameters (Table 7-1) and thus have sufficient flexibility to retain canal shape. However, in larger sizes, such as 30, 35, and 40, the files lose their flexibility very quickly, and alterations of canal shape may be devastating (Fig. 7-21).

To maintain shape in these curved systems, operators decided to keep canal preparation minimal, which may not have allowed for sufficient cleaning. Also, it was difficult to use a good condensation system to fill these minimally enlarged canals, so

Table 7-1. Diameters of standardized (.02 taper) and .04 taper instruments

Instrument no.	D₀ (original D₁)	Diameter (mm) at D₁₆ (original D₂)	.04 D₁₆
08	0.08	0.40	NA
10	0.10	0.42	0.74
15	0.15	0.47 *0.03 (48)*	0.79
20	0.20	0.52	0.84
25	0.25	0.57	0.89
30	0.30	0.62 *0.004.*	0.94
35	0.35	0.67	0.99
40	0.40	0.72	1.04
45	0.45	0.77	1.09
50	0.50	0.82	1.14
55	0.55	0.87	1.19
60	0.60	0.92	1.24
70	0.70	1.02	1.34
80	0.80	1.12	1.44
90	0.90	1.22	1.54
100	1.00	1.32	1.64
110	1.10	1.42	NA
120	1.20	1.52	NA
130	1.30	1.62	NA
140	1.40	1.72	NA

NA, Not available.

failures from inadequate filling were common. The result was that as an increased demand for treatment of these more complicated teeth occurred, it was necessary to develop new file systems.

In its first design change in more than 60 years, the Kerr Manufacturing Company modified its basic blank to develop the K-Flex file (Figs. 7-4, C, and 7-39). Rather than using a square or triangular blank, a diamond-shape blank was employed (Fig. 7-4, C) to decrease the cross-sectional diameter (the distance between the two "b"s in Fig. 7-4, C) and impart greater flexibility to the instrument. Because of this shape, only two angles of the K-Flex would cut into the dentin (angles "a" in Fig. 7-4, C). However, since these working angles were approximately 80 degrees, sharper than the 90-degree angles of the file, their cutting ability was compensated somewhat even though only two angles were present. Once the blank was twisted, there was an increased space between the working edges so more debris could be removed per outstroke.

The implication of instrument flexibility and other designs for flexible file systems will be discussed later in this chapter, dealing with preparation of curved canals.

Hedstrom files. Hedstrom files have flutes that resemble successively smaller triangles set one on another (Fig. 7-6, A and C). They are manufactured by means of a sharp rotating cutter that gouges triangular segments out of a round blank shaft in the same manner that wood screws are made. This produces a sharp edge that will cut on the removing stroke only. This process differs from that used for the standard reamers and files, which are made by twisting blades of triangular, square, or other shaped blanks. Several new designs have also been made by gouging, including the U-File and the Triocut.

The Hedstrom file, also called the H-file, has two serious drawbacks. It is weakened at each position of gouging during manufacture, resulting in a place for fracture if the flutes bind in dentin and the handle is rotated. Also, if it is handled incorrectly and rotated clockwise after binding in dentin, its screwlike configuration may further drive the instrument apically and crack the weakened and stressed root.

However, the Hedstrom file is an extremely effective cutting instrument because of the sharpness of the flutes. If used carefully, with filing action only, it will successfully plane the dentin walls much faster than the K type of files or reamers. The Hedstrom files are especially indicated in the instrumentation of immature teeth, where the

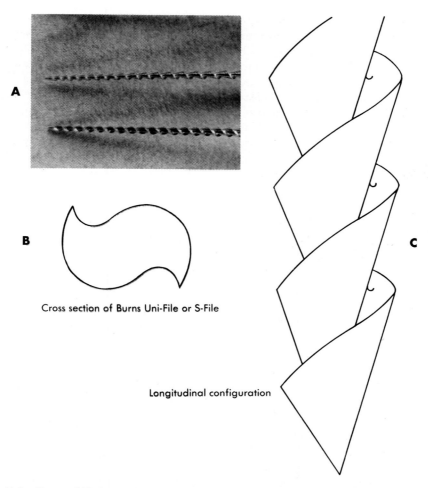

Fig. 7-6. Types of Hedstrom file systems, made from ground, not twisted, blanks. **A,** *Top,* Hedstrom file (also called the H-file), and, *bottom,* double Hedstrom design, originally called Burns Uni-File, now called S-File because of cross-sectional shape, **B,** indicating two rake angles for increased cutting ability. Wide cross-sectional diameter results in decreased flexibility for the S-File compared with the Hedstrom. **C,** Longitudinal configuration of the S-File demonstrates the design that allows it to cut deeply on the outstroke, minimizing packing of dentin into the apical portion of the preparation.

walls are irregular and may harbor considerable debris. These instruments are also useful in removing silver points or loose broken instruments from canals. The file is placed alongside the material to be removed, then rotated, and pulled toward the occlusal (or incisal) surface. If successful, the file flutes will hook into the point or broken instrument, break any retention within the canal, and deliver it. When the file is used to remove silver points, canal irrigation with chloroform to dissolve the root canal sealer should precede an attempt at dislodgement.

The Hedstrom and the other gouged instruments are strong, aggressive cutters. As such, they are potentially hazardous in the medium sizes of the apical portion of curved canals. For the same reason, however, they are excellent in widening straight canals or the straight, more coronal portion of curved canals. These files are well suited for performing preflaring or reverse flaring procedures, widening the orifices of any canals for easier placement of smaller instruments, and also in placing filling materials.

Burns and McSpadden applied the Hedstrom design by double-gouging, instead of placing a single groove, to create what they called the Uni-File, now referred to as the S-File because of its form in cross-section (Fig. 7-6, *B*). This instrument is even more aggressive than the Hedstrom file, so its cutting capacity is increased. It is excellent for reverse flaring, but since it has a wider diameter than the normal Hedstrom, it has less flexibility and can alter canal shape more quickly in curved canals. The S-File also was designed to have markings on the shaft to indicate working lengths of greater than 16 mm, an innovation now copied in several other instrument designs.

Styles of instruments. Files and reamers come in different lengths and widths and with various types of handles (Fig. 7-5). The shorter instruments are excellent for use in posterior teeth, but extremely long teeth, particularly maxillary cuspids, require those with the longest shaft. Long-handled instruments may be used for maxillary anterior teeth.

The measurement control handle (or test handle) may appear to be bulky and uncomfortable to use but is extremely useful for the dentist who confines endodontic efforts to single-rooted teeth. The length of instrument is governed by the handle, which physically stops the tip from penetrating too far past the cusp or incisal edge (Fig. 7-5, *C* and *D*). Once the working length of the tooth is correctly established, the files may be set and instrumentation carried out without fear of unintentional overinstrumentation due to misreading of the stop. The handle may also be used in the sectional method for silver points. (See Chapter 10.)

For many years it was common practice for any dentist, even a specialist, to use one type of endodontic file system. Whatever type or condition of canal was encountered, that one system had to do the job. Recent studies have indicated that if a large variety of teeth are to be treated, several types of file systems will be necessary, perhaps even including both hand and mechanical instruments. The more flexible files are best used in curved canals but take too long for work in wider, straight canals. Aggressive files or mechanical instruments are well suited for flaring but are dangerous at the tips of curved canals. New instruments of the future may have even more specific purposes.

Standardization. One of the most significant advances in endodontics has been the installation of a standardized system for intracanal instruments. As originally suggested by Ingle, this logical but long-overlooked development has been one of the greatest aids in bringing endodontic procedures within the scope and ability of the average dentist.

Prestandardization instruments. Before the establishment of standardization, endodontic instruments were numbered from 1 to 12. There was no system for determining instrument taper. The larger files and reamers usually had a greater taper than the smaller sizes, thereby causing great difficulty in uniformly enlarging the entire extent of the canal.

Gutta-percha cones and silver points similarly differed among manufacturers as to taper and length. Although the same numbering system was used for silver points as for files and reamers, these numbers did not necessarily correspond, even with the same manufacturer. Gutta-percha was identified by complicated descriptive terms— fine-fine, extra-fine, fine-medium, medium, fine, coarse, etc—that in no way really defined anything about the dimensions of the material.

Landmarks of standardized instruments, original and revised. In 1957 Ingle established a logical nomenclature for a standardized instrument so that all manufacturers could conform in length, width, and taper to a specific standard. Before this time, instruments were graduated from sizes 1 through 12, but these numbers meant very little. A size 3 meant that this instrument was larger than a size 2 and smaller than a size 4. The same number did not apply to different manufacturers, and in different years a specific manufacturer could alter any instrument size. Although canal filling materials were similarly loosely identified, this condition in enlarging instruments was devastating to the clinician.

In Ingle's system, which was endorsed and further developed by the International Standards Organization (ISO), the position where the cutting blades began on an instrument was called D_1, and the flutes extended up the shaft for 16 mm to stop at position D_2. The rest of the handle had no flutes, and its length was the difference between 16 mm and the total length from tip to handle. This length of cutting edges (length between D_1 and D_2) was to be 16 mm regardless of the length or style of instrument (Fig. 7-7, *top*).

Furthermore, the name of the instrument was to be its width at D_1 in hundredths of millimeters, instead of the antiquated 1 through 12 nomenclature. In addition, these standardized instruments all were given the same taper because D_1 plus .30 mm was established to be the width at D_2. This development of common taper made the placement of instruments in small or curved canals much easier.

Therefore, the name of each instrument gave considerable information about it. The operator knew how wide the instrument was at its working tip, how wide it was 16 mm up the shaft, and by dividing .30 by 16, it was calculated that each 1 mm of instrument length equaled 0.01875 mm (approximately 0.02 mm) of instrument width. To make this calculation easier and more useful, a slight accommodation was made several years later whereby the width between D_1 and D_2 was widened to .32 mm, or 0.02 mm of width per millimeter of length (Table 7-1). The standard ISO taper, therefore, was set at .02.

After many years of disagreement, several years ago an ISO committee made another change in standardization nomenclature. This change altered the name of the original site D_1 (where the cutting flutes begin) to become D_0, and 16 mm farther up the shaft was changed to D_{16} (Fig. 7-7, *bottom*). Several companies had begun to lengthen the cutting edges up the shaft to 18 mm or more, and the original designation of D_2 was not consistent enough (Fig. 7-7, *bottom*). The K-Flex file, for example, has cutting edges 18.5 mm up the shaft, which I consider to be beneficial.

Table 7-1 lists the widths of the instruments at the start of the cutting edges and at the 16 mm level (D_0 and D_{16}). It also indicates the widths of the non-ISO standard taper of .04, which is used for reverse flaring instruments and will be discussed later in this chapter.

In the prestandardized instruments it had been thought that there was often too great a difference in instrument width from one size to the next larger size. Therefore canal preparation became tedious and time consuming, since it frequently took great effort to reach the correct working length when using the next-sized-wider instrument. To rectify this problem, instrument widths were established so that only the differences of 0.05 mm would separate one size from the next in instruments smaller than size 60, with 0.10 mm between consecutive larger sizes. With experience in canal enlargement, the operator could anticipate the degree of looseness that must be felt with one instrument in the canal before the next-wider size could be placed.

Silver points and gutta-percha cones were similarly identified, sized, and shaped to conform more closely to the canals prepared with the standardized instruments.

Quality control. Materials and instruments manufactured under the specifications of the standardized system are certainly far superior to those previously available. However, it is difficult for companies to exert perfect quality control on their products, and discrepancies often are found. At present an instrument is still considered acceptable if it is within 0.02 mm of the standard. Therefore a size 30 file may be as small as 0.28 mm at D_1 or as wide as 0.32 mm. With the same assessment being

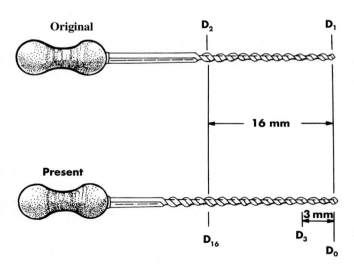

Original

D_2

D_1

Present

16 mm

3 mm

D_{16}

D_3

D_0

Fig. 7-7. Original and present (new) standardized instruments. The original standardized instrument *(top)* had the designation of D_1 at the beginning of the flutes and D_2 at the end of the flutes, 16 mm farther up the shaft. Originally the width at these sites was calculated to be D_1 + .30 mm = D_2, making the taper 0.01875 mm of width per millimeter of length, but this was soon altered to D_1 + .32 mm = D_2, or 0.02 mm of width per millimeter of length as the taper. In recent changes the new standardized instrument *(bottom)* was designed so that D_1 was changed to D_0 and 16 mm up the shaft was changed from D_2 to D_{16}, regardless if the flutes ended there or continued for several more millimeters farther. The standard taper remained as 0.02 mm of width per millimeter of length, but the new formula became D_0 + .32 mm = D_{16}.

made for filling materials, it is possible to attempt to use a 0.32 mm silver point in a canal enlarged by a 0.28 mm file, with unsatisfactory results.

Efforts are being made to tighten the degree of accuracy gained by the manufacturers to follow more exactly the originally suggested standardization methods. Until greater quality control is established, however, the operator should be aware of the possible inconsistencies and be able to anticipate the possibilities of a discrepancy and compensate correctly when one occurs. Filling materials must be tried into prepared canals and the correctness of apical fit verified by radiograph before final cementation. Such aids as a silver point gauge (Chapter 10) and customization of a master gutta-percha cone (Chapter 9) are often useful.

RULES FOR CANAL PREPARATION

For the best results in canal preparation, certain basic rules must be followed.

1. *Preparation must enlarge the canal while retaining the general form of the preoperative shape, but it also must develop the most desired shape to fill.* One of the most common faults occurring during canal preparation is an attempt by the operator to alter the canal's original shape. Overuse of reaming action, failure to precurve instruments, excessive use of chelating agents, and disregarding the path of the initial exploring instruments produce a preparation that does not include the original canal within its boundaries (Fig. 7-8).

The significance of retaining original canal shape may seem to be unimportant at first glance. So what if some variance occurs? How serious can that be? The entire problem may be seen in better perspective when one realizes that the original canal shape includes the apical foramen, the sealing of which is a prime objective of endodontic therapy. Because this site is at the tip of the root, a mild variance in the center portions of the root may lead to severe alteration at the tip, particularly if the canal is curved.

You may wonder how much alteration is permissible so the apical foramen remains within the final canal shape. Because of the minuscule dimensions with which we are dealing, there is not much room for error. Small canals may be negotiated initially with a size 10 file, which fits quite tightly at the apex. In other words, the narrowest diameter of the canal at that site is only 0.1 mm, and the total area of the file at that cross-sectional position is merely 0.00785 sq mm (Table 7-2). If the canal is enlarged apically to size 30, which is an average recommended size for such a small canal, the cross-sectional area there is 0.0707 sq mm. This means that the original canal of 0.00785 sq mm must be included in the final 0.0707 sq mm if the apex is to be sealed. If the canal deviates only a few tenths of a millimeter, this may cause serious problems.

The intracanal instruments must be used to enlarge the entire canal length to the apical foramen while still retaining the preoperative shape, not to produce a new or false canal. Obviously canal irregularities and large curvatures must be eliminated. However, if after preparation is completed the tooth could be superimposed over the preoperative configuration, the original canal shape must lie within the final preparation.

Based on these considerations and the physical principles involved, an ideal shape of preparation should be developed. This shape could be **as narrow as possible at the apex consistent with cleaning the canal and as wide as possible at the orifice consistent with not gutting the crown.**

Many of the procedures that are strongly encouraged in this chapter, such as flaring, reverse flaring, circumferential filing, and use of rasping action, enhance obtaining this desired shape.

2. *Once the working length of a tooth is determined, all instruments must be kept within the confines of the canal.* Overinstrumentation, or the continued passage of an intracanal instrument through the apical foramen, is a frequent cause of intratreatment pain. If the apical constriction is consistently broken during instrumentation, there will be no firm dentin against which to pack or place the canal filling material.

Therefore, as soon as the canal working length is determined, that measurement is recorded and adhered to during instrumentation. The only possible way to ensure that the canal length is observed during the preparation is to use a measurement indicator, or stop. It is impossible to tell by the eye alone the length that the instrument has penetrated beyond the tooth. The use of the measurement control handle has already been described. For those who prefer metal or plastic-handled instruments, stops made of rubber band, Styrofoam, silicone, or plastic are available.

3. *Instruments must be used in sequential order without skipping sizes.* Once the canal length is determined, the largest-size file that will reach the apical extent of the preparation will begin the

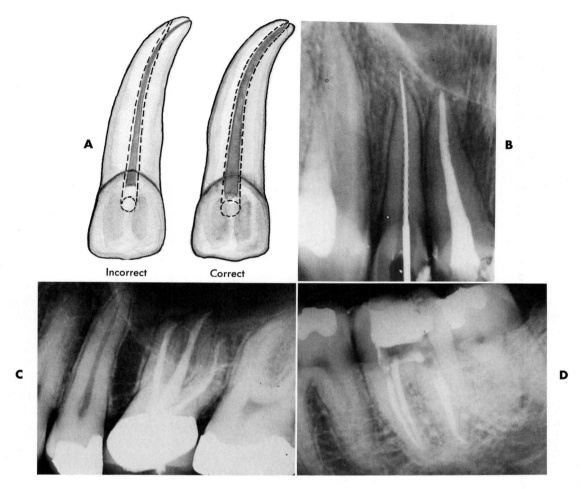

Fig. 7-8. Canal preparation must always retain original canal shape but allow for keeping the apex as narrow as possible consistent with cleaning the canal and the orifice as wide as possible consistent with not gutting the crown. **A** *(left),* Incorrect preparation *(dotted line)* does not include original canal *(shaded area);* correct preparation *(right)* enlarges original canal in all dimensions while retaining general original canal shape. **B,** Canal in lateral incisor has not been prepared correctly, and a false canal was produced. **C** and **D,** There are no straight canals in molar teeth, but rather canals with gradual gentle curves. Final filling radiographs must show that these curves have been enlarged along their entire lengths but that the general original shape has been retained.

Table 7-2. Correlation between files

Initial file that binds	Area at D_1 (sq mm)	Probable MAF	Area at D_1 (sq mm)	Final flare size
10	0.00785	25 or 30	0.0491 or 0.0707	40 or 45
15	0.01766	30	0.0707	45
20	0.0314	35	0.0962	50
25	0.0491	40	0.1256	55
30	0.0707	45	0.1590	60
35	0.0962	50	0.1963	70
40	0.1256	55	0.2375	80

removal of tissue from the dentin walls. Once this initial instrument becomes loose within the canal, indicating that it has enlarged the canal and completed the major portion of its effectiveness, the next-size-larger file must be used. This enlarging and then using the next-larger instrument is continued until the desired degree of preparation is obtained. At no time should file sizes be skipped. If a wider file is used out of sequence, it may be possible to gain the correct degree of apical penetration by rotary manipulation. However, such procedure may force the instrument to veer off from the true canal and start its own false canal or cause a ledge. Each instrument must fit smoothly into the apical portion of the preparation without forcing. If such is not the case, the next-smaller instrument should be used again or incremental instrumentation (discussed later in this chapter) should be employed.

4. *Instruments must be used extravagantly, particularly in the smaller sizes.* Every time a file or reamer is removed from the canal, it should be wiped clean of any debris with a cotton roll or other suitable material. At this time the flutes of the instrument must be examined for any sign of stress, fatigue, or alteration of shape (Fig. 7-9). If any doubt exists as to the condition of the instrument, it should be immediately discarded, particularly in breakage. There is no such thing as using too many instruments. When one considers the small cost of any instrument and compares this with the complications and aggravations that result from an instrument breaking within a canal, the plea for extravagant use is clearly defensible.

Sizes 8 and 10 should be used for a maximum of only one appointment and then discarded, regard-

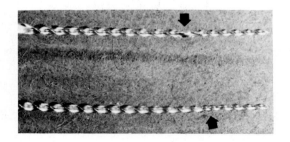

Fig. 7-9. Flutes with signs of fatigue or stress *(arrows)* must not be used in canal preparation. Instruments must be examined closely every time they are removed from canal for such telltale signs of danger.

less of the apparently normal-appearing flutes. If canals are very sclerotic and these small instruments are used for long periods, they should be replaced frequently at the same appointment.

Sizes 15 through 25 should be discarded after two appointments. To indicate when these instruments have been used once, so they may be discarded after the next appointment, a bur nick can be placed on the handle. When the tray is next cleaned, any instruments with nicks are known to have been used at one prior time and are thrown away. Those that were previously unmarred are then scored to indicate one use.

The flutes on instruments of size 30 or above are much larger and easier to see. These larger instruments should be replaced whenever any alteration from normal is noted.

5. *Canals must be prepared in a wet environment.* Heavy irrigation during canal preparation must always be observed. The preferred irrigating solutions are discussed later in this chapter.

Enlarging a dry canal may lead to packing of the area near the apical foramen with dentin chips that would prevent proper sealing. The use of an irrigant floats intracanal debris and dentin filings to the chamber, where they may be removed by aspiration or absorbent points. In addition, canal walls moistened by irrigants are much less likely to bind instruments, thereby reducing fatigue of the flutes and potential breakage.

DETERMINATION OF CORRECT WIDTH FOR CANAL PREPARATION

In addition to determining the correct length for canal preparation, a method for calculating the correct degree of enlargement must be clarified, both at individual appointments and by the time of canal filling.

Minimal instrumentation at any appointment— to reach size 25. The minimum degree of canal enlargement that will allow for the use of a broach to remove tissue bulk is that achieved by a size 25 instrument. Therefore this is the minimum degree of enlargement to obtain at the initial appointment for preparing any canal. The smaller-sized instruments begin to increase the canal diameter by removing hard tissue but merely shred vital pulp tissue, causing any remaining tissue to become inflamed. Tissue tags, debris, and other potential irritants are packed toward the apical portion of the canal during the initial phases of instrumentation. If these materials are not removed by broaching and irrigation before the end of the appointment, a chronic inflammation may occur, complicating subsequent procedures.

For these reasons, if it does not appear that an enlarging to at least size 25 is obtainable for a canal at any given appointment, it is best not to perform any enlargement on that canal. This means that in the treatment of molars, the first appointment would probably allow for access preparation, pulpotomy, and enlargement of the large canal. The smaller canals (mesial in mandibular molars and buccal in maxillary molars) are better untouched at this appointment, with even the taking of a radiograph for calculation of working length being avoided. At the next appointment, sufficient time will be available to enlarge the smaller canals to a minimum of size 25 and then allow for the broaching of the entire canal length.

This plan is possible in asymptomatic teeth or those where the inflammation is confined in the coronal pulp tissue. The medicament, usually some type of phenolic derivative, is placed over the orifices of the smaller canals and fixes the tissue and/or cauterizes the nerve endings. For symptomatic teeth with inflammation already spread to the smaller canals, sufficient time must be spent for proper debridement of the entire canal system.

Determination of apical width. The classic test for determining correct width of any canal preparation has been the finding of clean white dentin shavings on the flutes of the reamers and files. Although this is a seemingly objective and accurate test, I do not believe that it is correct. It does not necessarily indicate that there is a thorough removal of tissue, debris, and affected dentin; furthermore, it does not verify one very important requirement—that the canal is ready to fill.

Many canals are oval or ribbon shaped in cross section. Clean white dentin shavings are attainable from walls close to each other, but the far walls (poles) may be completely untouched while this sign is obtained. Figure 6-58, *A,* shows a central incisor with improper access cavity preparation, which forces the enlarging instruments against the labial wall of the canal without any preparation of the palatal portion. Clean white dentin shavings would be quickly noted, but almost half of the canal would be relatively untouched.

Bringing every canal to a similar size (e.g., size 40 in posterior teeth and size 80 in anterior teeth) is similarly incorrect, since some canals will be vastly overprepared and weakened, whereas others will not be sufficiently cleansed.

The optimal enlargement of each canal should be calculated separately; there is no hard and fast rule that is universally acceptable. However, I have used for some years a calculation based on the initial size of file that binds at the apical portion of the canal. In other words, if a size 10 file is put into a relatively small canal but is loose and does not remove dentin, it does not bind. In the same canal a size 20 or 25 files does work against the canal walls but does not reach the apical portion of the canal. A size 15 does reach the apical portion and does file the walls; thus it is the initial size of file that binds at the full working length. I then enlarge such a canal three full sizes larger than this initial file, or to size 30, using a circumferential filing technique. Obviously this calculation must be made for every case and will vary from canal to canal. The enlargement of the canal three full sizes larger than this is very standard, and the file thus used is a very important file to the remainder of the preparation. The file three sizes larger than the first file that binds is called the *master apical file* (MAF).

If the first file that binds is a size 10, a cross section of the canal conforming to D_1 of the file will have an area of about 0.00785 sq mm. The correct MAF will be size 25, and the cross-sectional area conforming to D_1 will be approximately 0.04909 sq mm or 6¼ times as large. This is a minimum degree of enlargement in even the tightest cases, yet going to this size of three files larger gives an increase near the apex of 6¼ times. Further up the canal the enlargement will be much greater. Table 7-2 lists initial binding file size, MAF size, and the respective diameters conforming to D_1 on the file.

Gaining sufficient enlargement for using guttapercha—the flared preparation. For many years the canal was enlarged at the apex and no further thought was given to the shape of the rest of the canal. Whatever shape it attained during the apical enlargement was not altered. However, many recent studies, particularly those by Walton and his group at Medical College of Georgia, indicated the great value of the flared preparation, in which the apical portion of the canal is enlarged to a specific degree and then the remainder of the canal is enlarged to even wider sizes to attain an exaggerated funnel shape.

There are many synonyms for flaring, including stepping and back-filling, but they all mean the same thing—proportionally greater enlargement away from the most apical portion of the canal. The studies investigating the use of flaring versus the classically taught method indicate that both degree of canal cleansing and ability to seal the apex are greatly enhanced by flaring. Those are very impressive reasons.

The flared preparation has several physical advantages:

1. The smaller, more flexible files are used in the apical portion, and the stiffer files need not be forced but are used short of the apex.
2. More apical dentin is available for the dentin matrix; thus if initial files are slightly too long, some dentin can retain gutta-percha within the canal.
3. Studies have shown that in curved canals, files often bind in the coronal portion and then become ineffective at the apex. With the coronal portion larger, files are more effective and may retain original canal shape better.
4. Because the canal is much wider, the intracanal irrigants have more room to gain access to the irritants and necrotic debris. This advantage and advantage 3 are reasons why reverse flaring works so well.
5. The wider coronal portion allows for easier placement of finger spreaders and gutta-percha cones.
6. The desired shape of a canal preparation is obtained: as narrow as possible at the apex consistent with cleaning the canal and as wide as possible at the orifice consistent with not gutting the crown.

Extremely large canals (i.e., canals that will accommodate a size 40 or larger) initially need minimal flaring after attainment of the MAF. The moderately wide and small canals, however, must receive flaring before using gutta-percha for filling.

Canal enlargement in moderately wide and/or straight canals.   Typical canals for this type of preparation are the maxillary anteriors, wider maxillary bicuspids, one-canaled mandibular cuspids and bicuspids, and the largest molar canal. Such canals will accommodate a size 25 or larger initial file and an MAF of 40 or larger (Fig. 7-10, *A* to *C*).

1. Enlarge the canal to the proper MAF according to Table 7-2. Making the MAF one or two sizes wider than the suggested instru-

ment is acceptable. However, if thorough rasping with circumferential filing is used, this is rarely necessary.
2. Select a file one size larger than the MAF and enlarge the canal 1 mm shorter than the working length.
3. Go back the full working length with the MAF.
4. Select a file two sizes larger than the MAF and enlarge the canal 2 mm shorter than the working length.
5. Go back the full working length with the MAF.
6. (Optional) Select a file three sizes larger than the MAF and enlarge the canal 3 mm shorter than the full working length.
7. Go back the full working length with the MAF.

Canal enlargement in smaller, relatively straight, canals.   Typical canals for this type of preparation are the mandibular incisors, bicanaled mandibular cuspids, and bicanaled maxillary bicuspids. The smaller molar canals and all narrow or curved canals also are suitable for this type of preparation, but they are better treated with reverse flaring, discussed later in this chapter. These require a size 10 or 15 as the initial file to bind at the full working length (Figs. 7-10, *D* to *G*, and 7-11).

1. Enlarge the canal slowly and carefully to size 30 at the full working length. Use incremental instrumentation (next section) if there is any difficulty in moving up to the next size. Use carbamide peroxide (Gly-Oxide) as irrigant up to size 20 and then switch to sodium hypochlorite. Emphasize rasping action. (Experienced operators may halt preparation at size 25 if the initial file that bound was no. 10. However, it is difficult to use size 25 gutta-percha, and I do not recommend it until many of the narrower canals have been successfully treated. Even size 30 may be difficult for many operators, and small canals will need enlargement to size 35 for gutta-percha; or silver points may be used for the smaller canals.)
2. Use size 35 file at 1 mm short of the working length and enlarge the canal.
3. Go back the full working length with the no. 30.
4. Use size 40 at 2 mm shorter than the full working length and enlarge the canal.

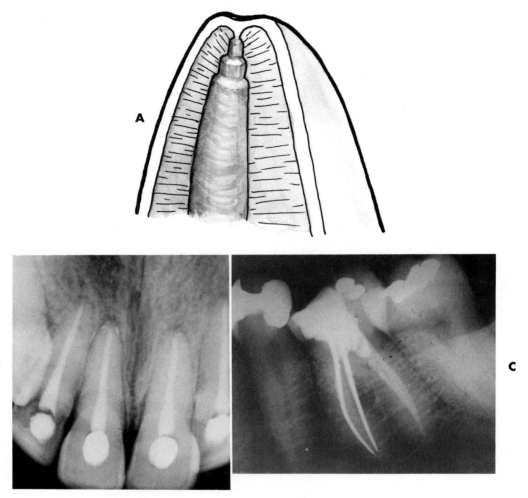

Fig. 7-10. Flared preparation that enhances keeping the apex as narrow as possible consistent with cleaning the canal and making the orifice as wide as possible without gutting the crown. **A,** Schematic drawing of flared preparation in a relatively straight canal. Apical area remains relatively small in order to retain the gutta-percha, whereas width increases toward coronal portion of preparation to allow for easier insertion of gutta-percha and finger spreaders. Each step is approximately 1 mm in length, with file widths one size wider than the more apical section. The MAF always is used after any wider file short of the full working length. **B,** Flared preparation in anterior teeth filled with gutta-percha. **C,** Flared preparation was used for distal canal of this mandibular molar, which was filled with gutta-percha. Mesial canals were filled with silver points; therefore no flaring.

Continued

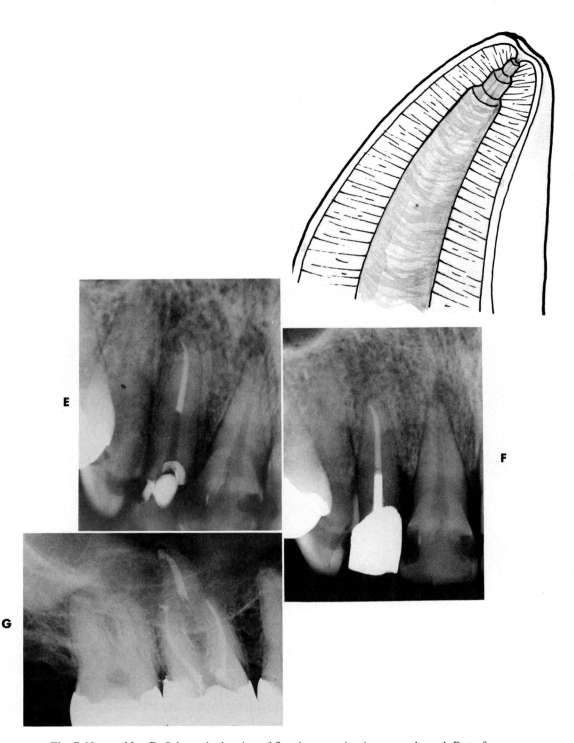

Fig. 7-10, cont'd. **D,** Schematic drawing of flared preparation in a curved canal. Part of preparation is at expense of inner portion of the curve. It is unwise to use more than three or four steps in the flaring because a strip perforation may result. This preparation will allow for placement and condensation of gutta-percha with finger spreaders. **E,** Maxillary lateral incisor enlarged apically to size 35 and flared to size 50, filled with laterally condensed gutta-percha and Wach's paste. (If I were to treat teeth similar to those in **E** and **G** now, I would use reverse flaring for greater ease of preparation.) **F,** Twelve years after treatment, area has maintained normal condition. **G,** Maxillary first molar with curved canals. Note well-retained original canal shape, filled with laterally condensed gutta-percha and Wach's paste. Palatal was enlarged to size 45 and flared to size 55, mesiobuccal was enlarged to size 30 and flared to size 40, and distobuccal was enlarged to size 30 and flared to size 45. (**F,** Restoration by Dr. Sherwin Strauss, Chicago.)

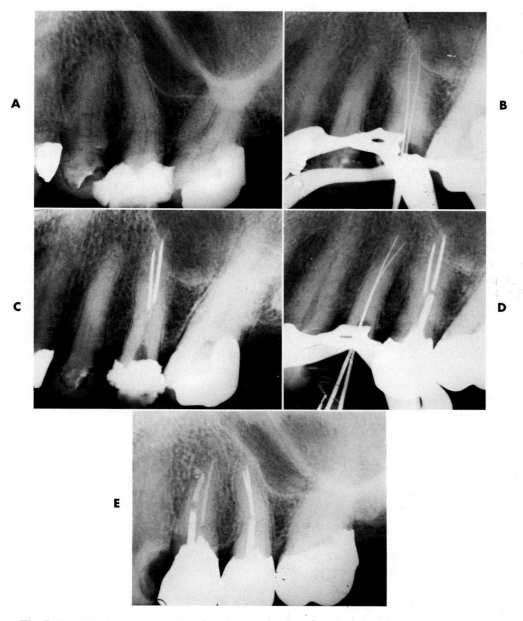

Fig. 7-11.   Flared preparation allows for use of gutta-percha. **A,** Radiograph of maxillary second bicuspid in a 71-year-old patient. **B,** Size 15 files in place to desired working lengths. **C,** Canals were enlarged with difficulty to size 25 and filled with sectioned silver points. **D,** Two years later the patient was referred for treatment of the first bicuspid. Again, size 15 files are in place to working lengths. **E,** Canals were enlarged apically to size 27 but were flared so gutta-percha, the preferable filling material, could be used. One year after treatment of the first bicuspid. (Restorations by Dr. Arnold Wax, Chicago.)

5. Go back the full working length with the no. 30.
6. Use size 45 at 3 mm shorter than the full working length and enlarge the canal.
7. Go back the full working length with the no. 30.

(For those who started preparation with the size 10 file and were comfortable with using no. 25 as the MAF, use files 30, 35, and 45 as the flaring files at 1 mm, 2 mm, and 3 mm shorter, respectively.)

Importance of using MAF as final instrument after using flaring files short of the working length. Failing to use the MAF the full working length as the last file in the canal will lead to serious errors, particularly in the smaller curved canals. Using the wider flaring files short of the working length leaves small ledges in the canal and may pack dentinal filings toward the apex. It is imperative that the MAF always be used last so a smooth passage for the gutta-percha is available the full working length.

Overuse and abuse of flaring. Just as with any technique that gives favorable results, flaring may be overused and abused. In smaller curved canals, only three steps or flaring files should be used. This is particularly true in the roots that are figure-eight in cross section, such as mandibular incisors, the mesial root of mandibular molars, and the mesiobuccal roots of maxillary molars. If these canals are flared too widely (Fig. 7-12, A to C), a perforation into the periodontal ligament space will result on the inner portion of the curve. This is called a *strip perforation* and may be several millimeters in length. If this stripped area is solidly filled with minimal extrusion of filling materials (not as in Fig. 7-12, A to C), the area may remain normal. However, in many cases the site breaks down, and a periodontal-type lesion results.

To minimize strip perforations, anticurvature filing should be employed. As investigated by Lim and Stock, this method is substituted for circumferential filing so that the wall toward the depression receives decreased rasping action (Fig. 7-12, D). In the mesiolingual canal of the mandibular molar, the rasping may be acceptable to the lingual and the mesial, but it is decreased to the distal and buccal because that is the position of the distal depression of the mesial root.

For the mesiobuccal canal of the maxillary and mandibular molars, the rasping may be acceptable to the mesial and buccal, but it is decreased to the distal and lingual. In narrow mandibular incisors, the rasping is acceptable to the buccal and lingual but minimized to the mesial and distal.

Final test for completion of canal preparation—placement of the finger spreader. When canals are filled with gutta-percha, it is imperative that the apical portion of the filling be condensed and deformed into the seat of the preparation. If the gutta-percha is not deformed at the apex, the canal filling will not achieve its function. Therefore the finger spreaders must be able to reach to within 1 mm of the working length.

To verify that the spreaders can reach that depth of penetration, they must be tried in the canal before the condensation procedure. If they do not reach too near the apex before placement of the cones, they surely will have no chance to reach that depth later when cones are in the canal. If they do not reach the desired length, the canal is not ready to receive the filling and further preparation is necessary.

The most consistent reason for spreaders to be short of the desired length is that insufficient flaring has taken place. The exact rationale for this statement appears later in this chapter in the discussion of the elbow. The clinical procedure to follow when the spreader is short is to use more rasping and circumferential filing with the flaring files, always going back to full working length with the MAF.

Completing canal preparation when using silver points. With silver point cases, canal flaring is not performed. It is desirable to keep the walls of the preparation only slightly tapered because that is the shape of the solid filling material. When flaring is performed, the taper is strongly accentuated. Then the silver cones have little adaptation to the canal walls, and this is contrary to the desired objective (Fig. 7-10, C).

AIDS FOR PREPARING DIFFICULT CANALS

At this point, I begin the discussion of preparation for the most difficult types of canals—those with considerable curves. For the clinician who does not desire to treat these types of teeth, preferring anterior teeth and the easier bicuspids, please skip this portion and go on to the discussion on p. 000, dealing with the use of ultrasonics.

It would be pleasant if only maxillary central incisors required endodontic therapy. Unfortunately, any tooth in the dental arch may require treatment, and in many cases the canal preparation may become complex. When canals are long, sclerotic,

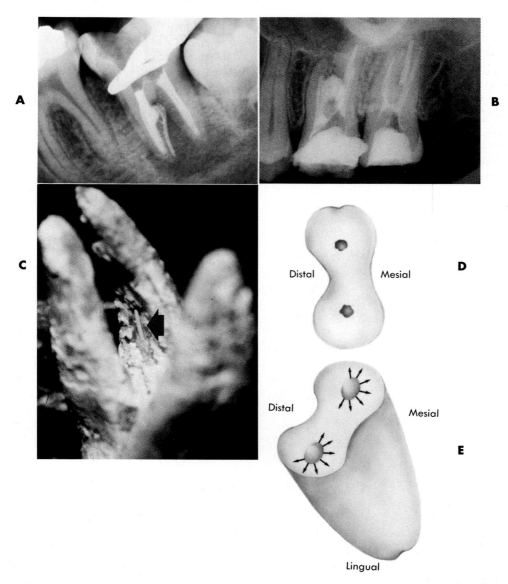

Fig. 7-12. Problems of strip perforations, often due to overzealous and inappropriate use of flaring. **A,** Mandibular second molar mesiobuccal canal was enlarged apically to size 40, but then was flared to size 90—much too widely—and perforation resulted because of the concavity on the distal surface of the mesial root. **B,** Radiograph of maxillary first molar with strip perforation of the mesiobuccal root. **C,** Photograph of an extracted maxillary first molar flared to size 70. A gutta-percha cone was placed into the canal, and the strip perforation is seen on the distal surface of the mesiobuccal root. *(arrow)* **D,** Diagram of mesial root of mandibular molar or mesiobuccal root of maxillary molar when two canals are present. There are depressions (concavities) on both surfaces, but they are much deeper on the distal surface. That fact plus the curve of these roots, first to the mesial and then to the distal, will cause a strip perforation when these canals are enlarged or flared too widely. **E,** To minimize the chances for strip perforations, final flare sizes must be restricted in these roots, and circumferential filing (Fig. 7-3) must be modified to avoid the dangerous distal depression. Instead of filing all around the circumference, the anticurvature method is used in these roots. For the mesiobuccal canal, filing to the distal and lingual directions is decreased; for the mesiolingual canal, filing to the distal and buccal directions is decreased.

or curved (and any combination of these difficulties may occur and cause even greater problems), only careful and meticulous technique will yield a safe and efficient enlargement.

Problems encountered in canal preparation. The most frequent problems occurring in canal preparation are root perforation, ledging, and instrument breakage (Fig. 7-13). Although any of these conditions may happen to even the best operator, it is important to develop the ability to keep such occurrences to an absolute minimum.

These problems usually occur as a result of forcing and driving the instrument, overuse of reaming action, and overreliance on chelating agents. To gain the full length of a sclerotic canal, it is often necessary to turn slightly, wiggle, or otherwise plunge with the initial exploring instrument. However, once the full working length has been obtained and the canal shown to be patent, all other instruments must go easily to place with a straight, inserting action. Because the endodontic enlarging instruments resemble wood screws, it is possible to force them into a canal and then, by using rotating or reaming action, to gain deeper penetration. It is precisely at this point, when the file is pushed against a wall, that a deviation from the original canal shape results, and then the operator creates his or her own shape. When files are

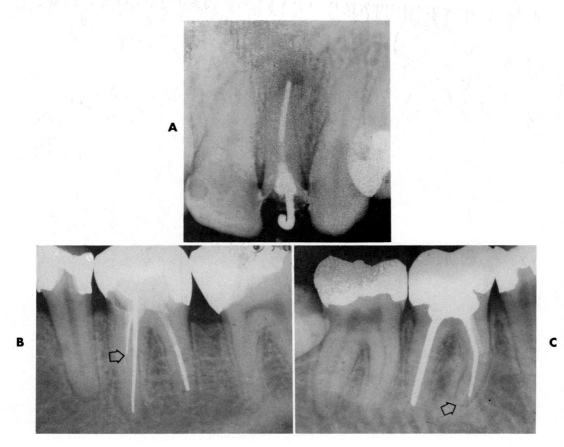

Fig. 7-13. Typical problems occurring during canal preparation. **A,** Root perforation following failure to retain original shape of canal. Although periapical tissue was normal before treatment, a radiolucency is now present, indicating failure. **B,** Ledging of one mesial canal prevented filling closer than half the distance to apex *(arrow)*. Radiolucency surrounding root, not present preoperatively, indicates probable failure. **C,** Broken file in one mesial canal *(arrow);* condensing osteitis around root indicates case is in jeopardy. (Although I treated none of these pictured teeth, occurrences of each of these types have been seen in my practice as well, but not since I altered my preparations as described here.)

forced into the dentin walls and bind, removal may result in breakage.

If chelating agents are heavily used, the canal walls are softened and may be penetrated and altered to even a greater extent by forced files used with reaming action.

Three important techniques may be utilized to prevent root perforation, ledging, and instrument breakage. When files are precurved, original canal shape is more easily maintained, root perforation is lessened, and reaming action must not be used. Incremental instrumentation allows instruments to be placed without forcing, and the correct working length is gained without the need to use forceful reaming action. With the step or flared preparation, the smaller, more flexible files are used to the full working length; however, the larger, more rigid instruments are kept away from the apex and confined to the straighter portions of the canal, where they do not significantly alter original canal shape.

Precurving of files. There are few straight root canals. Frequently the curvature is to the buccal or lingual aspect so that the routine radiographs give the false impression of a relatively straight canal. Palatal roots of maxillary molars often have a buccal curve, whereas maxillary lateral and mandibular incisors may have lingual curves that do not appear on the radiograph because the curve is perpendicular to the film.

In addition, as a result of eccentric dentin deposition or debris within the canal, the canal walls may have irregularities, projections, or other obstructions. When straight instruments are placed in such canals, they are stopped by the obstructions. If the file handle is rotated at this point, it will merely drive the tip of the instrument deeper into the impediment and create a ledge.

For these reasons it is best to enter canals only with files that have been precurved. When this is done, the file will have a better chance to traverse any canal curvatures. Also, if an obstruction is encountered, rotation of the handle will allow the tip to slide off and continue toward the apex.

There are two types of precurving. One is placing an extremely sharp curve near the tip of the instrument. This is used when the preoperative radiograph discloses a sharp apical dilaceration or when an obstruction is encountered. The degree of curvature to give the instrument may be estimated by holding the file over the preoperative radiograph and increasing the curvature until the configurations

of the file and the canal match. To avoid an obstruction, a short, sharper curve of approximately 30 to 40 degrees is usually sufficient. The other precurve is gradual for the entire length of the flutes and is to be used in all other cases (Fig. 7-14).

The sharper precurve is used when attempting to bypass a ledge from previous canal preparation and/or filling. When the dentist is re-treating a failing case that had short and straight canal fillings, the only hope for nonsurgical success is to reach the area of the apical foramen. Once the old fillings are removed or dissolved, using a straight file will merely continue the misdirection of the preparation. However, the sharply precurved instrument might be able to locate the correct direction and reclaim the case (Fig. 7-15, *B* to *D;* see also Fig. 10-4).

The curving may be imparted by drawing the instrument across a metal ruler, cotton pliers, or other sterile instrument (Fig. 7-15, *A*). The instrument must be resterilized before use if any nonsterile agent was used to give the curve.

Once the precurved file is placed into the canal, there is no way to tell in which direction the curve bends. To avoid this problem, the stop may be altered with a nick or flat end to indicate the curve. A rubber stop with a teardrop shape may be used, with the point showing the correct direction of the curve (Fig. 7-16).

The use of reverse flaring greatly enhances the ease by which precurved files may be inserted. The wider orifice will accommodate these instruments and prevent them from curling back onto themselves, which might happen when they are placed into narrow sites. Particularly in molar canals, without the orifice being widened, it is difficult to keep the curve intact, especially the type that is a sharp curve (Fig. 7-14, *A*).

Incremental instrumentation. The development of standardization increased the number of instrument diameters available for use, particularly in the smaller sizes. Therefore it became easier to place instruments to their correct working length, without the forcing or rotation that might cause breakage or prepare a false canal.

Even so, in difficult cases even the small increment of 0.05 mm between instruments is still too great. A new instrument may not achieve the same position that the previously used smaller size reached. The solution to this problem is to create new increments between the established widths by cutting off a portion of the file tip, thus making it slightly wider in diameter.

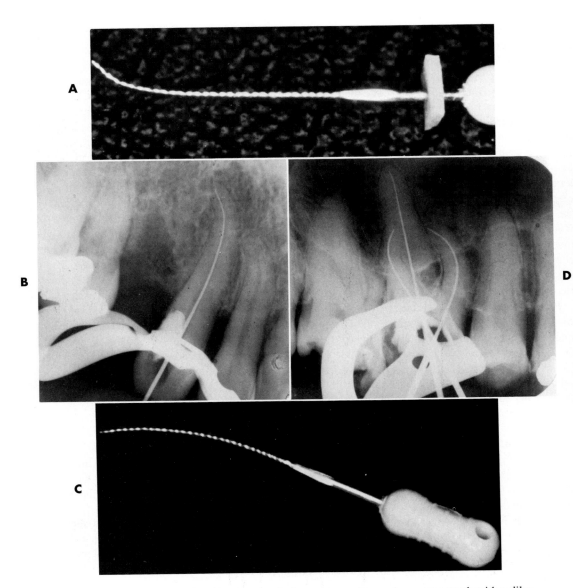

Fig. 7-14. Sharp bend at tip of instrument, **A,** is used to explore and prepare a tooth with a dilaceration, **B,** or to bypass an obstruction. A gradual bend, **C,** is given all other instruments. Use of straight instruments would make exploration of teeth similar to this maxillary molar, **D,** hazardous.

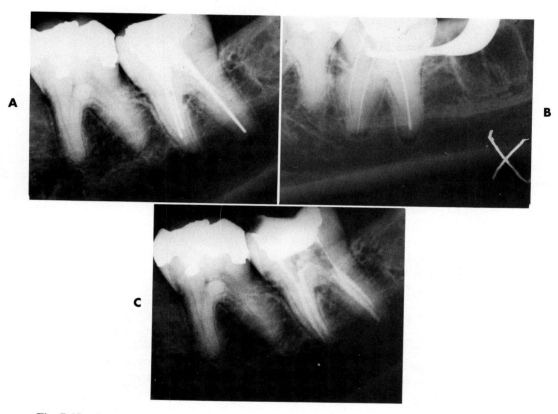

Fig. 7-15. Bypassing ledged canal by precurving files. **A,** Preoperative radiograph of mandibular second molar, 1 year after treatment with silver points. The tooth was tender to percussion, and the periodontal ligament space is thickened on the mesial root. Note that the fillings in the mesial root are very straight, even though the canals appear to be curved. **B,** The silver points were removed. If straight files were placed into the mesial canals, there would be no way to bypass the ledges. However, by sharply precurving the files, the correct position to terminate preparation was reached, according to this radiograph taken from the distal. **C,** Final filling of four canals with laterally condensed gutta-percha completes a successful re-treatment.

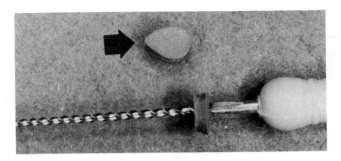

Fig. 7-16. Teardrop stop will aid in using the precurved file. Point of the stop *(arrow)* indicates direction of curve even when instrument is within canal. (Courtesy Dr. Arthur Rybeck, Jr., Wheeling, W. Va.)

As discussed earlier, the rule relating to standardized instruments has established that the distance between D_0 and D_{16} (the minimum length of flutes) is 16 mm and that the difference in diameter between these two points is .32 mm, or .02 mm of width per millimeter of length. Therefore, if a 1 mm segment is clipped from a size 10 file, the instrument becomes a size 12, etc.

To utilize this procedure in difficult cases, the dentist should routinely trim size 10, 15, 20, and 25 instruments to sizes 12, 17, 22, and 27, respectively, before going to the next larger size (Fig. 7-17). Because cutting the shaft imparts a flat tip, a metal nail file is used to smooth the end and reestablish a bevel after the removal of any segment.

In some extremely curved and very sclerotic canals, cutting off one full millimeter to widen the instrument by 0.02 mm is too great to enable the dentist to reach the full working length easily without forcing and/or using reaming action and thus potentially altering original canal shape. Therefore in these cases only 0.5 mm segments are trimmed, increasing the instrument width by 0.01 mm and making a size 10 into a size 11, etc. Again, the nail file is used after each trimming. In these extremely difficult cases, successive trimming of 0.5 mm and 1 mm segments can bring an initial instrument to a greater width than the next standard size. This works well, because of the possible variance in even quality-controlled instruments, to avoid the use of an incorrectly sized or marked second file, which might ledge a well-started difficult case. Unfortunately these successive cuttings reduce flute length; after 5 to 7 mm is removed, too little cutting distance remains to be effective.

New instruments with intermediate sizes. Because of the logic for making intermediate-sized instruments when treating the more difficult canals, several companies have now manufactured file systems that incorporate aspects of this technique.

Golden Mediums, made by Maillefer, are files made according to the standardized principles in the sizes that until now were available only by clipping. These files are available in sizes no. 12, 17, 22, 27, 32, and 37. They were manufactured so that the clinician did not have to clip files but instead had a readily available size in between the normally manufactured sizes.

The fallacy for this file system is that every file is not, nor need be, exactly what the D_0 designation indicates, but the standards allow a deviation of up to 0.02 mm to still be acceptable. Therefore a size no. 10 instrument may be as small as 0.08 or as large as 0.12 mm at D_0 and still be acceptable. This explains why sometimes the clinician may have great difficulty going from one size to the next larger in narrow, curved canals without using intermediate sizes. Perhaps the size no. 10, for instance, was in fact a size no. 8, and the size no. 15 to be used next was actually a size no. 17. In a narrow, curved canal it would be impossible to go from one size to the larger instrument without using an intermediate size.

By the same token, the intermediate sizes may almost overlap or even slightly overlap the standard sizes, even if manufactured with tight controls. A size no. 10 file may easily be size no. 11 and the size no. 12 (medium file) only slightly wider, perhaps no. 11.5. This would allow the medium file to go quite easily after the supposed size no. 10.

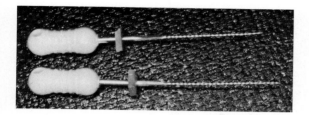

Fig. 7-17. Size 15 file *(top)* is compared to an instrument of similar size in which 1 mm has been removed from tip to produce a size 17 instrument. Note that stop has been moved toward handle of size 17 file to retain correct working length.

However, what if the no. 15 file was really size no. 16.5? It probably still would not go easily into a small, curved canal. What is available for the clinician to do? The answer is to clip the no. 12.

The only way to ensure that one size file is slightly larger than the previous file used is to clip the file. Any other method chances an error, no matter how tightly the manufacturing process is controlled.

Another recently introduced file system is the Series 29. Schilder has stated that even with the increased number of small-sized files introduced by the standardized system (sizes no. 08, 10, and 15) as opposed to the old 1 to 12 system (old no. 1 was usually slightly larger than new no. 10; old no. 2 was usually intermediate between new no. 15 and no. 20), more small sizes were needed in difficult canals. I certainly concur with the recommendation of intermediate files. Schilder proposed that instead of increasing each small file by 0.05 mm between sizes, they should be increased by 29%.

Therefore, if size no. 10 (D_0 to be 0.10 mm) were to be established as a key size, the file smaller than it would be 0.077 mm at D_0 and the file larger would be 0.129 mm at D_0. This system works well in these small sizes, but the difficulties begin after the fourth step, when one must go from a D_0 of 0.216 mm to that of 0.279 mm and then up to 0.360 mm. I do not believe this would be possible in a difficult, small, and curved canal. The only available solution, again, would be to clip the file to utilize intermediate sizes.

Need for remeasurement when preparing curved canals. As enlarging instruments are placed in and removed from curved canals, the flutes cut more deeply into the portion of inner surface of the bend. As preparation progresses, this tends to straighten out the canal to some degree (Fig. 7-18). In addition, through removal of this portion of the curve, the

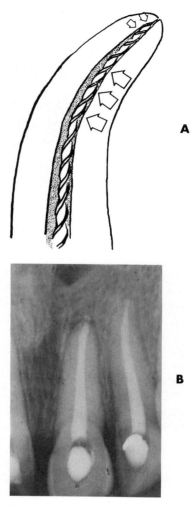

Fig. 7-18. **A,** When curved canal is being enlarged, flutes of enlarging instruments rasp more against inner border of curve *(large arrows)* and thus decrease working length. Because curved instrument tends to straighten, some pressure is also forced against opposite wall near apex *(small arrows)*. This may lead to a preparation that has an irregular taper with an elliptical apical portion, best filled by a condensation technique. **B,** Central incisor filled after an elliptical preparation. Note that from the access opening the canal tapers, but then it widens a few millimeters from apex. Drawing **A** closely resembles preparation of lateral incisor shown.

working length is effectively decreased because less length of file is required to go around the bend. Continuing to file at the original length will lead to overinstrumentation and resultant pericementitis. Since it is so important to have an apical matrix to pack the filling material against, failure to allow for this

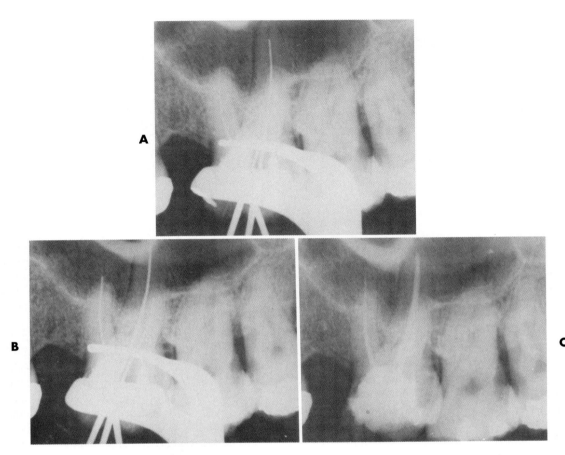

Fig. 7-19. **A,** Initial radiograph for length determination. Size 10 file in mesiobuccal canal measured 18.5 mm from mesiobuccal cusp and appeared to be in correct relation to apex. **B,** Verification after some canal enlargement. Size 25 file in mesiobuccal canal still 18.5 mm from mesiobuccal cusp. However, because of a decrease in working length by elimination of much of inner portion of the curve, file now passes through apical foramen. **C,** Since mesiobuccal apex was overinstrumented, no solid matrix of dentin was present to pack gutta-percha against, leading to overfill of that canal.

decrease in working length will complicate the filling of the canal (Fig. 7-19). Therefore, when curved canals are enlarged, radiographs to check for a new working length should be taken for every three increments of file width (e.g., if a size 15 file is the first instrument used, at size 25 a new radiograph is taken) and any decrease in working length calculated.

PREPARATION IN EXTREMELY CURVED CANALS

Many methods and techniques of canal preparation work well in the larger and relatively straight canals. However, when the canal curvature reaches 30 degrees or more, the complexity of the case increases markedly, and the techniques that render good results in the simpler cases may or may not be successful. This section will deal with the preparation of very curved canals.

Determination of canal curvature. Before the initiation of treatment, an estimate should be made as to the degree of curvature of the canals to be treated. As described originally by Schneider and then Jungman et al., the method for making this determination is quite simple (Fig. 7-20). Merely

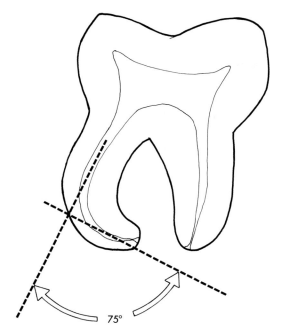

75°

Fig. 7-20. To estimate degree of curvature, imagine a straight line from orifice through more coronal portion of curve and another straight line from apex through apical portion of curve. The interior angle formed by intersection of these lines is the degree of curvature. Such an estimate is of mesiodistal curvature only and does not take into consideration any buccolingual curvature.

view the curved canal as having two segments, one extending from the floor of the chamber down the long axis of much of the coronal two thirds of the root and the second from the apex of the root extending back to the occlusal through the apical third of the root. These two lines will intersect and form four angles. The interior angle is the estimate of the degree of canal curvature.

This is merely an estimate and determines the mesiodistal curvature only without taking into consideration any buccolingual curvature. The operator should be aware of the teeth that typically have buccolingual curvature and take this into consideration. Common buccolingual curvatures are summarized in Table 7-3. The operator should also be aware of the shape of the initial files after they are removed from the tooth. Often some small, abrupt, or unnoticed curves will be indicated by an unusual shape in the file that corresponds to the true curvature within the canal. It is important to utilize this knowledge when further preparation is performed.

Observations that canal shape changes. As illustrated by Fig. 7-8, it is important to retain original canal shape. However it has been noticed for many years that the original canal shape may be ever so slightly altered with each file in a curved canal. Individually there is only a slight alteration between one file size and the next larger instrument, but the net change can be quite drastic (Fig. 7-21).

Performance of endodontic preparation has one significant disadvantage compared with that for operative or crown and bridge procedures. When preparing for inlays, onlays, crowns, amalgam, composites, or foils, the dentist may visualize the entire preparation at all times. However, during canal preparation in the course of endodontic treatment, only the orifice is visible; the critical apical areas are never seen by the naked eye. Only the radiograph gives some scant knowledge about what happens near the tip of the root.

In these more sharply curved canals, the shape changes more rapidly and may be undesirably altered, leading to potential failure (Fig. 7-22). Virtually everyone who has performed endodontic treatment on a number of extremely curved canals has observed these changes, which are more than merely subtle.

Plastic block studies. In an attempt to clarify the actions of the instrument during canal preparation, acrylic blocks were prepared that would simulate intracanal treatment conditions and allow for complete visualization of the procedures (Fig. 7-23, *A*). Small silver points were bent into a curve to simulate curved molar canals. The points were lubricated and placed in a mix of clear acrylic casting resin.* When the plastic hardened, the points were removed and a canal was left in the block. The Knoop hardness number of the blocks was 22, compared to 40 for dentin near the pulpal wall. According to Patterson, the number could be reduced to as low as 7 for dentin exposed to EDTA. The filing of the blocks felt similar to the filing of normal teeth.

These blocks were distributed to a number of endodontists and general dentists who had considerable endodontic experience. The practitioners were asked to prepare these canals in their routine manner. Some fascinating information was gleaned from analyzing these preparations (Fig. 7-23, *B*). For

*Dexter's clear polyester casting resin (no. 63-23505), Lee Ward's Creative Crafts, Elgin, IL 60120.

Table 7-3. Canal characteristics not seen on routine radiographs

Tooth	Buccolingual root curvatures	Buccolingual canal exiting
Maxillary teeth		
Central	Very rare	Short to buccal
Lateral	Distolingual common	To distolingual
Cuspid	Rare	Short to buccal
First bicuspid		
Buccal root	Buccal possible	Short to buccal
Palatal root	Buccal or palatal possible	—
Second bicuspid	—	—
First and second molars		
Mesiobuccal root	Distolingual common	Short to distolingual
Distobuccal root	—	—
Palatal root	Buccal very frequent	Short to buccal very common (Fig. 8-10, *E* and *F*)
Mandibular teeth		
Central	Distolingual possible	Many possibilities
Lateral	More frequently than central to distolingual	Same as central
Cuspid	Distolingual possible	Same as central
First bicuspid		Short to buccal possible
Second bicuspid		Short to buccal possible
First molar		
Mesiolingual canal	Initially to lingual, then to buccal	Almost always to distal
Mesiobuccal canal	Initially to buccal, then to lingual	Almost always to distal
Distal canals	Usually to mesial or distal	Any direction possible
Second molar		
Mesiolingual canal	Similar to first molar	Frequently to distal
Mesiobuccal canal	Similar to first molar	Frequently to distal
Distal canal	Similar to first molar	Similar to first molar

years it had been thought that after the completion of preparation, the narrowest point of the canal was at the apex. This was taken for granted, because it had to be true if endodontic therapy were to experience predictable successes. However, whereas the widest portion of the canals prepared in the blocks was at the orifice, *the narrowest site was never at the apex but was a few millimeters short of the apex.*

When the paper describing this study was reported by Weine, Kelly, and Lio, many strongly doubted its authenticity. They could not accept that in a curved canal which could be completely visualized at all times and with the file seemingly guided, as it could never be in a true clinical case,

it was impossible to gain a preparation narrowest at the apex. This cast considerable doubt over the veracity of the use of silver cones in curved canals because of the impossibility of the solid silver cone filling the biconcave shape. Even vertically or laterally condensed gutta-percha would have considerable problems here because a perfect funnel does not exist to allow for the packing down to the narrowest diameter at the tip.

In actuality, a study by Gutierrez and Garcia 7 years earlier on extracted teeth had reported many of these same observations, particularly concerning the tip of the preparation. These authors had stated that an hourglass shape existed at that site, whereby the narrowest point was not at the tip of

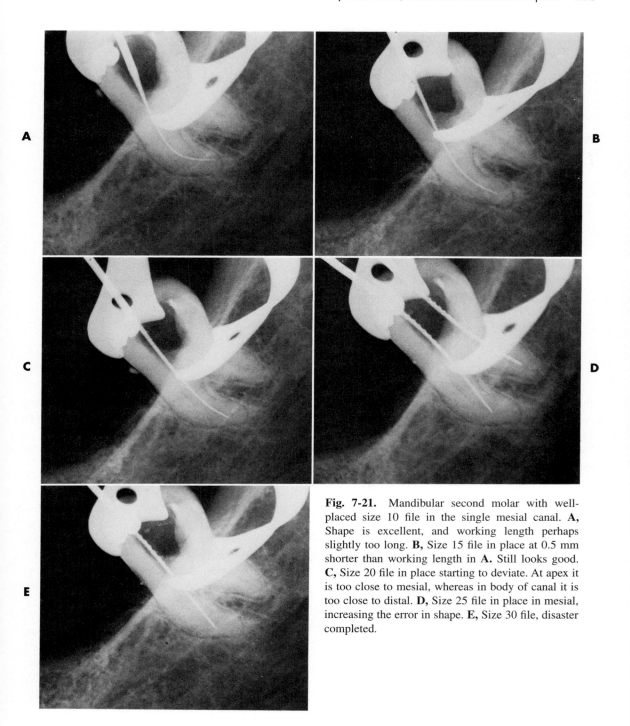

Fig. 7-21. Mandibular second molar with well-placed size 10 file in the single mesial canal. **A,** Shape is excellent, and working length perhaps slightly too long. **B,** Size 15 file in place at 0.5 mm shorter than working length in **A.** Still looks good. **C,** Size 20 file in place starting to deviate. At apex it is too close to mesial, whereas in body of canal it is too close to distal. **D,** Size 25 file in place in mesial, increasing the error in shape. **E,** Size 30 file, disaster completed.

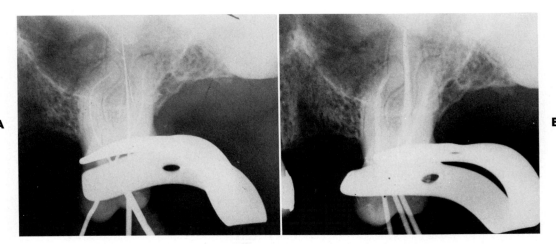

Fig. 7-22. **A,** Files in place to determine working lengths in maxillary first molar. Note that file in mesiobuccal canal *(left)* is perfectly centered in mesiobuccal root. **B,** When canals are filled, however, there has been an abrupt change in shape of filling in mesiobuccal canal. At apex, filling is too close to the mesial; in body of canal, filling is too close to distal. If this were to get too much closer on the distal, a strip perforation might occur. Fig. 7-24 explains this phenomenon.

the preparation but was several millimeters coronal from the tip. This was emphatically verified by the plastic block studies.

A further observation was made during the course of instrumentation in the curved plastic block canals (Fig. 7-23, *C*). During insertion or withdrawal, each file attempted to straighten within the canal, whether precurved or not. Therefore the file rode the inner portion of the canal between the orifice and the narrowest point of the preparation, whereas the file worked only on the outer wall between the narrowest point and the tip of the preparation. Between the narrowest point and the tip, each succeeding file went farther and farther away from the inner portion of the curve. It was impossible to avoid this tendency, even with increased precurving or attempting to redirect the file visually, which could be done with the transparent blocks but obviously not in a clinical case.

Viewing the base of the blocks, one could see that which would conform to the apical foramen gave an interesting perspective. In none of these blocks were the sites of exiting round, or even elliptical, but were teardrop shaped (Fig. 7-23, *D*). The narrowest portion of the teardrop was where the initial smallest files exited from the block with the sharpest portion of the curvature. As each

larger file exited farther and farther away from the inner portion of the curve, it widened the teardrop to that direction.

This situation may occur in a clinical case as well. When the final radiograph is viewed (Fig. 7-23, *F*), it might be assumed that the root tip had been perforated. In actuality, this is not a perforation but a slit or teardrop in the root tip. A perforation has two canals, the true canal and the false canal. In the apex that has been teardropped, the initial files made the curve but slightly overinstrumented the apex. Each succeeding file opened up slightly away from the curve, completing the error.

Because of this teardrop shape seen in Fig. 7-23, *D*, no possibility exists for such a preparation to be filled adequately by a silver cone. Condensed gutta-percha might be able to seal such a shape, but only at the cost of an overfill (Fig. 7-23, *E*), which will probably invoke a rather severe postoperative tenderness and cause problems in healing.

In addition to those critics who assailed the original Weine, Kelly, and Lio paper as inaccurate, many attacked the use of the plastic block as a substitute for extracted teeth studies or actual clinical cases. This view has now been reversed 180 degrees, and the use of plastic blocks has become quite dominant. In fact, if a new preparation technique

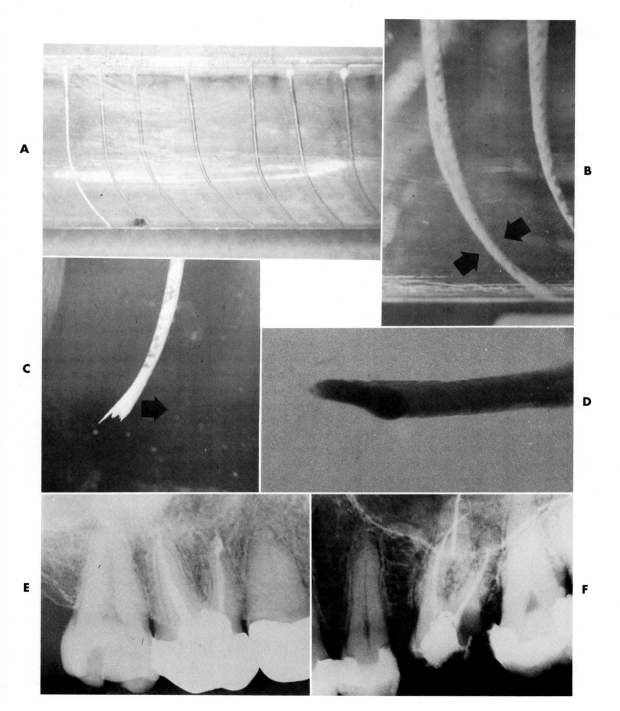

Fig. 7-23. **A,** Plastic block made to simulate curved canals prepared by curving silver points and pouring acrylic casting resin. **B,** Typical canal preparation *(left)*, which is not narrowest at apex but rather several millimeters from the apex *(arrows)*, illustrates hourglass shape. **C,** Canal prepared completely within block and enlarged to size 30. Path of the size 10 file was to the left and went perfectly around the curve. However, every file in canal after that went farther and farther away from curve in apical portion *(in direction of arrow)*. Even with a completely visualizable system, which is obviously impossible in a clinical case, it would be impossible to insert any file back down along the inner portion once the canal was enlarged to an appreciable extent. **D,** Cross section of block at level of arrow in **C,** demonstrating teardrop shape. *(left)* Position of size 10 file. Every instrument after that went farther to the right, with the 30 file farthest. **E,** Radiograph of maxillary first molar filled with laterally condensed gutta-percha. Sealer is exiting from mesiobuccal canal with a teardrop shape, demonstrating what has been done to tip of that root. **F,** Final radiograph of maxillary first molar. Note that mesiobuccal root was slightly overinstrumented and appears to be perforated. In actuality, apex has been moved severely to the mesial due to opening up of large files away from the curve.

or new endodontic instrument is introduced without an accompanying plastic block study, its veracity would remain in considerable question.

Standard preparation in the sharply curved canal. Observations of these block studies led to a number of interesting conclusions that were verified constantly, regardless of which operator was performing the preparations. The initial flexible files in a curved canal are able to make the curve and stay within the confines of the true canal (Fig. 7-24, *A*). However, as the larger, less flexible instruments are used, they do more work on the inner portion of most of the canal and on the outer portion of the canal near the tip (Fig. 7-24, *B*). The result is the misshapen canal that is so difficult to fill (Fig. 7-24, *C* and *D*). For want of any better names, the site where the canal is the narrowest was called the *elbow,* and the wider irregular area at the tip of the root was called the *zip.* A cross-sectional view of the tip is the teardrop-shaped site, and a canal prepared in this manner is considered *zipped.*

Applications on extracted teeth. To clarify their study further, Weine et al. slightly overprepared canals in teeth where the apical foramen came off shorter than routine, which therefore could be prone to such preparations. The results of these preparations verified that the plastic block studies were accurate. Custom mounts were prepared for these teeth so they could be rephotographed in virtually the same position before, during, and after preparation. The canals were prepared in a normal manner and the results analyzed (Fig. 7-25). In these teeth the teardrop shapes at the apices were clearly demonstrable. Radiographs taken during the course of treatment verified the existence of the apical zip, elbow, and hourglass shape. The correlation between these findings on extracted teeth and those of clinical cases is unfortunately true (Fig. 7-26).

Avoiding the apical zip and the elbow. Once these tendencies could be categorized and verified, potential solutions were devised. It seems obvious that in order to reduce the apical zip, we must prevent the file from opening up at the apex. The method I use employs the diamond-edged nail file, suggested for incremental instrumentation procedures (p. 325).

When the tip of the endodontic file is clipped to produce the intermediate sizes, the diamond-edged nail file is used to rebevel the tip of the instrument.

To avoid the apical zip, after the clip is made to gain an intermediate size, I drag the nail file

against the outer portion of the precurved endodontic file to remove the cutting flutes (Fig. 7-27) and thus produce a customized file—a file for that canal shape only. This should not be accomplished with a stone mounted in a handpiece. The distance between the elbow and the apex is estimated on the preoperative radiograph, and that length of flutes is removed from the outer surface of the endodontic instrument. I do this whenever the file is clipped to provide intermediate sizes. If it were done on every instrument in the canal, there would be no preparation on the outer portion of the curve near the apex, and the canal would be overprepared in the opposite direction.

The elimination of the elbow is much less difficult to accomplish. All that is needed is to provide adequate canal flaring. This opens up the bottleneck of the elbow and leads to a truly tapered canal (Fig. 7-28), which can be filled by a multiplicity of techniques and materials.

Application to clinical cases by using customized files. When these ideas and methods were applied to clinical cases, I found that the degree of apical zipping was tremendously reduced and that canal shape was retained in a high percentage of cases.

The curvature and the distance from the apex to the elbow must always be estimated in advance of the enlargement procedures. This is accomplished by measuring these distances on the preoperative radiograph and then verifying by the initial measurement films. On removing the first flexible file from the canal the operator should examine the configuration that the instrument has assumed. Frequently the curvature of the canal will be indicated by the curvature on this file.

When the canal has a curvature of 30 degrees or less, removal of flutes is not necessary. The canal should be prepared slowly and carefully, and if the curvature approaches 30 degrees, a flexible file system should be used to prepare the apical portion. In canals with curvatures of 30 to 45 degrees, one intermediate clip is required to minimize zipping, and a second clip may be used if there is any problem reaching the next full file size easily. In canals with 45 degrees or greater curvature, two or more intermediate clips are needed.

Use of reverse flaring. Reverse flaring, also known as preflaring, is the presently preferred development of flaring whereby the coronal portion of the preparation is flared before the completion of the apical portion. In the standard flaring technique, the apical portion of the tooth is prepared

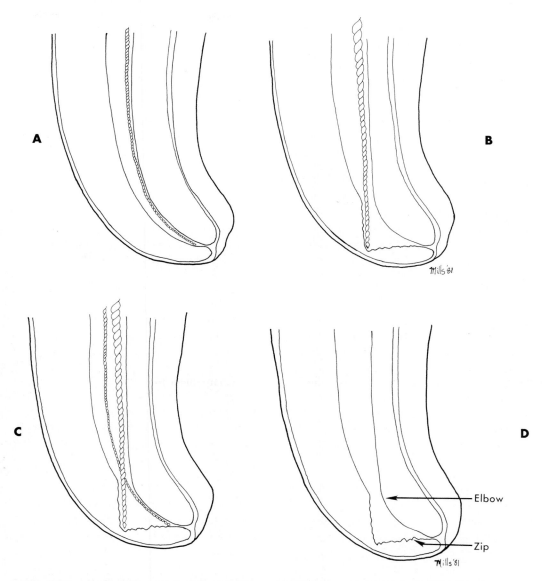

Fig. 7-24. **A,** Small files are flexible and able to traverse the curve with minimal difficulty. Virtually no alteration in canal shape results. **B,** As wider, stiffer files are used, each opens up away from curve near tip and gets closer to inside of curve between the tip and the orifice. **C,** Superimposition of **A** and **B** then results in **D,** the altered shape of a typical zipped canal. Preparation is not narrowest at tip but rather several millimeters from tip. This site is called the elbow. The zip, which is wider than the elbow, is the apical irregular area caused by opening up of files away from curve. A cross-sectional view near tip of zip is teardrop in shape.

Fig. 7-25. **A,** Apical view of mandibular incisor root with canal exiting short of apex to the buccal. This is a tooth that typically will be overinstrumented. **B,** Radiograph of file in place seems to be well within confines of the tooth. **C,** Profile radiograph of labiolingual view never seen with normal projection. Canal will be overinstrumented at a length that would seem satisfactory. **D,** Apical view after canal enlargement to size 35 at length indicated in **C.** This canal would be difficult to seal. **E,** Master gutta-percha cone size 35 appears to be approximately 0.5 mm too short. In fact, it was at least 0.5 mm too long.

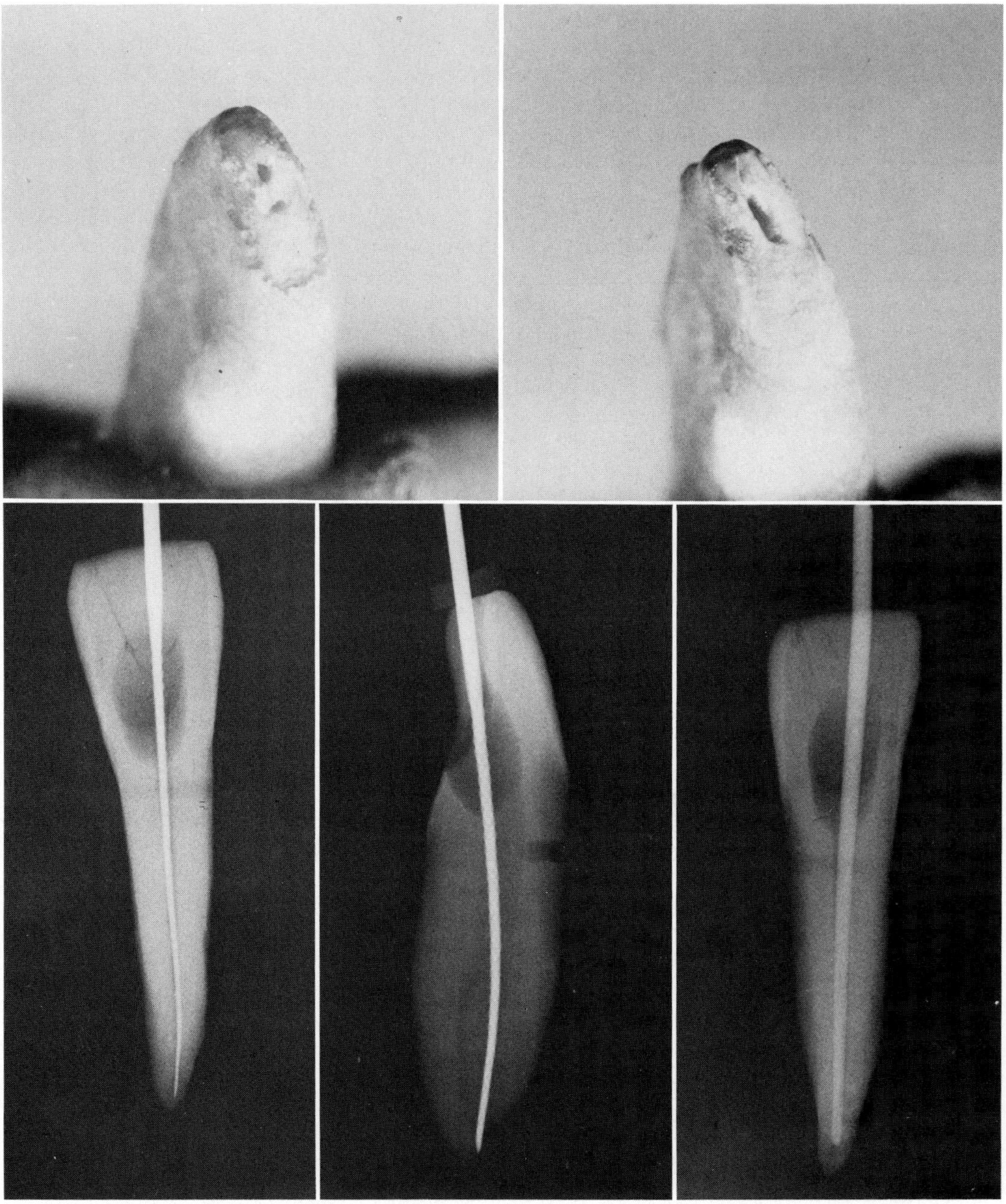

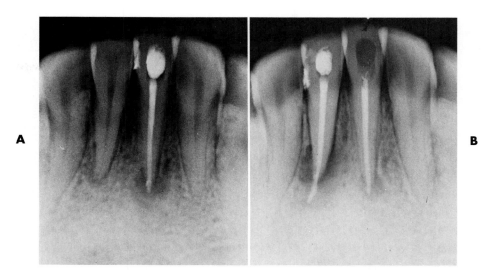

A   **B**

Fig. 7-26. Condition in Fig. 7-25 is not uncommon. **A,** After canal filling of tooth no. 24. Although I thought an apical dentin matrix was present, obviously I was incorrect; a considerable amount of sealer went past the apex. Poor as that case was, however, it was not as faulty as my attempt to fill no. 25 **(B),** in which I forced much sealer plus master and auxiliary cones past the nonexistent apical dentin matrix. Obviously these teeth both had apical configurations similar to those shown in Fig. 7-25.

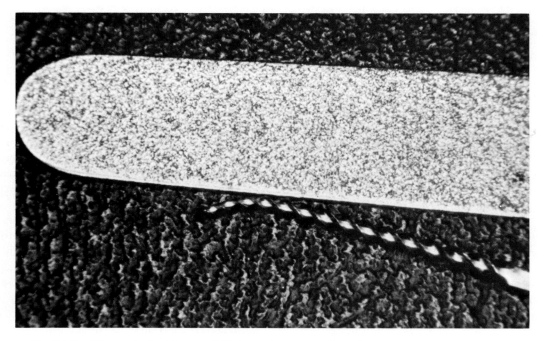

Fig. 7-27. Diamond-edged fingernail file is used to remove flutes from outside edge of instrument for intermediate sizes in treatment of curves of 30 degrees or greater. Flutes are removed from tip of file to approximate area of the elbow.

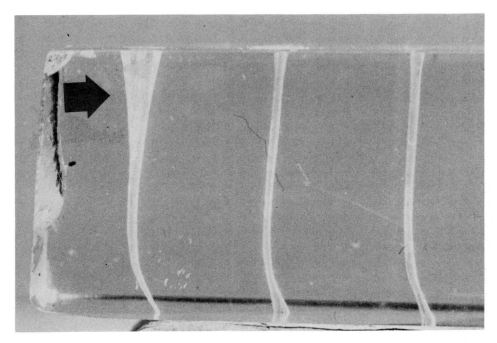

Fig. 7-28.   Plastic block canals enlarged with several techniques. Canal to left *(arrow)* was prepared by removing flutes for sizes 12, 17, 22, and 27 files, enlarging to size 30 apically, and flaring to size 45. Removal of flutes has prevented apical zipping, and the flaring has eliminated the elbow. This preparation is narrowest at apex, widest at orifice, and may be filled with many types of materials and techniques. Center canal was enlarged with a mechanical handpiece and has an elbow and zip. Canal at right was enlarged by reaming apically to size 30 and demonstrates an elbow and a zip.

completely before any filing is performed short of the tip. In the reverse flaring method, four aspects of preparation are carried out. First, minimal filing is done at the tip, followed by enlargement of the coronal portion. Then the apex is completed, and finally apical flaring is performed.

Although the final product would seem to be almost the exact same thing, this combination seems to have several advantages. As stated earlier, the irrigants are allowed to get down the canal earlier and farther to produce better cleaning. In curved canals (where this technique seems to be the most valuable), more effective preparation of the apical area is provided when the file has fewer obstructions in the coronal portion. Finally, files, pluggers, and filling material can penetrate to the apex more easily through a larger orifice.

The coronal portion of reverse flaring may be performed by hand instruments, ultrasonic devices, or mechanical instruments such as the Gates-Glidden bur or Peeso reamers. It seems to be accomplished quite well with some of the newer instruments

specifically designed for reverse flaring, which will be discussed in the next section.

Leeb reported finding a shape not generally considered in the curved mesial canals of molar teeth. Contrary to the belief that these canals were wide at the orifice before preparation, he found that a constriction often occurred at the orifice that made the canal quite narrow at this site. Thus the canal is narrow initially, becomes wider in the body of the canal and then narrows considerably as the apex is approached. Since these canals curve from the distal to the mesial in the coronal third, a triangle of dentin exists that guards the approach to the canal and must be removed to gain straight-line access to the apex. If this is not done, an artificially increased degree of zipping may result. Reverse flaring is a great aid in eliminating this problem.

The third edition of this textbook suggested reverse flaring only for canals with curvatures of 60 degrees or greater. Since that time I have used reverse flaring more and more, and now I recommend its use in every complex case. It may be used in all endodontic cases, even those that are relatively simple.

New instruments for reverse flaring. Because of the immediate popularity attained by reverse flaring, it was only a short time later that several new instruments were developed specifically for this technique. All of them have used deviations from the ISO taper of standardized instruments.

If one wants to enlarge only the coronal portion of the canal to a greater extent, earlier in the preparation procedure, examination of Fig. 7-10, *A* and *D,* suggests that a useful instrument would be one that is quite wide from the middle of the file up the shaft, but narrower as you approach the apex. Such an instrument would have an increase over the standard degree of tapering. This is exactly what has been accomplished with these new instruments that have been made with non-ISO standard tapers.

As described in the discussion of the standardized hand instrument, the taper of .02 mm of width per millimeter of length is present. For these instruments designed for reverse flaring, the taper has been increased (Fig. 7-29, *A*). The .04 tapers* are mechanical instruments produced to be used in a gear-reduction handpiece. They are made of nickel-titanium metal with a taper twice as wide as standardized instruments. The widths of the .04 tapers at D_0 and D_{16} are listed in Table 7-1.

The McXIM† (pronounced "maxim") is available in five instruments, all size no. 25, or 0.25 mm at D_0. The tapers are .03, .04, .045, .05, and .055 per millimeter. (To calculate the width at D_{16} of a .05 taper, merely add 0.16 mm to the column of .04 tapers in Table 7-1.) The McXIM is designed to be used in a gear-reduction handpiece as well, at approximately 340 rpm. The instrument is made from nickel-titanium in the Hedstrom style. It was designed by McSpadden, who advises always using a conventional file no. 25 down the canal before its use. Originally the McXIM series employed six tapered instruments with four file designs. After some use the technique was streamlined to the five tapers.

The Riitano files‡ are hand instruments made in several different tapers with a Hedstrom configuration. If these instruments are carried past the elbow, the potential for breakage greatly increases.

*Tulsa Dental Products, Tulsa, OK 74136.
†NT Company, Chattanooga, TN 37421.
‡Kerr Manufacturing Company, Romulus, MI 48174.

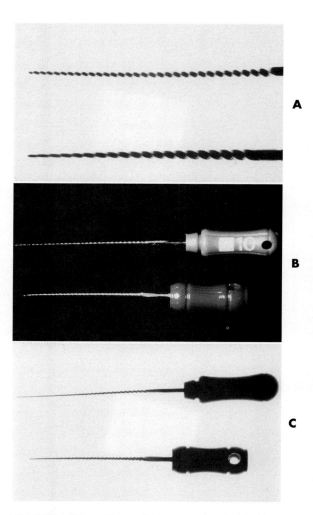

Fig. 7-29.   Files with non-ISO tapers. **A,** Shadowgraph of .04-taper instrument *(bottom),* approximately size 20 at the tip, but 0.84 mm at D16, compared to a size 20 Flex-o-file *(top),* which is 0.52 mm at D16. The. 04-taper instruments are made for a low-speed/high-torque mechanical handpiece out of nickel-titanium material. **B,** Riitano file *(bottom),* approximately 0.10 mm at the tip, 0.03 taper, and 19 mm length, compared to a standard size 10 file, 21 mm length. **C,** Shadowgraph of the two instruments. Even though both are 0.10 mm at D0, the Riitano file *(bottom)* is 0.58 mm at D16, compared to the standard file *(top),* which is 0.42 mm at that site. In these photos the Riitano file has a normal file configuration but will be using an H-type design.

Therefore the Riitano file is made in lengths shorter than the standard 21 mm (Fig. 7-29, *B*). The files are available in several different tapers.

When any of these instruments are used, it seems easier to prepare curved canals, and less

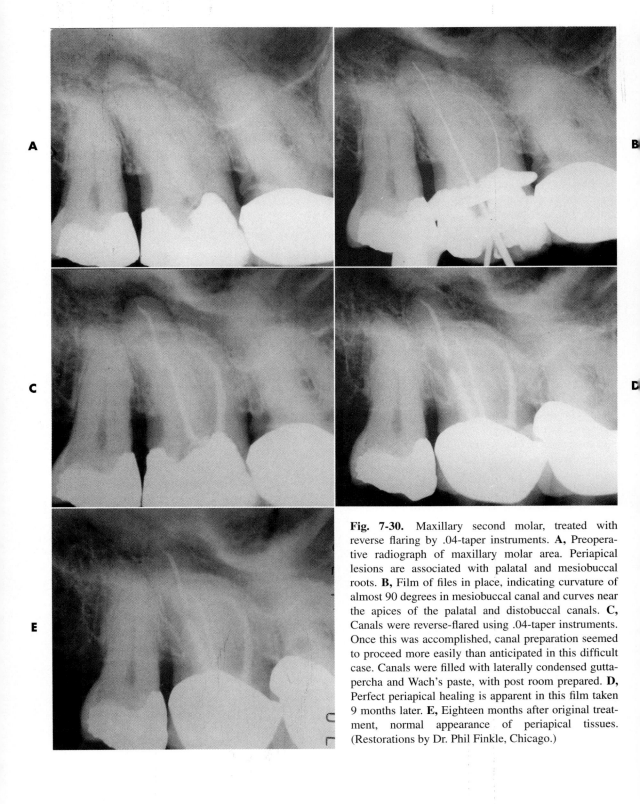

Fig. 7-30. Maxillary second molar, treated with reverse flaring by .04-taper instruments. **A,** Preoperative radiograph of maxillary molar area. Periapical lesions are associated with palatal and mesiobuccal roots. **B,** Film of files in place, indicating curvature of almost 90 degrees in mesiobuccal canal and curves near the apices of the palatal and distobuccal canals. **C,** Canals were reverse-flared using .04-taper instruments. Once this was accomplished, canal preparation seemed to proceed more easily than anticipated in this difficult case. Canals were filled with laterally condensed gutta-percha and Wach's paste, with post room prepared. **D,** Perfect periapical healing is apparent in this film taken 9 months later. **E,** Eighteen months after original treatment, normal appearance of periapical tissues. (Restorations by Dr. Phil Finkle, Chicago.)

time is required to accomplish this normally difficult task. Still the quality of treatment is maintained at a very high level (Fig. 7-30).

It is important to remember that if reverse flaring, or preflaring, is used early in the preparation and the flaring files do not reach to the apical third, the flaring described in Fig. 7-10 must be completed at the end of the preparation, as described in conjunction with Fig. 7-31 and 7-32.

The "crown-down" technique. This method involves starting preparation at the coronal portion with large instruments and then successively going farther down the canal with smaller instruments, in other words exactly the opposite of normal preparation. Although several studies have described and endorsed this technique, I have not found it to be useful or reliable. It is much safer to use an instrument the full working length (MAF) between every file short of that distance to verify that no ledge or stopping point is created.

Even if the crown-down does seem to work, I see no increased value over the reverse flaring procedure, and I do see many disadvantages if not used with exactness.

Typical cases. The instrumentation for typical cases is discussed next.

Curvatures of 30 to 45 degrees. This preparation was described in the third edition without reverse flaring as follows:

Maxillary first molar, mesiobuccal root (Fig. 7-31)
    Curvature = 40 degrees (Fig. 7-31, *A*)
    Distance from elbow to apex (estimated) = 6 to 7 mm
    Working length = 21 mm (verified by Fig. 7-31, *A*)
1. File with no. 10 file at 21 mm.
2. Clip 1 mm from no. 10 file (making a no. 12 file); remove 6 to 7 mm of flutes from outside of curve and file at 21 mm.
3. File with no. 15 file at 21 mm.
4. Clip 1 mm from no. 15 file (making a no. 17 file); remove 6 to 7 mm of flutes from outside of curve and file at 21 mm.
5. File with no. 20 file at 21 mm.
6. Clip 1 mm from no. 20 file (making a no. 22 file); remove 6 to 7 mm of flutes from outside of curve and file at 21 mm.
7. File with no. 25 file at 21 mm.
8. Clip 1 mm from no. 25 file (making a no. 27 file); remove 6 to 7 mm of flutes from outside of curve and file at 21 mm.
9. File with no. 30 file at 21 mm; this becomes MAF.
10. File with no. 35 at 20 mm; remove 5 to 6 mm of flutes from outside of curve before using this file.
11. Go back to no. 30 at 21 mm.

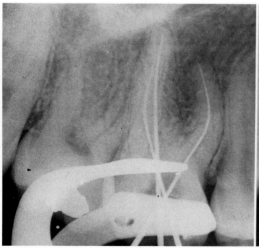 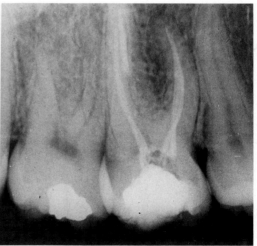

Fig. 7-31. **A,** Preoperative radiograph of maxillary first molar with mesiobuccal canal approximately 40 degrees curved. Distance to elbow is 6 to 7 mm. **B,** Mesiobuccal canal was enlarged apically to size 30 and flared to size 45. Flutes were removed in sizes 12, 17, 22, and 27. All canals filled with laterally condensed gutta-percha and Wach's paste, with post room prepared in palatal canal.

12. File with no. 40 at 19 mm; remove 4 to 5 mm of flutes from outside of curve before using this file.
13. Go back to no. 30 at 21 mm.
14. File with no. 45 at 18 mm; remove 3 to 4 mm of flutes from outside of curve before using this file.
15. Go back to no. 30 at 21 mm.
16. Verify completeness of preparation by fitting finger plugger and prepare for filling (Fig. 7-31, B).

If reverse flaring were to be used in this preparation schedule, it would be inserted after step 2 before continuing to step 3. For reverse flaring of curved canals, the key position is step 2, where

the no. 12 file is created by clipping 1 mm from the tip of the no. 10 file. This instrument *must* be inserted after every flaring size placed short of the tip, even if the flaring file went merely several millimeters into the coronal portion, to ensure that the canal remains patent to the apex. For that reason the no. 12 file becomes the *temporary master apical file* (TMAF) and is used to the full working length after each flaring file, or any other file, used short of that distance. This is done just as the MAF is used at the completion of the preparation in steps 9, 11, 13, and 15. Re-

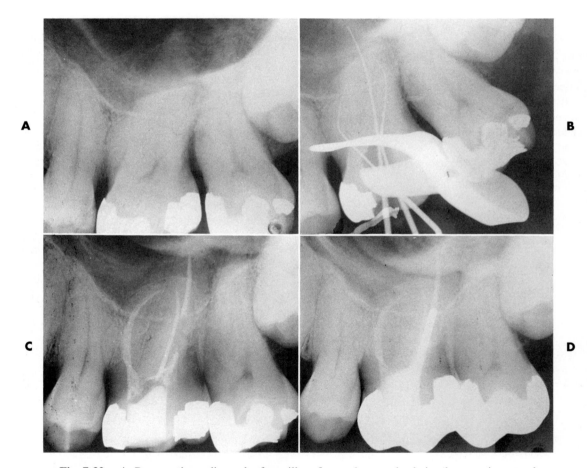

Fig. 7-32. **A,** Preoperative radiograph of maxillary first molar; canals obviously are quite curved. **B,** Files in place indicate a curvature in the mesiobuccal of approximately 55 degrees and an elbow at 7 to 8 mm. The curvature in the distobuccal is approximately 30 degrees. The curvature in the palatal appears much less because the root is curving directly toward the x-ray cone (Table 7-3), but it is probably greater than 30 degrees. To prepare the mesiobuccal canal, reverse flaring was used followed by customized files in sizes 12, 14, 17, 19, 22, and 24. **C,** The canals were filled with laterally condensed gutta-percha and Wach's paste. **D,** Three years later. (Restorations by Dr. Richard Lammermayer, Kenilworth, Ill.)

verse flaring with non-ISO standard instruments is included in the step-by-step preparations of the complex curved canal systems that follow.

Curvatures of 45 to 60 degrees. Instrumentation for these cases with reverse flaring is as follows:

Maxillary first molar, mesiobuccal canal (Fig. 7-32)
Curvature = 55 degrees (Fig. 7-32, *B*)
Distance from elbow to apex (estimated) = 7 to 8 mm
Working length = 22 mm (verified by Fig. 7-32, *B*)
1. File with no. 10 file at 22 mm.
2. Clip 1 mm from no. 10 file (making a no. 12 file); remove 7 to 8 mm of flutes from outside of curve and file at 22 mm. This file becomes the TMAF and will be used after each flaring file during reverse flaring procedure.
3. Select a no. 40 non-ISO taper, set the stop at 14 mm (working length of 22 mm minus 8 mm distance to elbow), and file the orifice portion of the canal. (File probably will not go more than 10 to 11 mm.)
4. Go back to TMAF, using no. 12 file at 22 mm.
5. Select a no. 35 non-ISO taper, set the stop at 14 mm, and file the orifice portion of the canal slightly deeper than step 3. (File probably will not go more than 11 to 12 mm.)
6. Go back to TMAF, using no. 12 file at 22 mm.
7. Select a no. 30 non-ISO taper, set the stop at 15 mm, and file the orifice portion of the canal slightly deeper than step 5. (File probably will not go more than 12 to 13 mm.)
8. Go back to TMAF, using no. 12 file at 22 mm. Reverse flaring is now completed: the apical portion of the canal has been minimally prepared without zipping, and the orifice portion has been widened considerably. The files now used at the apex will work more effectively, and the irrigants will penetrate throughout the canal.
9. File with a no. 15 flexible file at 22 mm (this is a normal no. 15 file of a flexible system as it comes from the manufacturer with no flutes removed or tip reduced). If this file does not go to the full working length easily, do not hesitate to reduce the size no. 12 an additional 1 mm and use it until the no. 15 will go.
10. Clip 1 mm from the no. 15 file (making a no. 17 file); remove 7 to 8 mm of flutes from the outside of the curve and file at 22 mm.
11. File with a no. 20 flexible file at 22 mm (this is a normal no. 20 file, with no flutes removed or tip reduced). If this file does not go easily, do not hesitate to reduce the size no. 17 an additional 1 mm and use it until the no. 20 will go.
12. Clip 1 mm from the no. 20 file (making a no. 22 file); remove 7 to 8 mm of flutes from the outside of the curve and file and 22 mm.
13. File with a no. 25 flexible file at 22 mm (this is a normal no. 25 file with no flutes removed or tip reduced). If this file does not go easily, do not hesitate to reduce the size no. 22 an additional 1 mm and use it until the no. 25 will go. After the size no. 25 is used and fits loosely within the canal, it becomes the MAF.
14. Take a size no. 30 flexible file, remove 6 to 7 mm of flutes from the outside of the curve, and file at 21 mm.
15. Go back to the no. 25 file at 22 mm.
16. Take a size no. 35 flexible file, remove 5 to 6 mm of flutes from the outside of the curve, and file at 20 mm.
17. Go back to the no. 25 file at 22 mm.
18. Take a size no. 40 flexible file, remove 4 to 5 mm of flutes from the outside of the curve, and file at 19 mm.
19. Go back to the no. 25 file at 22 mm.
20. Verify completeness of preparation by fitting figure plugger, and prepare for filling (Fig. 7-32, C).

Points to remember:
1. Keep all canals heavily irrigated. I prefer to irrigate up to size 20 with large amounts of carbamide peroxide (Gly-Oxide) and lesser amounts of sodium hypochlorite (NaOCl). Sizes 25 and above, I use mostly NaOCl, with lesser amounts of Gly-Oxide.
2. Be certain to set the indicator direction on your stop (Fig. 7-16), so you know where the flutes are removed when the file is within the canal.
3. Do *not* rotate the file, or you will distribute the flutes to portions of the canal where you do not want them.
4. Be prepared to make additional file clips if the next size of file does not go to place easily.
5. Proceed slowly.
6. Use flexible file systems only when working apical to the elbow (Table 7-4).

Curvatures of 60 to 90 degrees. Instrumentation for these cases is as follows:

Mandibular second molar, mesial canal (Fig. 7-33)
Curvature = 75 degrees (Fig. 7-33, *B*)
Distance from elbow to apex (estimated) = 5 to 6 mm
Working length = 19 mm (verified by Fig. 7-33, *B*)
1. File with no. 10 file at 19 mm.
2. Clip 0.5 mm from no. 10 file (making a no. 11 file); remove 5 to 6 mm of flutes from outside of curve and file at 19 mm. This becomes TMAF and will be used after each flaring file in reverse flaring procedure.

Table 7-4. Relative ability of file systems

Instrument type	Manufacturer	Process, blank	Penetrating ability	Flaring, reverse flaring	Use in curved canals	Best use; comments
Reamer	Many	Twisted, triangular	*	*	*1/2	Place sealer/medicaments, remove gutta-percha; 1st instrument
K-file	Kerr, then many	Twisted, square	Nos. 08 and 10* Nos. 15 and 20**	**	0	Straight canals, flaring above elbow; 1st improved instrument
Hedstrom	Many	Ground	1/2	***	Only small sizes	Aggressive cutting, flaring, irregular canals
Safety Hedstrom	Kerr	Double ground	1/2	**1/2	*** (Use with care)	Curved canals, must reverse to guard against strip
K-Flex	Kerr	Twisted, diamond	*	**Past elbow *Above elbow	***	Curved canals near apex, slow cutter; 1st instrument for curved canals
Flex-R-File	Union Broach	Ground, safety tip	0	**Past elbow, 1/2 Above elbow	***	Curved canals; 1st instrument with smooth tip
Profile 29 Regular	Tulsa Dental	Ground	*	*	0	Only one file between no. 21 and no. 36, important area of preparation
NiTi		Ground	0	0	***	
Canalmaster	Brasseler	Ground, pilot tip	0	0	?	Prone to breakage
Flex-o-file	Maillefer	Twisted, triangular	*	**Past elbow 1/2 Above elbow	***	Curved canal; may be slightly undersized
Golden Mediums	Maillefer	Twisted, triangular	*	**Past elbow 1/2 Above elbow	***	Intermediate sizes only, used for small curved canals
Pathfinder	Kerr	Twisted	***	0	*	To penetrate narrow sclerotic canals, non-ISO taper
.04 Taper	Tulsa Dental	29 series sizing, NiTi metal, ground	0	***	***	Extremely positive reports from excellent clinicians; combines NiTi, non-ISO taper, mechanical low speed/high torque
Riitano	Kerr	Hedstrom ground	0	***	0	Made for reverse flaring, cannot damage apical preparation
McXIM	NT	NiTi ground	0	***	*	Only 1 apical size, 5 tapers (.03 through .055); streamlined from 6 tapers and 4 file designs

3. Select a no. 40 non-ISO taper, set the stop at 13 mm (working length of 19 mm minus 6 mm distance to elbow), and file orifice portion of the canal. (File probably will not go more than 7 to 8 mm.)
4. Go back to TMAF, using no. 11 file at 19 mm.
5. Select a no. 35 non-ISO taper, set the stop at 13 mm, and file orifice portion of the canal slightly deeper than step 3. (File probably will not go more than 8 to 9 mm).
6. Go back to TMAF, using no. 11 file at 19 mm.
7. Select a no. 30 non-ISO taper, set the stop at 13 mm, and file orifice portion of the canal slightly

deeper than step 5. (File probably will not go more than 9 to 10 mm.)

8. Go back to TMAF, using no. 11 file at 19 mm. Reverse flaring is now completed: the apical portion of the canal has been minimally prepared without zipping, and the orifice portion has been widened considerably.
9. Clip additional 1 mm from no. 10 file (making a no. 13 file); remove additional 1 mm of flutes from the outside of the curve and file at 19 mm.
10. Clip additional 1 mm from no. 10 file (this becomes a no. 15 file that you have customized, not a normal

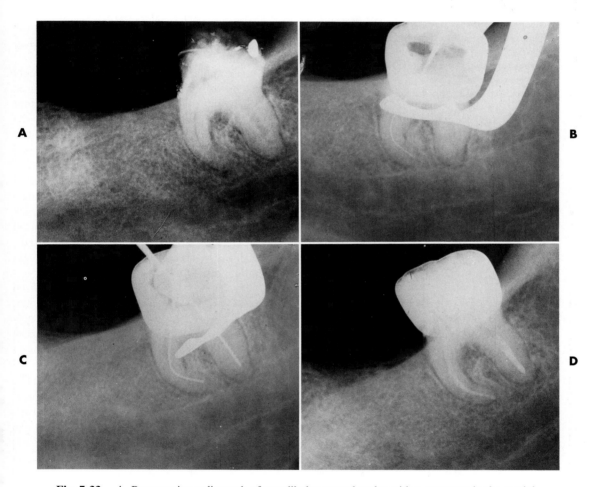

Fig. 7-33. **A,** Preoperative radiograph of mandibular second molar with a curvature in the mesial root of at least 60 degrees. **B,** Film of size no. 10 file in place in single mesial canal indicates curvature of approximately 75 degrees (this tooth is the model for the diagram shown in Fig. 7-20) and distance to the elbow of 5 to 6 mm. It is difficult to tell the curvature without a file in place. This canal was prepared with reverse flaring and customized files in sizes 11, 13, 15, 16, 18, 20, 21, 23, and 25. The distal canal was enlarged apically to size 40 and flared to size 50. **C,** Size 25 file in mesial canal in exactly the same position as was the no. 10 file in **B. D,** Canals filled with laterally condensed gutta-percha and Wach's paste.

no. 15 that comes from the manufacturer); remove additional 1 mm of flutes from the outside of the curve and file at 19 mm.

11. File with a flexible no. 15 file at 19 mm (this is a normal no. 15 that comes from the manufacturer).

12. Clip 0.5 mm from this no. 15 file (making a no. 16 file); remove 5 to 6 mm of flutes from the outside of the curve and file at 19 mm.

13. Clip additional 1 mm from no. 15 file (making a no. 18 file); remove additional 1 mm of flutes from the outside of the curve and file at 19 mm.

14. Clip additional 1 mm from no. 15 file (making a customized no. 20 file, not a normal no. 20 that comes from the manufacturer); remove additional 1 mm of flutes from the outside of the curve and file at 19 mm.

15. File with a flexible no. 20 file at 19 mm (this is a normal no. 20 that comes from the manufacturer).

16. Clip 0.5 mm from this no. 20 file (making a no. 21 file); remove 5 to 6 mm of flutes from the outside of the curve and file at 19 mm.

17. Clip additional 1 mm from no. 20 file (making a no. 23 file); remove additional 1 mm of flutes from the outside of the curve and file at 19 mm.

18. Clip additional 1 mm from no. 20 file (making it a customized no. 25, not a normal no. 25 that comes from the manufacturer); remove additional 1 mm of flutes from the outside of the curve and file at 19 mm.

19. File with a flexible no. 25 file (this is a normal no. 25, not a customized file) at 19 mm; when this fits loosely with the canal, it becomes the MAF (Fig. 7-33, C).

20. Take a no. 30 flexible file, remove 4 to 5 mm of flutes from the outside of the curve, and file at 18 mm.

21. Go back to no. 25 at 19 mm.

22. Take a no. 35 flexible file, remove 3 to 4 mm of flutes from the outside of the curve, and file at 17 mm.

23. Go back to no. 25 at 19 mm.

24. Take a no. 40 flexible file, remove 2 to 4 mm of flutes from the outside of the curve, and file at 16 mm.

25. Go back to no. 25 at 19 mm.

26. Verify completeness of preparation by fitting finger plugger, and prepare for filling (Fig. 7-33, D).

Curvatures of greater than 90 degrees. The previous three sample preparation schedules can be modified for curvatures of 30 to 90 degrees. In canals with curvatures even greater, it is still possible to gain a desirable result (Fig. 7-34) by clipping 0.5 mm increments and removing flutes to

produce many customized files. Cases of this type should not be attempted unless the operator has had considerable experience in curved canals and has mastered completely the techniques for curvatures of 30 to 90 degrees. Also, it is virtually impossible to enlarge these canals apically beyond size 25. Therefore, in order to fill these canals, the dentist must be able to manipulate gutta-percha cones for that narrow diameter.

The critical portion of the preparation technique recommended for curvatures of 60 degrees and greater is the very small amount of increase in file tip width for successive files used to widen the apical portion. It has long been known that in these very difficult canals, everything may seem to be going smoothly, but suddenly, when a new file is introduced, a ledge, zip, or other undesired incident results.

To accommodate for this possibility, it is strongly suggested that incremental instrumentation be used scrupulously in such canals so that only minor increases of apical file tips result. Also, in the instrumentation suggested for Fig. 7-33, illustrating preparation for curvatures of 60 degrees and greater, files tips are clipped so that when new files are introduced (steps 11, 15, and 19) there is very little, if any, difference in width between the new file and the previous file in the canal (steps 10, 14, and 18, respectively). That means that customized files of sizes no. 15, 20, and 25 are used immediately before regular manufacturer's sizes no. 15, 20, and 25, respectively.

My preference would be that the customized files be slightly wider than the manufacturer's sizes to follow. This would virtually ensure that the new files would always go right to place easily, without loss of working length, because the slightly larger file has already been seated properly.

Consequence of position of the elbow. The objective for using a customized file technique is to prepare an instrument for the individual variabilities of a canal. The position of the elbow can vary tremendously, from only 1 or 2 mm (Fig. 7-35) to 6 mm or more. This calculation must be made in each case and retained throughout the preparation phase for optimal results.

Preparation of bayonet-curved canals. The bayonet, or double-curved, canal often poses considerable problems during endodontic therapy, and not without cause (Fig. 7-36 and 7-37). In actual-

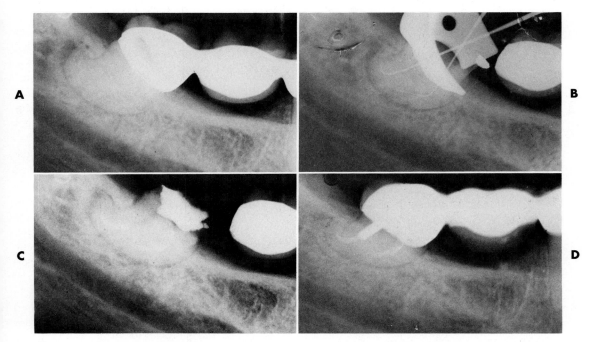

Fig. 7-34. **A,** Mandibular third molar with extreme curvature of both roots, distal apical radiolucency, and distal bridge abutment. **B,** Files in place, indicating curve on mesial of 85 degrees and on distal of 120 degrees. Both canals were prepared with clips of 0.5 mm and enlarged apically to size 25 with flaring to size 40. **C,** Canals filled with laterally condensed gutta-percha and Wach's paste; post room in distal. **D,** Excellent healing 1 year later. (Restorations by Dr. Steve Mele, formerly of Oakbrook, Ill.)

ity, it is not as complicated as it appears and can be safely enlarged and filled as long as several factors are kept in mind:

1. Protect against the zip in the area of the more apical curve, but the more coronal curve is straightened to gain better access to the apex. The distance to the elbow and the angle of curvature are calculated as before. Flutes will be removed from the outer side of the curve accordingly.

2. Once the working length is established with a small file, that file must not be totally removed from the canal until it is very loose. In many instances the initial small flexible file will reach to the apical portion of the canal. However, if the file is removed prematurely, it becomes extremely difficult to gain the correct length with another file, even one of the same size. Therefore, once the correct working length is established by radiograph, the file is not removed but is worked up and down only several millimeters per movement until minimal resistance is felt. Only then may the instrument be removed.

3. Clip minimal increments from each file, working up at not more than 0.5 mm removals and then only when that file is very loose within the canal. The danger of enlarging the bayonet curve is that the file becomes stuck at the first curve and ledges or starts to perforate at that site. If the operator panics and attempts to force the instrument, the condition will quickly worsen. Working up too rapidly through the sizes only increases the chances for this undesired ledging.

4. Flare very carefully. Because the more coronal curve is greatly straightened, that portion of the canal is not enlarged evenly, and it

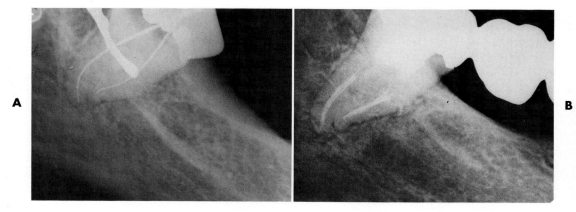

Fig. 7-35. **A,** Files in place in mandibular second molar, extremely curved distal canal with elbow of approximately 2 mm. **B,** Two years after completion of endodontic treatment. (Restorations by Dr. Steve Labkon, Kenilworth, Ill.)

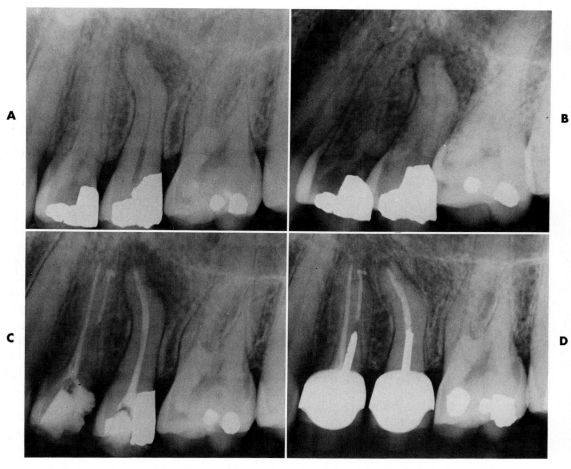

Fig. 7-36. Maxillary bicuspid area. Note periapical lesion associated with no. 13, which has a bayonet-curved canal; no. 12 also needs endodontics. **A,** Preoperative radiograph. **B,** Preoperative angled view. **C,** Postoperative radiograph. Canals filled with laterally condensed gutta-percha and Wach's paste, keeping original canal shape; post room prepared. **D,** Excellent healing 1 year later. (Restorations by Dr. Robert Salk, Chicago.)

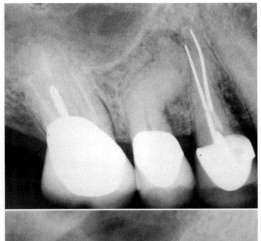

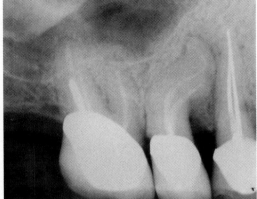

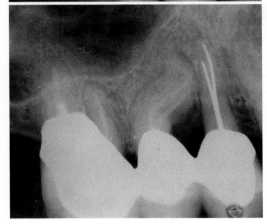

A

B

C

Fig. 7-37. Double-curve successfully treated. **A,** Preoperative radiograph of maxillary posterior area. Treatment had been performed on the first bicuspid 12 years earlier and on the first molar 7 years earlier. A periapical lesion is seen associated with the second bicuspid, and a double curvature is present in that root. **B,** Maximal reverse flaring was performed for the two canals, and flutes were removed for 4 mm on the mesial side of customized files to protect against mesial opening of the file at the tip. Canals were filled with vertical condensation using a modified chloropercha technique (Chapter 9). I removed the crown during treatment and did not cement it correctly. Periapical lesion has decreased considerably since the treatment was started 1 month earlier. **C,** Nine months later, periapical lesion has healed and a splint is in place. Periodontal surgery had been performed on the mesial of the second bicuspid. (Restorations by Morton Schreiber, Highland Park, Ill.)

NEW FILE SYSTEMS FOR PREPARATION OF CURVED CANALS

In the past 10 years a plethora of new file system designs have been introduced for preparation of curved canals. As usual with most new products, several of these have been very useful and efficacious, but others have been worthless and some have been potentially detrimental. Table 7-4 provides a listing of older and newer file systems and their usefulness for various aspects of canal preparation.

There have been three major areas of development for these systems: (1) increase in flexibility by changes in file designs, (2) increase in flexibility by changes in file metals, and (3) files that do not zip because of flute removal or modified tips.

Effects of increased flexibility on final canal shape. One of the major reasons why larger files alter canal shape so quickly as opposed to the smaller sizes is that the instruments decrease in flexibility as the sizes increase. In this context, I am defining the word *flexibility* to mean the ability to stay bent in a curved canal and not attempt to straighten. The degree of flexibility may differ from manufacturer to manufacturer and even among batches of instruments by the same manufacturer.

In general, when a difference in flexibility is present in the same size of files by different companies, the more flexible files will alter canal shape less than will the less flexible files of the same sizes (Fig. 7-38). By the same token, the

does not retain its original shape. This means that the inner portion of the first curve (the mesial of tooth 13 in Fig. 7-36, C) could become strip-perforated if flaring to a size too wide is attempted.

more flexible files remove less tooth structure than do the less flexible files. When one uses the more flexible files, which seem more desired in the curved canals, the aspect of flaring must receive particular attention so the more coronal portions of the canal are made wide enough to allow for the filling procedures.

Flexible file systems. As mentioned earlier in this chapter, the first flexible file to be introduced as an aid for preparation of curved canals was the K-Flex (Figs. 7-4, *C,* and 7-39, *bottom*). These files quickly increased in popularity, since it was clearly seen that they minimized drastic change in the shape of canals with moderate curves (approximately 30 degrees). Examination of plastic blocks (Fig. 7-38) and cases treated with these new instruments (Fig. 7-40) clearly indicated their usefulness.

The success of the K-Flex led to further attempts to design more flexible file systems, and the next

entrant into this field was the Flex-o-file.* This instrument utilized a triangular blank, as used for the reamer (Figs. 7-4, *A,* and 7-39, *top*), with the flutes twisted more tightly to give more cutting edges but maintaining the same narrow cross-sectional diameter for increased flexibility.

Nickel-titanium files. More flexible systems were also developed by changes in the metal from which the files were made. Instead of the carbon steel (used for the old 1 to 12 designations and in a few of the more modern systems) or stainless steel (used in most file systems presently), nickel-titanium was introduced for endodontic use. Called NiTi files, these instruments have the ability to return to their original shape, even if bent severely and held in this position for a long time (Fig. 7-41, *A*). They have minimal resistance to pressure, and thus have been considered to be "flexible." Whether or not they are

*Caulk/Dentsply, Milford, DE 19963.

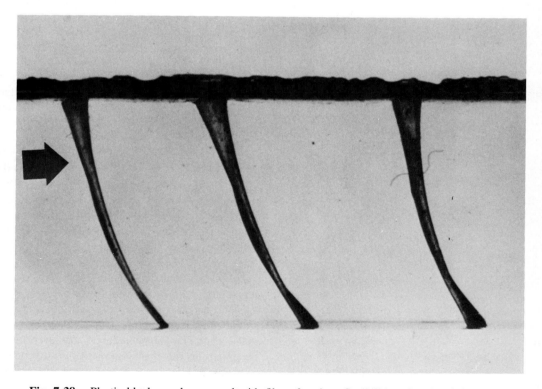

Fig. 7-38. Plastic block canals prepared with files of various flexibilities. Canal at left *(arrow)* was prepared with Kerr K-Flex files to size 30 and no removal of flutes. Minimal elbow and virtually no zip. Center canal was prepared with files to size 30 from a company that manufactures very inflexible files. Narrow elbow and wide zip. Right canal was prepared to size 30 by the most inflexible files I could find, regardless of the manufacturer. Considerable zipping and constricted elbow.

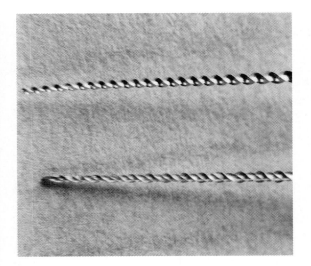

Fig. 7-39. Flutes of two popular flexible file systems. The K-Flex file *(bottom)* is the result of twisting a diamond blank (Fig. 7-4, *C*) to give cutting edges. Close examination reveals that only every other edge is a true cutting edge. However, this skip of cutting edges helps to remove more dentin and debris from the canal. The Flexo-file *(top)* uses a triangular blank (Fig. 7-4, *A*), as typically used for reamers, but it is twisted more tightly to give more cutting edges. The triangular shape yields the narrowest cross-sectional diameter among the variously shaped blanks for twisting.

truly "flexible" is a matter of semantics. I believe they have great "memory" and usually will return to their original (straight) shape. If this happens at the tip or through the apex of the tooth, overinstrumenting the canal, the result may be undesirable. Files that straighten at the apex or through the tip of the canal will produce zipping (Fig. 7-18, *A*).

Because they have so little resistance to pressures, the NiTi files cause little change in canal shape when they are used by hand. However, by the same token, when used by hand, these files do very minimal preparation for given time periods. Therefore, it has been suggested that they be used in mechanical handpieces to complete preparation in a reasonable amount of time (Fig. 7-41, *B*).

Minimizing zipping by flute removal and modification of tips.   The first article dealing with flute removal, by Weine, Kelly and Lio, was published in 1975. Although the paper indicated that the technique was effective in reducing alteration of canal shape in curved canals of both plastic blocks and clinical cases, only a small number of dentists were moved sufficiently to utilize the method in their own endodontic treatments.

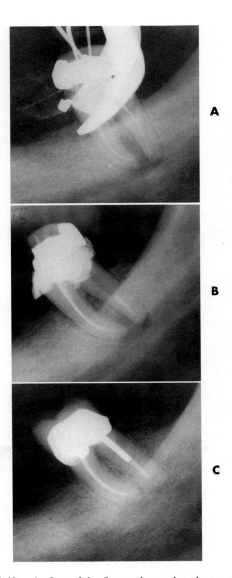

Fig. 7-40.   A, One of the first molar teeth to be treated with a flexible file system. Film of files in place of mandibular second molar, indicating curves of approximately 30 degrees in the mesial canals and large periapical lesion. Canals were prepared with K-Flex files to the full working lengths and apical to the elbow, incremental instrumentation used to create intermediate sizes, and Hedstrom files for flaring coronal to the elbow. **B,** Film taken after canal filling with laterally condensed guttapercha and Wach's paste, with post room prepared. Minimal zipping despite no flutes removed during preparation. **C,** Eight years after treatment, excellent healing. (Restoration by Dr. John Davis, Park Ridge, Ill.)

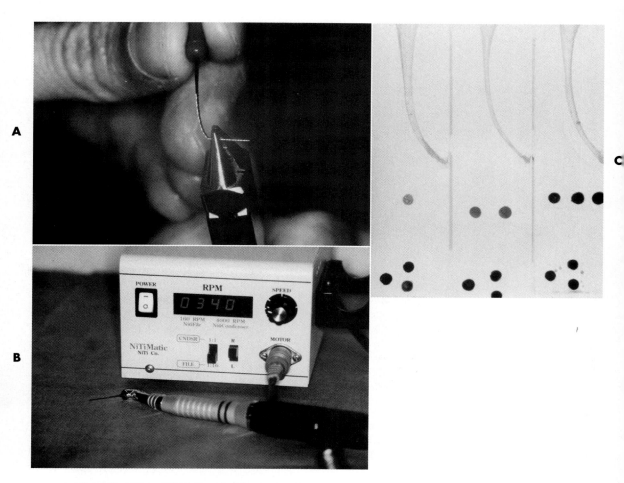

Fig. 7-41. Use of NiTi files. **A,** Files made of nickel-titanium have been described as "superelastic" because of their ability to return to their original shape. This NiTi was bent with a pliers at 90 degrees for 1 hour, but when released, it returned to being straight. **B,** Because the NiTi instruments are slow cutters, canal preparation is very slow and removes minimal amounts of tooth structure unless the instrument is used with a mechanical handpiece. **C,** Three plastic blocks, all prepared for the same length of time, all with reverse flaring. *Left,* NiTi with mechanical handpiece; *center,* NiTi by hand; *right,* customized files with flutes removed (similar to Fig. 7-50, *C*). *Center,* NiTi by hand indicates a minimally prepared canal. The two side blocks are fairly similar, with the mechanical NiTi canal *(left)* having a smoother taper than the hand-prepared canal *(right),* with a more irregular taper. (Courtesy Dr. Mary Campbell, Milwaukee.)

This original paper did spark a number of investigations, virtually all of which endorsed its conclusions. Gradually, more techniques and modifications were introduced that attempted to alter the shape, position, or presence of file-cutting ability to maintain canal shape.

In 1985 and 1986, papers were written by Roane, Sabala, Powell et al., and others from the group at the University of Oklahoma, suggesting a new preparation technique, called "balanced forces." Among other aspects of therapy, this method recommended use of file rotation, filing to the radiographic apex, and the use of only three preparation regimens to cover every type of canal width, length, or degree of curvature. These theories are all completely contrary to my own. In these reports, however, a new type of file was suggested for use with this technique, the Flex-R-File.* This file had its tip modified so that there were no cutting edges or surfaces present (Fig. 7-42). Studies indicated that this new shape reduced ledging and root perforation because the nonworking tip acted

*Union Broach Co., New York, NY 10010.

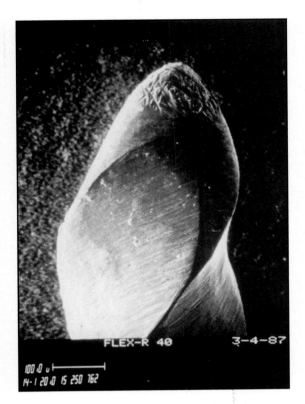

Fig. 7-42. Tip of the Flex-R-File, indicating total absence of cutting ability, which should eliminate ledging and greatly diminish zipping. (Courtesy Union Broach Co., New York.)

merely as a guide for the instrument to pass through the curved portion of a canal without removing dentin. Since that time, many companies have changed their file tips to this new shape.

In theory, tip modification is the next step after removal of flutes, since the cutting ability in the apical area is restricted and therefore zipping is reduced. I believe that it is the Flex-R-File, not the theory of balanced forces, that has enabled cases treated with that technique to be successful. Benenati et al. addressed iatrogenic strip perforations treated successfully at the University of Oklahoma. To obtain the sample size necessary to report on this procedure, a huge number of molar teeth had to be available with strip perforations, a common problem with the file rotation recommended in balanced forces but uncommon in a rasping-only method. Sabala et al. also reported that in a technique course using balanced forces at that school, instrument breakage was 17%. This number is incredibly high

but, again, typical of a rotation technique, although unheard of when using rasping.

A similar modification recently introduced is the pilot tip, used for the Canal Master,* where a noncutting tip of 1.5 mm is present, followed by several millimeters of cutting flutes and then a more narrow smooth shaft. Several other instruments have pilot tips.

Buchanan designed the Safety Hedstrom,† for which the flute removal has been already made on the instrument by the manufacturer. Also, the flute removal is not merely from the tip to the point of the elbow, but along the entire instrument, from the tip through the handle. The handle is scored as well so that the operator knows where the spatial position of the flute removal is found, even when the file itself is well within the confines of the canal. Without this knowledge, the flutes might be distributed where they are not wanted. This feature is also provided by the eccentric silicone stops (Fig. 7-16). This instrument may also be used by reversing the position of the flute removal 180 degrees to file the area away from the wall where a strip perforation might occur.

Disadvantages of flexible files

When the new flexible instruments were introduced for treatment, they became very popular almost immediately for use in small, curved canals because they performed the function of enlargement very well. However, some portions of this type of preparation were not clearly understood.

Three different functions must be performed by instruments for treating curved canals, and a single file system rarely performs all of these. They are (1) penetration, the ability to gain access to the tip of a narrow canal; (2) need for flaring and reverse flaring; and (3) maintaining the shape of the curve. The flexible file systems, while being excellent for maintaining curves, are very poor in penetrating to the tip of these channels, often lined by sclerotic dentin deposits that make the walls very irregular. When flexible files were used in an attempt to traverse such canals, many would buckle, just like a wet noodle, particularly when the small sizes (nos. 08 and 10) were used. Clearly, for this function, another type of file was necessary. The files available with their primary functions are listed in Table 7-4.

*Brasseler USA, Savannah, GA 31419.
†Kerr Manufacturing Co., Romulus, MI 48174.

Non-ISO taper file for penetration. To perform the function of reaching the apex of a curved, sclerotic canal, another type of file was needed. In the old 1 to 12 system, Kerr had manufactured such an instrument as its no. 1.

The old Kerr no. 1, not having been manufactured with any thought of accordance with a standardized taper, in fact had a very narrow taper of approximately 0.015 per millimeter of width for every 1 mm of length. With a tip size of approximately 0.12, the D_{16} width was only 0.40 mm. However, this non-ISO taper gave it better ability to be twisted and forced into a small, tortuous canal than the flexible instruments, particularly because the metal used was carbon steel. The instrument was called the Pathfinder* (Fig. 7-43).

PREPARATION OF TYPE II CANAL SYSTEMS

As shown in Fig. 6-2, four common canal configurations are possible. The Type II system consists of two canal orifices exiting the chamber, then merging within the body of the root into a single canal to the site of exiting. This system is most frequently found in the mesial roots of mandibular molars and maxillary second bicuspids, but it also may occur in any bicuspid, the distal root of mandibular molars, and mesiobuccal root of maxillary molars.

The most difficult root with a Type II system is the mesial of the mandibular molar, where curvatures complicate the relationship of the two canals. However, a Type II system still is easier to prepare and fill than a Type III system of similar canal width and curvature.

The standard method for preparation of a Type II system is to select one of the branches to be the master canal, prepare that completely, and then file the other, dependent, canal merging into it. Although that is not difficult in most bicuspids, the mesial root of the mandibular molar may cause problems (Fig. 7-44). In the mandibular first molar the mesiolingual should always be selected as the master canal. In the mandibular second molar the mesiolingual usually is preferable as the master canal but in some cases the mesiobuccal is the better choice. In bicuspids the choice varies between the buccal and palatal canals. The master canal is chosen on the basis of being the canal most consistent with the root curvature.

*Kerr Manufacturing Co., Romulus, MI 48174.

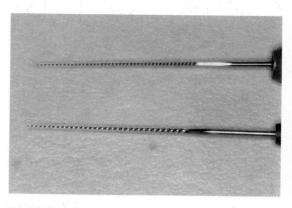

Fig. 7-43. Pathfinder instrument, very useful for penetrating to the apex in sclerotic, narrow canals. Note that the Pathfinder *(top)* has much less taper than the standardized size 10 file *(bottom)*. (Courtesy Kerr Manufacturing Co., Romulus, Mich.)

It may seem logical to file the master canal to its entirety, then file the dependent canal to the site of merging. Doing that, however, may cause dentin shavings from the dependent canal to block off the master canal at the point of confluence and prevent filling to the desired end point.

The correct method involves alternating preparation between the two canals, starting and ending in the master canal but also enlarging the dependent canal between work on the master. A typical case of this type is shown in Fig. 7-45; the working length of the mesiolingual (master canal) was verified at 19 mm, and the site of confluence (working length of the dependent mesiobuccal canal) was 17 mm. The mesiolingual was enlarged with a size 10 file to 19 mm, then the mesiobuccal with a size 10 to 17 mm, and then the mesiolingual again to 19 mm to prevent dentin from packing at the point of confluence. When a size 15 could be used, it was passed down the mesiolingual to 19 mm, then into the mesiobuccal to 17 mm, and back into the mesiolingual at 19 mm. This system was continued until the MAF was reached and until flaring was performed similarly. Reverse flaring, removal of flutes, or customized files might be used as necessary.

The key step in these preparations is to pass the file the full working length in the master canal following every file used in the dependent canal to ensure patency to the apex. Type IV canal systems (see Fig. 6-2), one main canal that branches into two separate and distinct canals at the apex, are very complicated to prepare. Once each branch

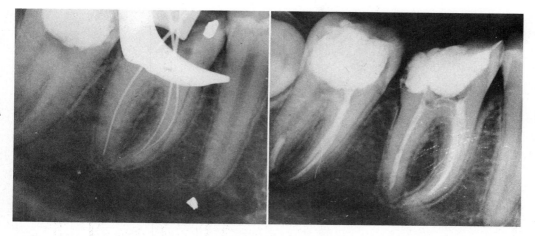

Fig. 7-44. Incorrect method for preparation of Type II canal system. **A,** Radiograph of files in place for treatment of mandibular first molar. The file in the mesiolingual went 20 mm, and the file in the mesiobuccal canal joined it at 18 mm (this view was slightly from the distal). The mesiolingual was made the master canal and was enlarged to size 30 at that length and flared to size 45. Then the mesiobuccal canal was enlarged apically to size 30 at 18 mm and flared to size 40. Unfortunately the filing from the mesiobuccal canal packed off the mesiolingual canal at the point of confluence. **B,** When the canals were filled, a ledge was created at 18 mm, and no filling material could be packed past that site. The case was jeopardized by the error in preparation.

(buccal and lingual) have been located and measured, preparation will be easier if the main segment is widened buccolingually so that the files will find the apical branches more readily. This may be accomplished by preflaring.

COMPLETE ENDODONTIC TREATMENT OF PRIMARY TEETH

In most instances complete endodontic treatment—that is, total canal preparation and filling with gutta-percha—is not required in primary teeth. Pulpal involvement without apical spread of inflammation or infection may be treated by pulpotomy, and even if the periapical tissues do become involved, the canals may be prepared routinely but filled with a medicated cement (Chapter 16). However, if a primary tooth with no permanent successor develops pulpal or periapical involvement, I prefer to treat with complete routine methods of therapy (Fig. 7-46).

In single-canaled teeth this is usually no problem (Fig. 7-47) because the canals are relatively large and straight, although shorter than those of the permanent teeth. Even though permanent successors are absent, the primary teeth may still display some apical resorption; thus preparation of

the dentin matrix must be carefully done. Because the roots are not large, canal preparation wider than size 40 is discouraged. Flaring may be minimal because the roots are so short and straight.

However, complete treatment of primary molars is as complex as any procedure in endodontics. The canals may be quite wide buccolingually yet narrow mesiodistally (Fig. 7-48, *B*). The roots are much more curved than in permanent teeth because they have the shape that is supposed to act as a crypt for the permanent tooth. In the maxillary second primary molar the curve of the mesiobuccal root first to the mesial and then to the distal is readily seen on the radiograph, as is the curve of the distal root first to the distal and then to the mesial (Fig. 7-46, *B*). However, unseen on the film is the curve of the palatal root first to the palatal and then to the buccal and the buccal roots curving initially to the buccal and then to the palatal. These curves may be quite severe, and the chances of zipping at the apex and/or strip perforating in the center of the curves are always present.

To prepare these canals properly, the practitioner must use small increments of file clips and remove flutes to protect against the zip. Fortunately the roots are fairly short so apical pressures on the files

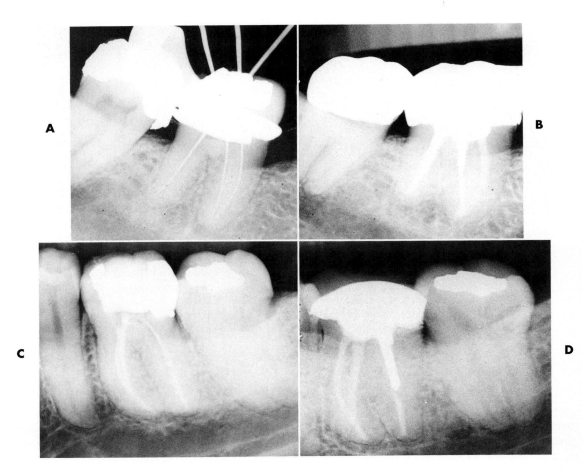

Fig. 7-45. Correct preparations for Type II canal systems. **A,** Radiograph of mandibular second molar with files in place, angled from mesial. Canals merged short of the apex, and the mesiolingual was made the master canal. It was filed to the apex with a no. 10 file, the mesiobuccal canal was filed to the point of confluence with the no. 10 file, and then the mesiolingual was filed the full length with the no. 10 file. This procedure was continued through size 30 to the full working length and flared to size 45, alternating between the mesiolingual and the mesiobuccal and always ending with the mesiolingual. **B,** One year after treatment, very extreme angle from the mesial indicates that the mesial canals have been filled to their full lengths. **C,** Mandibular first molar, similarly treated, straight-on film immediately after filling. **D,** Extreme angle from the mesial 1 year after treatment, indicating that the canals in the mesial root have been filled to their full lengths. (Restorations by Dr. Robert Salk, Chicago.)

are minimized. Radiographs of the maxillary molars are quite difficult to evaluate because of the angles of the projections and the overlapping of radiopaque structures. Because of the strangely shaped canals, much irrigant is needed because it is doubtful whether the files themselves would be able to clean the canal sufficiently.

Lateral condensation of gutta-percha is suggested for filling (Chapter 9), but vertical conden-

sation should not be attempted because the roots are so thin and susceptible to fracture. Excess sealer and cones are common due to the frequency of apical resorption (Fig. 7-48, *C*).

USE OF ENGINE-DRIVEN INSTRUMENTS

Because of the tedium that some dentists associate with canal preparation and the considerable length of time involved in the use of files and ream-

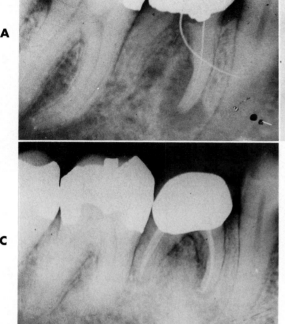
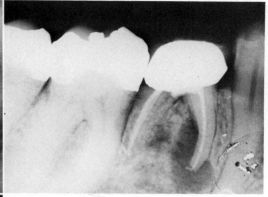

Fig. 7-46. A, Radiographs of initial files in place after referral from a general dentist for treatment of primary second molar without permanent successor. Perforation into furcation and a large apical radiolucency of mesial root. **B,** Completed treatment. Canals filled with laterally condensed gutta-percha and furcation perforation sealed with ZOE. **C,** Excellent healing 2 years later. (Endodontics by Dr. Gene R. Palmer, Escondido, Calif.)

ers in some difficult cases, engine-driven instruments have been used to save time and effort.

Engine-driven reamers. Reamers have been mounted in handpiece mandrels or built with a latch-type end so that they can be used as rotary instruments in handpieces used for ordinary operative procedures. Although such engine-driven reamers can be used satisfactorily when preparing perfectly straight canals, their use in posterior teeth, where canals all have some degree of curvature, will lead to complete alteration of original canal shape (Fig. 7-49) and often lead to root perforation. Because of the pressures that are often used to gain penetration to the tip of the canal, instrument breakage might be a serious problem as well.

Endodontic handpieces. The most frequently used engine-driven instruments have been the Giromatic* and the Dynatrak.

In reporting on the Giromatic, Frank stated that he did not think that the instrument saved a great deal of time, but he suggested that it could well be incorporated into the endodontic armamentarium under certain conditions. O'Connell and Brayton prepared canals in extracted teeth with the two automated handpieces and by hand instrumentation. They compared them by making impressions of the interiors of the prepared canals. However, they reported that the hand preparation was superior in quality of surface smoothness, apical preparation, shape of preparation, and elimination of morphologic aberrations. Time involved in the use of the various techniques was not compared.

Weine et al. reported that the W. & H. Endodontic Contra Angle* greatly deviated from the original canal and was capable of ledging and apical zipping. They stated that the Giromatic did not perforate

*Micro-Mega Suisse, Geneva, Switzerland.

*Pfingst & Co., Inc., New York, NY 10003.

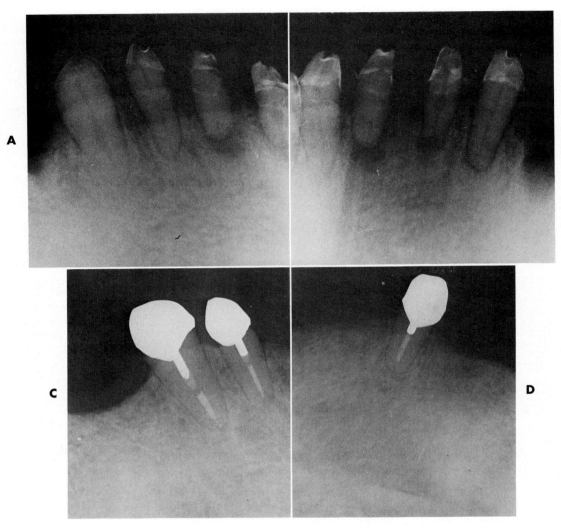

Fig. 7-47. Mandibular incisor area. Although patient was 30 years old, only primary incisors were present without permanent successors. Because of the resorptive defect on one tooth and the large lesion on the other, two incisors were extracted. **A** and **B,** Preoperative radiographs. **C** and **D,** One year later, endodontics completed. Canals are filled with laterally condensed gutta-percha and Wach's paste; post rooms prepared. Teeth are supporting overpartial.

through the side of the root but did greatly change the apical anatomy should the rotating instruments extend beyond the site of exiting of the canal. Furthermore, they believed that neither saved time compared with hand instrumentation (Fig. 7-50), although physical fatigue and tedium were minimized.

Because of these reports, I am not in favor of using automated handpieces, particularly for the full working length of the canal. It would appear that the Giromatic may have value in producing the flared type of preparation after hand instrumentation in the apical regions. If dentists want to use a Giromatic in curved canals because of the ease and convenience that it offers, they must remember that the apical portion should be prepared with hand instruments using suitable removal of flutes. This method will retain the general shape of the canal in the critical apical area, whereas the efforts of the Giromatic will be confined to the more coronal site, where some straightening normally occurs.

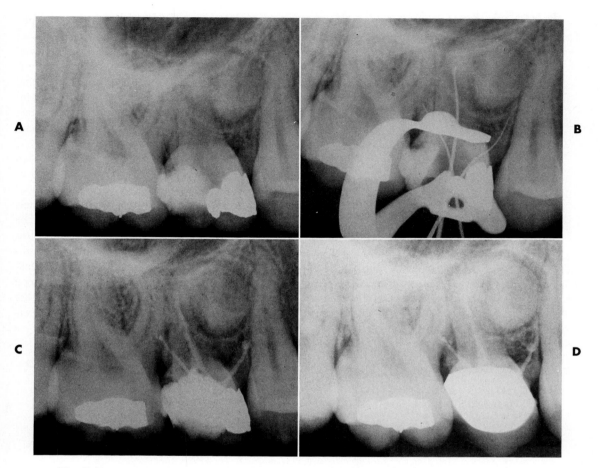

Fig. 7-48. Maxillary posterior area of an 18-year-old patient with primary second molar and merely bud of the permanent successor. **A,** Preoperative radiograph. **B,** Files in place give some indication of mesiodistal curves but no sign of considerable buccolingual curvatures. **C,** Canals filled with laterally condensed gutta-percha and Wach's paste. Some excess sealer has been expressed. **D,** Eighteen months later.

The W. & H. Endodontic Contra Angle is not widely used and should never be employed except in very straight canals. The Dynatrak is an engine-driven instrument with a safe-tipped feature that does not produce apical zipping. Unfortunately, since there is no tip-cutting capacity, it does not cut at the apical portion. If the Dynatrak is forced into a portion of the canal where apical binding occurs, it will fracture in many instances. The Dynatrak is excellent for flaring and reverse flaring procedures. However, it only should be used where it moves freely within the body of the canal with no binding at the tip. Forcing it into apical areas will produce no preparation and can only lead to disasters.

Gates-Glidden burs and Peeso reamers. Gates-Glidden burs and Peeso reamers must only be used with the withdrawal motion to remove tooth structure at very slow speeds with irrigation. Active tooth removal by forceful insertion is absolutely undesirable. Because of their design, any breakage in these instruments will occur so that a long stem protrudes from the canal for relatively easy removal rather than separating at the tip, where removal is almost impossible.

The functions of the Gates-Glidden burs and Peeso reamers are as follows: (1) to gain more direct access to the apical portion of the canal by removing the curvatures at the orifice that might cause

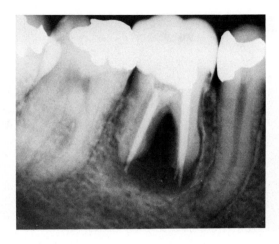

Fig. 7-49. Mandibular first molar prepared with engine-driven reamer. Canal fillings are perfectly straight, indicating that original canal shape has been considerably altered. Pulp was vital but inflamed before treatment, with normal periapical regions, but case is now obviously failing.

deflection of the enlarging instruments; (2) to open the canal orifice and eliminate filing of the cervical portion of the canal, thus allowing for ease in placement of curved enlarging instruments, filling materials, and condensing and plugging instruments; and (3) to allow for the use of coronally wider nonstandardized master gutta-percha cones (some operators believe that they are easier to place than the thinner standardized gutta-percha cones).

For many years these instruments have been used mounted in a standard handpiece for procedures similar to reverse flaring (Fig. 7-51). It was recommended that minimal preparation of the apical portion be performed first and that a TMAF be used the full working length between these instruments used coronally. With the advent of the non-ISO taper files, I believe that the use of the Gates-Glidden and Peeso reamers will be greatly reduced for this function. Being much more flexible, the non-ISO tapers are less prone to cause a strip per-

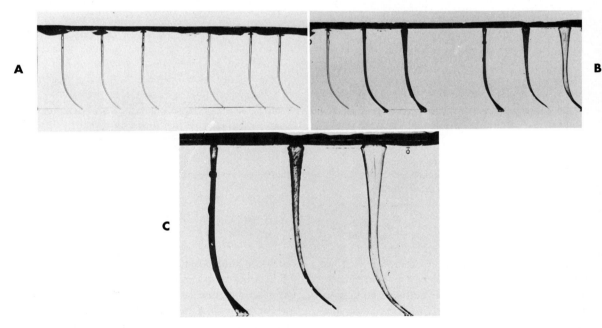

Fig. 7-50. Plastic block, **A,** before canal preparation. **B,** After completion of preparations. *From left,* Unprepared canal, reamed canal, canal prepared with W. & H. Contra Angle, canal prepared with Giromatic, canal that ledged with W. & H., canal prepared with removal of flutes and flared. All canals were enlarged apically to size 30. Reamed canal took the least amount of time, followed by canals prepared with flute removal and Giromatic (which were approximately equal), and finally by canal prepared with the W. & H. (by far the slowest). Reamed canal has small zip and slight elbow, whereas W. & H. has severe zip and very narrow elbow. **C,** Enlargement of right side of the plastic block. Canal prepared with removal of flutes *(right)* has no zip and no elbow. Canal prepared with Giromatic has significant zip and narrow elbow. (From Weine FS, Kelly RF, Bray KE: *J Endod* 2:298, 1976.)

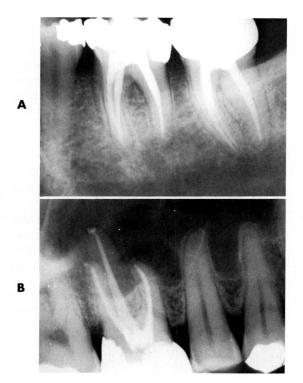

Fig. 7-51. Mandibular molars, **A,** and maxillary first molar, **B,** in which flaring of canals was produced by Peeso reamers. Radiographic appearance of canals as wide in cervical third, then abruptly tapering down, is clearly visible. (Courtesy Dr. Jeffrey Woodson, Dallas.)

foration. With many more available sizes, greater control is available. With the tip size graded in standard endodontic file terms, use with hand instruments is easier.

Restorative dentists may continue to use Gates-Glidden and Peeso instruments for preparation of post space, although I prefer that heated hand pluggers followed by hand instruments be used for that purpose (Chapter 9).

ULTRASONICS

History of ultrasonics in dentistry. Ultrasonic devices have been used in industry to remove unwanted materials and debris for many years. In 1957 Richman reported on the use of a barbed broach connected to an ultrasonic delivery system for use in canal preparation and apical resection. Other applications in endodontics were not reported for more than 20 years, but vibrations at

ultrasonic levels (20 to 30 kHz) were used in medicine and dentistry for cleaning instruments during this period.

Then, beginning in 1980, Martin and Cunningham and their group in the Washington, D.C./ Bethesda Naval Hospital area started to report studies on many aspects of ultrasonic treatment. At this same time, Miyahara and others in Japan evaluated ultrasonic use, most specifically in canal preparation and cleaning, but also with removal of unwanted items from the canal space and as a method for thermoplasticizing gutta-percha for canal filling.

These innovators sparked many additional investigations into newer techniques, wider ranges for use, and improved delivery systems. Research in the area of ultrasonics has been constant since then, and many teeth are now saved that could not be treated successfully otherwise. This is particularly true for many endodontic specialists who find much of their practice being devoted to re-treatments. Removal of canal fillings and posts from failing cases (Figs. 10-45 and 10-49) facilitates successful nonsurgical retreatment in many instances where surgery had been the only choice. Even if surgery were ultimately necessary, the resection could be performed down to solidly filled canals, where the chance for success was higher than with apically placed fillings.

Method for action. Martin and Cunningham have coined the term *endosonics* to refer to endodontic treatment by supersonic, sonic, or subsonic systems. They also have stated that the use of this equipment creates a *synergistic system* whereby canal preparation and cleaning, irrigation and disinfection, and canal packing and filling are all accomplished with the same group of devices.

Ultrasonic cleaning was described initially as implosion or cavitation. *Cavitation* occurs when the ultrasonic file vibrates in a liquid to produce alternating compressions and rarefactions of pressure. A negative pressure develops within the exposed cells of the intracanal materials (pulp tissue, bacteria, debris, metabolites, substrates, etc.). This causes an *implosion,* or inward explosion, that breaks these cells apart inwardly and leads to their destruction. Since an irrigation/aspiration system is employed in the endodontic equipment for ultrasonics, the broken cell parts are washed out and then removed from the canal system. The atomic bomb also works by the implosion principle, as do other methods for destruction and removal of materials.

Recently, Ahmad and her group from Guy's Hospital published papers that offered another mechanism for ultrasonic cleaning. They stated that the power setting used to energize the endodontic unit was too low to produce cavitation and that the width of the canal space was too small to allow for this condition. They suggested that the principle was that of *acoustical streaming,* a process by which the vibrating file generates a stream of liquid to produce eddies and flows of oscillation. The dimensions of these eddies and flows around the file are consistent and reproducible. Other studies have indicated that the dimensions produced will destroy or disrupt mammalian tissues.

Whichever of these principles is responsible, it seems that ultrasonics does work and will allow for many desirable and effective procedures. Removal of dentin for canal preparation, elimination of unwanted intracanal materials, and improved cleaning of the canal all may be accomplished, often in less time than by hand and with better efficiency than by other machines.

The energy from ultrasonic devices is derived from instruments vibrating at levels of 20 to 30 kHz by either electromagnetic or piezoelectric power sources. Both of these are power sources that convert other forms of energy into electric energy. Electromagnetic energy is produced by rotary generation and is typical of the electric power used in homes and industries. The most frequently used ultrasonic electromagnetic unit is the Cavi-endo,* the instrument used in the investigations by Martin and Cunningham. Piezoelectric energy is induced by subjecting crystals of certain materials, such as quartz or Rochelle salts, to physical force or pressure, as typically used in phonographs and microphones. For dental use, piezoelectric units (Fig. 7-52, *A*) are much more powerful than electromagnetic units. Thus they are most effective in removing unwanted items, such as silver points and posts, from the root canal space. The most frequently used piezoelectric unit is the Enac.† Lower levels of power are also available, in the so-called sonic or subsonic range, for handpieces.

Techniques for use. The ultrasonic systems involve a power source (Fig. 7-52, *A*) to which an endodontic file is attached with a holder and an adapter (Fig. 7-52, *B*). Irrigants are emitted from cords on the power source and travel down the file into the canal to be energized by the vibrations. A wide range of files is available with varying abilities, including those with safe-ended tips and instruments of diamond particles. The latter reputedly have enhanced properties for conducting ultrasonic energy.

The irrigants may be either water or sodium hypochlorite. Sodium hypochlorite may cause a problem with these units because of clogging or corrosion. Evacuation devices must also be used to remove the irrigants and debris from the canal.

Initial articles have indicated that ultrasonics give better canal debridement than does preparation by hand instruments. More recent papers have cast some doubt on those claims. Removal of the smear layer may be accomplished more readily with ultrasonics, but the sites where the tip actually touches the canal wall produce a new smear layer. Therefore Camp recommends that the ultrasonic device be used after canal preparation by hand has been completed and that the file should remain in the center of the canal away from the walls. No one knows the true significance of removing the smear layer, but Cameron recommends its elimination so that the filling material may enter into the superficial layers of dentin tubules.

Because the intracanal irritants are blown apart by the ultrasonic system and then removed from the canal by the evacuator, some claim that fewer noxious agents are pushed through the apex of the tooth into the periapical tissues. This decrease was found to lead to fewer postoperative flare-ups with the ultrasonic device than with routine therapy.

Canal filling with the ultrasonic system involves the file being replaced with a noncutting endosonic plugger. Energizing the plugger allows for a heating of the gutta-percha so that the latter can be compacted, condensed, and welded together to gain increased three-dimensional obturation of the prepared canal system. This may be augmented by cold hand plugging as well.

Removal of posts, silver points, cements, and other unwanted materials in the canal have been reported with the ultrasonic systems (Chapter 10). The larger items (posts, silver points) are loosened with instruments usually involved with scaling and gross debris removal, whereas the cements require the endosonic files. Dentistry in eastern Europe often involves filling canals with cements that have

---

*Caulk/Dentsply, Milford, DE 19963.
†Osada Electric, Tokyo, Japan.

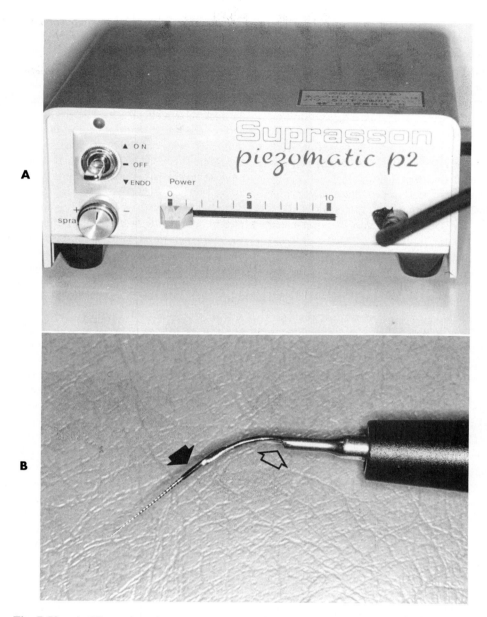

Fig. 7-52.   A, Ultrasonic unit powered by piezoelectricity. **B,** Ultrasonic tip with file attached to pictured unit. A plastic sleeve *(solid arrow)* has been placed to indicate working length because a rubber stop would prevent the movement of liquids from the unit *(open arrow)* into the canal. The plastic sleeve may lessen the effectiveness of acoustical streaming.

no solvents. To re-treat failing cases, it becomes necessary to drill out the cement, which often leads to root perforation. The ultrasonic unit offers an extremely favorable alternative.

Canal preparation. Some studies with the ultrasonic device have indicated minimal or no zipping when the instrument was used for preparation of curved canals. My initial investigations indicated that this was not consistently true (Fig. 7-53, D and E). In their first report in 1985, Chenail and Teplitsky stated that the instrument could safely prepare curved canals. However, they stayed with minimal sizes, and zipping rarely occurs at these small sizes. By 1988, when they had evaluated enlargement to size 30 and greater, they also found that zipping was a constant feature.

Schulz-Bongert et al. recently described the use of a piezoelectric source* for preparation of curved canals alone and in combination with hand preparation, including flute removal, at the apex (Fig. 7-54). They reported that when used alone in canals with curvatures of 30 degrees and greater, severe zipping occurred (Fig. 7-54, A and B). However, when the ultrasonic unit was used above the elbow only for reverse flaring and flaring, in combination with hand filing at the apex, minimal zipping resulted (Fig. 7-54, C and D). Stripping (Fig. 7-12, C) also occurred with ultrasonics alone, but not in the combination-treated cases.

Because the electromagnetic units are not as powerful as the piezoelectric sources, the former may cause less zipping than the latter in the same amount of time. The process of retaining the working length is quite important when using these machines, because when the tip goes through into the periapical tissues, the degree of destruction that it causes is considerable and the degree of zipping greatly increased (Fig. 7-53, E).

It is impossible to use rubber stops for length control because they would interfere with the passage of irrigants up the files. Therefore length control can be a problem even when using miniature rubber sleeves that fit on the files (Fig. 7-52, B) or using the files with millimeter serration indicators on the shaft. Some of the sonic systems have wire length indicators for working length that come off the handpiece and thus allow for free passage of fluids in both directions.

My preference for the use of ultrasonic and sonic units in curved canals is to limit them to flaring and reverse flaring, leaving the apical portion to be pre-

*Electro Medical Systems SA, Le Sentier, Switzerland.

pared by hand files with flexible properties. Camp and Zakariasen believe that the MM1500* is especially well adapted for this function.

Related uses for ultrasonics. The advent of ultrasonics has improved the ability of the dentist to treat successfully a wider variety of cases. Despite the lack of agreement as to the degree of cleaning ability compared with nonultrasonic use, I am impressed with the amount of debris removed by ultrasonic use in teeth with open apices and necrotic pulps (Chapter 16), those with chronic lesions (Fig. 7-55), and teeth that have been left open for long periods that need to be reclosed. After completing preparation of the walls and gaining the desired shape in such cases, either with or without the use of mechanical aids, I allow for several minutes of ultrasonic cleaning, leaving the tip centered in the canal during that time with the sodium hypochlorite passing freely within the canal.

The ultrasonic unit is quite useful in preparing teeth for re-treatment because of its ability to gain a cleaner environment (Fig. 7-56). Failing cases requiring the retrieval of silver points are particularly easier to re-treat since the advent of ultrasonics. Generally in these cases, some cements are on the chamber floor around the previous canal fillings. If a bur is used to clean the chamber, the portion of the points protruding from the canal is cut away, and re-treatment is severely hampered by inability to pull out the materials. However, if an endosonic file is used around and into the cement, the chamber contents are removed cleanly, and the protruding silver point segments remain in the same position that is favorable for removal. The entire floor is much cleaner, and unwanted debris is eliminated if locating an additional canal becomes necessary.

In addition to disposing of unwanted filling materials, ultrasonic devices have a good chance to remove broken instruments and amalgam shavings packed into the apical portion of the canal from coronal restorations.

As these devices are used more and more, further clinical evaluations will be made to delineate the exact areas of effectiveness and prospects for the future. These machines are very powerful and are able to perform tasks that were very difficult or even impossible in the past. By the same token, this power makes them potentially dangerous if not used correctly. At present it is safe to say that endosonics have improved the quality, number,

*Medidenta, Geneva, Switzerland.

A   **B**   **C**

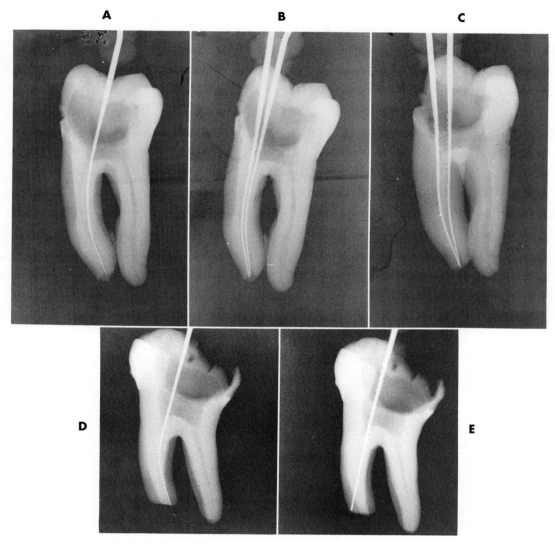

D   **E**

Fig. 7-53. Initial studies on retaining original canal shape using a piezoelectric ultrasonic unit. **A,** Hand file in one of the mesial canals of an extracted mandibular molar to indicate original canal shape. **B** and **C,** Two views of size 30 files in place after only 1 minute of ultrasonic preparation. This was rated as an excellent preparation. **D,** Hand file in one of the mesial canals of another mandibular molar to indicate original canal shape. **E,** Size 30 file in place after only 30 seconds of ultrasonic preparation. This was rated as an unacceptable preparation.

and types of treatable cases but that considerable care is required for proper use.

IRRIGANTS AND CHELATING AGENTS

Functions of irrigants. Irrigants perform important physical and biologic functions during endodontic therapy. Their action is unquestionably more significant than that supplied by the use of intracanal medicaments. When there is a wet environment dur-

ing canal preparation, the dentin shavings are floated to the chamber, where they may be removed by aspiration or paper points. Therefore they do not pack near the apex to prevent proper canal filling. Files and reamers are much less likely to break when the canal walls are lubricated by the irrigants.

Many liquids would provide these aids, but in addition the irrigants that are typically used have the function of being necrotic tissue solvents.

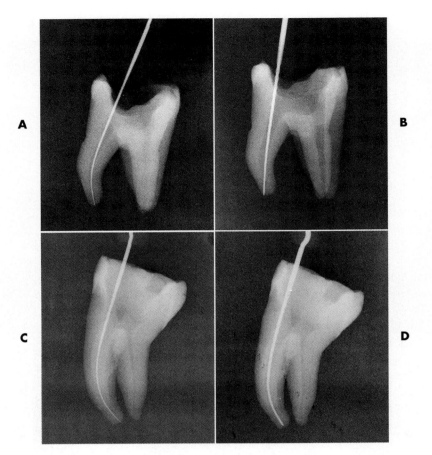

Fig. 7-54. Use of the ultrasonic unit for preparation of curved canals. Extracted teeth were prepared with ultrasonic use only or with a combination of ultrasonics coronal to the elbow and hand filing with flute removal apical to the elbow. **A,** Example of use of ultrasonics only, size no. 10 file in place to the working length, indicating curvature of approximately 30 degrees. **B,** After use of ultrasonic preparation only, size no. 30 file was placed, indicating complete straightening of the canal with apical zip. **C,** Example of combination of ultrasonics coronal to the elbow and hand filing with flutes removed apical to the elbow, size 10 file in place indicating curvature of approximately 50 degrees. **D,** After completion of preparation, size no. 30 file in place in virtually the same position as was the no. 10 file, with minimal straightening or zipping. (Reprinted with permission from Schulz-Bongert U, Weine FS, Schulz-Bongert J: *Compend Contin Educ Dent* 16:270, 1995.)

When used with canal instrumentation, the irrigants loosen debris, pulp tissue, and microorganisms from the irregular dentin walls so that they can be removed from the canal. Because reamers and files are much too small to fit into accessory canals, it is the solvents' action that removes the tissue remaining there so that the subsequently used filling materials may be packed or pushed into these areas.

Most irrigants are germicidal but have further antibacterial effect by ridding the canal of the necrotic debris. With reduced substrate present, the microorganisms have less chance for survival. Irrigants also have a bleaching action to lighten teeth discolored by trauma or extensive silver amalgam restorations and decrease the chance of postoperative darkening.

The commonly used irrigants are capable of causing inflammation of periapical tissue. Therefore instrumentation must be confined within the canal to limit the forcing of irrigants through the apical foramen. Unquestionably, solution frequently does

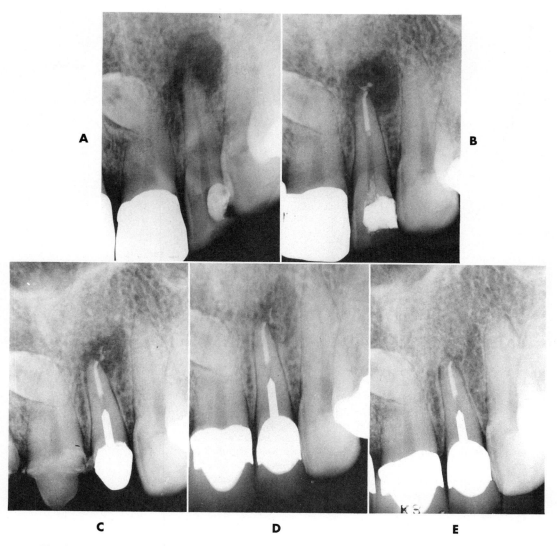

Fig. 7-55. Typical case where ultrasonic unit was used to aid in cleaning canal rather than preparing canal. **A,** Preoperative view of maxillary lateral incisor, periapical lesion present, temporary restoration leaking badly, apical soreness, and history of several exacerbations. Canal was enlarged apically to size 35 and flared to size 50, sodium hypochlorite used as irrigant, and ultrasonic unit left in the center of the canal to aid in debridement and cleaning after preparation was completed. **B,** Canal filled at second appointment with laterally condensed gutta-percha and Wach's paste, with post room prepared. There were no symptoms after initial appointment. **C,** Six months after treatment. **D,** One year after treatment. **E,** Eighteen months after original treatment, lesion has healed perfectly. (Restorations by Dr. Sherwin Strauss, Chicago.)

reach the periapical tissue and some inflammation results. Since the stronger solvents produce greater inflammatory response, the strength of the solutions should be kept to the lowest level that will be effective in debridement.

Useful irrigants. Sodium hypochlorite (NaOCl), NF, is the most widely used irrigant in endodontics and has effectively aided canal preparation proce-

dures for many years (Fig. 7-57). A 5% solution provides excellent solvent action but is dilute enough to cause only mild irritation when contacting periapical tissue. Household liquid bleach (Clorox, Linco) has 5.25% NaOCl and therefore requires slight addition of distilled water to lower the incidence of periapical inflammation. For those who perform endodontic treatment frequently,

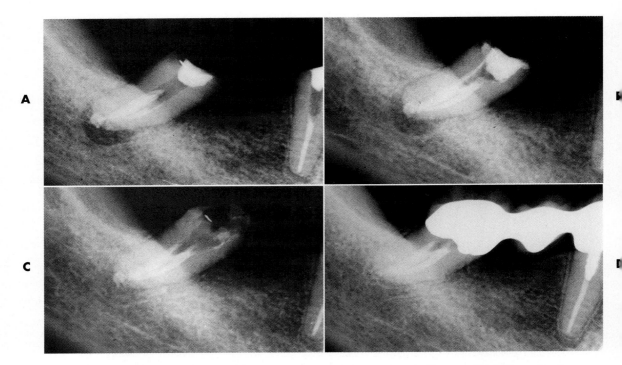

Fig. 7-56. Improved cleaning ability by ultrasonic preparation. **A,** Preoperative radiograph of mandibular posterior area. The second molar had been treated 1 year earlier and had a vital pulp with no periapical lesion at that time. Now it is tender to percussion and slightly mobile, and a periapical lesion is present. The treatment seemed satisfactory, and I was reluctant to attempt re-treatment. Because the involved tooth was a posterior abutment and without it no fixed prosthesis could be placed, I agreed to attempt redoing the therapy but stressed to the patient the questionable prognosis. **B,** I discovered that the original treatment was performed at only one appointment, which is difficult on a C-shaped second molar. My repreparation included the use of a solvent to remove the old gutta-percha and ultrasonic cleaning, which had not been used earlier. At the second appointment, I filled the canals with laterally condensed gutta-percha and Wach's paste. My filling really appears to be no different than the original filling shown in **A.** I advised the referring dentist to place a temporary bridge to evaluate healing. **C,** Six months later, the periapical lesion has healed and the tooth is firm and comfortable. I advised the restorative dentist to go ahead with the permanent bridge. **D,** Two years later, a fixed bridge has been constructed and the posterior abutment is comfortable and functioning well. (Restorations by Dr. Kerry Voit, Chicago.) (Reprinted with permission from Schulz-Bongert U, Weine FS, Schulz-Bongert J: *Compend Contin Educ Dent* 16:270, 1995.)

these solutions are easier utilized than preparation of the irrigant by dissolving sodium carbonate and chlorinated lime.

In a tissue culture study, Spangberg suggested that NaOCl be diluted with distilled H_2O to a concentration not in excess of 0.5% for endodontic irrigation. He stated that this solution still was an effective necrotic solvent, although having a less detrimental effect on periapical tissues should any material pass through the apex. One additional advantage to using a preparation that develops an apical dentin matrix is that it reduces passage of

materials into the periapical tissues when compared with those techniques that recommend complete patency.

Hydrogen peroxide solution (H_2O_2), USP, is also widely used in endodontics, with two modes of action. The bubbling of the solution when in contact with tissue and certain chemicals physically foams debris from the canal. In addition, the liberation of oxygen destroys strictly anaerobic microorganisms.

The solvent action of H_2O_2 is much less than that of NaOCl. However, many clinicians use the solu-

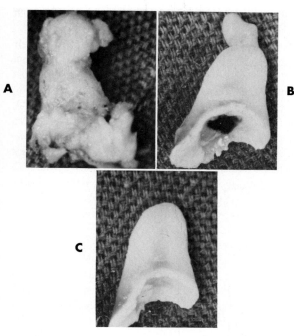

Fig. 7-57. Solvent action of 5% sodium hypochlorite solution. **A,** Maxillary bicuspid with granulomatous mass attached, shortly after extraction. **B,** After exposure to the NaOCl for 30 minutes, much of tissue has dissolved, leaving only a small portion of the lesion attached to the apex. **C,** After 60 minutes of exposure, all soft tissue has been dissolved.

tions alternately during treatment. This method is strongly suggested for irrigating canals of teeth that have been left open for drainage, since the effervescence is effective in dislodging food particles as well as other debris that may have packed the canal.

Being less effective as a solvent, H_2O_2 is also less damaging to periapical tissues. Therefore, when procedural accidents have caused either root or floor of chamber perforation or when the apical constriction has been destroyed with severe pericementitis present, it is the preferred irrigant. However, peroxide should not be the last irrigant used in a canal, since nascent oxygen may remain after access preparation closure and build up pressure. Therefore NaOCl should be used to react with the H_2O_2 and liberate the oxygen remaining; then the canal is dried with paper points and closed.

Carbamide peroxide is available in any anhydrous glycerol base (Gly-Oxide*) to prevent decomposition

*SmithKline Beecham Consumer Healthcare, L.P., Pittsburgh, PA 15230.

and is a useful irrigant. It is better tolerated by periapical tissue than NaOCl yet has greater solvent action and is more germicidal than H_2O_2. Therefore it is an excellent irrigant for treating canals with normal periapical tissue and wide apices, in which the more irritating solutions would cause severe inflammation when forced out of the canal. The best use for Gly-Oxide is in narrow and/or curved canals, utilizing the slippery effect of the glycerol. Whereas chelating agents react with dentin and may cause root perforation or ledging in the softened walls, this action will not occur with Gly-Oxide, where only lubrication is enhanced. Because the canal walls are slippery, they are easier to prepare but are less likely to be gouged or perforated (Fig. 7-58).

Method of irrigation. Disposable plastic syringes of 2.5 or 5 ml capacity with 25-gauge blunted needles are useful for endodontic irrigation. Glass syringes with metal tips are also satisfactory but are much more expensive and more easily broken. A bend of approximately 30 degrees is made in the center of the needle so the canals of both anterior and posterior teeth are reachable (Fig. 7-59).

Irrigants must never be forcibly inserted into the periapical tissue but gently placed within the canal. It is the action of the intracanal instruments that distributes the irrigant to the nooks and crannies of the canal rather than the injecting syringe. For relatively large canals the tip of the syringe is placed until resistance from the canal walls is felt, then the tip is withdrawn a few millimeters. The solution is expressed very slowly until much of the chamber is filled. In the treatment of posterior teeth and/or small canals, the solution is deposited in the chamber. The files will carry the irrigant into the canal, and the capillary action of the narrow canal diameter will retain much of the solution. Excess irrigant is carried away by aspiration with a small tip, of approximately 16 gauge, if available. Otherwise, a folded gauze pad (2 × 2 inches) is held near the tooth to absorb the excess. To dry a canal in a case where aspiration is not available, the plunger of the irrigating syringe may be withdrawn, and the bulk of the solution will be aspirated in that manner. Paper points are then used to remove residual liquid.

Kahn et al. have described the use of the Irrivac, which provides both aspiration and irrigation with the same instrument. A 25-gauge needle is inserted through Teflon tubing attached by way of a bypass to the saliva ejector. The irrigant is expressed

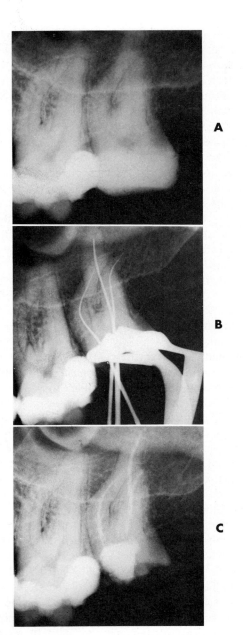

Fig. 7-58. Typical case treated with carbamide peroxide (Gly-Oxide) as irrigant. (Gly-Oxide is available in ½- and 2-ounce bottles and disposable plastic ampules.) **A,** Maxillary second molar with curved canals, verified by radiograph, **B,** with files in place to determine working lengths. **C,** By careful preparation, using precurved files, incremental instrumentation, removal of flutes, and lubricating properties of Gly-Oxide, canals were prepared sufficiently to fill with gutta-percha.

through a syringe into the canal and aspirated out the tubing (Fig. 7-60).

Recent studies concerning irrigants and their clinical implications. For many years intracanal irrigants were considered to be among the most mundane of the entities involved in endodontic therapy. Almost every case involved either NaOCl, H_2O_2, or both, and relatively little thought was given to their use. The medicaments were considered to have better antimicrobial action, and their names, formulae, and odors were more exotic.

Then, in the last decade or so, a plethora of articles investigating the actions and uses of irrigants has appeared, and some significant differences in endodontic therapy have resulted.

Baker et al. studied the effectiveness of various strengths and volumes of saline, NaOCl, H_2O_2, Gly-Oxide, and chelates. They reported no irrigant better than any other in dissolving necrotic debris or making canals cleaner. Therefore these clinicians recommended that the most biologically acceptable material be used as an intracanal irrigant—physiologic saline. The study received considerable attention, and many clinicians switched to saline. However, these clinicians failed to analyze the study carefully. The canals were considered to be well prepared when clean white dentin shavings were produced—not a good criterion. Also, no canal flaring was performed. Thus the canals were not well prepared, and the conclusion of the study should have been that when canals are poorly prepared, no solution will do a superior job in irrigation.

Two years later Svec and Harrison, using better methods of canal preparation, found that the combination of 5.25% NaOCl and 3% H_2O_2 gave a superior preparation to one utilizing normal saline or either irrigant alone. The following year Harrison et al. reported that in a study of 253 cases there was no statistical difference in incidence and degree of pain among groups irrigated with saline, 5.25% NaOCl, or NaOCl and H_2O_2.

Daughenbaugh and Schilder have reported a scanning electron microscopic study using various concentrations and combinations of irrigants. Their canals were widely enlarged at the orifices and flared. This change in preparation method alone gave generally much better results than those reported by Baker et al. The conclusion of the study was that 5.25% NaOCl alone produces clean canals, free of organic tissue, but that the walls have fewer open tubules than those prepared

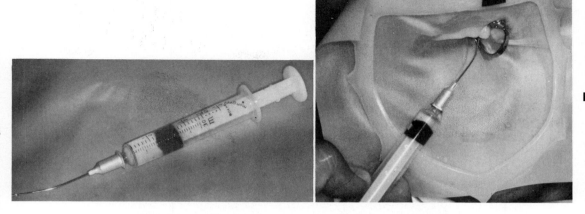

Fig. 7-59. **A,** Disposable syringe filled with the irrigant of choice. **B,** With a 30-degree angled bend placed in center of needle, the tip can be easily inserted into access preparation of any anterior or posterior tooth.

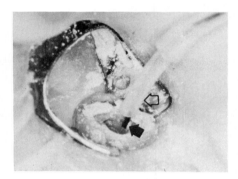

Fig. 7-60. As designed by Kahn, the Irrivac is a syringe with tip placed through tubing attached to an aspiration system, thus providing aspiration and irrigation simultaneously with a single device. Solution is placed in access cavity through needle tip *(solid arrow)*, and excess is aspirated through tubing *(open arrow)*, which is attached to a shunt through the saliva ejector.

with a combination of 2.5% NaOCl and 3% H_2O_2 (Fig. 7-61). The open tubules were considered to be desirable because they allowed for penetration by the medicaments and better adhesion for the sealers.

I believe that these studies make it clear that alternating irrigants gives a cleaner canal with less organic debris and more desirable walls. Considering the studies by Sundqvist (Chapter 15) on the potentially destructive anaerobes, I find the additional value of liberated oxygen to be also quite appealing (Fig. 7-62). One other study, by Senia et al., also enters in my choice of irrigants. They had reported that NaOCl does not reach the apex of small canals until the canals are enlarged to size 20 or greater. However, Gly-Oxide, being more viscous with a high surface tension, can be manipulated into very small canals and will liberate oxygen in even these deep recesses. Therefore I prefer to use Gly-Oxide as the major irrigant in small canals until size 20 is reached and then switch to NaOCl (Fig. 7-63). In larger canals I merely alternate irrigants. In teeth with periapical lesions I make considerable effort to allow for free exchange between the irrigants so the oxygen will be liberated and will kill the anaerobes.

Function of chelating agents. The problems of enlarging very sclerotic canals nagged even the earliest practitioners in endodontics. Phenolsulphonic acid, reverse aqua regia, and other severely caustic chemicals were advocated to aid in the enlargement of canals with narrow diameter. These chemicals were nonselective and therefore destroyed anything in contact, including periapical tissue.

Chelating agents provide an excellent alternative, since they act on calcified tissues only and have little effect on periapical tissue. Their action is to substitute sodium ions, which combine with the dentin to give soluble salts, for the calcium ions that are bound in less soluble combination. The edges of the canal are thus softer, and canal enlargement is facilitated.

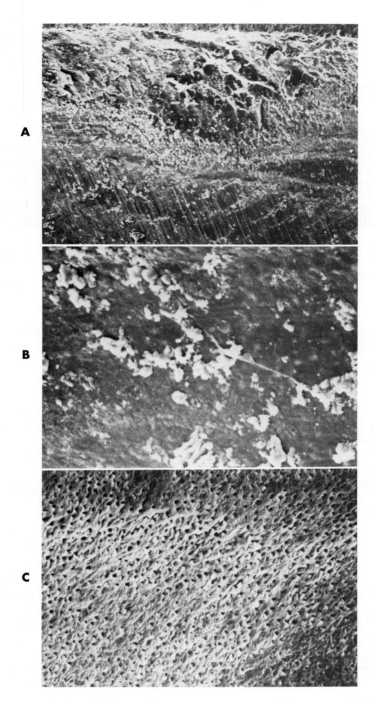

Fig. 7-61. Photomicrographs of in vitro specimen prepared as follows. **A,** Saline irrigant. Much organic tissue present. (×56.) **B,** 1% NaOCl. Smearing of dentin surface, and organic debris present. (×560.) **C,** 2.5% NaOCl alternated with 3% H_2O_2. Beautifully clean and smooth canal. (×560.) (Courtesy Dr. Jeffery A. Daughenbaugh, Salinas, Calif.)

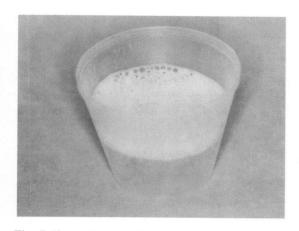

Fig. 7-62. A few milliliters of sodium hypochlorite (NaOCl) were placed in this dappen dish, and then a few milliliters of Gly-Oxide were added. A bubbling and foaming reaction immediately took place. The same reaction occurs in the canal when these two chemicals are mixed. The bubbling is the oxygen escaping, which will kill anaerobes. The foaming helps to wash out unwanted debris.

Chelating agents are placed in the orifice of a canal to be enlarged on the tip of the endodontic explorer or on the flutes of the enlarging instrument if the agent is foamy (as is RC-Prep) or by plastic irrigating syringe if liquid (e.g., EDTA). EDTA reacts with glass, so syringes of that material may not be used.

Chelating agents may be useful in the location of a difficult-to-find orifice by sealing in the chamber between appointments. Because the orifices are less calcified than the surrounding dentin, sufficient softening may allow it to be located with the sharp tip of the endodontic explorer at the next appointment.

If misused, chelating agents may cause problems during endodontic therapy. They should not be used in a ledged or blocked canal to aid in reaching the apex. If a sharp instrument is forced or rotated against a wall softened by the chelate, a new but false canal will be started. The operator may erroneously believe that the canal has been

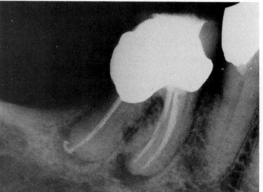

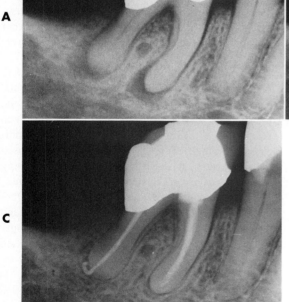

Fig. 7-63. Radiograph of mandibular first molar with periapical lesions on both roots and extremely narrow canals, particularly in mesial root. Canals were enlarged to size 20 with carbamide peroxide and then alternated with NaOCl. **B,** Filled with laterally condensed gutta-percha and Kerr's antiseptic sealer. **C,** Excellent healing 3 years later.

located and continue the preparation, thus losing any chance for finding the true canal.

Chelating agents are dangerous in curved canals once the larger-sized instruments (size 30 or greater) are being used. These instruments are not as flexible as the smaller sizes and, with the canal walls softened, may produce an elliptication of the apex or root perforation.

The best use of these agents is to aid and simplify preparation for very sclerotic canals after the apex has already been reached with a fine instrument.

EDTA. Patterson did much research on the disodium salt of ethylenediaminetetraacetic acid (EDTA). He reported that a 10% solution lowered the Knoop hardness number of treated dentin to 7, from a normal reading of 25 near the dentinoenamel junction up to 70 at approximately one third of the distance from the dentinoenamel junction to the canal wall when untreated. Next to the lumen of the untreated canal, where canal instrumentation is initiated, the Knoop hardness number was found to be 42. Reduction to a reading of 7 significantly reduces the difficulty encountered in using the smaller-size instruments to begin canal preparation.

Patterson further states that a 10% solution of EDTA did produce bacteriologic inhibition comparable to that of beechwood creosote against alpha-hemolytic streptococci and *Staphylococcus aureus.* Injection of 0.1 ml of 10% EDTA in the back muscle of albino rats produced moderate inflammation, whereas injections of distilled water and eugenol produced inflammation described as slight.

EDTA will remain active within the canal for 5 days if not inactivated. If the apical constriction has been opened, the chelate may seep out into the tissue and damage the periapical bone. For this reason, at the completion of the appointment the canal must be irrigated with a sodium hypochlorite–containing solution, a small file being placed into each canal where EDTA was used to ensure penetration of the inactivator.

Some research seems to indicate that the use of EDTA in canal preparation aids in the removal of the smear layer on the dentin wall. This might allow for better surface contact between the canal filling and the dentin wall and better potential penetration of the sealer into the dentinal tubules.

EDTAC. The addition of Cetavlon, a quaternary ammonium compound, to EDTA produces a solution called EDTAC, which has greater germicidal activity. However, it has greater inflammatory potential to tissue as well. The inactivator for EDTAC is NaOCl.

RC-Prep.* As developed by Stewart, RC-Prep combines the functions of EDTA plus urea peroxide to provide both chelation and irrigation. The foamy solution has a natural effervescence that is increased by irrigation with NaOCl to aid in the removal of debris. RC-Prep may be placed in the canal on the flutes of a file by plastic irrigating syringe (Fig. 7-64).

INTRACANAL MEDICAMENTS

Originally endodontics was mainly a therapeutic procedure in which drugs were used to destroy microorganisms, fix or mummify vital tissue, and effect a sealing of the root canal space. The drugs used were generally caustics, such as phenol and its derivatives, and periapical tissues were frequently adversely affected.

Gradually the reliance on drugs has been replaced by emphasis on debridement. It cannot be argued that what is removed from the canal has a greater significance in endodontic success than what is placed in the canal. Even so, drugs are still used as intertreatment dressings, although an ever-increasing number of endodontists use them only for symptomatic cases.

Function of intracanal medicaments. Most medicaments are effective antimicrobial agents. With the number of microorganisms reduced by irrigation and instrumentation, the medicament destroys those remaining and limits the growth of any new arrivals.

Corticosteroid-antibiotic combinations are useful in treating apical periodontitis, occurring either as a pretreatment symptom or as a result of over-instrumentation.

Volatile medicaments should never be used to determine, through retention of their scent on the cotton pellet taken from the chamber, whether the material used to seal the access cavity has been effective. Culturing is a much more reliable indicator, although many practitioners cannot resist the opportunity to sniff the dressing after opening the access cavity at the start of each appointment.

Phenol and related volatile compounds. Phenol was used for many years for its disinfectant and caustic action. However, because it has strongly inflammatory potential, at present it is rarely used as an intracanal medicament. Phenol is used for disinfection before periapical surgery (Chapter 11) and for cauterizing tissue tags that resist removal with broaches or files.

*Premier Dental Products, Norristown, PA 19401.

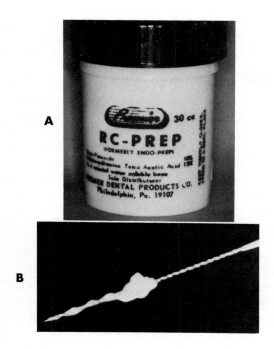

Fig. 7-64. **A,** RC-Prep (developed by Stewart) provides for chelation and irrigation by using a combination of EDTA and urea peroxide. **B,** Because it is foamy, RC-Prep is placed on flutes of a file and carried directly to walls of canal being prepared.

Eugenol also has been used in endodontics for many years. It is a constituent of most root canal sealers and is used as a part of many temporary sealing agents. Although the compound has a high irritating potential when evaluated histologically, it seems to be extremely soothing clinically to vital tissue, probably from some type of caustic action to irritated nerve endings. It is used as an intracanal medicament after partial or complete pulpectomy.

Camphorated monoparachlorophenol (CMCP) is probably the most widely used medicament in endodontics presently, even though its use has decreased considerably in the past few years. It has a wide antibacterial spectrum and is effective against fungi as well. CMCP is much less irritating to periapical tissue than either phenol or eugenol without sacrificing antimicrobial action. It is inexpensive, has a long shelf life, and does not appear to yield false-negative cultures if carried to the medium on a paper point.

Metacresyl acetate (Cresatin) was reported by Schilder and Amsterdam to have the same desirable qualities and actions as CMCP yet be even less irritating to periapical tissues. It has excellent

anodynic qualities for vital tissue and therefore is useful after pulpectomy.

Formocresol, a combination of formalin and cresol, is used as a dressing for pulpotomy to fix the retained pulpal tissue. It may also be used as an intratreatment medicament when a pulpotomy is performed as emergency treatment to relieve pain, in situations where pulp inflammation is confined to the pulp chamber.

Other similar compounds used as medicaments are cresol, beechwood creosote, and thymol. All are more irritating to periapical tissue than CMCP but have various adherents among clinicians.

The efficacy of medicaments in endodontic therapy has undergone many changes. In recent years there has been a strong impetus to use the best-tolerated medications regardless of their antimicrobial efficiency. An extremely impressive series of studies by Makkes et al. in Amsterdam has further weakened the position of the pro-medication faction among endodontists, particularly when treating teeth with nonvital pulps. They studied the tissue response to sterile dead muscle and necrotic muscle tissue treated by fixation. The two groups are analogous to pulp tissue that became necrotic by physical or chemical trauma and necrotic tissue onto which chemical fixative medicaments had been placed.

For many years it was assumed that the necrotic pulp tissue was a source of serious irritation to the local area, even without ingress by microorganisms, and that this reaction was responsible for the initial development of a granuloma. On the other hand, many practitioners believed that treatment of this necrotic tissue with fixatives such as formaldehyde will render the pulp remnants harmless. However, Makkes et al. reported a very contrary finding. Tissue reaction to the sterile dead muscle was minimal and self-limiting, whereas the response to fixed muscle tissue by formaldehyde or glutaraldehyde was a severe chronic inflammation, even in the absence of microorganisms.

Many clinicians reserve the strongest medicaments (e.g., formocresol) for treatment in necrotic cases. Although these medications do have an impressive antibacterial spectrum, they also often contain elements that cause fixation of the necrotic pulp remnants. Under these circumstances, I believe that the canals of teeth with necrotic pulps should be well cleansed and heavily irrigated to reduce tissue remnants and substrate but that the mildest medication or no medication at all should be used. In fact, more than 90% of the cases illustrated in this textbook were managed without any intracanal medicament.

My use of formocresol is limited solely to pulpotomy dressing as emergency treatment (Chapter 5) when there is no apical spread of inflammation or infection, so the medicament is placed on vital tissue a long distance from the periapical tissues.

All the phenolics and similar compounds are highly volatile with low surface tension. Therefore, if they are placed on a cotton pellet in the chamber of a tooth in treatment, the vapors will permeate the entire canal preparation, and placement on a paper point is unnecessary. Only a tiny quantity of medication is needed for effectiveness—a fact always to be remembered, since periapical irritation must be avoided. The proper way to apply these volatile medicaments is to invert the bottle containing the medication to allow the liquid to cling to the side near the mouth of the jar. The cover is removed and a sterile cotton pellet lightly wiped on the inside, picking up some of the liquid. The amount absorbed on the cotton will be more than enough for use.

PBSC. As mentioned by Grossman, PBSC has enjoyed wide use among dentists trained at the University of Pennsylvania and those who have participated in postgraduate courses at that institution. The constituents of the paste are as follows:

Penicillin—effective against gram-positive microorganisms
Bacitracin—effective against penicillin-resistant microorganisms
Streptomycin—effective against the gram-negative microorganisms
Caprylate—as the sodium salt, effective against fungi

Nystatin replaces sodium caprylate as the antifungal agent in a similar medicament, PBSN. Both are available in a paste form that may be injected into root canals or impregnated on paper points. Because there is no volatility, the drug must be placed in the canal to have effect in that area.

PBSC may interfere with subsequent culturing procedures, and penicillinase may be added to culture media to inactivate penicillin should it be transferred on the paper point taken to incubate. Reports of allergic reaction to the drug have been presented, although considering the wide use on patients who might have had sensitivity, it seems to be a minor point. However, if the patient reports history of allergy to any of the constituents, the drug should not be used.

With the decline in popularity of intracanal drugs in general, and because of the potential for sensitivity due to topical use of antibiotics, PBSN largely has fallen into disuse.

Sulfonamides. Sulfanilamide and sulfathiazole are used as medicaments by mixing with sterile distilled water or by placing a moistened paper point into a fluffed jar containing the powder. Yellowish tooth discoloration has been reported after use. The medication is suggested for use when closing teeth that had been left open after an acute periapical abscess. (See Chapter 5.)

Corticosteroid-antibiotic combinations. Medications that combine antibiotic and corticosteroid elements are highly effective in the treatment of overinstrumentation; they must be placed into the inflamed periapical tissue by a paper point or reamer to be effective (Chapter 5). Terra-Cortril, Corti-Sporin, Mycolog, and other combinations are available as salves or ophthalmic ointments for use in endodontics.

The corticosteroid constituent reduces the periapical inflammation and gives almost instant relief of pain to the patient who has complained of extreme tenderness to percussion after canal instrumentation. The antibiotic constituents are present so that no overgrowth of microorganisms will occur with the inflammatory response diminished.

Calcium hydroxide as a medicament for "weeping" cases. One of the most perplexing conditions to treat is the tooth with constant clear or reddish exudation associated with a large apical radiolucency. The tooth often is asymptomatic, but it may be tender to percussion or sensitive to digital pressure over the apex. If cultured, the drainage generally will not support bacterial growth. When opened at the start of the endodontic appointment, a reddish discharge may well up, whereas at a succeeding appointment the exudate will be clear (Fig. 7-65). Some pressure is present, but not nearly as much as with an acute periapical abscess. If the tooth is left open under a rubber dam for 15 to 30 minutes, it may be closed up by absorbing the exudate with an aspirator and paper points; however, a similar condition will still be present at the next appointment. The canal has already been enlarged to a more than acceptable size. This is referred to as a *weeping canal.*

One is always in a quandary as to the correct method for treating such a canal. Classically those with exudates were not considered to be ready for filling (Chapter 9). Should surgery be

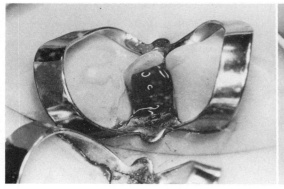
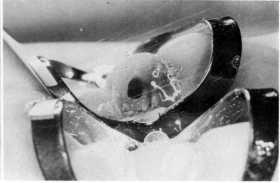

A

B

Fig. 7-65. **A,** Maxillary lateral incisor with large periapical lesion opened for drainage, allowing heavy bloody exudate to discharge. **B,** Several appointments later, a clear exudate (shiny area to right of access cavity) discharged.

performed to curette the area of pathosis at the same appointment at which the canal is filled? Perhaps it would be best merely to fill the canal and see whether surgery could be avoided. The problem with this regimen is that because of the apical oozing, it is very difficult to fill weeping canals adequately. Prescribing antibiotics for the patient seems foolish because of the frequency of negative cultures.

The answer to this recalcitrant problem is to dry the canal with sterile absorbent paper points and place calcium hydroxide paste in the canal, similar to what is done to gain apexification in teeth with open apices and nonvital pulps (Chapter 16). It is absolutely astonishing to see a perfectly dry clean canal at the next appointment that is simple to fill after minimal further preparation (Fig. 7-66).

The exact mechanism for the action of calcium hydroxide in this type of case is an object of much conjecture. I believe that it is closely related to the pH of the periapical tissues, which must be acidic in the weeping stage. The pH is converted by the paste to a more basic environment. Others believe that the calcifying potential of the medicament starts to build up bone in the lesion. Still others suggest that the caustic action of the calcium hydroxide burns residual chronic inflamed tissue.

Whatever the reason, I have used this technique in several cases that healed magnificently and were followed up for significant time periods (Figs. 7-67 and 7-68).

• • •

Many dentists presently select calcium hydroxide as the intracanal medicament of choice for rou-

tine cases, replacing the phenolic derivatives. This is particularly true in the Scandinavian countries, where a considerable amount of research on this material has been reported. It has advocates in the United States as well.

Because of its pH, few microorganisms can survive in calcium hydroxide's presence. The material has an excellent record of helping to heal radiolucencies. Unlike the phenolic derivatives, calcium hydroxide leads, at worst, to a minimal number of immunologic reactions.

I still believe that the functions of medicaments should be sublimated to use of excellent debridement and that they should be employed only in those few cases where other aspects of therapy have not worked. Ultrasonic use has given us cleaner canals; healing of radiolucencies will occur without employing calcium hydroxide; and using no medicament is even more likely to avoid an immunologic reaction.

SEALING AGENTS FOR INTERTREATMENT DRESSINGS

Need for sealing agents. Because endodontic treatment usually takes two or more appointments, some type of temporary sealing agent is needed to close the access cavity between visits. The material selected must provide for effective closure against microorganisms and salivary contamination, which would bring irritants to the periapical tissue if allowed free passage. The access-sealing agent must also retain the intracanal medicament, if used, within the tooth to allow effectiveness for the drug.

Types of available sealing agents. According to radioisotope studies, silver amalgam plus cavity

A   **B**   **C**

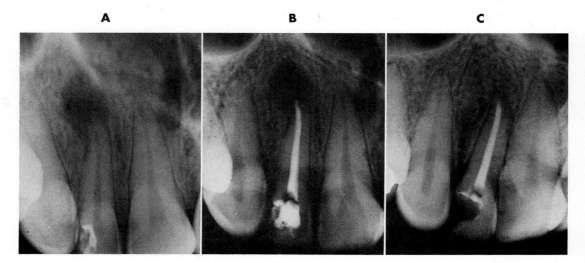

Fig. 7-66.   Case similar to that shown in Fig. 7-65. Maxillary lateral with large periapical lesion. **A,** Preoperative radiograph. First time canal was opened, a large bloody exudate welled up; at subsequent appointments and after several negative cultures, calcium hydroxide paste was placed. **B,** Exudates ceased by the next appointment, and the canal was filled. **C,** Excellent healing 6 months later.

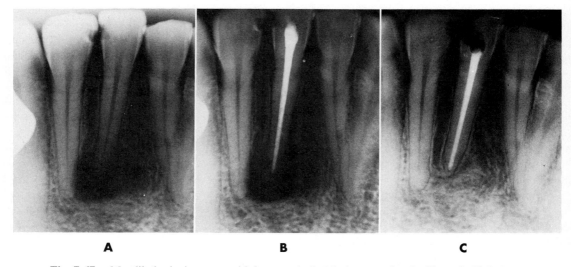

A   **B**   **C**

Fig. 7-67.   Mandibular incisor area with large periapical lesion associated with tooth 25 that gave persistent discharges. **A,** Preoperative radiograph. **B,** Calcium hydroxide paste was used to stop exudation, and canal was filled. **C,** Six years after treatment.

varnish is the most effective sealant available in dentistry. Unfortunately, it would be difficult and time consuming to use those materials at the conclusion of each appointment and then have to drill everything out at the next visit.

Fortunately, zinc oxide powder with eugenol (ZOE) provides an excellent seal and is much easier to place and remove than amalgam. The addition of zinc acetate crystals speeds the set of ZOE without decreasing the sealing properties.

A large, thick mix of ZOE may be prepared each morning by the dental assistant and placed into the well of an empty ink bottle. A desiccating chemical, such as those included in bottles of medicines that may be altered by moisture, is placed in the bottom of the jar to retain the ZOE in usable condition for the entire day (Fig. 7-69). Placement of the jar in the refrigerator will further retain the properties of the temporary sealer in workable form for a few additional days. When the

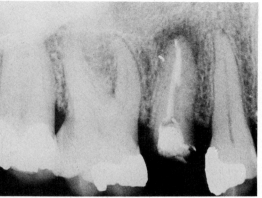

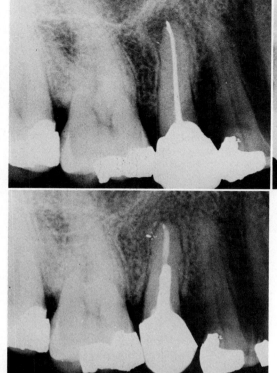

Fig. 7-68.   Similar history to those in Figs. 7-66 and 7-67. Failing silver point case. **A,** Preoperative radiograph. **B,** Canal filling with gutta-percha after using calcium hydroxide paste. **C,** Two years after original treatment. (Restorations by Dr. R. Ceisel, Evanston, Ill.)

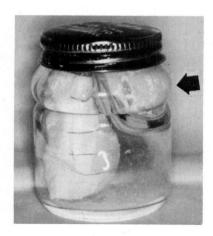

Fig. 7-69. Empty ink bottle is used to store zinc oxide–eugenol cement for use throughout the day. ZOE is mixed in morning and placed in well *(arrow).* Bottom of jar has desiccating crystals to inhibit set of cement. One mixing will provide cement for as long as a week if jar is kept in refrigerator.

temporary seal is needed, a suitable amount is removed from the jar and the acetate added.

Cavit and Cavit G* were introduced for use in endodontics. Both are easy to apply, and Cavit G may be removed with a spoon excavator, not even requiring a bur. Unfortunately the response of these two materials on radioautographic studies has been poor (Fig. 7-70). However, many practitioners use them and report a significantly high number of negative cultures, indicating that even if the isotopes penetrate, the microorganisms do not. As long as ZOE is available, these remain second choices in my opinion.

The use of a double seal of zinc oxyphosphate cement over gutta-percha was advocated for many years. However, neither of these materials alone or in combination has been shown to be resistant to either isotope or dye penetration.

The use of gutta-percha as an intermediate layer beneath ZOE is acceptable, not as a sealing agent but to prevent the temporary filling from falling into and blocking canals—an accident that might occur in mandibular teeth, particularly molars, when a fragment of hardened ZOE falls into the chamber

*Premier Dental Products, Norristown, PA 19401.

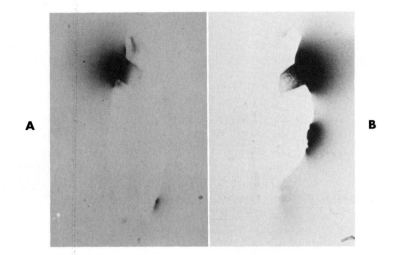

Fig. 7-70. Radioautograms of central incisor access cavities closed with, **A,** Cavit and, **B,** Cavit G, both with considerable marginal leakage.

and is forced into a thin canal by the explorer or an intracanal instrument. To avoid this problem, at the time of closure the dentist places the cotton pellet in the chamber and covers it by heated and softened gutta-percha, over which the ZOE is placed as a seal. At the next appointment the seal is removed and the access examined for loose particles before the gutta-percha is touched. Then a hot instrument can be used to remove the gutta-percha and cotton without fear of blocking a canal.

Recently a light-cured material, TERM (Temporary Endodontic Restorative Material),* has been introduced. Its major advantages are the ease with which it may be used, since it may be placed with a syringe from sterile prepacked compules, and it is set by exposure to visible light for 20 seconds.

The leakage studies have indicated a variety of results, from superior to poor. However, even the manufacturer advises that TERM be used only for 1 month or less because of several reports that its sealing ability decreases rapidly after 2 months.

TREATMENT OF OPERATIVE PERFORATIONS

Endodontic cases are increasing in complexity to a considerable degree. Cases are managed now that only a decade ago would have been thought to be hopeless. This has encouraged dentists to undertake

*Cault/Dentsply, Milford, DE 19963.

therapy in more and more complicated cases; and, unfortunately, some of the teeth become involved in procedural misadventures—one of the most aggravating of which is the operative perforation. Adding to the problem is that the average age of the population is increasing, and septagenarians and octagenerians often display canals of extremely small size.

Operative perforations are defined here as a procedural accident whereby an artificial opening is created in a tooth so that a communication exists between the pulp canal space and the periodontal tissues. They may occur during an attempt to locate or enlarge a canal or when preparing room for a post or similar retentive device. Perforations may be due to trauma or to an altered state of pulpal or periodontal ligament tissue. These are inflammatory, not operative, perforations; their treatment is discussed in detail in Chapter 16, and to a lesser degree in Chapter 11. Many inflammatory perforations are treatable with calcium hydroxide pastes as an interim dressing, but our experience with that medicament in operative perforations is rather poor.

The indication of a perforation is generally a slow but steady seeping of blood. Because this symptom also often occurs during the extirpation of a vital pulp from a small canal, it may not immediately inform the operator of the procedural problem. However, as the false canal is enlarged, the seepage does not diminish but may increase. Drying attempts with paper points are futile. Ultimately a radiograph from at least two directions will confirm the problem.

General rules for treating operative perforations. The dentist always feels some guilt when an operative perforation occurs. Although I readily sympathize with that attitude, it should be put in the correct frame of reference. If the tooth did not need endodontics, the perforation would not have resulted. Therefore the etiology of the perforation transcends the appointment when the accident occurred. This may seem simplistic, but there is a very good reason for what I say. For the best prognosis *a perforation must be sealed as soon as possible* (Fig. 7-71). The chances for success diminish greatly when the perforation is closed at an appointment subsequent to the occurrence. When a perforation occurs, the operator must stay calm and make the repair immediately, hoping for the best.

Even in the best circumstances a perforation does limit the degree of success for an endodontic case. Although I have had some perforated teeth remain normal and asymptomatic for years, some suddenly develop serious periodontal lesions. Therefore I prefer to retain perforated teeth when they are surrounded by sound adjacent teeth. If the treated tooth goes bad, it may be extracted and a fixed bridge used as a replacement. Attempting to use a perforated tooth as a bridge or splint abutment is very hazardous. If the treated tooth develops further problems, the complex restoration will have to be seriously compromised or scrapped. It is not worth the chance. It is better to face the music, extract the perforated tooth, and utilize other abutment teeth.

Inform the patient what has transpired. Perforations occur during the course of treating complicated teeth. The patient must be informed for legal purposes and also to understand the further choices of therapy available. Sooner or later the patient will discover what has happened; it is far better to learn it from you at the time of the occurrence.

Treatment of furcation perforations by packing the chamber. This type of perforation is very common and has a fairly good prognosis when the perforation is sealed off immediately and when the patient's periodontal condition is good. It generally occurs when searching for a small canal that is diminished by irritation dentin (Fig. 7-72, *A* and *B*). On occasion the operator will think that the missing canal has been located. However, the telltale sign of seeping bleeding may be verified by the placement of a file and taking of a radiograph (Fig. 7-72 *B*) from two angles.

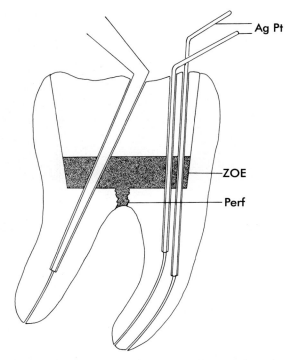

Fig. 7-71. Diagram of perforation repair. Following perforation the true canal must be found. Silver points (or endodontic files) are placed well into the canals, protruding through the access cavity, to keep patency during the packing procedure. A heavy mix of ZOE is prepared and packed into the defect with a cotton pellet or cotton-tipped swab. Several more millimeters of ZOE are packed over the floor to provide a bulk of material for the closing of the perforation. When the cement has set, the silver points (or files) are removed, patency verified, and treatment completed (Figs. 7-72, *E,* and 7-73, *E*).

The correct course of action at this point is to continue to search for the missing canal. If it cannot be located, an extraction or root amputation is indicated and there is no need to take the time to make the repair. Very frequently the true canal will be located (Fig. 7-72, *D*) immediately after the perforation is verified by radiograph. The x-ray film will indicate the relationship between the true canal and the perforation, and the operator has another reference point to use in making the corrected location. All the canals should be enlarged to at least a minimum degree (i.e., size 25 or larger) at the correct working length. Use the least irritating irrigant for this procedure—saline would be fine—because there must be minimal irritation

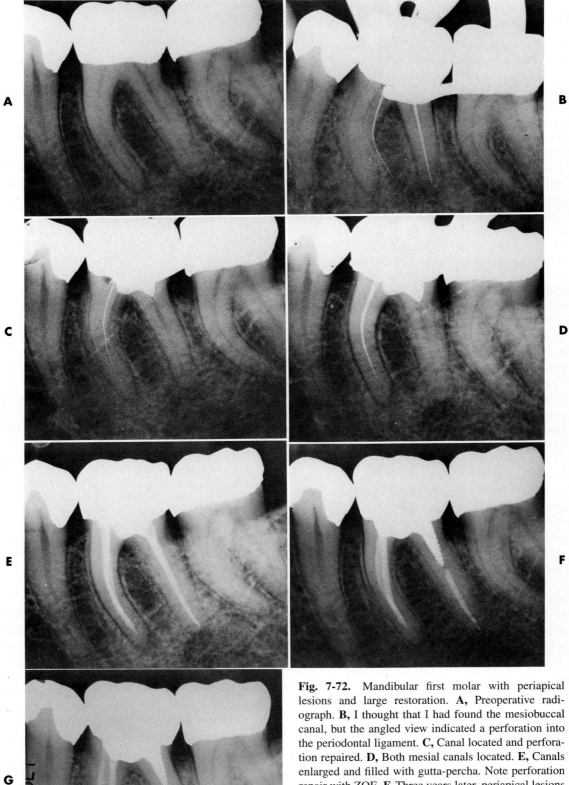

Fig. 7-72. Mandibular first molar with periapical lesions and large restoration. **A,** Preoperative radiograph. **B,** I thought that I had found the mesiobuccal canal, but the angled view indicated a perforation into the periodontal ligament. **C,** Canal located and perforation repaired. **D,** Both mesial canals located. **E,** Canals enlarged and filled with gutta-percha. Note perforation repair with ZOE. **F,** Three years later, periapical lesions have healed and furcation has remained normal. **G,** Fourteen years after original treatment, perforation repair still present, furcation area still closed, and all tissues appear normal. (Restorations by Dr. Sherwin Strauss, Chicago.)

to the injured periodontal ligament adjacent to the perforation. A small inverted cone bur is used to slightly widen the most occlusal portion of the perforation. This also creates a somewhat retentive lock for the sealing material.

A silver point (or endodontic file) is placed in each canal. It need not bind at the apex but should bind several millimeters short of the apex and protrude through the access opening. These points will keep the filling material from going into the canals during packing of the chamber. This method is similar to that shown in Fig. 6-63. Then a heavy mix of ZOE is prepared. A small portion of the cement is placed over the perforation and gently but firmly packed down. A larger portion of ZOE is placed over this area and again packed down (Fig. 7-71). Once the cement is hardened, the silver points are removed from the canals. A slight amount of enlargement of these canals is performed to verify their patency.

The case is then completed in the routine manner (Fig. 7-72, *E,* and 7-73, *E*). The patient should be recalled initially at 6-month intervals. In addition to radiographs, the area of repair should be examined for any periodontal defects and the presence of mobility. One hopes that the repair will remain as a tight seal against leakage and that the periodontal structures retain a normal condition (Figs. 7-72, *F* and *G,* and 7-73, *F* and *G*).

Treatment of perforations by enlargement and filling as an additional canal. The disadvantage of sealing perforations by packing is that the operator has no true control over the movement of the ZOE cement. Some perforations may be overpacked and may cause extreme inflammation to the periodontal ligament, which is what we are trying to keep in a healthy state. On the other hand, if the cement is not packed to seal off most of the defect, the empty space will be an area to harbor bacteria and tissue breakdown products.

Accordingly, if the distance between the pulp canal space and the periodontal ligament is quite long and consequently difficult to pack off, the perforation may be enlarged and filled as an additional canal. There are some serious difficulties encountered in this technique as well. Many perforations extend to the buccal or lingual rather than proximal, however, and it is difficult to judge the exact site at which the defect reaches the periodontal ligament. Those that extend to the proximal can be measured with greater accuracy.

Again, it is wise to attempt to complete the sealing of the perforation as soon as possible after the misadventure is discovered. A measurement film is taken (Fig. 7-74, *C*) and the canal prepared as in a routine case. The canal is filled with gutta-percha and lateral condensation. The periodontal ligament area should then remain in a relatively normal state (Fig. 7-74, *E*) or heal (Fig. 7-75, *F*).

Lateral perforations treated by packing gutta-percha adjacent to the defect. Cases falling into this category generally have quite wide perforations that cannot be filled at all by further preparation, as discussed in the previous section. Also, my experience with recalcification of operative perforations using calcium hydroxide is quite poor. Surgical repair is a viable alternative but almost impossible if the defect is to the lingual. Also, surgical access demands a considerable removal of bone, which probably will not heal back to the original topography. Some strip perforations (Fig. 7-12) are sealed in this manner.

The canal must be enlarged (Fig. 7-76, *C*), and fitting of a customized master cone (Chapter 9) is preferable (Fig. 7-76, *D*). The canal is filled with a routine lateral condensation procedure (Fig. 7-76, *F* to *H*). It is hoped the filling material will remain essentially within the confines of the tooth and seal off the defect. Then the adjacent periodontal ligament will heal satisfactorily, and the area will remain in a normal condition (Fig. 7-76, *J* and *K*).

Perforations eliminated by surgery. If the perforation is near enough to the gingival margin, it may be eliminated completely with a relatively simple surgical procedure (Fig. 7-77). A small tissue flap is raised so the base of the flap is apical to the perforation. If the perforation is apical to the height of the bone, the hard tissue must be removed so no bone is coronal to the defect. The remaining bone is recontoured to allow for correct bony architecture.

If the perforation is completely coronal to the height of the crestal bone, the defect may be eliminated by removal of tooth structure coronal to it or by packing with ZOE. As long as sufficient periodontal support for the tooth remains after surgery, these defects generally heal beautifully and cause no further problem.

Perforations treated surgically or orthodontically. These entities will be described in Chapters 11 and 14, respectively.

New materials for perforation repair. Many studies on perforation repair have investigated the

Text continued on p. 392.

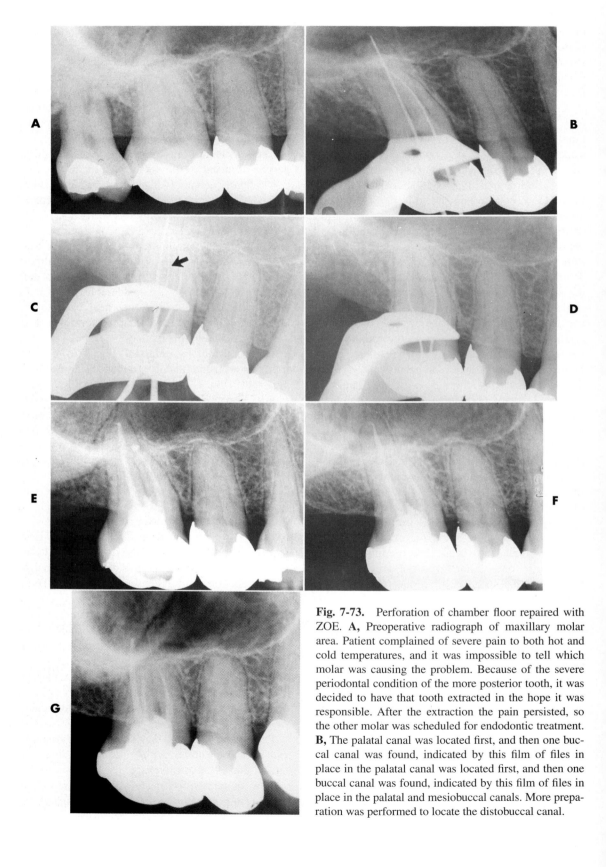

Fig. 7-73. Perforation of chamber floor repaired with ZOE. **A,** Preoperative radiograph of maxillary molar area. Patient complained of severe pain to both hot and cold temperatures, and it was impossible to tell which molar was causing the problem. Because of the severe periodontal condition of the more posterior tooth, it was decided to have that tooth extracted in the hope it was responsible. After the extraction the pain persisted, so the other molar was scheduled for endodontic treatment. **B,** The palatal canal was located first, and then one buccal canal was found, indicated by this film of files in place in the palatal canal was located first, and then one buccal canal was found, indicated by this film of files in place in the palatal and mesiobuccal canals. More preparation was performed to locate the distobuccal canal.

Fig. 7-73, cont'd. C, I thought that I had located it, so I placed files and took this radiograph. The file with the arrow had perforated the floor of the chamber rather than being placed in the distobuccal canal. **D,** The distobuccal canal was located slightly more to the distal. Files were placed into the canals to keep them patent during the repair. The orifice portion of the perforation was slightly widened with an inverted cone bur. Then the entire chamber floor was packed with ZOE. When the cement had set, the files were removed and patency verified. **E,** Treatment was completed, with canals filled with laterally condensed gutta-percha. **F,** Three years after original treatment. The tooth is comfortable, no pocket can be probed, and the area has retained a normal condition. **G,** Thirteen years after original treatment, all tissues appear normal.

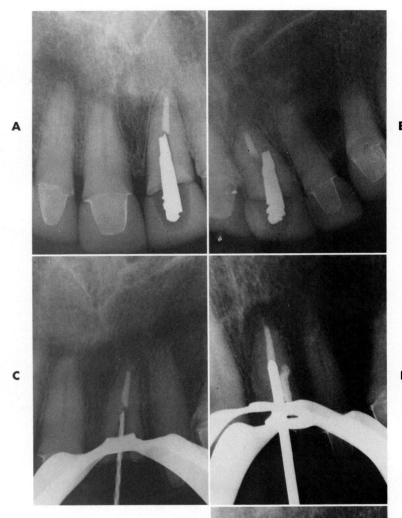

Fig. 7-74. A, Radiograph of anterior area with post and porcelain jacket crown. Post appears to be in canal, but the patient had a sinus tract on the palate, and I suspected a perforation. **B,** Angled view from distal verifies perforation to the palate. **C,** Crown and post were removed, and distance to perforation was measured with a file to slightly short of sensitivity by the patient. **D,** That false canal was filled with laterally condensed gutta-percha and Wach's paste, and an Endopost measured adjacent to it. **E,** Two years later the tract has not returned, and the tooth is comfortable. (Restorations by Dr. Don Hackman, formerly of Chicago.)

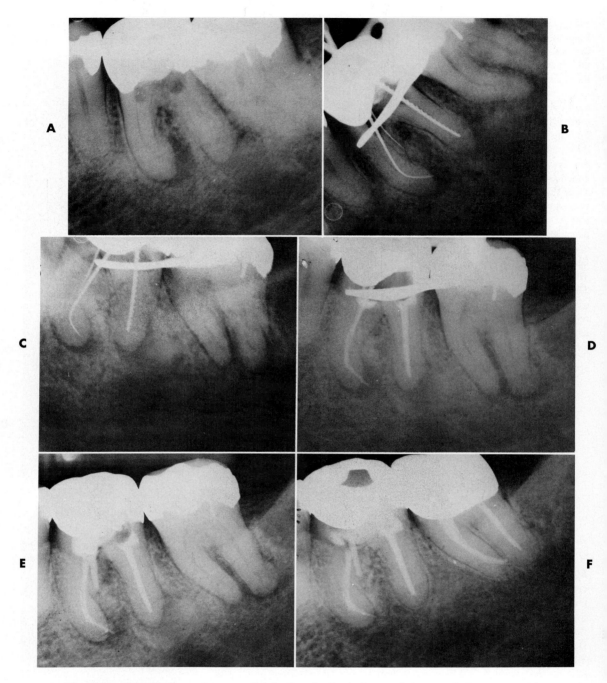

Fig. 7-75. Mandibular molar area. Originating dentist had started the case but was uncertain whether canals were located or a perforation was present. **A,** Preoperative radiograph. Periapical lesions present on both root apices of first molar. **B,** Files in place indicate perforation in area of mesiobuccal. **C,** Two mesials located and joined far short of apex. **D,** Mesial and distal canals filled with laterally condensed gutta-percha. **E,** Perforation sealed by enlargement and filling as an additional canal. Second molar had periapical lesions and also required treatment. **F,** Two years later, all areas are healed.

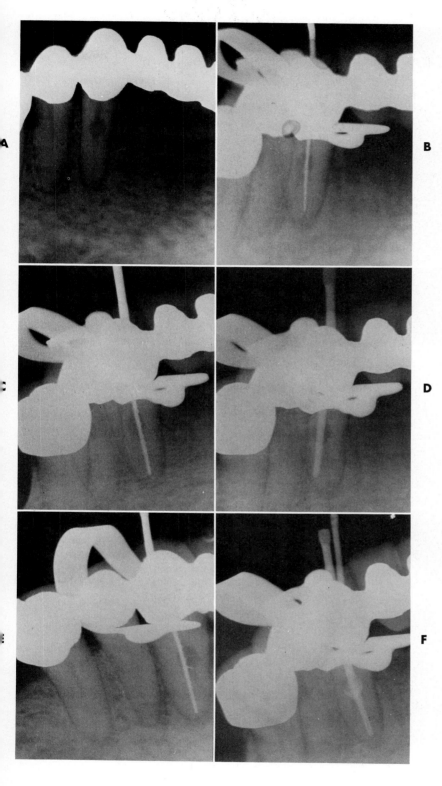

Fig. 7-76. Mandibular cuspid with operative perforation by originating dentist. **A,** Preoperative radiograph. **B,** True canal located. **C,** Enlarged to size 50 and flared. **D,** In the attempt to gain a customized master cone, the perforation was again located. **E,** Canal relocated, enlarged further, and closed to fill at next appointment. **F,** Master cone and one auxiliary cone placed, indicating that all are in the true canal.

Continued

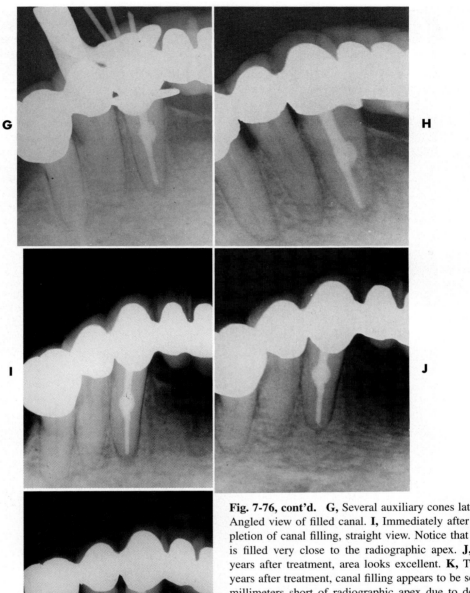

Fig. 7-76, cont'd.   G, Several auxiliary cones later. **H,** Angled view of filled canal. **I,** Immediately after completion of canal filling, straight view. Notice that canal is filled very close to the radiographic apex. **J,** Two years after treatment, area looks excellent. **K,** Twelve years after treatment, canal filling appears to be several millimeters short of radiographic apex due to deposition of cementum. Tooth is firm and comfortable.

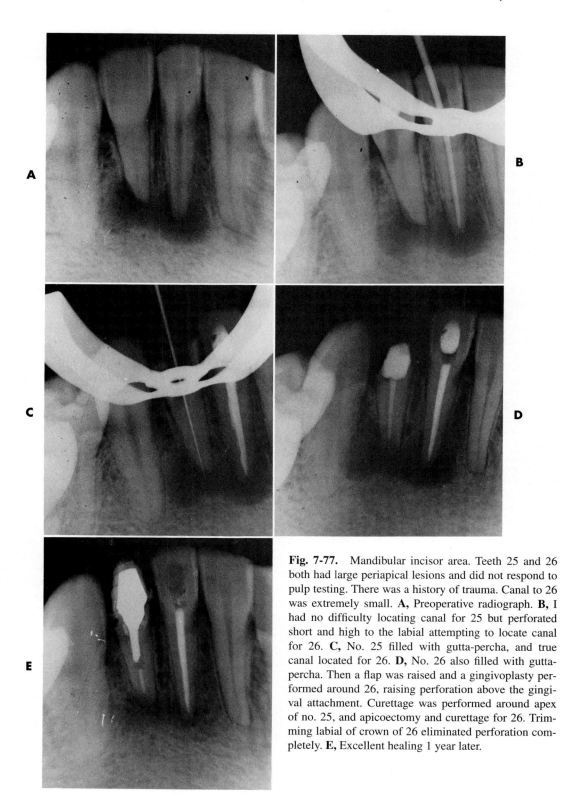

Fig. 7-77. Mandibular incisor area. Teeth 25 and 26 both had large periapical lesions and did not respond to pulp testing. There was a history of trauma. Canal to 26 was extremely small. **A,** Preoperative radiograph. **B,** I had no difficulty locating canal for 25 but perforated short and high to the labial attempting to locate canal for 26. **C,** No. 25 filled with gutta-percha, and true canal located for 26. **D,** No. 26 also filled with gutta-percha. Then a flap was raised and a gingivoplasty performed around 26, raising perforation above the gingival attachment. Curettage was performed around apex of no. 25, and apicoectomy and curettage for 26. Trimming labial of crown of 26 eliminated perforation completely. **E,** Excellent healing 1 year later.

use of amalgam. I have found this material deficient for this use, particularly if any excess material is expressed into the periodontium. If that occurs, a defect results almost immediately. Excess ZOE, on the other hand, usually is resorbed without the creation of a defect.

Recently, Torabinejad and his group from Loma Linda University have investigated the use of mineral trioxide aggregate (MTA) for use as a repair material for perforations, as a reverse filling material in periapical surgery, and in several other endodontic areas. The material seems to be very easy to use. Even though initial reports seem very favorable, more time is needed for evaluation.

REFERENCES

Adams WR, Patterson SS, Swartz ML: The effect of the apical dentinal plug on broken endodontic instruments, *J Endod* 5:121, 1979.

Allison DA, Weber CR, Walton RE: The influence of the method of canal preparation on the quality of apical and coronal obturation, *J Endod* 5:298, 1979.

Baker NA, Eleazer PD, Auerbach RE, Seltzer S: Scanning electron microscopic study of the efficacy of various irrigation solutions, *J Endod* 1:127, 1975.

Benenati FW, Roane JB, Biggs JT, Simon JH: Recall evaluation of iatrogenic root perforations repaired with amalgam and gutta-percha, *J Endod* 12:161, 1986.

Brian JD Jr, Ranly DM, Fulton RS, Madden RM: Reaction of rat connective tissue to unfixed and formaldehyde-fixed autogenous implants enclosed in tubes, *J Endod* 6:628, 1980.

Briseno BM, Sonnabend E: The influence of different root canal instruments on root canal preparation: an in vitro study, *Int Endod J* 23:15, 1991.

Campos JM, delRio C: Comparison of mechanical and standard hand instrumentation techniques in curved canals, *J Endod* 16:230, 1990.

Canales ML, Montgomery S, delRio CE: Root canal instrumentation with Unitek and K-Flex files, *J Endod* 10:12, 1984.

Clem WH: Endodontics: the adolescent patient, *Dent Clin North Am* 13:483, 1969.

Coffae KP, Brilliant JD: The effect of serial preparation versus nonserial preparation on tissue removal in the root canals of extracted mandibular molars, *J Endod* 1:211, 1975.

Council on Dental Materials and Devices: New American Dental Association specification no. 28 for endodontic files and reamers, *J Am Dent Assoc* 93:813, 1976.

Daughenbaugh JA, Schiler S: A scanning electron microscopic evaluation of sodium hypochlorite in the cleaning and shaping of human root canal systems, master's thesis, Boston, 1982, Boston University.

Dolan DW, Craig RG: Bending and torsion of endodontic files with rhombus cross sections, *J Endod* 8:260, 1982.

ElDeeb ME, Boraas JC: The effect of different files on the preparation shape of severely curved canals, *Int Endod J* 18:1, 1985.

Felt RA, Moser JB, Heuer MA: Flute design of endodontic instruments: its influence in cutting efficiency, *J Endod* 8:253, 1982.

Frank AL: An evaluation of the Giromatic endodontic handpiece, *Oral Surg* 24:419, 1967.

Frank AL: Calcium hydroxide: the ultimate medicament? *Dent Clin North Am* 23:691, 1979.

Genet JM, Hart AAM, Wesselink PR, van Velzen SK: Preoperative and operative factors associated with pain after the first endodontic visit, *Int Endod J* 20:53, 1987.

Green D: Stereomicroscopic study of 700 root apices of maxillary and mandibular teeth, *Oral Surg* 13:314, 1965.

Gutierrez JH, Garcia J: Microscopic and macroscopic investigation on results of mechanical preparation of root canals, *Oral Surg* 25:108, 1968.

Haga C: Microscopic measurements of root canal preparations following instrumentation, *Northwest Univ Bull Dent Res Grad Study,* Fall 1967, p 11.

Haikel Y, Alleman C: Effectiveness of four methods for preparing root canals: a scanning electron microscopic evaluation, *J Endod* 14:340, 1988.

Harris WE: A simplified method of treatment for endodontic perforations, *J Endod* 2:126, 1976.

Harrison JW, Baumgartner JC, Svec TA: Incidence of pain associated with clinical factors during and after root canal therapy. Part 1. Interappointment pain, *J Endod* 9:384, 1983.

Harrison JW, Svec TA, Baumgartner JC: Analysis of clinical toxicity of endodontic irrigants, *J Endod* 4:6, 1978.

Harty FJ, Stock CJR: The Giromatic system compared with hand instrumentation in endodontics, *Br Dent J* 137:239, 1974.

Heuer MA: The biomechanics of endodontic therapy, *Dent Clin North Am,* July 1963, p 341.

Hulsman M, Stryga F: Comparison of root canal preparation using different automated devices and hand instrumentation, *J Endod* 19:141, 1993.

Ingle JI: A standardized endodontic technique using newly designed instruments and filling materials, *Oral Surg* 14:83, 1961.

Jungman CL, Uchin RA, Bucher JF: Effect of instrumentation on the shape of the root canal, *J Endod* 1:66, 1975.

Kahn H et al: An improved endodontic irrigation technique, *Oral Surg* 36:887, 1973.

Kessler JR, Peters DD, Lorton L: Comparison of the relative risk of molar root perforations using various endodontic instrumentation techniques, *J Endod* 9:439, 1983.

Kyomen SM, Caputo AA, White SM: Critical analysis of the balanced force technique in endodontics, *J Endod* 20:332, 1994.

Lee SJ, Monset M, Torabinejad M: Sealing ability of a mineral trioxide aggregate for repair of lateral perforations, *J Endod* 19:541, 1993.

Leeb J: Canal orifice enlargement as related to biomechanical preparation, *J Endod* 9:463, 1983.

Lim SS, Stock CJR: The risk of perforation in the curved canal: anticurvature filing compared with the stepback technique, *Int Endod J* 20:33, 1987.

Littman SH: Evaluation of root canal debridement by use of a radiopaque medium, *J Endod* 3:135, 1977.

Luiten DJ, Morgan LA, Baumgartner JC, Marshall JG: A comparison of four instrumentation techniques on apical canal transportation, *J Endod* 21:26, 1995.

Luks S: An analysis of root canal instruments, *J Am Dent Assoc* 58:85, 1959.

Madison S, Anderson RW: Medications and temporaries in endodontic treatment, *Dent Clin North Am* 36:343, 1992.

Makkes PC, Thoden van Velzen SK, Wesselink PR: Reactions of the living organism to dead and fixed dead tissue, *J Endod* 4:17, 1978.

Mizrahi SJ, Tucker JW, Seltzer S: A scanning electron microscopic study of the efficacy of various endodontic instruments, *J Endod* 1:324, 1975.

Morgan LF, Montgomery S: An evaluation of the crown-down pressureless technique, *J Endod* 10:491, 1984.

Mullaney TP: Instrumentation of finely curved canals, *Dent Clin North Am* 23:575, 1979.

Newman JG, Brantley WA, Gerstein H: A study of the cutting efficiency of seven brands of endodontic files in linear motion, *J Endod* 9:316, 1983.

O'Connell DT, Brayton SM: Evaluation of root canal preparation with two automated endodontic handpieces, *Oral Surg* 39:298, 1975.

Orahood JP, Cochran MA, Swartz M, Newton CW: In vitro study of marginal leakage between temporary sealing materials and recently placed restorative materials, *J Endod* 12:523, 1986.

Patterson SS: In vivo and in vitro studies of the effect of the disodium salt of ethylenediamine tetraacetate on human dentine and its endodontic implications, *Oral Surg* 18:83, 1963.

Penick EC, Osetek EM: Intracanal medications in endodontic therapy. *Dent Clin North Am* 14:743, 1970.

Roane JB, Sabala CL, Duncanson MG: The "balanced force" concept for instrumentation of curved canals, *J Endod* 11:203, 1985.

Roth WC, Gough RW, Grandich RA, Walker WA: A study of the strength of endodontic files: potential for torsional breakage and relative flexibility, *J Endod* 9:228, 1983.

Sabala CL, Biggs, JT: A standard predetermined endodontic preparation concept, *Compend Contin Educ Dent* 12:656, 1991.

Sabala CL, Roane RB, Southard LZ: Instrumentation of curved canals using a modified tipped instrument: a comparison study, *J Endod* 14:59, 1988.

Sampeck AJ: Instruments of endodontics: their manufacture, use, and abuse, *Dent Clin North Am,* Nov 1967, p 579.

Saunders WP, Saunders EM: Comparison of three instruments in the preparation of the curved root canal using the modified double-flared technique, *J Endod* 20:440, 1994.

Schafer E, Tepel J, Hoppe W: A comparison of nickel-titanium and stainless steel root canal instruments, *Endodontie* 3:185, 1994.

Schilder H: Filling root canals in three dimensions, *Dent Clin North Am,* Nov 1967, p 723.

Schilder H: Cleaning and shaping the root canal, *Dent Clin North Am* 18:269, 1974.

Schilder H, Amsterdam M: Inflammatory potential of root canal medicaments, *Oral Surg* 12:211, 1959

Schneider SW: A comparison of canal preparation in straight and curved root canals, *Oral Surg* 32:271, 1971.

Seltzer S et al: Biologic aspects of endodontics. III. Periapical tissue reactions to root canal instrumentation, *Oral Surg* 26:534, 1968.

Seltzer S, Soltanoff W, Sinai I, Smith J: Biologic aspects of endodontics. IV. Periapical tissue reactions to root-filled teeth whose canals had been instrumented short of their apices, *Oral Surg* 28:724, 1969.

Senia ES, Marshall JF, Rosen S: The solvent action of sodium hypochlorite on pulp tissue of extracted teeth, *Oral Surg* 31:96, 1971.

Sinai I: Endodontic perforations: their prognosis and treatment, *J Am Dent Assoc* 95:90, 1977.

Southard DW, Oswald RJ, Natkin E: Instrumentation of curved molar root canals with the Roane technique, *J Endod* 13:479, 1987.

Spangberg L: Cellular reaction to intracanal medicaments. In Grossman LI, editor: *Transactions of the Fifth International Conference on Endodontics,* Philadelphia, 1973, University of Pennsylvania.

Stewart GG, Cobe HM, Rappaport H: A study of a new medicament in the chemomechanical preparation of infected root canals, *J Am Dent Assoc* 63:33, 1961.

Stewart GG, Kapsimalas P, Rappaport H: EDTA and urea peroxide for root canal preparation, *J Am Dent Assoc* 78:335, 1969.

Svec TA, Harrison JW: Chemomechanical removal of pulpal and dentinal debris with sodium hypochlorite and hydrogen peroxide vs. normal saline solution, *J Endod* 3:49, 1977.

Walton RE: Histologic evaluation of different methods of enlarging the pulp canal space, *J Endod* 2:304, 1976.

Walton RE: Current concepts of canal preparation, *Dent Clin North Am* 36:309, 1992.

Webber J, Moser JB, Heuer MA: A method to determine the cutting efficiency of root canal instruments in linear motion, *J Endod* 6:829, 1980.

Weine FS, Healey HJ, Gerstein H, Evanson L: Precurved files and incremental instrumentation for root canal enlargement, *J Can Dent Assoc* 36:155, 1970.

Weine FS, Kelly RF, Bray KE: The effect of preparation with endodontic handpieces on original canal shape, *J Endod* 2:298, 1976.

Weine FS, Kelly RF, Lio PJ: The effect of preparation procedures on original canal shape and on apical foramen shape, *J Endod* 1:255, 1975.

Zakariasen KL, Zakariasen KA, McMinn MM: Today's sonics, *J Am Dent Assoc* 123:67, 1992.

Uses for ultrasonics

Ahmad M, Pitt Ford TR, Crum LA: Ultrasonic debridement of root canals: an insight into the mechanisms involved, *J Endod* 13:93, 1987.

Ahmad M, Pitt Ford TR, Crum LA, Walton AJ: Ultrasonic debridement of root canals: acoustic cavitation and its relevance, *J Endod* 14:486, 1988.

Baker MC, Ashrafi SH, VanCura JE, Remeikis NA: Ultrasonic compared with hand instrumentation: a scanning microscopic evaluation, *J Endod* 14:435, 1988.

Barnett F, Trope M, Tronstad L: Bacteriologic status of the root canal after sonic, ultrasonic, and hand instrumentation, *Endod Dent Traumatol* 1:228, 1985.

Cameron JA: The use of ultrasonics in the removal of the smear layer: a scanning electron microscope study, *J Endod* 9:289, 1983.

Cameron JA: The use of sodium hypochlorite activated by ultrasound for the debridement of infected, immature root canals, *J Endod* 12:550, 1986.

Camp J: Clinical perspectives in sonic and ultrasonic canal cleaning and shaping. Presented at Controversies in Dentistry, Chicago, Oct 25, 1987.

Chenail BL, Teplitsky PE: Endosonics in curved root canals, *J Endod* 11:369, 1985.

Chenail BL, Teplitsky PE: Endosonics in curved canals. Part II, *J Endod* 14:214, 1988.

Cunningham WT, Joseph SW: Effect of temperature on the bactericidal action of sodium hypochlorite endodontic irrigant, *Oral Surg Oral Med Oral Pathol* 50:569, 1980.

Cunningham W, Martin H, Forest W: Evaluation of root canal debridement by the endodontic synergistic system, *Oral Surg* 53:401, 1982.

Cymerman JJ, Jerome LA, Moodnik RM: A scanning electron microscope study comparing the efficacy of hand instrumentation with ultrasonic instrumentation of the root canal, *J Endod* 9:327, 1983.

Fairbourn D, McWalter G, Montgomery S: The effect of four preparation techniques on the amount of apically extruded debris, *J Endod* 13:102, 1987.

Goon WWY: Innovative uses of ultrasonic energy for the elimination of problematic root canal obstructions, *Compend Contin Educ Dent* 13:650, 1992.

Johnson TA, Zelikow R: Ultrasonic endodontics: a clinical review, *J Am Dent Assoc* 114:655, 1987.

Kielt L, Montgomery S: The effect of endosonic instrumentation in simulated curved root canals, *J Endod* 13:215, 1987.

Krell KV, Johnson R: Irrigation patterns of ultrasonic diamond coated files, *J Endod* 12:129, 1986.

Langeland K, Liao K, Pascon EA: Work-saving devices in endodontics: efficacy of sonic and ultrasonic techniques, *J Endod* 11:449, 1985.

Martin H, Cunningham W: Endosonic endodontics: the ultrasonic synergistic system, *Int Dent J* 34:198, 1984.

Martin H, Cunningham W, Norris JP: A quantitative comparison of the ability of diamond and K-files to remove dentin, *Oral Surg* 50:566, 1980.

Martin H, Cunningham W, Norris J, Cotton W: Ultrasonic versus hand filing of dentin: a quantitative study, *Oral Surg Oral Med Oral Pathol* 49:79, 1980.

Miyahara A: *Ultrasonic endodontics,* ed 2, Osaka, Japan.

Pedicord D, ElDeeb ME, Messer HH: Hand versus ultrasonic instrumentation: its effect on canal shape and instrumentation time, *J Endod* 12:375, 1986.

Reynolds MA et al: An in vitro histologic comparison of the step-back, sonic, and ultrasonic instrumentation techniques in small, curved root canals, *J Endod* 13:307, 1987.

Richman MJ: Use of ultrasonics in root canal therapy and root resection, *J Dent Med* 12:12, 1957.

Schulz-Bongert U, Weine FS, Schulz-Bongert J: Preparation of curved canals using a combined hand-filing, ultrasonic technique, *Compend Contin Educ Dent* 16:270, 1995.

Stamos DE, Sadeghi EM, Haasch GC, Gerstein H: An in vitro comparison study to quantitate the debridement ability of hand, sonic, and ultrasonic instrumentation, *J Endod* 13:434, 1987.

Walmsley AD: Ultrasound and root canal treatment: the need for scientific evaluation, *Int Endod J* 20:105, 1987.

Weller RN, Brady JM, Bernier WE: Efficacy of ultrasonic cleaning, *J Endod* 6:740, 1980.

Yahya AS, ElDeeb ME: Effect of sonic versus ultrasonic instrumentation on canal preparation, *J Endod* 15:235, 1989.

Zakariasen KL: Sonics and lasers. Presented at E.D. Coolidge Study Club, Chicago, Sept 30, 1987.

8 Calculation of working length

As stated in Chapter 7, the most important segment of endodontic treatment is canal preparation. Carrying this a bit further, one of the most important steps in canal preparation is the calculation of working length. The significances of this procedure are the following:

1. The calculation determines how far into the canal the instruments are placed and worked and thus how deeply into the tooth the tissues, debris, metabolites, end products, and other unwanted items are removed from the canal.
2. It will limit the depth to which the canal filling may be placed.
3. It will affect the degree of pain and discomfort that the patient will feel following the appointment.
4. If calculated within correct limits, it will play an important role in determining the success of the treatment and, conversely, if calculated incorrectly may doom the treatment to failure.

Therefore it can be seen quite clearly that the procedure for calculation of working length should be performed with skill, using techniques that have been proven to give valuable and accurate results and by methods that are practical and efficacious. If performed in this manner, dentists will produce many treatments of high quality and considerable longevity.

However, if this step is performed perfunctorily, without thought and skill, using techniques of dubious accuracy, many teeth so treated will be failures.

To emphasize the importance of this procedure and to give sufficient depth for a full discussion, this fifth edition of my textbook will devote a full chapter to the subject.

Most experts agree that, theoretically, the canal preparation and, thus, the canal filling, should terminate at the cementodentinal junction (CDJ). The term "theoretically" is applied here because the CDJ is a histologic site and a microscope must be used to find it. In the clinical setting, it is impossible to use a microscope in this area. Therefore methods must be applied that will allow the clinician to ascertain this critical position during endodontic treatment.

HISTORICAL PERSPECTIVES

In the early days of endodontic treatment, at the end of the nineteenth century, radiographs had not yet been applied to dentistry, and working length was usually calculated to the site where the patient experienced feeling for an instrument placed into the canal. Obviously this led to a multiplicity of errors. If vital tissue were left in the canal unextirpated, the resulting calculation would be too short. If a periapical lesion were present, the calculation could be much too long. Teeth with more than one canal in a root could also give inaccurate information.

Then, with the advent of application of x-rays to dentistry by Kells in 1899, teeth treated without the benefit of radiographs, but evaluated by dental films, indicated these miscalculations. This was part of the disillusionment with endodontic treatment that was common in the early twentieth century.

There can be no question that the refutation of the focal infection theory and the introduction of aseptic techniques did much to enhance the attitude of the members of the health sciences toward endodontics. However, the introduction of a calculated working length, even though it still was in error at that time, was also a significant step in the acceptance of endodontic treatment.

In this early portion of the 1900s, the popular opinion was that the dental pulp extended through the tooth, past the apical foramen into the periapical tissue, and that the narrowest diameter of the apical portion of the root canal was precisely at the site where the canal exits the tooth at the extreme apex. These views fostered the then-prevailing technique to calculate to the tip of the root on the radiograph—the radiographic apex—as the correct site to terminate canal preparation and fill the canal. Thus the radiograph apex replaced the feeling of the patient as the apical position for the calculation of working length.

In the 1920s, considerable study of the apex of the tooth led Grove, Hatton, Blayney, Coolidge, and others to offer reports that contradicted this position. Grove concluded that pulp tissue could not extend beyond the CDJ because the cell unique to the dental pulp, the odontoblast, was not found past the CDJ. Hatton, and Grove, again, advised that preparation beyond the natural constriction of the CDJ would result in injury to the periapical tissues. Blayney and Coolidge offered cases and histologic evaluations indicating that filling slightly short of the root tip gave the best results.

It finally fell to Kuttler, an endodontist from Mexico City, to report on the most comprehensive anatomic microscopic study of the root tip in 1955. Even those who disagree with his application of the results of his study do agree with his description of the root tip. Empirically, Kuttler decided that filing to the radiographic apex was an unwise clinical procedure, contributing to postoperative pain and lowering the production of successful cases. He undertook research on the anatomy of the apex, studying several thousand teeth under a light microscope and reporting a myriad of measurements from this area.

Soon thereafter, other studies of the root tip, including histologic studies involving the soft and hard tissues of the apex, were reported and lent tremendous support to Kuttler's views. Not everyone immediately embraced his methods, but many decided to file specific distances away from the root tip in an effort to stop filing into the periapical tissues.

Some aspects of Kuttler's study have been questioned. The teeth that he studied had no caries, either no restorations or minimal restorations, and no periapical lesions. These are hardly the type of teeth that are treated endodontically. However, many other authors have verified his anatomic descriptions of the root tip and have agreed with his statistics in regard to the complex measurements of various sites and distances in this area. Also, his view that the canal or canals exit short of the root tip in a very high percentage of cases has been confirmed in studies by Coolidge, Hess, Green, and many others.

For these past forty + years, Kuttler's study has continued to regal the students of endodontic the-

ory and practice. Unquestionably, it is one of the most important papers that set proper standards for sophisticated, successful endodontic treatment, despite some minor errors. His dedication and determination in continuing to pursue results through thousands of calculations stands unmatched in the annals of endodontic research.

METHODS FOR CALCULATION OF WORKING LENGTH

Currently there are four major, specific methods for calculation of working length, that is, four methods that have enough adherents that result in many teeth being treated according to the theory of choice. They are the following:

1. *Radiographic apex*—filing to the tip of the root as seen on the x-ray film.
2. *A specific distance from the radiographic apex*—accepting that filing to the radiographic apex is too long, a distance short of that, most often 1.0 mm, is selected.
3. *According to the studies of Kuttler*—examination of the preoperative radiograph to locate the major or minor diameter.
4. *Use of an electronic apex locator*—by using the difference in electrical charge between the tissues of the periodontal ligament and the sites within the canal.

Results. Interestingly, even though each of these methods often will give different numeric calculations, excellent results have been reported using any and all of these four techniques! This undoubtedly explains why each has its supporters and adherents. Although I have my own choice, I accept that all the methods may yield good results when supported by other aspects of therapy that are sound physically and biologically.

Some methods of treatment match up better with certain of these methods. For instance, as stated in Chapter 10, users of silver points who filed and filled to the radiographic apex probably would have a greater percentage of failures than would those using packed gutta-percha. The stiff points seemingly would tend to create more problems for periapical tissues than would the better tolerated gutta-percha.

USE OF THE RADIOGRAPHIC APEX AS TERMINATION POINT

Although used many years ago and refuted by many studies, there still remain a number of excellent clinicians who utilize the radiographic apex as the site to terminate canal preparation. Graduates of the endodontic program at Boston University and their disciples are the most active proponents of this technique. Many teeth so treated, either accidentally or purposely, have indicated perfect healing (Fig. 8-1).

Those who endorse this concept state that it is impossible to locate the CDJ clinically and that the radiographic apex is the only reproducible site available in this area. They state that by calculating the length of the tooth to the radiographic apex, keeping this distance patent, and using larger files a bit shorter (within the body of the tooth), the most ideal preparation is developed. A patent root tip and larger files kept within the tooth may be excellent

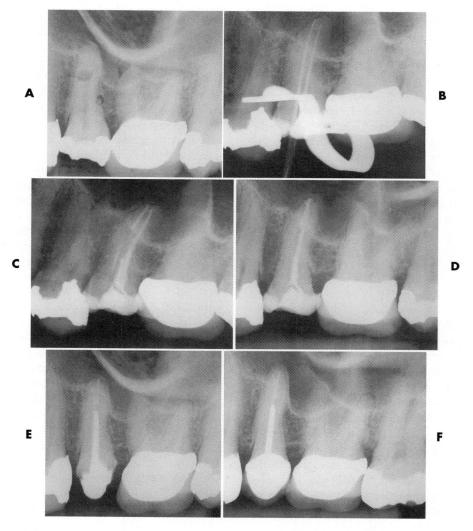

Fig. 8-1. Successful treatment, canals filled to radiographic apex. **A,** Preoperative radiograph (straight view) of maxillary second bicuspid (film was not fixed properly and several water spots remain). **B,** Following canal preparation, master cones were fit and this angled view taken from the mesial. Cone in palatal canal is obviously a bit too long, but cone in buccal canal seemed correct. Length of palatal canal was shortened 1 mm, and a new cone refit to that length. **C,** Immediate post-filling angled view, and **D,** straight-view films following lateral condensation of gutta-percha and Wach's paste. Some sealer and gutta-percha are at the radiographic apex of each canal. **E,** One year later, post has been made and temporary acrylic crown was used because the patient did not have time to complete the restoration. **F,** Ten years after original treatment, the canal fillings appear to be well within the confines of the canals, and the periapical regions are perfectly normal. (Restoration by Dr. Arnold Wax, Chicago.)

treatment, but filing to the radiographic apex can be only one thing—IT IS TOO LONG! Fig. 8-2 is taken from a study by Palmer et al. in which extracted teeth were selected at random, their apices covered with cotton, then radiographed with a file in place to the radiographic apex. The cotton was removed and the root tips were photographed. Of the 40 teeth surveyed, half indicated that the file was extending 1.0 mm or more through the apical foramen. Grove, Green, and Kuttler, among others, also reported on the common finding of the apical foramen exiting at distances from 1 to 3 mm from the root tip.

Is the radiographic apex reproducible?   This question is very significant if one uses this technique. The supporters obviously believe that it is reproducible, but many clinical experiences indicate the fallacy of that belief. The position of the radiographic apex depends on many factors: the angulation of the tooth, the position of the film, the holding agent for the film (finger, x-ray holder, hemostat, cotton roll), the length of the x-ray cone, the horizontal and vertical positioning of the cone, the use of intentional distortions of the cone (for angled views), the anatomic structure adjacent to the tooth, as well as many other factors.

In Fig. 8-3, teeth are radiographed from two horizontal angles. In each one the straight view indicates the file to be short of the radiographic apex. If one follows the use of the radiographic apex for working length calculation, these two teeth should be filed at least 1 mm closer to the tip. However, in each case the angled view indicates that the file or canal filling is already too long.

Taking angled radiographs in addition to the normal file measurement view (Fig. 8-3) will give further important information. Relying on merely the routine straight-on radiograph may cause a considerable error in determining the position of the apical foramen. In answer to the question posed at the beginning of this section, the radiograph is accurate, but the interpretation may be incorrect or insufficient views may give a false impression.

Advantages.   Many dentists are compulsive and actively seek to eliminate unwanted, possibly diseased materials. In operative dentistry, all caries must be removed. In periodontal treatment, all calculus must be removed. Similarly, in endodontic treatment, all materials, tissues, and debris from the canal must be removed. Many of the clinicians who believe this are not satisfied unless some excess material is pushed through the apical foramen, to indicate that the apical portion of the canal has been filled and thus has been sufficiently cleaned. They

know that they are filing a bit too long, but they are willing to make this accommodation for the greater good of completely cleaning the canal.

Another advantage of filing to the radiographic apex is that a small error in length calculation will not lead to an undesirably short filling with an apical segment of unprepared canal. By keeping the apical segment of the canal patent, the operator can go back to any portion of the canal and widen the preparation, if necessary. The "short fill," which is despised by the compulsive dentist, rarely occurs.

Disadvantages.   Studies on success and failure, including those by Strindberg, Seltzer et al., and many others, have reported on the decrease in success when filling materials are passed into the periapical tissues, as is commonly seen in this method. The paper by Davis et al. also corroborated this view. Reports on postoperative pain also indicate an increase when canals are filed and filled to this site as compared to within the body of the canal. Many of the complaints that endodontic patients had in the past with treatment was the postoperative pain that was so common when filing to the radiographic apex was the prevalent view.

In addition, the physical studies (see Chapter 7) have indicated that when the canal exits eccentrically short of the root (very common in molar teeth, much less common in maxillary anterior teeth), as described by Levy and Glatt as well as others, preparation to the radiographic apex leads to an undesirable shape—a teardrop—which is very difficult to seal by any technique (see Figs. 7-23, 7-25, and 7-26). This is probably why teeth with long fills have a lowered success ratio.

Another point made by Levy and Glatt was that canal exit deviation occurs toward the buccal or lingual aspect of the tooth twice as often as toward the mesial or distal aspect. This confirms the importance of taking angled radiographs, which may suggest this deviation to the buccal or lingual aspect. It certainly would not be possible to visualize anything but mesial or distal deviation on a nonangled (straight) view.

Even so, filing to this site is still endorsed by many, successful cases are displayed using it, and, I am certain, this view will always be followed by some.

SPECIFIC DISTANCES SHORT OF THE RADIOGRAPHIC APEX

Many clinicians noted that teeth filled to the radiographic apex were, in fact, filled too long. This awareness could have occurred when performing an apicoectomy (Fig. 8-4), viewing a previously treated

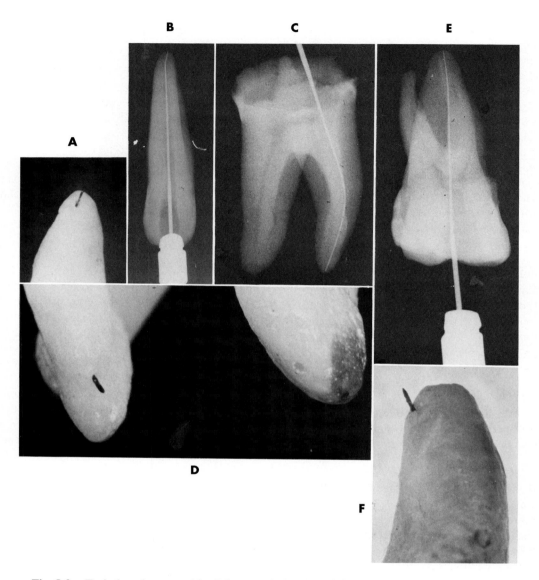

Fig. 8-2. Typical teeth surveyed by Palmer et al., in which cotton was placed over the apices of extracted teeth, and then files were placed so that they appeared to be at the radiographic apex on the films. In the study, 50% of the teeth radiographed had files protruding 1 mm or more through the apical foramen when viewed with the cotton removed. **A** and **B,** File in maxillary cuspid. **C** and **D,** File in mesiobuccal canal of mandibular first molar. **E** and **F,** File in palatal canal of maxillary first molar, an extremely common finding on this root, and present in each of the maxillary molars surveyed. Also the film shown in **E** was taken from an angle exactly parallel to the root. In clinical conditions this root is usually radiographed with the cone superior, pointed down. With that cone placement, it would appear that the file in this tooth was approximately 1 mm short of the radiographic apex! (From Palmer MJ, Weine FS, Healey HJ: *J Can Dent Assoc* 37:305, 1971; with permission of the Canadian Dental Association.)

extracted tooth, examining the root tip of an untreated tooth with mild magnification, and so forth. These findings were sufficient to encourage some dentists to file a specific distance short of the apex.

The method for calculating this termination site was to locate the radiographic apex and then back

off a specific measurement from that length. At first this distance short was calculated to be 0.5 mm by many, but often it was lengthened ultimately to 1.0 mm when microscopic studies indicated that the CDJ usually was more than 0.5 mm from the root tip.

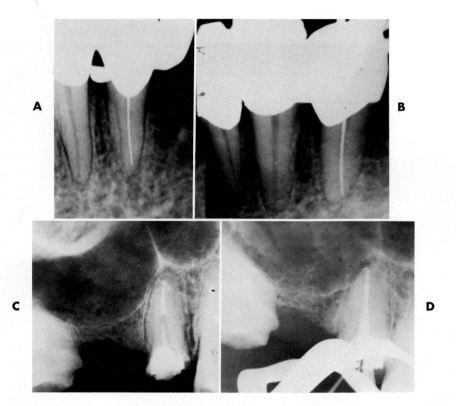

Fig. 8-3. **A,** Straight-on radiograph seems to indicate that file is at least 1 mm from radiographic apex. **B,** Angled view discloses that the file has already reached the periodontal ligament space. **C,** Immediate postfilling film taken straight on seems to indicate that canal filling is quite short of apex, leading to consternation that area of unfilled canal may lead to failure. **D,** Examination of intrafilling film taken from an angle shows that canal is completely filled. In fact, the button of sealer at apex is excess, past the minor diameter.

Filing to this position does give many excellent cases. Postoperative pain after filing and filling will be decreased. A very high percentage of teeth have canals exiting between 0.5 and 1.0 mm from the apex, and in all these cases the measurement will be as close to perfect as could be accomplished by any technique. The only problem occurs when the canal exits more than 1.0 mm from the radiographic apex, usually eccentrically from the root tip, and the problems of teardrop shape and overfilling without sealing will occur.

If the clinician who favors this technique can examine the preoperative radiographs and search for clues to short exiting (see next section of this chapter), then make the correct accommodation in these cases, even better results will accrue.

ACCORDING TO THE STUDIES OF KUTTLER

According to Kuttler, the narrowest diameter of the canal is definitely not at the site of exiting of the canal from the tooth but usually occurs within the dentin, just prior to the initial layers of cementum. He referred to this position as the *minor diameter* of the canal, although others call it the apical constriction (Fig. 8-5, *A*). It is at this site that I prefer to terminate canal preparation and build up the apical dentin matrix. The diameter of the canal at the site of exiting from the tooth (*major diameter*) was found to be approximately twice as wide as the minor diameter. The average distances between the minor and major diameters were 0.524 mm in teeth examined in an 18-to-25-year-old group and 0.659 mm in a 55-year-old and older age group. This means that the longitudinal view of the canal as a tapering funnel to the tip of the root is incorrect. The funnel tapers to a distance short of the site of exiting and then widens again (Fig. 8-5, *A*). Because the adjacent walls of cementum are slightly convex or hyperbolic or funnel shaped when viewed in long section, the

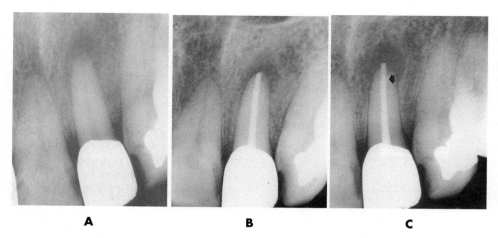

A   **B**   **C**

Fig. 8-4. **A,** Preoperative radiograph of maxillary lateral incisor, indicating periapical lesion with apical resorption. **B,** This tooth was treated in 1964, when filling to the radiographic apex was in vogue. The immediate postfilling film indicates that the gutta-percha has been packed exactly to that site, and for 1964, this is an excellent result. **C,** The radiolucency increased in size and symptoms of apical tenderness were present 1 year later. The tooth was treated surgically by apicoectomy and reverse filling (Chapter 11). Even though the gutta-percha still seems to be at or close to the radiographic apex, when the tooth was flapped, it was noted that the gutta-percha apical to the arrow was out of the root in the periapical tissues.

configuration of the area between the minor and major diameters resembles that of a morning-glory flower. On viewing postfilling radiographs when sealer has been slightly extruded past the apical constriction, the morning-glory configuration is often clearly visualized (Fig. 8-5, *B* to *D*).

In his original English language publication, reported in 1955, Kuttler measured the distances among 20 different anatomic positions. These calculations, for example, were from the major diameter to the minor diameter or the widths of either diameter. One measurement that he did not make was the distance from the minor diameter to the root tip, because he was unequivocal in his opposition to filing to the radiographic apex.

The exact method for utilizing Kuttler's theories to calculate working length will be presented later in this chapter.

Advantages.   Utilizing the studies of Kuttler, in my opinion, is the most scientific method for calculation of working length. In itself, Kuttler's measurements produced a physical-anatomic study. However, they have been reinforced by many histologic studies and proven to be accurate in use with a huge number of very successful cases, accompanied by pain-free treatment in a high percentage of treated teeth.

If slight errors are made, less than 1 mm in either direction (too long, too short), the variance

rarely causes serious problems and usually will give a calculation similar to the other methods of working length calculation. For instance, a slightly long calculation may cause a filling to the radiographic apex or a slightly short calculation may end up 1 mm from the radiographic apex.

A major advantage of this method is it allows the rapid development of a solid apical dentin matrix. This will enhance the possibilities for retaining the filling materials within the canal, a most desirable situation, and one that has yielded very high success percentages in reported studies (Figs. 8-6 and 8-7). It improves the opportunity for demonstrating lateral canals. The dense matrix does not allow excess sealer to exit through the tip during condensation. Therefore the sealer that is squeezed by the gutta-percha cones and condensing instruments is forced up the walls and through the lateral canals, allowing identification on the radiographs.

Disadvantages.   This calculation method is the most complicated of those listed, takes the most time, and requires radiographs of excellent quality with magnification. Many dentists are not willing to make these concessions, especially when they are convinced that other, easier techniques also give acceptable results. Errors do occur with this method, as well, although, as stated earlier, these errors are usually quite minimal. When an error does occur and, for

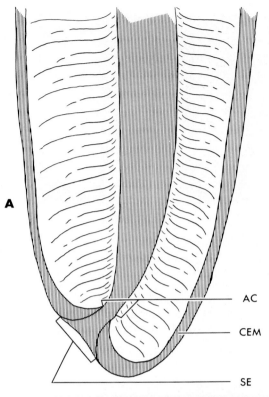

Fig. 8-5. Anatomy of the apex, taken from the studies of Kuttler. **A,** Long-section diagram of the root. The apical constriction *(AC),* the narrowest place in the canal, was referred to by Kuttler as the *minor diameter.* It lies within the dentin, just before the first layers of the cementum *(CEM).* From the crown, the canal tapers down to the *minor diameter* and then widens again as it approaches the site of exiting from the root *(SE),* which was referred to by Kuttler as the *major diameter.* The space between AC and SE is hyperbolic or funnel shaped; Kuttler referred to it as the shape of a morning-glory flower (the walls get wider very quickly). **B,** Preoperative radiograph of mandibular incisor with periapical radiolucency. **C,** Canal filling with laterally condensed gutta-percha and Wach's paste. Note that excess sealer past AC has outlined the funnel, morningglory shape. **D,** Perfect healing 1 year later. Note that canal definitely did not exit at the radiographic apex and that it did exit shorter than 1 mm from the radiographic apex.

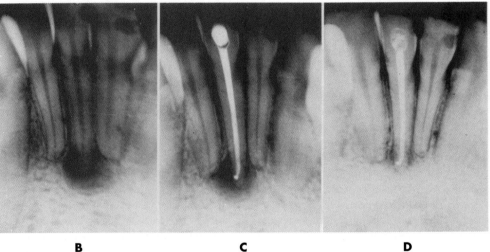

instance, filling materials are expressed into the periapical tissues (Fig. 8-8), the operator may become upset and blame the technique. No method can guarantee perfect results each time, and every clinician must decide the direction that is most comfortable.

Technique for calculating working length. As stated in Chapter 6, *before* starting endodontic treatment, the dentist must identify the probable canal *con-*figuration present and any common variants that might be present, the estimated *l*ength of the root(s), the site of *e*xiting of the canal(s), and the estimated *w*idth of the canal(s) (the mnemonic, C-L-E-W). This is done by analyzing the preoperative radiographs available, usually both straight—for site(s) of exiting, root(s) length, and canal(s) width—and angled views—for canal configuration and site(s) of exiting. This analysis will be

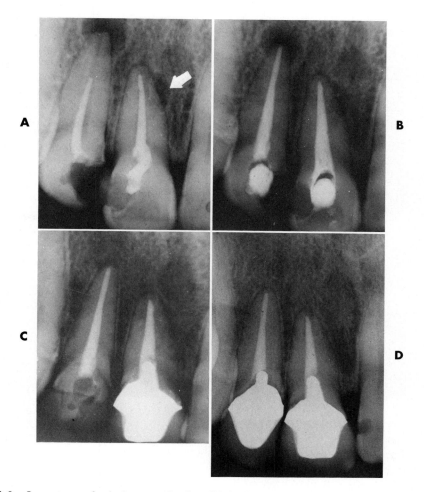

Fig. 8-6. Importance of apical preparation in solid dentin. **A,** Preoperative radiograph of maxillary central and lateral incisors with poor canal fillings. Note that improper initial access has severely hampered any procedures to follow. Lateral incisor has radiolucency around the apex, whereas central incisor has radiolucency on mesial aspect *(arrow),* suggestive of significant lateral canal. **B,** At the time canals were filled. Preparation in solid dentin provided matrix for packing of gutta-percha. Sealer extruded through lateral canal to radiolucency adjacent to central incisor. **C,** Healing almost completed 1 year after treatment. **D,** Twelve years after original treatment, area has retained normal appearance. (**A** to **C** from Palmer MJ, Weine FS, Healey HJ: *J Can Dent Assoc* 37:305, 1971; with permission of the Canadian Dental Association.)

aided by use of magnification or projection. The calculations dealing with the site of exiting of the canal(s) lengths and widths will help to identify the major and often the minor diameter. The calculations dealing with the widths and lengths are invaluable in making the calculation for working length (Figs. 8-9 and 8-10).

The basis for this method's value are the measurements provided by Kuttler relating to the distance between the major diameter (site of exiting of the canal) and the minor diameter (CDJ). In younger patients the distance between these two

positions is approximately 0.5 mm, and in older patients, due to increased buildup of cementum, the distance is approximately 0.67 mm. Using the radiograph, the dentist must locate the major diameter, then interpolate the position of the minor diameter or locate the minor diameter by seeing the funneled shape into the tooth from the site of exiting. These sites of exiting can be seen if they exit in the mesial or distal direction on the straight films.

It is not always possible to locate either of these positions. Thus, attempts must be made to find

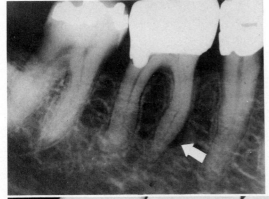

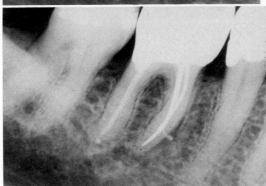

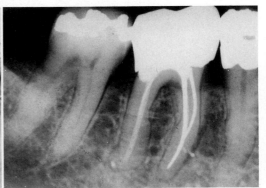

Fig. 8-7. Silver point filling also requires preparation in solid dentin. **A,** Mandibular first molar with radiolucency on mesial border of mesial root *(arrow).* **B,** Sealer is prevented from being pushed out of apex so it is forced up the canal to fill discrepancies between canal preparation and perfectly round silver point. Extrusion of sealer toward radiolucency demonstrates that this has occurred. **C,** Healing 1 year after treatment. (From Palmer MJ, Weine FS, Healey HJ: *J Can Dent Assoc* 37:305, 1971; with permission of the Canadian Dental Association.)

either of these positions by other than direct identification. If a periapical radiolucency is noted, generally the canal exits to the center of the lesion (Figs. 8-9 and 8-10). If the radiolucent line of the pulp canal space stops near the tip of the root, it usually indicates that the canal is exiting to the buccal or lingual direction at that level (Fig. 8-11).

The step-by-step technique for using Kuttler's method for calculation of working length is as follows:

1. Using the information from the straight and angled radiographs about the expected canal configuration of the tooth, prepare the correct access cavity, as described in Chapter 6. Be certain to place the rubber dam as soon as the canal orifice(s) is (are) located. Remove whatever pulp tissue or debris that you believe should be removed prior to taking the length.

2. Locate the major diameter or minor diameter on the preoperative radiograph. In some cases the exact site may not be seen (Fig. 8-11, *A*), only that the radiolucent line of the pulp canal space stops near the tip of the root.

3. Estimate the length of the root(s), either by measuring the length with a millimeter ruler on the preoperative radiographs (without

projection, but may use magnification) or using Tables 6-1, 6-2, or 6-3. (If the tooth is longer than average, use the 95th percentile; if average, use the average length; if shorter than average, use the 5th percentile.)

4. Estimate the width of the canal(s) on the radiographs. If the canal being estimated is narrow, consider using a size 10 or 15 file; if average, select a size 20 or 25 file; if wide, choose a size 30 or 35; if very wide, select a size 50 or larger.

5. Using the file selected by step 4, set the stop for the working length according to the measurement estimated in step 3. Place the file into the access cavity and take an initial radiograph. If the file seems to stop at a length that could be accurate, stop and take a radiograph (Figs. 8-11, *B,* and 8-12, *A*), rather than force the file too far into the periapical tissues.

6. If the file appears too long or too short by more than 1 mm from the minor diameter, make the interpolation, adjust the file accordingly, and retake the film to verify accuracy (Figs. 8-11, *C* and *D,* and 8-12, *B*).

7. If the file appears too long or too short from the minor diameter by less than 1 mm, make

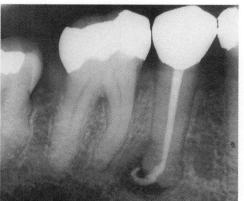

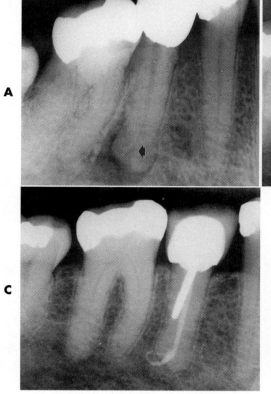

Fig. 8-8.   A, Preoperative radiograph of mandibular second bicuspid with periapical lesion, apical resorption, and heavy apical cementum deposition. The minor diameter is seen 2 mm from the site of exiting *(arrow).* **B,** Immediate postfilling film indicates that a solid apical dentin matrix was not present and that the canal was prepared with a slightly long working length. A considerable amount of sealer (Kerr's Antiseptic Root Canal Sealer) is seen pushed past the major diameter into the lesion. The shape between the minor and major diameters is clearly that of a funnel or morning-glory flower. **C,** Film taken 12 years later indicates perfect healing of the radiolucency and resorption of much of the sealer. The post is not in the canal but, luckily, seemed to still be within the root.

the interpolation and use that as the calculated working length. If it is exactly where you want it to be, use that distance as the calculated working length.

8. If your file reaches the major diameter exactly, subtract 0.5 mm from that length if the patient is 35 years old or younger or 0.67 mm from that length if the patient is older. If the file reaches the site that you believe is exactly at the minor diameter, use that as the calculated working length. (If it is obvious that a great deal of cementum has been deposited at the root tip, subtract a greater amount from the site of the major diameter to rectify the increased distance.)

Additional considerations. *Short exiting.* Do not be shocked if your analysis indicates that there is a very short exiting to the canal, either by radiograph examination of the preoperative film or film with file in place. Exiting short may occur in many roots at levels as far as 4 mm from the radiographic apex (Figs. 8-10, *B,* and 8-13).

Effect of periapical radiolucency with resorption. Radiolucent areas are present in some teeth with nonvital pulps because of destruction of periapical bone by phagocytic cells. Due to the similarity in composition of bone, cementum, and dentin, it is obvious that these destructive cells will destroy tooth structure in addition to bone, causing root resorption (Fig. 8-14). This fact was emphasized in a study by Bhaskar and Rappaport.

Therefore, whenever a tooth with a large periapical radiolucency is treated, it may be assumed that resorption is present. If a definite periapical radiolucency is present with radiographic indication of apical resorption, the apical preparation must end an additional 0.5 mm from the calculated working length. If radiographically visible apical root resorption is extensive, it might be necessary to shorten this length by as much as 2 mm or more to allow for the dentin matrix (Fig. 8-14, *C* through *E*).

Symptoms of overinstrumentation. If the patient returns at the appointment after canal preparation and reports that the treated tooth has been very tender to percussion, it may be assumed that the canal was overinstrumented. There is a method that may be used to see whether this presumption is correct. After the rubber dam is placed and the

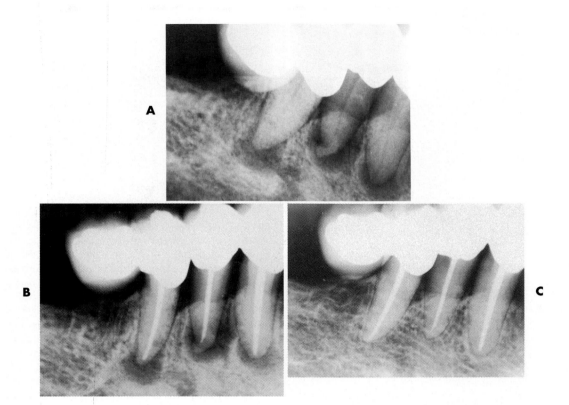

Fig. 8-9. **A,** Preoperative radiograph of mandibular cuspid (right) and bicuspids with periapical lesions and some resorption. On the second bicuspid *(left)* the canal can be seen exiting *(major diameter),* just slightly to the distal. The first bicuspid has a site of exiting short to the distal. The site of exiting of the cuspid is near the tip. **B,** With this information, calculation of working length was made easily and laterally condensed gutta-percha placed to these calculated sites. **C,** The referring dentist was of the training that fillings for teeth with necrotic pulps and apical lesions needed to be placed to the radiographic apex. The patient was 73 years old and had some systemic illnesses. He was disturbed with my results, fearing I had left necrotic tissue behind. However, the correctness of treatment was verified by this radiograph taken 2 years later, indicating perfect healing. If necrotic tissue had been left behind, results probably would not have been successful.

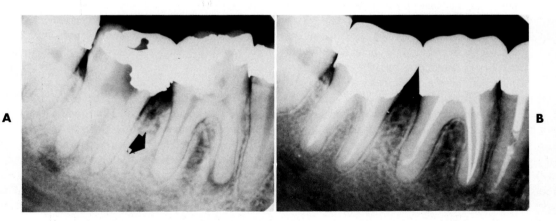

Fig. 8-10.   See legend on opposite page.

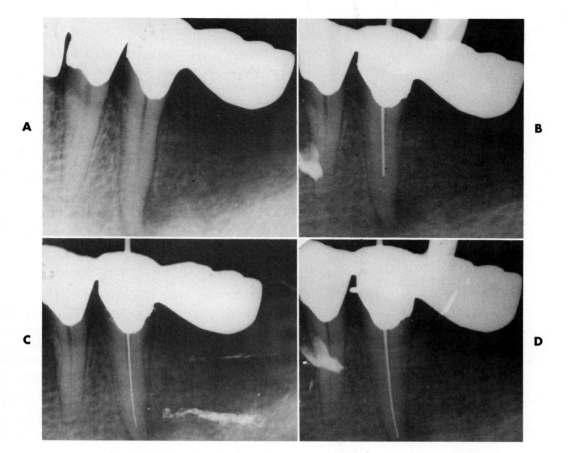

Fig. 8-11.   Use of radiographs and trial placement of files to calculate working length. **A,** Preoperative radiograph of mandibular second bicuspid with periapical lesion. The canal seems to stop near the apex, indicating a slightly short exit to the buccal or lingual direction. The canal seems to be average in width and measured 24 mm long on the radiograph, longer than average. I selected a size 25 file, setting the stop at 22.5 mm because of the lesion and some resorption. **B,** As I inserted the file, I felt some resistance at 18 mm, very close to the average length for this tooth (perhaps the tooth was elongated on the film?). Rather than continuing to push and causing a ledge or forcing the file into the periapical tissues, I took this film to see the relative positions of the root and file tips. Obviously I was quite short. **C,** I calculated that the file was 4 to 5 mm short, so I set the stop at 22.5 mm on a size 15 file and took this film. **D,** It appears that I am more than 1 mm from the tip, so I made an interpolation of the variance, set the stop at 23.5, and took this film. This position seems accurate for calculation of working length.

Fig. 8-10.   **A,** Preoperative radiograph of mandibular molar area. On the distal root of the first molar, the canal exits *(major diameter)* quite sharply to the distal *(arrow)*. Note the radiolucency adjacent to this position of the root, approximately 4 mm from the radiographic apex. **B,** One year after treatment, the canal was filled to the site of exiting indicated, and the excess sealer indicates the funnel, morning-glory shape of the place between the minor and major diameters, indicating that the filling is not too short, even though 4 mm from the radiographic apex. Note excellent healing.

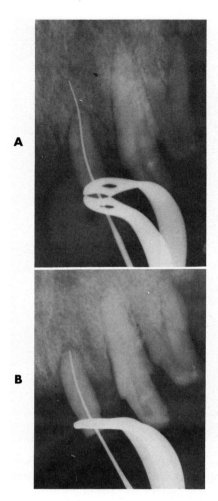

Fig. 8-12. **A,** Because of a provisional plastic splint, it was difficult to obtain an accurate estimated working length from the radiograph. I set a size 20 file at 22 mm and took this film. I estimated the file to be 4 mm too long. **B,** A size 30 file was set at 18 mm and this film was taken. The tip of the file appeared to be slightly short of the site of exiting, so I calculated the working length to be 17.5 mm.

temporary seal removed, a sterile paper point narrow enough to reach the apical portion of the preparation is picked up with cotton pliers at slightly more than the working length and inserted into the canal. If the canal has been overinstrumented, the paper point will pass easily past the previously determined measured length. When the point is withdrawn, a reddish brown discoloration indicates the seeping inflamed tissue of the periapical area. When the apical preparation stops in solid dentin, the paper point will be stopped short

of the periapical tissue. Treatment of this problem is discussed in Chapter 5.

A new shorter working length must be calculated to prevent the repeated irritation of the periapical tissues and to provide for a proper apical preparation.

Conclusions. In my opinion Kuttler's method is an excellent, reproducible, reliable technique to use to calculate working length. It is time consuming and not always perfect (Fig. 8-8). However, in the vast preponderance of treated teeth, it will produce superior results, as seen in the many clinical cases shown in this textbook.

If you know you have used it correctly, and yet the results seem to indicate that you have filled farther from the radiographic apex than might be correct (Figs. 8-15 through 8-18), do not fret. You will be very pleased with the results.

USE OF THE APEX LOCATOR

The three previously discussed current methods for working length calculation require the operator to use radiographs to locate certain sites and then perform certain numeric calculations to determine where the filing should be terminated. Depending on the technique being used, visualization of some areas (radiographic apex, site of exiting of the canals, apical constriction, etc.) may be aided by magnification or projection, but still the final result is accomplished with a subjective assessment of information by an individual, which may or may not turn out to be accurate.

In this day of electronically inspired calculators and computers, it was only a matter of time before a device would be developed that indicated an objective determination for this information. The result is the electronic apex locator.

Despite the positive method of judgment provided by the locators—a sound or movement of a dial or indicator when the correct position is reached—as opposed to the obvious potential for flaw in the individual calculation, the apex locators have been far from being universally accepted. Some sophisticated practitioners in Europe and Japan use them, and they are popular in some geographic areas in the United States. However, at this time they are used much less often than the other methods of working length calculation. Still, apex locators are surely an ingenious product, and the thought processes involved in their development should be applauded by anyone performing endodontic treatment, whether or not the dentist uses them.

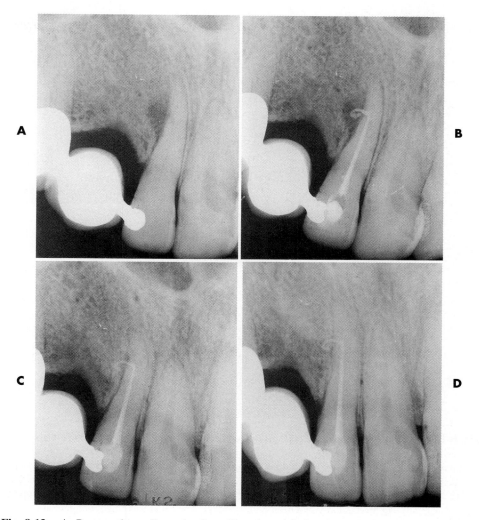

Fig. 8-13.   A, Preoperative radiograph of maxillary lateral incisor area. Traumatic incident several years earlier had avulsed the cuspid and obviously damaged the lateral incisor. The canal space is extremely narrow and seems to stop several millimeters from the apex. A lateral radiolucency is noted to the distal, and this position is sore when touched. There do not seem to be any areas of pathosis at the apex of the tooth, which is comfortable when touched. I advised the patient of the strong possibility of needing surgery due to the difficulty in locating the canal first and then the possibility of not reaching the apex later. I opened up the access and, fortunately, was able to find the canal space. However, my small-sized files could not reach within 4.5 mm of the apex. **B,** After the appointment for canal preparation, the area adjacent to the distal side of the tooth was no longer sore to the touch. However, I informed the patient that surgery was now necessary because I could not reach the apex. I enlarged the canal as far as I could and then filled the prepared space with laterally condensed gutta-percha and Tubliseal. This film was taken. Is it possible that the canal might be exiting at this point? Rather than go directly to surgery and cut off 4 or more mm of root tip, I decided to observe for 6 months. **C,** Six months later, this radiograph confirmed that the lesion was decreasing. **D,** Three years later, the lesion has healed and the tooth has been totally asymptomatic. (Restoration by Dr. Steven Fishman, Chicago.)

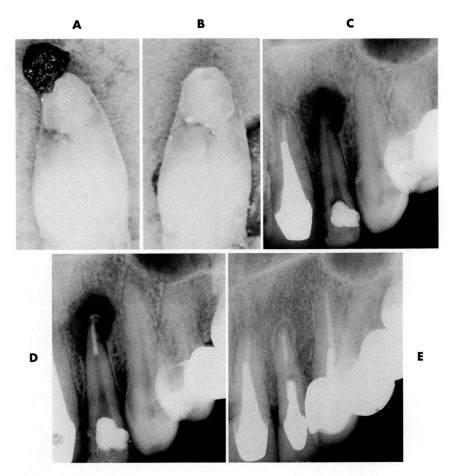

Fig. 8-14. **A,** Extracted tooth with periapical lesion attached. **B,** I carefully dissected the soft tissue lesion away, revealing a cup-shaped area of apical resorption. **C,** Preoperative radiograph of maxillary lateral incisor, indicating a larger periapical lesion with obvious resorption at the apex and distal side of the root. The tooth measured 24 mm on the film, but my calculated working length was 22.5 mm. The adjacent central incisor had periapical surgery 2 years earlier. It appears that a diagonally cut apicoectomy had been performed. **D,** The canal was filled with lateral condensation of a customized cone and Wach's paste, and some excess sealer pushed into the periapical tissues. **E,** Radiograph taken 8 years later, indicating excellent periapical healing. A very small radiolucency is seen, but probably is fibrous tissue, common on large lesions as well as lateral incisors. Note the rounded tip now seen on the adjacent central incisor.

History. Suzuki reported his study on ionophoresis of ammoniated silver nitrate in the teeth of dogs. The silver solution was placed in the root canals and then totally dispersed by a negative electrode in contact with the oral mucous membrane. The conclusion of this experiment was that the electrical resistance of the periodontal ligament, which could only be measured by passing through the root canal, was equal to the electrical resistance of the oral mucous membrane, which could be measured directly on any patient by access into the oral cavity.

Suzuki went no further in his report, but in 1962 Sunada used a simple ohmmeter to study the electrical resistance between these two sites. When the reamer attached to the ohmmeter was in various places in the root canal, the ohmmeter gave differing readings. However, once the reamer reached the periodontal ligament, the ohmmeter registered 6.5 kiloohms on a consistent basis. This was not only true during placement through the root canal, but also during placement through perforations of the walls. These resistance readings were consistent in the individual in every portion of the peri-

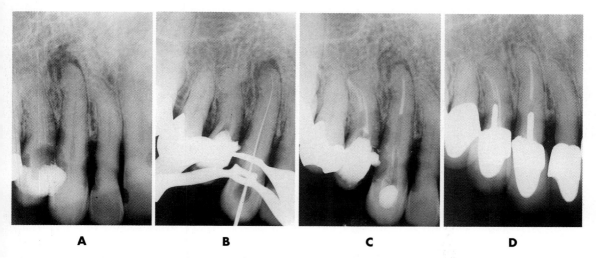

| A | B | C | D |

Fig. 8-15.   A, Preoperative film of maxillary cuspid with periapical lesion, obvious apical resorption, and probable short exiting to labial. **B,** Radiograph of a file in place to site that seems desirable for calculated working length of 27 mm. **C,** Final canal filling with laterally condensed gutta-percha and Wach's paste to 27 mm, post room prepared. Those who desire canal filling at or close to radiographic apex would not be happy with this result. **D,** Radiograph taken 8 years later indicates perfect healing and remodeling of resorbed apex. Canal filling in adjacent first bicuspid also appears short, although at the time of filling (see **C**), some excess sealer is seen past apex to the distal point.

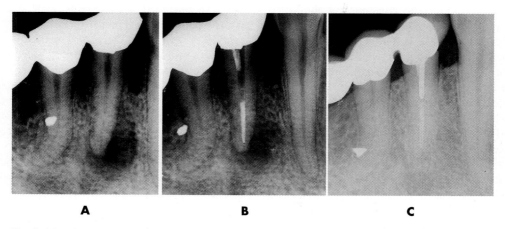

| A | B | C |

Fig. 8-16.   A, Preoperative radiograph of mandibular first bicuspid with large apical radiolucency mainly to the mesial and site of the exiting probably short to the mesial as well. **B,** Radiograph after canal filling with laterally condensed gutta-percha and Wach's paste, post room prepared. Canal filling is several millimeters from radiographic apex. **C,** Radiograph 18 years later. The reconstruction is different, but the radiopaque mass near the second bicuspid attests that it is the same patient. Perfect healing is obvious. (Restoration by Dr. Kerry Voit, Chicago.)

odontal structures and by passing through teeth varying in type and shape.

Then, in 1969 Inoue regaled those attending the annual meeting of the American Association of Endodontists in Atlanta with his demonstration of electronic calculation of working length, using a resistance-type instrument, the first generation of apex locators. Since then, many researchers have conducted experiments with electrical resistent locators and their progeny, the impedance and frequency locators. A partial list of these studies may be found in Table 8-1. (Suzuki, Sunada, and Inoue are all

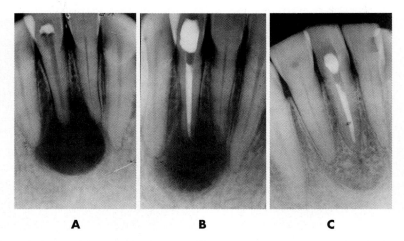

Fig. 8-17. **A,** Preoperative radiograph of mandibular incisor with large periapical lesion and obvious apical resorption. The tooth had been under treatment for almost 2 years, had exacerbated several times, and, at the time of this film, had access cavity left open for drainage. **B,** Canal filling accomplished by laterally condensed customized gutta-percha and Wach's paste. **C,** Radiograph taken 21 years later, canal filling 3 mm short of radiographic apex and perfect healing.

Japanese, with whom electronic developments are closely associated. Ever since these early days, experiments with apex locators are still dominated by Japanese researchers.)

When examining Table 8-1, one can see that the apex locators are far from perfect, despite their ultra-sophisticated developments. Also, the indication that the use of these aids would eliminate the need for radiographs in endodontics is absolutely incorrect, as will be discussed later in this section. However, when used correctly and where indicated, in concert with accurate radiographic evaluations, apex locators offer a significant aid during endodontic treatment. I would also predict that considering the advances made and improvement in these products during the past 20+ years, it is fair to expect that further refinements will continue to improve the ability of these devices to calculate with accuracy.

Development of differing types of apex locators. After their introduction, those dentists who started using the locators began to report inconsistent results. Several of the earlier products had to undergo refinement and upgrading to produce reliable results with some degree of consistency. The Mark IV,* illustrated in Fig. 8-19, for instance, is the third upgrading of the original product. Blood, pus, chelating agents, irrigants, other materials used within the canal, and contact with metallic restorations could give false readings. Problems occurred when the batteries in the

systems were low, but gave no indication of this to the operator. The lip clip, needed to complete the electrical circuit, could be annoying to the patient, so it might not be fastened properly.

Even though corrections were made to counteract these problems (e.g., insulating sleeves were made for the coronal portion of the file so that no contact could be made with the restorations present), different types of apex locators were developed to overcome these difficulties. The second generation, based on the principle of impedance, was developed, such as the Endocater.*

Impedance systems are based on the theory that the root canal, a long, hollow tube, develops an electrical impedance, caused by transparent dentin deposition, which exhibits a sharp decrease at the CDJ. This sudden drop can be measured electrically.

The impedance systems complete the circuit with a hand-held electrode, which does not pinch the patient as the lip clip might. The probes are insulated and can detect canal bifurcations, perforations, and perhaps even auxiliary canals. On the deficit side, they work poorly in young patients (transparent dentin starts to develop in the patient's late teen years), the insulation is bulky and prevents insertion in narrow, curved canals, and the unit is more complicated to use than its counterparts.

The third generation is the frequency-dependent machine. Christie et al. recently described

---

*Union Broach, New York.

*Hygenic Corporation, Akron, Ohio.

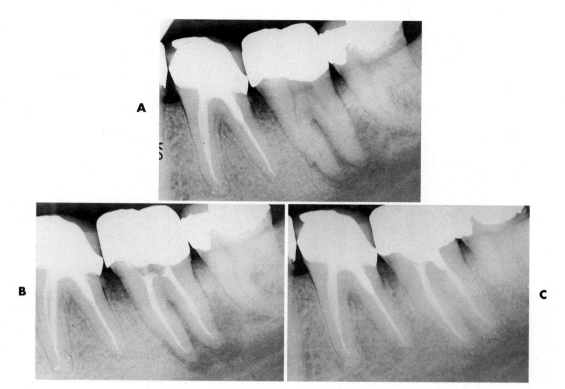

Fig. 8-18. **A,** Preoperative film of mandibular molar area. The first molar had been treated several years earlier, but now there is a large periapical lesion associated with the second molar. **B,** Immediate postfilling film following canal filling with laterally condensed gutta-percha and Wach's paste. Working lengths for this tooth were calculated to be more than 1 mm from the radiographic apex for each canal and filled to those distances. **C,** Two years later, perfect periapical healing of the second molar is evident. The adjacent first molar, also with canal fillings short of the radiographic apices, now 5 years after treatment, also indicates retention of a normal situation. (Restoration by Dr. Morton Schreiber, Highland Park, Ill.)

the use of the Root ZX* machine, which works similarly to the Endex.† They described the effectiveness of these machines and endorsed them for the office, and particularly for dental school situations. The basis for the frequency-dependent locators lies in the fact that sites in the canal give differences in impedance between high (8 kHz) and low (400 Hz) frequencies. After calibration, again with lip clip, the coronal portion of the canal gives minimal difference between these two frequencies. As the probe goes deeper into the canal, however, the difference in frequencies increases and is the greatest at the CDJ. This system requires liquid in the canal, so irrigants and

blood not only have no negative effect, but, in fact, are necessary. Problems with this type of unit include the presence of too much liquid in the canal and remaining gutta-percha (an insulator), such as when performing the re-treatment of a failing case.

Technique for calculating working length using the resistance locators. Each instrument works differently, even among the same generation of locators. Before using the machines, the instructions must be read carefully and understood clearly. Even better is to find a colleague who uses a locator, even if another model or generation machine, and observe its use in a clinical case. The method suggested here is for electronic use concomitantly with high-quality radiographs. The resistance type of locator is described because I am the most familiar with the unit developed by Inoue.

*J. Morita Corp, Osaka, Japan.
†Osada Electric Co., Tokyo.

Table 8-1. Studies on the effectiveness of apex locators

Author(s), year	Sample	Method of investigation	Results
Inoue, 1972	101 canals	EL verified by Rad	92% accuracy
Bramante and Berbert, 1974	224 anterior and posterior teeth	EL and Rad verified by AL	Rad superior, except in palatals
O'Neill, 1974	32 teeth	EL verified by AL	83% correct, 17% 0.5 mm short
Seidberg, Alibrandi, Fine, and Logue, 1975	100 single-rooted teeth	DT compared with EL, verified by Rad	DT 64% accurate, EL 48% accurate
Busch et al., 1976	72 single-rooted teeth	EL verified by Rad	93.3% accurate to radiographic apex
Becker, Lankelma, Wesselink, and Thoden van Velzen, 1980	41 canals in molars of pigs	EL and Rad verified by AL	Rad superior
Chunn, Zardiackas, and Menke, 1981	20 canals	EL and Rad verified by AL	EL 35%, Rad 60% accurate
Trope, Rabie, and Tronstad, 1985	127 anterior and posterior canals	EL verified by Rad	90.6% within 0.5 mm of tooth outline
Fouad et al., 1990	20 single-rooted teeth	5 locators, EL verified by AL	55%–75% within 0.5 mm of apical foramen
McDonald and Hovland, 1990	67 canals	EL verified by AL	93.4% within 0.5 mm of apical constriction
Keller, Brown, and Newton, 1991	69 teeth with 99 canals	EL and Rad verified by AL	EL 51.5%, Rad 80.2% accurate
Hembrough, Weine, Pisano & Eskoz, 1993	26 DB and palatal canals in maxillary 1st molars	EL verified by AL	EL 88.5% within 0.5 mm of major diameter

EL, Electronic length; *Rad*, radiographic length; *DT*, digital, tactile length; *AL*, direct anatomic length.

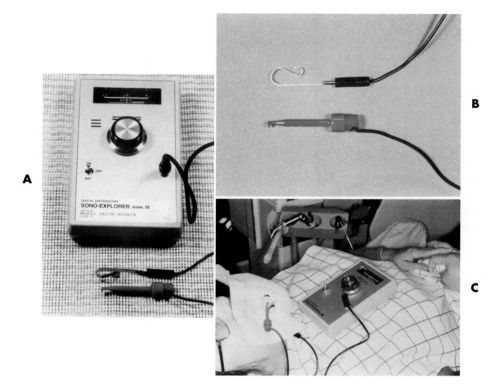

Fig. 8-19. Mark IV Sono-Explorer, updated version of the apex locator that shocked the endodontic community when first demonstrated by Inoue at 1969 meeting of the American Association of Endodontists. **A,** Close-up of machine. Window at top indicates site in center where reference needle will indicate that probe has entered oral mucous membrane or periodontal tissues. Control knob beneath window is to adjust needle to center point after placement of file into sulcus. On-off-bat button is to turn on, turn off, or test battery. At bottom is lip clip, and beneath it is reamer/file holder. **B,** Close-up of lip clip *(top)* and reamer/file holder *(bottom)*. **C,** SonoExplorer pinned on patient's napkin, lip clip lead seen beneath rubber dam, reamer/file holder attached to file in tooth. If the operator wishes, the machine may be placed on the bracket tray, adjacent table, or any nearby receptacle. (Courtesy Dr. N. Inoue, Tokyo.)

The step-by-step technique for using a Mark IV apex locator for calculation of working length is as follows:

1. Turn on the device and attach the lip clip near the arch being treated. Place a size 15 file into the reamer/file holder. Use a file with a plastic handle (metal handled files need insulators) that is 25 mm long, unless the tooth is very short, so that you have enough metal protruding through the tooth to attach the file clip (for very long teeth, use a 31 mm file). Insert the tip of the file approximately 0.5 mm into the sulcus of the tooth to be treated, similar to the placing of a periodontal probe. Adjust the control knob until the reference needle is centered on the meter scale and produces audible beeps. Set the holder aside until needed to record the measurement.

2. Using the preoperative straight and angled radiographs for information about the expected canal configuration of the tooth, prepare the proper access cavity, as described in Chapter 6. Place the rubber dam as soon as the orifice(s) is (are) located. Irrigate the canal and remove any pulp tissue, debris, foreign material, unwanted items, and so forth that are present with broaches and Hedstrom files.

3. Using the preoperative radiographs, estimate the working length and canal width as described in the section on applying Kuttler's

studies. Using the instrument calculated as correct for width, set the stop at the estimated length. The canal should be slightly wet with irrigant (hydrogen peroxide or sterile water is better here than hypochlorite solutions, which are ionizing). If bleeding from a vital extirpation is excessive, dry with paper points until it recedes.

4. Insert the file slowly into the canal until the reference needle moves from the extreme left to the center of the scale and the alarm bleeps sound. This should happen near the site where you have placed the stop if your estimate has been accurate. Reset the stop at the reference point (later this chapter), remove the file, and record the length.

5. Take a radiograph with the file in place at the length indicated by the locator and examine the resulting film. If the suggested length is considerably longer or shorter than your estimate, it is possible that the preoperative films were elongated or foreshortened, or that the apex locator has been inaccurate. Using the film with the file in place, attempt to reconcile the differences and arrive at a logical working length. If the length suggested by the locator still seems too short, consider a short exiting of the canal (Figs. 8-9, 8-10, and 8-13). If the length suggested indicates the file is out of the root, it is obviously too long, and this is a situation where the locator has provided inaccurate information.

Advantages.   The major advantage of the apex locator is that it supplies objective information with a high degree of accuracy. It is particularly useful for the dentist who was taught in dental school that it is best to fill to the radiographic apex, but knows that such a procedure is wrong and often results in postoperative pain. In this way the crutch of the locator gives the information as to where the preparation should end.

The best use for the apex locator is where radiographs are difficult to read accurately for calculation of working length. Such a situation often exists in maxillary molars, where the radiopaque structures of the malar process or floor of the maxillary sinus may superimpose the apices of the teeth, making radiographic calculation difficult. Mandibular tori may do the same for mandibular bicuspids and molars.

It is also useful for the dentist who requires a number of radiographs to arrive at an acceptable length. In these cases, the locator may be used as an estimating tool and then confirmed with a file in place for a radiograph. Patients who gag easily with radiographs also profit from preliminary use.

Locators also may be useful in verifying perforations of the root.

Disadvantages.   The major disadvantage of the apex locators is that, at best, the accuracy is somewhere in the low 90 percentiles. In the study by Hembrough et al., it was reported that when the locator tested was in error, the miscalculation tended to be on the long side. This meant that without a confirming radiograph, filing done to the incorrect length could cause an increase in postoperative pain and a decrease in success.

There are a multiplicity of problems that may cause these machines to give incorrect or inaccurate readings. The battery may be low (check battery and replace frequently), too much tissue may remain in the canal (broach canal and use a Hedstrom file to verify that gross tissue is gone), the canal may be too wet (dry mildly with paper points) or too dry (irrigate mildly with peroxide or sterile water), the file may be too narrow (use a file that is slightly loose in the canal, not a size 10 each time; estimate first to chose the proper width), a blockage may be present (try to bypass CAREFULLY!), the lip clip may fall off (check that it is in place), and other conditions.

Apex locators will seem to function best when used frequently, but seem inaccurate when used rarely. What really is happening is that clinicians using them gain better success with experience. When used by a novice, an individual who could profit by this aid, a multiplicity of errors may creep up unnoticed, which would not occur when used by one experienced in the procedure. If you are interested in using an apex locator in your endodontic treatments, use it for every case for several weeks to a month, being aware of the possibilities for error, and include radiographs when indicated. At the end of that time, assess your results and decide if it is useful in your practice. If so, continue using it frequently and you will enjoy the results.

If, on the other hand, you are not satisfied, return to your previous technique. Many excellently treated cases do not involve apex location use.

Apex locators versus radiographs.   It is a mistake to think that apex locators will eliminate radiographs during endodontic treatment. Excellent preoperative films must always be taken prior to any active treatment on the tooth. Apex locators cannot help the dentist determine canal width, canal curvature, or number of canals, and they can only partially help with sites of canal division. These must be determined by radiograph. Fouad et al. stated that apex locators were not meant to replace radiographs, but to add to the information obtained by radiographs. This is a wise statement.

Conclusions. Apex locators have a definite use in endodontics, but their use is not mandatory for all. They are most effective when used by those who use them often and must be combined with high-quality radiographs.

There are three types of locators at present. The oldest, resistance locators, work because the electrical resistance of the periodontal ligament equals that of the oral mucous membrane, and they identify when a probe goes through the tooth to reach the ligament. The newest two, impedance and frequency locators, indicate where the canal is the narrowest.

All the locators agree that filing to the radiographic apex is incorrect, either by being past the narrowest constriction of the canal or into the periodontal ligament.

USE OF REFERENCE POINTS

Any measurement of length refers to the distance between two points. Whereas one point of the measurement of a working length refers to the end point of the preparation, the other point may vary considerably. In anterior teeth the other reference point is usually the incisal edge, but broken-down teeth may be measured from adjacent teeth or from some projecting portion of the remaining tooth structure. In bicanaled bicuspids the buccal canal is generally measured to the buccal cusp tip, but the palatal canal may use either cusp tip as reference. There may be a variance of at least 1 mm in length, depending on which reference point is used in measuring. Similarly, buccal canals of maxillary molars may be measured from either buccal cusp, mesial canals of mandibular molars from either mesial cusp, and so forth.

Therefore, in addition to recording the working length of any canal, the reference point from which it is measured must be similarly recorded (Fig. 8-20).

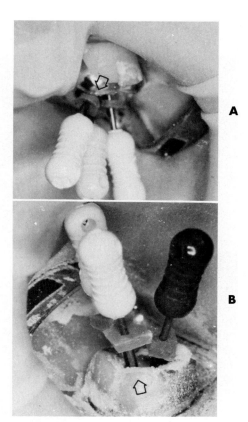

Fig. 8-20. **A,** Maxillary first molar with files in place for taking radiograph to measure working length. File at left goes into distobuccal canal, whereas file at right inserts into mesiobuccal canal. Crossing of the files frequently occurs in small canals of molars because of angulation of canals. Mesiobuccal cusp *(arrow)* acts as reference point for files in each buccal canal. **B,** Mandibular second molar with files in place. File in foreground inserts into mesiolingual canal but will use mesiobuccal cusp as reference point *(arrow).* File with the dark handle *(at right)* is in mesiobuccal canal and may be measured from either mesial cusp. Small files are photographed here. By the time the canals have been widened to any appreciable extent, the files tend to straighten and no longer cross.

USING THE BUCCAL OBJECT RULE AND DETERMINING WORKING LENGTHS FOR POSTERIOR TEETH

It has already been stated that radiographs taken to determine working length must be taken from a straight-on and an angled direction to determine apical foramen deviation. This method also allows canal identification and measurement

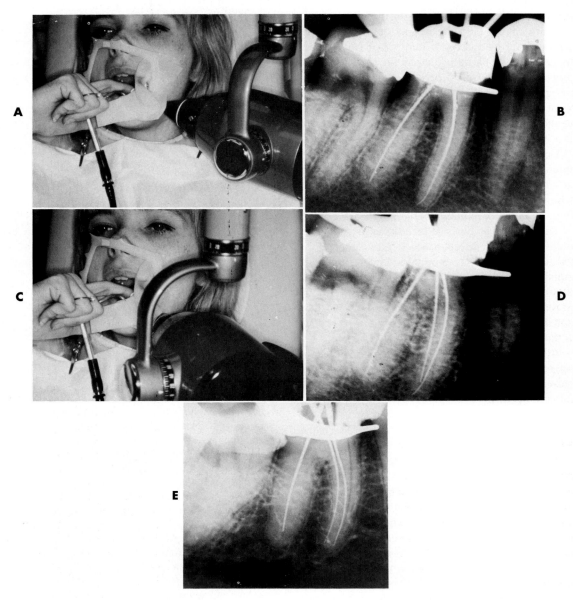

Fig. 8-21.   Radiographic technique for determination of working length in mandibular molars. **A,** Cone is in position to take straight-on view. **B,** Typical radiograph as a result of such angulation, showing position of file in distal canal but superimposing instruments in mesial canals. **C,** For the angled view from the mesial, the cone is pointed to the distal at an angle of 25 degrees to 35 degrees as compared to the straight-on film. **D,** Typical radiograph as a result of such an angulation. Files in the mesial canal are now seen separately and seem to join short of the apex. The canal to the right, the master canal, is the mesiolingual, and the mesial canal to the left is the mesiobuccal. **E,** Another typical radiograph as a result of such an angulation. This is a different tooth than shown in **D,** and in this case the mesial canals are both separate and distinct to the apex; that is, they do not join. In both views **D** and **E** the accurate angled view indicates that the file in the distal canal is well centered in that root. That generally means that only one distal canal is present. Contrast with Fig. 8-24.

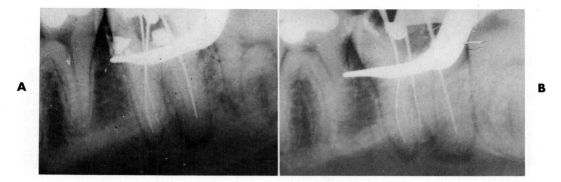

Fig. 8-22. Straight-on radiograph, **A,** discloses that file in distal canal is at least 1 mm short of desired end point. Because tooth is rotated, files in mesial canals are not superimposed; but it is still impossible to make an accurate differentiation between them. Angled view toward distal, **B,** definitely shows file in mesiolingual canal as mesial to instrument in mesiobuccal canal.

for multicanaled teeth through the buccal object rule; this rule states that the root or canal farthest from the film (the buccal) moves the greatest distance on a radiograph taken with the cone angled in the horizontal plane. This means that if the cone is pointed from the mesial aspect toward the distal when a bicanaled bicuspid is radiographed, the buccal root and/or canal image will move more than the palatal and appear distal to the palatal root and/or canal image on the film. If the cone is pointed from the distal surface toward the mesial, the buccal root and/or canal will appear mesially. In mandibular molars the same process will separate the images of the two mesial canals. When the cone is pointed toward the distal direction, the mesiobuccal canal moves the greater distance and appears distal to the mesiolingual canal (Fig. 8-21). If the cone is pointed mesially, the position of the two canals is reversed.

For most teeth, cone angulation from the mesial aspect to the distal will produce highly satisfactory results. If this direction is used routinely, roots and canals on angled films will always be easily identifiable when examined at a later date, with the buccal root and/or canal located distally. When the distal-to-mesial angulation is used, an X or other identifying mark may be placed on the crown or elsewhere on the film during the processing to indicate that the buccal root and/or canal appears to the mesial aspect.

To determine the working length of mandibular molars, the dentist places the files to the estimated length. A straight-on view and an angled view toward the distal are taken. The straight-on view will allow for calculation of the working length of

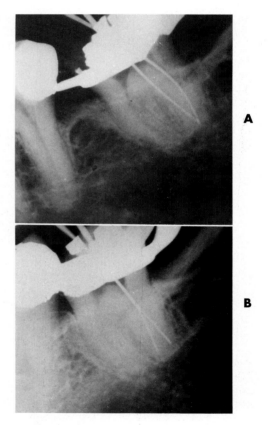

Fig. 8-23. From straight-on view, **A,** it appears that distal canals merge in this mandibular second molar. However, angled view, **B,** discloses that two separate and distinct distal canals are present. If one were to rely on the configuration shown in **A,** the preparation and filling of that canal system could lead to failure. The canals must be prepared as being separate and distinct, as shown in **B.**

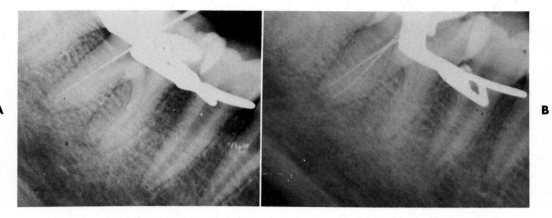

Fig. 8-24. **A,** On angled view, file in distal canal is not in center of root. Radiolucent line is seen mesial to it, indicating presence of a second canal. Line may be second canal in some cases, but here it is periodontal ligament space of inner portion of a root having a figure-eight shape. **B,** Further exploration to lingual aspect disclosed another separate canal, confirmed by angled radiograph.

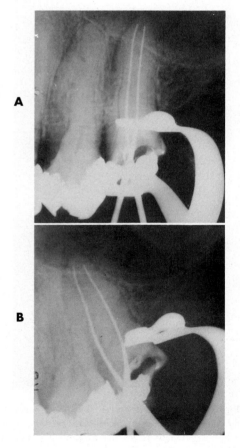

Fig. 8-25. **A,** Straight-on radiograph of maxillary second bicuspid fails to separate canals sufficiently because of rotation of tooth. **B,** View toward distal allows excellent visualization of both canals, with buccal root toward distal aspect.

the distal root and show any unusual deviation of the apical foramina of the mesial canals. The angled view will allow for calculation of the working lengths for the mesial canals and will show unusual deviation of the apical foramen of the distal root (Fig. 8-22 on p. 419). When two distal canals are present, their working lengths will be calculated in the same manner as the mesial canals. The two views are necessary to determine when there is a Type II canal configuration (two orifices merging to form one apical foramen). One radiograph may indicate that canals merge, but this finding must be confirmed by both views. (See Fig. 8-23 on p. 419.) Also, the angled radiograph will aid in detecting an undiscovered additional distal canal. If only one distal canal is present, the file appears in the exact center of the root. However, if the file appears in the distal portion of the root and a view from the mesial was taken, a second distal canal should be anticipated to the lingual side (Fig. 8-24).

Bicanaled bicuspids are radiographed from the mesial direction and in straight-on view after the files are placed to the estimated working lengths. The films are examined to determine position of each apical foramen, with the buccal canal identified to the distal side on the view from the mesial (Fig. 8-25).

Because of potential confusion in using the buccal object rule, other methods have been suggested as alternatives in determining working lengths in multicanaled teeth. One technique involves taking separate films with one file in place per film. This involves more exposure to the patient and is much

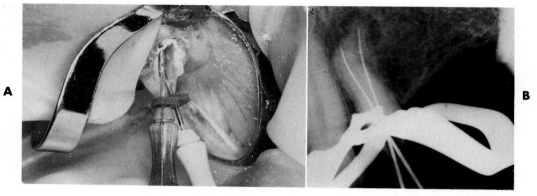

Fig. 8-26.   A, To avoid using buccal object rule to determine identification of canals, I placed a size 25 reamer in the buccal and a size 15 file in the palatal canal. **B,** Radiograph fails to distinguish clearly between the sizes or types of instruments used.

more time consuming. Another suggestion is to identify specific canals in teeth or roots with two canals by using a reamer in one canal and a file in the other or by using a large instrument in one canal and a smaller instrument in the other (Fig. 8-26). Although these methods can be useful, I believe that it is best to learn and master the buccal object rule.

As is the case for all teeth, the estimated working lengths for the posterior teeth must be verified to be within 1 mm of the apical foramen for the length to be recorded. If any measurements are off by more than 1 mm, an interpolation is made, the files readjusted accordingly, and two new views taken for confirmation.

REFERENCES

Becker CJ, Lankelma P, Wesselink PR, Thoden van Velzen SK: Electronic determination of root canal length, *J Endod* 6:876, 1980.

Berman LH, Fleischman SB: Evaluation of the accuracy of the Neosono-D electronic apex locator, *J Endod* 10:164, 1984.

Bhaskar SN, Rappaport HM: Histologic evaluation of endodontic procedures in dogs, *Oral Surg Oral Med Oral Pathol* 31:526, 1971.

Blank LW, Tenca JI, Pelleu GB: Reliability of electronic measuring devices in endodontic therapy, *J Endod* 1:141, 1975.

Bramante CM, Berbert A: A critical evaluation of some methods of determining tooth length, *Oral Surg Oral Med Oral Pathol* 37:463, 1974.

Bramante CM, Berbert A, Borges RP: A methodology for evaluation of root canal instrumentation, *J Endod* 13:243, 1987.

Busch LR et al: Determination of the accuracy of the Sono-Explorer for establishing endodontic measurement control, *J Endod* 2:295, 1976.

Caldwell JL: Change in working length following instrumentation of molar canals, *Oral Surg Oral Med Oral Pathol* 41:114, 1976.

Christie WH, Peikoff MD, Hawrish CE: Clinical observations on a newly designed electronic apex locator, *J Can Dent Assoc* 59:765, 1993.

Chunn CB, Zardiakas LD, Menke RA: In vivo root canal length determination using the forameter, *J Endod* 7:515, 1981.

Coolidge ED: Anatomy of the root apex in relation to treatment problems, *J Am Dent Assoc* 16:1456, 1929.

Cox VS, Brown CE, Bricker SL, Newton CW: Radiographic interpretation of endodontic file length, *Oral Surg Oral Med Oral Pathol* 72:340, 1991.

Davis MS, Joseph SW, Bucher JF: Periapical and intracanal healing following root canal fillings in dogs, *Oral Surg Oral Med Oral Pathol* 31:662, 1971.

Dummer PMH, McGinn JH, Rees DG: The position and topography of the apical canal constriction and apical foramen, *Int Endod J* 17:192, 1984.

Einbinder AB, Kratchman SI: Apex locators: a systematic approach for usage, *Compend Contin Educ Dent* 14:34, 1993.

Fouad AF et al: A clinical evaluation of five electronic root canal measuring instruments, *J Endod* 16:446, 1990.

Grove CJ: Faulty technic in investigations of the apices of pulpless teeth, *J Am Dent Assoc* 13:746, 1926.

Hasselgren G: Where shall the root filling end? *NY State Dent J* 60:34, 1994.

Hatton EH: Microscopic studies of diseased peridental tissues, *JAMA* 71:1549, 1918.

Hembrough JH, Weine FS, Pisano JV, Eskoz N: Accuracy of an electronic apex locator: a clinical evaluation in maxillary molars, *J Endod* 19:242, 1993.

Inoue N: Dental "stethoscope" measures root canal, *Dent Surv* 48:38, 1972.

Inoue N: An audiometric method for determining the length of root canals, *J Can Dent Assoc* 50:6306, 1973.

Keller ME, Brown CE, Newton CW: A clinical evaluation of the Endocater—an electronic apex locator, *J Endod* 17:6, 1991.

Kuttler Y: Microscopic investigation of root apexes, *J Am Dent Assoc* 50:544, 1955.

Levy AB, Glatt L: Deviation of the apical foramen from the radiographic apex, *J NJ Dent Soc* 41:12, 1970.

McDonald NJ: The electronic determination of working length, *Dent Clin North Am* 36:293, 1992.

McDonald NJ, Hovland EJ: An evaluation of the apex endocater, *J Endod* 16:5, 1990.

O'Neil LJ: A clinical evaluation of electronic root canal measurement, *Oral Surg Oral Med Oral Pathol* 38:469, 1974.

Palmer MJ, Weine FS, Healey HJ: Position of the apical foramen in relation to endodontic therapy, *J Can Dent Assoc* 37:305, 1971.

Seidberg BH, Alibrandi BV, Fine H, Logue B: Clinical investigation of measuring working lengths of root canals with an electronic device and with digital-tactile sense, *J Am Dent Assoc* 90:379, 1975.

Seltzer S, Bender IB, Turkenkopf S: Factors affecting successful repair after root canal therapy, *J Am Dent Assoc* 67:651, 1963.

Stein J, Corcoran JF: Nonionizing method of locating the apical constriction (minor foramen) in root canals, *Oral Surg Oral Med Oral Pathol* 71:96, 1991.

Strindberg L: The dependence of the results of pulp therapy on certain factors: an analytic study based on radiographic and clinic follow-up examinations, *Acta Odontol Scand* 14 (suppl 1):1, 1956.

Sunada I: New method for measuring the length of the root canal, *J Dent Res* 41:375, 1962.

Swartz DB, Skidmore AE, Griffin JA: Twenty years of endodontic success and failure, *J Endod* 9:198, 1983.

Trope M, Rabie G, Tronstad L: Accuracy of an electronic apex locator under controlled clinical conditions, *Endod Dent Traumatol* 1:142, 1985.

Vande Voorde HE, Bjorndahl AM: Estimating endodontic "working length" with paralleling radiographs, *Oral Surg Oral Med Oral Pathol* 27:106, 1969.

9 Canal filling with semisolid materials

The final step in endodontic treatment has been stated to be the sealing of the apical foramen at the cementodentinal junction with an inert material (Fig. 9-1). In this chapter the semisolid materials used to seal canals will be discussed, and the next chapter will discuss the solid materials.

The solid materials have gradually fallen into disfavor, and at present gutta-percha techniques are quite dominant, even in the smaller curved canals (Figs. 7-31 to 7-35 and 7-37). Research goes on to uncover an even more acceptable filling material, whether solid or semisolid, and views may change as to the preferred choice for the future.

READINESS OF THE CANAL FOR FILLING

Regardless of the material used, established criteria must be met before the canal is considered ready for filling. Obviously the canal must be completely prepared to the acceptable depth and width prior to even considering readiness for filling. For many years most authorities agreed that four conditions must be satisfied: (1) negative culture test, (2) no excessive exudate from the canal, (3) absence of foul odor, and (4) lack of periapical sensitivity.

This list has undergone periodic revision, and several of the conditions have been given more credence form time to time. Presently, however, at least one condition—gaining of a negative culture—has been eliminated from the list.

Problems stemming from reliance on negative culture. This was a dominant criterion for many years for two major reasons. First, it was the only criterion that was completely objective. The culture test was either positive or negative, and no degree of "slightly" positive was possible in such a qualitative test. Second, the pioneers of endodontics were aware of the potential dangers of bacteria in the apical portions of the canal and the periapical tissues. They took pride in their ability to rid these areas of microorganisms, even if it took a number of appointments, and they were able to point to the negative culture test as proof of their efforts. This demonstration of a bacteria-free canal greatly enhanced the stature of endodontics in both the dental and the medical communities.

The reliance on the negative culture test decreased when important studies indicated that false negatives could give an inaccurate assessment of the microbial population in the critical areas. In addition, even a positive culture did not vouch for the potential pathogenicity of the offending microorganisms. Even more serious was the fact that some of the most pathogenic organisms were grown only with great difficulty by the culture methods then in vogue (Chapter 15).

This is not meant to infer that a contaminated canal should be filled with impunity. On the contrary, the presence of bacteria due to a faulty temporary seal or frank intracanal infection on opening the canal are obvious contraindications for completion.

Significance of foul odor. For many years it was common practice for dentists to smell the paper points then used in the closing of the canal, particularly as a substitute for culturing. The absence of odor supposedly was an indication that no infection was present and the canal could be filled.

Grossman reported a poor correlation between canal odor and culture results—positive cultures were found in canals free of odor. In addition, a foul odor has been associated with anaerobic growth, which is difficult to verify with routine culturing techniques.

For these reasons, absence of canal odor is rarely considered as an indication for filling.

No excessive exudate. In regard to the finding of exudate, the word *excessive* presents a problem of semantics. A tooth with a flaring apex is almost impossible to rid of tissue fluids without resorting

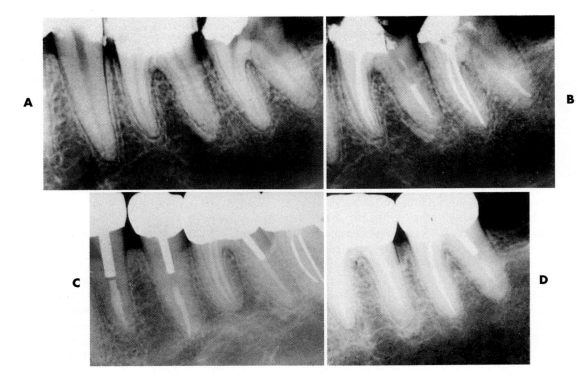

Fig. 9-1. **A,** Preoperative view of mandibular posterior area indicating bicuspid and molar teeth that had been decimated by decay and poor restorations, now temporized and requiring endodontic treatment. **B,** Angled view following completion of endodontic treatment of molars in 1969. The first molar and distal root of the second molar were filled with semisolid materials—gutta-percha—whereas the mesial canals of the second molar were sealed with solid materials—silver points. Kerr's antiseptic sealer also was used. The bicuspids were filled with gutta-percha as well. **C** and **D,** Radiographs taken in 1987, 18 years later, indicating perfect healing of the four teeth. Without the intervention of endodontic treatment, this patient would have lost these teeth with resultant problems extending to other areas of the mouth and jaws. Both the solid and the semisolid materials have held up well, and there is no reason to believe that these teeth will not continue to last for many more years. (Restorations by Dr. Sherwin Strauss, Chicago.)

to caustic chemicals that might cause periapical inflammation. On the other hand, the presence of even a slight purulent exudate may indicate the possibility of an incipient exacerbation.

Lack of periapical sensitivity. Since the previously discussed criteria may be difficult to assess, the lack of periapical sensitivity retains the strongest cogency. The amount of sensitivity is determined by lightly tapping the treated tooth with the butt end of a mouth mirror and by digital manipulation of the buccal and lingual plates of bone surrounding the tooth. In a tooth ready for filling, the result should be the same as for an adjacent or a contralateral nontreated tooth. The presence of sensitivity indicates retained inflammation in the periodontal membrane space, most frequently as a result of overinstrumentation. If the

canal is filled before the inflammation has dissipated, the additive inflammation that normally results from the packing of the canal with filling materials and sealer will often cause an extremely painful episode, which may prompt the patient to insist on an extraction or require heavy administration of pain relievers. Unless tissue resistance is strong enough to overcome this considerable increase of inflammatory potential, an area of periapical inflammation (granuloma) will result or a previously existing lesion will be perpetuated.

NEED FOR FILLING CANALS

The emphasis in Chapter 7 consistently enforced the importance of canal preparation as the most critical phase of endodontic treatment. To emphasize this fact, Fig. 7-1 stated and demon-

A   **B**   **C**

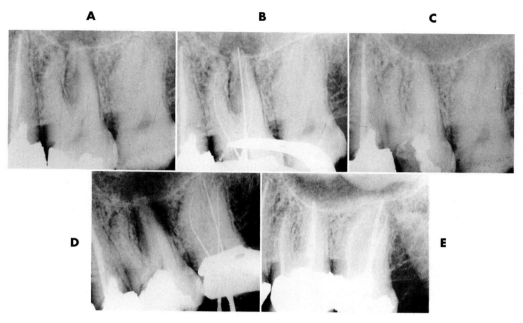

D   **E**

Fig. 9-2.   A, Radiograph of posterior maxillary area. The second bicuspid had been treated several years earlier, but now there was a periapical lesion associated with the first molar that also required therapy. In my interest to treat the first molar, I neglected to notice the carious lesion on the mesial surface of the second molar, which was symptom free at that time. **B,** Radiograph taken at the first appointment for treating the first molar, files in place (too long in palatal root, seemingly correct in buccal roots). **C,** The patient did not return for his second appointment for *over 1 year!* At that time he complained of pain to hot and cold in the area, but obviously it could not come from the treated second bicuspid or pulpless first molar. I took this film and noted the deep caries on the mesial surface of the second molar. Even more surprisingly, the periapical lesion associated with the first molar had healed, despite the absence of canal filling. Compare this with Fig. 7-1. I performed a pulpotomy as emergency treatment for the second molar and replaced the partially lost temporary restoration in the access cavity for the first molar. Also, I instructed the patient on the importance of keeping his appointments on a regular schedule. **D,** Despite my admonition, the patient failed to return for *over 1 more year!* Now the second molar was tender to percussion, so I opened it and performed a complete pulpectomy. This radiograph was taken during that appointment to determine working lengths. It also demonstrates that a periapical lesion has returned to the first molar. **E,** Film taken 3 years after the completion of treatment, 4 years after the initiation of therapy in those two teeth, demonstrating complete healing.

strated that following canal preparation, a periapical lesion could be healing before the canal filling was placed.

This should not be misconstrued to imply that canal filling is unimportant and perhaps not even necessary. If a periapical lesion heals *without* a canal filling, what is the function of the placement of that filling, other than to indicate that endodontic therapy had been performed? This question is answered by Fig. 9-2, illustrating the treatment of a maxillary molar with an associated periapical lesion present prior to therapy. The canals were prepared properly (Fig. 9-2, *B*), and a subsequent

film indicated that the lesion had healed without canal filling (Fig. 9-2, *C*). However, the patient failed to return for other appointments for 1 year. Radiographs taken then revealed the return of the lesion (Fig. 9-2, *D*). Fortunately, when the treatment schedule was followed correctly, healing resulted (Fig. 9-2, *E*).

This case clearly endorses the concept that canals must be filled to retain the periapical tissues at their most desirable condition. Healing is initiated once the canals are prepared properly. However, unless the canal space is closed by filling, the irritants, metabolites, microorganisms, and so forth, that may cause periapical breakdown have the opportunity to return. This may lead to a recurrence of the lesion, as depicted in Fig. 9-2, *D*.

RATIONALE FOR USING SEMISOLID MATERIALS

Effect of canal preparation. Semisolid materials have the important quality of being compressible and thus may be packed into an irregularly shaped prepared cavity. As stated previously, the objective of canal preparation is to remove the irregularities of the walls and enable the canal to receive the sealing materials. Even though gross irregularities are usually removed, the canal preparation will produce some of its own.

The different types of instruments used in canal enlargement produce different general shapes. Reaming will result in a relatively circular preparation, whereas filing gives an elliptical shape when viewed in cross section. Hedstrom files gouge and give more irregular shapes than do other instruments.

Effect of original shape. The original shape and degree of curvature of the canal are factors in determining what shape results at the completion of preparation. Some canals are irregularly shaped and can never be enlarged to give a completely circular preparation. Among these are the kidney bean–shaped distal canals of mandibular molars, the oval canals of mandibular anterior teeth and palatal canals of maxillary molars, the figure

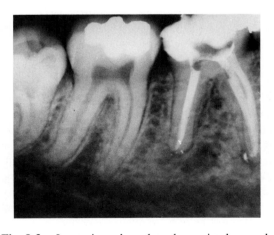

Fig. 9-3. Large, irregularly shaped, noncircular canals are indications for use of semisolid filling materials. All canals in this mandibular first molar of a 17-year-old patient are filled with gutta-percha.

eight–shaped canals of single-rooted maxillary premolars, and most teeth treated on young patients.

The result of canal preparation and its effect on original canal shape yields a final canal shape that is generally quite irregular in cross section. One of the objectives of canal preparation is to create a tapering funnel longitudinally, so diameters from the orifice to the apex are successively smaller. However, again it is probably impossible to gain this in every case, particularly in curved canals. Therefore even ideal preparations do have many irregularities, which are best filled with condensible materials that may be packed against these walls.

Indications. Semisolids are the filling materials of choice in the following instances:

1. Whenever it is anticipated that irregular walls or noncircular shape is present, either because of canal anatomy or as a result of preparation (Fig. 9-3).
2. Whenever a condensation technique may be utilized, usually requiring a flared preparation to size 30 or greater.
3. When a lateral or an auxiliary canal is anticipated or when it is determined that multiple apical foramina are present (Fig. 9-4).
4. Whenever the strong possibility of an overfilling is present, as in apical resorption or destruction of apical constriction by overinstrumentation, since the semisolids are well tolerated in periapical tissue (Fig. 9-5).
5. In cases of internal resorption (Fig. 9-6).
6. When periapical surgery is to be performed.

On the basis of these indications, semisolid materials should be routinely used to fill virtually every conceivable case. This might require slightly greater final canal width for the preparation than was formerly gained when silver points were commonly used, but with careful preparation and proper flaring this objective is attainable. Flaring (Chapter 7) is especially important in the smaller canals so that the condensing instruments are able to reach the apical few millimeters. Unless the gutta-percha is condensed and deformed at the tip, it has few, if any, advantages over the solid canal filling materials.

GUTTA-PERCHA

The most popularly used semisolid material is gutta-percha, which has enjoyed acceptance as a dental material for more than 100 years. When

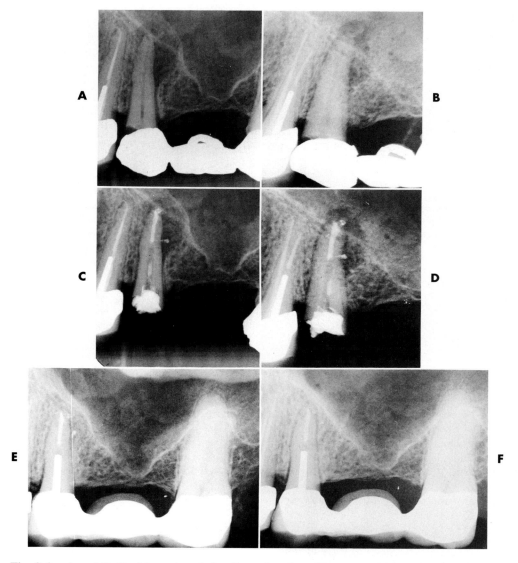

Fig. 9-4. **A** and **B,** Straight and angled radiographs of maxillary second bicuspid with periapical lesion encircling the root. **C** and **D,** Straight and angled views immediately after filling with laterally condensed gutta-percha and Kerr's Antiseptic Root Canal Sealer. Multiple lateral canals can be noted. The radiopaque line mesial to the fill on the angled view is a scratch. **E,** Two years after treatment. **F,** Four years after treatment. (Restorations by Dr. Ascher Jacobs, formerly of Chicago.) (From Weine FS: *Dent Clin North Am* 28:833, 1984. With permission.)

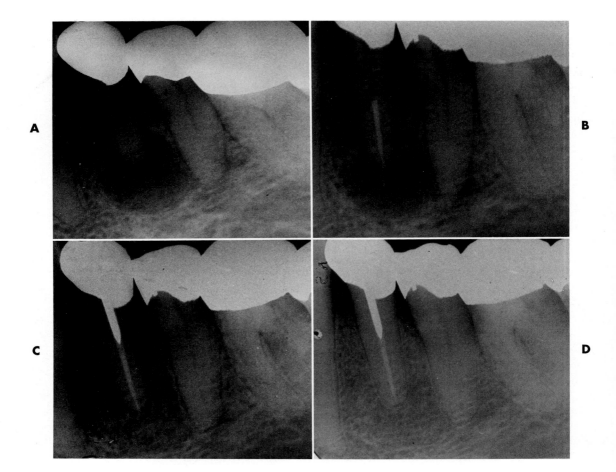

Fig. 9-5. **A,** Preoperative radiograph of mandibular first bicuspid with large periapical radiolucency and probable apical resorption. **B,** Canal filled with laterally condensed gutta-percha and Wach's paste as sealer. Master cone and some sealer are past apex, probably because of failure to account for degree of apical resorption in calculating the working length. **C,** Three years after canal filling, much of excess has been absorbed. **D,** Eleven years after canal filling, entire excess has been absorbed. Apical extent of canal filling is several millimeters short of radiographic apex, probably due to apical deposition of cementum. (Restorations by Dr. Rod Nystul, formerly of Park Ridge, Ill.)

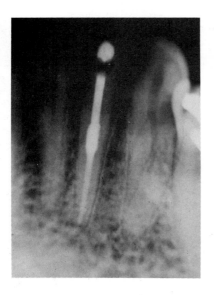

Fig. 9-6. Lower incisor 2 years postoperatively with internal resorption, filled with semisolid materials.

used as a temporary filling material in operative dentistry or endodontics, gutta-percha is a poor sealant, according to radioisotope and dye studies. However, Marshall and Massler showed by way of isotopes that in a lateral condensation procedure, gutta-percha gives the best apical seal among the commonly used canal-filling techniques.

In its pure molecular structure, gutta-percha is the *trans* isomer of polyisoprene and has an approximately 60% crystalline form. The *cis* isomer is natural rubber, which has a largely amorphous form. The very close molecular structure of gutta-percha and rubber accounts for a number of similarities in physical properties, but the crucial difference in form makes the mechanical behavior of gutta-percha more like that of the partially crystalline polymers.

Other polyisoprene products besides gutta-percha and natural rubber are chicle, used as the base for chewing gum, and balata, used in the production of golf balls. Both these substances have physical properties very similar to the other polyisoprene derivatives. For many years it was reported that gutta-percha was taken from the sap of the Indian rubber trees indigenous to the Malaysian archipelago. Although this may have been true prior to World War II, it is untrue now. Because of its greater commercial value, the rubber tree sap from the areas of Malaysia, Borneo, and Indonesia is almost exclusively used as the *cis* isomer and turned into natural rubber and similar products. Gutta-percha now comes from central South America.

As it comes from the tree, gutta-percha is white in color. By the addition of dyes, gutta-percha may be turned any color of the rainbow. For many years it was dyed pink or red for endodontic use because that was the color of the pulp, which it replaced.

Phase transitions of *trans*-polyisoprene. Many chemical formulas are available as different substances, depending on their temperature, by virtue of being susceptible to phase changes. Depending on the temperature, H_2O may be ice, water, or steam. Gutta-percha, similarly, has three possible phase changes as well.

In the unheated tree or in the cone at room or body temperature, gutta-percha is considered to be in the *beta* phase. In this phase, gutta-percha is solid, compactible, and elongatible; may become brittle when aged; and does not stick to anything. When heated to temperatures of 42° to 49° C, gutta-percha undergoes a phase change to the *alpha* phase. In this phase it is runny, tacky, sticky,

noncompactible, and nonelongatible. The third, or *gamma* phase, occurs when heating is raised to 56° to 62° C, but the properties at this level are not well known and seem to be similar to that of the *alpha* phase.

The significance of these phases, in addition to the changes in physical properties, is that the materials expand when heated from the *beta* to the *alpha* or *gamma* phases, from less than 1% to almost 3%. When cooled down to the *beta* phase, a shrinkage takes place, of similar percentiles, but the degree of shrinkage almost always is greater than the degree of expansion and may differ by as much as 2%. That means that if gutta-percha is heated above 42° to 49° C (108° to 120° F) and then inserted into a prepared canal, a condensation procedure should be applied or some method used to lessen the problem of shrinkage.

Advantages.   Gutta-percha in the *beta* phase has a number of advantages as a canal filling material:

1. *Compressibility.* Gutta-percha allows for excellent adaptation to the walls of a canal preparation by a packing technique. In fact, this is not compressibility but *compactability.* Compressibility means that the atoms of the gutta-percha molecule are pushed closer together in a spatial relationship during condensation; this does not occur. However, the term compressibility has been used for many years in regard to gutta-percha, and I will honor the traditional description even if it is not perfectly accurate on a molecular level.

2. *Inertness.* Of all the materials used in clinical dentistry, gutta-percha is almost the least reactive and is considerably less reactive than silver or gold.

3. *Dimensional stability.* Gutta-percha undergoes almost no dimensional change after completion of condensation in the canal.

4. *Tissue tolerance.* According to studies performed by embedding gutta-percha in the back of the rat and the periodontium of the hamster, gutta-percha is well tolerated in tissue.

5. *Radiopacity.* Gutta-percha is radiopaque and therefore is easily recognizable on a dental x-ray film, as are most of the other endodontic filling materials, including silver points.

6. *Becomes plastic when warmed.* As stated earlier, when heated above 42° to 49° C, *beta* phase gutta-percha will undergo

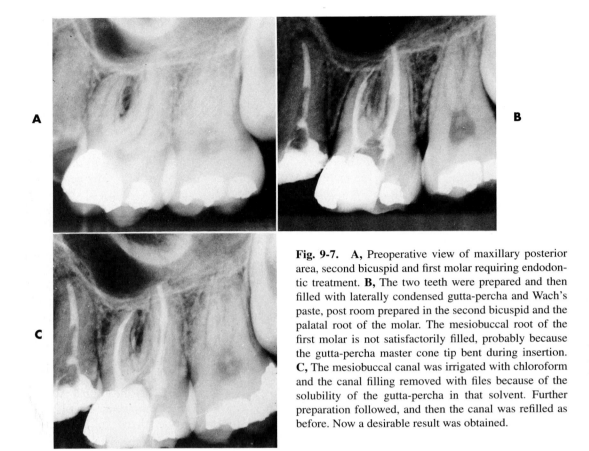

Fig. 9-7. **A,** Preoperative view of maxillary posterior area, second bicuspid and first molar requiring endodontic treatment. **B,** The two teeth were prepared and then filled with laterally condensed gutta-percha and Wach's paste, post room prepared in the second bicuspid and the palatal root of the molar. The mesiobuccal root of the first molar is not satisfactorily filled, probably because the gutta-percha master cone tip bent during insertion. **C,** The mesiobuccal canal was irrigated with chloroform and the canal filling removed with files because of the solubility of the gutta-percha in that solvent. Further preparation followed, and then the canal was refilled as before. Now a desirable result was obtained.

changes in some physical properties that are useful during endodontic treatment. Marlin and Schilder reported that after heating, gutta-percha could be packed with pluggers and its mass increased in a given volume. This allows use of the thermoplastic techniques that will be discussed more fully later in this chapter.

7. *Has known solvents.* Gutta-percha may be dissolved by several known solvents, the most common being chloroform and xylene. This gives it a significant advantage over the other commonly used canal filling material— silver points—which may be only physically removed if the need for re-treatment occurs (Figs. 9-7 and 9-42 to 9-45). By having these solvents, gutta-percha also allows itself to be more versatile as a canal filling material. It may be dissolved completely by chloroform and used as chloropercha or be partially dissolved by eucalyptol and used as eucapercha. Also, it may be softened by chloroform and used to take an interior canal imprint in larger canals.

8. *Elongatible when fresh, brittle when old.* A mild relationship exists between the ability for gutta-percha to be elongated and to be compacted. When gutta-percha is fresh, it may be stretched by pulling the ends of a cone between thumb and forefinger. If, however, the cone snaps quickly when this is done, it indicates that the cone is old and probably will not compact as well as a fresher cone. Since the ability to compact is important for the cold condensation procedures, it is good to have this test available to predict the compactability of the product.

Disadvantages.   There are two significant disadvantages to the use of gutta-percha, both of which should be borne in mind when contemplating its use:

1. *Lack of rigidity.* Gutta-percha will bend rather easily when subjected to lateral pressure, which makes it more difficult to use in the smaller sizes (i.e., less than 35).
2. *Lack of length control.* In addition to its compressibility, gutta-percha permits vertical distortion by stretching; unless it meets an obstruction or is packed against a definite matrix or stopping point, there is little control over what depth it will reach. To ensure against overfilling with gutta-percha requires a meticulous preparation that affords a definite stop in the apical portion. (Fig. 9-8). Fortunately, since gutta-percha is so well tolerated by periapical tissue, only rarely is a posttreatment failure noted in conjunction with an overfilling. Most instances show no abnormal radiographic evidence, and in some cases there is an actual amputation of the overfilling with phagocytosis of the extra mass (Fig. 9-9).

Composition of gutta-percha cones. Friedman et al. reported several exhaustive studies on the physical properties of gutta-percha as used in endodontic procedures. Analysis of the available brands indicated that the composition of any individual cone varied between manufacturers, sometimes to a significant extent. The constituents and their percentages in the brands tested are listed in Table 9-1.

Because of these differences, there are variances in some of the properties of gutta-percha cones (e.g., yield strength, resilience, tensile strength, elasticity, flexibility, elongation). The authors stated that no one brand of gutta-percha presently on the market possesses all the most desirable properties, such as ease of insertion into small canals and flow into canal crevices.

Importance of canal preparation. These potential weaknesses in the properties of gutta-percha as a canal filling material merely underscore the importance of canal preparation prior to the condensation procedure. When using gutta-percha, the dentist must enlarge the orifice of a small canal sufficiently to allow easy insertion of a relatively flexible small master cone. Proper flaring must be performed so the condensing instruments can reach to the deepest portions of the preparation in order to deform the gutta-percha and pack it against the apical dentin matrix to fill in the crevices and irregularities. The apical dentin matrix must be correctly prepared so it will retain the semisolid materials within the confines of the canal.

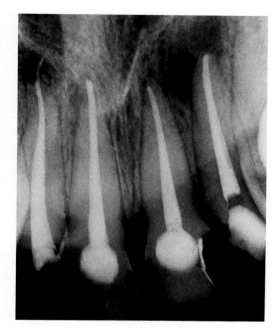

Fig. 9-8. Prior to standard use of apical dentin matrix, apical position of the canal filling was extremely variable. Here, on one radiograph in a single area of one patient's mouth, are four possibilities for apical extent of canal filling. *Left to right,* Lateral incisor, auxiliary cones past apex whereas master cone remains in tooth; central incisor, master and auxiliary cones past apex; central incisor, apical extent to approximately minor diameter, apical dentin matrix present; lateral incisor, canal filling at radiographic apex, site that was desirable when this case was filled.

Availability of cones. Gutta-percha is available in two styles. The easier to use for a master cone is the standardized style, available in sizes 25 through 140, conforming in apical width and taper to standardized instruments. The other style has an increased taper and is available by descriptive size, ranging from smallest to largest as extrafine, fine-fine, medium-fine, fine, medium, and coarse. These cones are used in canals of unusual shape and as auxiliaries in condensation techniques (Fig. 9-10).

Recently, color coding has entered into the area of gutta-percha cones. Several manufacturers have painted the wide end with colors (white, yellow, red, blue, green, or black) to indicate the appropriate size. The Spectrapoint* system was also introduced by Hygenic Corporation. As stated earlier, gutta-percha is white and may be colored to any

*Hygenic Corporation, Akron, OH 44310.

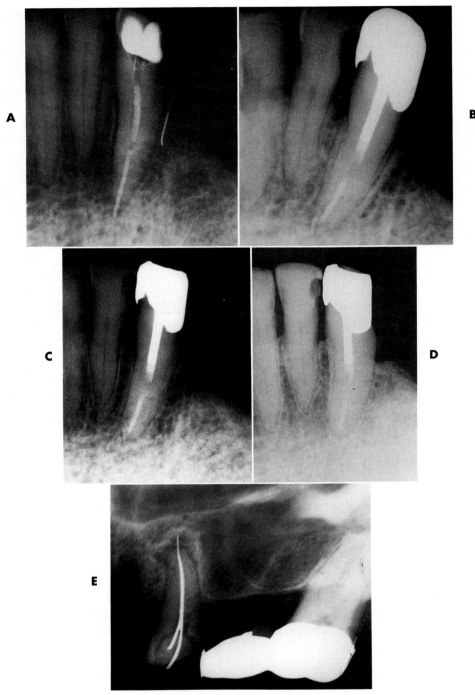

Fig. 9-9. Fate of excess gutta-percha when apex is sealed. **A,** Mandibular cuspid was filled with gutta-percha and Wach's paste. During lateral condensation, excess materials were pushed through apex. **B,** Two years postoperatively, excess filling materials appear to be amputated and healing is evident. No surgery was performed. **C,** Eight years after treatment, only a small shred of material remains just mesial to apex. **D,** Fourteen years after original treatment, no gutta-percha remains. (**A** to **D,** Restoration by Dr. Jacob Lippert, formerly of Chicago.) **E,** Endodontic treatment had been performed 2 years earlier, but apex was apparently not sealed by poorly fitting silver points.

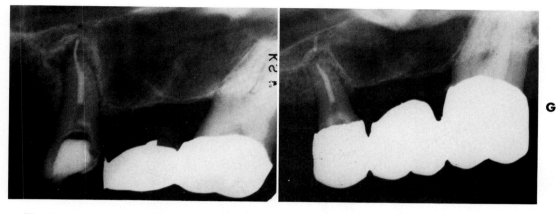

F   G

Fig. 9-9, cont'd.   F, Maxillary second bicuspid canal was filled with gutta-percha and Rickert's formula sealer. Again materials were pushed through into periapical tissues. No surgery was performed. **G,** Three years after treatment, no surgery performed, excess materials have been amputated and periapical radiolucency has healed. Although same degree of overextension occurred with both materials, case was successful after gutta-percha filling because the canal was apparently well sealed.

Table 9-1.   Constituents of commercial gutta-percha cones

Material	Percentage	Function
Gutta-percha	18 to 22	Matrix
Zinc oxide	59 to 76	Filler
Waxes/resins	1 to 4	Plasticizer
Metal sulfates	1 to 18	Radiopaquer

hue. Spectrapoints have the entire cone, not just the tip, in the above colors.

The advantage of colored cones (entire cone or tip) is that most clinicians store the various sizes until use in long boxes with separations to compartmentalize each size. But what happens if the box is shaken or falls, and some cones fall or slide into the incorrect compartment? Even worse, what if the box is upset during a filling with the top off and many cones of varying sizes become mixed up? It is a very difficult project to remeasure the cones and return them to the proper space. Color coding allows instant identification.

CANAL FILLING IN NONCOMPLICATED CASES

The filling of most anterior and bicuspid teeth with gutta-percha is usually relatively simple and noncomplicated. However, molars, displaying multiple canals that are generally small and often curved, necessitate a much more complex procedure requiring different handling and planning. This section will address the less complicated cases.

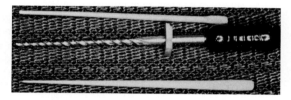

Fig. 9-10.   Standardized gutta-percha cones *(top)* have taper similar to that of enlarging instruments and are available by same numbering system. Old-style cones *(bottom)* have greater taper and may be used as auxiliaries with widely tapered spreaders or in unusually shaped canals.

Filling large, relatively straight canals

Obtaining master cone.   Once the canal is verified as ready for filling, a suitable master cone should be obtained. The rubber dam is placed, the contents of the canal removed, and the final master apical size is obtained by preparation. Even if the final size was achieved at the previous appointment some filing should still be performed at the time of filling. This will remove any debris that might have gathered between appointments and freshens the canal walls to better receive the sealer. The canal is irrigated with sodium hypochlorite (NaOCl), which will act as a lubricant for the trying-in of a master cone. A cone the size of the master apical file (MAF) is selected and placed to the predetermined length. It need not have a resistance to removal, referred to as

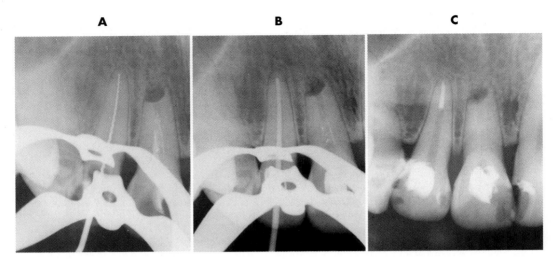

Fig. 9-11.   Filling large canal with customized gutta-percha master cone. **A,** Radiograph of maxillary lateral incisor with initial apical file, size 25 Hedstrom, in place at calculated working length of 22.5 mm. Canal was enlarged to size 40 and flared to size 55. (The adjacent central incisor had previous surgery with poor canal filling and will be re-treated with calcium hydroxide to gain apical closure.) **B,** After completion of preparation, a customized gutta-percha cone was fit, according to Fig. 9-15. **C,** Film taken after filling canal with customized cone, lateral condensation with Wach's paste, and post room prepared. Filling is at exactly the same position as was the file in **A,** with "Washington Monument" configuration at tip of filling. (Central incisor now filled with calcium hydroxide paste, lesion decreasing, see Chapter 16.)

"tug-back." Tugback is rarely obtainable in smaller canals properly flared because there is just a small area of close approximation between the cone and the canal walls. However, the cone should be the widest that will go the full working length. If the proper-size cone does not go the full working length, further apical preparation, and specifically flaring, will be required.

Once satisfactory apical positioning appears to be obtained, a radiograph is taken to verify cone positioning. If an accurate canal length determination and careful enlargement have been performed, the radiograph will show that the master cone reaches to the most apical position of the preparation or to a point slightly (less than 0.5 mm) short of it (Fig. 9-11). When the cone is slightly short, the added pressure of condensation plus the increased lubrication afforded by the sealer will be sufficient to produce complete seating.

If the master cone goes to the correct length but is ascertained to be too far short of the apex, according to the radiograph, the canal must be reprepared to an increased length by going back to files of the smallest size and continuing through to the desired degree of enlargement.

However, if a radiolucent line is noted between the master cone and the apical portion of the preparation, adjustment is likewise needed, since the master cone is evidently not reaching the greatest depth of the preparation (Fig. 9-12). The apical portion should be reinstrumented with the last two files used to allow for sufficient removal of dentin to grant complete seating of the cone.

Another possibility is that the cone passes through the apical foramen, usually as a result of improper canal length determination or incorrect apical preparation. If the amount of excess gutta-percha is determined and then clipped off the master cone, it is possible that a satisfactory filling will be obtained. However, the lubricating action of the sealer and the force of condensation will usually produce an overfill. What has happened in this case is that there is no apical dentin matrix to pack against. The proper procedure is to recalculate a corrected working length. The canal is reinstrumented several sizes to prepare an apical dentin matrix (Fig. 9-13). A new master cone should be obtained, preferably by the customized method, and radiographed to verify correctness.

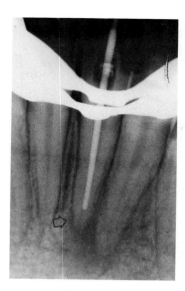

Fig. 9-12. Radiolucent line *(arrow)* apical to master cone reveals that the cone is not reaching far enough apically.

Customized master cone development. A cone developed by the preceding method, going to the correct length, will usually produce an excellent final result. However, in canals that are enlarged to sizes 50 and greater, eccentricities and irregularities of cross-sectional shape frequently occur. Since the object of filling is to seal the apical portion of the preparation, it is obvious that a preparation produced by a file that comes to a point at its tip, which may gouge the walls and produce an eccentric shape, will be difficult to seal with a round, smooth-surfaced, blunt-tipped master cone (Fig. 9-14, *A*). The ideal answer would be to gain an impression of the apical portion of the canal and from it to fabricate a master cone. From a practical standpoint this is impossible.

However, an imprint of the apical portion can be obtained by using a solvent, and a master cone can be developed as described.

The suggested solvent is chloroform, preferred because it is more volatile than xylol or oil of eucalyptol, and no solvent adhering to the cone is desired during condensation.

Cotton pliers with a lock or a hemostat (Fig. 9-14, *B*) are also mandatory in this technique, since the cone must be inserted into the canal several times in exactly the same spatial relationship. By holding the cone with a locking device and using some portion of the tooth—usually a cusp tip or

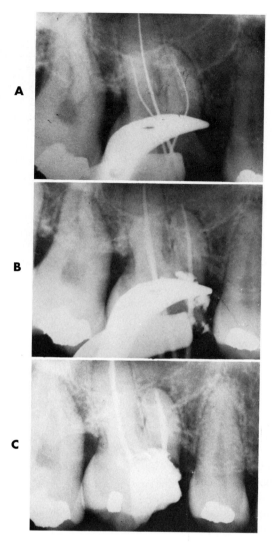

Fig. 9-13. **A,** Files in place to determine working length for maxillary first molar. Mesiobuccal canal was prepared 1 mm longer than distance of file in that canal. **B,** Master gutta-percha cones in place. Probably because of lost working length, apical portion was overprepared and gutta-percha cone is too long in the mesiobuccal canal. **C,** Mesiobuccal canal was prepared two sizes larger at 1.5 mm short length, and a new cone was fitted. Final radiograph shows a desirable result.

incisal edge—as a landmark, the dentist can reinsert the cone in the same path as frequently as necessary to obtain a satisfactory imprint.

A master cone that has correct length and width is seized with the pliers at the predetermined length and dipped into a dappen dish containing chloroform (Fig. 9-15, *A*). Only the apical 5 mm

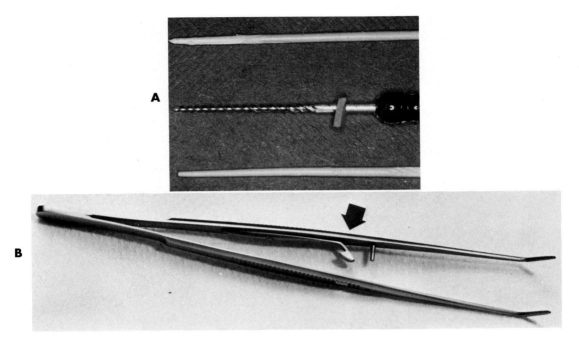

Fig. 9-14. **A,** Standardized cone *(bottom)* is round, has smooth surface and blunt tip, and cannot perfectly fill canal preparation made with sharp-tipped file *(middle)*. Customized master cone *(top)* can be developed to recapitulate the shape of the canal. **B,** Cotton pliers with locking device *(arrow)* permits reinsertion of a customized master cone in same spatial relationship as often as needed for gaining satisfactory imprint. A hemostat could be used as well.

of the cone is dipped, for 1 to 2 seconds. The softened cone is then placed into the prepared canal with slight apical pressure, held for a few seconds, and withdrawn (Fig. 9-15, *B*). This procedure should be repeated at least one more time or until a satisfactory imprint is obtained. If a correct preparation has been made, the cone will assume a pointed tip and striations will be noted along the lateral portion, recapitulating the canal interior (Fig. 9-15, *C*).

It is advisable to have the canal filled with irrigant while the imprint is taken. Either NaOCl or anesthetic solution is very good for this purpose. Otherwise, some of the softened gutta-percha might stick to the dried dentin walls and cause distortion of the cone.

When the cone has assumed what appears to be an accurate shape, a radiograph is taken to verify the correctness of the apical position (Figs. 9-11, *B* and 9-16, *A*). During the time that the radiograph is being developed, the cone should be removed from the canal and retained in the locking pliers so it may be correctly reinserted during filling. At this

time any residual solvent will volatilize and the cone will regain its original rigidity.

If the cone is found to be too long, the dentist usually can easily tell at which point it passes through the apical foramen. A constriction in the cone is seen, with the area past this constriction being irregular and frequently having residual blood (Fig. 9-15, *D*). As in Fig. 9-13, the error in working length is calculated and corrected to the site of the constriction. The apical portion of the canal is enlarged one or two more sizes and another customized cone obtained.

Once its correct length is verified, the cone is used in one of the acceptable cementing techniques (Fig. 9-11, *C,* and 9-16, *B*).

Lateral condensation in larger canals

Does lateral condensation really condense laterally? The technique for lateral condensation of gutta-percha has been used for many, many years, and surveys have indicated that it is the most popular method for canal filling among the Diplomates of the American Board of Endodontists.

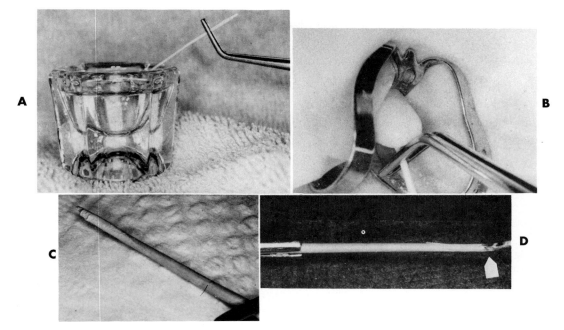

Fig. 9-15. Taking an imprint for a customized cone. **A,** Chloroform is poured into a dappen dish. A master cone with correct length and width is grasped with the locking cotton pliers (Fig. 9-14, *B*) at the working length and dipped into the chloroform for a few seconds. **B,** While being held with the cotton pliers, the cone (tip softened by the chloroform) is inserted into the canal with slight apical pressure. The canal has been irrigated with NaOCl for lubrication. **C,** The cone assumes the shape of the interior of the canal. Note the pointed tip and lateral striations. The customized master cone of Fig. 9-16 looked like this. **D,** If the cone passes through the apex into periapical tissue, residual blood is seen near the tip. The true apical foramen *(arrow)* is indicated by the constriction prior to the indication of bleeding. To correct this problem, measure the distance to the true apex, enlarge several sizes, and then take a new custom cone.

Most of the cases in this textbook were filled with this method, and many were followed for long periods of time to verify healing and the efficacy of the preparation and filling techniques.

Still, many other filling techniques are employed, and some of their advocates have denigrated the effectiveness of lateral condensation. Schilder, in particular, has been especially vociferous in his opposition to lateral condensation. In his chapter from Gerstein's book, Schilder stated and presented an illustration to demonstrate that lateral condensation did not really produce a dense mass of gutta-percha, but that the individual cones were merely suspended in a sea of cement. I tried several times to disprove this assertion and in previous editions of this textbook attempted to illustrate that lateral condensation was effective in sealing canals in three dimensions. He, and many of his former students, did not accept my proof.

A major problem in my attempts to indicate the quality of filling by lateral condensation with horizontal sections (Fig. 9-17, *A* and *B*) of extracted teeth was due to the gutta-percha cones all being pink, both master and auxiliary cones. There was no way to prove that the various cones were deformed and condensed to fill the prepared canal spaces in three dimensions.

However, several years ago, Sakkal et al. were able to demonstrate without equivocation that lateral condensation DID condense laterally and truly produce a three dimensional filling. They prepared plastic blocks with 30° curves to size 30, flared to size 55. Canals were filled using a size B finger plugger, pink master gutta-percha cones, and Wach's paste, as well as other sealers.

Hygenic Corporation accommodated the investigators by producing size 20 Spectrapoint auxiliary cones (normally colored yellow only) in all

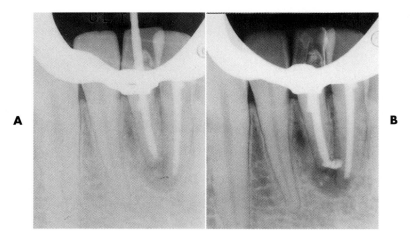

Fig. 9-16. Filling of a very large canal with a customized cone. **A,** Mandibular incisors had been treated surgically, with chronic draining sinus indicating failure of incisor to the left (rubber dam clamp is placed on it) with apical constriction totally destroyed. Tooth was treated with calcium hydroxide (see Chapter 16), with both sinus healing and radiolucency decreasing soon thereafter. Canal had been enlarged to size 100, but now a new constriction is obviously present, although probably not complete. (Note how the tip of the cone is tapered, similar to Fig. 9-15, *C*). **B,** Film taken after filling with customized cone, lateral condensation, and Wach's paste. Some sealer has been pushed through due to incomplete apical closure, but it is only a minimal amount.

Fig. 9-17. Illustrations of canal filling with lateral condensation that refutes statements that cones are suspended in a sea of cement. **A,** Sections 1.5 mm and **B,** 2.0 mm from tip of preparation in the distal root of an extracted mandibular molar enlarged apically to size 70 without flaring and filled with laterally condensed gutta-percha and Wach's paste. These sections indicate that the canal is oval, not round, even this close to the tip, but that the canal appeared to be well filled. Because the master cone and the auxiliary cones are all pink, it is difficult to tell what portion of the canal is filled with what type of cone. To clarify this further, canals in plastic blocks with curvatures of 30° were enlarged to size 30, flared to size 55, and filled with laterally condensed gutta-percha and Wach's paste, using a size B finger plugger. Horizontal sections were made starting at 0.5 mm from the tip of the filling at 1.0 mm intervals. The master cone used was pink, the first auxiliary cone was white, the second was yellow, the third was red, the fourth was blue, the fifth was green, and the sixth was black. **C,** At the 1.5 mm level, the master cone has been deformed by the first auxiliary cone which is seen at the 12 o'clock position. No sealer is seen and the canal appears to be well filled. **D,** At the 2.5 mm level, the master cone *(arrow)* is being squeezed out by the first three auxiliary cones, no sealer is seen, and the canal is well condensed. **E,** At the 3.4 mm level, the master cone has been completely squeezed out by the condensation of the first four auxiliary cones. Some sealer is seen at both the 2 and 10 o'clock positions. **F,** At the 4.5 mm level, five auxiliary cones are seen, all deformed, still no master cone, and sealer is seen at the 1 and 10 o'clock positions. **G,** At the 5.5 mm level, the master cone has returned *(arrow)*, surrounded by six auxiliary cones, starting at 5 to 7 o'clock positions by the red cone, 7 to 8 o'clock positions by the blue, and 9 o'clock position by the yellow. The white cone goes laterally from the 10 to 2 o'clock positions, enveloping the green and black cones at the top, no sealer present. **H,** At the 6.5 mm level, the master cone *(arrow)* and all the auxiliary cones are deformed, they completely fill the preparation, and no sealer—let alone a sea of sealer—is seen. (*C* to *H* are at 40×; *C* to *G* reprinted with permission from Sakkal S, Weine FS, Lemian L: *Compend Contin Educ Dent* 12:796, 1991.)

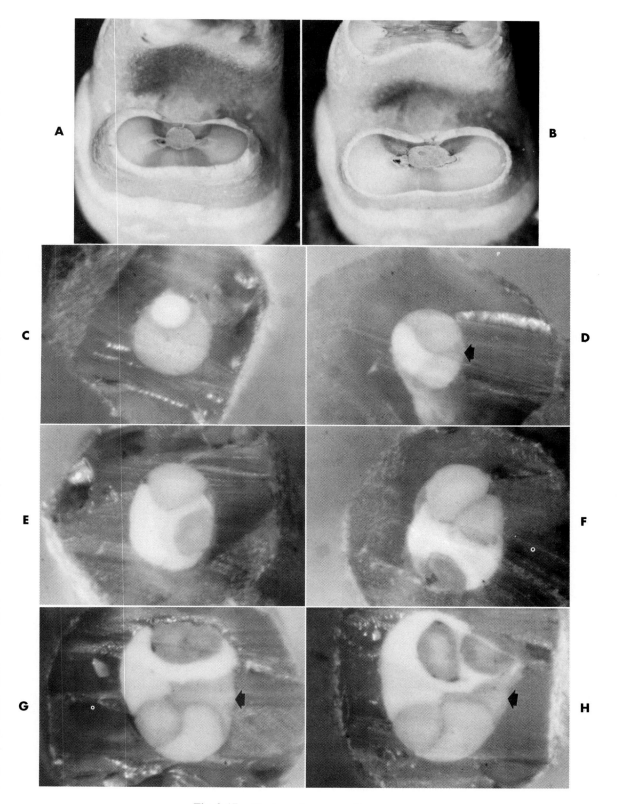

Fig. 9-17. For legend see opposite page.

six standard colors. The auxiliary cones were used in their normal standardized order, that is, the first auxiliary cone used was white, the second was yellow, the third was red, and so on. Horizontal sections were made at 1.0 mm intervals without heat using a scalpel blade starting at 0.5 mm from the tip of the filling. Because of the difference in color, it was obvious which cones were seen in each section (Fig. 9-17, *D* through *H*).

Photos were made of approximately 360 sections with a stereomicroscope at 40X enlargement. When viewed, they demonstrated well-filled canals, with excellent condensation and deformation of both the master and auxiliary cones. Very minimal amounts of sealer were seen (Fig. 9-17, *F* and *G*), but nowhere near what Schilder had described or drawn.

Yes, friends, lateral condensation condenses laterally! And quite well, at that.

Armamentarium. The tray setup for use with the lateral condensation method is illustrated in Fig. 9-18, and a brief discussion of the pertinent instruments follows:

Hand spreader—long tapered instrument, used to compress the gutta-percha toward the periphery of the prepared canal and into the irregularities of the canal walls, leaving a void for the insertion of an auxiliary cone; because of its relatively wide diameter, generally used in canals that have been enlarged to size 60 or larger.

Finger spreaders*—same shape and function as the hand spreader, only available for smaller canals or for placing the initial auxiliary cones in larger canals (Fig. 9-19); because of smaller length as well as

*L.D. Caulk Co., Division of Caulk/Dentsply, Milford, DE 19963.

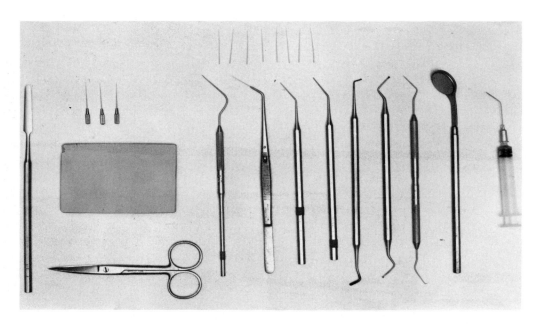

Fig. 9-18. Tray setup for canal filling with gutta-percha using the lateral condensation method. *(from left)* Cement spatula, glass slab, Kerr no. 3 spreader, locking cotton pliers with master cone in position, Luks pluggers nos. 2 and 3, plastic instrument, excavator, endodontic explorer, front surface mirror, irrigating syringe. Finger spreaders are above the mixing slab, prepared auxiliary points above pluggers, and scissors under slab.

Fig. 9-19. **A,** As suggested by Luks, finger spreaders are available in four sizes, three pictured here to show relationship to endodontic file *(top)*. **B,** Proximal view of prepared extracted mandibular bicuspid. Kerr no. 3 spreader reaches only to middle third of root. **C,** No further preparation was performed, but size B finger spreader reaches to apical few millimeters. **D,** Maxillary central incisor during canal filling. Kerr no. 3 spreader was used and four auxiliary cones were placed, but apical portion of canal is poorly condensed. **E,** Gutta-percha was removed and canal refilled using finger spreaders. Now apical portion of canal is well condensed because deeper penetration was gained with finger spreaders.

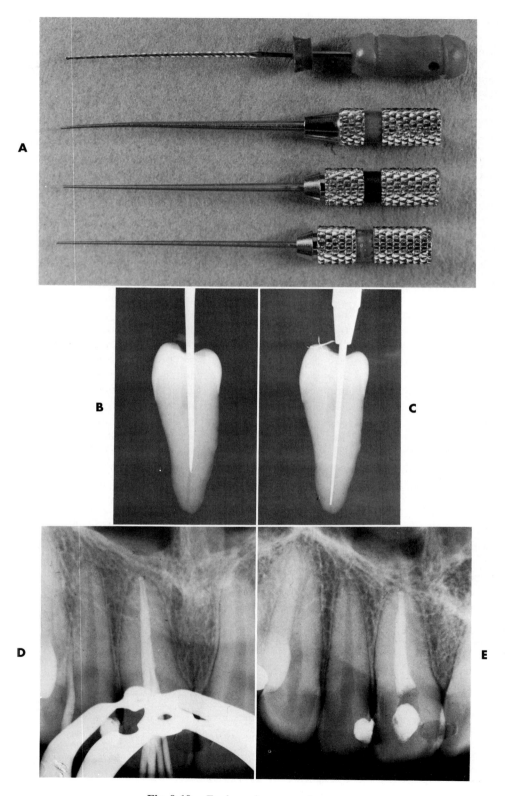

Fig. 9-19.   For legend see opposite page.

diameter, finger spreaders are much easier to use in posterior teeth; because of shape, similar to that of a file, the finger spreader's angle of insertion for condensation is same as angle of insertion for the enlarging instruments

A finger spreader (yellow stripe)

B finger spreader (red stripe)

C finger spreader (blue stripe)

D finger spreader (green stripe)—optional

Auxiliary cones—available in sizes conforming to the spreaders as listed in Table 9-2.

Because the gutta-percha cones have wide blunt ends that may interfere with seeing their site of insertion, it is advisable to clip the coronal 4 mm (Fig. 9-20).

Mixing slab—presterilized by any of the accepted methods and available for the mixing of the sealer

Pluggers—for vertical condensation techniques and for preparing dowel room

Plastic instrument—for removing excess gutta-percha and for placing of the temporary filling.

In addition to the instruments shown and discussed, a suitable heat source, such as a Bunsen burner or alcohol lamp, is necessary to remove the excess cones and/or for use in warm techniques.

Technique.   The canal is dried of any residual irrigant, washed with 95% alcohol solution, and dried with absorbent paper points. This final irrigant acts as a desiccating agent to remove residual materials and moisture from the canal walls and gain better adhesion for the cones. A suitable sealer is spatulated to the desired consistency. A reamer one size smaller than the MAF is selected, the correct length marked, and a small amount of sealer picked up with the tip. The reamer is placed to its correct length in the canal and turned counterclockwise, spinning the sealer into the canal. For large irregular canals at least two coatings should be applied. The tip of the master cone is dipped into the sealer and placed into its correct position within the canal. Even when a customized cone is not used, it is wise to hold the master cone with locking cotton pliers at a point even with the

incisal edge or cusp height so it will be easy to tell when the cone has reached the correct depth at the apical portion of the canal preparation.

Once the correct depth is reached, a spreader is placed alongside the master cone and, with both apical and lateral pressure applied, forced toward the apex. If a noncustomized cone is used, the first spreader should reach to within the apical 1 to 2 mm of the canal, since it is the apical area that requires considerable density to seal. When a customized cone is used, this depth of penetration is rarely possible to reach. Once the correct depth is reached, the spreader is rotated counterclockwise out of the canal, leaving a void into which an auxiliary cone is placed. To give the auxiliary cones sufficient lubrication to reach the space prepared for them, the cones are dipped into the sealer, which has been made slightly thinner than the original mass by addition of liquid. The action of the spreader not only creates a space into which new cones are introduced, but also laterally pushes the previously placed cones into the recesses and irregularities of the canal (Fig. 9-21).

The number of auxiliary cones needed varies with each case; but as more and more cones are placed, the spreader has shallower penetration. When it is determined that no cones are reaching past the cervical third of the canal, condensation is terminated.

If there is any question as to the continued fit of the apical portion of the master cone, an intrafilling radiograph should be taken after the placement of the first auxiliary cone. At this time, if improper apical preparation has failed to give adequate resistance to the condensation, the radiograph will reveal that gutta-percha has emerged into the periapical tissue (Fig. 9-22). Since the sealer still has considerably plasticity, the cones usually are easy to remove; then further apical preparation may be performed or a new and more tightly fitting master cone selected. If this checking radiograph is taken after the condensation is completed, the dense

Table 9-2.   Correspondence of finger spreaders to apical canal width and auxiliary cones

MAF size	Finger spreader	Auxiliary cone*
25	A	No. 20
30 to 35	B	Clip 2 mm from tip of no. 20
40 to 50	C	No. 25, perhaps larger
Larger than 50	D or hand spreader	Varies

*To be used as a guide only. Sizes change from time to time and are not truly standardized from manufacturer to manufacturer.

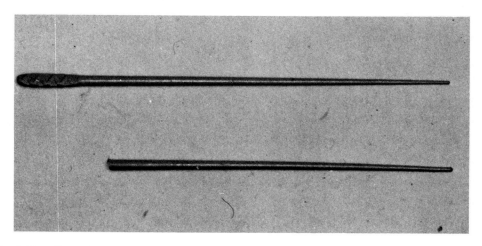

Fig. 9-20. Coronal portion of auxiliary cone is clipped *(bottom)* so ends will not protrude too far through access and make visualization difficult. An unclipped auxiliary cone is at top.

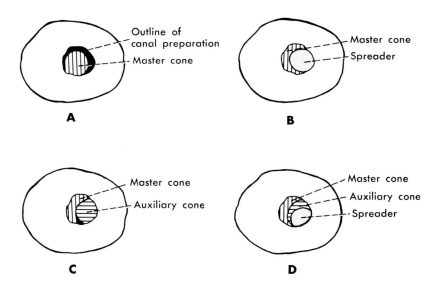

Fig. 9-21. Diagrammatic representation of lateral condensation—cross sections of a prepared canal approximately 3 mm from apical foramen. **A,** Master cone has been placed in preparation, but because of irregular oval outline of canal, the cone does not completely fill the void. **B,** Spreader is introduced, forcing master cone into a U shape against canal walls and leaving room for placement of an auxiliary cone. **C,** Auxiliary cone has been placed, but some void still exists. **D,** Spreader is reintroduced, forcing both master cone and auxiliary cone against walls, leaving room for additional auxiliary cones. This process is repeated until prepared canal is obliterated by filling material (Fig. 9-17, *G* and *H*).

mass plus the initial set of the sealer makes it difficult to withdraw the cones in the event of an overfill. Rarely does an overfill result subsequent to the placement of the first or second auxiliary cone. The time of this placement is therefore the ideal time for making the intrafilling radiograph.

If this radiograph shows that the cones have failed to reach the desired penetration, the cones and sealer should be removed and a new master cone fabricated and verified. This occurs on occasion when the cone tip catches at the orifice or in the canal during insertion and bends over.

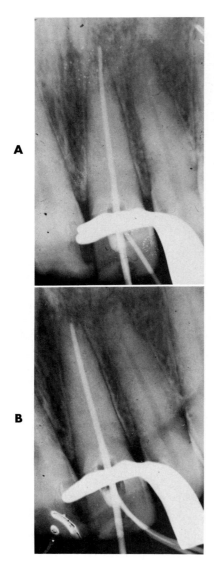

Fig. 9-22. **A,** Intrafilling radiograph reveals that cones have passed into periapical tissue. **B,** By adjustment, a satisfactory filling is obtained.

CANAL FILLING IN COMPLICATED CASES
Filling smaller curved canals

The armamentarium for filling teeth with smaller curved canals is the same as for those that are less complex, but the key instruments become the finger spreaders. Because of their narrower diameter as opposed to the hand spreader, these instruments will gain deeper penetration in the curved canals, where preparation must be kept to minimal sizes in order to preserve original canal

shape. (See Chapter 7.) In addition, the smaller length of the finger spreaders allows easier insertion into the molars, particularly into the mesial canals of these teeth.

Fitting the finger spreader. Contrary to the technique used in larger canals, the fit of the finger spreader is verified *prior* to that of the master gutta-percha cone. The reason for this is to ensure that the spreader will reach the apical few millimeters of the prepared canal in order to deform the gutta-percha and condense it against the walls and into the seat of the apical dentin matrix. In the larger straighter canals this condensation is much simpler to accomplish. The matching of finger spreader to canal size and auxiliary cone is listed in Table 9-2.

Once the canal is deemed ready for filling, the appropriate finger spreader is selected according to the information given in Table 9-2. A rubber stop is placed to indicate working length, and the spreader is tried in the canal (Fig. 9-23, *B*). It should fit to within 1 mm of the working length; if it does, it need not be verified by radiograph. If it seems quite loose, the next-larger size may be tried but only substituted if the fit to the apical millimeter is obtained.

If the seemingly appropriate finger spreader is selected but stops several millimeters short of the desired penetration, this is a sign that insufficient flaring of the canal is present. The spreader is hanging up at the elbow (Chapter 7), and the canal filling should not be performed yet. Further flaring of the canal must be instituted, always being certain to go back the full working length with the MAF. At this point, if sufficient flaring has been accomplished, the spreader should go to place correctly.

Obtaining the master cone. After the fit of the finger spreader is verified, a gutta-percha cone is selected the same size as the MAF. The canal is irrigated to give additional lubrication, since dry canal walls tend to cause too much friction with the dry cone. Tugback is not significant in flared canals and often does not occur. However, the cone must be the widest that goes to within 1 mm of the working length (Fig. 9-23, *C*) and must not pigtail (Fig. 9-24). A radiograph is taken to verify cone positioning (Fig. 9-23, *D*). Problems with cones too long or too short are handled as described earlier in this chapter.

Customized master cones are not used in these cases because insufficient width is available in the smaller preparations. The solvents necessary for customizing make the cones too plastic to be placed firmly into the canal.

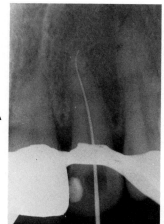

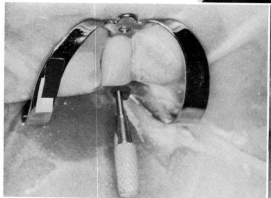

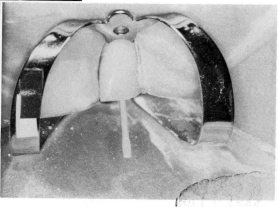

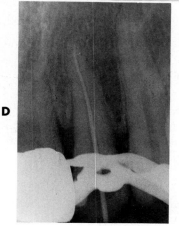

Fig. 9-23. **A,** Radiograph of file in place in a maxillary lateral incisor to indicate verified working length and initial canal shape. The canal was enlarged apically to size 30 and flared to size 45. **B,** When canal preparation is completed, finger spreader is fit first, prior to fitting of the master gutta-percha cone. Spreader must fit to within 1 mm of working length. Then rubber stop is moved to coincide with incisal edge. **C,** After finger spreader is fit, master gutta-percha cone is tried into an irrigated canal. **D,** This position is verified by radiograph. Cone must fit to within 1 mm of working length.

Continued

Lateral condensation. The canal is irrigated with 95% alcohol and then dried with absorbent paper points. The sealer is mixed to the proper consistency (Fig. 9-23, *E*) and placed in the prepared canal by means of a reamer one size smaller than the MAF utilizing counterclockwise motion (Fig. 9-23, *F*). The tip of the master cone is dipped into the sealer (Fig. 9-23, *G*) and placed in its cor-

rect position within the canal; locking cotton pliers are used if necessary.

A thinner mix of sealer may be used with the auxiliary cones. The previously fit finger spreader is placed in the canal alongside the master cone and should go to within 1 mm of the rubber stop (Fig. 9-23, *H*). *There should be no rush to remove the spreader because it must deform*

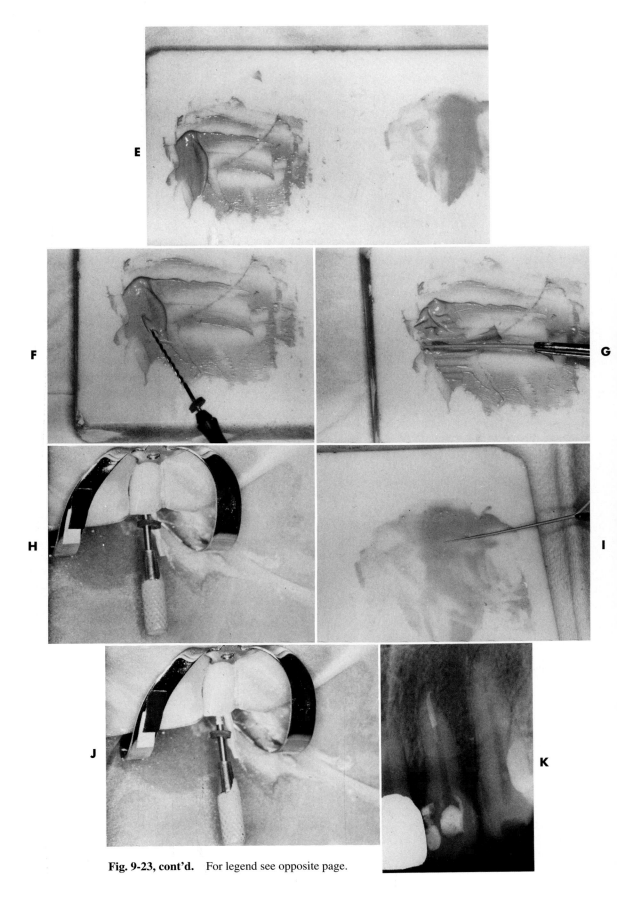

Fig. 9-23, cont'd. For legend see opposite page.

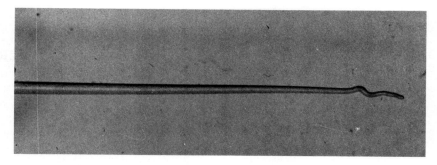

Fig. 9-24.   Pigtail appearance of an ill-fitting master cone. This cone is too narrow for preparation and buckled when placed against apical dentin matrix.

the gutta-percha. Due to the resilience of gutta-percha, some spring-back of the material will occur when the spreader is removed. If the spreader is placed for too brief a duration, maximum deformity of the gutta-percha will not be obtained. The appropriate auxiliary cone is selected (using Table 9-2), the spreader is removed, and the cone is inserted into the void thus created after being dipped into the thin mix of sealer (Fig. 9-23, *I*). The depth of penetration of the spreader should be measured, and the auxiliary cone should go to that depth.

This is continued until the canal is filled into the coronal third. In these smaller canals, generally from four to eight auxiliary cones are sufficient to gain the desired filling. In the middle and coronal third of the canal, the next larger finger spreader and the appropriate auxiliary cone may be used because of the greater width available in this portion of the canal. Post room may be prepared at this point and a final radiograph is taken (Fig. 9-23, *K*).

Filling molar teeth

Molar teeth require all the techniques used in filling small curved canals, as previously described, but are yet more complicated and demanding since there are three or more canals to be filled at the same time.

Fitting the finger spreader. Once the canals are deemed ready for filling, the finger spreader is fit as described in the previous section, using Table 9-2 as a guide. A separate spreader should be fit for each canal. If two canals require the same-sized spreader, some indicator must be used to identify the specific canal (e.g., putting two stops on the spreader for the mesiobuccal canal).

Again, great care must be taken to verify that the spreaders reach to within 1 mm of the working length; and increased flaring must be performed if this is not the case.

Obtaining the master cone. As previously described, the master cones are selected and placed in the canal; intracanal irrigant can be used for additional lubrication (Fig. 9-25, *A*). The position is verified by radiograph (Fig. 9-25, *B*). In mandibular molars several radiographs (straight and angled) may be necessary (Fig. 9-25, *C*). In some molars the largest canal—single distal of the mandibular or palatal of the maxiliary—may require the use of a customized cone, whereas the cones in the small curved canals are fit as

Fig. 9-23, cont'd.   **E,** Two thicknesses of sealer are mixed, a thick mix *(left)* and a thinner mix *(right),* for auxiliary cones. **F,** Some of thick sealer is picked up on tip of a reamer one size smaller than MAF. This is placed into canal with a counterclockwise motion. **G,** Master cone, gripped in locking cotton pliers, is dipped into thick mix and then placed in canal. **H,** Previously fit finger spreader is placed alongside master cone and inserted. It should go to within 1 mm of rubber stop. **I,** Suitable auxiliary cone is dipped into thinner mix of sealer and placed into the void created by removal of the spreader. **J,** Spreader is reinserted and now will be still shorter than last penetration. **K,** Radiograph following canal filling and post room preparation. Canal shape has been well maintained, and an excellent result is anticipated.

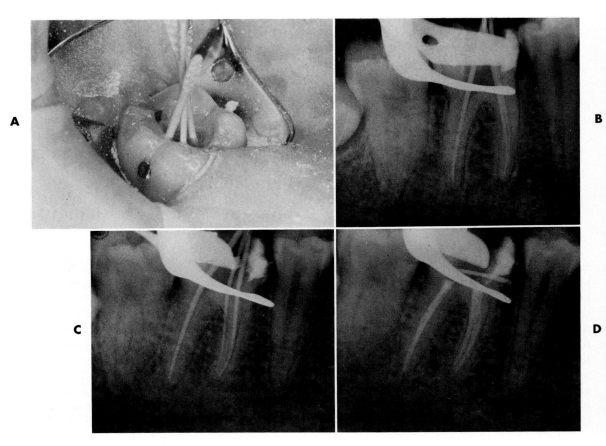

Fig. 9-25.   Fitting master cones for a mandibular molar is performed after fit of the finger spreaders is verified. **A,** Master gutta-percha cones in place. Note intracanal irrigant for added lubrication. **B,** Straight view. **C,** Angled view. **D,** At conclusion of condensation.

indicated in this section. If a custom cone is used in these molars be certain to remove it from the tooth while waiting for the development of the radiograph.

Lateral condensation.   In mandibular molars I prefer to fill completely the distal canal or canals first (Fig. 9-26) and then condense the mesials. Similarly, in three-canaled maxillary molars I first completely fill the palatal canal and then the buccals. When four canals are present, generally I will first fill the palatal and the distobuccal, then the two mesiobuccals. Two canals in one root should always be filled together, even if the operator is very certain that the canals do not join at the apex. Some of the faster-setting sealers will not be usable for the entire condensation, and two batches will be necessary.

Once the master cones are verified by radiograph (Fig. 9-27, *C*), they are removed from the

canals and set on the pack in a definite order so the operator knows which cone goes into which canal. Multiple locking cotton pliers are useful to hold these at their working lengths. The canals are irrigated with 95% alcohol and dried with absorbent paper points (Fig. 9-27, *D*). The sealer is placed in the largest canal by a reamer one size smaller than the MAF with counterclockwise motion. The master cone is dipped into the sealer and placed in its correct position (Fig. 9-27, *E*). The spreader is placed alongside the master cone (Fig. 9-27, *F*) and should go to within 1 mm of the previously determined length. An auxiliary cone is measured at slightly less than the working length, dipped into the thinner mix of sealer, and placed in the void created when the spreader is removed (Fig. 9-27, *G*). Again, there should be no great haste to remove the spreader because the maximum deformity is needed. The spreader is cleaned

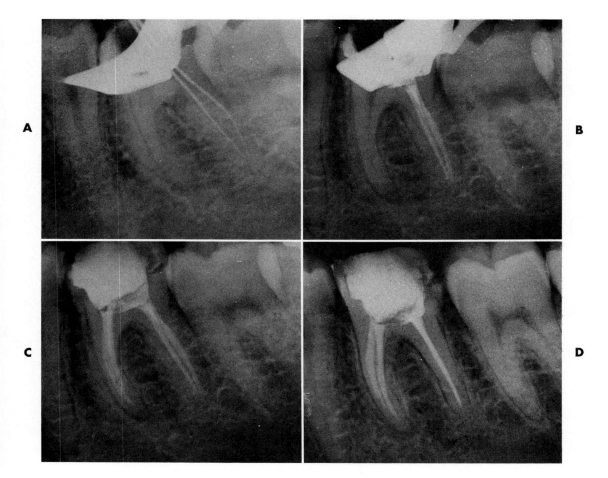

Fig. 9-26. Filling four-canaled mandibular molars. **A,** Angled view demonstrating two distal canals. **B,** After canal preparation completion the patient is reappointed for canal filling procedure. At that sitting, distal canals are filled first. **C,** With those canals completely condensed, mesial canals are filled; straight view. **D,** Final film, angled view.

of residual sealer and replaced into the canal. It will not go quite as far this time as it did during the initial insertion (Fig. 9-27, *H*). The depth of the spreader is estimated, and an auxiliary cone is selected and grasped at approximately that length. It is dipped into the thinner mix of sealer and placed in the void left when the spreader is removed. When several auxiliary cones protrude from the canal, they and the excess master cone should be removed with a heated instrument to allow for better visualization of the area (Fig. 9-27, *I*). This process of inserting auxiliary cones after spreader placement is repeated until the canal is filled into the coronal third. The floor of the chamber is cleansed to verify that the orifices of the smaller canals are patent.

The sealer is placed in the smaller canals with a reamer one size smaller than the MAF, and the previously measured master cones are inserted to their correct lengths (Fig. 9-27, *J*). One of the previously fitted finger spreaders is placed in its canal and should go to within 1 mm of the previously determined depth (Fig. 9-27, *K*). A suitable auxiliary cone is selected at approximately that length, dipped into the thinner mix of sealer, and placed in the void created when the spreader is removed (Fig. 9-27, *L*). This is continued until these canals, too, are filled (Figs. 9-27, *M* to *O*). Post room may be prepared at this point (Fig. 9-27, *P* and *Q*), and final radiographs are taken (Fig. 9-27, *R*).

Arrangement for restoration.   When the same dentist who has performed the endodontic therapy

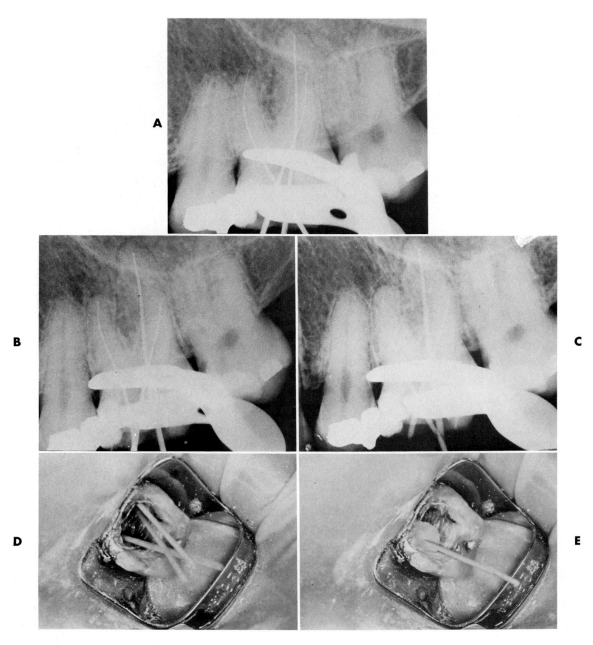

Fig. 9-27.   Canal filling for a maxillary molar. **A,** Initial files in place, mesiobuccal too long. **B,** Corrected files in place. Canal preparation was completed, and the patient reappointed for canal filling. **C,** After fitting of finger spreaders, fitting of master gutta-percha cones is verified by radiograph. **D,** Canals are dried with absorbent paper points. **E,** Sealer is placed into palatal canal, and a master cone previously dipped into the sealer is inserted to place.

is to restore the tooth, suitable appointments for the restoration should be arranged at the time of filling. Although it is usually best to wait a brief period after canal filling to start on the restoration, an observation period to determine success may cause further damage should the tooth fracture during that period. A reasonable waiting period before the restoration is commenced would be 1 to 3 weeks. If the endodontic situation is highly questionable, a properly contoured temporary

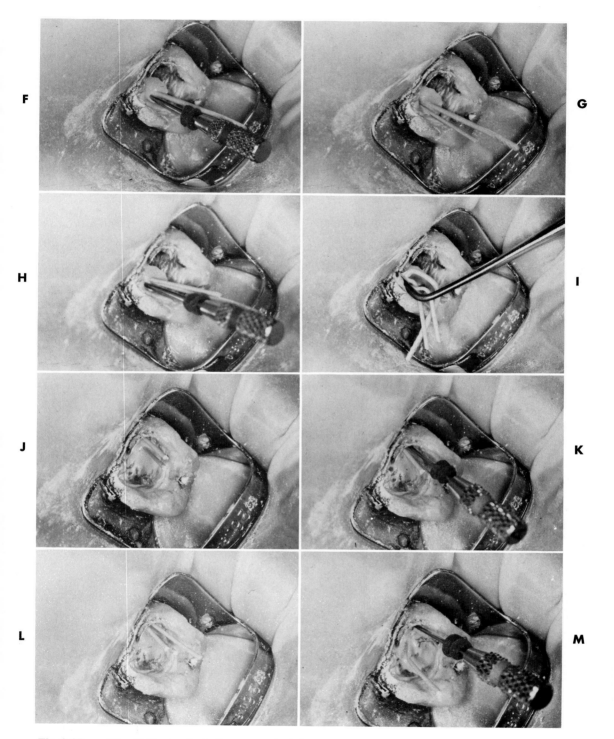

Fig. 9-27, cont'd. **F,** Previously fit finger spreader is inserted to place and should go to within 1 mm of its previously determined length. **G,** Auxiliary cone is placed into void created by removal of the spreader. **H,** Spreader is placed again, and this time it does not go as deeply as it did in **F. I,** Excess master and auxiliary cones are removed with a heated plastic instrument to give better visualization of the area. **J,** After palatal canal has been completely condensed, sealer is placed into buccal canals, followed by the previously fit master cones. **K,** Finger spreader is placed into mesiobuccal canal, going to within 1 mm of its previously fit length. **L,** Auxiliary cone is placed into void created by removal of spreader. **M,** This is repeated several more times.

Continued

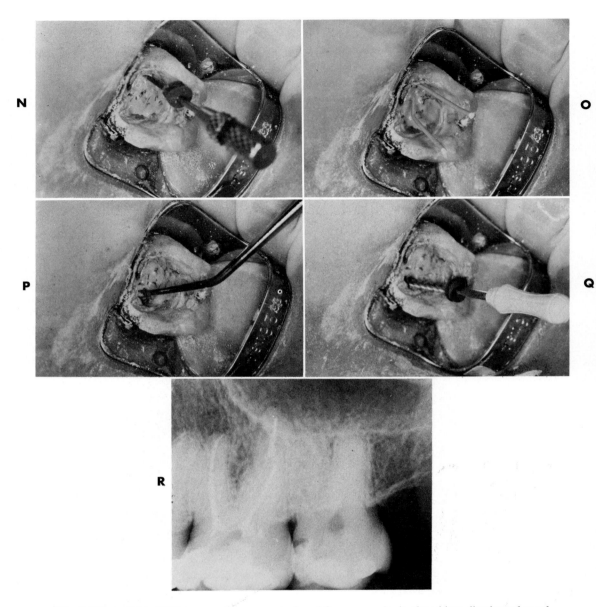

Fig. 9-27, cont'd. **N,** Excess cones are removed, and finger spreader is placed into distobuccal canal. **O,** Several auxiliary cones in distobuccal canal. **P,** Heated Luks hand plugger is placed into palatal canal. This is done several times to gain proper depth for post preparation. **Q,** Once that depth is established, hand instruments are used to widen the canal. In this case a size 90 is being used. **R,** Final radiograph indicating well-filled canals with original canal shape maintained (compare to **B**) and post room in the palatal canal.

crown capable of retaining adjacent and occluding teeth in correct position should be constructed. This may be accomplished by using quick-curing acrylic, celluloid crown forms, or, in the posterior teeth, stainless steel crowns.

Whenever endodontic therapy has been performed on a referral basis, the endodontist must make it very clear to the patient that treatment in this case must be completed with a proper restoration by the referring dentist. The patient should be told to contact and advise the referring dentist of the completion of the endodontic therapy and to arrange appointments for construction of the restoration. The endodontist should send pretreatment and posttreatment radiographs to the referring dentist, with a note describing the canal contents, temporary filling material, post room preparation dimensions if made, and any other pertinent information.

Care of finger spreaders

Finger spreaders are excellent aids to better endodontic treatment, particularly when smaller canals are being filled. They compact and deform gutta-percha very well and are much easier to insert in molar teeth than the bulkier hand spreaders. However, some practitioners have problems with the previously placed cones being pulled out of the canal when the finger spreader is removed. This has happened to me only rarely and always when one of two things has happened:

1. The spreader has not been cleaned prior to insertion. Caked sealer from a previous case or excess sealer may form on the spreader during condensation. This roughness is sufficient to cause the smaller cones to cling to the spreader and be pulled out of the canal. Be certain that all spreaders are carefully cleaned with a suitable sealer solvent, such as chloroform, prior to use. Also, during condensation, be certain that the spreader is carefully wiped clean prior to each reinsertion into the canal.
2. The spreader has become bent or corkscrewed. The finger spreader may be given a gentle curve prior to use so it will traverse a curved canal. However, sometimes the apical portion becomes bent or assumes the shape of a corkscrew. When such a spreader is removed from a canal, it may impale the previously placed cones and eject them from the canal.

The small size A finger spreaders are quite thin and cannot be used and reused as can the other sizes. In most molars I have six size A spreaders ready for use and generally use them all during the course of the canal filling. Any twisted, bent, or corkscrewed spreaders should be thrown away immediately and never reused.

In some cases the tip of the finger spreader may separate during the condensation procedure. This causes great consternation to the operator. However, the spreaders are sterilized in the salt sterilizer prior to use and thus are not harboring any bacteria. When they separate, they merely become a portion of the filled canal, recognizable by being an area of greater radiopacity on the film.

The only potentially serious drawback for the separated spreader is if it protrudes into the periapical tissues and causes a physical irritation as well as contributes to a corrosive process. This should not occur because the spreader has been prefit prior to the canal filling and has already been tested to ensure that it will not go past the apical portion of the preparation.

ALTERNATIVE CANAL FILLING METHODS
Warm gutta-percha

Rationale. Sectional filling or vertical condensation of the root canal has been used only sparingly, as a result of the considerable time required for the technique. Schilder has popularized this method by way of lectures and publications, referring to it as "warm gutta-percha, or filling canals in three dimensions." He believes that vertical condensation yields superior apical density when compared with lateral condensation. As proof of the increased density of this method, Schilder has produced radiographs displaying multiple filled lateral canals and apical foramina.

Technique. The technique requires that a master cone wider than the apical diameter of the prepared canal be selected, verified by radiograph, and placed in the canal after minimal sealer application. Since this cone is wider than the canal, it will bind a few millimeters short of the apical portion of the preparation. The coronal portion of the master cone is seared off, and a spreader is heated and applied apically to soften the cone. A cold plugger (condenser) then forces the softened mass toward the apex. Continued heatings and condensations eventually force the gutta-percha into the varying irregularities, lateral canals, and foramina that it could not fill in its original state. After the apical portion is filled, sections of gutta-percha are introduced and, with continued heating and condensing, the remainder of the canal is filled.

Comparison with other methods. Whereas the warm gutta-percha method obviously gives a more dense filling than any single-cone technique, the lateral condensation method using a customized master cone, as previously illustrated, successfully fills the canal irregularities and peculiarities, at

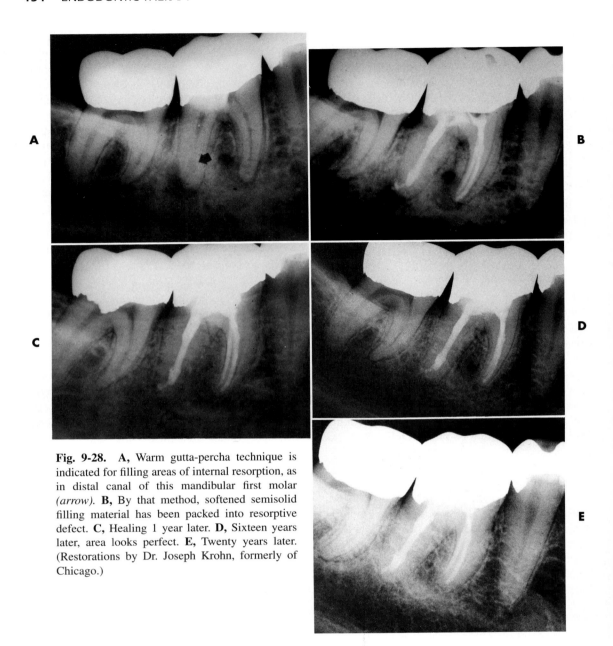

Fig. 9-28. **A,** Warm gutta-percha technique is indicated for filling areas of internal resorption, as in distal canal of this mandibular first molar *(arrow)*. **B,** By that method, softened semisolid filling material has been packed into resorptive defect. **C,** Healing 1 year later. **D,** Sixteen years later, area looks perfect. **E,** Twenty years later. (Restorations by Dr. Joseph Krohn, formerly of Chicago.)

least on a macroscopic basis. Lateral canals and multiple apical foramina are filled by many methods, even those employing single cones.

Tremendous emphasis on any filling technique fails to recognize that the most important phase of endodontic therapy is the preparatoryø phase, which rids the canal of irritants, substrates, gross irregularities, pupal debris, etc. When great care is used in preparation, any of the popularly used filling methods will yield successful results in an extremely high percentage of cases.

Indications. The warm gutta-percha method and the other vertical condensation method that will be described shortly, utilizing chloropercha, have excellent indications in certain specific instances. They are best used when the fitting of a conventional master cone to the apical portion of a canal is impossible, as when there is ledge formation, perforation, or unusual canal curvature. These vertical condensation methods then afford the operator a chance to gain success in a case that might fail if any other kind of treatment were used.

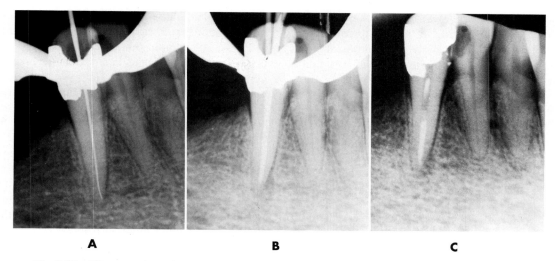

Fig. 9-29. Warm condensation after lateral condensation. **A,** Radiograph of mandibular cuspid showing canal exiting to mesial side of the root. **B,** Laterally condensed gutta-percha has been packed straight down into canal, but has not been moved toward the site of exiting. **C,** Heated pluggers were used to remove gutta-percha down to apical few millimeters and to repack canal with warmed segments. Warmed filling material now points toward area of exiting, and room for a post is available.

The warm gutta-percha method is specifically indicated when maximum condensation is desired, the most frequent uses being to fill a tooth with internal resorption or with a large lateral canal (Fig. 9-28).

Warm condensation may be used after routine lateral condensation if the postfilling radiograph indicates that the entire prepared canal has not been filled (Fig. 9-29, *A* and *B*). Using heated pluggers, the canal filling is removed down to the apical few millimeters and recondensed; then warmed gutta-percha segments are repacked down into the prepared canal to gain a more desirable result (Fig. 9-29, *C*).

THERMOPLASTIC GUTTA-PERCHA DELIVERY SYSTEMS

Taking advantage of the phase changes of gutta-percha and the resultant differences in physical properties, recent developments in gutta-percha delivery systems have dealt with heating or thermoplasticizing the material to temperatures of 42°C and higher. At these temperatures, gutta-percha changes from solid to being runny and tacky, will stick to the canal walls even without sealer, and will be in the *alpha* or *gamma* phase. It is important to remember that at body temperature, the gutta-percha returns to the *beta* phase, will no longer stick to the call walls, and suffers some shrinkage.

The delivery systems employed for thermoplastics take cold gutta-percha, heat it by electricity or a rotating instrument, and then distribute the softened material into the canal, often with an injection tip. Depending upon the technique being used, the gutta-percha may be packed into position with pluggers. In the *alpha* or *gamma* phase, condensation accomplishes little. However, as the gutta-percha cools into the *beta* phase, condensation is effective.

Heating the gutta-percha seems to increase the fusion of the material into a single mass, developing homogeneity, and, hopefully, decreasing voids. A large number of papers have been written during the past 10 years testing various aspects of filling with the thermoplastics, usually against each other or against lateral condensation. No unbiased, well controlled study has ever shown any of these newer techniques to be superior to lateral condensation, although some claims have been made that a particular system approaches or is equal to it.

Before switching from a standard canal filling technique to a thermoplastic system, the clinician should practice on a number of canals prior to using it on a patient. Extracted teeth or plastic blocks (Chapter 7) offer excellent means for analyzing and attempting various aspects of filling.

The thermoplastic techniques listed here—McSpadden method, Obtura II, Ultrafil, and

Endotec—all utilize placement of heated gutta-percha only. Thermafil is also a thermoplastic, but because of the necessity of a central core, it is discussed in Chapter 10 with the solid-core filling materials.

Compacted gutta-percha

The McSpadden or compacted gutta-percha method was a cousin of the warm gutta-percha technique. A large cone of gutta-percha was placed in the prepared canal, and a special bur—the compactor—was used in a low-speed handpiece to both plasticize it and pack it against the canal walls. The compactor was similar to a reverse Hedstrom file that drives material back into the canal rather than removes it. The fills thus obtained were quite dense and had a close relationship to the canal walls. Furthermore, it took only a few seconds to fill a canal with this method.

Presently, the McSpadden method is only of historical interest because very few dentists, if any, use it any longer. It did have an effect on the obturation methods used by many dentists because it offered a new method of inserting the gutta-percha, by quickly heating it, and then packing it to place. Although similar in philosophy to Schilder's method for using warm gutta-percha, the time required to fill a canal was much, much less and, thus, more attractive to many dentists.

The major disadvantage was that the compactor was best used in canals of size 50 and larger and in those which were relatively straight. Most dentists did not have much of a problem in filling large, straight canals. However, in smaller, curved canals, where all dentists could use help, the compactor was very difficult to use. Other difficulties included separation of compactor tips (not difficult to remove, but it did take time) or driving the compactor through the root tip if the edges of the instrument contacted the canal walls and the compactor was turning in the wrong direction.

Because of the ability to fill very irregular spaces, the McSpadden method was popular for use in filling teeth with resorptive defects (Fig. 9-30), which were difficult to fill properly with a cold lateral condensation technique. The McSpadden compaction gave a dense fill to the very irregular canal space (Fig. 9-30, *D*). Interestingly, the sole indication now for using a compactor seems to be in placement of calcium hydroxide pastes in teeth requiring apexification or resorption repair (see Chapter 16).

McSpadden, himself, continues to develop new instruments for both canal preparation and filling. The nickle-titanium instruments for canal preparation (Chapter 7) have been improved and marketed largely through his efforts. However, his work with phase changes in gutta-percha and alternative pluggers systems has been relatively unproductive.

Injection-molded techniques

Obtura II. The original Obtura was produced by Unitek, but the instrument (called the Gutta-Gun) and the technique did not take hold as the company anticipated, so the product was cut loose. A few improvements were made, and now the Obtura II* is manufactured by Texceed.

The delivery system is very similar to that used for hydrocoloid impression materials. Cold gutta-percha is placed in a gunlike injector (Fig. 9-31) and heated to approximately 80° C (180° F). A light goes on when the correct temperature has been reached. The "trigger" is squeezed and a few millimeters of thermoplastic gutta-percha is injected into the preparation and condensed with pluggers. This is continued—injection and condensing—until the preparation is filled (Fig. 9-32, *D*). During the placement of the filling, the gutta-percha is being injected at a temperature of approximately 55° to 60° C.

In my experience, this technique is very valuable in very wide and irregular canals, where selecting a suitable master gutta-percha cone would be very difficult, as demonstrated in Fig. 9-32. Also, I have used it with success in extremely narrow, minimally prepared canals (Fig. 9-33). In Fig. 9-33, even though the canal has virtually no preparation whatsoever, the gutta-percha could be injected for several millimeters. I make no claim that the canal has been filled and no sealer was used, but I find it quite remarkable that the material was able to be forced into the canal.

A few tips should be passed along to make Obtura use better. You may not use routine gutta-percha sticks that come in boxes or tubes for normal condensation, but, rather, the gutta-percha made for the Obtura II, which has a high-molecular-weight. Once the gutta-percha is heated in the chamber, it should be used within 15 minutes. A slow-setting sealer, not affected by heat, should be used (NOT Wach's paste or Tubliseal). Before

---

*Texceed Corporation, Costa Mesa, Calif.

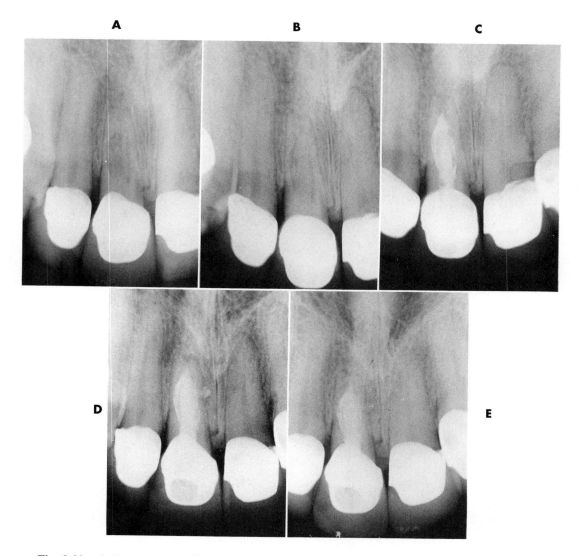

Fig. 9-30. **A,** Preoperative radiograph of maxillary central incisor with internal resorption defects causing unusual canal shape. **B,** The canal was cleaned, and calcium hydroxide was placed to halt the resorption. **C,** A chronic draining sinus to the mesial healed, so 6 months later the canal was reprepared, and then gutta-percha was vertically condensed with Kerr's antiseptic sealer. I was disappointed with the quality of fill, even though it took almost 1 hour to condense. **D,** I dissolved the filling with chloroform, reprepared the canal, and then filled the canal by the McSpadden method with Kerr's sealer again. This time the canal filling seems more satisfactory, even though it took only several minutes to place. Note some filling material expressed toward the mesial. **E,** Two years later, area appears normal.

starting the injection into the prepared canal, squirt out several inches onto the bracket table to ensure that the flow and plasticity are correct. Use a plastic stop on the tip to indicate the working length. The gutta-percha will inject about 3 millimeters around a canal curvature of approximately 30° and may be condensed several millimeters more.

Because of its ability to fill small and large canals, to allow condensation with pluggers, and to go around at least medium-sized curvatures, I feel that this product is the most useful of the thermoplastic techniques. However, these delivery systems are very individually oriented. What appeals to me may not be enjoyed by everyone.

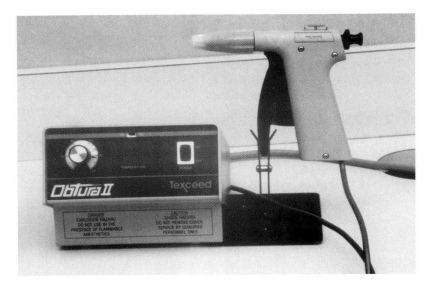

Fig. 9-31.   Obtura II machine for plasticizing gutta-percha. The injector is in its holder attached to the control box. The silver applicator needle has not yet been placed into the injector. Controls include on/off button, centigrade or Fahrenheit reading, and temperature control.

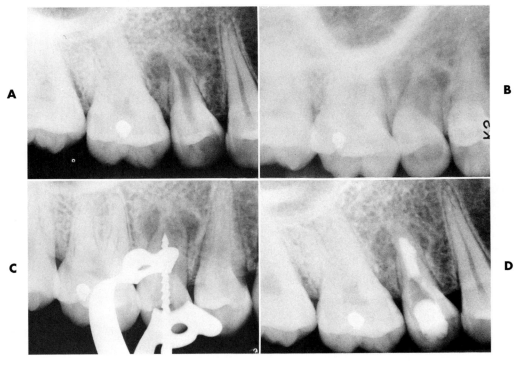

Fig. 9-32.   **A,** Preoperative view of maxillary second bicuspid with large periapical lesion, undeveloped apex, and two chronic draining sinus tracts. **B,** Angled view. **C,** Calcium hydroxide was used to stimulate apical development successfully, and sinus tracts closed. File in place is 17 mm, at which length the canal was prepared prior to placement of the paste. This canal shape is very difficult to fill adequately. **D,** Immediate postfilling film, canal filled with Obtura injectable technique, Kerr's antiseptic sealer, and vertical condensation.

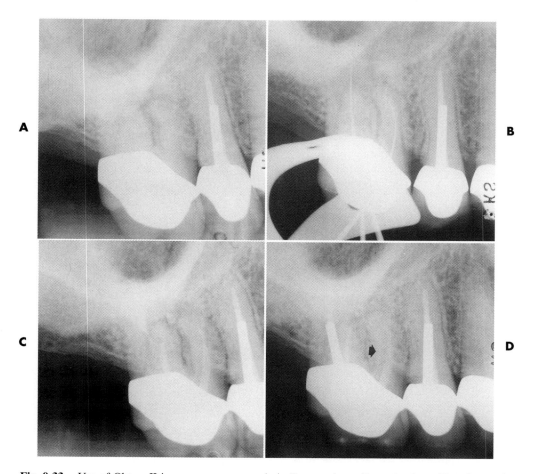

Fig. 9-33.   Use of Obtura II in a very narrow canal. **A,** Preoperative radiograph of maxillary first molar indicating periapical lesions associated with the mesiobuccal and palatal roots and apical tenderness on the buccal bone overlying the tooth. **B,** Film of files in place to acceptable positions in the mesiobuccal, distobuccal, and palatal canals. Although not pictured here, I was able to locate the second canal in the mesiobuccal root, the mesiolingual canal (ML), and placed a size 10 in it to a reasonable length. However, I made a serious mistake and withdrew the file immediately thereafter, without any preparation or orifice enlargement. When I tried to reenter the ML a bit later, I could not get the file to penetrate at all, even though I spent one hour trying to do so. **C,** At the next appointment, I completed preparation of the three other canals and tried unsuccessfully to get down the ML. At the third (filling) appointment, I filled the three prepared canals with laterally condensed gutta-percha and Wach's paste. Then I put the tip of the Obtura II in the area where I thought the ML opened and squeezed the trigger. Imagine my surprise when viewing this immediate post-filling film to see some radiopaque material in the ML! **D,** Three years after treatment, the lesions have healed, the tooth is comfortable and material can be clearly seen in the ML *(arrow).*

Ultrafil.   The Ultrafil* system uses a metal syringe that will accommodate any of three different types of gutta-percha in a cannule with attached needle (Fig. 9-34, *A*) to inject into the prepared canal. The cannules are warmed in a heating unit

(resembles a glass-bead sterilizer, Fig. 9-34, *B*) for approximately 15 minutes to bring the temperature of the gutta-percha to 70° C (160° F) and then placed into the injector. The injector/cannule combination may be returned to the heating unit (Fig. 9-34, *C*) during the course of the filling to keep the gutta-percha softened during condensation of

*Hygenic Corporation, Akron, OH 44310.

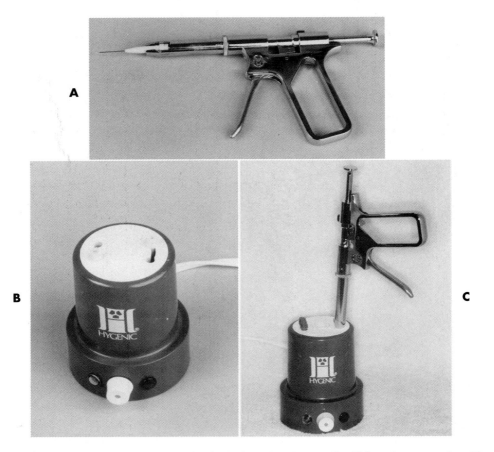

Fig. 9-34. Instruments for using Ultrafil. **A,** Syringe for placing Ultrafil into the preparation. The white cannule (regular set) has been inserted. **B,** Heating unit, resembling glass-bead sterilizer, has two white cannules heating. **C,** Knob in center turns unit on and off. One light on indicates that the unit is heating and both lights on indicate that the heating temperature (70° C) has been reached.

already-placed mass. The material is injected into the preparation at 42° to 45° C.

The three different types of gutta-percha for this system are:

1. Regular set (white cannule), low viscosity, not requiring condensation.
2. Firm (blue cannule), condensation possible, but not required.
3. Endoset (green cannule), must be condensed.

As stated earlier, I believe that all thermoplastics should be condensed, so I would only use the Endoset.

The technique for Endoset, according to the manufacturers, is to place the heated cannule into the preparation and extrude several millimeters of gutta-percha. (The technique requires a fairly wide apical preparation, an enlargement of size 70 at 7

mm from the tip.) This is packed with a plugger until the gutta-percha resists further condensation. This sequence is repeated—packing and plugging—until the preparation is filled.

I do not use the instrument in that manner. After placing the sealer into the prepared canal, I use the injector as a delivery system for the apical few millimeters of gutta-percha. After packing that segment as well as possible, I place a plugger as far as possible and then continue to use lateral condensation with auxiliary cones until the preparation is filled (Fig. 9-35, *A* and *B*).

Both of the injection-molded methods are useful for treating teeth with resorptive defects (Fig. 9-35, *C*) and backfilling and certainly are easier to use in wide, relatively straight canals. Dentists who have enjoyed using paste-type canal fillings or other noncondensation techniques generally

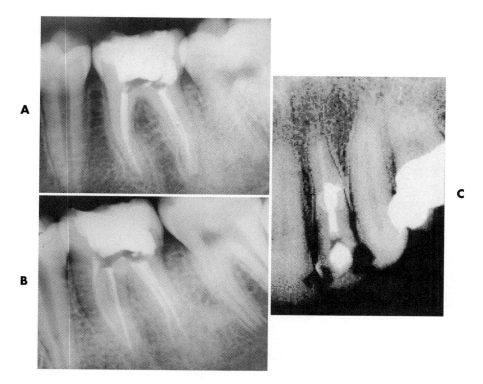

Fig. 9-35. Use of Ultrafil. Straight (**A**) and angled (**B**) views immediately after canal filling of four-canaled mandibular first molar with Ultrafil Endoset, lateral condensation of gutta-percha, and Grossman's formula sealer. A few mm of Endoset were injected into each canal, condensed with a plugger, and the rest of the canal was filled with auxiliary cones laterally condensed. **C,** Internal resorptive defects are well treated with thermoplastics. In this lateral incisor, calcium hydroxide had been used to seal an internal resorption defect that had perforated (see Chapter 16). The apical portion, above the resorption, was enlarged to size 30 and filled with laterally condensed gutta-percha and Wach's paste. The remainder of the canal was enlarged to size 80, the Ultrafil syringe was loaded with an Endoset cannule and vertical condensation was used to fill the remainder of the canal and the defect.

enjoy using the regular or firm Ultrafil without any condensation. A danger of this is to remove the injector prematurely, which usually will pull out most, if not all, of the filling material. The operator must allow the material to push out the injector.

Several other techniques may be used with the Ultrafil system, including the so-called Trifecta, where thermoplasticized gutta-percha is placed on the tip of a file or reamer, spun into the apical portion of the canal, condensed, and then this combination of three steps (tri-portion of Trifecta) is repeated until the canal is filled.

Endotec. Thermoplastic, but not injection-molded, the Endotec* technique employs a spreader-like instrument that is attached to a heating element. Following sealer and master cone placement, this spreader is inserted alongside the cone and the heat turned on. The master cone is thus softened and distorted, allowing deeper spreader penetration. When the spreader is removed, a space is created for the placement of an auxiliary cone. This process is repeated with another heated spread, followed by auxiliary cone placement, and so on until the canal is filled.

A potentially useful alternative to this method allows for routine canal filling by lateral condensation with cold spreaders. If there is some concern about the adequacy of the fill, a radiograph is taken with the rubber dam still in place, before temporization. If the film indicates that a satisfactory result has been obtained, the temporary is placed and the dam removed. If, however, the fill

*L.D. Caulk Co., Division of Caulk/Dentsply, Milford, DE 19963.

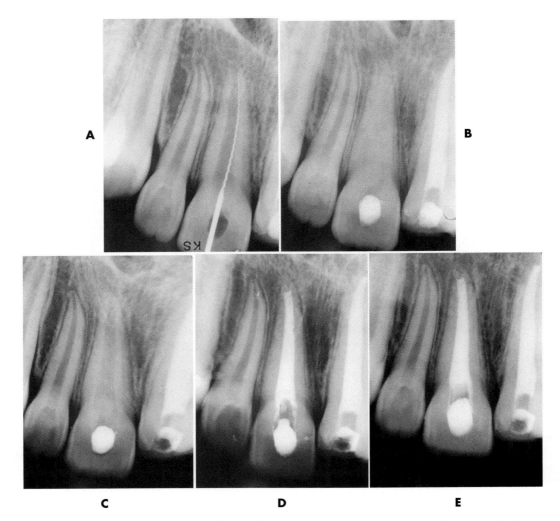

Fig. 9-36. Use of the Endotec. **A,** Film of file in place indicates that the central incisor to the left (tooth 8) has an open apex that will require apexification procedures (Chapter 16) to gain apical closure prior to completing canal filling. On the other hand, the central incisor to the right (tooth 9) could be treated routinely because the apex had sufficient closure to pack gutta-percha. **B,** Tooth 8 received canal preparation and then placement of calcium hydroxide paste, tooth 9 had been successfully filled with laterally condensed gutta-percha and Wach's paste. **C,** The apex of tooth 9 had closed sufficiently and may now may be filled. Both centrals were quite long—32 mm. **D,** During the filling of tooth 8, due to the length of the tooth and the fact that it was a very humid day (Wach's paste sets quickly in high humidity), the apical portion of the fill exhibited many voids and other signs of incomplete filling, although the coronal portion was quite dense. **E,** Rather than remove the entire filling and attempt to refill similarly (and probably make the same mistakes), the Endotec was used to remove most of the old filling, which was then repacked and recondensed with gutta-percha. A more desirable fill has been obtained. This result is similar to that seen in Fig. 9-29.

is inadequate (Fig. 9-36, *D*), the Endotec may be used to remove much of the old filling quickly, without solvents, heat the apical portion, and allow recondensation. Hopefully a desirable result will follow (Fig. 9-36, *E*).

Use of sealers with thermoplastics. It would appear that sealers are not needed in conjunction with thermoplastic gutta-percha filling. Because the filling material is injected into place, and in some cases further packed to the apex, it seems logical that any sealer placed before the gutta-percha would merely pool at the apex and do little to improve the sealing ability for such a technique.

On the contrary, studies on using each of these techniques have unanimously concluded that the sealing ability is enhanced considerably when root canal sealer *is* used in conjunction with the thermoplastics. Therefore, contrary to the manufacturers' instructions with the units, root canal sealer *should* be used with any of these devices.

Need for apical dentin matrix. As stated in Chapter 7, the techniques espoused in this textbook strongly encourage the use of an apical dentin matrix, most desirably at the cementodentinal junction. Not all authorities agree on the need for or type of such a matrix. Some suggest that a patency be established through it into the periapical tissues, whereas others prefer a collar or shoulder to pack against. When using sticks of gutta-percha as canal filling components, some degree of patency is tolerable and overfills may not result because the cone may jam into the apical walls and not extrude.

On the contrary, when thermoplastics are injected, unless a solid matrix is present, extrusions are almost impossible to prevent. Because of the softened form used, complete lack of matrix may cause immense extrusions not possible with stick material.

Therefore, if the operator has a strong suspicion that the apical matrix is absent, alternatives to thermoplastics should be utilized. With the increase in popularity of the thermoplastic filling systems, and the indications that many of the filling techniques of the future will involve thermoplastics, it is advised that those operators who have been reluctant to utilize a preparation with a solid dentin matrix should reconsider their position. Thermoplastics may be able to do things that stick gutta-percha cannot. The sooner that the entire technique can be mastered, including the

solid matrix, the better the clinician will be able to handle different types of filling situations.

Partially dissolved gutta-percha

Callahan and Johnston suggested techniques using solvents with gutta-percha to fill canals. The solvents were chloroform or oil of eucalyptol, which were placed into the canal with a syringe; then cones of gutta-percha were plunged into the solvent. From the evaporation of the solvent and dissolving of the soluble gutta-percha, a thick creamy mass developed, which solidified to form a canal filling.

Disadvantages. Subsequent studies revealed that a considerable amount of contraction developed in the filling after solidification. This dimensional change amounted to as much as 7%, which could possibly destroy the apical seal. Other studies indicated that the solvents used were more irritating to periapical tissue than were most root canal sealers. For these reasons, the techniques were only rarely employed, although students of the originators, most of whom practiced in the southeastern portion of the United States, remained as adherents.

Modified chloropercha

Other authors, notably Ostby of Norway, were impressed by the fact that if the sealing materials

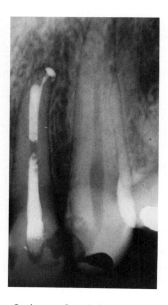

Fig. 9-37. Incisor referred for treatment after ledge formation. Ledge was bypassed and canal filled by a chloropercha technique.

could be altered from the completely solid state while being placed, they could be formed more easily to the irregularities of the canal preparation. Therefore sealers were devised that acted to partially dissolve the central core and allow it to be compressed into the cavity.

As described by Kahn, small segments of gutta-percha are placed into a 5 ml covered container of chloroform and periodically mixed until a cream of chloropercha is developed. A master cone is selected that will reach to approximately 2 mm from the apex but will not completely seat in the apical portion of the preparation. The chloropercha is placed into the canal in the same manner as sealers are placed in other methods, that is, with a reamer rotated counterclockwise. The master cone is dipped into the chloropercha, and then forceful vertical condensation is exerted toward the apex, pushing the partially dissolved tip of the master cone to its apical seat. Auxiliary cones, first dipped into the chloropercha, are packed into the canal until a satisfactory filling is obtained.

Indications. As previously mentioned, excellent indications for this method are found in ledge formation, perforation, unusual curvatures, or any cases in which the apical foramen cannot successfully be sealed by other methods (Figs. 9-37 on p. 463 and 9-38).

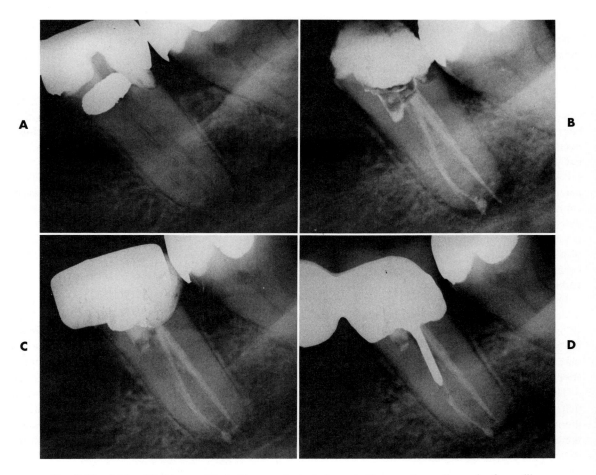

Fig. 9-38. Molar filled by modified chloropercha technique. **A,** Preoperative radiograph of mandibular second molar with periapical lesion adjacent to distal portion of root and an unusual canal shape. (Perhaps C shaped, Chapter 6.) **B,** It was difficult to clean and enlarge these canals satisfactorily, and I thought that filling the canals with laterally condensed gutta-percha would not give a desirable result. Accordingly, I used a modified chloropercha technique. **C,** Tooth was temporized briefly to verify that healing was taking place. **D,** Eighteen months after treatment, area has healed and tooth is comfortably serving as a distal abutment for a fixed bridge. (Restorations by Dr. Arnold Wax, Chicago.)

RE-TREATING FAILING GUTTA-PERCHA CASES

First, analyze the failure. Before any re-treatment is performed, the dentist must determine the cause of the failure. Some failures cannot be retreated, and any attempts to do so will only lead to wasted time and antagonism between the patient and the dentist. Some failures will require surgery, whereas others merely need the removal of the old canal filling followed by repreparation and refilling.

If the failure is indicated by a radiolucency along a lateral border of one root extending for much of the root length, there is a strong possibility of a vertical root fracture and re-treatment is useless (see Fig. 2-28, *D*). If a radiolucency is present in a tooth in which treatment seems adequate and the canal filling seems well condensed, the possibility of a second canal should be explored (Fig. 9-39). This is particularly true if the failure is occurring in a tooth in which recent studies indicate that a second canal has a significant chance of being present. The most common teeth for this are mandibular incisors and first bicuspids, maxillary second bicuspids, mesiobuccal roots of maxillary first molars, and distal roots of mandibular molars.

Whenever possible, the failing tooth should be re-treated nonsurgically prior to any move toward more aggressive therapy. Even if this requires entry through an existing complex restorative effort (Fig. 9-40, *A*) including removal of existing post-and-core types of restorations, it is best to attempt treatment from this position. It is surprising how often repreparation of the canals, often with the aid of the ultrasonic treatment (see Chapter 7) for adding cleansing action, and refilling will give a successful result (Fig. 9-40, *E*).

Even if this leads to continued failure, and indeed surgery becomes necessary, you can be certain that there is a dense canal filling present that may be cut back to, which avoids the need for reverse filling.

Some failing cases are best managed surgically. Among these are teeth with post-and-core type of crowns in place; canals whose original shape has been badly altered during preparation and the chances of returning to the true canal shape are poor; teeth in which overinstrumentation has caused apical zipping; and Type IV canals in which the bifurcation occurs near the apex, but only one apical portion has been prepared and filled (Fig. 9-41). Also, failures originally treated surgically often are best retreated with surgery (Fig. 9-42).

Cases that respond most favorably to re-treatment without surgery are those in which the canals have fillings far short of the apex and those in which insufficient canal preparation and/or condensation have prevented apical seal.

Re-treating short fills. Short canal fillings usually offer no serious problem in re-treatment. Either chloroform or xylene is used to irrigate the canal and soften the coronal portion of the canal filling. That the gutta-percha has begun to soften may be verified by forceful insertion of the endodontic explorer or an ultrasonic tip. Upon removal, the tip of the explorer should be tinged with the pink dissolving canal filling. At this point a small file of moderate flexibility—size 20 or 25—is inserted and worked into the filling with a back-and-forth motion. For increased penetration, further irrigation with the solvent should be performed.

The distance of canal filling to be bypassed should be estimated in advance. Once this distance is reached, a film may be taken to verify that a file extends beyond the old canal filling. When this is accomplished, the canal should be heavily irrigated with sodium hypochlorite to remove any residual solvent that might irritate the periapical tissues.

The full working length of the canal is now calculated and verified by radiograph with a file in place. In the smaller curved canals this is accomplished by going down to a smaller-sized file—10 or 15. The preparation of the canal is now continued as in a normal case and the filling placed at a subsequent appointment in accordance with Chapter 19 (Figs. 9-43 and 9-44).

Many times such re-treatment cases end with canal fillings short of the desired distance. This is often unavoidable because the canal has been ledged during the previous effort and the ledge cannot be bypassed. The correct procedure is to fill as far as possible with densely condensed gutta-percha and observe for healing. If healing does not take place, periapical surgery may be performed, cutting the root tip back to the gutta-percha filling.

Re-treating for insufficient canal preparation and/or condensation. Usually these two entities go hand in hand. If a canal is insufficiently condensed, it is generally due to insufficient canal preparation. If a canal is prepared insufficiently, it is virtually impossible to gain a good condensation.

It is assumed, however, that these canals have been enlarged so the working length is close to accurate. As before, the canal filling is removed

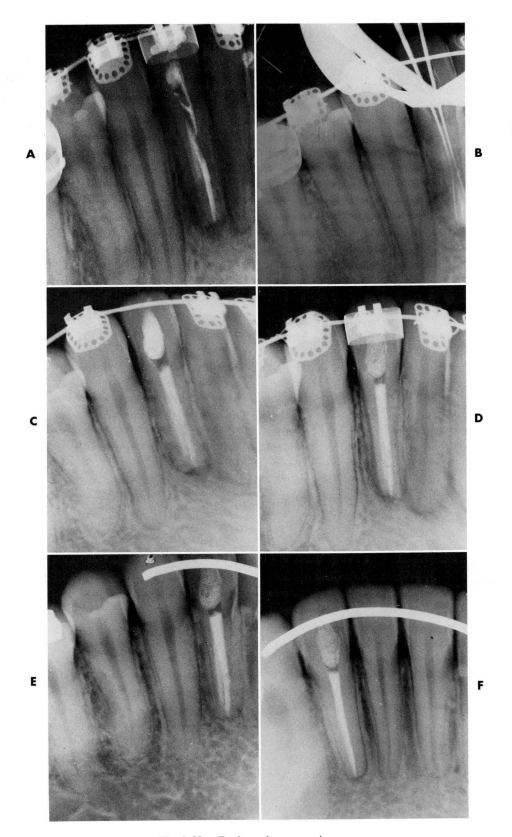

Fig. 9-39.   For legend see opposite page.

with a suitable solvent and the working length is radiographically verified with a file in place. In the very curved canals care must be exercised to avoid zipping (Chapter 7) since these are the canals that often are poorly prepared and filled initially. They must be given adequate flaring (Chapter 7) so a canal filling of desirable density can be placed to gain optimal seal. The failure to flare adequately is a frequent major problem in cases of this type because insufficient flaring prevents proper placement of the spreaders and does not allow for apical deformation of the gutta-percha.

After repreparation the canal is filled at a subsequent appointment, as stated earlier in this chapter (Fig. 9-45).

It is truly amazing that cases of this type respond beautifully to correct re-treatment. One of the greatest satisfactions I have in endodontics is to take a case that has failed and reclaim it with proper re-treatment. The patient is often initially antagonistic to endodontic therapy, but this attitude quickly turns to appreciation when the tooth is saved.

SEALERS WITH SEMISOLID MATERIALS

Most root canal sealers are some type of zinc oxide–eugenol cement, although certain resins have also been utilized. To be an acceptable root canal sealer, the material must be capable of producing a seal while being well tolerated by periapical tissue. All the sealers presently used appear to have good sealing ability. However, all do produce periapical inflammation, raging from mild to severe, in the initial few days after cementation. Fortunately, the inflammatory process does appear to resolve completely and healing follows.

Functions. Root canal sealers are used in conjunction with filling materials for four purposes. All the popularly used sealers contain some antibacterial agent, and so a germicidal quality is exerted in the period of time immediately after its placement. The sealer is needed to fill in the discrepancies between the fit of the filling material and the dentin walls. Since the sealers are in the plastic or semiliquid state when placed in the canal and then harden to a solid consistency, they are able to form a bond between the filling material and the dentin walls in the same manner as a cement holds a dental casting.

With the use of semisolid materials, the most important function for the sealer to perform is its action of lubrication. Having little rigidity, gutta-percha must have considerable lubrication when it is placed to reach its desired position in the apical portion of the preparation. Therefore, to some extent, the choice of sealer used in any particular case should be predicated on what degree of lubrication is desired, since there are a number of sealers available with varying physical properties.

All sealers display some degree of radiopacity; therefore their presence can be demonstrated on a radiograph. This is an important property, since it may disclose the presence of auxiliary canals, resorptive areas, root fractures, and the shape of the apical foramen and other structures of interest.

Certain techniques dictate the use of a particular sealer. The chloropercha technique, for instance, uses that material as a sealer as well as a solvent for the master cone, allowing the shape of a previously machine-made cone to be altered to conform to the prepared canal.

Rickert's formula. As described by Schilder, the warm gutta-percha method uses Rickert's formula, also known as Kerr's Antiseptic Root Canal Sealer*, as a sealer. This sealer has been the material of choice in many other methods and has been suggested by many clinicians as it has stood the test of time for over 50 years. The formula contains zinc oxide powder, resin, thymol iodide, and precipitated silver in the powder, with oil of cloves as the major constituent of the liquid. The sealer has excellent lubricating qualities, allows a working

Text continued on p. 471.

---

*Kerr Manufacturing Company, Romulus, Mich.

Fig. 9-39. Nonsurgical retreatment of failing mandibular incisor with unfilled second canal. **A,** Unfilled canal by earlier endodontic effort with periapical and lateral lesions, slightly angled preoperative film. **B,** Projection from distal demonstrates file to apical portion of lingual canal *(to left)* and other file to seemingly solid portion of labial canal filling. **C,** Lingual canal filled with laterally condensed gutta-percha and Wach's paste. Remainder of labial canal has been refilled. **D,** Three months later, lateral lesion has healed and periapical lesion is considerably reduced. **E,** Eighteen months after original treatment, healing is complete; angled view. **F,** Straight view.

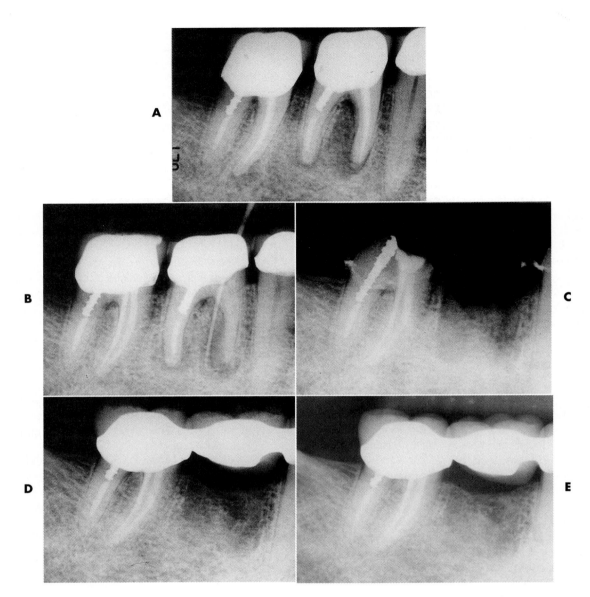

Fig. 9-40. A, Preoperative radiograph of mandibular molar area. Endodontic treatment had been performed several years earlier, but both molars were sensitive to percussion, and the first molar was slightly mobile with a chronic draining sinus tract tracing to its mesial apex. I believed that the first molar had a crack, but I wanted to try to attempt retreatment on the mesial canals of both teeth. **B,** I opened into the mesial canals of the first molar, dissolved the old fillings, and cleaned the canals as well as I could. However, when the patient returned for the next appointment, the tract still traced to the mesial root. Therefore, I referred the patient to an oral surgeon who would expose the apices of the first molar. If the crack went through both roots, the tooth would be extracted. If only the mesial root was involved, that root would be amputated and I would retreat the distal root. **C,** The crack involved both roots of the first molar, so it was extracted. I retreated the mesial canals of the second molar, but my fills (laterally condensed gutta-percha and Wach's paste) did not appear to be any better than the previous attempt. **D,** However, 9 months later, the lesion was healing well. **E,** Two years after treatment, the tooth is comfortable and the lesion is gone. (Restorations by Dr. Howard Paule, Highland Park, Ill.)

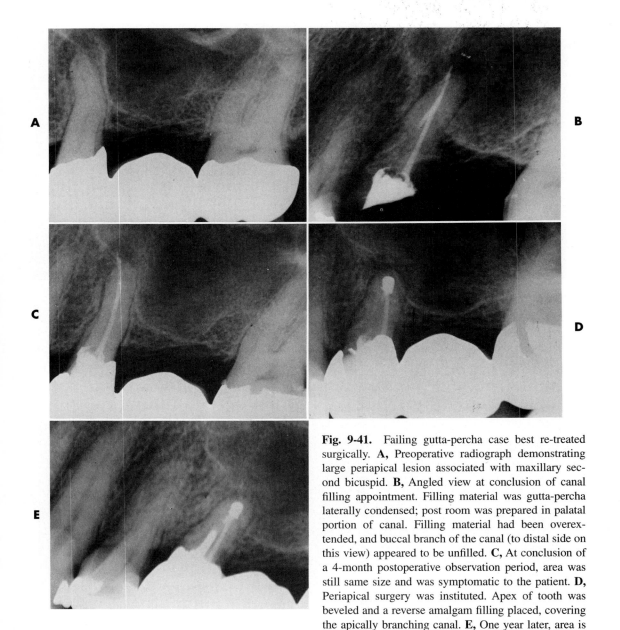

Fig. 9-41. Failing gutta-percha case best re-treated surgically. **A,** Preoperative radiograph demonstrating large periapical lesion associated with maxillary second bicuspid. **B,** Angled view at conclusion of canal filling appointment. Filling material was gutta-percha laterally condensed; post room was prepared in palatal portion of canal. Filling material had been overextended, and buccal branch of the canal (to distal side on this view) appeared to be unfilled. **C,** At conclusion of a 4-month postoperative observation period, area was still same size and was symptomatic to the patient. **D,** Periapical surgery was instituted. Apex of tooth was beveled and a reverse amalgam filling placed, covering the apically branching canal. **E,** One year later, area is healing well and all symptoms have subsided.

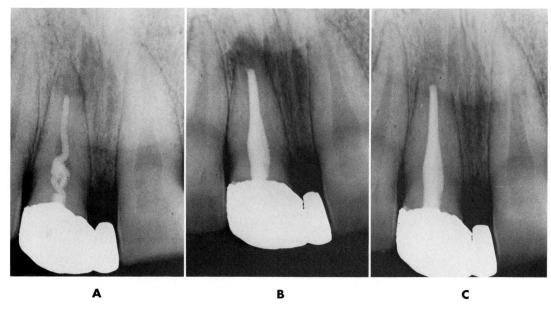

Fig. 9-42. Failing surgical case filled with gutta-percha, best re-treated surgically. **A,** Maxillary central incisor, treated surgically 1 year earlier, with extremely poor gutta-percha filling. Patient had had a chronic draining sinus tract. **B,** Gutta-percha was removed, and canal refilled with laterally condensed gutta-percha and Tubliseal. Area was flapped, and an apicoectomy performed down to densely filled portion of canal. **C,** One year later, area has healed perfectly.

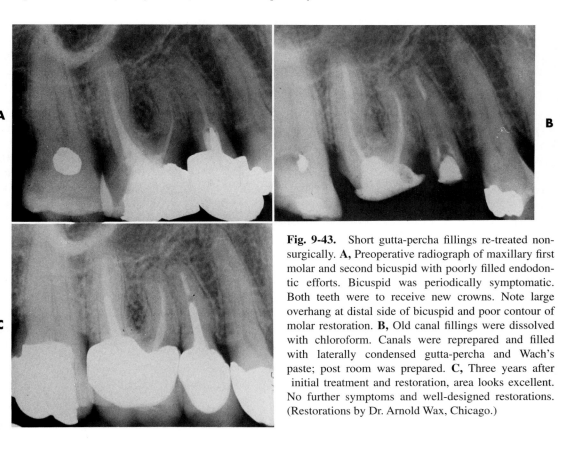

Fig. 9-43. Short gutta-percha fillings re-treated nonsurgically. **A,** Preoperative radiograph of maxillary first molar and second bicuspid with poorly filled endodontic efforts. Bicuspid was periodically symptomatic. Both teeth were to receive new crowns. Note large overhang at distal side of bicuspid and poor contour of molar restoration. **B,** Old canal fillings were dissolved with chloroform. Canals were reprepared and filled with laterally condensed gutta-percha and Wach's paste; post room was prepared. **C,** Three years after initial treatment and restoration, area looks excellent. No further symptoms and well-designed restorations. (Restorations by Dr. Arnold Wax, Chicago.)

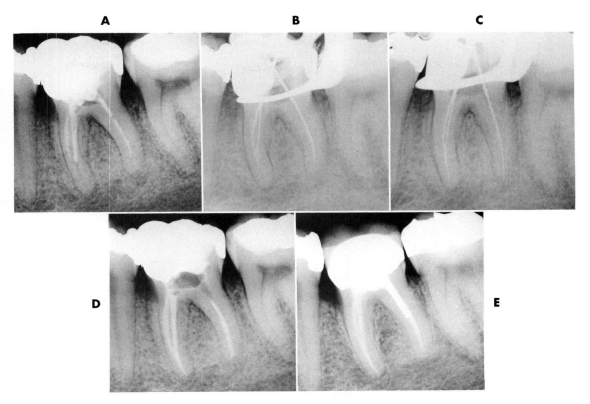

Fig. 9-44.   A, Preoperative radiograph of mandibular first molar with short canal fillings, tenderness to percussion, and periapical lesions developing. **B,** The initial files in place went to the sites of the original preparation. This is often the problem, because the canal is ledged at the depth of the earlier preparation. **C,** Fortunately, these sites were bypassed to more desirable depths. **D,** Canals filled with laterally condensed gutta-percha and Wach's paste. **E,** Eight years later, periapical areas have healed. (Restoration by Dr. Steven Potashnick, Chicago.)

time of more than 30 minutes when mixed in a 1:1 powder-to-liquid ratio, and has germicidal action. The major advantage of this sealer is that it has greater bulk than any other sealer. This makes it ideal for condensation techniques, since the sealer then may be pushed into voids and irregularities, such as may remain lateral to gutta-percha cones, and into auxiliary canals.

The major disadvantage of Rickert's formula is that the presence of silver makes the sealer extremely staining if any of the material enters the tubules of the crown (Fig. 9-46). Since posterior teeth are restored with complete cuspal coverage and frequently a full crown, discoloration is rarely a problem in bicuspids or molars. However, when used in anterior teeth, considerable care should be exercised to wash out the pulp chamber with xylol after condensation of the gutta-percha to ensure the removal of any residual sealer.

I have found Kerr's antiseptic sealer to be the material of choice when a lateral canal is anticipated. Many of the lateral canal cases shown in Chapter 2 were filled using this sealer. Schilder claims that his warm gutta-percha technique demonstrates more lateral canals than any other method, and he uses this sealer routinely. I believe that lateral canals can be demonstrated by virtually every technique, and many cases in this book involve the indication of lateral canals, with a variety of sealers and filling techniques used.

However, the ability to increase the body of Kerr's sealer by adding more powder allows for a greater bulk that will move during condensation into these branching areas. Also, the precipitated silver present in the powder is very radiopaque. It may be that what is seen in demonstrated lateral canals with this sealer is the silver rather than the mass of sealer mix or any softened gutta-percha.

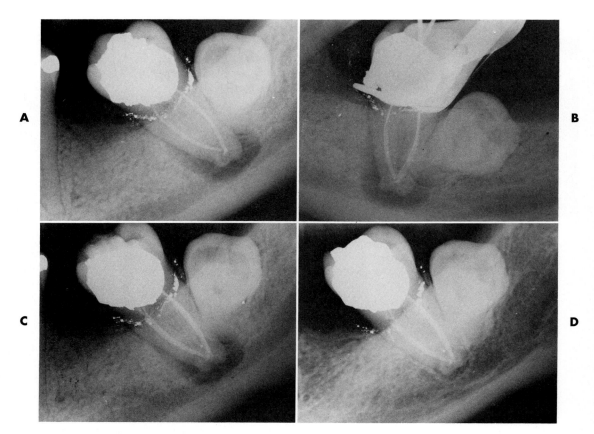

Fig. 9-45. Re-treating cases with insufficient canal preparation and/or condensation. **A,** Radiograph of mandibular second molar. Endodontic treatment had been performed 2 years earlier, and history from the patient indicated that pulp had been vital at that time. Very large periapical radiolucency is now present. Canals are obviously underprepared and consequently insufficiently condensed. Radiopaque lines near gingiva are amalgam tattoo from gingival amalgam restoration. **B,** Radiograph of files in place. They offered little resistance to placement at this length. **C,** Canals reprepared, flared, and filled with laterally condensed gutta-percha and Wach's paste. **D,** One year later, periapical lesion is almost completely healed.

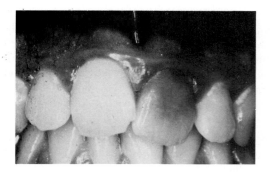

Fig. 9-46. Well-filled treated tooth has considerable discoloration because of failure to remove excess sealer from tubules of the crown.

Interestingly, I have observed that lateral canals demonstrated with Kerr's sealer remain observable radiographically far longer than do such canals with Wach's paste (Figs. 9-47 and 9-48).

The Kerr Manufacturing Company packages Rickert's formula with the powder contained in a pellet or bulk and the liquid in a dropper bottle. For use with gutta-percha, one drop of liquid is added to one pellet of powder (1:1 ratio) and mixed with a heavy spatula until relative homogeneity is obtained. Because of the precipitated silver, some granular appearance remains even when the spatulation is completed.

Tubliseal. Slight modifications have been made in Rickert's formula to eliminate the staining

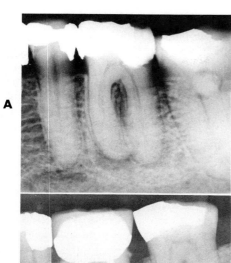

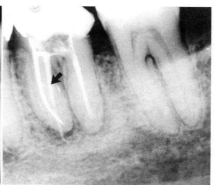

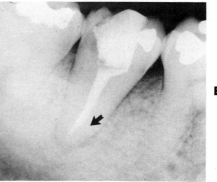

Fig. 9-47. This case was originally published to indicate that silver cones may be used in canal filling where lateral canals are demonstrated. **A,** Preoperative radiograph of mandibular first molar with periapical lesions on both roots. **B,** Immediate postfilling angled view, with distal and mesiolingual canals filled with gutta-percha and mesiobuccal with silver cone; Kerr's antiseptic sealer used for all three canals. The lateral canal *(arrow)* extends from the canal with the silver cone. **C,** After 16 years the periapical areas healed and remained normal, and some of the sealer *(arrow)* can still be seen on the radiograph. (From Weine FS: *Dent Clin North Am* 28:833, 1984. With permission.)

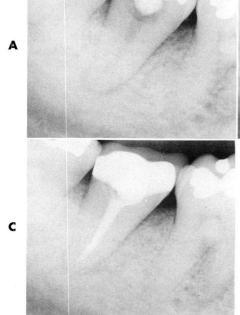

Fig. 9-48. **A,** Preoperative radiograph of mandibular second molar with a single large canal, periapical lesion, and tenderness to percussion. **B,** Film immediately following canal filling with laterally condensed gutta-percha and Wach's paste. Note the later canal *(arrow)* indicated by the sealer. **C,** One year later, the periapical lesion has healed completely, but the sealer in the lateral canal is no longer apparent.

property, and the result was the manufacture of Tubliseal. This sealer is easy to mix, does not stain tooth structure, and is extremely lubricating. For this reason Tubliseal is indicated when apical surgery is to be performed immediately after canal filling. In cases of this type the canal may be intentionally overfilled with very heavy condensation and the excess removed when the area is curetted. Tubliseal allows maximal condensation and packing, is white in color with good contrast to the flapped tissue during the surgical procedure, and as a result of its rapid setting time is easily removed from periapical tissue.

Because of its great lubricating qualities, Tubliseal is a good choice for use when it becomes difficult for a master cone to reach the last millimeter of preparation.

The major disadvantage of Tubliseal is that it appears to be irritating to periapical tissue, causing considerable periapical sensitivity when used in teeth where the pulp was vital and the periapical tissue normal before treatment. This same irritating quality may be turned to an advantage when it is used in teeth where a large radiolucency is present, since the sealer may act as a stimulant to periapical healing. The Kerr Manufacturing Company is doing considerable research to determine why the sealer has this irritating potential and how to lessen the response.

Another disadvantage for Tubliseal is that its working time is less than 30 minutes and even shorter in the presence of moisture. In multirooted teeth for which a longer working time is necessary, plans should be made to use more than one mix. Additionally, great care should be exercised to ensure that all canals are as dry as possible

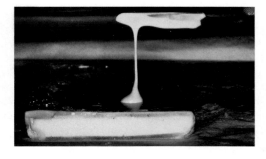

Fig. 9-49. For Wach's paste to be at correct consistency, a spatula must draw 1 inch of sealer when raised from the mass.

prior to sealer insertion, and extra wipings with paper points provide additional insurance against moisture.

Tubliseal is packaged with base and accelerator tubes so that equal lengths of each (about 1/2 inch being sufficient in most cases) are spatulated into a creamy mix.

Wach's paste. A highly desirable sealer for use with gutta-percha is Wach's paste.* The powder contains zinc oxide and some minor constituents to give radiopaque qualities, whereas the liquid contains Canada balsam with a lesser amount of oil of cloves. Wach's paste has a medium working time, has much less lubricating quality than most sealers, causes minimal periapical sensitivity even when a great deal is expressed through the canal, and is germicidal. Because of its limited lubricating property and its excellent acceptance by periapical tissue, this material is ideal for use when any chance of an overfilled canal is present. Increasing the thickness of the sealer lessens its lubricating effect; thus when an overfilling appears possible, a maximal degree of thickness should be employed.

Wach's paste is especially useful in small curved canals of minimal caliber. It has such a light body that it does not deflect the small master gutta-percha cones used to fill these canals. By the same token, due to the presence of Canada balsam it is very sticky. Therefore the paste will remain on the reamer during placement until it is spun off in the apical portion of the preparation and does not completely rub off on the canal walls during insertion. Also, a small amount of sealer is placed on the apical portion of the master cone and this, similarly, stays in position due to its tackiness at an important site at the tip of the cone.

Powder and liquid are packaged separately, and one drop of liquid is used with an appropriate amount of powder. No measuring device is included with the powder, so sample batches should be mixed to enable the mixer to tell what amounts give desired results. The mass spatulates to a smooth, creamy consistency. The correct thickness is obtained when the spatula can be raised from the mass and can draw 1 inch of sealer with it (Fig. 9-49). Large canals generally require a slightly thicker mix.

Procosol. Grossman has developed a sealer with eugenol as the liquid that has properties similar to those of Wach's paste. It is indicated in the same types of cases and is similarly packaged and

*Balas Pharmaceuticals, Chicago, IL 60602.

mixed. The formula for this sealer is similar to Rickert's, but the precipitated silver has been removed to make it non-staining.

This sealer is much slower setting than Wach's paste or Tubliseal. Therefore it is recommended for use with the thermoplastics (Fig. 9-35, *A* and *B*) and for molar teeth with clinicians who are a bit slow. Because of the rapid set of Wach's paste in humid weather, this sealer is often used as an alternative in summer months.

Other sealers. There are other sealers available for endodontic use in addition to those listed in Table 9-3. Those to which I have already made reference I use constantly in practice, and they cover every type of treatment.

Among the other sealers are Diaket (a polyketone widely used in Europe), Nogenol (a noneugenol combination), and polycarboxylate cement, commonly used for cementation of castings in operative dentistry.

Calcium hydroxide sealers. Recently sealers with significant amounts of calcium hydroxide have been introduced as a replacement for the typical zinc oxide–eugenol cements. The theory behind such a development was the documented osteogenic potential of calcium hydroxide being used to gain more desirable healing in the periapical area. Cox and associates at the University of Michigan studied Sealapex* and reported bony repair following its use to seal both canals and perforations.

There are serious questions that must be answered before such sealers gain popular acceptance. Whereas there is no doubt that calcium hydroxide expressed into periradicular tissues will lead to adjacent bone formation, how much chemical is needed for this to occur? For how long must the chemical be in an active state to gain osteogenesis? When used in a paste with free calcium

*Kerr Manufacturing Company, Romulus, Mich.

Table 9-3. Sealers

Name	Indications	Contraindications	Packaging	Mixing
Wach's paste	All lateral condensation methods, especially when chance of over-filling is present	When heavy lubrication is needed, as with short master cone	Liquid and powder in separate bottles	Mixed to creamy consistency, mass to draw 1 inch from raised spatula; thicker for larger canals and if chance of overfill
Rickert's formula	Vertical condensation of "warm" gutta-percha, when large bulk of sealer is needed or when lateral canals are anticipated	Has staining qualities; care needed to remove from crown	Liquid in dropper bottle; pre-measured powder in pellet	One pellet of powder to one drop of liquid (1:1)
	For silver points	When sealer cannot be placed to apical portion of preparation	Same as above	Two pellets of powder to one drop of liquid
Tubliseal	When extreme lubrication is needed, as in slightly short master cone, before apical surgery	Irritating to periapical tissue; not to be used if overfill probable with normal periapical tissue; sets very rapidly when wet	Two tubes, base and accelerator	Mixed, equal lengths, to creamy consistency
Chloropercha	After ledge formation, perforation, unusual curvatures	May be irritating to periapical tissue; chance of contraction	Made up before use	Chloroform plus gutta-percha, segments mixed
AH-26	Had been used in Europe as paste filling; packaged with Thermafil as ThermaSeal	None reported	Liquid and powder in separate bottles	Mixed to creamy consistency

hydroxide available, the effect of the chemical persists for some time, but is that the same as using it in a cement that must harden? If the cement hardens very slowly, will that allow for more distribution of calcium hydroxide? Will a very-slow-setting cement be effective in sealing the canal?

It would seem that the need for setting for sealing purposes would offset the potential osteogenic properties of such a sealer. If the calcium hydroxide is continuously given off for long periods, the sealing properties are weakened. Placement of calcium hydroxide pastes to gain apical closure, repair perforated resorptions (Chapter 16), and avert lateral resorption following replantation of avulsed teeth (Chapter 5) is much different than use in a permanent sealer. In the former three cases the paste is in place for several weeks to several months, never sets hard, and is present to induce short-term alteration of periapical tissue condition. In a root canal sealer extreme longevity is required, and unless long-term sealing is obtained, whatever short-term effectiveness is gained will be offset by loss of apical seal.

I have used calcium hydroxide sealers in teeth with middle-third root fractures and severe apical resorption, but my cases are recently completed and require further observation before any conclusions may be drawn.

Selection of sealer. For use with gutta-percha, appropriate sealers should be selected to aid in the filling of the canal. The operator should determine the amount of lubrication needed, the length of working time estimated, and the filling material to be used before deciding which sealer or sealers would best perform the necessary functions.

In lateral condensation methods the use of sealer should be minimal, since the compressible filling material will be able to fill most irregularities. All the sealers have resorbable properties when expressed into periapical tissue, although rarely has resorption of the sealer within the canal been noted. Still, it is preferable to seal a canal with the packed solid-core material, which is largely unresorbable, as compared to the sealer.

Table 9-3 lists various sealers, with their advantages, disadvantages, and packaging and mixing instructions summarized.

REFERENCES

Brayton SM, Davis SR, Goldman M: Gutta-percha root canal fillings; an in vitro analysis, *Oral Surg* 35:226, 1973.

Callahan JR: Rosin solution for the sealing of the dentinal tubuli and as an adjuvant in the filling of root canals, *J Allied Dent Soc* 9:53, 1914.

Cox CF, Beavers RA, Bergenholtz G: *The histopathologic evaluation of a calcium hydroxide medicament to promote healing of periapical, lateral and bifurcation lesions of the periodontium,* University of Michigan, Ann Arbor.

Czonstkowsky M, Michanowicz A, Vazquez J: Evaluation of an injection-thermoplasticized low-temperature gutta-percha using radioactive isotopes, *J Endod* 11:71, 1985.

Davis SR, Brayton SM, Goldman M: The morphology of the prepared root canal: a study utilizing injectable silicone, *Oral Surg* 34:642, 1972.

ElDeeb ME: The sealing ability of injection molded thermoplasticized gutta-percha, *J Endod* 11:84, 1985.

Feldmann G, Nyborg H: Tissue reactions to root filling materials. I. Comparison between gutta-percha and silver amalgam implanted in rabbit, *Odontol Rev* 13:1, 1962.

Feldman G, Solomon C, Notaro PJ: Resorption of gutta-percha in the apical region, *Oral Surg* 20:102, 1965.

Friedman CE, Sandrik JL, Heuer MA, Rapp GW: Composition and physical properties of gutta-percha endodontic filling materials, *J Endod* 3:304, 1977.

Glickman GN, Gutman JL: Contemporary perspectives on canal obturation, *Dent Clin North Am* 36:327, 1992.

Goodman A, Schilder H, Aldrich W: The thermomechanical properties of gutta-percha. II. The history and molecular chemistry of gutta-percha, *Oral Surg* 37:954, 1974.

Guttuso J: Histopathologic study of rat connective tissue response to endodontic materials, *Oral Surg* 16:713, 1963.

Higginbotham TL: A comparative study of the physical properties of five commonly used root canal sealers, *Oral Surg* 24:89, 1967.

Hunter HA: The effect of gutta-percha, silver points and Rickert's root sealer on bone healing, *J Can Dent Assoc* 23:385, 1957.

Ingle JL: Root canal obturation, *J Am Dent Assoc* 53:47, 1956.

Jacobsen EL, BeGole EA, Vitkus DD, Daniel JC: An evaluation of two newly formulated calcium hydroxide cements: a leakage study, *J Endod* 13:164, 1987.

Kahn H: Modified chloropercha technique. In Levy S, editor: Syllabus of Michael Reese Hospital and Medical Center Dental internship program, Chicago, 1968.

Kapsimalis P, Evans R: Sealing properties of endodontic filling materials using radioactive polar and nonpolar isotopes, *Oral Surg* 22:386, 1966.

Luccy CT, Weller RN, Kulild JC: An evaluation of the apical seal produced by lateral and warm lateral condensation techniques, *J Endod* 16:170, 1990.

Luks S: Gutta-percha versus silver points in the practice of endodontics, *NY State Dent J* 31:341, 1965.

Maisto OA, Erausquin J: Reacción de los tejidos periapicales del molar de la rata a las pastas de obturación reabsorbibles, *Rev Assoc Odontol Argent* 53:12, 1965.

Marlin J, Schilder H: Physical properties of gutta-percha when subjected to heat and vertical condensation, *Oral Surg* 36:872, 1973.

Marshall FJ, Massler M: The sealing of pulpless teeth evaluated with radioisotopes, *J Dent Med* 16:172, 1961.

Maurice CG, Kroeger AV, Krieger M: Antimicrobial activity of root canal sealing agents, *J Dent Med* 20:7, 1965.

McElroy DL: Physical properties of root canal filling materials, *J Am Dent Assoc* 50:433, 1955.

McElroy DL, Wach EC: Endodontic treatment with a zinc oxide–Canada balsam filling material, *J Am Dent Assoc* 56:801, 1958.

Michanowicz A, Czonstkowsky M, Piesco N: Low-temperature injection gutta-percha: a scanning electron microscopic investigation, *J Endod* 12:64, 1986.

Negm MM, Lilley JD, Combe EC: A study of the viscosity and working time of resin-based root canal sealers, *J Endod* 11:442, 1985.

Rappaport HM, Lily GE, Kapsimalis P: Toxicity of endodontic filling materials, *Oral Surg* 18:785, 1964.

Rising DW, Goldman M, Brayton SM: Histologic appraisal of three experimental root canal filling materials, *J Endod* 1:172, 1975.

Sakkal S, Weine FS, Lemian L: Lateral condensation: inside view, *Compend Contin Educ Dent* 12:796, 1991.

Schilder H: Filling root canals in three dimensions, *Dent Clin North Am,* Nov 1967, p 723.

Schilder HS: Vertical compaction of warm gutta-percha. In Gerstein H, editor: *Techniques in clinical endodontics,* Philadelphia, 1983, Saunders.

Schilder H, Goodman A, Aldrich W: The thermomechanical properties of gutta-percha. III. Determination of phase transition temperatures for gutta-percha, *Oral Surg* 38:109, 1974.

Stewart GG: A comparative study of three root canal sealing agents, *Oral Surg* 11:1029, 1174, 1958.

Sweet C Sr.: Procedures for treatment of exposed pulpless deciduous teeth, *J Am Dent Assoc* 17:1150, 1930.

Weine FS: The enigma of the lateral canal, *Dent Clin North Am* 28:833, 1984.

Weiner BH, Schilder H: A comparative study of important physical properties of various root canal sealers. I. Evaluation of setting times, *Oral Surg* 32:768, 1971.

Weiner BH, Schilder H: A comparative study of important physical properties of various root canal sealers. II. Evaluation of dimensional changes, *Oral Surg* 32:928, 1971.

Winford TE, Gutman JL, Henry CA: Microbiological evaluation of the Unitek Obtura heated gutta-percha delivery system, *J Endod* 13:351, 1987.

Zeldow LL: Pre-shaping of the gutta-percha master point by an internal impression method for precise obturation, *NY State Dent J* 41:286, 1975.

10 Solid-core canal filling materials: theory, technique, and re-treatment

When I was preparing this chapter for the fourth edition of this book in 1987, I wrote that solid-core filling materials (meaning silver cones) had fallen into disfavor, with few practitioners using them and virtually no dental schools teaching the technique. This was certainly true then and is still accurate. I further wrote, "I believe, however, that in the future an improved type of solid-core filling material will become available and will be used successfully in certain cases when an exacting technique is followed." This statement was proven to be most accurate within several years of that writing, as the Thermafil technique became widely used.

The other introductory remarks from the fourth edition are still accurate, with only slight revisions. When silver cones are involved in current endodontic therapy, it is to remove them during re-treatment and then reprepare and refill. However, successful re-treatment necessarily requires knowledge of how the technique was performed originally.

Therefore a condensed version of canal filling with silver cones will be presented in this chapter, followed by solid-core filling of middle-root fractures, and then suggested methods for re-treatment of solid-core filling failures. New material on the use of the Thermafil and Thermafil types of canal filling materials will be presented in the final segment of this chapter. The history and theories for solid-core fillings, still important as applicable in using Thermafil, will still be discussed.

HISTORY OF SOLID-CORE FILLINGS

The first solid-core filling materials were used unintentionally—they were endodontic instruments that separated within the canal. When the canal had been enlarged to at least some minimal size and the periapical tissues then were normal

prior to treatment, observation indicated that many cases involving instruments separating in the canal remained symptom free and normal radiographically. Generally these misadventures occurred in small curved canals, which had a poor prognosis in many cases at that time even using routine therapy. It certainly was not the desired form of therapy, but some of these cases remained comfortable and radiographically normal over very long periods. Extraction at the time of instrument fracture did not seem to be the correct treatment.

This prompted a number of dentists to separate instruments intentionally within the canal, usually in the presence of a root canal sealer, as a canal filling material. The typical technique involved use in a small curved canal where the apical enlargement was to a size 20 or 25. The shaft of the last instrument used (either file or reamer) in preparation was weakened with a bur short of the working length, sealer was placed in the canal, and then the instrument was forced apically and twisted. The file, or reamer, thus became the apical canal filling. Although most of these cases failed, some met with success (Fig. 10-1). In the cases of failure the metal tended to corrode after exposure to the periapical fluids, causing a dissolving of the filling and consequent loss of seal.

Even though the advent of stainless steel offered an instrument much less susceptible to corrosion, the use of an instrument has an inherent disadvantage. When the sealer is placed in the canal, the excess will collect in the flutes of the instrument rather than being forced against the canal walls to fill voids and discrepancies.

Gutta-percha had been used to fill canals for almost 100 years when silver points were introduced to endodontics in the 1930s. In attempts to fill small, thin, and/or curved canals, gutta-percha was very difficult to use. Since the enlargement needed for use of gutta-percha was frequently time consuming and tedious to obtain, many dentists tended to avoid endodontic treatment of teeth having canals difficult to enlarge, particularly the molars. Even when therapy was undertaken, many gutta-percha fillings were necessarily terminated considerably short of the apex. The search for a truly acceptable filling material that could be forced through a thin canal to a considerable depth continued until 1941 when Jasper introduced silver wires. Available in varying widths, with some relationship in size and shape to the enlarging instruments, silver points or cones, as they were later called, took the endodontic community by storm.

The total length of time required to treat complex cases was decreased, since the degree of enlargement needed for gutta-percha condensation was unnecessary. Operators were able to face difficult cases with greater confidence, since a new filling material was available for successful use in those canals not conducive to the use of gutta-percha.

Overuse of silver points. Unfortunately, as with any new and useful filling material, silver points were subjected to overuse; this led to inappropriate changes in therapy by some. Since smaller canals could be filled by silver points, often the degree of enlargement normally attainable in a given case was not reached. Sublimating the more important debridement procedures for the use of the easier filling material, many users of silver points felt justified in doing minimal enlargement. This led to frequent failures, since necrotic and pulpal debris and affected dentinal tubules were not removed; thus a nidus of irritated material was left to cause posttreatment periapical inflammation and failure. Additionally, incomplete preparation failed to gain a proper apical seat, needed to give a seal between the silver point and the canal walls.

Similarly, the solidly radiopaque appearance of the silver points compared with gutta-percha on the dental radiograph made it appear that a root canal was densely filled when the solid material was used. This could lead to a false security, since the silver point could merely thread rather than fill a canal and still appear satisfactory on a radiograph. Most teeth in the dental arch have root canals wider buccolingually than mesiodistally. However, routine dental radiographs show only the mesiodistal dimension. Therefore a canal could appear well filled from this vantage point,

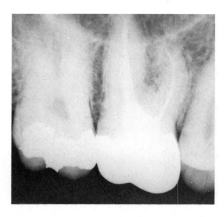

Fig. 10-1. Many years ago, endodontic files were purposely separated with a sealer in the canal as a filling material. This technique is no longer used and generally led to failure. The maxillary first molar shown was treated 4 years earlier with gutta-percha placed in the distobuccal and palatal canals and a stainless steel size 25 file in the mesiobuccal canal with Kerr's antiseptic sealer. The tooth was asymptomatic when the film was taken. (Restoration by Dr. Morton Rosen, Chicago.)

although a great deal of space would be noted if a proximal view were taken (Fig. 10-2).

Instead of following a meticulous preparatory and sealing technique, as is required in all endodontic procedures, it was believed by some that silver points provided a shortcut to success, which they did not.

Errors were made in choice of filling materials, which added to the burden of damage with silver point use. Silver points are round in cross section and perform best when filling canals that can be prepared to be round. The easiest canal to prepare round is the maxillary central incisor, but silver points were rarely, if ever, used there. The most difficult canal to prepare round is the single mesiobuccal canal of the maxillary first molar. At the zenith of their use, silver points were frequently used in those canals. Out-of-round canals were really contraindications for silver point use (Fig. 10-3).

Binding of silver points into dentin. Considerable discussion has revolved around the method by which silver points seal canals. It seems logical to assume that sealer is placed into a prepared canal and then the solid core point is forced apically, squeezing the sealer against the canal walls and sealing off the apical foramen. This action is

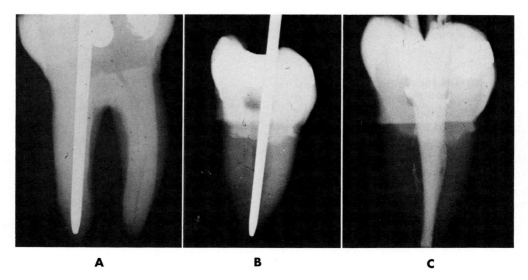

Fig. 10-2. **A,** Buccal view, mandibular molar with size 80 silver point in distal canal. Point seems to fill preparation completely. **B,** Mesial view of distal root, never seen in an actual clinical case. Radiolucencies adjacent to point disclose that preparation will not be completely filled in buccolingual dimension. **C,** Mesial view of same preparation filled with gutta-percha (lateral condensation technique). In this dimension canal is well filled. Note greater width of canal filling compared with that of silver point. The preparation used was not flared. If flaring were employed, an even greater discrepancy would be seen in **B,** and an even wider canal filling with gutta-percha in **C.**

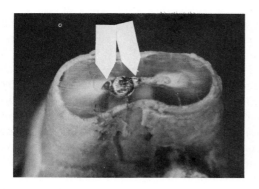

Fig. 10-3. Cross section of distal root of mandibular molar, 1 mm from apex. Canal was enlarged to size 60 and filled with a silver point of same width. Preparation was not perfectly round, and sealer was required to fill the eccentricities *(arrows)*.

similar to the placement of an inlay into a cavity preparation with oxyphosphate cement acting to fill the voids between the tooth and the casting.

However, it has been suggested that an actual bind of the point into the canal walls may take place. The Knoop hardness number of silver points is higher than that of dentin. Therefore it is possible that with the use of sufficient pressure the dentin may give slightly and grip the forced point. This is similar to the ductility of dentin allowing pounded gold foil to gain an actual grip into the cavity preparation.

Corrosion potential of silver points. Being metal, silver cones may corrode by oxidation to form a surface compound on the point of silver amine sulfate amide hydrate. This was reported in a scanning electron microscope and electron probe analysis study by Seltzer et al. Furthermore, using silver points from failing endodontic cases, Seltzer et al. found that these cones had a cytotoxic effect on tissue culture, whereas fresh unused cones caused no damage.

Although deformation by cutting and trimming the silver points could cause the initiation of some of the corrosion noted, it was necessary to have some sulfur present to react with the silver to form the cytotoxic product. Sulfur is present in amino acids, heparin, thiamine, and other compounds in blood, cementum, bone, and saliva. Therefore the corrosive product probably resulted from an inadequate apical seal of the canal, an

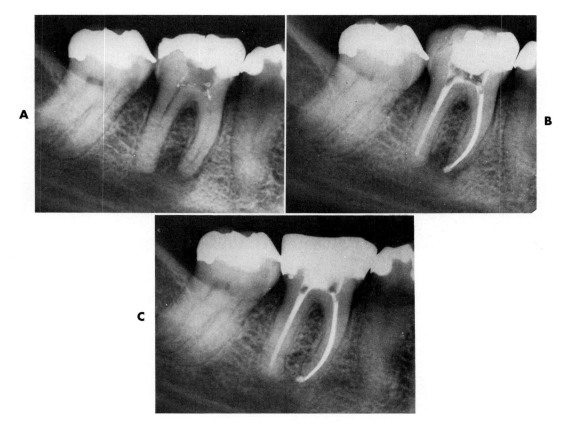

Fig. 10-4. Successful long-term cases utilizing silver points as canal filling material are shown in Figs. 10-4 to 10-11. **A,** Preoperative radiograph of mandibular first molar with large periapical radiolucency. **B,** After filling appointment. Distal canal filled with laterally condensed gutta-percha and mesial canals with silver points. Some sealer was expressed past apex. **C,** Five years postoperatively, perfect healing. (Restoration by Dr. Gerald Jaffee, formerly of Olympia Fields, Ill.)

overextension of the cone into the periapical tissues, or an improper coronal seal. If the canal were truly sealed at both ends by a cone completely within the canal, it is questionable whether the high degree of corrosion could exist or cause the type of reaction reported. Since this reaction unquestionably could occur, it was important that great care be used when silver cones were utilized to ensure that the filling material remain within the canal. However, the termination point of canal preparation for most dentists between 1942 and 1965, when silver points were enjoying their most usage, overwhelmingly was to the radiographic apex. Even though some dentists still use the radiographic apex as reference point for canal filling (see Chapter 8), present-day dentists are filling with some form of gutta-percha as master cone. Overextension of that material will not cause a cytotoxic reaction. When silver points were

placed so that the tip of the filling was to the radiographic apex, the silver was unquestionably in contact with the periapical tissues and thus susceptible to development of the silver amine sulfate amide hydrate corrosion product.

Evaluation of well-treated silver point cases. Because of problems with corrosion and many long-term failures, silver points fell out of favor in the endodontic community. Although these were not truly a fair reason for change, there has been a concomitant improvement in preparation and gutta-percha filling techniques that has enhanced the utilization of the semisolid filling materials. The silver point cases that failed, in general, were those that were poorly treated. Poorly treated gutta-percha cases will have too high a percentage of failures as well.

Many cases using silver points have lasted well and saved teeth, whereas treatment might not have been successful with the prevalent preparation and

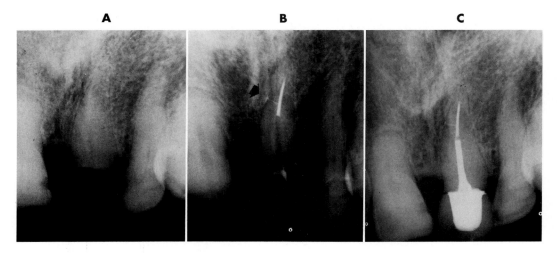

Fig. 10-5.   A, Preoperative radiograph of maxillary central incisor broken off at gingival margin. **B,** Canal filled with sectioned silver point. Note sealer forced into lateral canal *(arrow).* **C,** Four years after treatment, area has remained normal. (Restoration by Dr. Don Hackman, formerly of Chicago.)

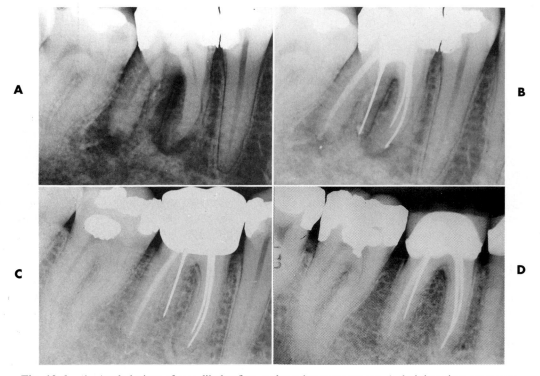

Fig. 10-6.   A, Angled view of mandibular first molar prior to treatment. A draining sinus tract was present in the furcation, and a pocket could be probed to the apex of the mesial root. This case was originally shown in the section on treating endo/perio problems in the first edition of this textbook. **B,** The distal canal was filled with laterally condensed gutta-percha, whereas the distolingual and both mesial canals were filled with silver points. The sinus tract had healed soon after canal preparation. **C,** Nineteen years after original treatment. **D,** Twenty-seven years after original treatment, crown has been changed, but all radiolucencies have healed, no sinus tract is present, and no probing is possible.

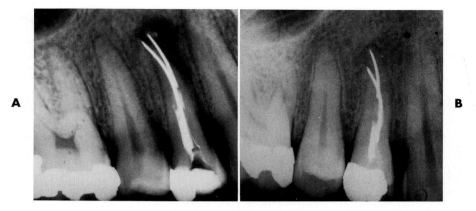

Fig. 10-7. **A,** Maxillary first bicuspid filled with sectioned silver points. Extensive radiolucency involved almost half of the mesial portion of the roots. **B,** Three years after treatment, areas have healed perfectly.

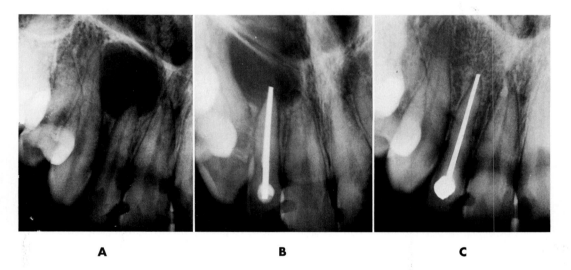

Fig. 10-8. **A,** Preoperative radiograph of maxillary lateral incisor with extensive periapical radiolucency. **B,** Canal was filled with a silver point. At the time of treatment, November 1957, the technique for sectioning of silver points was unknown. Because of persistent positive cultures, 12 appointments were required for treatment, but no surgery was performed. **C,** Film taken in May 1975, 18 years after original treatment. The periapical area has healed perfectly and remained all this time in a normal condition.

filling techniques then in vogue. In these well-treated cases, if large radiolucencies were present prior to treatment, the lesions healed and the tissues remained normal (Figs. 10-4, 10-6, 10-7, 10-8, and 10-10). When the periapical tissues were normal prior to treatment, long-term postoperative views indicated the maintenance of the normalcy (Figs. 10-5, 10-9, and 10-11). These cases, and many others in this book, testify to the ability of silver cones to give desirable results when properly used. When canal preparation was carefully performed, a good seal obtained, and the cones retained within the canal, the result was frequently successful.

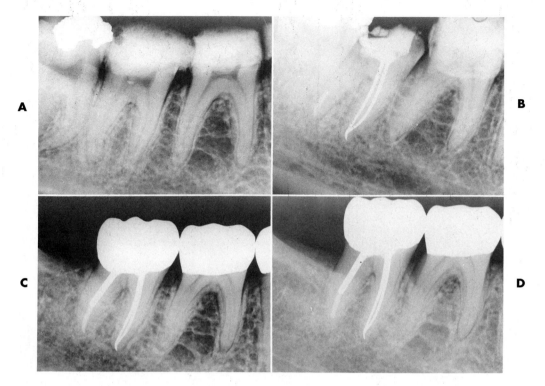

Fig. 10-9. **A,** Preoperative view of mandibular second molar requiring endodontic treatment. **B,** Angled view, immediately after canal filling. Distal canal was filled with laterally condensed gutta-percha (post room prepared) and mesial canals with silver points. The mesial canals merged short of the apex. **C,** One year later, tooth has been restored with post-and-core and crown. **D,** Eighteen years after original treatment, area has remained normal. (Restorations by Dr. Sherwin Strauss, Chicago.)

In some curved canals, an attempt to enlarge the preparation to a size large enough to use gutta-percha might lead to a severe alteration of original canal shape. Even when a well-condensed compressible material was used, the prognosis might be poor if the original apical portion of the canal was not closed by the final canal filling. Perhaps, if preparation were halted a size or two earlier and silver points were used, there would have been no need to use the less flexible, larger files and a desirable result would have occurred (Fig. 10-12).

Future for solid-core filling materials. There has been some effort to investigate new and efficacious solid-core filling materials that do not have corrosion potential. Among the tested materials with desirable results have been the titanium-aluminum-vanadium alloys, which have

been found to corrode as little as 176 times more slowly than stainless steel, and with minimal inflammatory potential. As the semisolid filling materials have increased in popularity, research in dentistry with the solid materials has been minimized. However, medical research continues in the area of implantology and orthopedics. In the future a new and better-tolerated solid endodontic filling material may again receive clinical acceptance.

TECHNIQUE FOR FILLING WITH SILVER POINTS

Readiness of the canal for filling. As discussed in the previous chapter, it must be determined that the canal is ready for filling. The criteria for readiness are the same when solid materials are to be used as they are when semisolids are the filling of choice.

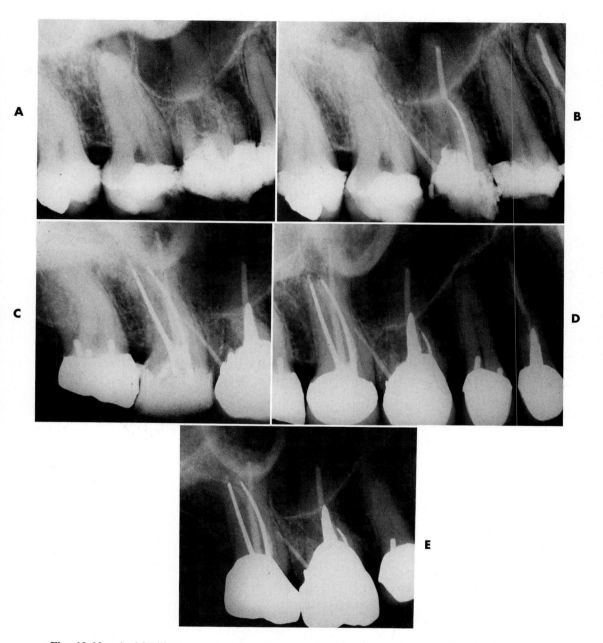

Fig. 10-10.   A, Maxillary posterior area, large excavations temporarily restored with zinc oxide–eugenol following pulp exposures of first and second molars. Large periapical area is present on palatal root of first molar. **B,** Endodontics completed on first molar, as palatal root is filled with gutta-percha and buccals with silver points. **C,** Endodontics completed on second molar, using same type of canal filling materials as were used in first molar. **D,** Five years postoperatively, all areas well healed. **E,** Seventeen years after treatment was initiated, third molar has been extracted but all other teeth continue to look excellent. (Restorations by Dr. Sherwin Laff, Chicago.)

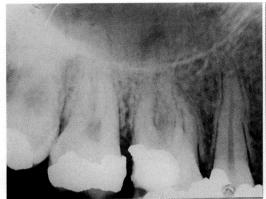

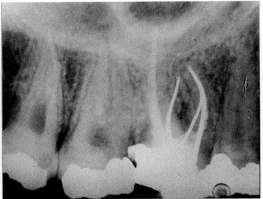

A

B

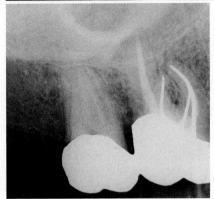

C

Fig. 10-11. **A,** Preoperative radiograph of maxillary molar area. The first molar has a very deep restoration, some caries, and a periapical lesion associated with the palatal root. **B,** Immediate postoperative film with three buccal canals filled with silver points and palatal canal filled with laterally condensed gutta-percha, all four canals with Kerr's Antiseptic Root Canal Sealer. This tooth was treated in 1967—one of the first cases I treated by filling four canals in a maxillary first molar. Note that the canal filling in the palatal root is relatively flat at the apex, indicating a slight overfill. **C,** Radiograph taken in 1994, 27 years after original treatment. The third molar has been extracted, but the configuration of the buccal fills indicates unmistakably that this is the same case. However, observe the configuration of the filling in the palatal root—it has been completely remodeled over all these years and has the appearance of the Washington Monument!

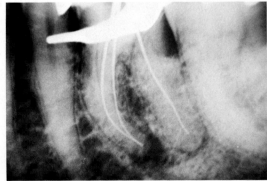

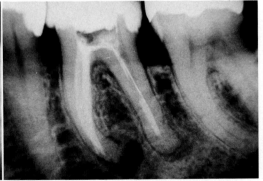

A

B

Fig. 10-12. **A,** Measurement radiograph of mandibular first molar, showing files in excellent position in mesial canals following the curves perfectly. **B,** Because the operator wanted to use gutta-percha, canals were enlarged to size 40. Stiffer instruments have altered the original canal shape severely and the tooth is now in jeopardy.

Before insertion of the trial points, some enlargement should be performed at the filling appointment. This final enlargement removes any dentin that has been softened by irrigants or medicaments retained between appointments. It also removes any temporary filling material that may have fallen into the preparation.

Armamentarium. The tray setup and additional materials necessary for use in filling with silver points are illustrated (Figs. 10-13 and 10-14), and a brief discussion of the pertinent instruments follows:

Silver point forceps or pliers—used to place forcibly the point to the most apical position in the canal prepara-tion; when improved silver points are used, these instruments are not necessary for insertion but should still be available

Silver point gauge—several types available, used to select a point that conforms approximately to width of the last enlarging instrument

Selection of silver points—desirable that all sizes commonly used be available, since variation may exist in sizes of enlarging instruments as well as points and since frequently the size anticipated for use is not the correct size finally determined as best

Mixing slab—presterilized by any accepted method and ready for use in the mixing of the sealer

Cement spatula—heavier and thicker than usual handle and mixing portion needed, since sealer for use with silver points is mixed very thickly

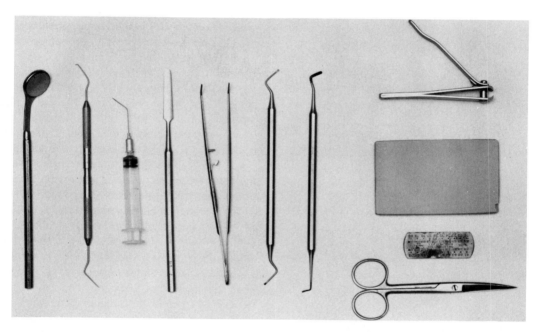

Fig. 10-13.   Tray setup for using silver points. *(from left)* Front surface mirror, endodontic explorer, irrigating syringe, cement spatula, locking cotton pliers, excavator, plastic instrument. *(at right, from top)* Silver point notcher, mixing slab, silver point gauge, scissors.

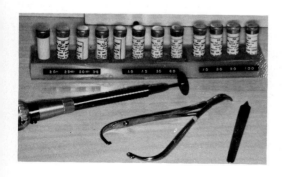

Fig. 10-14.   Additional materials needed for canal filling with silver points. *(at top)* Selection of silver points. *(at bottom, from left)* Slow-speed handpiece with Joe Dandy disk mounted, silver point pliers, metal fingernail file.

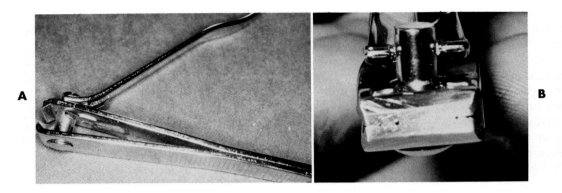

Fig. 10-15. **A,** Silver point notcher, made by modifying toenail clipper. **B,** When jaws of notcher are closed, serrations allow for weakening of silver point without cutting through completely.

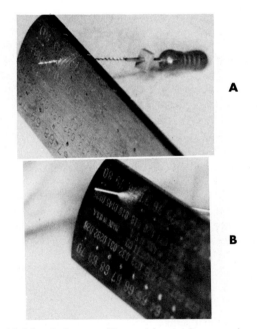

Fig. 10-16. **A,** Largest file used in canal preparation is placed with a hole in gauge so the tip protrudes a few millimeters. **B,** Silver point is selected that will protrude through same hole approximately the same distance.

Joe Dandy disk—mounted on a straight handpiece mandrel, to be used in giving apical taper to the silver point

Silver point notcher—for weakening the point when a sectional technique is used; may be made by modifying toenail clipper (Fig. 10-15) or be purchased already prepared for notching.

Selection of the trial point. The largest file used in preparing the apical portion of the canal is used also as a guide in selection of the trial silver point, since the diameter of the apical portion of this file will be only slightly smaller than the apical diameter of the preparation. The file is placed through one of the holes in the silver point gauge so that approximately 2 to 3 mm of the tip protrudes (Fig. 10-16, *A*). If a gauge is used that has been specifically manufactured for endodontic use, the holes in the gauge are marked with the appropriate standardized numbers.

When incremental instrumentation is employed in the smaller canals, the last used file may not conform well to any of the holes if standardized sizes only are provided for.

However, a machinist's gauge is satisfactory, is generally much less expensive, and has a greater number of holes in the smaller sizes, where silver points are most frequently used. The numbers on a gauge of this type do not refer to the metric system, on which standardized sizes are based. Therefore, before this type of gauge is used for the first time, files of the smaller sizes, plus the commonly used incremental instrumentation files, should be placed in the various holes to determine metric system equivalents. Once the corresponding endodontic size has been identified for each hole, the correct designation may be engraved on the back side of the gauge, which comes unmarked, using a small round bur.

Once the correct hole for the file has been determined, the file is removed from the gauge and a silver point of the same size is selected and placed in the same hole (Fig. 10-16, *B*). If incremental instrumentation has been used and the largest file is not a manufactured size, the next smaller silver point is selected. By using the gauge, it immediately becomes obvious if the silver point will approximately fit the prepared canal.

If the silver point extends much farther through the hole than the file did, the point will fit the canal too loosely. This is rectified by clipping the tip off the point so approximately the same length of point protrudes through the same hole in the gauge as did the file.

If the point selected does not fit through the hole at all or just slightly through, the point is too wide and will not reach the apical portion of the preparation. If this occurs, another point should be selected that is the next size smaller, tried in the gauge, and if necessary modified until it protrudes the correct distance through the gauge.

It should be emphasized that this method is intended merely to ascertain if a point has approximately the same diameter as the canal preparation. The correctness of the fit must be determined by placement into the canal and verified by radiograph. Points that are obviously too wide or too narrow are never placed in the canal, since the gauge acts as a screening device to eliminate points of unsuitable diameter rapidly and simply.

Preparation of the trial point. If the canal preparation has been properly accomplished, a definite stop has been placed within solid dentin. Since the instruments used in canal preparation come to a point, this preparation also comes to a point. However, silver points that come from the manufacturer have either blunted or sharply flat-tened ends (Fig. 10-17, *A*). Obviously, such a point will not fit directly into a preparation that comes to a point. Additionally, points with sharply flattened ends may have tiny burs at the tip. When the point is placed into the prepared canal, these burs may catch on the side walls and cause a buckling or curling of the point. The burs may also catch dentin filings and pack them into the apical portion of the preparation, preventing complete seating of the point.

For this reason the apical portion of the point is beveled with a Joe Dandy disk mounted on a straight handpiece mandrel. With the silver point held at an angle, the disk is run at slow speed. The point is turned into it until a bevel approximately the same as the bevel of the enlarging instru-ment's tip is imparted (Fig. 10-17, *B*.). This, how-ever, does increase slightly the corrosion potential of the point.

Placement of the trial point. The method of placement that will be described here is for the conventional silver points that have been in use for many years. Notching and twist-off techniques will be discussed later.

The silver point that has now been determined by use of the gauge to be approximately the cor-rect size has been beveled with the Joe Dandy disk. The point is seized by the silver point pliers so that the beak of the pliers grasps the point at the length to which the canal has been prepared.

The point is placed into the prepared canal. Once the correct depth has been reached, which is indicated by the pliers' tip coinciding with the

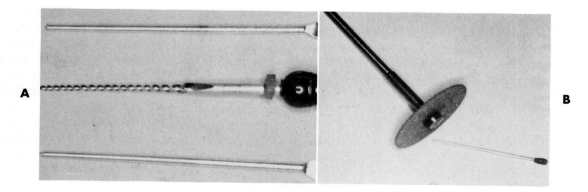

Fig. 10-17. A, Silver points are manufactured with a blunt tip *(top)*. However, because file used for canal enlargement comes to a point *(middle)*, so will preparation. Therefore silver point must be modi-fied to come to a point, too *(bottom)*. **B,** Joe Dandy disk is run at slow speed to impart a bevel to silver point. Note that point must be held at an angle to the disk.

reference cusp or incisal edge at the proper length, the degree of tightness of fit should be determined. When fitting properly, the point should require a definite pull of the pliers for removal and should completely resist removal by cotton pliers or fingers.

If the point is too easily removed, a 0.5 mm segment should be cut off the apical portion, the point rebeveled, and retried into the canal. This process should be repeated until the desired retention is obtained. When the gauge is used, this step is only rarely needed, but the tightness of the apical fit is important and must be verified in every case.

If the point does not stop at the correct depth but goes farther than the measured canal length, the point should be pushed until binding is felt and then be regrasped by the pliers adjacent to the reference cusp or incisal edge. It is obvious that no apical stop is present and the point is passing into the periapical tissue, a very undesirable situation. The correct procedure now is to recalculate the working length, reprepare the canal to a wider size creating an apical stop, and utilize gutta-percha as the canal-filling material.

If the point does not reach the desired penetration, further slight apical preparation generally will allow the distance to be reached. If that becomes difficult, a new point—one size smaller than that previously used—should be selected, adjusted by use of the gauge, beveled, and tried for fit.

Once a point has been tried in and found to have good retention at the desired depth, a radiograph should be taken to verify the apical position. In multirooted teeth where silver points are to be used in more than one canal, one pliers is needed for each canal. After each point is fitted, it is set aside while being held at the correct length in the pliers until all the points are ready, at which time all are replaced for the radiograph. In mandibular molars two radiographs should be taken, with angles similar to those used in the taking of measurement x-ray films for determining the initial canal length, as discussed in Chapter 8 (Fig. 10-18).

If the radiograph shows that the silver point does not reach the desired position near the apex but is at the measured depth, further canal enlargement should be performed to the corrected length. This requires going back to the smaller files and reenlarging the apical portion until a silver point is obtained that does reach the proper position. In some cases, particularly when the canal has a curvature, the small files are unable to

reach the corrected length but are halted by the ledge produced by the original preparation. In those cases it is best to increase the width of the preparation to a minimum of size 30 and use gutta-percha with lateral condensation as the filling method for superior sealing qualities compared with a silver point.

Filling the canal. After a satisfactory fit has been verified, the silver point—or points in multiple canals—while being retained in pliers at the correct length, is set aside. The canals are dried with paper points to remove any remaining irrigant; then the canals are irrigated with 95% alcohol and again dried with paper points to desiccate the dentinal tubules.

Rickert's formula, available as Kerr's Antiseptic Root Canal Sealer, is the preferred sealer for use with silver points. Although a 1:1 powder-to-liquid ratio is used with gutta-percha, for silver points the ratio should be thickened to 2:1. The thicker sealer is necessary for filling voids and discrepancies that are not filled by the solid materials. Also, the solid filling materials may be forced through the thicker mass, which is not possible with the softer gutta-percha. A very heavy cement spatula is needed to spatulate this thicker mix.

A reamer one size smaller than the last enlarging instrument used, with the correct canal length marked with a suitable stop or marker, is dipped into the mass of sealer (Fig. 10-19) and placed into the canal with a counterclockwise rotation. This coats the prepared walls, particularly in the apical portion. Two applications of sealer are usually necessary to coat the walls properly.

A small amount of sealer is placed on the tip of the silver point. The point is firmly placed into the canal until it reaches its apical seat. If multiple canals are to be filled, the same procedure is followed for each. If any question exists as to the proper placement of any point, a radiograph may be taken with the rubber dam still in place and the occlusal portion of the point still protruding up into the access so that the point may be easily removed, if necessary.

Final temporary filling with silver points. A cotton pellet is dipped into xylene and wiped around the floor of the chamber to remove any excess sealer. This sealer might cause discoloration and prevent complete gripping of the cement placement that follows. Excess xylene is volatilized by a blast from the air syringe.

A thick mix of oxyphosphate cement is prepared and forced into the chamber so the cement

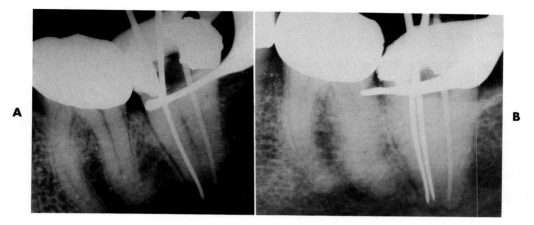

Fig. 10-18. Two radiographs taken to verify positions of cones for sealing mandibular molar. **A,** Straight-on view shows position of gutta-percha cone in distal root, but silver points in mesial root are superimposed. **B,** Angled view shows positions of silver points in mesial root.

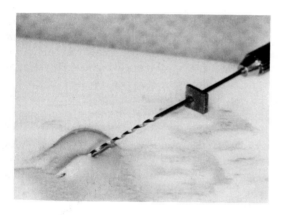

Fig. 10-19. Reamer one size smaller than largest file used is dipped into mix of Rickert's formula (Kerr's Antiseptic Root Canal Sealer) root canal sealer. For use with silver points, thick mix has approximately 2:1 powder-to-liquid ratio.

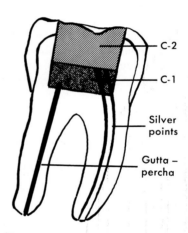

Fig. 10-20. Diagram of mandibular molar at conclusion of canal filling appointment. Distal canal was filled with gutta-percha, and two mesial canals were filled with silver points. Entire chamber was filled with oxyphosphate cement, and after set the excess points and cement were removed with a no. 37 inverted cone bur to slightly short of floor chamber *(C-1).* Fresh batch of cement was used to close access opening *(C-2).* This is merely a temporary restoration and must be replaced by full cuspal coverage.

completely surrounds the point. Once the cement has set, the excess point protruding through the access preparation is clipped with sharp scissors. By means of a sharp no. 37 inverted cone bur in high speed, the silver point and its surrounding cement are removed with a brush stroke to slightly short of the chamber floor. Once this has been accomplished, a fresh batch of cement is mixed and placed in the preparation (Fig. 10-20).

The occlusion must be carefully checked with articulating paper after the second placement of cement. Teeth are often tender to percussion after

canal filling, and this would be severely accentuated in the present of a high temporary filling. Also, contact points should be checked and any excess temporary material removed to guard against periodontal damage in the interim before a restoration is placed.

Two final radiographs should be taken and carefully examined to make sure that a desirable result has been obtained. The patient should be advised that slight pain, particularly to percussion, is normal and no cause for concern. If a considerable amount of sealer has been extruded past the apex, particularly in cases where normal periapical tissue was present preoperatively, the patient should be given a prescription for moderate relief of pain.

Suitable arrangements are made for restoration, as outlined in Chapter 9.

IMPROVED SILVER POINTS

Improved silver points were developed and introduced into endodontics by me in 1968—shortly before silver points fell into disrepute. These improved points were easier to use in routine cases and much easier to use with various types of sectional procedures (see next segment of this chapter) than the types of points previously available. Although they are no longer manufactured, some still exist deep in the drawers of endodontic offices. A condensed version of their use follows.

Specifications. Improved silver points differ from the conventional points described earlier in this chapter in that they resemble the enlarging instrument of corresponding size as closely as possible. Therefore the point has a color-coded plastic handle attached at 25 mm from the tip and has a standardized taper, which is equivalent to that of the enlarging instrument (so $D_0 + 0.32$ mm $= D_{16}$) and extends 16 mm up the shaft of the point (Figs. 7-7 and 10-21).

Advantages. Conventional silver points are inserted with pliers or a hemostat, which is held in the operator's hand. This differs from the method of insertion of the enlarging instruments, which are held in the more sensitive fingers. If the silver point being placed by pliers encounters an obstruction, curvature, or irregularity, forceful apical pressure will often cause a buckling or bending of the point (Fig. 10-22). With the improved silver point these hazards are immediately felt by the fingers, and a slight back-and-forth rotation along the long axis of the point will frequently enable the problem to be bypassed and the apex reached.

Additionally, the force needed for seating with pliers is not applied along the long axis of the point but merely parallel to it. Only a method of insertion similar to the digital placement of any enlarging instrument distributes the forces along the long axis. Point placement along the long axis allows greater pressure to be developed at the tip of the point than when the pressure is applied parallel to the long axis. Clinically this means that an extremely thick sealer may be used without fear of preventing the point from reaching its intended seat. Also, because of the greater pressure that may be used to seat the improved silver point, the factor of difference in hardness between the point and the dentin is taken advantage of. With the greater pressure the point may force its penetration into the softer dentin walls so that the latter actually gain a grip on the point.

The angle for insertion of the point when pliers are used differs from the angle of insertion for

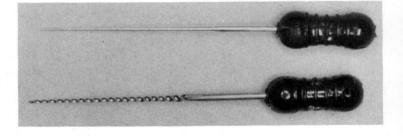

Fig. 10-21. Improved silver point *(top)* has same size, shape, and handle as file of corresponding size *(bottom)*.

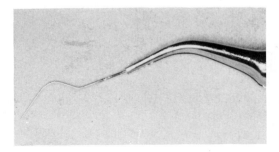

Fig. 10-22. Forceful apical pressure may buckle a silver point being inserted by pliers or hemostat.

placing the instruments used in canal preparation. This is an important factor in treating molars, in which the angle of insertion is tricky to reproduce consistently. However, by the time sufficient enlargement is gained so that the canal is ready for filling, this angle has been mastered. When the improved silver points are used, this same angle of insertion is utilized for point placement.

Since the handles of the improved silver points are color coded, the size is immediately recognizable. These points are extremely adaptable and are especially suitable for the sectional or twist-off method, which will be described next.

SECTIONAL OR "TWIST-OFF" TECHNIQUE

Problems of gaining room for a post. It is mandatory that posterior teeth be restored with complete cuspal coverage after endodontic therapy. Anterior teeth should be restored with jacket crowns after endodontic treatment when caries or proximal restorations are present. The use of a core in connection with the restoration of choice is optional. The core may utilize some sort of post or dowel extending into the root canal. When the root canal has been filled with gutta-percha, it is a simple matter to remove a sufficient portion of the filling material to allow for dowel placement. This may be accomplished by using a heated plugger or a suitable solvent and then enlarging the space with reamers.

However, if the canal is filled with a silver point, neither heat nor solvents will have any effect. Some of the cervical portion of the point may be removed by using a high-speed bur. Since the distance between the bur flutes and the head of the handpiece rarely is long enough to prepare a sufficient depth of dowel space, this method is seldom satisfactory. Also, with this method, it is possible that the flutes of the bur may catch the silver point and loosen or even whip it from the canal. Using a bur within the canal may be very hazardous, since a root perforation may occur if the bur fails to follow the outline of the canal and veers off into the dentin.

Indications for sectional technique. The treatment plan may not call for the use of a post-and-core type of restoration for the treated tooth. However, there is always the possibility that a post and core may be needed at some later date. This may occur if a new carious lesion develops, if a portion of the tooth fractures, if the treated tooth becomes a bridge or partial denture abutment, or in any other case where greater retention within the tooth

is needed. To provide for such a contingency, whenever a silver point is used in a single-root tooth, a twist-off or sectional technique should be utilized. If silver points are used to fill all the canals in a posterior tooth, a sectional technique should be used in at least one canal to allow for that canal's carrying a post, if needed. In molars the canal selected for the twist-off is generally the largest: the palatal canal in maxillary molars and the distal canal in mandibular molars.

Technique. Selection, preparation, and verification of apical fit for a trial point are obtained in the same manner as for a conventional case. The sectional method has been described, with the silver point pliers or hemostat used as the instrument to perform the twisting off. However, these instruments are bulky and difficult to use in posterior teeth.

Unless improved silver points are being used, it is suggested that measurement control handles, which are called test handles by some manufacturers, be used to replace the bulkier pliers. Once the apical fit has been determined to be satisfactory, the handle is attached to the point at the verified canal length (Fig. 10-23, *A*). A set of measurement control handles always comes with a tightening wrench. This wrench must be used to tighten the point to the handle securely at the correct length so no slippage is possible when pressure is used to force the point to its correct seat in the apical portion of the canal. At this point the silver cone and handle combination acts exactly the same as an improved silver point.

The point notcher (Fig. 10-15) is used to cut partially through and weaken the silver point at the desired position (Fig. 10-23, *B*). As manufactured, the notcher has four slots to accommodate various point widths. A little practice will soon enable the user to recognize which notch is correct to use for each of the point sizes.

The sealer is mixed and placed in the canal in the same manner as previously described. The tip of the notched point is dipped into the sealer mass, and the point is forced with apical pressure to its seat (Fig. 10-23, *C*). By having the handle or marker set at the correct canal length, the operator is constantly aware of the distance to the apex. Once the correct depth is reached, the handle or marker will be contacting the reference cusp or incisal edge. With continuing apical pressure the handle is rotated until a decrease in resistance to the rotation is felt. This indicates

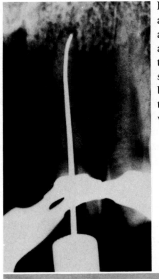

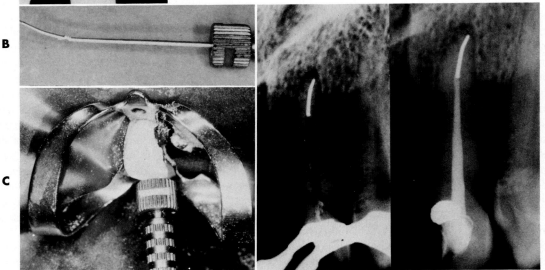

Fig. 10-23. **A,** Radiograph used to verify apical fit of silver point attached to measurement control handle. **B,** Point is weakened by notcher at junction of middle and apical thirds of root. Note precurving of point and apical bevel. **C,** Point is inserted to its apical seat. Handle is now twisted to gain separation. **D,** Radiograph confirms correct position of the sectioned point. **E,** After sectioning of point, the remainder of canal has been filled with gutta-percha. When tooth is restored with a post and core type of crown, much of gutta-percha will be removed with a hot instrument without disturbing apical seal.

that the apical portion has separated. If any doubt exists as to the position of the sectioned segment, a radiograph may be taken to verify the correctness (Fig. 10-23, *D*).

Determination of position for notching. Indications for using the sectional silver point method anticipate the need for a portion of the root canal space to accommodate a dowel or post. For that reason, before the silver point is notched, a calculation is made to determine what length of canal must be made available for the dowel. Although there are several methods for determining this length, a relatively simple way is to measure the length of the clinical crown and use this as the minimal dowel length. In long-rooted teeth a calculation of one and one-half times the length of the clinical crown is even more desirable, but this is a maximum.

In most cases, using the length of the clinical crown as the desired dowel length will coincide with using the cervical two thirds of the root for the dowel and confining the silver point to the apical third of the root. The only instances in which this method does not work satisfactorily occur when teeth have shorter than average roots or when the crown-root ratio has been considerably altered by periodontal disease. In these cases, using the length of the clinical crown as a guide for the length of the dowel room may reveal that the dowel needs to be longer than the root canal filing, which is, of course, an impossibility. Therefore a compromise must be worked out whereby the available dowel room length is decreased and the silver point is confined to the apical one fourth or one fifth of the root.

As a general rule, most cases will be satisfactory if the total root length is determined and divided by three and the quotient is used as the distance from the tip of the point where the notching is to be placed.

Use of twist-off to terminate at chamber floor. A twist-off technique may be utilized to amputate the point within the canal near the floor of the chamber when the need for a dowel is absent. This can be particularly useful when the buccal canals of maxillary molars and the mesial canals of mandibular molars are filled with silver points while the large canal in each tooth is filled with gutta-percha and will retain a dowel. The smaller canals need not retain a dowel, but using a sectional technique with their filling saves the step of packing the chamber with cement and amputating the point with a bur.

Where desired, the notching is placed at a point corresponding to the floor of the chamber. The technique for sealer and point placement is identical to that described for confining the point to the apical third, except that the point separates even with the chamber floor. No gutta-percha need be packed above or adjacent to the point.

Finishing and temporization. If a post-and-core type of crown is to be constructed after completion of the endodontic therapy, the preparation for the post is best made immediately after placement of the sectioned point by the dentist performing the endodontic treatment, who is the most familiar with the angulation and width of the canal. This minimizes the chances for perforation in preparing the post room at a later date. For use with the Endopost, Endowel, or similar techniques, reamers are used to enlarge the unfilled portion of the canal to a minimum of size 80. The length and width of the post preparation must be recorded on the patient's record so that the information will be available when the time comes for placement of the post. If the endodontic therapy is performed on a referral basis, this information is sent to the referring dentist, together with the preoperative and postoperative radiographs.

An easy-to-remove temporary filling should be employed with these cases, since the entire temporary seal will soon be removed at the time that the post-core and crown are prepared. To accomplish this, cotton is placed over the canal orifice, and cement is used to close the access preparation. Easy to remove, cement allows for mastication and prevents packing of food into the endodontic opening.

If a post-and-core type of restoration is not to be used after endodontic therapy, but the sectional method has been employed to provide for the contingency of such a restoration at a later date, a different method of finishing is employed. Rather than leave a large segment of the canal completely unfilled, gutta-percha is laterally condensed to fill the remaining canal space (Fig. 10-23, *E*). Since the total canal length has been decreased by the presence of the sectioned silver point, a new working length must be calculated by inserting a file into the canal until it butts against the point, adjusting the stop or marker to the reference cusp or incisal edge, and then measuring the new length. This segment is enlarged to a minimum of size 40 and then filled with a master gutta-percha cone with lateral condensation of auxiliary cones. A verification radiograph of the master cone is unnecessary as long as the cone reaches the adjusted working length. The excess gutta-percha is removed by a hot plastic instrument, and any suitable temporary filling material is placed to close the access preparation. A final radiograph is taken and arrangements made for restoration.

TREATMENT OF FRACTURES OF MIDDLE THIRD OF ROOT

Therapy for horizontal fractures of the root always involves considerable difficulty. Endodontic treatment is not indicated if the fracture sites remain in proximity and if the pulp retains its vitality. However, if clinical symptoms develop or the segments appear to be separating according to the radiograph, some treatment is needed.

Fractures of the apical third requiring therapy are treated surgically (Chapter 11). If a cervical third fracture needs treatment, the supragingival segment of the tooth is removed, alveoloplasty or orthodontic extrusion (Chapter 14) is performed with endodontic therapy, and the tooth is restored with a post, core, and jacket crown.

Fractures of the middle third have long been considered hopeless, since surgical removal of the apical segment creates an undesirable crown-root ratio, whereas too little is left to support a jacket crown if the coronal portion is removed. However, the use of an endodontic stabilizer will enable such teeth to be retained for many years, thus avoiding the use of a removable partial denture or the hazardous abutment preparation for fixed replacement (Figs. 10-24 to 26).

Local anesthetic is administered and the rubber dam applied. The working length is established and the canal prepared. In relatively straight canals, the apical portion may be enlarged several sizes more than in routine cases, that is, to five or six sizes larger than the initial apical file, rather than only three sizes. In these straight canals, reaming action may be used to produce a relatively round preparation. In canals with initial apical curvature, routine enlargement of the apical area is correct. Incremental instrumentation is used so minimal binding of the files occurs. If the file binds too tightly, the use of reaming may tend to separate the segments further. After completion of preparation, sterile cotton is placed as dressing and the access sealed with zinc oxide–eugenol.

The patient is seen 1 to 4 weeks later. Anesthesia is obtained. The rubber dam is applied and the dressing removed. Minimal rasping will remove

any residual debris and freshen up canal walls. A properly fitting master gutta-percha cone is obtained using a customized cone method (Chapter 9) if wide enough, and is verified by radiograph. The canal is filled with the lateral condensation method, at least to the level of the junction of the middle and cervical thirds of the root, that is, well past the fracture line. Then a heated hand spreader is used to remove the gutta-percha in a manner similar to making room for a post. Three to five millimeters of gutta-percha should remain at the apex, and the canal should now be empty from a site in the middle of the fractured segment to the access. Some combination of softened gutta-percha and sealer may extrude through the fracture site.

The empty portion of the canal is reprepared to a minimum of size 100. A chrome-cobalt pin—the same size as the last file used—is selected, and the apical portion is beveled with a Joe Dandy disk. It is sterilized in the salt sterilizer while being held in a hemostat, cooled in alcohol, and then tried in the preparation. If the pin is too loose, 0.5 mm segments of the apical portion of the alloy are removed until binding is obtained. If the pin is too tight, further enlargement is performed or a smaller pin is selected. It is quite important that the pin bind into both the apical and the cervical

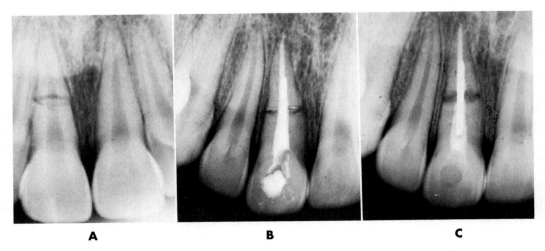

A   **B**   **C**

Fig. 10-24. A, Maxillary central incisor with fracture of middle third of root and mobility of coronal segment. **B,** Canal was filled with gutta-percha and lateral condensation. Then all but apical few millimeters of the filling was removed with a heated Luks plugger. Canal was further enlarged and a chrome-cobalt alloy pin placed to immobilize segments. **C,** Two years later the tooth is much tighter, and both apical and lateral areas appear normal. Note increased deposition of apical cementum. (Restoration by Dr. Fred Hill, River Forest, Ill.)

segments so that true support is obtained. A radiograph is taken to verify the fit of the pin and the binding into both segments.

Once the desired fit is confirmed, the procedure for seating is similar to that used for a silver point twist-off. The pin is severely weakened with an inverted cone bur at a point corresponding to the middle of the cervical segment of the root. A very thick mix of Kerr's Antiseptic Root Canal Sealer is prepared and placed into the desiccated and dried portion of the canal with a reamer. The pin is inserted to its apical seat, and then a twist-off-

procedure is performed. The remaining segment of the pin is used as a plugger to ensure correct depth of placement, a suitable temporary is placed, and a radiograph is taken (Fig. 10-24, *B,* and 10-25, *B*).

Periodic radiographs should indicate that the segments remain in proximity (Fig. 10-24, *C*) and that no lateral or apical areas of rarefaction develop. Ideal healing is seen when a cementoid callus around the fracture site (Fig. 10-25, *D* and Fig. 10-26, *C*) appears, which is known as cementogenic repair.

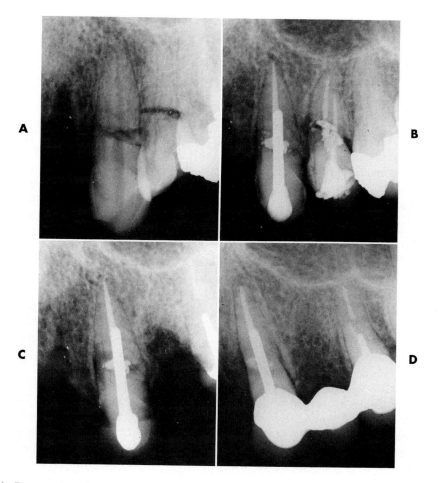

Fig. 10-25. **A,** Preoperative view of maxillary cuspid and first bicuspid area, demonstrating midroot fractures on both teeth. Both teeth were tender to percussion and mobile. **B,** Postoperative view. Cuspid (no. 11) was filled apically with laterally condensed gutta-percha and a chrome-cobalt pin used to stabilize the sections. First bicuspid (no. 12) was also filled with laterally condensed gutta-percha, but no stabilizer was placed. **C,** Nine months later, no. 11 has stabilized and is tight and asymptomatic. No. 12 continued to be sore and the coronal portion was still mobile, so it was extracted. **D,** Seven years after original treatment, cementogenic repair is apparent, particularly on the distal portion of no. 11. It acts as the anterior abutment of a fixed bridge and the posterior abutment of a removable partial denture. (Restorations by Dr. Robert Wheeler, Chicago.) (From Weine FS, Wenckus CS: *CDS Rev* 79:33, 1985.)

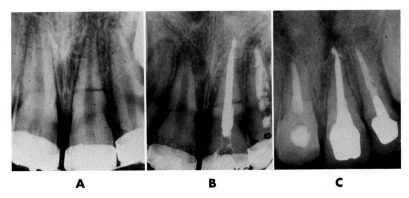

Fig. 10-26. **A,** Fracture in middle third of root in right central incisor accompanied by clinical symptoms requiring endodontic treatment. Removal of apical segment to place implant would leave too little remaining tooth structure. **B,** Chrome-cobalt alloy pin is used to fill canal and provide stabilization of segments. **C,** Eighteen months postoperatively the segments are close, and it appears that a cementum-like callus has formed across fracture site. Trauma that caused root fracture also resulted in need for endodontic treatment of adjacent teeth. (From Weine FS, Altman A, Healey HJ: *J Dent Child* 38:215, 1971.)

This method replaces the previously used technique whereby the alloy pin acts as both the apical canal filling and the stabilizer (Fig. 10-26). The use of gutta-percha provides for the better sealing material in the apical portion and allows for increased central preparation to use the stronger stabilizer.

THERMOPLASTIC SEMISOLID + SOLID-CORE = THERMAFIL*†

It could be a humorous television commercial. A dentist is working in his office in a large metropolitan medical building. He is trying to get a small gutta-percha cone into a curved canal of a mandibular molar without success and is obviously becoming agitated. He thinks, "Why isn't there a way to put something solid into this cone so I can get it to place?"

Across the hall in another office, another dentist is treating another mandibular molar. By using a silver cone, she has gotten her filling to the root tip, but, in fact, she has pushed it slightly too far, with the tip of the cone in the periapex. She, too, is

now agitated, and thinks, "Why isn't there a way to put some gutta-percha on the tip of this cone so that a slight overfill would still be well tolerated by the body?"

Ta da! Through their respective windows, in flies the answer—Thermafil—the marriage of a solid-center central obturator with gutta-percha completely surrounding that portion to be placed into the canal.

Of course, another solution to this scenario would be for the dentist to use some of the techniques described in Chapter 8 for preparation of curved canals. But Thermafil was introduced to combine the best properties of both the semisolid and solid-core filling materials and many teeth have been saved because of its availability (Fig. 10-27).

History. After using it in his practice for several years, W. Ben Johnson of Tulsa, Oklahoma, published an article in the *Journal of Endodontics* in 1978 describing this technique. He used the widest endodontic file to the tip of his preparation (MAF), coated it with heated, softened gutta-percha, and placed it into the prepared canal that had been coated with sealer.

Johnson was trained in graduate school at Baylor University, where silver points were used predominantly, but he was also well versed in the use of gutta-percha. He knew that gutta-percha was superior to silver cones for sealing and was better tolerated by the body, but he also was conversant

*Tulsa Dental Products, Tulsa, OK 74136.

†I acknowledge the assistance of Mark Oliver, CEO of Tulsa Dental Products, in the development of the material on Thermafil. I thank Dr. W. Ben Johnson, Tulsa, Oklahoma, for his kindness in allowing me to use his cases to illustrate Thermafil treatments, shown as Figs. 10-35 through 10-38. Teeth shown in Fig. 10-28 were definitely *not* treated by Dr. Johnson!

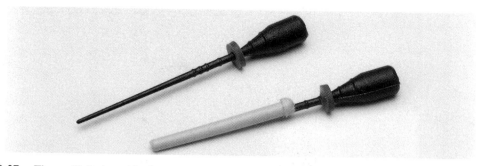

Fig. 10-27.   Thermafil device with plastic obturator *(top)* and gutta-percha added *(bottom)*. The obturator, even when plastic is used, still is stiff enough to force the device into small, curved, properly prepared canals. When the gutta-percha is heated to the correct temperature and remains apical to the plastic, the softened mass will produce apical sealing of the preparation in combination with the sealer.

with the ability of silver cones to traverse through small canals more easily and to have better length control. He believed that this new development could combine the best of both worlds.

For the most part, very little interest was paid to this technique, and it gained only a small number of adherents. Then, in 1989, a company was formed to manufacture and distribute this product, which was named Thermafil (it is also distributed as Densfil*). Immediately it received wide attention and interest, particularly among general practitioners.

Basis for success. Because of the ease with which it could be placed into the canal, abuse of Thermafil did occur, very similarly to what happened with silver points (Fig. 10-28). Some dentists minimized or misapplied the canal preparation procedures, others failed to understand the theory of its method to seal with the gutta-percha, and some failed to practice the technique sufficiently before using it in clinical cases. For these reasons, some serious failures occurred, which made some members of the dental community very opposed to its use.

Johnson and others from Tulsa Dental made a number of refinements in the technique. The metal core was replaced by a plastic core (Fig. 10-29) that allowed post room to be made more simply and re-treatment, if necessary, to be performed more easily, particularly in the larger sizes. Courses were given that emphasized canal preparation and offered tips on usage. A specific sealer was suggested for use and sold with the product (Fig. 10-30). For new users, plastic

blocks were recommended for practice prior to use on patients.

A very important element for successful Thermafil use is to learn to insert the handle so that the gutta-percha always remains apical to the obturator. The canal can be filled successfully by the softened gutta-percha. Sealing by the obturator alone, if pushed through the gutta-percha, is much less likely. By using the plastic blocks, new adherents to the technique could learn the methods for insertion of the obturators to ensure that this could happen.

A particularly important innovation was the introduction of the ThermaPrep oven* (Fig. 10-31). When first introduced, the devices were to be heated over a Bunsen burner. One of three things could happen, two of which were bad. The gutta-percha was supposed to be heated by rotation in the heat until a shiny coat developed on the gutta-percha. If it were not heated sufficiently before placement, the obturator did not go to place and the metal would push through the gutta-percha. This made the entire unit unusable, and it had to be discarded.

A new unit was taken, and obviously this time the dentist would be certain to heat it enough, and might tend to overheat, causing the gutta-percha to conflagrate, again becoming unusable. Only the exact amount of heat, not easy to obtain with the Bunsen burner, produced a desirable result.

The introduction of the oven now enables the operator to have a consistently reliable temperature of the obturator, giving the best chance for smooth, complete placement.

*Caulk Division/Dentsply, Milford, DE 19963.

*Tulsa Dental Products, Tulsa, OK 74136

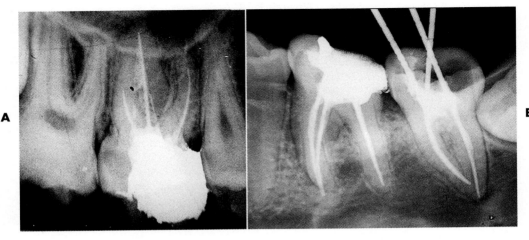

A

B

Fig. 10-28. Improper use of Thermafil. **A,** Maxillary first molar with Thermafil obturators used to complete case, but the patient now has symptoms of tenderness to percussion and temperature changes. The material has been used poorly, with only a size no. 25 filling used in the very wide palatal canal. Considerable working length has been lost in both buccal canals, and it appears that a second canal is present in the mesiobuccal root. **B,** Intrafilling film of the mandibular second molar. It appears that the gutta-percha has not been pushed ahead of the obturator in the distal canal, leading to potential failure in that root. In the first molar, filled a few days earlier, the obturators are apparent in the periapical tissues of the mesial root with straightening of the mesial canals and probable zipping of their apices. This tooth, too, is a potential failure. Of course, such results could occur with gutta-percha or silver points as canal filling materials with poor canal preparation and are not found in Thermafil cases only.

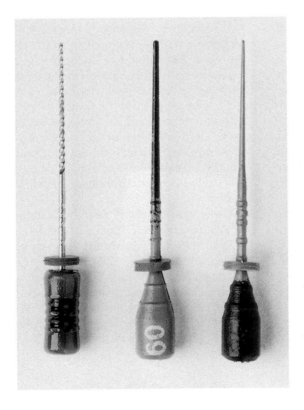

Fig. 10-29. Metal core for obturator (*left,* used in Fig. 10-28) has been replaced by plastic core to allow easier preparation of post room and retreatment, if needed. In the larger canals, the material used is a polysulfone polymer *(center)* and has several solvents. In the smaller canals, a stiffer material—liquid crystal polymer *(right)*—is used, which is resistant to solvents.

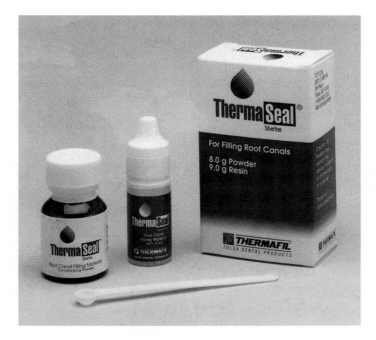

Fig. 10-30. ThermaSeal, using a resin-based liquid, is the preferred sealer for use with Thermafil, although other sealers may also be employed. This formula is very similar to AH-26, which is widely used in central Europe, often as a paste filler without core filling material, and has been widely investigated with good results.

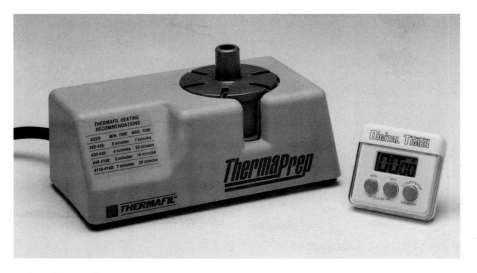

Fig. 10-31. ThermaPrep oven offers an excellent improvement to the formerly used heating by a Bunsen burner. When used according to directions, the gutta-percha portion of the obturator will be heated to the correct consistency, allowing proper placement and flow ahead of the carrier. It is wise to heat an extra obturator for each canal, in case a problem occurs during filling, after the sealer has already been placed. Heated but cooled obturators may be heated again without damage.

Size verification.   One of the deficiencies, as compared with stick gutta-percha, is that there is no way to test if the master cone fits properly and check by radiograph when using Thermafil. This is true for the other thermoplastic techniques (see Chapter 9), as well. For this reason, it was suggested in Chapter 9 that a finger spreader be fit, as it would be when using stick gutta-

percha, when using thermoplastics, so that the presence of an apical dentin matrix and removal of the elbow is verified prior to insertion of the softened mass.

For use with Thermafil, a size verification kit (Fig. 10-32) is available to perform this function. This kit is a collection of the plastic obturators only, without the gutta-percha portion. If the obtu-

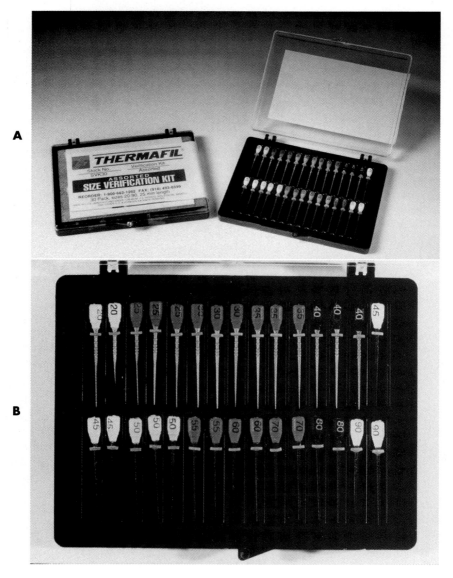

Fig. 10-32.   A, Size verification kit will allow the anticipated proper placement of obturator because radiograph of master cone in place (see Chapter 9) is not possible with Thermafil. This procedure is similar to placement of finger plugger prior to the fitting of master cone in lateral condensation cases. (See Fig. 10-35, *C.*) **B,** Kit contains several plastic carriers of each size from no. 20 through no. 90. In addition to placement of carrier of the same size as the MAF, it is suggested that a smaller verifier also be used to ensure that an apical dentin matrix is present to prevent over-filling of the carrier.

rator will seat into the apical millimeter of the preparation, then, it is assumed, the softened gutta-percha coating can be packed to the correct position. Fitting an obturator of the same size will provide this feature, but it might not verify the presence of an apical dentin matrix. To accomplish that purpose, it is suggested that a verification obturator two or three sizes smaller than the MAF be tried in. If this stops at the working length, the matrix is confirmed.

Importance of canal preparation. As stated a number of times in this textbook, canal preparation, regardless of the type of filling technique used, remains the most significant segment of endodontic treatment. Users of Thermafil should never be deluded into thinking that this filling technique has any inherent advantages in sealing that might overcome errors or insufficient steps in canal preparation.

If anything, canal preparation should be performed even more carefully, especially in curved canals, when using Thermafil. If a significant elbow (see Chapter 7) is present, this will constrict the softened gutta-percha as it is pressed through this area. Even with the residual springback that occurs whenever gutta-percha is compressed, the filling material probably will not be able to return to a sufficient width to seal off the area apical to the elbow, leaving some voids at this crucial site (Fig. 10-33).

Stick or injected thermoplastic gutta-percha may be condensed in the apical few millimeters, but may also require the elimination or, at least, the minimization of the elbow. For use with Thermafil, the elbow may cause a more serious problem, if present, in diminishing the bulk of gutta-percha apical to it.

Carriers. The carrier used in the original technique was a file used for preparation. Following the production of Thermafil, manufactured stainless steel files were coated with softened gutta-percha, shaped and cooled, and then boxed for delivery. These files had not been involved in the preparation of the canal to be filled, but corresponded to the master apical file (MAF). In cases where a post was required for restoration, a significant amount of this metal file needed to be removed, as with a sectioned silver point (see earlier in this chapter). This was not easy to accomplish, and there was fear that attempts at "twisting-off" or partial removal might decrease the apical seal.

Several years ago, the metal carrier was replaced by plastic. This material could be more

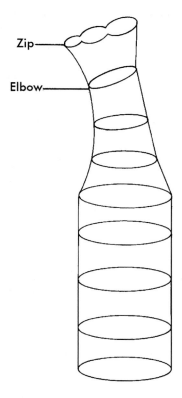

Fig. 10-33. An improperly prepared curved canal would be very difficult to fill with any filling material or technique. Thermafil is particularly susceptible to failure to eliminate, or even minimize, a problem with an elbow and apical zip. As the gutta-percha mass is forced by the obturator into the apical portion of the preparation, the widest diameter of the material is constricted by the narrowest diameter of the preparation—the elbow. Even with some springback by the gutta-percha, it will never fill completely the area between the elbow and the tip of the preparation if the discrepancy between the widths at these two sites is more than minimal. Furthermore, if the most apical portion of the preparation is enlarged past the tip of the root, the zip will occur without a matrix to pack against. When using Thermafil, the operator should make every attempt to minimize the discrepancy at the elbow and to ensure a good matrix to pack against.

easily removed after being placed in a canal with the Preppi bur,* a smooth round, noncutting bur (Fig. 10-34) that removed the plastic by heat—much easier and safer than attempting the twist-off with stainless steel.

*Tulsa Dental Products, Tulsa, OK 74136.

Plastic obturators sizes #25 through #40 are composed of liquid crystal plastic (Fig. 10-29, *right*), sizes #45 and larger are made from polysulfone polymer (Fig. 10-29, *center*). Both plastics are nontoxic, highly stable polymers, which are well tolerated by the body. The liquid crystal plastic is quite resistant to solvents, but the polysulfone is susceptible to most of the solvents used in dentistry, including chloroform. This means that when plastic carrier fillings are re-treated, the larger canals do not offer much problem. For the smaller canals, the gutta-percha may be dissolved easily by solvents, then the trick is to hook the carrier with a Hedstrom file for removal.

Sealer with Thermafil. As with other thermoplastics, sealer must be used for best results, as reported in a study by Hata et al. For use with Thermafil, the sealer aids in the lubrication of the heated gutta-percha mass to funnel into the apical portion of the preparation, and it allows for an interface between the filling material and the canal walls to close any spaces or gaps.

Thermafil kits come with their own sealer—ThermaSeal*, which has a formulation very similar to that of AH-26 (Fig. 10-30). This sealer is widely used in central Europe as a paste filler to fill the entire canal. It has been tested in several studies in the United States and is highly rated for both sealing ability and periapical tolerance. ThermaSeal may be used with condensation techniques other than merely Thermafil.

Steps for Thermafil obturation. It is important to follow these steps in the correct order to gain the best results for the material:

*Tulsa Dental Products, Tulsa, OK 74136.

1. Prepare a proper access cavity to get straight line access to the canal space. This is even more important than with a stick gutta-percha case because the solid-core is so much more rigid. (See Chapter 6.)

2. Calculate and confirm by radiograph the correct working length—to the apical constriction (minor diameter), not to the radiographic apex. (See Chapter 8.)

3. Prepare a funneled canal preparation with a smoothly tapering flare and a definite stop at the apical constriction. (See Chapter 7.) (I believe that a solid dentin matrix is even more important with Thermafil than with stick gutta-percha, because pushing the obturator through the mass into the periapical tissues gives the poorest chance for seal. Johnson, the founder of the Thermafil technique, desires a matrix to pack against, but prefers using a small file (no larger than no. 15) to keep patency at the apex, which might allow a small passage of gutta-percha and/or sealer.) Make every effort to minimize the width of the elbow in curved canals.

4. Select the Thermafil verification device (Fig. 10-32) of the same size as the largest file used to the apex (MAF). insert the device into the canal to verify that the carrier will reach the proper length without binding prematurely. Select a size verification device several sizes smaller than the MAF to confirm the presence of the apical dentin matrix.

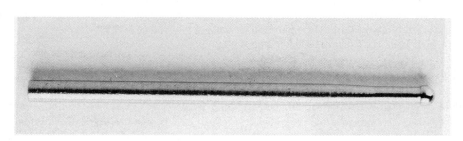

Fig. 10-34. Preppi bur for use in preparing postroom in teeth filled with plastic carrier. This round, noncutting tipped bur removes gutta-percha and plastic by heat alone and will not perforate or cause ledges in the canal walls.

5. Preheat the ThermaPrep oven (Fig. 10-31) for 20 minutes. Select an obturator for each canal the same size as the MAF and the verification device that was confirmed.
6. Set the working length and mark it with a rubber stop, using the calibrations on the carrier for measurement, not a ruler measured from the tip of the gutta-percha. The calibration rings are measured from the tip of the carrier, not the tip of the gutta-percha.
7. Disinfect the obturator in a 5.25% sodium hypochlorite solution for 1 minute, rinse in 70% alcohol, and dry.
8. Place an obturator for each canal in the oven. You may place an extra obturator for each canal in the oven, measured as before, in case any problems develop with the original.
9. Heat the obturators in the ThermaPrep oven, observing the maximum and minimum times.
10. Dry the canals with paper points. Mix the sealer of choice. Although ThermaSeal is

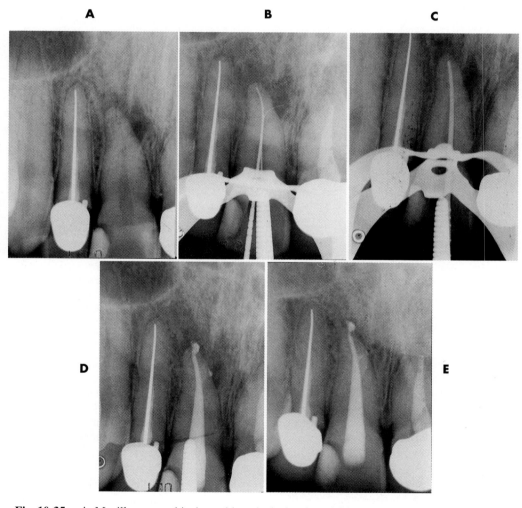

Fig. 10-35. **A,** Maxillary central incisor with periapical and mesial lateral radiolucent lesions present. The pulp did not respond to electrical or temperature tests. **B,** Radiograph of no. 20 file in place in the main canal and a no. 8 file in the lateral canal. **C,** Size verification instrument present, indicating that the length of the preparation is correct and that some stop at the apex is present. **D,** Immediate postfilling film, with Thermafil plastic obturator and ThermaSeal. Puffs of sealer indicate that the filling materials have been forced into the mesial lateral canal and through the apical foramen. **E,** One year later, lesions have decreased considerably in size.

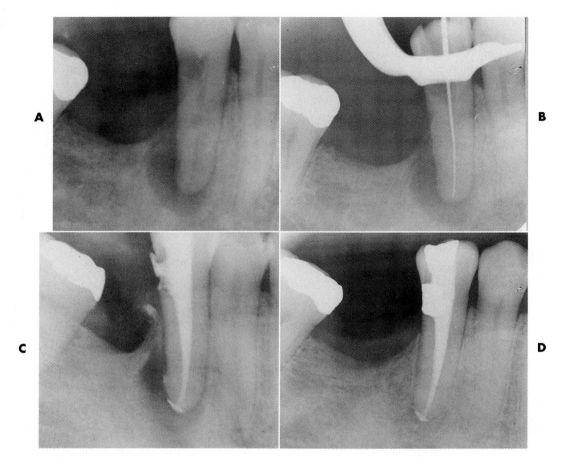

Fig. 10-36. **A,** Preoperative radiograph of mandibular second bicuspid with large periapical lesion extending coronally along the distal surface. A large composite filling is present at the distogingival, and the tooth does not respond to electrical or temperature testing. **B,** Access was prepared, pulp was totally necrotic, and no. 25 file placed to determine working length. **C,** Immediate postfilling film with Thermafil plastic obturator and ThermaSeal sealer. **D,** Radiograph one year later with lesion almost totally healed.

suggested, many other sealers will work well. Apply sealer to the walls of each canal using a reamer one size smaller than the appropriate MAF.

11. Remove the obturator from the oven and insert it into the canal using firm apical pressure.

12. Using a round or inverted cone bur, trim the plastic carrier shaft to just below the level of the canal orifice.

13. Remove the gutta-percha and carrier to the desired depth using the Preppi bur (Fig. 10-34). Pack the remaining gutta-percha around the severed shaft.

14. Radiograph to verify correctness of the fill and make arrangements for prompt restoration, or, if restoration is to be delayed, appropriate temporization to ensure safety of the remaining tooth structure.

When these instructions are followed carefully, Thermafil cases give excellent results (Figs. 10-35 through 10-38). Recent studies in the endodontic literature (listed in the reference section after the conclusion of Chapter 10) have, in general, been favorable.

SEALERS WITH SOLID MATERIALS

Filling of voids. As mentioned frequently in this chapter, the sealer performs the important

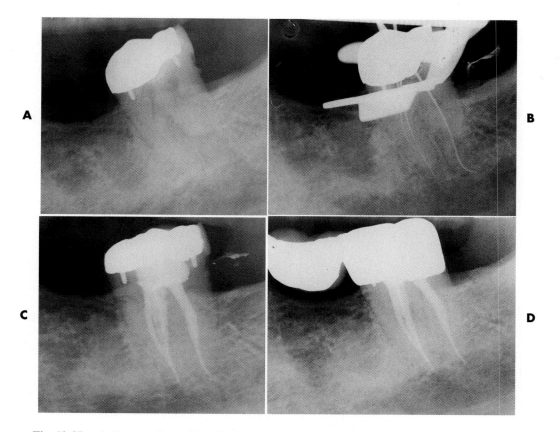

Fig. 10-37.   A, Preoperative radiograph of mandibular second molar. The tooth was painful to percussion and sensitive to heat. The large restoration and pins are in proximity to the pulp. **B,** Radiograph for calculation of working lengths, no. 10 files in mesial canals and no. 15 file in distal root indicating sharp curve to the distal. **C,** Immediate postfilling film, angled view, indicating canals filled with Thermafil plastic obturator and ThermaSeal. Mesial canals merged short of the apex (type II canal system), but filling material is noted coronally between the canals, indicating a third mesial canal or communication between the canals. **D,** One year after treatment, symptoms are long gone and the tooth serves as the posterior abutment for a fixed bridge. Radiolucency noted apical to the roots unquestionably is a lingual salivary gland depression (see Chapter 2).

function of filling voids and discrepancies between the canal walls and the filling when solid materials are used. The thickest possible sealer, with a heavy puttylike consistency, is indicated for use so that the bulk of the sealer may pack throughout the canal when the point is forcefully placed. Rickert's formula, mixed two parts powder to one part liquid, has been demonstrated to perform this function most satisfactorily.

Other functions of sealer.   Just as described for use with gutta-percha, the sealer continues to exert an antibacterial action in the period immediately after its placement. Although important

for use with gutta-percha, the quality of lubrication provided by the sealer is not as significant for use with solid materials. Because they are not flexible, the solid materials require little lubrication to reach the apical portion of the preparation.

The final function of the sealer is to provide radiopacity to the filling. Again, although useful with the less dense gutta-percha, solid materials are themselves quite radiopaque. The radiopaque feature is important to view the excess sealer that has been forced through the apical foramen or into lateral canals.

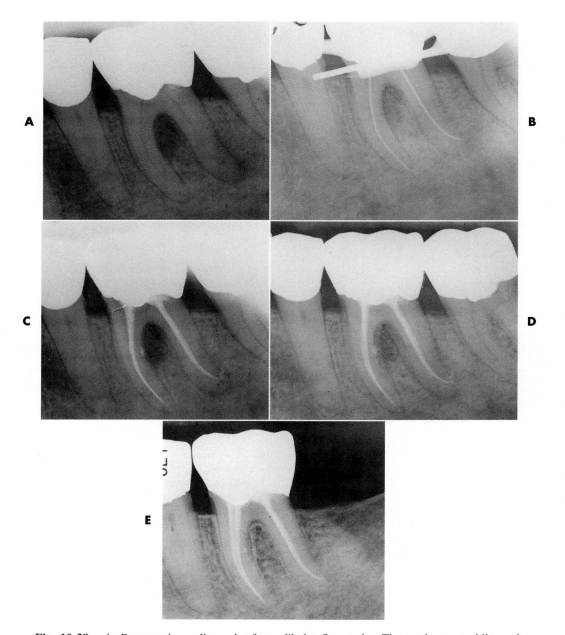

Fig. 10-38. A, Preoperative radiograph of mandibular first molar. The tooth was mobile, and a chronic draining sinus tract was present draining near the furcation area. Radiolucencies are present near the apex and up the distal surface of the distal root, and in the bone of the furcation, and there is a slight thickening of the periodontal ligament space of the mesial root. There was no response to heat or cold applied to the restoration, but it was not possible to test with electricity. **B,** Files in place, slightly long on one of the mesial canals. In the distal root, the canal is seen exiting short of the apex to the distal surface. The sinus tract closed shortly after the preparation appointment. **C,** Straight view following canal filling, the three canals filled with Thermafil plastic obturators and ThermaSeal. Note the lateral canal indicated on the distal surface of the mesial root, directly to the lateral radiolucency. The canal filling in the distal root exits towards the lesion on the distal surface with some excess sealer. **D,** Six months after treatment, the tooth is firm, the sinus tract is gone, and the radiolucencies are greatly reduced. **E,** One year after original treatment, healing is already complete according to the radiograph.

RE-TREATMENT OF SILVER POINT CASES

No filling material or technique yet devised has a perfect track record. Because of certain inherent problems plus their too frequent abuse, silver point canal fillings must be removed and the teeth re-treated in certain cases. For the most part, these re-treatments become necessary when the endo-dontically treated teeth are failing, either with symptoms or as determined by radiograph (Figs. 10-39 to 10-51). In some cases, however, re-treatment is needed for prosthetic reasons, generally to accommodate a post-and-core type of restoration (Fig. 10-42).

The major problem that can occur in re-treating silver point cases is that there is no solvent for the filling material. Therefore the point must be grasped or impaled in order to be removed. In some cases the removal offers no problem; in others it is quite complicated.

Points that offer no problem in removal. Re-treatment is generally very simple when the point protrudes well past its canal orifice. It then may be easily gripped by the silver point pliers (Fig. 10-14) and removed. Whereas the filling material itself has no solvent, virtually all the root canal sealers can be dissolved by chloro-form or xylene. When a point is easily grasped but cannot be delivered, irrigate the canal around it with one of these solvents. The residual sealer is softened, and often the point can be removed.

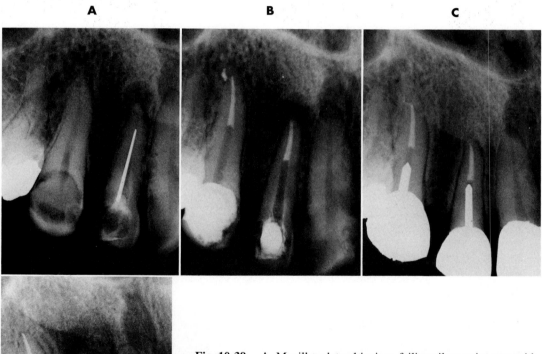

Fig. 10-39. **A,** Maxillary lateral incisor, failing silver point case with periapical lesion. **B,** Silver point protruded sufficiently through orifice so it could be grasped with silver point pliers. Canal was reprepared and filled with laterally condensed gutta-percha, and post room was provided. **C,** Four years later, lesion has healed. **D,** Nine years after original treatment. (Restorations by Dr. Sherwin Strauss, Chicago.)

The correct working length is established, and the canal reprepared and filled, preferably with gutta-percha (Fig. 10-39). In re-treating obviously failing cases, prepare the canals at one appointment and fill at a subsequent visit, as stated in the discussion of teeth with periapical involvement (Chapter 4). There is always a chance that a periapical area will exacerbate. When the canal is both prepared and filled at the same appointment, the only way to dissipate pressures or exudate must be via a surgical approach.

Many instances requiring re-treating of obviously failing cases involve points that have been placed into canals following insufficient canal preparation (Fig. 10-40). These points flick out easily, often with an endodontic excavator or when merely jarred by the bur during access cavity preparation.

Points that cannot be easily gripped. Some silver points defy normal dislodgment procedures. When the cones are placed by the sectional method at the apex, only a surgical approach (Chapter 11) is available to retain a failing case.

Some points are sectioned at or slightly below the canal orifice, making it impossible to be grasped by a silver point pliers. Several methods for removal of these have been suggested, including engagement with a Hedstrom file or using a Masseran trepan bur to drill a circular trench similar to the method for removing a broken file. Trenching will usually give enough room for a thin-nosed pliers (e.g., a Stieglitz) to be placed around the point. However, most small round or fissure burs gouge or cut the silver point during the trenching preparation, which causes a deeper separation when the point is pulled.

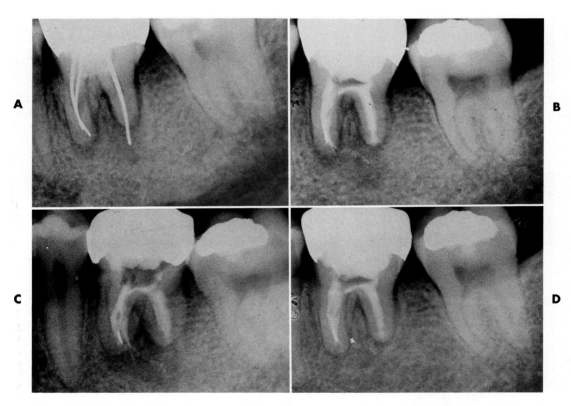

Fig. 10-40. **A,** Mandibular first molar, failing silver point case with periapical lesions. **B,** Silver points had been placed after obviously insufficient canal preparation. Points flicked out easily with an endodontic excavator, although a small portion of one of the mesial points remained. Canals were reprepared and filled with laterally condensed gutta-percha. **C,** Angled view, filling materials condensed apical to small remaining tip of silver point. **D,** Three years after treatment, areas have healed.

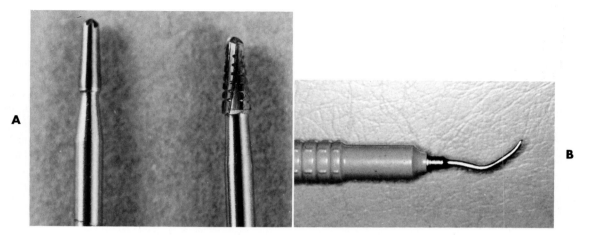

Fig. 10-41. **A,** Specially prepared bur *(left)* has a half-circle round cutting end for making trough around silver point without any gouging or nicking of the protruding metal. Contrasted on right is a 702R. (Courtesy Premier Dental Products Co., Norristown, Pa.) **B,** Larger scaler used with ultrasonic device to remove tightly fitting silver point and posts.

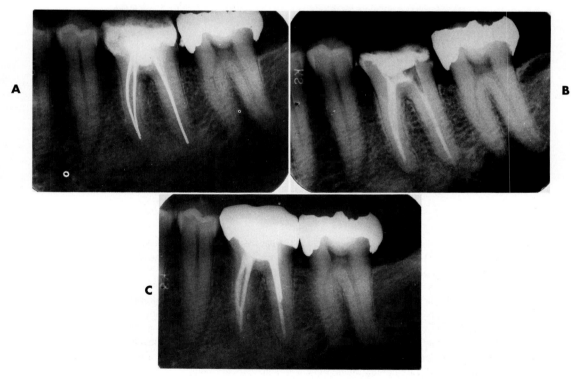

Fig. 10-42. **A,** Mandibular first molar was restored with amalgam several years earlier after canal fillings with silver points. Amalgam and a portion of the tooth cracked, necessitating construction of a full gold crown with a post and core. **B,** In an attempt to remove the distal silver point, the mesiobuccal point was dislodged. Distal point could not be grasped, but special bur was used to make a trough. Points were removed, canals were reprepared and filled with laterally condensed gutta-percha, and post room was prepared. **C,** One year later, canal fillings and new restoration. (Restorations by Dr. Larry Perlis, formerly of Highland Park, Ill.)

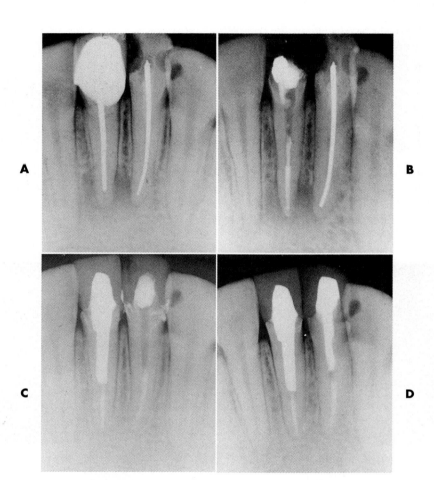

Fig. 10-43. **A,** Preoperative view of mandibular central incisors. There is a silver point in each tooth and a periapical area definitely associated with the central to the left, and perhaps involving the central incisor to the right as well. The originating dentist attempted to remove the points but was unsuccessful. Therefore he recommended periapical surgery as the only alternative. However, the patient had a serious clotting problem, which would make surgery an extremely hazardous undertaking. **B,** I removed the crown on the central at left and, using an ultrasonic device, was able to remove the silver point. The canal was reprepared and then filled with laterally condensed gutta-percha (post room prepared). **C,** The other tooth was similarly treated, using ultrasonics to remove the silver point. This film was taken 6 months after completion of treatment, and the periapical area is closing rapidly. **D,** Two years after completion of treatment, the periapical area appears normal.

The correct bur to gain the trenching is a pure end-cutting bur of the tapered fissure series with a half-circle round cutting end. It can be made by trimming the sides of a 700R series or is available already trimmed (Fig. 10-41, *A*). Such a bur works around the periphery of the point to be removed until a sufficient trench is prepared. During the initial stages of preparation, great care should be exercised so the tip of the bur does not touch the point, because then further gouging may result. However, as the tip of the bur begins to make the trench and the tip is working on the dentin adjacent to the point, the bald portion of the bur may

be brought close to the point. The friction created by this contact may be sufficient to unseat the point. Under any circumstances, with careful use and analysis of the dimensions of the root that holds the point, a sufficiently deep trough can be prepared without nicking, gouging, or reducing the silver point. Then the thin-necked pliers is placed firmly around the point to gain removal.

This method may be used for successful cases when a post-and-core type of restoration is necessary, but the presence of a nonsectioned silver point prevents post room preparation by the routine method (Fig. 10-42). These specially

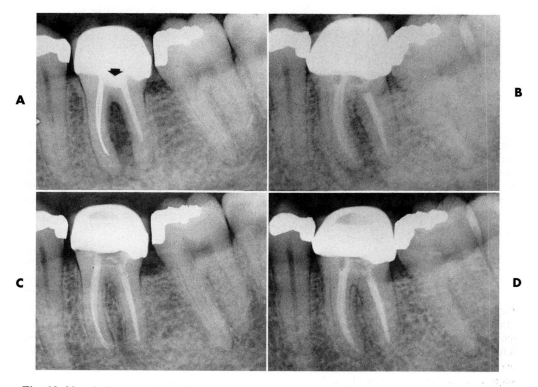

Fig. 10-44. **A,** Preoperative radiograph, straight view, of mandibular first molar. Tooth had been treated over 2 years earlier, but now it was mobile and a sinus tract was present in the furcation area. When the chamber was entered, cement had been packed around protruding silver points *(arrow)*. I was afraid to drill down with a bur, so I used an ultrasonic file to remove all the cement, leaving the points available for access. Using the scaler tip, the points were removed from the mesial canals and chloroform was used to remove the gutta-percha from the distal canal. **B,** Angled view of immediate postfilling film. The canals were filled with laterally condensed gutta-percha. The sinus tract had healed, and the tooth had tightened following canal preparation. **C,** Straight and **D,** angled view 3 years following retreatment. The intrafurcal area has healed, and the tooth is tight and comfortable.

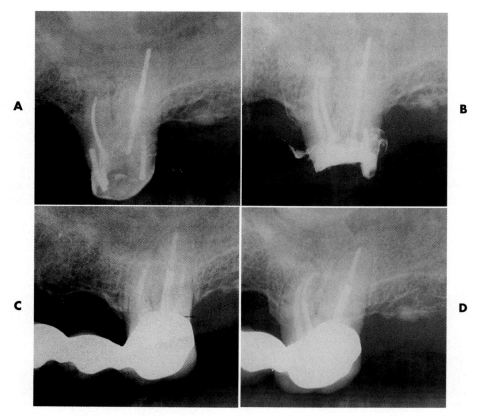

Fig. 10-45. **A,** Preoperative radiograph of maxillary first molar, previously filled with silver points, periapical lesion associated with mesiobuccal root, soreness felt by patient at the root tip. Canal fillings were removed with ultrasonic use. Area palatal to the mesiobuccal orifice was carefully cleaned with an ultrasonic tip and another orifice uncovered. **B,** Immediate postfilling film, view from the distal, indicating four canals filled with gutta-percha and Wach's paste, post room prepared in palatal root. Two years later **C,** (straight view) and **D,** (angled from distal) indicates excellent healing. (Restoration by Dr. Steven Potashnick, Chicago.)

Fig. 10-46. Very difficult re-treatment greatly aided by ultrasonic treatment. **A,** Preoperative radiograph indicates mesial root with overextended silver point, associated with periapical lesion and apical tenderness, and poorly treated distal root with small amount of gutta-percha. The patient had been referred to an oral surgeon, but preferred not to have periapical surgery due to the possibility of a paresthesia. I doubted that the overextended point could be retrieved, but was willing to try to avert surgery. **B,** The tooth was opened and the distal gutta-percha easily removed. One of the silver points from mesial root was easily removed, and this view taken from the distal to determine where the point was still present. **C,** The ultrasonic was used on the remaining point, which came out straight! I took this film to verify that the entire point had been removed and that the tip had not broken off. **D** (straight view) and **E** (angled view from mesial), Film taken after canal filling with gutta-percha and Wach's paste. Even though I knew that the mesial root had apical resorption, I pushed some filling material through the tip into the periapical tissue. The silver point had left a path in the tissue, and excess sealer followed the same position as noted in **A. F,** After one year, the periapical lesion has healed and no apical tenderness was present. **G,** Three years after treatment, the excess sealer has resorbed totally and the tooth is firm and comfortable. (Restoration by Dr. Steven Potashnick, Chicago.)

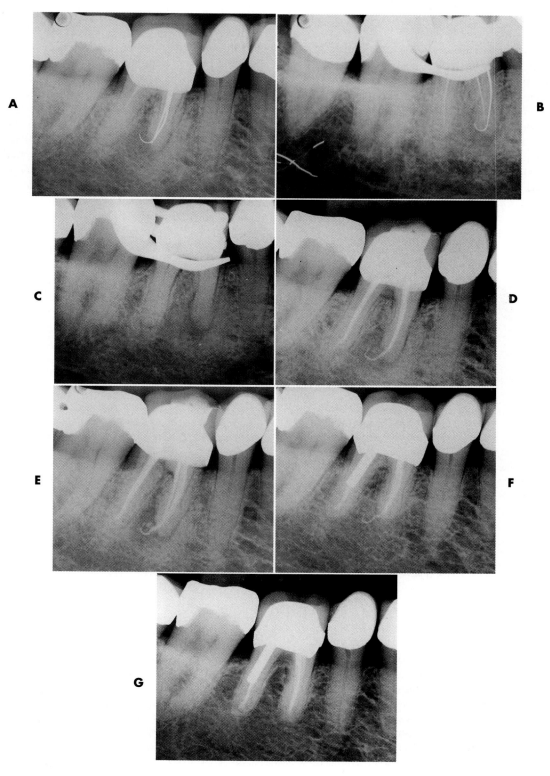

Fig. 10-46.   For legend see opposite page.

prepared burs are useful in removal of broken posts as well, usually in conjunction with an ultrasonic device.

Ultrasonic treatment to remove tightly fitting points and posts. Ultrasonics were used to remove silver points and posts prior to their use in endodontic canal preparation (Chapter 7). Ditching around the material to be removed with a bur and then touching the metal with an ultrasonic scaler tip (Fig. 10-41, *B*) has yielded excellent results on cases that resisted re-treatment by any other method (Figs. 10-43 through 10-49).

Now that ultrasonic preparation has been adapted for routine endodontic use, more instruments are available for even more efficient removal of unwanted materials. When cement is used to surround the points, as shown in Fig. 10-20, it is difficult to remove the cement without clipping the silver points in the process. This shortens the amount protruding, an undesirable condition with which to deal.

A regular endodontic ultrasonic tip may be used to penetrate and then remove the cement without damage to the points (Fig. 10-44), and then removal by the ultrasonic scaler tip is facilitated.

When re-treating maxillary molars and removing materials from the mesiobuccal root, the operator should always examine that root for the possibility of a second canal, which is present in approximately 50% of these teeth (see Chapter 6).

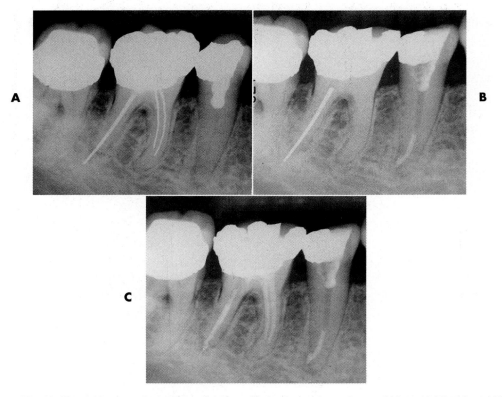

Fig. 10-47. **A,** Preoperative radiograph of mandibular first molar and second bicuspid. The bicuspid has old vital pulp therapy and a periapical lesion. The molar has short silver point fillings in the mesial root, but no lesion is present. The distal root, however, has an overextended silver point and apical tenderness. Successful periapical surgery and reverse filling would be very difficult on this distal root. **B,** The silver points were easily removed from the mesial canals, but it was not possible to pull the distal point out with a silver point forceps or engage it with Hedstrom files. An endodontic explorer was placed in contact with the point, and the ultrasonic was energized on the handle of the explorer. A bit later, the point was loosened and removed. **C,** The bicuspid was completed. The molar mesial canals could not be prepared any further due to ledging, and all canals were filled with gutta-percha. The tooth will be observed for healing.

It would be a shame to re-treat this tooth and miss this often present canal, thus continuing the failure potential. The ultrasonic may be used to aid in the location by cleaning up the floor of the chamber and exposing the entrance to the mesiolingual orifice (Fig. 10-45).

By gaining experience using the ultrasonic, I have re-treated more and more complicated cases nonsurgically than I could have imagined before the availability of this excellent machine. Failures that would be most difficult to re-treat with surgery have succumbed to ultrasonic procedures (Figs. 10-46 and 10-47).

Fig. 10-47 describes a case where the silver point had been sectioned beneath the floor of the chamber—a most difficult condition to re-treat. Unfortunately, the point went past the apex of the root by several millimeters and was causing constant pain during mastication. Re-treatment was mandatory.

To re-treat surgically, the distal root (more difficult to reach through the bone than the mesial root because it is farther from the buccal bone) would require an apicoectomy to remove the overextended point and then, in all probability, a reverse filling. Recent evaluations of reverse fillings seem to indicate the presence of a relatively high failure rate (see Chapter 11). A nonsurgical approach would be best, if possible.

After access preparation, the gingival portion of the point was located, but it could not be engaged

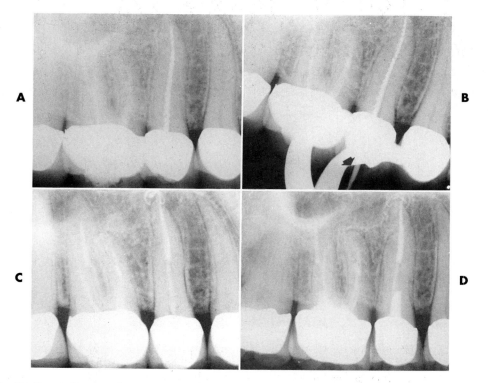

Fig. 10-48. **A,** Preoperative view of maxillary second bicuspid, periapical lesion present; evidently a Hedstrom file had been used to fill the canal. Apical tenderness was also present. I tried many techniques for over 1 hour in an attempt to remove the file, but to no avail. After 10 minutes of using an ultrasonic device, a size 40 Hedstrom file was delivered. **B,** Assuming that the canal was now clear, I enlarged to size 50 and placed a master gutta-percha cone to be verified by radiograph (coronal portion of the master cone is indicated by arrow). Imagine my chagrin when I viewed this film and then realized that *two* Hedstrom files had been used to fill the canal! **C,** I easily removed the other file, enlarged further, and then filled the canal with laterally condensed gutta-percha (post room prepared). Some excess sealer has been extruded into the periapical area. **D,** Eighteen months later, the lesion is decreased considerably, and the tooth is comfortable and functioning well.

with a silver point forceps. Attempts were made to insert Hedstrom files alongside the point to pull it out, but, after 10 minutes of effort, no progress was perceived. An endodontic explorer was inserted adjacent to and in contact with the point. The ultrasonic tip (Fig. 10-41, *B*) was energized onto the handle of the explorer for approximately 20 minutes, and the point was loosened and delivered.

Broken instruments often pose serious problems in removal. My own batting average at successful re-treatment has always been extremely low in these conditions. Ultrasonics at least give the operator a fighting chance at removal of

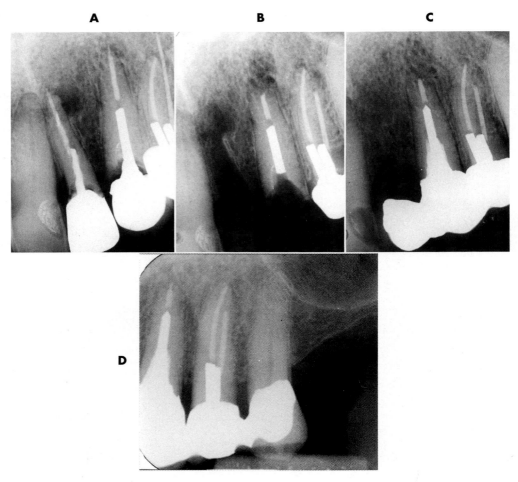

Fig. 10-49. **A,** Preoperative film of maxillary left anterior and first bicuspid areas, periapical surgery to be performed. There is a large periapical lesion distal to the lateral incisor (no. 10), a poor post and poor canal filling. The cuspid (no. 11) has decay around the post, a periapical lesion, and apical tenderness. The first bicuspid (no. 12) had a badly overextended filling from the buccal canal with apical tenderness. In retrospect, I suppose that best treatment would have been to remove the posts first from nos. 10 and 11, but I was uncertain of what I would find during surgery. After the flap was raised, I located a very large perforation at the distal of no. 10, so it was extracted. The excess fillings on nos. 11 and 12 were trimmed, areas curetted, and apicoectomies performed down to well-filled portions of the canals. **B,** The restorative dentist had trouble removing the post from no. 11, and after drilling a portion of it away, decided that he would put a superstructure over the root without a post. I knew that would never work. Using an ultrasonic device, I easily removed the post. **C,** Six months later, the case looks promising. Note the new post in no. 11 is of sufficient length. **D,** Twelve years after original treatment, area continues to function well and no problems have occurred. Anterior abutment is holding well. (Restoration by Dr. Richard Lammermayer, Kenilworth, Ill).

instruments, whether they were purposely segmented as canal filling materials (Fig. 10-48) or merely were broken as a result of a procedural accident.

Similarly, posts, which often defy removal by any other means, are subject to coming out with the larger ultrasonic scaler. This is much preferable to attempting to drill a post out with a bur, where there is a danger of sliding off the dense metal and severely gouging tooth structure or, even worse, causing a perforation. Attempting to pull posts out using a pliers or pressure devices may cause root fracture.

The ultrasonic technique is very safe compared to these methods. Ditching is accomplished with the tip-cutting bur (Fig. 10-41, *A*). Then the ultrasonic scaler tip is used at a higher-than-normal level of energy to work around the periphery. Much water must be used as irrigant because of

the considerable increase in temperature of the metal and potential overheating of surrounding structures. The use of irrigant as coolant is similarly important when removing silver points that protrude into the periapical tissues and may cause blistering of these vital structures.

When the posts are quite large and retentive, it may take several appointments to gain removal. However, if the case is potentially hopeless unless the metal is removed, the extra time involved is well spent and frequently a happy ending follows (Fig. 10-49).

Potential danger of the ultrasonic.   That the ultrasonic unit is valuable and extremely useful in re-treating failing endodontic cases cannot be denied. By the same token, failure to recognize that the instrument is extremely powerful and might cause damage if not used with great care is also true.

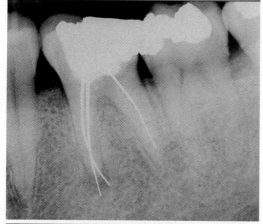

A

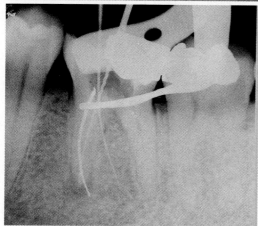

B

Fig. 10-50.   A, Preoperative radiograph of mandibular molar, indicating failing silver points in both mesial and distal roots. Patient had been to an oral surgeon, but did not wish to chance possible paresthesia from periapical surgery and was referred to me for evaluation and treatment. I thought that nonsurgical retreatment was possible and suggested that method of therapy. **B,** I opened the tooth and easily removed the distal and mesiobuccal silver points. However, I could not engage the point in the mesiolingual canal. I decided to try to use a file with the ultrasonic unit to get alongside of the point. The patient was not given any anesthetic and felt nothing as I proceeded. In a few seconds, the ultrasonic file seemed to go easily down the mesiolingual canal to the apex. I placed a file into the pathway that had been made and took this film. Imagine my surprise and my chagrin when I examined the film and saw this devastating perforation!

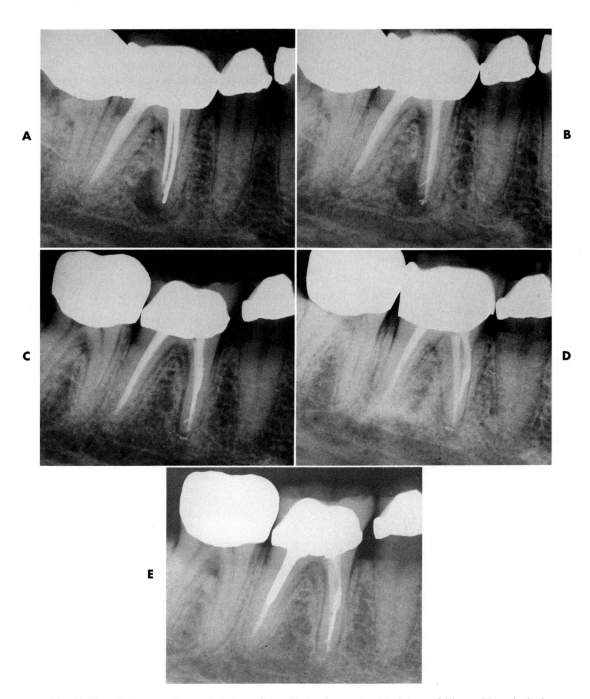

Fig. 10-51. **A,** Preoperative angled view of mandibular first molar. Mesial root failing, with periapical lesion. Distal canal seems fine. It is impossible to ascertain which mesial canal is failing, so both must be re-treated. Points could not be grasped by silver point pliers, so a trough was cut around them with a specially prepared bur. **B,** Canals were reprepared and filled with gutta-percha. **C,** Straight-on view 4 years after treatment shows healing of periapical lesion. **D,** Angled view. **E,** Eight years after original treatment. Distal canal was never re-treated. (Restorations by Dr. Steve Labkon, Kenilworth, Ill.)

Because of the tremendous power that is inherent in the ultrasonic machine, the drilling potential may easily cause the file to pass completely through the dentin very quickly and cause a horrible perforation (Fig. 10-50). Ultrasonic energy should be used only under strict and total control by the operator. High risk procedures should be undertaken only when the tooth is hopeless unless this small chance is successful. In the more routine cases, safety must constantly be a primary consideration.

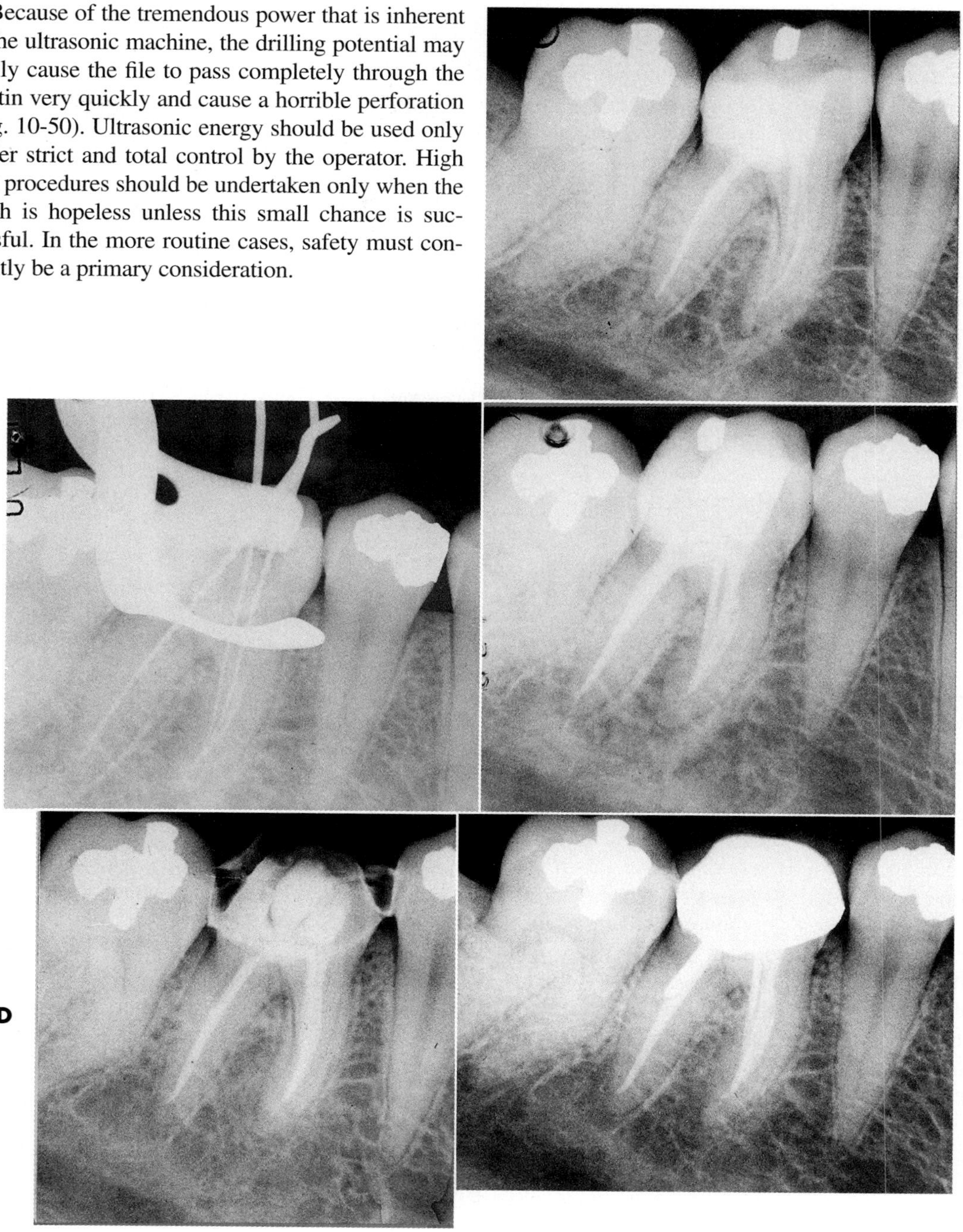

Fig. 10-52. **A,** Preoperative radiograph, angled view from the mesial, of mandibular first molar. A periapical lesion is present associated with the mesial root and the tooth is tender to percussion. Gutta-percha is present in the distal root, but the material in the mesial root has another substance in it. **B,** The tooth was opened, the gutta-percha in the distal root removed and a Thermafil type of filling removed from the mesiobuccal. Another device is still in the mesiolingual, but it, too, was removed with Hedstrom files. **C,** After repreparation, the canals were filled with laterally condensed gutta-percha and Wach's paste. **D,** Six months later, a temporary crown had been fabricated, the tooth was comfortable, and the lesion almost gone. **E,** Two years later, with perfect healing. (Restoration by Dr. Arnold Wax, Chicago.)

Re-treating a portion rather than the entire tooth. In failing cases of multirooted teeth, the entire tooth need not be retreated if the failure is confined to one root. When silver points were at the height of their popularity, many mandibular molars received gutta-percha fillings in the distal root and silver points in the mesial canals. Similarly, in maxillary molars, gutta-percha was used in the palatal root and silver points in the buccal roots. When failing cases are analyzed, if one root is satisfactory and the other is the failing portion, re-treatment of only the root that is failing is necessary. In mandibular molars it may be difficult to decide which of the mesial canals is failing when there is a periapical lesion on the mesial root. In that case, it is best to re-treat both canals if possible (Fig. 10-51).

Re-treating Thermafil failures. Failures from teeth where Thermafil was used for canal filling generally are not difficult to re-treat. Many of these failures occur when insufficient canal preparation was performed and/or undersized obturators were used (Fig. 10-28, *B*). In these instances, the canal fillings may be removed relatively easily to allow proper preparation and refilling.

Another advantage for re-treatment of Thermafil is that gutta-percha, with many available solvents, is surrounding much of the obturator. Once the gutta-percha is dissolved, Hedstrom files or ultrasonic treatment, or both, will remove the canal contents to allow successful repreparation and refilling (Fig. 10-52). As stated earlier, if the canal filling utilized a plastic obturator, the larger fillings have plastics that also may be dissolved. The canals with obturators of less than size no. 40 may offer difficulty, especially if much of the gutta-percha is rubbed off prematurely and the coronal portion of the filling was removed for post preparation.

REFERENCES

Gerstein H, Weine FS: Specially prepared burs to remove silver cones and fractured dowels, *J Endod* 3:408, 1977.

Jasper EA: Adaptation and tissue tolerance of silver point canal fillings, *J Dent Res* 4:355, 1941.

Morse D, Barnett A, Maggio J: A scanning electron microscopic examination of endodontic implants, *Oral Implantol* 3:139, 1972.

Palmer GR, Weine FS, Palmer MJ, Healey HJ: A study of the tissue reaction to silver cones and Ti-6A1-4V in the rhesus monkey, *J Endod* 5:116, 1979.

Seltzer S, Green DB, Weiner N, DeRenzis F: A scanning electron microscope examination of silver cones removed from endodontically treated teeth, *Oral Surg* 33:589, 1972.

Soltanoff W, Parris L: Controlled silver point filling technic for endodontically involved teeth, *J Am Dent Assoc* 65:301, 1962.

Weine FS, Altman A, Healey HJ: Treatment of fractures of the middle third of the root, *J Dent Child* 38:215, 1971.

Weine FS, Healey HJ, Lippert JL: Use of silver points with improved digital control, *J Am Dent Assoc* 83:125, 1971.

Weine FS, Rice RT: Handling previously treated silver point cases: removal, retreatment and tooth retention, *Compend Contin Educ Dent* 7:652, 1986.

Weine FS, Wenckus CS: Treatment of horizontal midroot fracture: 3 case reports, *CDS Rev* 79:33, 1985.

Thermafil

Chohayeb AA: Comparison of a conventional root canal obliteration technique with Thermafil obturators, *J Endod* 18:10, 1992.

Gencoglu N, Samani S, Gunday M: Evaluation of sealing properties of Thermafil and Ultrafil techniques in the absence and presence of smear layer, *J Endod* 19:599, 1993.

Hata G, Kawazoe S, Toda T, Weine FS: Sealing ability of Thermafil with and without sealer, *J Endod* 18:322, 1992.

Ibarrola JL, Knowles KI, Ludlow MO: Retrievability of Thermafil plastic cores using organic solvents, *J Endod* 19:417, 1993.

Johnson WB: A new gutta-percha technique, *J Endod* 4:184, 1978.

Juhlin JJ, Walton RE, Dovgan JS: Adaptation of Thermafil components to canal walls, *J Endod* 19:130, 1993.

Lares C, ElDeeb ME: The sealing ability of the Thermafil obturation technique, *J Endod* 16:474, 1990.

McMurtry LG, Krell KV, Wilcox LR: A comparison between Thermafil and lateral condensation in highly curved canals, *J Endod* 18:68, 1992.

Scott AC, Vire DE, Swanson R: An evaluation of the Thermafil obturation technique, *J Endod* 18:340, 1992.

Franklin S. Weine • Manuel A. Bustamante

11 Periapical surgery

According to the strictest definition of the word *surgery,* most endodontic treatment falls into the category of a surgical procedure, since a removal of tissues, such as vital pulp, necrotic debris, or dentin, is involved. However, as commonly used, the term *endodontic surgery* refers to the removal of tissues other than the contents of the root canal space to retain a tooth with pulpal and/or periapical involvement.

Currently, endodontic surgery falls into more than one domain. Many general practitioners and most oral surgeons routinely perform various types of endodontic surgery. Endodontists should be able to perform periapical surgery on any root in the dental arch, including mandibular molars. Periodontists may become involved in endodontic surgery, periapical or amputational, when a tooth requiring periodontal surgery has a periapical problem of pulpal origin in addition.

Depending on the abilities, desires, or philosophies of their dentists, patients requiring endodontic surgery may be referred to and from general practitioners, oral surgeons, and endodontists. Some of the situations and techniques that will be described in this chapter are beyond the abilities of certain members of each group. They are presented here so the reader will be aware of the fact that such procedures are possible and can be utilized to retain involved teeth and so a proper referral may be made.

Also, considerable space will be given to a list of situations that do not require surgical treatment so the patient may be spared the more traumatic treatment whenever possible.

There are two major areas of endodontic surgery at this time: periapical and amputational. The two have certain basic similarities but have considerable differences as well. This chapter will will deal with periapical surgery, and the next chapter will discuss root amputations.

For many years the term *conservative treatment* has been used as a synonym for nonsurgical treatment. Chivian correctly protested that using *conservative* to mean "without surgery" would indicate that surgery is radical treatment. Since periapical surgery usually saves a tooth that could not be retained by other methods, it too is conservative. We also agree that periapical surgery should not be considered radical therapy; in contrast, tooth retention by any method is conservative. However, in this chapter the long-honored tradition of using the terms *nonsurgical* and *conservative* interchangeably will be followed.

FALSE INDICATIONS

Various methods of endodontic surgery have been described since late in the nineteenth century. At one time most of the endodontic treatment practiced was in conjunction with a surgical procedure, and the indications for surgery included almost every type of case. However, studies in the basic sciences were applied to clinical situations, and

---

Authors' note: We are aware that many cases presented in this chapter include the placement of an amalgam reverse filling. Many are illustrated with long-term success, and a few indicate failure. We have emphasized in this edition, however, that amalgam should no longer be used in this procedure. Why, then, do we show these cases and only a few with alternatives to amalgam? In the already classic study of Frank, Glick, Patterson, and Weine, it was shown that amalgam reverse fills may indicate total healing, but revert to failure in 10 years or less. Virtually all the cases that we have treated with amalgam substitutes (other than gutta-percha) are of 10 years or less. Therefore, we are reluctant to print too many, because they, too, may be failures in a few more years. We hope that the readers of this chapter will understand this dichotomy between illustrations presented and current philosophy of treatment.

considerable experience with nonsurgical treatments resulted in a high degree of success. Therefore it soon became obvious that many cases would succeed without surgical intervention, and the list of indications for surgery has shrunk considerably.

Any periapical surgery involves the laying of flaps and the removal of tissues from outside the root canal space, including bone, periodontal membrane, and periosteum. It usually produces postoperative pain, edema, and discoloration. This is in contrast to nonsurgical treatment, which rarely produces postoperative sequelae and which is confined to the root canal space. As such, conservative treatment should always be preferred to surgical intervention and the latter used only when no other course of therapy remains. Even so, many elements in the dental literature suggest as indications for surgery conditions that may be successfully treated nonsurgically with excellent results. A list of these false indications for surgery, accompanied by the rationale for nonsurgical treatment, follows.

1. *Presence of an incompletely formed apex, making hermetic sealing of the apex impossible.* Nonsurgical endodontic treatment of a tooth with an undeveloped, open, or "blunderbuss" apex has long been a difficult problem. Since the greatest width of the canal in a tooth of this type is at the apex, there appeared no way to prepare and seal the tooth successfully in the apical portion with anything but an apical approach.

Since these cases generally involved young patients, the use of a surgical procedure with its attendant discomfort and need for excellent patient cooperation often resulted in a less than desirable outcome, the production of a management problem for further dental treatment of the patient, or both. Hospital procedures were suggested so these youngsters would be given a general anesthetic and thus would not remember the trauma involved while allowing the surgeon to execute the procedure properly. Even when performed in this manner, the final result produced a tooth with extremely thin dentin walls, often complicated by a decreased crown-root ratio if an apicoectomy was required in addition to curettage.

Happily, the advent of the apexification techniques to gain apical closure after pulpal death has allowed nonsurgical treatment to be performed in most cases. This technique, discussed in Chapter 16 has yielded successful results in most instances. If pulpal death has not occurred but trauma has exposed the pulp on a tooth with incomplete closure, pulpotomy procedures may be performed to complete apexification.

Although little clinical research or evidence has been presented in the area, there also exists the possibility that periapical healing may result in open apex cases where the canal is prepared and filled to the narrowest aperture of the root, even if this point is some distance from the apex. Fig. 11-1 illustrates a case in which the canal was filled to that position, anticipating that a surgical procedure

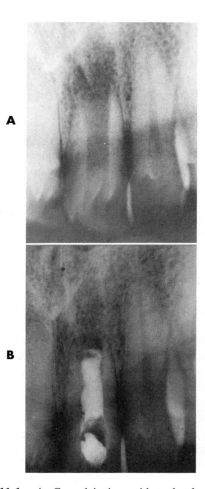

Fig. 11-1. **A,** Central incisor with undeveloped apex required treatment because of large periapical radiolucency. Case was treated prior to report of apexification procedures, and treatment plan called for canal filling through access opening to be followed by a reverse filling placed surgically. **B,** Gutta-percha canal filling was placed, but surgery was canceled because of illness. Four years later this radiograph was taken and showed healing of lesion without further treatment.

would follow to pack amalgam from an apical approach against the gutta-percha matrix that had been placed. The surgery was not performed, however, and the large preoperative radiolucency healed without further treatment.

Since procedures are now available to gain apical closure and since surgery on young patients is difficult to perform and may produce a future problem dental patient, the open apex case should not be an indication for surgery.

2. *Marked overfilling.* From the discussion on the variation of the position of the apical foramen in relation to the radiographic apex (Chapter 7), it is obvious that a tremendous number of successful cases are in fact overfilled. This overfilling may extend as much as 2 mm past the apical foramen into the periapical tissues yet appear to be within the canal when viewed on the radiograph. Therefore some degree of overfilling is tolerable to periapical tissue.

Since many texts and articles indicate that marked overfilling is an indication for endodontic surgery, at what point is a canal overfilled sufficiently to require that type of intervention? The correct answer to that question would seem to be as follows: when an overfilled case appears to be failing according to postoperative recheck radiographs and/or clinical symptoms, surgery is indicated. Also, if persistent tenderness remains after an overfilling, surgery is indicated to relieve the subjective symptoms.

However, if an overfill is present and a periapical radiolucency that was present before treatment is healing or no such area has developed in a tooth that had a normal periapical region preoperatively, there is absolutely no indication for surgery despite the degree of overfilling.

In fact, the degree of overfilling probably has little if any direct causative influence toward periapical inflammation if gutta-percha is used as the canal filling material, since gutta-percha is so well tolerated by periapical tissue and is nonrigid. Silver is well tolerated by periapical tissue, but an overextended silver point may cause physical irritation because of its rigidity. The constant gouging of the rigid metal into periapical tissue during mastication and other occlusal contacts may cause a chronic inflammation.

The major factor of overfilled teeth causing problems may be due not to the overfilling as such but rather to one or both of two other consequences. An overfilled canal may in reality be an underfilling with an overextension. This may seem to be a contradiction; but, lacking a matrix to pack against, the filling material may extrude past the apex yet not seal all segments of the opening. In that case the cause of the failure is not the overfilling but the lack of apical seal.

Another problem of overfilling that may contribute to failure is that overfilling is almost always preceded by overinstrumentation. When the preparation is so finished as to terminate in solid dentin, it is almost impossible to produce an overfilling. For an overfilling to occur, the preparation of the canal must have destroyed the natural apical constriction and allowed the filling to extend into the periapical tissues. Thus it may be the preceding overinstrumentation rather than the overfilling that causes the failure.

3. *Persistent pain.* The rationale for assuming that persistent pain indicated a need for endodontic surgery was the impression that the pain was due either to inflammation in the periapical tissue, which would not respond to conservative treatment, or to retained irritants within the root canal foramina that could not be removed with instrumentation. Therefore the surgical treatment was advocated, which would remove the irritated periapical tissue and a portion of the apex of the tooth where the irritants resided.

Unquestionably this method successfully resolved the problem in most instances. However, a greater understanding of apical anatomy and a desire to prevent problems rather than have to solve them offer a nonsurgical solution. The major cause of persistent pain is overinstrumentation due to the operator's inability to locate the elusive apical constriction correctly. The proper philosophy of treatment is to radiograph from various angles to determine the position and therefore preserve the apical constriction.

If, however, through error or inability to determine its location, the apical constriction is violated, pain will probably occur. Instead of immediately going to a surgical procedure, the proper treatment involves the utilization of a corticosteroid-antibiotic combination to treat this secondary pericementitis. A number of combinations of anti-inflammatory drugs plus broad-spectrum antibiotics to prevent microorganism overgrowth are currently available. When a patient complains of persistent pain, one of these combinations should be used as a medicament. The exact method for use of a medicament of this type is described in Chapter 5. If the operator determines that a great deal of overinstrumentation has been performed at any particular appointment, the anti-inflammatory-antibiotic combination should be used prophylactically to prevent the pain from occurring.

Second to overinstrumentation as a cause of persistent pain during treatment is the presence of an additional, unexpected canal. Mesiobuccal roots of maxillary first molars and buccal roots of maxillary first bicuspids, mandibular bicuspids, cuspids, and incisors usually have only one canal but may have two canals. If only one canal is cleansed, the irritation of the solvents and medicaments may cause a pulpitis in the uninstrumented canal. Pretreatment radiographs from various angles usually will reveal the presence of an additional canal. If an anti-inflammatory-antibiotic combination is first used to grant relief of persistent pain yet is unsuccessful in alleviation for teeth that frequently have additional canals, an exploratory procedure plus additional radiographs should be undertaken before surgery is recommended.

4. *Failure of previous treatment.* Retreatment of failures constitutes a large segment of surgical cases. Before surgery is undertaken, however, a careful evaluation of the etiology of the failure should be made. Once the cause of the failure is determined, further evaluation should be made to see if conservative re-treatment could be performed rather than surgery.

Common causes of failure amenable to nonsurgical re-treatment include the following:

Presence of additional canal—particularly prevalent in mesiobuccal roots of maxillary first molars, maxillary and mandibular bicuspids, mandibular anterior teeth, and distal roots of mandibular molars; may be determined by taking radiographs from various angles.

Lack of apical seal—particularly when silver points or poorly condensed gutta-percha has been used as canal filling material or if canal is filled considerably short of the apex; may be treated nonsurgically if the filling can be removed or dissolved; possible then for canal to be reprepared and properly filled.

Insufficient instrumentation—noted when a filling of minimal size is present, which is readily removable.

Specific treatment for nonsurgical therapy of failing cases is found at the ends of Chapter 9 and 10.

In each of the instances cited the canal has been either poorly filled or not filled at all. These cases should be treated conservatively, to place a satisfactory canal filling. If the case still appears to be failing after a suitable observation period, surgery may be undertaken. But now the surgery is performed with a good canal filling in place, which is easier to work with if an apicoectomy is deemed necessary.

5. *Extensive destruction of periapical tissue and bone involving one third or more of the root apex.* The rationale for surgery here was the belief that if a radiolucency extended for over one third of the distance down the size of the root, there would be insufficient effect of irrigants and medicaments to bring about healing without curettage of the involved area. Areas of this type, which may hug the proximal surface of the root, as opposed to those that balloon out apically, are difficult to curette without removing a segment of the root for access. For that reason an altered crown-root-ratio occurs, which often is undesirable. Therefore it behooves the dentist to evaluate the probable postoperative configuration and the possibility for conservative treatment before instituting surgery in cases of this type.

Careful postoperative evaluation of nonsurgical treatment of such cases reveals a high degree of success. Since the irritants are intracanalicular in origin, instrumentation of the canal removes the source and allows the body to resorb the products of inflammation. This is true no matter what configuration appears radiographically.

6. *Root apex that appears to be involved in a cystic condition.* There is no way to differentiate between a cyst and a granuloma except by histopathologic study of biopsy material. Although some authors claim to be able to distinguish between the two on the basis of radiographic appearance, such differentiations have been shown to be no more accurate than a pure guess. Many radiolucencies having a distinct border, supposedly indicative of a cyst, have on biopsy revealed a granuloma. On the other hand, some diffuse radiolucencies, resembling granulomas in configuration, have been given the diagnosis of cyst after specimen examination under the microscope.

Therefore, since it is impossible to predetermine the presence of a cyst, it is wrong to advise surgical treatment purely on the basis of radiographic appearance. Even if a tooth appears to have a cyst, nonsurgical treatment may yield success if, in fact, a granuloma is present.

Two separate theories of granuloma and cyst percentages have been published. One study, published by Wais and supported by Patterson et al., stated that approximately 13% of periapical lesions are cystic. The opposing theory, originally made by Bhaskar and supported by Lalonde and Luebke, stated that the percentage of periapical radiolucencies that are cysts is closer to 45%. The latter theory further contends that many cysts will respond and heal after nonsurgical endodontic therapy, since much less than 45% of periapical lesions fail to heal after conservative treatment.

Regardless of which theory is correct, it appears evident that nonsurgical treatment has little to lose, since the root canal must be cleansed and filled in any case (Fig. 11-2). Only after a suitable observation period, if periapical healing fails to occur, should surgery then be initiated (Fig. 11-3).

7. *Presence of crater-shaped erosion of the root apex, indicating destruction of apical cementum and dentin.* The original rationale for resorting to surgery in this instance was that if resorption of the apical dentin and cementum was occurring, the pathologic process was too severe to be halted by nonsurgical treatment. However, once again the experience gained from observation of completed cases indicates that a high percentage of teeth with this condition may be successfully treated without surgery. In some cases after nonsurgical treatment the apical resorptive area is remodeled, and new cementum

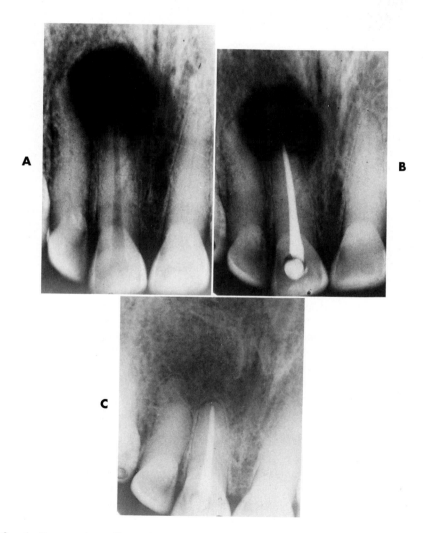

Fig. 11-2. **A,** Preoperative radiograph showed appearance suggestive of a periapical cyst, including deflection of root of adjacent tooth, sclerotic border of a lesion, and very radiolucent area. **B,** Canal filled by lateral condensation procedure. No attempt was made to overinstrument area. **C,** Two years later, area has healed without surgery.

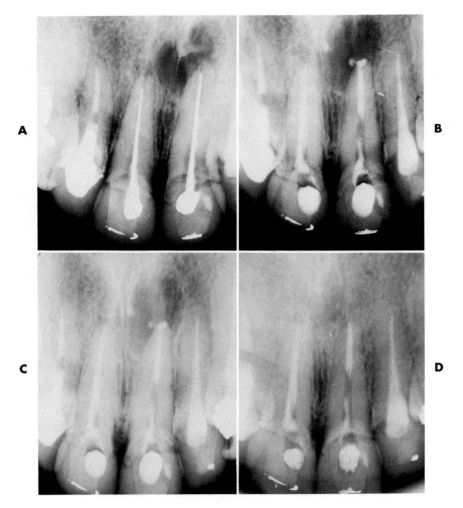

Fig. 11-3. **A,** Radiograph of maxillary anteriors 3 years after endodontic treatment with silver point fillings in central incisors. Central incisor to left (no. 8) had small periapical radiolucency, whereas central incisor to the right (no. 9) had much larger lesion. **B,** Canals were reprepared and refilled with gutta-percha and lateral condensation. **C,** Six months later, lesion on no. 9 appears the same in size, whereas area on no. 8 has healed. **D,** Periapical surgery was performed on no. 9, with the area curetted. Apical fill was checked during surgery and appeared good, so no reverse filling was placed. Biopsy report was for an apical periodontal cyst. Radiograph taken 9 months later shows excellent healing.

or cementoid material is deposited to give a different posttreatment apical configuration (Fig. 11-4).

In fact, in most cases there is apical root resorption when a periapical radiolucency is present, even if none is discernible on the radiograph. The osteoclastic cells that engulf periapical bone and cause the radiolucency cannot differentiate between the bone they are resorbing and the adjacent cementum and/or dentin. As the bone is resorbed by those phagocytic cells, so is some tooth structure. For this reason it was suggested that roots with radiolucencies be instrumented a greater distance from the radiographic apex than nonradiolucent cases. In the former case some apical resorption should always be anticipated.

A tooth with advanced apical resorption (Fig. 11-4, *A*) usually still contains the ability to heal with nonsurgical treatment, which should be

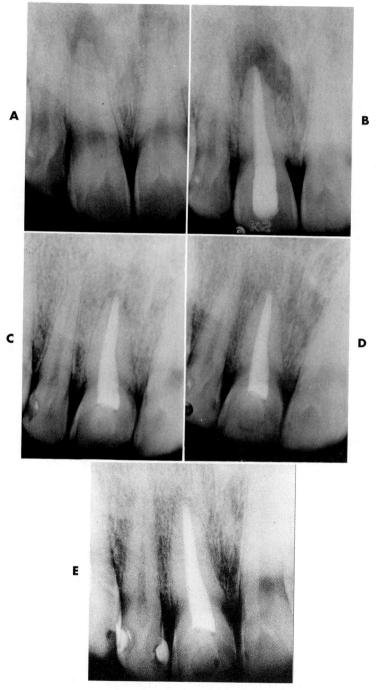

Fig. 11-4. Nonsurgical treatment despite crater-shaped erosion at root apex. **A,** Preoperative radiograph of maxillary anterior area. Central incisor to the left has periapical lesion, plus crater-shaped erosion on the mesial side of the root apex. Tooth was to be treated with routine, nonsurgical therapy. **B,** At the conclusion of the second appointment, canal preparation was completed and the canal was filled with laterally condensed gutta-percha and Wach's paste, custom cone developed as described in Chapter 9. **C,** One year after treatment, lesion is greatly reduced. **D,** Five years after treatment, periapical lesion is gone and there is complete repair of mesial erosion as well. **E,** Eleven years after original treatment, entire area looks excellent. (Restoration by Dr. Harold Brill, Chicago.)

attempted before any thoughts of surgical intervention. Proper canal preparation will produce a periapical region conducive to healing. A well-filled canal with a solid matrix of dentin short of the radiographic apex will ensure that, should surgery be needed later, the root may be beveled back to the well-condensed gutta-percha.

8. *Inability to gain negative culture.* The problems and implications of a negative culture are discussed in Chapter 15. Culturing is rarely utilized in clinical practice at this time under any circumstances. A number of studies have indicated that canal filling after a negative culture is gained shows increased chances for endodontic success as opposed to filling after a positive culture. However, even in teeth whose canals were sealed in the presence of a positive culture, success resulted in a minimum of 80% of the cases.

This indicates that bacteria as such do not cause endodontic failure. If every case that does not yield a negative culture were treated surgically and if the previously stated statistics were reliable, 80% of the so-treated cases could have responded to nonsurgical treatment. Those patients treated surgically were put through the added discomfort and inconvenience of surgery unnecessarily.

Additionally, some teeth filled after negative culture result in failure. Therefore the gaining of a negative culture does not guarantee success any more than a positive culture obligates failure.

After a suitable postoperative observation period, a tooth that has been filled after a positive culture should be evaluated clinically and radiographically. If desired healing has not transpired or if increased bone destruction or symptoms are present, only then should surgery be recommended. This is true whether a positive, a negative, or no culture was obtained before canal filling.

9. *Internal resorption.* There is no question that severe internal resorption cases often require surgery for sealing to occur. The defects may be so large that the cells responsible could not be removed by intracanal instrumentation but only by the curettage that can be performed with the area exposed surgically.

However, many cases with internal resorption (see Fig. 9-35, *C*), especially those with no or minimal perforation into the periodontal ligament space, may be successfully treated nonsurgically. In those cases, heavy irrigation with hypochlorite and subsequent canal enlargement with rasping instruments to relatively large sizes will remove the osteoclastic cells causing the resorption. Heavy condensation or thermoplastic techniques, described in Chapter 9, should be utilized to fill the canal and seal the defects by packing material into the irregular spaces.

Even patients with extremely large perforative resorptive defects may be treated without surgery by placing initially a calcium hydroxide paste following canal preparation and then, after a suitable observation period, filling the canal with heavily condensed gutta-percha (Chapter 16).

Even if surgery must be performed subsequently, there is little to lose by cleansing and filling the canal in the previously suggested manner. The cells responsible must be removed if the resorptive process is to be halted. The canal filling with a heavy condensation technique will force the sealer and filling materials to protrude through the defects and make them more apparent during the surgery.

Based on these considerations, it appears to be a justifiable procedure to attempt to treat cases with internal resorption by nonsurgical means, except in severe defect cases.

10. *Extreme apical curvature.* Most apical curvatures, even those that are extreme, may be safely enlarged and filled with the aids suggested in Chapter 7. Precurved files, incremental instrumentation, removal of flutes, new file systems, and heavy irrigation are of utmost importance. With slow but meticulous preparation and increased use of incremental instruments of intermediate size, beyond normal usage, many abruptly curving canals lend themselves to filling.

When no periapical inflammation is present before treatment, canals that are enlarged and filled shorter than normally desirable will often respond favorably. In these cases the majority of the pulp tissue is removed and the remainder receives pulpotomy-like treatment by the use of intracanal medicaments and sealers.

When a periapical radiolucency is present before treatment and the apical foramen is not reached for debridement, the remaining nidus of inflamed necrotic pulpal tissue may be sufficient to perpetuate the damage. In these cases, when apical curvature is severe, surgery may be required to gain success. However, if instrumentation and filling are carried out close to the apical foramen, a brief postoperative observation period will frequently reveal the initiation of healing and circumvent the need for surgery.

11. *Fracture of root apex with pulpal death.* Roots may fracture without pulpal death occurring if the pulp tissue is able to withstand the injury and not sever at the apical foramen or within the pulp canal space. If pulpal death does occur or if sensitivity to percussion or temperature changes persists, some type of endodontic treatment is mandatory to retain the injured tooth.

For reasons of classification, fractures are categorized according to the position on the root where the break occurs—that is, apical, middle, or cervical third. Many papers recommend surgical treatment for fractures in the apical third and extraction for fractures of the middle third as well as for those in the cervical third when sufficient root face cannot be exposed by means of an alveoloplasty.

At present there are a variety of methods for treating root fractures that become symptomatic. Cervical third fractures may be treated by removal of the coronal segment and forced eruption (Chapter 16) with only periodontal surgery. Fractures further apically may be treated nonsurgically if both segments can be instrumented. The apical few millimeters of the prepared canal are packed with gutta-percha, and then a chrome-cobalt pin is used to stabilize the fracture segments (Chapter 10).

If both halves cannot be instrumented together, there is still a chance to avoid surgery by treating the coronal portion only (Fig. 11-5). The pulp in the apical segment may have retained its vitality and the trauma disturbed the pulp in the coronal section only. If the coronal section is prepared and filled satisfactorily, the area may be observed. If no symptoms occur and the radiograph indicates no abnormal lesions, surgery may be averted. If surgery does become necessary at a later date, the apical portion may be removed and the root trimmed back to the well-condensed gutta-percha filling.

Apical third fractures may be treated similarly—by treating the coronal segment only. For many years, following the treatment of the coronal segment, the fractured root tip would then be removed surgically (Figs. 11-57 and 11-58). However, this view has been altered recently, and the apical segment may be left and then observed. It has been found that in many cases the apical fragment causes no problems (any lesion heals, the unfilled segment remains normal) or, in fact, the apical segment resorbs, leaving only the treated coronal portion (Fig. 11-6).

SURGERY FOR CONVENIENCE OF TREATMENT

With so many false indications listed, it appears obvious that a relatively low number of cases truly require surgical treatment. However, where needed, surgery is a most important adjunct to successful therapy, and a number of cases definitely require surgery to reach a desired result. One general purpose for which surgery may be need is greater convenience of treatment. This refers to the cases in which surgery offers the simplest and swiftest successful result. Specific examples in this area include teeth with periapical radiolucencies and a very short period of time available for completion of therapy, cases with recurrent acute exacerbations, root configurations that present a strong possibility of failure if nonsurgical treatment is followed, and cases in which the most convenient access is available by way of the apex. In addition, a surgical approach is needed to gain relief in cases requiring immediate drainage that is impossible or inconvenient to gain through the root canal, although further therapy, either surgical or nonsurgical, is still necessary.

Teeth with radiolucencies and brief period of time available for completion of therapy. Radiolucencies are often amenable to nonsurgical treatment when time for more than one appointment is available and when the patient may be recalled at a later date for evaluation of healing. However, if time for only one appointment exists, teeth with radiolucencies should be treated by canal enlargement and filling followed by apical surgery. One-appointment nonsurgical treatment of teeth with radiolucencies will lead to a tremendous number of postoperative exacerbations, which then must be treated by surgery or extraction but under acute conditions. To avoid this, elective surgery is frequently used for military personnel and others who are brought considerable distances to dental dispensaries with the proviso that all necessary work must be completed in the shortest possible period of time.

Although one-visit nonsurgical treatment may be performed without severe periapical reaction on teeth with vital pulps, that method is not recommended. If even 2 days are available for treatment, the canals may be enlarged at the first and filled at the second appointment. The need for the second appointment is to allow the intracanal medicaments to fix any retained pulp tissue, to arrest the

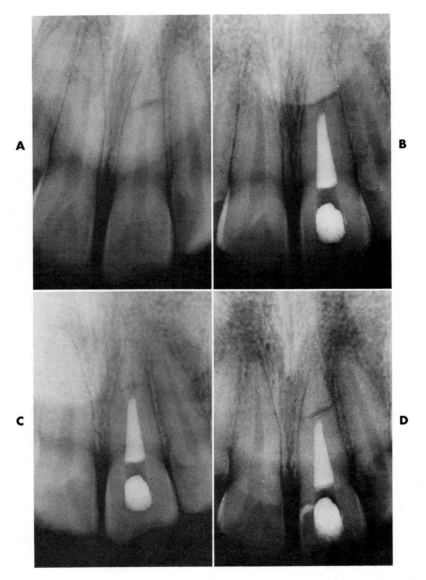

Fig. 11-5.   Treatment of tooth with root fracture by endodontics on coronal portion only. **A,** Maxillary central incisor with midroot horizontal fracture. Coronal portion is mobile and tender to percussion. **B,** Apical segment could not be instrumented. Accordingly, coronal portion is prepared and filled with gutta-percha. If surgery does become necessary later, root may be trimmed back to the well-condensed filling, so nothing is lost by this effort. Tooth is no longer tender to percussion and is much less mobile despite no stabilization. **C,** Three months later. **D,** Eighteen months later, tooth is tight and not tender to percussion. Apical segment has remained normal radiographically. (Courtesy Dr. Chris Wenckus, Chicago.)

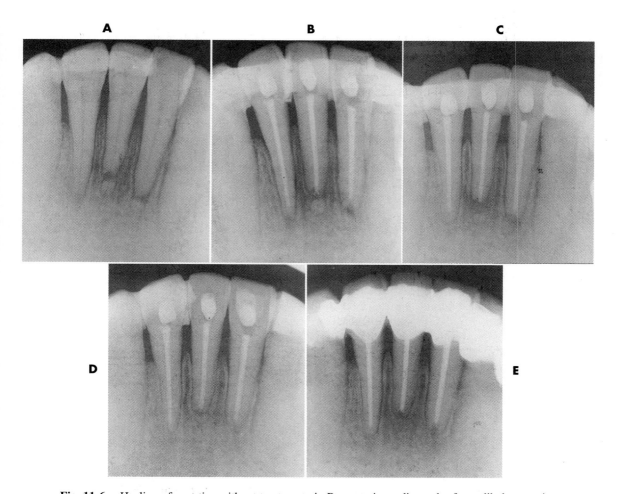

Fig. 11-6. Healing of root tips without treatment. **A,** Preoperative radiograph of mandibular anterior area. Mandibular lateral incisor to the left (tooth no. 26) was exquisitely sensitive to percussion, slightly mobile, and responded to electric pulp testing. Adjacent central incisor (no. 25) was mildly tender to percussion, nonresponsive to pulp testing, and slightly mobile. Central incisor to the right (no. 24) was not tender to percussion nor mobile and did not respond to pulp testing. It was decided to treat all three teeth, wait for some healing and then enter surgically to remove the root tips for no. 24 and no. 25. If any problem existed with the healing of any of the three teeth, it would be addressed at the same time with curettage, reverse filling, or whatever else was deemed to be appropriate. **B,** Teeth no. 24 and no. 25 responded to treatment rapidly and were filled with laterally condensed gutta-percha and Wach's paste after two appointments each. On the other hand, no. 26 was tender to percussion throughout treatment, despite placement of a corticosteroid/antibiotic combination apically and further splinting with composite. After five appointments, it improved and was filled in the same manner as were the others. Note that on the postfilling film, the root tip for no. 25 seems to have rotated 90 degrees. **C,** Six months later, all three teeth are comfortable, with composite splint still in place. Root tip of no. 25 has moved further away from the rest of the tooth, root tip for no. 24 has moved to mesial, and the periapical lesion for no. 26 seems to be healing. The patient was advised that surgery seemed to be necessary for no. 24 and no. 25, but that no. 26 seemed to be better. Therefore, we decided to wait another 6 months to evaluate healing further. **D,** One year after original treatment, splint has broken, but teeth are firm, comfortable, and lesions seem to be decreasing in size. Even more interestingly, the root tips for no. 24 and no. 25 seem to be decreasing considerably! **E,** Six years after original treatment, all teeth are comfortable and firm (cast splint may be responsible for this), and there is virtually no sign of the root tips! No surgery was ever performed.

hemorrhage in the apical pulpal vessels, and to allow for easier removal of the elements of the predentin layer that had been packed against the walls of the preparation. Although some authors suggest the use of periapical surgery whenever a one-visit endodontic filling procedure is employed, regardless of the condition of the periapical tissue, that theory does not appear to be consistent with biologic principles and clinical experience. When the periapical tissues appears to be normal, surgery is rarely needed. On the other hand, if a periapical radiolucency is evident, surgery is suggested.

Recurrent acute exacerbations. Even the most experienced endodontists are faced with the distress of acute exacerbations. Whether the result of overinstrumentation, anaerobic bacteria, lowered resistance of the patient, virulence of the microorganisms, or some other reason, the exacerbations cause extreme pain, discomfort, and inflammatory sequelae. In addition, recurrent exacerbations may cause psychological as well as physical damage.

Most exacerbations respond quickly and easily to nonsurgical therapy. However, in some cases the exacerbation may repeat itself; when this occurs, a decision must be made concerning possible alteration of the treatment plan. It has been stated earlier that surgery is much more painful and destructive to tissue compared with nonsurgical treatment, but this factor must be weighed against the damage that may result from future exacerbations if conventional treatment is pursued. The most reliable rule to follow appears to be that if surgery would be extremely difficult, as with posterior teeth, with teeth bordering on vital structures, or with patients suffering from debilitating diseases, further efforts with nonsurgical treatment should be attempted. If the area to be treated surgically is relatively easy to manipulate, as in anterior teeth or buccal roots of maxillary molars, and the patient is in good health, then surgery obviously would be the choice of treatment.

The frequency with which acute exacerbations now occur is much less than it was several years ago. Because of recent studies and basic science knowledge, canals are overinstrumented less often and teeth are left open for drainage less frequently, which results in fewer problems in closing, too. Subculturing of exudates has promptly determined the susceptibility of causative microorganisms and reduced their actions. Calcium hydroxide treatment has been shown effective in chronic "weep-ing" cases (Chapter 7). Soon the indication of recurrent acute exacerbations may join the others as a nonviable condition.

Root configurations presenting a strong possibility of failure if treated nonsurgically. The most common type of case falling into this category is the tooth with a sharp apical dilaceration plus a periapical radiolucency. In general, teeth with periapical radiolucencies must be instrumented to the apical foramen to rid the canal of necrotic debris, metabolites, bacteria, and other irritants causing the adjacent bone inflammation and then filled to that point to prevent recurrence. However, if because of a sharp apical dilaceration the apical foramen is not reached in cases showing radiolucency, nonsurgical treatment would yield a strong possibility of failure. To circumvent this, the dentist should perform surgery when the problem is recognized rather than wait. Although postponing the surgery may result in a small percentage of healing cases, it also may allow an acute exacerbation to occur, increasing the size of the lesion so it approaches an important adjacent structure; or postponement may permit the patient, thinking that the case is successful, to leave the area of control of the treating dentist.

In the cases with a vital pulp and normal periapical tissue, if the apical foramen cannot be reached for enlarging and filling, treatment may be successfully carried out by terminating as close to the apex as is physically possible. If the tissue left within the canal is able to remain relatively uninflamed, success will follow filling to that point.

Teeth with canal bifurcations in the middle or apical third may present considerable problems, similar to those found in teeth with sharp dilacerations. Although one of the two canals, the one most continuous with the large, main passage, usually is amenable to adequate enlarging and filling procedures, it is often extremely difficult to prepare and fill the other canal. If vital tissue remains in the inadequately treated canal and retains a noninflamed condition, success may result. However, if this untreated canal has necrotic tissue or is associated with a radiolucency, it is unlikely that success will be gained unless surgery is performed. The procedure during surgery would involve the removal or filling of the additional canal from apical access.

Dens in dente and other root anomalies present problems that are difficult to solve without periapical surgery. In these cases the peculiar shape and angulation of the canals prevent the normal routine debridement and filling procedures. By resorting to periapical surgery, the canal apices are sealed by reverse filling methods, or apicoectomies are performed to remove root substance down to the position where a canal filling has been placed.

Teeth with most convenient access available by way of the apex. The most common types of cases falling into this category are (1) the problem of calcific degeneration and (2) the post-and-core crown associated with developing periapical pathosis or clinical symptoms (Fig. 11-7).

As previously discussed, *calcific degeneration* has many synonyms, is generally caused by trauma, and rarely, if ever, leads to complete, microscopic obliteration of the root canal space (Fig. 11-8). Despite the radiographic appearance, somewhere inside the dentin a root canal space exists, probably containing pulp tissue with some degree of inflammation, degeneration, or necrosis. This entity has been called *nature's root canal filling,* and statistics have been presented to indicate that calcification often occurs without clinical or radiographic evidence of disease. However, a certain percentage of cases with no apparent root canal space do require endodontic treatment because of pain, usually to percussion, and/or radiographic evidence of periapical breakdown. Even if a very faint canal confined to the root portion of the tooth is noted on the radiograph, routine endodontic therapy becomes hazardous. An attempt to prepare the access cavity usually results in a considerable gutting of the tooth, leaving the remaining portion extremely fragile, or may even lead to root perforation. As a result, an increase rather than a decrease of problems transpires.

The removal of a large, well-fitting *post and core* is difficult and may be dangerous, since the possibility of root fracture exists. If a satisfactory post and core is present on a tooth requiring endodontic treatment, an alternative access should be utilized rather than one through the root canal space. The need for therapy may be periapical breakdown after the failure of a previously placed canal filling or, unusual as it may seem, a post and core having been placed in the absence of a canal filling.

In my opinion, if a poor, failing root canal filling is present, even when the post, core, and crown are satisfactory, it is best to *disassemble the restoration and re-treat, even if surgery may still be necessary.* Without re-treating prior to surgery, it is almost always necessary to use a reverse filling when the post-and-core remains to improve the apical seal. With recent studies questioning the reliability of reverse fillings, especially those employed amalgam, it is best to re-treat through the canal. This alone will yield a number of successful cases, without resorting to surgery. Even if surgery still becomes necessary later, the apical portion of the filling can be cut

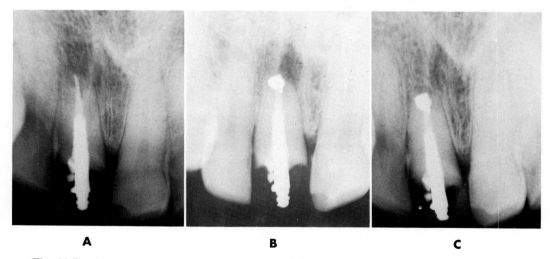

A   **B**   **C**

Fig. 11-7. Surgery where most convenient access is by way of apex. **A,** Large post could not be removed, but a periapical lesion is present **B,** Apical surgery was performed and reverse filling placed. **C,** Excellent healing 1 year later.

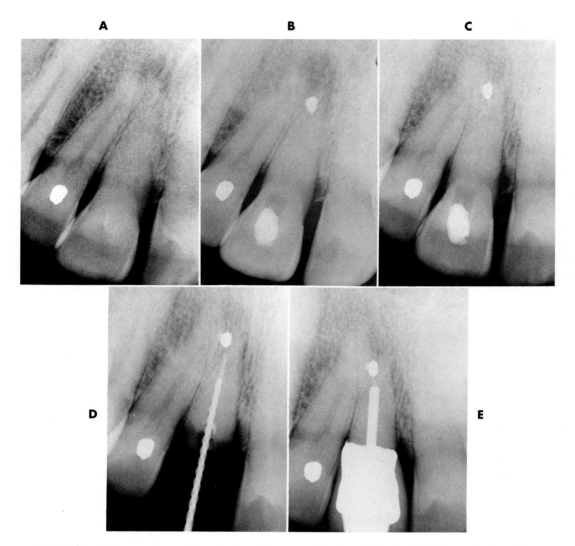

Fig. 11-8. **A,** Preoperative radiograph of maxillary central incisor with periapical lesion, apical sensitivity, and no apparent canal. **B,** An attempt was made to locate the canal, but after drilling into the tooth to a level beneath the gingival line, it was decided to treat surgically only, for fear of perforating while looking for the canal. Consequently an apicoectomy and reverse filling with amalgam were performed, and the periapical lesion curetted. **C,** One year later, all apical sensitivity was gone and periapical lesion has healed. **D,** Six months later, the crown broke off at the gingival margin. The dentist started to prepare room for a post and uncovered the canal! A gutta-percha filling was placed into the prepared canal and room for a post provided. **E,** Three years after original treatment, a post-core, and crown have been placed, the periapical region has remained normal, and no apical sensitivity is present. Even though it appeared that no canal was present, as determined by radiograph and access preparation, several millimeters of canal length were present. (Restoration by Dr. Steve Potashnick, Chicago.)

back to well packed gutta-percha rather than relying on a reverse filling technique.

Apical surgery is still chosen by many as the first choice in these conditions. Some prefer surgery to locate and fill the apical foramen by access from the apex rather than through the root canal. The definition of a root canal filling is stated to be the sealing of the apical foramen with an inert material and does not specify the direction from which the filling is placed. The reverse or retrograde filling technique, either with amalgam, gutta-percha, or other material, may be successfully utilized in cases of considerable dentinal obliteration or in teeth with post and core in position. It is important to emphasize that in treating cases with calcific degeneration, a reverse filling should always be placed, even if no canal is evident. Since a microscopically small canal may be present, failure to place an apical filling will allow the inflamed tissue present to perpetuate the problem and prevent healing. The exact method of surgery will be discussed later in this chapter.

SURGERY TO RE-TREAT A FAILURE OR SYMPTOMATIC CASE

It has been strongly suggested that conservative endodontic therapy should be carried out whenever possible, before instituting a surgical procedure, even if the conservative treatment has a definite chance of failure. However, if nonsurgical treatment fails to gain the desired result, surgery is waiting in the wings to avert extraction. Endodontics is fortunate that, rather than be saddled with only one method of therapy, it has a second method of therapy available to reclaim a tooth and allow it to continue functioning as an integral portion of the dental arch. Specific types of cases falling into the category of failing or symptomatic conservative cases to be re-treated surgically will be discussed next.

Failure of an incompletely formed apex to close. If the use of apexification methods fails to gain the desired apical closure, surgery may be performed. The exact method for treating this type of case surgically will be discussed in the section concerning the use of reverse fill procedures. However, if an open apex case fails to continue apexification after one attempt to debride and place the effective paste, it is usually desirable to pursue a second or even third apexification attempt before resorting to surgery, since internal weakness of the tooth is a usual result because of the minimal amount of dentin and cementum in the underdeveloped tooth treated surgically. The position for placement of a post and core at a later date must be considered before placing the canal filling prior to surgery. Also, the crown-to-root ratio that will result after surgery should be estimated to ensure that an acceptable ratio will be present.

Open apex cases usually occur in youngsters. Since the surgical procedure may be traumatic to a child, a suitable premedicament may be necessary.

Marked overfilling associated with failure. Any tooth with marked overfilling, whether gutta-percha or silver point, that fails to heal after conservative treatment is a good candidate for periapical surgery. The overfilling protrudes through the bone to give an excellent landmark for finding the apex of the tooth. Often the reason for failure of an overfilling is that the fill was preceded by overinstrumentation, which in turn caused a severe inflammation in the adjacent periapical tissue. When the excess filling material is removed by curettage with a hand instrument or by bur, the inflamed adjacent tissue is also removed, allowing for excellent healing in most cases.

Many overfilled canals are in reality underfilled with overextended filling materials failing to seal the apical foramen. Removal of the overextended filling materials will not give the canal a seal at the apex. In fact, a probable cause for the failure is the incompleteness of the seal rather than the overextended material. In most cases with gutta-percha as the filling material, there will be a site within several millimeters of the apex where the canal is densely filled. For surgery in these cases, an apicoectomy down to the site of dense filling should be accomplished whenever such a reduction does not jeopardize the crown-to-root ratio.

For overextended silver points or when there are no sites near the apex where gutta-percha is densely sealed, some type of reverse filling must be placed to ensure apical seal, either by reverse filing and filling with gutta-percha or by reverse filling.

Persistent pain. Since the advent of the corticosteroid-antibiotic combinations and the decrease in use of caustic intracanal medicaments, rarely does intratreatment pain persist. Therefore the need for periapical surgery to correct this problem is infrequent. However, surgery may be needed when pain after canal filling persists.

The complaint of pain after canal filling is not unusual. In most cases the tenderness dissipates after a few days and rarely lasts for more than 1 week. The few instances in which pain persists beyond that length of time frequently are difficult to comprehend when radiographs reveal no apparent fault. When posttreatment pain fails to subside, surgery is usually suggested so that an accurate examination of the periapical tissues where the pain resides can be made and any discrepancies corrected. Often the flapping of the tissue reveals an unexpected picture, much unlike that indicated by radiographs alone, and the cause of the pain becomes apparent. Examples of teeth that appear satisfactory on radiographs but have an obvious problem when exposed surgically are those with apical fenestrations and root fractures.

A fenestration is a "window" in the bone through which the apex protrudes; this commonly occurs in maxillary central incisors, cuspids, and the buccal roots of the maxillary first bicuspid and molar when the apical foramen exits labially. If the root canal filling extends any distance past the apical foramen, the movable connective tissue covering the apical portion of the root remains in an inflamed condition. In surgical treatment of these cases, it is simple to locate the apex, since the root has no bony covering. The excess filling is trimmed, and some of the labial portion of the root is reduced so the remainder falls within the bony housing, where it will probably be covered by bone after the healing process (Fig. 11-9).

Persistent pain will follow the fracture of a root during canal filling whether due to excessive forces used in condensation of gutta-percha, placement of a silver point, or insertion of a dowel. Because these fractures are usually vertical rather than horizontal, the line of fracture is rarely discernible on the radiograph, although the typically large, diffuse radiolucency along the lateral surface of the root begins to develop soon after the accident. When the affected root is exposed by surgical means, the fracture line may be visualized. Unfortunately, the prognosis for such a condition is usually hopeless, and extraction is indicated.

Rarely does pain persist in cases where incomplete debridement of a portion of the apex has left inflamed material in contact with periapical tissue. However, when a canal is found to have been enlarged and filled short and pain remains after treatment, the unfilled portion of the canal is removed, down to where the canal filling is sealing satisfactorily.

Overinstrumentation, particularly at the canal filling appointment, may cause persistent postoperative pain. Usually this will be eliminated before causing consideration of surgery, but it may not.

As in the case of treating an overfilling by surgery, the locating and trimming of the apex of the tooth will remove the inflamed periapical tissue causing the pain.

If the root can be trimmed down to a solid gutta-percha site that seals the canal, no reverse filling is needed. Otherwise, reinforcement of seal will be required.

Acute exacerbation after canal filling. Much more serious than merely persistent pain is the occurrence of an acute exacerbation after canal filling. The etiology of such a reaction is probably the inoculation of the periapical tissues with a microorganism of high virulence. If the root canal is well filled, surgery must be performed to retain the tooth and grant relief from the typical symptoms of pain, mobility, and swelling.

Since it is highly desirable to control the infection before performing periapical surgery, the proper therapy is to prescribe antibiotics and obtain drainage by incision into the periapical tissue. After the symptoms subside, periapical surgery is scheduled, with the antibiotic that proved to be effective represcribed. In some cases the surgical procedure may be little more complicated than obtaining drainage through the soft tissues and bone. If that is the situation, the apical surgery may be performed under acute conditions, but only with heavy antibiotic coverage.

Drainage through the root canal is almost always preferable to incision through periapical tissue to the apex, especially when an acute infection is present. Therefore, if it appears that a gutta-percha canal filling could be dissolved by solvents and the periapical tissues reached through the canal, that is the better route to choose. If the canal is filled with a silver point, the filling must extend to a position where it can be retrieved in order to go through the canal to the periapex. If the canal seems to be ledged or communication to the infected periapical space impossible to gain by

---

Fig. 11-9.   Surgery to treat apical fenestration. **A,** Maxillary first bicuspid 3 months after completion of endodontic treatment. Tooth had needed therapy due to carious exposure of a vital pulp, but immediately after completion of treatment a very sore area developed at the site approximating tip of the buccal root. **B,** Old canal fillings were dissolved, and canals were reprepared and filled with laterally condensed gutta-percha. Fillings seemed more densely and better filled, but apical tenderness persisted. **C,** Area was flapped surgically, and a "window" in the bone was noted immediately *(arrow)* without removal of any hard tissue. **D,** Root tip was merely trimmed back so it was completely within bony housing. **E,** Postsurgical radiograph. **F,** Eleven months later, symptoms had vanished immediately, never to return.

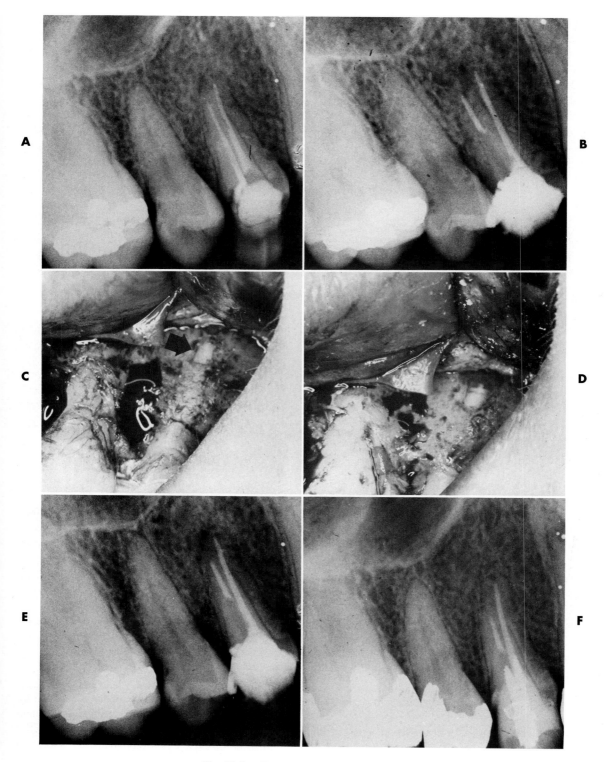

Fig. 11-9. For legend see opposite page.

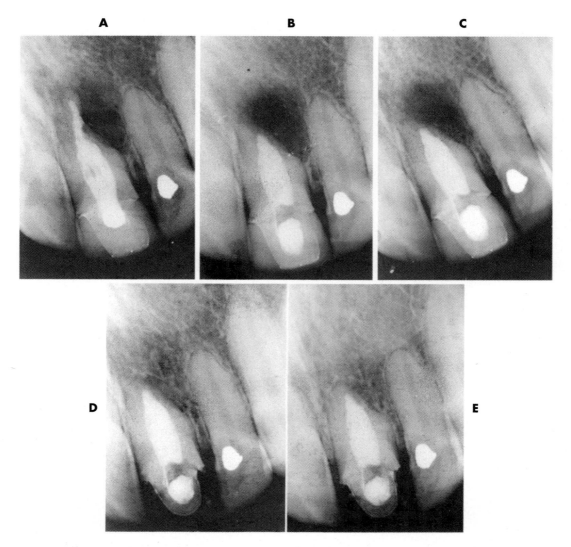

Fig. 11-10. A, Preoperative radiograph of maxillary central incisor. Tooth had been treated initially with apexification procedure, but when that failed, periapical surgery was performed. A periapical lesion and a chronic draining sinus tract were present. **B,** It was decided that another surgical procedure was needed. The access was opened and the old gutta-percha removed. A new gutta-percha filling was placed using lateral condensation and Tubliseal. The periapical lesion was curetted and part of the root tip removed. **C,** Six months later. **D,** Eighteen months later. **E,** Thirty months after original treatment, the lesion has healed and the tooth is tight, with no tracts present. A temporary crown had been in place up to this time, but now the referring dentist was informed that completion of the restoration could be undertaken. (Temporization by Dr. Kerry Voit, Chicago.)

that route, surgical incision may be the best solution. Another attempt at nonsurgical treatment is justifiable if the area requiring the surgery is considered to be a difficult one in which to operate.

Lack of apical seal. Ingle stated that the most frequent cause—58% of failing cases—was lack of apical seal. Although we believe the stated percentage is much too high, there is no question that

lack of apical seal is a frequent cause of failure and must be taken into consideration when apical surgery is done to re-treat a failure.

In some of these cases the canal may appear to be well filled radiographically and within the confines of the root. However, when the case is flapped and the seal examined carefully, voids around the filling are discovered. In gutta-percha

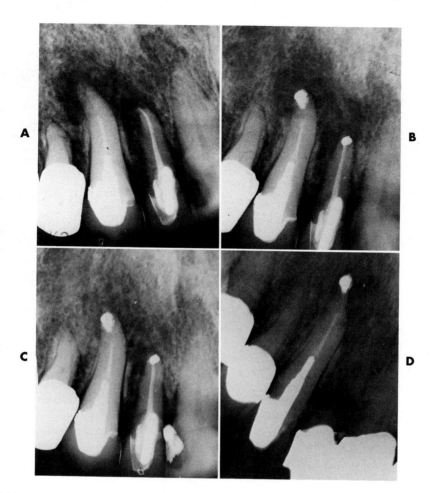

Fig. 11-11. **A,** Maxillary cuspid and lateral with poor canal fillings and large periapical lesions. **B,** Rather than refill the teeth, only apical reverse fills were placed after curettage. In retrospect, posts probably should have been removed and the canals reprepared and refilled. **C,** Six months later, some healing is evident. **D,** Nine years later, lateral has been extracted, and there is a return area of pathosis around apex of cuspid. It is doubtful whether amalgam is still within confines of the root; it probably has been exfoliated due to apical resorption.

cases this may be due to failure to flare the canal sufficiently, inability to condense the apical portion of the filling, or failure to place auxiliary cones in the space created by the spreader. In silver point cases this results because the round filling material fails to close the irregularly shaped canal (see Fig. 11-48). Small crevices or voids around the sealing material may be sufficient to harbor irritants capable of perpetuating apical inflammation.

If a case involving incomplete apical seal is to be re-treated surgically, every effort should be made to remove the previous canal filling and replace it with well-condensed gutta-percha prior to the surgery (Fig. 11-10). This method may demonstrate the presence of lateral canals, give more information concerning the

shape of the canal, or suggest the presence of additional main canals that had been uninstrumented earlier. This initial refilling may make the surgical entry unnecessary but surely makes the knowledge gained in filling useful in the surgical approach.

If a poorly filled canal is merely reverse filled, the surgery will probably remove the irritated tissue and seal up the source of damage. However, several factors may occur later to cause a renewal of the problem. If the tooth so treated later requires a post-and-core crown, the removal of a portion of the poor filling may dislodge the apical seal and recreate the problem. If apical resorption occurs around the reverse filling, the apically placed material may lose seal or, even worse, be exfoliated (Fig. 11-11).

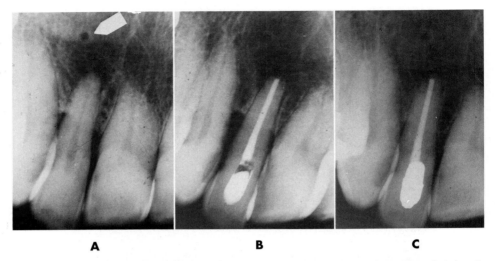

A   **B**   **C**

Fig. 11-12. **A,** Patient was referred for treatment of the lateral incisor. History revealed that three "operations for cyst removal over the tooth" had been performed, but canal was never filled. Note small fibrous tissue defect *(arrow)*. **B,** Canal was filled and area curetted. Biopsy report was apical periodontal cyst. **C,** Area healed 18 months later. Fibrous tissue defect will not heal any further radiographically.

Although it seems difficult to believe, the philosophy of placing a canal filling in a tooth during a surgical effort is a policy not always adhered to. In some cases no canal filling whatever is present (Fig. 11-12). These cases may often be successfully treated without any further surgery, merely by cleansing and then filling the canal.

Unfilled portion of the canal. Failure resulting from an unfilled portion of the canal really is another type of case involving lack of apical seal. The tissue in the untreated portion of the canal breaks down and, with apical seal lacking, causes an inflammatory process in the adjacent periapical tissue. Usually the portion is left unfilled because it was not recognized to be present, as in a canal with a bifurcation in the apical third, or because it was impossible to instrument, as with a sharp dilaceration.

Many cases with an unfilled portion of the canal do not fail, and careful evaluation of the radiographic and clinical situation must be made before further therapy in the form of surgery is suggested. However, if a radiolucency is present in a tooth that had normal periapical tissue preoperatively, if there is no decrease in an area that was present preoperatively, if a chronic draining sinus is associated with the tooth in question, or if tenderness to percussion is present, surgery is indicated. Attempting to re-treat such teeth conservatively usually is a futile exercise, since it is

rarely possible to bypass the ledge formed during the initial instrumentation at the point of bifurcation or dilaceration.

The method of therapy varies according to the anatomic position of the problem. Reverse fill procedures may be used from the apex to seal the canal, or the unfilled portion of the root may be removed down to the point at which the canal was previously filled.

Failures for unknown clinical reason. Some cases defy categorization as to failure from a clinical standpoint. The canals appear to be well prepared and filled. Angled radiographs reveal no additional unfilled canals. Repreparation and refilling do not appear to offer a better chance, so surgery is performed. With the apex flapped, the filling appears to be quite adequate.

In these cases, if the operator is positive that the seal is adequate, curettage of the periapical pathologic area only is indicated. A high percentage of these cases will heal well without reverse filling (Figs. 11-13 and 11-14).

Since this type of failure is reclaimed after surgery without altering the canal filing, it is obvious that the failure is not due to lack of apical seal. In fact, there appears to be no clinical reason why the case has failed. The only possible reason for the failure could be due to something explainable by basic science.

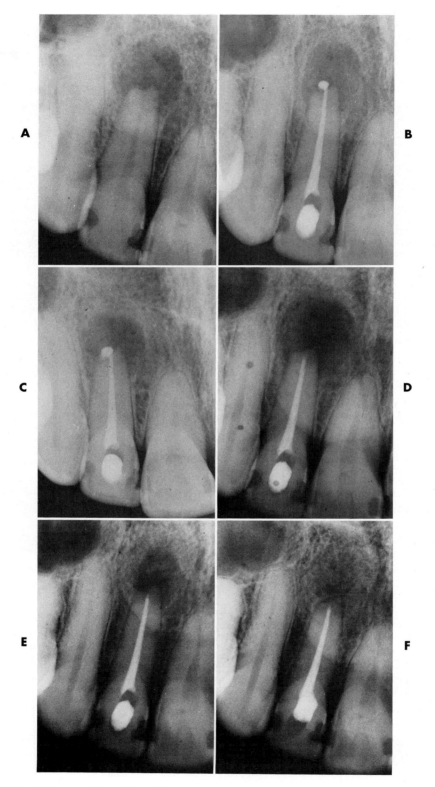

Fig. 11-13. **A,** Preoperative radiograph of maxillary lateral incisor with larger periapical lesion. **B,** Canal filling with laterally condensed gutta-percha. **C,** One year later, no decrease in size of the lesion. **D,** Periapical surgery was performed and the area curetted. Canal filling appeared good at time of surgery, and no reverse filling was placed. Biopsy indicated apical granuloma. **E,** Six months later, area is decreasing. **F,** Eighteen months after surgery, area has almost disappeared.

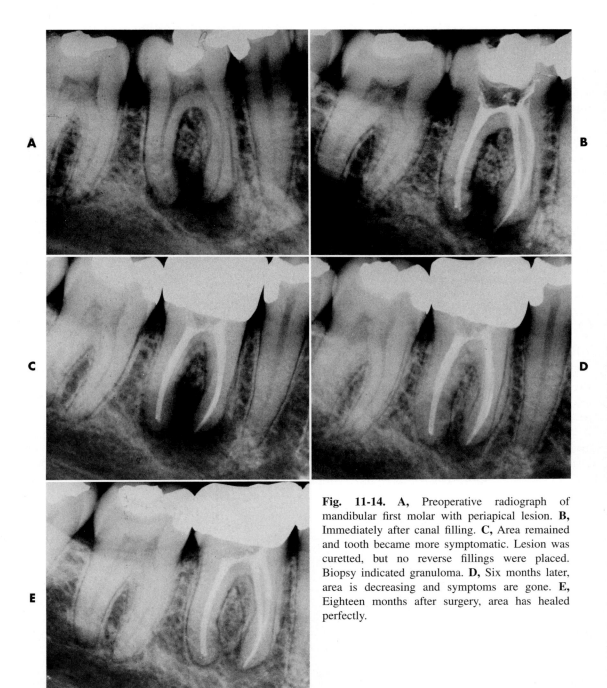

Fig. 11-14. A, Preoperative radiograph of mandibular first molar with periapical lesion. **B,** Immediately after canal filling. **C,** Area remained and tooth became more symptomatic. Lesion was curetted, but no reverse fillings were placed. Biopsy indicated granuloma. **D,** Six months later, area is decreasing and symptoms are gone. **E,** Eighteen months after surgery, area has healed perfectly.

If the lesion were a cyst, the presence of that lesion could be responsible for the failure to heal. There are several acceptable theories that give convincing evidence for the nonsurgical healing of cystic lesions. Even so, some cysts do not heal. The pathologic report on some curetted nonhealed periapical lesions indicate that a granuloma was present, not a cyst. It would appear that in some conditions, granulomas also do not heal without surgical curettage (Fig. 11-13).

The cause for such failure may be that the virulence of the microorganisms present is too great for the resistance of the patient. Only the physical removal of the well-entrenched microorganisms and associated substrate by curettage would lead to healing. Another possible explanation may be the presence of an intense inflammatory reaction that has a perpetuating rather than a healing potential. There are several immunologic explanations that dovetail with this situation.

Under any circumstances, it is fortunate that surgical procedures are present that allow for these perplexing conditions in which a failure is present for no apparent clinical reason.

SURGERY AFTER PROCEDURAL ACCIDENT

The most common procedural accidents encountered during endodontic therapy are breakage of instruments and filling materials, ledging, and root perforations. The major cause of endodontic failure is lack of apical seal, and any of these accidents may prevent the obtaining of a desirable seal. Therefore, although the teeth of some patients with these problems will heal without surgical treatment, even in the most favorable conditions all are potential candidates for surgery. If surgery is not immediately undertaken in the hope that some chance for healing is present, suitable recording must be made on the patient's chart and periodic recall examinations must be arranged to evaluate repair.

Broken instruments. The position of broken instruments in relation to the root apex, the width of the shaft, the degree of enlargement, and the pretreatment condition of the periapical tissues must be evaluated before any further course of therapy is decided. In many cases, periapical surgery may be postponed until after a suitable observation period for determining the postoperative progress. This is particularly true in cases where the preexisting periapical tissue was normal, where the broken instrument was very close to the apical foramen, or where a periapical radiolucency was present but a considerable degree of canal enlargement had been accomplished. In a significant number of these cases healing will occur without surgical intervention.

However, when a strong possibility for failure exists, surgery should be undertaken. As a general rule, when a broken instrument protrudes past the apex, surgery should be performed to remove the constant irritant. If a periapical radiolucency is present and minimal canal enlargement has been performed before the accident, surgery is indicated, since the periapical tissues have had little opportunity for healing to be stimulated. When the instrument breaks far from the apical foramen, leaving a large portion of the canal apically or laterally unfilled, particularly when a periapical radiolucency is present, surgery is needed. However, in a limited number of cases when instruments break off some distance from the apex, they may be bypassed with smaller files. Then further instrumentation will either remove the fragment or enable the operator to fill the apical portion of the canal properly and obtain a desirable result without surgery.

The type of surgical procedure to be used varies with the position of the broken instrument. When the fragment is at or near the apical foramen, the remaining unfilled portion of the canal is filled with gutta-percha by the lateral condensation method; then a suitable flap is used to expose the apex and an apicoectomy performed to the site of the well condensed gutta-percha.

A similar technique may be followed when the broken instrument extends past the apical foramen, since the excess material will be removed when the apical bevel is placed prior to the apicoectomy. However, the postresection filling technique, or "two open ends," which will be explained later in this chapter, is usually best when a fragment extends past the apex. In this method the broken instrument is surgically removed, and then the entire canal is filled with laterally condensed gutta-percha.

Broken filling materials. Broken filling materials rarely require the use of surgery. If the filling material is gutta-percha, a suitable solvent, such as xylene or chloroform, may be used to dissolve the undesired material. If a silver point breaks off in the apical portion of a canal without sealer coating the canal walls, there is always a possibility that the point may still give sufficient seal to the apical foramen. When the point seems to be in a desirable position, an observation period is used to determine the need for further intervention. If a

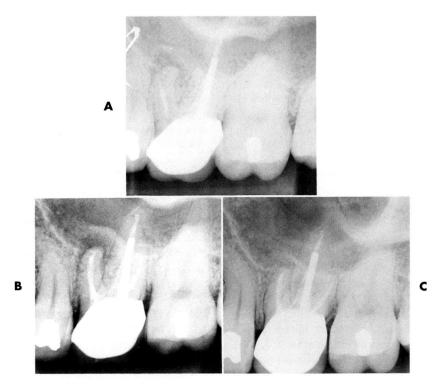

Fig. 11-15. A, Preoperative radiograph of maxillary first molar. Endodontic therapy had been attempted, but a ledge was present in the mesiobuccal root; a periapical lesion and apical sensitivity also represent. Periapical surgery could have been performed, but it would be better to refill the mesiobuccal canal first under any circumstances. **B,** The ledge was bypassed with a small instrument, and the canal prepared to its correct length. Filling with laterally condensed gutta-percha and Wach's paste followed, and the area was observed for healing. **C,** One year later, the lesion is considerably decreased in size. Probably no surgery will be needed. If surgery does become necessary, the root may be resected down to the well-filled canal rather than relying on a reverse filling to a poorly filled canal.

silver point breaks off short of the apex, it is possible to bypass the filling with a file and either remove the filling material or properly prepare and fill the canal past the broken point.

The fact that a canal is ready for filling considerably improves the prognosis after such a procedural accident. The irritants within the canal have been removed, and the periapical tissues are either noninflamed or in a condition conducive to healing.

Therefore teeth with broken filling materials require surgery with even less frequency than do those with broken instruments. However, if a silver point breaks off past the apex and there is indication that the point does not seal the apical foramen, surgery is suggested. Just as in treatment of a tooth in which an instrument is broken past the apex, the postresection filling technique should be used first to remove the fragment surgically and

then to fill the root canal. If a silver point separates within the canal confines short of the apex and no instrument can bypass it, apical surgery with a reverse fill procedure should be performed.

Ledging. The use of radiographs to determine canal length, heavy irrigation, precurved files, and incremental instrumentation greatly reduces the chances for ledging. When ledges do occur, some may be bypassed with smaller instruments (Fig. 11-15) or a filling inserted past the ledge by a partially dissolved filling method. However, in most instances ledging prevents the obtaining of a satisfactory apical seal and thus frequently leads to endodontic failure.

If the periapical tissue was normal preoperatively and if the ledging occurs relatively close to the apical foramen, the canal should be further enlarged and filled with a heavy condensation technique.

After an observation period, further evaluation will determine whether or not surgery is necessary.

When a preoperative periapical radiolucency is present or when the ledging occurs far short of the apex, periapical surgery is suggested to save the tooth. In cases of this type, reverse filling procedures coupled with periapical curettage remove the inflamed tissue and seal the canal. If the ledge occurs only slightly short of the apex, the unfilled portion of the root may be removed, and if a tight seal is provided by the gutta-percha, no reverse filling is needed. However, if a considerable amount of root requires removal in order to get to the previously placed canal filling, an undesirable crown-to-root ratio would result. Reverse filling is therefore preferable.

If periapical surgery is needed but impractical because of tooth position or local factors, an extraction should be considered. When this situation prevails in a multirooted tooth, root amputation is preferable to extraction. The offending root is removed, and the remaining root or roots are left in the arch to prevent the need for a fixed or removable replacement.

Root perforation. In addition to procedural accidents during attempts to locate a canal or follow its configuration, perforations may occur as pathologic entities in internal or external resorption. Not all perforations require surgery for repair, since many are sealed satisfactorily by heavy condensation procedures or by additional packing through the root canal. Massive perforations, either pathologic or man-made, may contraindicate endodontic therapy entirely. As with ledging, careful canal enlargement procedures usually prevent root perforations. When they do occur, the use of heavy condensation or partially dissolved gutta-percha techniques (Fig. 9-37) may enable the operator to seal the perforation as well as the true root canal and obtain satisfactory results without surgery.

When a root perforation does occur, there is a point of separation at which the two canals divide. When the division occurs close to the apex or on a relatively long tooth, an apicoectomy may be performed to this point of separation. Since it is usually no problem to fill the canal tightly up to that point, the unfilled canal and the false canal are removed but the canal sealed at the point of surgery. This technique is easier to perform than two separate reverse fills and may be used whenever a satisfactory crown-root ratio would remain after surgery.

If the point of separation is in a less favorable position or if the true canal is not sealed, surgery becomes more complex. In order to seal the true and the man-made canals, two separate reverse fillings may be necessary. The root must be cut down and beveled toward the operator's view so that the entire root face may be examined for the location of any unfilled canals. Preparations for the reverse fillings must be placed very carefully so that sufficient dentin remains to retain the reverse filling materials and provide for a margin of solid dentin on the periphery. The damaged area might well be an apical "zip" rather than a perforation (Chapter 7), which will require the repair of a slotted tear-drop-shaped defect. The root bevel must be sufficient to provide the operator with a view of the complete root face so that the correct treatment can be made.

SURGERY TO GAIN INFORMATION FROM A BIOPSY

Reports on histopathologic examination of periapical lesions indicate that approximately 99% are related to the loss of vitality of the pulp and thus are either granulomas, cysts, or chronic abscesses. Of the remaining 1%, lesions such as apical scar, cementoma, foreign-body reaction, and giant cell lesion have been reported. The traumatic bone cyst will also be found on surgical exposure of a lesion, but no tissue is available for biopsy in this condition. Of the many possibilities, the chance of a malignancy being present associated with a tooth is extremely rare. Even a serious nonmalignant condition, such as an ameloblastoma, resembling a periapical granuloma or cyst, is also extremely rare.

Even so, on rare occasions a serious lesion masquerading as a granuloma or cyst might be present. Performing nonsurgical treatment and waiting to see if expected healing would transpire might lose precious time and cause spread or metastasis. Schlagel et al. reported a case of adenoid cystic carcinoma, a malignant glandular tumor, associated with maxillary anterior teeth. Although the preoperative diagnosis of the surgeon was that of chronic periapical abscess, because of the lack of response to the electric pulp tester by the lateral and cuspid, an apicoectomy was fortunately performed. The authors suggested that periapical curettage and microscopic examination of the lesion should be used more routinely to arrive at a diagnosis rather than merely being used as a last resort for the retention of an involved tooth.

Some articles have been written suggesting that a biopsy should be done on every periapical lesion on the chance that a malignancy might be present, even if the odds were 1 million to one (still probably a low fade). This seems to be an extremely barbaric philosophy, particularly when one considers the potential complications of periapical surgery on mandibular molars, palatal roots of maxillary molars, and bicuspids, as well as the normal discomfort in even the more accessible areas. However, if certain criteria are present, periapical surgery to gain tissue for a biopsy sample might well be justified.

Fig. 1-13 illustrates a case where a systemic condition or a lesion more serious than one due to the loss of pulpal vitality was suspected. In this instance the histopathologic examination confirmed that the lesion was not serious, and healing followed uneventfully. Surgery with this in mind was not difficult to justify because of the suspicion of another condition. However, we would not consider it as a routine procedure for all lesions because of the problems inherent with mandibular posterior surgery.

Medical history of a malignancy. Doing surgery on every periapical lesion for a patient

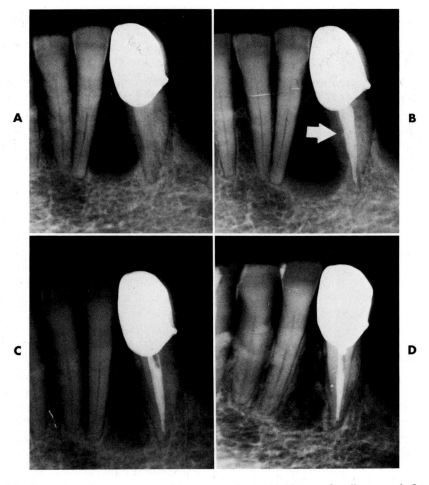

Fig. 11-16. Surgery performed to gain a biopsy on patient with history of malignancy. **A,** Lesion on mesial of cuspid appeared to be lateral periodontal cyst, but tooth did not respond to heat test on lingual surface or crown. **B,** Endodontic treatment was performed, including canal filling, with gutta-percha and lateral condensation. Some Tubliseal extends toward mesial *(arrow)*. Area was curetted, and biopsy report was for a granuloma. **C,** Because of patient's history, area was radiographed and examined at 3-month intervals. **D,** Excellent healing 1 year after surgery.

with a medical history of malignancy probably is unwarranted, as long as the associated tooth, topography and configuration of the lesion, and diagnostic tests are well within the expected range. When the responses to vitality tests are negative, when the periapical lesion is adjacent to the site of exiting of the apical foramen, and when the etiology of pulpal involvement is obvious, it would seem safe to treat the tooth with routine nonsurgical procedures. Of course, careful periodic examinations are mandatory.

On the other hand, if the pulp appears vital, if there are no deep restorations or carious lesions in the tooth, and/or if the lesion is not at the common periapical sites for patients with a history of malignancy, periapical surgery should be strongly considered (Fig. 11-16).

Findings of a periapical lesion, vital pulp, and extensive apical resorption. Those reported malignant lesions in proximity to the root of a tooth seem to share a common characteristic. Because of their aggressive and invasive action, active root resorption is noted frequently, and the associated tooth has a vital pulp. This combination of circumstances would seem to warrant microscopic examination of the tissue. (See Fig. 11-17.)

Lip paresthesia. Malignancies of the mandible may be associated with lip paresthesia. Again the key finding of a vital pulp in the associated tooth plus no reason for the paresthesia (trauma, recent mandibular or mental block injection) might make the dentist suspicious of a possible malignant lesion.

All tissues removed must be examined microscopically. There is no excuse for failure to submit a biopsy specimen for histopathologic examination on any tissue removed from the oral cavity or jaws, including curetted periapical tissue. Almost every dental school and many hospitals have competent oral pathologists available to examine and report on the samples, and the charges for such services are minimal. The most innocent-appearing tissue may be merely masquerading and in fact be a serious, invasive, lethal lesion. Failure to submit such tissue properly certainly should be considered malpractice.

Small bottles half-filled with 10% formalin can easily be prepared in advance and kept ready at the time of periapical surgery. The tissues removed are placed into the fixative and may be kept for a relatively long time while still retaining their histologic integrity. The specimens should be submitted as soon as practical, along with a clinical description, and, if possible, a preoperative radiograph.

FLAPS AND INCISIONS

By definition, surgery involves the cutting into and/or removal of tissue, and therefore some type of incision must always be made. Usually the incision results in a flap to be raised for exposure of underlying tissue. Although there are relatively few types of incisions and resultant flaps used in endodontic surgery, considerable thought must be given to the type, position, and method of tissue retraction before the scalpel is even lifted. Thorough analysis before the surgery is begun saves time and anguish during the procedure and leads to optimal and uneventful healing postoperatively. Such factors as number of teeth involved, position and shape of teeth and roots, amount of attached gingiva, degree of pocket depth, adjacent vital structures, restorations present or planned for, and type of surgery to be performed all have an impact on the selection of type, shape, and extent of flap to be utilized.

At this point the functions of a flap, the requirements for an acceptable flap, and the types of flaps commonly used in endodontic surgery will be discussed.

Functions of a flap. The most important function of a flap is to raise the soft tissue overlying the surgical site to give the best possible view to the operator and sufficient exposure of the area to be operated on. Since the free and attached gingiva and the underlying mucosa have considerable vascularity, attempting to work through them would lead to increased blood loss and obstructed view.

Endodontic surgery has had a great advantage over gingivectomy, gingivoplasty, and push-back procedures—methods of periodontal surgery that were in vogue for some time and until recently. These types of surgery left raw, bleeding tissues in addition to uncovered bone in some cases. They were characterized by considerable postoperative pain and required surgical pack placement. In endodontic surgery the overlying tissue was stripped back and could be replaced after the procedure to give the best possible covering to the surgical site.

Therefore the second important function of a flap is to provide healthy tissue that will cover the area of surgery, decrease pain by eliminating bone exposure, and aid in obtaining optimal healing.

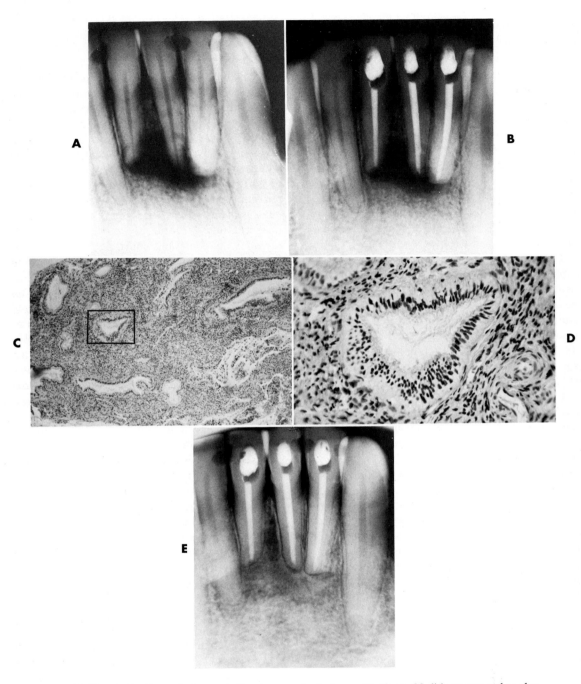

Fig. 11-17. **A,** Radiograph demonstrating large periapical area. Tooth no. 23 did not respond to electric pulp tester, but teeth nos. 24 and 25 responded normally, despite considerable apical resorption. **B,** It was decided to fill canals and curette area for biopsy examination. **C,** Lowpower view of lesion. **D,** Higher-power view. Slides were submitted to four oral pathologists, each of whom gave a different diagnosis—adenoameloblastoma, metastatic carcinoma, median mandibular cyst, and granuloma with acinar arrangement. **E,** One year after surgery, perfect healing. (Surgery by Dr. Howard Adilman, formerly of Chicago.)

It is no wonder that sophisticated periodontal surgery has incorporated the use of flaps, and most operations now involve that type of approach. The split-thickness flap, apically repositioned flap, sliding flap, and others have been found invaluable in the treatment of periodontal disease. Many of the new improvements in endodontic flap design and methods of flap retraction have been gleaned from the experiences of periodontists. Whenever endodontic surgery is to be performed, an extremely careful periodontal evaluation must be made to ascertain the most desirable flap. Additionally, when the site is opened for endodontic surgery, the operator should concomitantly perform any periodontal surgery necessary in the area. In many cases the exposure afforded by flap retraction for endodontic surgery exposes periodontal defects that would otherwise remain undetected.

Requirements of an ideal flap. The requirements for an ideal flap in endodontics are the same as for an ideal flap in oral surgery, periodontics, or any other phase of dentistry. Many of the requirements have been presented in lectures and described and preached in articles and textbooks for a considerable period. Yet it is surprising how frequently even the most basic principles are violated. Even the most skillful surgeons may discover that their flap design is inadequate or incorrect because of some problem that could not be normally anticipated. However, error in flap design because of inadequate preoperative preparation or examination is definitely preventable. Close adherence to the suggestions that follow and cognizance of these entities in every preoperative examination will minimize problems during surgery.

Making sure base is widest point of flap. Of all the requirements for flap design, the most important is that the base be the widest point of the flap. The obvious need for the width at the base is to afford sufficient circulation to the raised portion of the flap so that the edges do not become ischemic and later slough.

To be sure of incorporating this requirement in the flap, the operator should outline the entire flap on the mucosa before making any incision with the scalpel. Such outlining may be performed with an indelible pencil that has been presterilized in dry heat or by using the sharp point of the endodontic explorer to penetrate the mucosa and leave a series of dots. This outline should then be examined to be sure that it satisfies the desired requirement. The pencil marks are wiped away before making the incision so that only a faint outline is left as a guide. If excess dye from the pencil remains, it may tattoo the tissue at the line of incision and leave an undesirable discoloration after healing.

It is extremely important to draw the incision lines with indelible pencil and examine the area before cutting the tissues so the operator is certain that all the requirements of a proper flap have been fulfilled. Once it has been determined that the incision lines are in the most desirable position, the flap is prepared with the scalpel, using care to avoid sharp points at the edge.

When this is not done and the individual incisions are made without considering the entire flap, it is surprising how frequently the base ends up more narrow than other portions of the flap. After the incisions are already made, there is no way to correct this deficiency.

Avoiding incision over a bony defect. The lines of incision must not overlie any defect in the bone that is present preoperatively or will be produced by the surgical procedure. One of the major advantages in the use of vertical flaps is that the defect is easily avoided, since the horizontal portion of the flap is at the gingival margin, where the bone usually remains intact, whereas the vertical incisions are placed a minimum of one tooth over from the tooth with the lesion.

When only a horizontal incision is used, the problem of avoiding the bony lesion is a bit more difficult. The gingival extension of the lesion must be estimated; if the extent is considerable, an alternate type of flap should be used.

Including the full extent of the lesion. When the lesion appears to be extensive, as when a large diffuse radiolucency is present, or if considerable bone needs removal before the lesion is reached, as in a palatally inclined maxillary lateral incisor, the vertical incisions may be better placed two teeth over from the tooth with the lesion. It should always be remembered that in many areas of the mouth, the extent of a periapical radiolucency visualized on a radiograph is less than the actual bone destruction present. Extending the flap farther laterally to avoid incision over a bony defect or to afford better visualization of the surgical site should never be considered overly destructive, since it usually allows for improved healing and thus is more conservative.

A specific need for extending the incision is to gain optimal healing. When a maxillary or mandibular lateral incisor is treated by using double vertical incisions, the mesial incision normally would adjoin or dissect the frenum. When this attachment is tight or extensive, any movement of the lip during the postoperative period will tend to displace the segments and lead to retarded healing and/or scar formation. It is better to extend the vertical extension of the flap to the distal aspect of the opposite central incisor and lift the entire frenum for most desirable healing.

Avoiding sharp corners. The tips of sharp corners of a flap have a tendency to become ischemic in the few days after the surgery before collateral circulation across the sutured tissues becomes established. Ischemia will lead to sloughing of these tips and to retarded healing. Scar formation would develop as the area heals by other than primary intention.

Avoiding incision across a bony eminence. Bony eminences are usually found in the maxillary cuspid area but may be present on the labial bony covering of other teeth. Since the mucosa covering the eminence is thinner than that covering the interdental bone, less circulation is available to provide nutrition to the edges of a flap placed on the eminence. Also, if unesthetic scar formation develops, these unsightly areas will be prominently displayed on patients with high lip lines. The lines of incision are better placed in the trough between the eminence and the next distal tooth, typically between the cuspid and first bicuspid. An incision so placed has a better healing prospect and remains unnoticed.

Guarding against possible dehiscence. If the mucosa covering a dehiscence is stripped away during the raising of a flap, there is a strong possibility that the tissue will reattach poorly after the surgery, resulting in a periodontal pocket or at least a dimpling of the marginal gingiva. Certain roots, such as those of cuspids and the buccal roots of maxillary molars and first bicuspids, are especially likely to have a dehiscence. Whenever these teeth are to be included in the flap, the possibility of a dehiscence is present. Any other tooth in the arch may have a dehiscence, which might be deduced by radiographic and/or periodontal examination.

Three types of flaps are useful when a dehiscence appears likely. The semilunar or horizontal flap is placed near the apex of the tooth to be treated and avoids the problem of exposing a dehiscence. However, as will be discussed shortly, there are many disadvantages in this type

of flap, particularly when compared with the vertical flaps. If the operator is using a double vertical flap but suspects a dehiscence, a split-thickness flap may be used at the gingival half of the exposure, leaving tissue attached to that area, whereas a full-thickness flap is used to uncover the bone around the apex of the tooth requiring surgery. The Ochsenbein-Luebke flap avoids contact with the covering over the gingival third of the root and is safe for use when a dehiscence appears likely.

Placing a horizontal incision in the gingival sulcus or keeping it away from the gingival margin. In conjunction with a single or double vertical incision, a horizontal incision may be placed in the gingival sulcus. When the gingival tissue is retracted, a scalloped effect is obtained that allows for excellent visualization of the area of surgery, enables correction of local periodontal defects, and provides for desirable gingival healing. If it is decided to place the horizontal incision away from the gingival margin for reasons that will be discussed later, there must be a minimum of 2 mm of attached gingiva around each tooth to be flapped. If the incision is any closer and encroaches on the depth of the gingival sulcus, tissue retraction during the healing process may cause a dimpling of the gingival tissue in the area or an alteration in the normal gingival architecture.

To avoid this, the sulcus depth of each tooth to be flapped should be determined by a periodontal probe and marked with a pocket marker or other suitable instruments. Sufficient width of attached gingiva then may be provided for. If an area of considerable pocket depth is found, an alternative incision should be utilized.

Avoiding incisions in the mucogingival junction. The worst possible place to put any portion of the incision is in the mucogingival junction. This junction of the attached gingiva and the alveolar mucosa has extremely friable tissue and must exert frequent movement during talking and eating. Incisions placed here take a much longer time to heal and frequently lead to residual discomfort and scarring many months after the surgical procedure (Fig. 11-18).

One of the problems involved in the use of the semilunar type of horizontal incision was that the entire incision was often placed in the mucogingival junction, particularly if the patient had a minimal width of attached gingiva. Similarly, by using vertical incisions placed one or two teeth distant

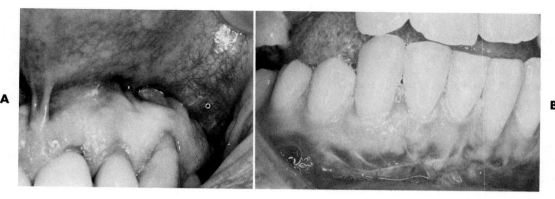

Fig. 11-18.   Poor healing of horizontal incisions placed in mucogingival junction. **A,** Maxillary cuspid, treated 1 year earlier. **B,** Mandibular anteriors, treated 2 years earlier. Contrast these with postoperative appearances of cases later in this chapter in which horizontal incisions were placed in attached gingiva or gingival sulcus.

from the tooth to be operated on, the dentist could avoid the mucogingival junction completely.

Avoiding improper treatment of periosteum. A periosteal covering for bone is necessary to achieve optimal healing and to diminish postsurgical pain. In most surgical endodontic procedures a full-thickness flap is used. Therefore the periosteum must be lifted together with the covering mucosa. Firm incisions must be made with sharp scalpels to penetrate all the soft tissue layers instantly and directly to the bone. A sharp periosteal elevator must be used to separate the periosteum from the bone so that the periosteum remains in contact with the mucosa.

If a split-thickness flap is to be utilized, sharp scalpels must be used to dissect the periosteum from the mucosa so that the periosteum remains intact to cover the bone.

The use of sharp instruments prevents shredding and tearing of the manipulated tissue. This in turn promotes healing by primary intention, since the tissues may be replaced in close contact immediately after the surgery. Scalpel blades are disposable and should be discarded after every procedure so a new sharp blade will be ready to start every surgical case. If several incisions may be needed during one procedure, alternative blades should be available to give the sharpest possible edge for each penetration. Periosteal elevators must be checked for sharpness before sterilization for any procedure and sharpened by mounted stones or with a sharpening block if necessary.

Taking care during retraction.   After the flap is opened, the tissue retracted from the underlying bone must be held away from the surgical site. Care should be exercised so that the retractor is placed beneath the tissue and supports the tissue from that position. The retracted tissue must not be mashed by the retractor or the patient's lip; if it is, the blood supply of the flap will be diminished and the healing retarded.

The retractor should be kept under the tissue to avoid manipulation of the edges to be sutured. If considerable manipulation of the edges occurs, alteration of the topography of the area takes place and it becomes difficult to suture the tissues into close contact.

Types of flaps.   The flaps that will be discussed in this section are the semilunar, full vertical, palatal, and Ochsenbein-Luebke flaps. The full vertical types include single and double vertical incisions and modified envelope flaps. The following paragraphs will discuss the advantages, disadvantages, indications, and techniques for each flap.

Semilunar flap.   The semilunar flap has been used for many years in endodontic surgery. The chief advantage of this flap is its simplicity, requiring merely a straight, horizontal incision firmly through the soft tissues to the underlying bone. Because the incision is placed away from the gingival margin, the semilunar flap does not cause the uncovering of gingiva from the gingival margin of crown restorations or disturb the healing of gingiva after periodontal surgery. It is referred to as *semilunar* because the horizontal incision is slightly modified to have a dip toward the incisal aspect in the center of the flap, giving a resemblance to a half-moon.

The disadvantages of this flap have caused it to be replaced by types of vertical incisions. Among these disadvantages are the following:

1. Considerable lateral extension is required to expose sufficient area at the surgical site.
2. If sufficient lateral extension is not provided, the incision may tear at the edges during retraction and create areas that heal poorly and with considerable scar formation.
3. If minimal attached gingiva is present, the flap may encroach on the sulcus depth of the teeth to be flapped.
4. Since the edges to be sutured are held apart during surgery, the healing is not as rapid as healing with other flaps and may result in considerable scar formation.
5. If the lesion is larger than anticipated, the incision may end up being over the surgical defect.
6. When the cuspid or adjacent tooth is involved in the surgery, the cuspid eminence is violated by the incision.
7. This flap usually originates in or is placed in the mucogingival junction, often leading to retarded healing and scar formation (Fig. 11-19, *E*).

Indications for use of the semilunar incision are situations in which the contour and shape of the marginal gingiva must be preserved, as in patients with complete jacket crowns in the area or for use after periodontal surgery. This type of flap is contraindicated where deep periodontal pockets are present, where minimal attached gingiva is present, when a very large lesion is anticipated, and when other types of flaps are deemed to be more desirable.

It is especially important that the gingival sulcus of all teeth involved in a semilunar flap be explored with a periodontal probe before the incision is made. The horizontal incision must be made a minimum of 2 mm from the greatest sulcus depth.

Vertical flaps. Although referred to as vertical flaps because of the vertical incisions made to aid in the raising of the tissues, these flaps are always made in conjunction with a horizontal incision. The horizontal incision is usually placed in the gingival sulcus. This portion of the incision is developed by cutting the epithelial attachment around the necks of the teeth and across the interdental papillae. When pushed back by a periosteal elevator, the gingival edge of the flap has a scalloped border. When periodontal surgery is to be performed in addition to the endodontic surgery, a reverse bevel may be used to remove the diseased gingival tissue around the necks of the teeth and to return more healthy tissue to that area during closure.

If one vertical incision is used, the flap is referred to as a *single vertical,* whereas the term *double vertical* implies the use of two vertical incisions. The vertical incisions greatly aid in the retraction of the tissue overlying the defect and have been recommended for use by periodontists. If the Ochsenbein-Luebke incision is considered to be a vertical type, which it truly is, vertical flaps have taken over almost completely as the most desirable type in endodontic surgery. The chief advantages of vertical flaps are that optimal healing usually occurs, since no edges of the flap are manipulated during surgery, and the visualization of the surgical site is excellent because of the maximal uncovering of the area. In addition, any necessary minor periodontal surgery may be performed at the same time. The disadvantages are that the gingival areas of many teeth are uncovered, the possibility of opening a dehiscence is present, careful flap design must be adhered to in order to avert having the base too small, and sharp corners may be present at the junction with the horizontal portion of the incision.

The only contraindication for the use of vertical flaps are the cases in which the shrinkage that may occur during gingival healing might lead to the uncovering of gingival margins of crowns or cases in which gingival tissues are still healing after periodontal surgery. If the possibility of a dehiscence is present, the gingival portion of the flap may be prepared to be a splitthickness flap, leaving the periosteum covering undisturbed. Since vertical flaps are much more complicated to prepare and reflect than the semilunar flaps, only those familiar with periodontal and surgical techniques should utilize them during the initial attempts at endodontic surgery. As greater experience and confidence are gained, improved results may accrue with the use of the vertical flaps.

In the typical flap, double vertical incisions are used when anterior teeth are treated. The incisions are placed to the farthest edge of each tooth adjacent to the tooth to be treated. If the defect is expected to be very large or if the terminal end of the incision would normally approximate an attachment to be avoided, the vertical incisions may be placed two teeth over from the surgical site (Fig. 11-19). In the posterior areas, generally only one vertical incision is used, located mesially to the tooth one or two teeth anterior to the one to be treated (Fig. 11-20).

In mandibular molars a scalloped incision is developed around the necks of the adjacent teeth, extending anteriorly to the first bicuspid or cuspid, in which a short, single vertical incision is placed to relax the flap and aid in visualization of the area of defect.

Some vertical flaps suggested for use are designed with an extremely wide base compared to the edge of the flap. This is to ensure that there will be sufficient blood circulating to all portions of the flap, which may be a problem if a vertical flap is not correctly designed. The base extends the width of two adjacent teeth, with two vertical incisions coming down at an oblique diagonal angle to the mesial and distal edges of only the tooth with the defect. Although this method does minimize the area of bone uncovered during the surgery, it may prove to be too restrictive if the bone defect is larger than anticipated. This type of flap is often referred to as an envelope flap since it resembles the back of an envelope.

Palatal flaps. The use of a flap to retract the palatal tissues of the maxilla may be needed in

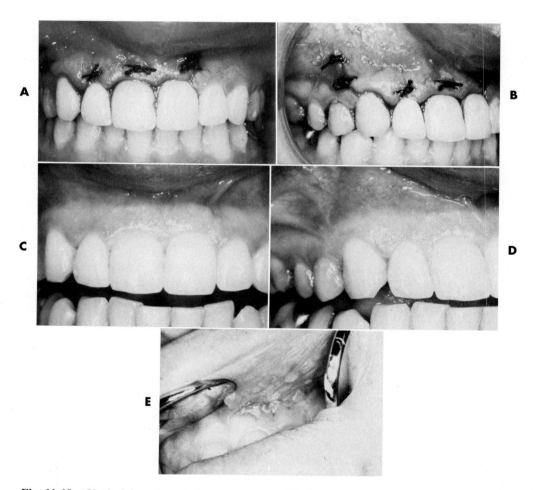

Fig. 11-19. Vertical flaps for anterior surgery. **A,** and **B,** Suturing after double vertical flap for periapical surgery on lateral incisor on the left. Vertical flaps were placed distal to adjacent cuspid and opposite central incisor with horizontal incision in gingival sulcus. **C,** and **D,** Excellent healing 6 months later. **E,** Contrast with healing of semilunar flap 1 year after treatment in a similar case.

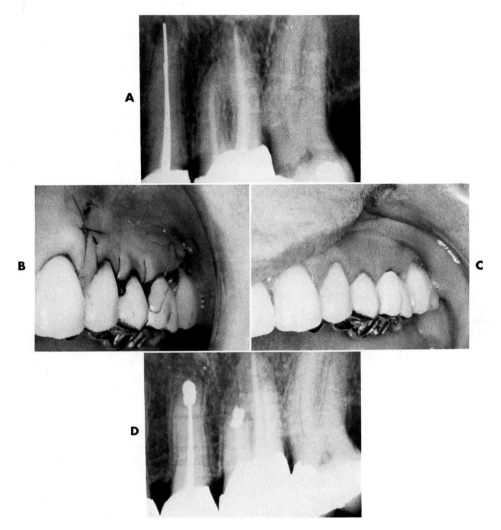

Fig. 11-20. Vertical flap for posterior surgery. **A,** Preoperative radiograph of maxillary bicuspid and molar areas. Second bicuspid has failing treatment, and a periapical lesion is present at apex of mesiobuccal root of first molar. **B,** Suturing after periapical surgery. Vertical incision was placed mesial to first bicuspid with horizontal incision in gingival sulcus to distal of second molar. Circumferential suture was placed around second bicuspid. **C,** Excellent tissue response 3 months after surgery. **D,** Radiograph taken 6 months after surgery demonstrates excellent healing.

certain cases. These include reverse filling, perforation repair, apicoectomy or root amputation of the palatal root of a maxillary bicuspid or molar, and perforation or resorption repair of the palatal surface of anterior teeth. As in any flap, all rules for flap design must be satisfied for best results. However, the rich vascular supply of the palatal area provides for excellent healing in most instances.

The typical palatal flap is prepared with a scalloped incision around the gingival margins. Nor-

mally at least two teeth to the mesial and to the distal aspects of the tooth that is to be operated on must be included in the flap retraction for desirable visualization. Relaxing incisions are best placed between the first bicuspid and cuspid to diminish the chance for severance of the palatal blood vessels and resultant hemorrhage problems. The blood vessels from the incisive canal and greater palatine foramen anastomose in this area and are not as large as they are farther anteriorly or posteriorly.

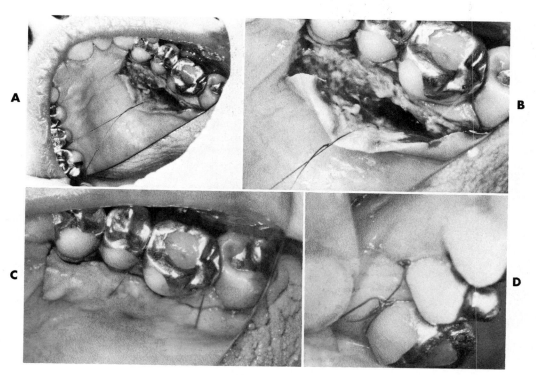

Fig. 11-21. Palatal flap. **A,** Vertical incision between cuspid and first bicuspid and scalloping of gingival margin for surgery on palatal root of maxillary first molar. Suture is tied through retracted tissue and then looped around opposite molar to give increased visualization. **B,** Close-up of area of surgery. **C,** Suture placed to mesial and distal of molar and looped around labial without being tied to buccal tissue. **D,** Completion of this case is seen in Fig. 11-32.

The bone topography in the posterior area of the palate is inclined to be more pebbly than the labial or buccal surface of either the maxilla or mandible. This makes periosteum elevation more difficult as the elevator strikes humps or peduncles of bone during retraction. The scalpel may be used to partially dissect the tissue for a modified split-thickness flap in these cases.

Even with the mucosa retracted, examination of the surgical site with a palatal flap is difficult. Even with assistance it is very complex to retract the flap, use a mouth mirror for visualization of the area, and use a handpiece or hand instrument for preparation, curettage, or filling. Therefore it is wise to obtain retraction by placing a suture at the edge of the flap and tying it tightly to the teeth on the opposite side of the arch (Fig. 11-21). The tissue on the opposite side need not be penetrated, but the suture material is merely tied around the gingival margin of a bicuspid or molar. When the surgery is completed, the suture is cut and routine replacement afforded to the flap.

Ochsenbein-Luebke flap. Developed by a periodontist and an endodontist, this flap has been designed to combine the advantages of the vertical flaps with those of the semilunar flaps. Since the horizontal portion of this flap is placed a minimum of 2 mm from the depth of the gingival sulcus, those gingival tissues covering jacket crowns or healing after periodontal surgery are unaffected. The site of surgery has excellent exposure and yet less tissue is reflected, since the flap does not extend to the marginal gingiva. The exact width of the flap may have greater variability, since the flap does not have to terminate at a particular edge of any tooth. The edges of the flap are not manipulated during the surgery; therefore the blood supply to the area of suture margins remains excellent. Suturing is easier than when the horizontal incision lies in the gingival sulcus. There is no chance of opening a dehiscence (Fig. 11-22).

The main disadvantage of this flap is that extreme care must be exercised so no sharp points occur at the junction of the vertical and horizontal incisions.

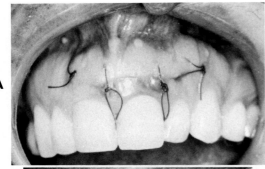

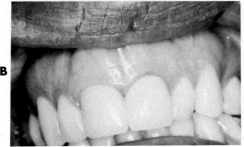

Fig. 11-22. Healing after Ochsenbein-Luebke type of flap. **A,** Because of recently constructed esthetic jacket crowns on both central incisors, it was decided not to place a horizontal incision in gingival sulcus, thus avoiding any excessive shrinkage to open the line of margin. Five days after reverse filling procedure on central incisor to the right. **B,** Four months later, excellent tissue response.

There are only a few contraindications to this type of flap. If minor periodontal surgery is to be performed around the gingival sulcus, the double or single vertical incisions will expose that area. If the horizontal incision is to be placed across a prominent eminence, vertical incisions avert the problem. If minimal attached gingiva is present, the horizontal incision may approach the mucogingival junction.

ARMAMENTARIUM

The instruments used in endodontic surgery are similar to those used in any surgical procedure. The standard tray should include the following items (Fig. 11-23):

Scalpel—size 15 blade, mounted (size 12 optional, in addition)
Periosteal elevator
Surgical curettes of various sizes—three, one possibly a spoon excavator
Periodontal curettes—two, right and left of same type (Fig. 11-24)

Hemostats—two, one miniature
Scissors—two, one suture and one tissue
Endodontic explorer
Front surface mirror
Cotton forceps, with lock
Irrigating syringe
Metal millimeter gauge ruler
Suturing material—two packages
Anesthetic syringe—with one Carpule mounted and extra Carpules
Flap retractor
Surgical length burs—nos. 700, 701, 557, 558, 4, 6
Regular length burs—nos. 33½, 557, 700

For reverse amalgam fillings the following instruments are needed in an additional pack (Fig. 11-25):

Reverse fill carriers—two, one large and one small
Reverse fill pluggers—two, one large and one small
Amalgam squeeze cloths (used if amalgam is being employed as reverse filling material)
Stellate plastic instrument
Miniature reverse fill mirrors
Miniature head aspirator tips—to fit on surgical aspirator, but much smaller than normal size; may be fabricated by cutting the beveled tip from a 16-gauge needle and using an adapter on the usual aspirator tip holder
Ultrasonic holder and appropriate tips

In the preparation of these packs, the needed instruments are scrubbed with surgical soap, dried, and packed in taped towels or metal containers. Dry-heat sterilization is used, and the instruments are kept in a sterile condition until needed. All the instruments just listed may be kept ready for use in this manner, except for the anesthetic Carpules, which are kept in a disinfecting solution and added to the tray at the time of the surgery. The additional armamentarium needed for root amputation will be listed in Chapter 12.

In addition to the instruments required in the packs, the following materials and supplies should be available for possible use during surgery:

Sterile distilled water—for irrigation of surgical cavity; when sterile saline is needed, possible to use the solution from the syringe with the mounted anesthetic Carpule
Hemostatic agents—such as Gelfoam or Adaptic (the hemostatic, not the filling, material); may be needed when performing reverse fills
Additional suture material—two packages possibly insufficient
Heat source—alcohol lamp or Bunsen burner, for cauterizing seeping blood vessels or searing gutta-percha

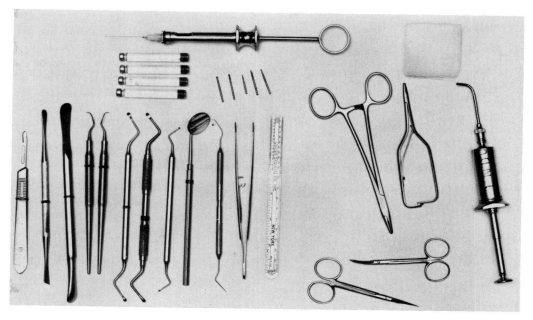

Fig. 11-23.   Tray setup for periapical surgery. *(from left)* Scalpel, periosteal elevator, flap retractor, curettes (two periodontal and three surgical), front surface mirror, endodontic explorer, cotton forceps, metal ruler. *(at right, top)* Two hemostats; at bottom: two scissors, irrigating syringe. *(top, left)* Anesthetic syringe with extra Carpules, burs, sterile gauze.

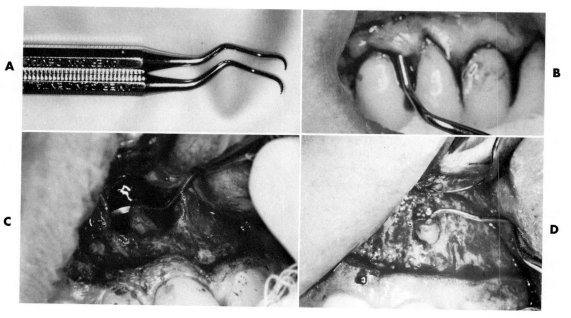

Fig. 11-24.   Use of periodontal curettes in endodontic surgery. **A,** Pair of periodontal curettes *(right* and *left)* are included in surgical setup. **B,** After initial incisions these curettes are used to strip gingival attachment and free gingival margins. This initiates lifting of tissue prior to use of periosteal elevator. **C,** Curettes can clean inflamed tissue from bony walls and curette tissue from back to root tip. **D,** Carving of excess amalgam during reverse filling procedure.

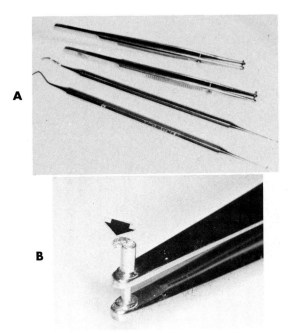

Fig. 11-25. A, Reverse filling instruments. Miniature carriers *(top)* and pluggers of same diameters *(bottom)*. Originally designed for use with amalgam, these instruments will carry and pack any of the reverse filling materials. **B,** When carrier is packed with filling material, no excessive material must be allowed beyond barrel. Excess here *(arrow)* will not be pushed into preparation at apex but probably will fall adjacent to the tooth and remain after surgery.

Biopsy bottle—filled half with formalin, for sending specimen to pathologist for histopathologic report

Additional aspirator tips—both small and large, in case blood or materials clog the mounted tip

Premeasured file—during periapical surgery on a tooth of known length, a file with the stop set at the correct length kept sterilized and available for use; when needed, may be placed across buccal plate to indicate approximate position of apex (see Fig. 11-28)

Vaseline in a Dappen dish—petroleum jelly is sterilized and made available to be placed on suture material, thus preventing premature knotting of the strands and allowing for tighter ties

Individual philosophies, desires, and techniques may dictate the need for other instruments to be added to these lists. Although it is better to have more instruments than usually needed, in case a particular instrument is required for a special need, too much clutter on a tray becomes a hazard. It is best to keep a minimum number of standard instruments on the basic tray. Additional trays are kept available to hold instruments that are used with some frequency but not routinely, as for reverse fills. Also, additional individual instruments used only rarely are retained sterile in autoclave bags. If their use becomes necessary, they may be added to the tray by cutting the bag fold and dropping onto the sterile tray.

OPERATORY AND PATIENT PRESURGICAL PREPARATION

Controversy exists concerning the need for special presurgical preparation of the patient and/or operatory prior to any dental surgery. Although some maintain that the same conditions required for any nonsurgical method are sufficient for surgery, others believe that direct incision into the tissues, exposing the blood vasculature to the environment, demands prior disinfecting procedures.

There is no question that skill and careful manipulation of the surgical site are much more important than merely aseptic technique. However, it is not too complicated to arrange for presurgical preparation of the patient and operatory in order to follow a relatively aseptic technique. Although the methods that follow are strongly suggested and appear simple to incorporate in any surgical technique, they are by no means mandatory and may be decreased or enlarged on as the surgeon wishes.

Operatory preparation. Many presurgical scrub solutions are available to aid in the preparation of the operatory. These solutions are used in the disinfection of military field hospital units as well as in hospitals and in surgeons' offices. Instructions for handling and application must be carefully followed. Usually these solutions are caustic, and rubber gloves should be worn by whomever is performing the disinfection.

The areas to be scrubbed are those onto which the surgical instruments are to be placed, such as counter tops, mobile units, and surgical stands. Also, anything that might be touched by the operator or the assistant during surgery—such as the dental unit, the seat and headrest portions of the dental chair, the x-ray machine, and the water faucets—requires scrubbing. Cloth cover-gloves that can be presterilized by dry heat are available to place over the handles of the x-ray machine and the operatory light.

Once the disinfecting solution has been used where needed, sterile towels are placed and the presterilized surgical packs opened. The instruments needed for the procedure to be performed are placed on the sterile towels with a sterile lifting instrument. When the surgical instruments are in the desired position, a sterile covering towel is placed. All this preparation is done before the patient enters the operatory to be used for surgery. Ideally, it should be started so the room is ready just before the time for the surgical procedure. When the two-step technique is to be utilized, the canal enlarging, disinfection, and filling are performed in one operatory while another is prepared for surgery. When the postresection filling technique is to be performed or apical surgery is required on a previously filled canal, the room preparation is started while the surgeon is treating the patient prior to the surgery.

Patient preparation. When the surgical room is ready, the patient is brought in by an assistant and requested not to touch anything. A surgical gown of the appropriate size is placed over the patient's clothing. These gowns are available on a rental basis from linen supply companies, and disposable gowns are sold by paper supply companies.

The patient should not wear any excessively warm or bulky clothing underneath the gown, which would tend to increase the perspiration normally present because of anxiety. Men are instructed to remove their jackets, vests, sweaters, and ties prior to gown placement. Even their shirt may be removed and the gown worn over the undershirt. The articles of clothing are placed in the patients' closet and brought back into the room by the assistant to be again worn after the procedure is completed. In this way no blood, water, or irrigants get on the patient's clothing during the surgery, and the patient's own fresh, dry apparel is ready to wear when he leaves the office. Similarly, women may wish to remove a dress, sweater, or blouse, in addition to the jacket and coat, prior to donning the surgical gown.

After the patient has been dressed in the gown and the other clothing removed from the room, the patient is seated in the dental chair. A sterile towel is draped around the patient's head and pinned. A sterile towel is placed across the patient's chest and pinned to encompass the neck tightly to absorb any solutions or liquids that reach this area.

Towelettes are available that are manufactured with a disinfecting solution, and these are used to wash the patient's face, with considerable time spent in washing the area around the lips and mouth. The patient is instructed to rinse with 4 ounces of full-strength mouthwash to reduce the number of microorganisms.

All these preparations have been made without the surgeon being present. The surgeon now enters the operatory and administers the necessary local anesthetic or the additional amounts needed to potentiate any previously given injections. The patient again rinses with full-strength mouthwash while the surgeon prepares.

Surgeon preparation. The surgeon washes his face and then puts on glasses, a mask, and a cap. Glasses should be worn whenever any rotary instrument is used to protect the eyes from potential damage by flying debris. If prescription glasses are not ordinarily worn, plain glass spectacles or those with a slight magnification may be used.

A short-sleeved gown is worn by the surgeon, which permits a scrubbing procedure from the elbow down. A disinfecting soap is used with a scrub brush. pHisoHex and Betadine are the choices of most hospitals and are satisfactory for the dental office. After scrubbing, the arms and hands are rinsed with tap water and dried with a sterile towel. Sterile gloves are worn during the surgery. Powder or salve may be used on the hands to aid in donning the gloves. The surgical assistant goes through the same preparation. All is now ready to commence the surgery.

First we will discuss the two-step operation and then the postresection filling technique.

TWO-STEP OR FILLING-FIRST TECHNIQUE

Two types of cases require canal filling prior to periapical surgery. One type is the failing case with a canal filing that may be removed, whereas in the other the need for surgery had become apparent during the course of routine therapy before the filling appointment. The re-treatment of failing cases involves a considerable percentage of surgical cases. Whenever it is possible to remove the previously placed filling in a failing case and fill it prior to surgery, such a method should be followed. It is surprising how frequently a heavy condensation technique will give important additional information helpful during the surgery. Such disclosures may include the position of the apical foramen, existence of significant lateral canals, resorptive defects, and bifurcated canals.

If a canal needs filling before surgery, the proper time for this filling is either immediately before the surgery or during the surgical exposure. When a canal is filled more than a day before the surgery, the chances for presurgical exacerbation or inflammation are increased. This is especially true if the indications for surgery are persistent exacerbations or intratreatment pain.

Two methods are available for canal filling in conjunction with a surgical procedure. The two-step or filling-first method involves the placement of the rubber dam and canal filling just as in the routine, nonsurgical type of case. The surgery then becomes the second step after the canal filing has been placed and the dam removed. The second method is the postresection filling technique, in which the flap is opened, the apex of the tooth exposed, and the canal filled.

Canal preparation before filling. When possible, canal preparation is performed at the appointment preceding the surgical procedure. Depending on the tooth involved, a maximal degree of enlargement should be gained so that the tightest possible seal is obtained. The master gutta-percha cone or cones to be used to fill the canal(s) may also be selected at this appointment and the correctness of fit verified by radiograph. This makes the surgery appointment shorter than when everything is done at once and usually affords better patient cooperation. If any doubt exists as to the possibility of an acute exacerbation before the surgery, the tooth should be left open.

If it is not convenient to prepare the canals at a prior appointment, all instrumentation may be performed at the surgical appointment, to be followed by canal filling and surgery.

Intentional overfilling of a canal prior to apical surgery has been advocated by many. It was thought that this overfilling would afford a landmark during the removal of bone to aid in the discovery of the canal apex and ensure that the canal was tightly sealed. Rather than intentionally overfill in every case, it is now considered better to evaluate each individual case and then decide on the method of canal preparation and filling.

If it is thought that an apex may be difficult to locate, overinstrumentation of the apex is performed so that the canal will be overfilled. This occurs most frequently during performance of apical surgery on teeth having no radiolucencies and thus having no perforation of the overlying bone to aid in apex location (see Fig. 11-27). In treating lateral incisors, which often have palatal inclination, and posterior teeth, the dentist may overinstrument to gain an overfilling.

However, in a canal whose apex is overinstrumented, it is much more difficult to gain a very dense fill when compared with a case that has firm dentin to pack against. Therefore intentional overfilling should not be employed when a very dense fill is necessary.

In teeth with large radiolucencies, rarely is there any problem in finding the apex. Teeth with large radiolucencies often display many lateral canals when a heavy condensation canal filling technique is used and may have apical resorption that alters the position of the exiting of the apical foramen. For these reasons, it is better to enlarge such cases slightly short of the point where the apical foramen is determined to be exiting so that a definite matrix in solid dentin is obtained. Then, when a heavy condensation technique is used for canal filling, a good apical seal will be ensured and lateral canals may be picked up by sealer extrusion. Lateral canals of significant size may be reverse filled during the surgical procedure and are much easier to locate when the button of sealer is present (Fig. 11-26).

If after filling it becomes apparent that the canal has been prepared farther from the apex than anticipated and that a segment of unfilled canal is present, no great problem exists. During the surgery this unfilled portion may be removed by apicoectomy down to the densely filled gutta-percha.

Disinfection immediately prior to filling. Both the need and the method for performing immediate disinfection are subject to dispute. When the postresection filling technique is used, no immediate disinfection is possible and excellent results still are routinely reported. Even when the fill-first method of surgery is utilized, many operators believe that no disinfection is needed before filling the canal.

Despite these objections, immediate disinfection requires only a few minutes to perform and may well be time beneficially spent. This is particularly true when a canal had been left open before being filled and therefore is heavily contaminated, as is the surrounding periapical tissue. Just as the area of surgery is swabbed with a disinfectant prior to the opening of a flap, the rationale for immediate disinfection is to minimize the population of microorganisms, to lessen the chance for inoculating the remaining tissues during surgery, and to decrease the possibility of postoperative infection.

In addition, when phenol is to be used as canal disinfectant, that chemical acts as a coagulant of protein and therefore will halt periapical bleeding that may occur as a result of overinstrumentation

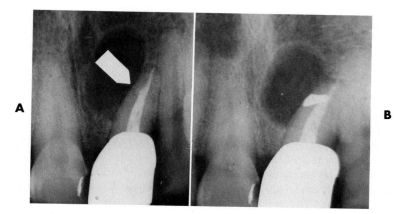

Fig. 11-26. **A,** Radiograph taken after canal filling in which heavy condensation technique was performed, using apical stop to prevent overfilling. Lateral canal going right to the radiolucency picked up by the sealer *(arrow).* **B,** Lateral canal reverse filled. (Surgery by Dr. Howard Adilman, formerly of Chicago.)

during canal preparation of serous exudate that is a result of an inflammatory process. It is difficult to seal a canal properly when blood or serous fluids creep in from the periapical tissues, and the tight seal is mandatory in all cases. By the same process of protein coagulation, the phenol cauterizes any remaining viable tissue within the confines of the canal and aids in its removal during subsequent irrigation. This enables the filling materials to gain a tighter fit against the walls of the canal and may increase the possibility of picking up lateral canals during the condensation. After the use of phenol, the canal will be irrigated with 95% alcohol, which is hydrophilic and further makes the canal quite free of water. This is followed by the use of absorbent paper points. The net result is a canal that is free of moisture, is ideal for a sealer such as Tubliseal, and should be able to be densely filled.

Grossman has suggested the use of electrosterilization for immediate disinfection. Although this method has been proven to be effective in disinfecting the canal, it has certain disadvantages. It involves equipment rarely used in other areas of dentistry, cases of hand burns associated with its use have been reported, and the electrical makeup of the unit may be psychologically distressing to patients. The increased influence on healing that electrical sterilization has been said to provide has never been proven.

On the other hand, phenol has also been shown to be effective. Although the study reporting its success in providing immediate disinfection involved the use of 8 minutes of application, this slight increase in time required when compared with electrosterilization is offset by other advantages. The chemical is inexpensive, additional equipment not normally used in endodontics is not required, and the patient is unaware of its use, either physically or mentally. The caution of avoiding direct contact with the chemical by the operator or patient must, of course, be observed. Also, only the interior of the canal and the periapical tissues that will be removed by the subsequent surgery should be allowed to come in contact with the phenol.

Technique for using phenol. A local anesthetic must be administered prior to the disinfection. All of the injections required for the surgical treatment may be given at this time or merely the anesthetic needed to block the nerve endings in the immediate area of the treated tooth administered. The latter method is sufficient for performing the disinfection and canal filling and is preferable because when more anesthetic solution is deposited in the adjacent areas, which will be required for opening the flap, some degree of analgesia is already present in the tissues.

A rubber dam is applied and the treatment site swabbed with a local disinfectant. If the endodontic opening had been sealed, it is reopened by a sterile bur and the medicaments and other contents of the canal removed. If the access cavity had been left open, the canal is irrigated with hypochlorite, broached to remove any food debris, and then dried with sterile, absorbent paper points.

A sterile, dry paper point, slightly smaller than the largest file used in the canal enlargement, is dipped in liquefied phenol and placed into the canal to extend to the apex. The point is rotated with cotton pliers to contact a maximal area of dentin walls for approximately 1 minute. The point is discarded, a new saturated point placed, and the procedure repeated until 8 minutes of disinfecting action is gained. The canal is irrigated with 95% alcohol to neutralize the phenol and then dried with paper points.

It must be emphasized that canal disinfection with phenol should be used only prior to periapical surgery. This method is not indicated for nonsurgical cases because the chemical is caustic and causes considerable damage to periapical tissue. In surgical cases the necrotized tissue is curetted from the area and need not be phagocytized before replacement with new viable tissue. Leaving tissues exposed to phenol, as if used in nonsurgical cases, might attract saprophytic bacteria to the site and thus increase rather than decrease the bacterial population.

Canal filling. The root canal sealer suggested for use in canal filling prior to surgery is Tubliseal. This material is very lubricating and aids in gaining a dense fill. It has an excellent coefficient of film thickness and thus has a good chance to extrude into lateral canals. It is strongly radiopaque and therefore shows up well on radiographs. One of the disadvantages of this sealer is that it is irritating to periapical tissue, but this has no significance if surgery is to be performed since the tissue in contact with it will be removed with curettage. The other major disadvantage of Tubliseal is that it sets rapidly if the canal is wet. When phenol is used for immediate disinfection, apical bleeding and exudation are minimized. However, considerable care must be exercised to ensure that the canal is dry prior to insertion of this sealer to avoid premature setting.

The canal filling method used is lateral condensation with gutta-percha, as described in Chapter 9. A maximal number of auxiliary cones are

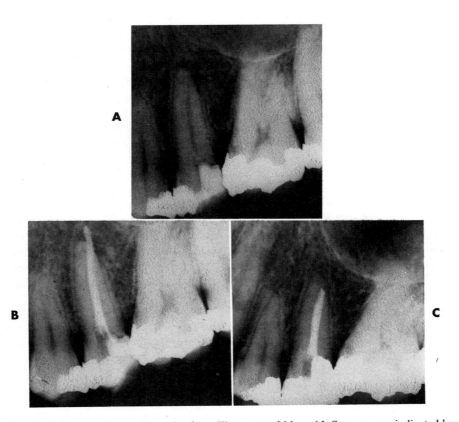

Fig. 11-27. **A,** Preoperative radiograph of maxillary second bicuspid. Surgery was indicated by persistent exacerbations, probably due to overinstrumentation. **B,** Canals were enlarged, disinfected with phenol, and intentionally overfilled to provide aid in apex location. **C,** Healing 1 year later.

employed with deep penetration of the spreader after each cone insertion. This is particularly important if the canal has been overinstrumented to gain an overfilling. The lack of apical stop in this case makes a dense filling more difficult to produce. After the canal has been filled, post room may be prepared and a suitable temporary seal placed. The rubber dam is removed and a postfilling radiograph taken. Depending on the method of instrumentation employed, the canal should be either overfilled or filled short of the apex, as desired (Fig. 11-27).

CURETTAGE AND APICOECTOMY

With the canal and periapical tissue immediately surrounding the tooth disinfected and the canal densely filled, the apical surgery may now be performed. The postfilling radiograph must be carefully examined for any additional information not noted on the preoperative radiographs that might influence the surgical procedure.

Preparation of the surgical site. If only the tooth being filled has been anesthetized, further injections are administered to ensure that the entire area involved in the flap and surgery will cause no discomfort to the patient. Where possible, the hard tissues such as teeth and bone should be anesthetized by block injections. Mandibular, mental, and posterior superior block injections are effective in eliminating operative pain and have a prolonged effect that allows analgesic drugs to be taken to lessen postoperative pain. In addition, when blocks are used, less solution is needed to anesthetize a large area and thus less tissue distention occurs compared with use of multiple infiltrations. However, after the symptoms of anesthesia are obtained by blocks, local infiltrations should be given to obtain hemostasis afforded by the vasoconstrictor drugs in the anesthetic solution. It is important to wait until the proper symptoms are present before giving the infiltrations because the latter may mimic the lip and tissue symptoms that blocks produce but may give far less depth of anesthesia.

The saliva ejector is placed in the patient's mouth, two 2-by-2–inch folded gauze sponges are placed between the patient's teeth in the area of the surgery, and instructions are given the patient to close firmly until contact is made. The saliva ejector serves to keep the patient's mouth free of excess saliva and water from the irrigation used during surgery and from the water spray from the handpiece, whereas the gauze provides greater comfort in keeping the jaws closed during the length of the surgical procedure and absorbs any excess bleeding from the surgical site.

The area of surgery is scrubbed with the surface disinfectant of choice, and sterile gauze sponges are placed on each side of the site when an anterior tooth is being treated and anterior to the site when a posterior tooth is treated.

The sterile indelible pencil is used to draw the outline of the planned flap, and this is carefully examined to be sure that all the requirements for a desirable flap are satisfied. In initial surgical cases the operator may want to have a checklist of these requirements typed out on a small sheet of paper unobtrusively placed on a cabinet or counter top behind the patient. Before these procedures a certain degree of nervousness is not unusual in even the most experienced operator, and an important flap requirement may be forgotten that complicates the entire procedure to follow.

Once the surgeon is satisfied that the flap has the proper outlines, a gauze sponge saturated with the surface disinfectant is swabbed across the site to redisinfect the area and remove any excess pencil marks, still leaving some width of the lines as reference.

Opening the flap. By means of the scalpel with the size 15 blade mounted, a firm incision is made through the periosteum to the bone, first along the vertical lines of incision and then along the horizontal lines. If a split-thickness flap is to be utilized, the necessary modifications are followed at this point to dissect the periosteum from the overlying mucosa.

A periodontal curette is passed along the incision lines to free the edges from the bone (Fig. 11-24, *B*). This is especially important when the horizontal flap is in the gingival sulcus so the epithelial attachment is stripped from the tooth. The periosteal elevator is used to peel the periosteum from the bone. Short, firm strokes toward the apical portion of the flap are necessary to avoid tearing the tissue.

Once the flap has been raised with the periosteal elevator to the desired extent, the retractor is placed beneath the raised tissue with its edge against the bone. If the edge of the retractor pinches any portion of the flap, maceration of the tissue will occur. The raised tissue gently lies along the length of the retractor, with its edges free and blood supply unaffected.

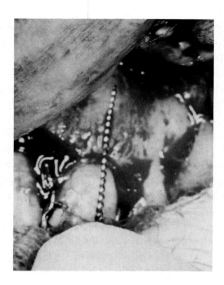

Fig. 11-28. Prior to surgery, a file is set to indicate canal working length, if known. When no defect is present in periapical bone, file is laid alongside tooth to locate correct position for beginning bone removal. Tip of file should correspond to position of apex of the tooth.

Locating the root apex. If a defect is obviously present, the smallest surgical curette is used to begin the removal of the granulation tissue and the uncovering of the root apex. If a defect is not readily apparent, the sharp tip of the endodontic explorer is forcibly placed on the bone in the area where the defect is expected. Often only a thin layer of bone covers the area of pathosis, and the pressure of the explorer breaks the covering and discloses the defect. In some cases a tiny hole in the bone leads to the defect. The bone in the suspect area should be heavily aspirated and any holes explored to determine if the defect lies beneath.

In cases where no defect can be found or no radiolucency is present, the premeasured file is placed along the buccal bone at the estimated angulation of the tooth. This estimate of angulation may be aided by the topography of the overlying bone, since a hump in the bone usually corresponds to the buccal surface of the root (Fig. 11-28). The scalpel with a size 15 blade mounted is placed just apical to the premeasured file, and some of the periapical bone is peeled off. This will often expose the root tip or the lesion (Fig. 11-29). Even if its does not, the bone bur next used to begin bone penetration will have an

indentation to penetrate rather than the possibility of sliding off the smooth bone of the cortical plate and tearing adjacent tissue. A no. 557 or 700 bur is placed in the airotor and, by using a brush stroke with water spray, the bone is removed in the area estimated to be overlying the root apex. The motion of the handpiece to remove bone is similar to that used for crown preparation: a gliding motion with light pressure and heavy water spray. The water keeps the bone cool and washes away the debris.

If a defect or the apex is not found after a few minutes of bone removal, an estimate radiograph must be taken. A radiopaque material, such as the tip from the wide end of a gutta-percha cone, a small segment of a silver point, or a square from the lead foil backing of an x-ray film packet, is placed in the bone preparation and radiographed (Fig. 11-30). The processed film is examined for the relationship between the radiopaque object and the root apex. Any discrepancy is corrected and more bone removed. A second estimate radiograph may be taken if the apex is not readily noted, but usually only a slight initial correction is needed before the desired point is reached.

Curettage. Once the area of pathosis is located, the smallest curette is used to begin the removal of the inflamed tissues. At this time the total extent of the lesion may be determined by working the curette with a sweeping motion along the bone at the periphery of the lesion. The biopsy bottle must be kept open to receive tissue samples for histopathologic examination. If the lesion is large, the larger curettes are used for tissue removal.

When the gross removal of tissue is accomplished, the tip of the root is cleansed with the surgical curette or the periodontal curette. Any excess gutta-percha and/or sealer is removed, and the tightness of the apical seal is examined with the endodontic explorer. The possibility of an additional canal or root should be investigated.

If a reverse filling is to be placed, the final scraping of the cavity wall is delayed until after the amalgam placement to remove any excess filling materials. If no reverse filling is to be placed, the smallest curette is now used to complete the removal of tissue, leaving solid bone to outline the cavity.

Curettage as opposed to apicoectomy. For many years, whenever surgical endodontic therapy was performed, it was advocated to do an apicoectomy (i.e., to cut off the apical portion of the root). The rationale for such procedure was the belief

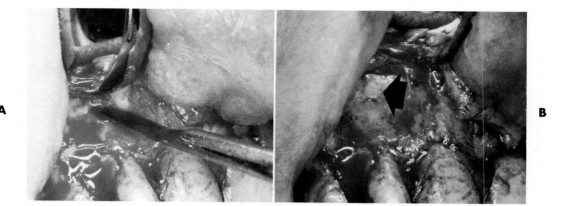

Fig. 11-29. **A,** Scalpel with size 15 blade is used to peel back bone at estimated apex. **B,** Small indentation is made, and a portion of root *(arrow)* is exposed.

that the apical portion retained necrotic cementum, which would delay healing, and was the location of unfilled and uncleansed lateral canals that would perpetuate the inflamed condition.

This attitude is no longer considered to be valid. Most of the necrotic cementum may be removed during apical surgery with a periodontal curette without cutting off segments of the root. If the crown-root ratio reaches an undesirable point should portions of the root be removed, root conservation must be observed. Successful cases are routinely reported with no reduction of tooth length.

Another formerly advocated practice was performance of an apicoectomy down to the greatest depth of pathosis, if such an area extended laterally alongside the root. It is true that in cases where the inflamed tissue extends laterally, palatally, or lingually along the side of the root, some tooth reduction is necessary to provide for access to gain adequate curettage. However, reduction to the level of pathosis is absolutely unnecessary, and only the amount of tooth reduction needed for access is advised. If the area of pathosis is predominantly confined to a single surface and some root reduction is necessary to gain access for curettage, such reduction may be diagonal rather than horizontal. In this way only the portion of the root that interferes with inflammatory tissue elimination is removed, whereas the maximum amount of root length is maintained.

Whenever a reverse filling procedure is to be used, apicoectomy is mandatory to provide a table into which the preparation and filling will be placed.

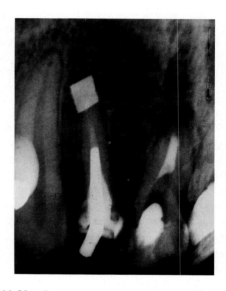

Fig. 11-30. In some cases apex may still not be located, even after considerable bone removal. To reveal proximity of entry to desired position, the lead foil backing from an x-ray packet was placed in bone preparation and the area was radiographed. In this case preparation was slightly too far to distal of apex.

Completing the surgery. At this point the operator determines if a reverse filling is necessary. The indications and methods for reverse fillings will be discussed later in this chapter. If no reverse filling is needed and the surgery is considered to be completed except for suturing, a radiograph is taken. This film must be carefully examined to ensure that no excess canal filling material

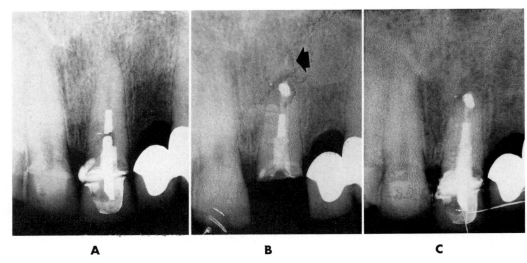

Fig. 11-31. Necessity for taking a radiograph prior to completion of a surgical case. **A,** Maxillary central incisor with a broken bur that could not be removed in canal, preventing proper canal preparation and filling. **B,** Canal was filled as well as possible with intent to reverse fill after surgical exposure of apex. Case seemed to be well done, but immediate postoperative film taken while patient was still in the operating room and the flap was still opened showed apical portion of root *(arrow)* remaining. **C,** Root tip was removed, and area seemed well on the way to healing 4 months later. (Temporary splint by Dr. Harold Brill, Chicago, to evaluate degree of healing prior to final bridge construction.)

or root fragments remain in the bony cavity, that the root tip has no sharp spicules, and that no unfilled portions of canal are near the apex (Fig. 11-31). The film must always be taken before suturing is started so any of the preceding problems may be corrected. If everything appears satisfactory, the flap is replaced and sutured.

Surgery from palatal access. The flap used with a palatal access has already been described (Fig. 11-21). Palatal roots are extremely difficult to reverse fill, usually leading to misplaced filling materials and a poor final result. Therefore the most desirable cases are those in which an apicoectomy can be performed and the root is cut back to a place where the canal is correctly filled. Following this necessity, if the canal filling for a palatal root is poor, it should be removed, the canal reprepared, and a well condensed gutta-percha filling placed if at all possible.

Access to the root tip is very difficult in these cases because the vault of the palate gets wider toward the apex of the palatal root, whereas the root itself generally curves to the buccal. This means that as the surgeon approaches the apex of the palatal root, there is more bone to penetrate and the root tip goes in the opposite direction.

Therefore the operator must make a diagonal cut that goes through the palatal bone a few millimeters apical to the gingival margin of bone and direct this cut apically and buccally to intersect with the root a few millimeters from the tip. The gingival margin of bone must be protected as in all surgical cases to prevent a periodontal defect from occurring.

If the cut is made properly, the pink of the gutta-percha canal filling is visualized. The root tip is removed by pulling from the buccal to the palatal with a scaler or periodontal curette and is examined to verify the correctness of the cut (Fig. 11-32, *C*). The apical tissues are curetted and retained for biopsy, the root tip beveled, and after a confirming radiograph, the area is sutured (Fig. 11-21, *C* and *D*).

Satisfactory healing should result (Fig. 11-32, *E*), and the tooth should return to health. This treatment is quite complicated but seemingly more desirable than extraction or root amputation. Some authors have suggested intentional replantation to reverse fill palatal root in the hand and then return the tooth to its socket. We, however, tend to try to avoid intentional replantation whenever possible (Chapter 5) and prefer this method.

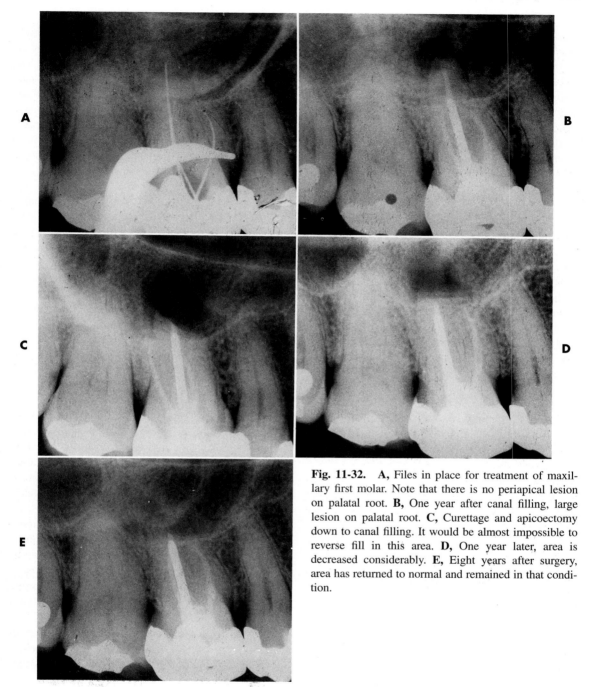

Fig. 11-32. **A,** Files in place for treatment of maxillary first molar. Note that there is no periapical lesion on palatal root. **B,** One year after canal filling, large lesion on palatal root. **C,** Curettage and apicoectomy down to canal filling. It would be almost impossible to reverse fill in this area. **D,** One year later, area is decreased considerably. **E,** Eight years after surgery, area has returned to normal and remained in that condition.

POSTRESECTION FILLING TECHNIQUE

Although many oral surgeons and endodontists prefer the postresection filling technique in surgical endodontics, it has certain inherent disadvantages.

Disadvantages and advantages. Probably the major disadvantage of the postresection filling method is that the time spent with the tissue reflected and bone uncovered is greater than with the two-step technique, since both the canal filling and the curettage are performed after the flap is opened. Since the degree of pain and edema is usually proportional to the time that the flap is retracted, this method would appear to cause greater postoperative problems. However, the total time involved for the canal filling and curettage is usually less for the postresection method than the two-step treatment. Time for the total procedure is lessened because no immediate disinfection is performed, no application of rubber dam is necessary, and no master gutta-percha cones need be verified radiographically.

There are other disadvantages, including the presence of blood from the periapical tissues interfering with the condensation of the cones and the usually less dense filling, since there is no solid dentinal matrix to pack against. The additional information derived from viewing the radiograph of the canal filling is not available. Also, since no rubber dam is placed, it is possible for the patient to taste any of the canal irrigants, such as chlorinated soda or 95% alcohol, and begin coughing because of the irritation. Even worse, the possibility of swallowing or aspirating a file or reamer is present.

The major advantage of the postresection method is that it is easier to locate a difficult-to-find apex, since a large instrument may be placed through the canal and into the periapical tissue as a landmark. Also, if an instrument or filling material is broken off in the apical portion of the canal or partially into the periapical tissues, the fragment may be surgically removed before canal filling. Then the entire canal receives a filling, and the original crown-root ratio is maintained.

Armamentarium. In addition to the surgical instruments listed earlier in this chapter, canal enlarging instruments and the tray needed for canal filling are required.

Technique. If convenient, the canal preparation may be accomplished at an appointment before the surgical visit, but no master gutta-percha cone need be obtained. If any chance for a between-appointment exacerbation exists, the canal should be left open.

The patient is prepared for surgery in the routine manner and the necessary local anesthetic administered. The surgical site is examined for the most desirable flap preparation. As before, the indelible pencil outline method is used. The incisions are made with the size 15 scalpel; tissue is reflected with the periosteal elevator and retracted (Fig. 11-33, *B*). If a surgical defect is not apparent, bone removal and apex uncovering are performed in the manner previously described. A large file may be placed through the lingual opening into the periapical tissues to aid in the location of apex (Fig. 11-33, *C*).

Once the apex is found, it is uncovered by high-speed preparation if surrounded by bone or by curettage if covered by granulation tissue. The canal is enlarged to the desired width, with care taken to prevent irrigants from falling into the patient's mouth. A gutta-percha cone one size smaller than the largest file used in canal preparation is placed into the canal. It should extend a maximum of 2 mm past the apex but have some retention within the canal (Fig. 11-33, *D*).

The canal is irrigated with 95% alcohol and dried as well as possible with absorbent paper points. It is usually difficult to gain complete dryness since the fluids from the apical tissues may seep into the canal. For this reason, Tubliseal is not used, and Wach's paste or a similar product is the preferable root canal sealer. The sealer is mixed on the heavy side and applied to the canal walls with a reamer turned counterclockwise. The previously obtained master cone is placed in the canal through the lingual opening so the tip extends past the apex. This protruding portion of the cone is seized with the locking cotton pliers (Fig. 11-33, *E*) and pulled apically to gain as tight a fit as possible within the canal. This apical portion of the cone should be seated with a tugging motion and short strokes. Attempting to pull the cone too strongly will distort the semisolid gutta-percha, resulting in stretching of the cone and a change in the dimensional shape of the key apical portion. Lateral condensation with auxiliary gutta-percha cones completes the canal filling procedure (Fig. 11-33, *F*).

A sharp scalpel is used to cut through the excess gutta-percha and remove it. The apical portion of the filling is cold condensed with a burnisher or amalgam plugger. Attempting to sear the apex with a hot instrument has been found to improve the seal on one side of the cone but to distort and decrease the seal on the opposite side.

Any remaining inflammatory tissue is curetted and a radiograph taken to ensure all is in order before suturing (Fig. 11-33, *G*). After any necessary corrections are carried out, the flap is sutured to place.

Removing broken instruments and filling materials. As previously stated, the postresection filling method is superior to the two-step procedure in treating cases with broken instruments and filling materials.

The procedure is identical to that just described for the postresection method in patient preparation and flap retraction. No file may be placed in the

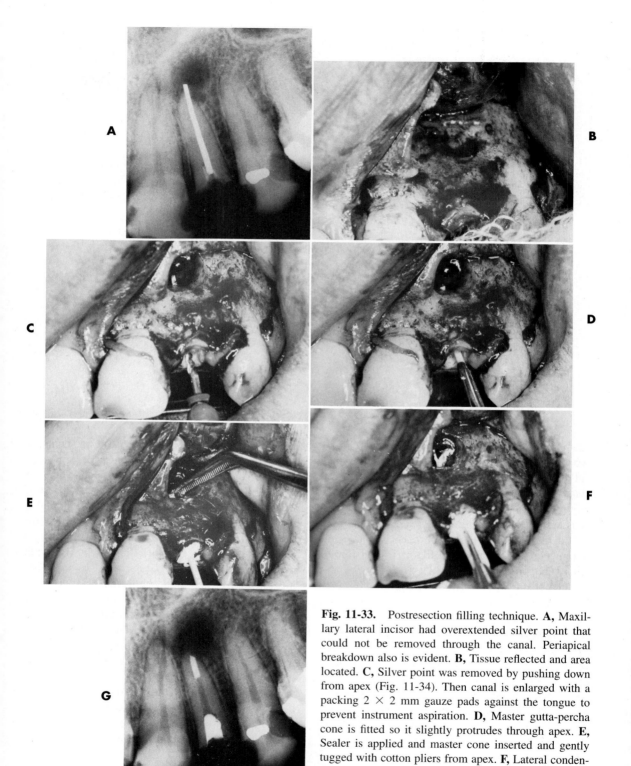

Fig. 11-33.   Postresection filling technique. **A,** Maxillary lateral incisor had overextended silver point that could not be removed through the canal. Periapical breakdown also is evident. **B,** Tissue reflected and area located. **C,** Silver point was removed by pushing down from apex (Fig. 11-34). Then canal is enlarged with a packing 2 × 2 mm gauze pads against the tongue to prevent instrument aspiration. **D,** Master gutta-percha cone is fitted so it slightly protrudes through apex. **E,** Sealer is applied and master cone inserted and gently tugged with cotton pliers from apex. **F,** Lateral condensation is completed with auxiliary cones, excess is removed, and post room is prepared. **G,** Radiograph taken after surgery.

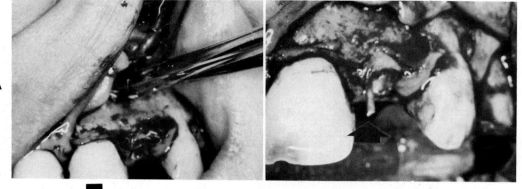

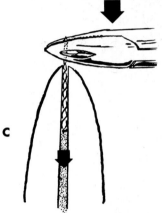

Fig. 11-34. Removal of a broken instrument or silver point slightly through apex. **A,** Hemostat grabs extended point, pictured in Fig. 11-33, and slightly twists and forces it back into canal. **B,** Point *(arrow)* is delivered back down canal and removed through canal opening. **C,** Attempting to pull point or broken instrument out will only cause more binding in canal because of taper.

tooth to aid in the location of the apex, since it would be blocked by the retained fragment. Careful exploration is used to uncover the apex by searching for the defect or by taking estimate radiographs with radiopaque materials in the bone preparation. If the fragment extends into the periapical tissues, care should be exercised to avoid cutting it off with a bur during bone preparation, since that complicates removal.

Since this method varies only slightly according to whether the fragment is broken off within the canal or extends past the apex, for the moment let us assume that we are dealing with an instrument that does extend into the periapical tissues. Once the apex and fragment are located, a cotton pellet is placed into the lingual opening to prevent the swallowing of the delivered piece. A sharp-tipped hemostat is used to seize the fragment, and a firm incisal push is exerted in an attempt to dislodge the instrument and return it down the canal (Fig. 11-34, *A* and *B*). Because both the instrument and the preparation are tapered toward the apex, attempting to pull the instrument out apically merely binds it farther in the canal in most instances (Fig. 11-34, *C*). Only if a tiny amount of

the fragment is retained within the canal will an apical pull remove it.

In cases where the fragment does not budge, a no. 557 or 700 bur in the airotor is used to trim off a portion of the root and then dislodgement is attempted. If the broken material still remains, or if it did not extend into the periapical tissues initially, approximately 1 mm of root apex is removed. Then the endodontic explorer is used to push into the canal in an effort to gain dislodging incisally. If the material is not delivered after this attempt, the method may be repeated after removal of an additional 1 mm of root. When a considerable length of fragment remains tightly in the canal after 2 mm of root has been removed, a decision must be made as to whether an undesirable crown-root ratio would result from continued root reduction. In such a case it would be better to place a reverse filling in the apex and pack the unfilled portion of the canal from the access opening with gutta-percha.

In most cases the broken instrument or filling material is easily pushed out after one or two attempts. When this is accomplished, the cotton pellet from the access opening is removed and the fragment usually comes with it. If the separated portion remains within the body of the canal, it is easily removed with a broach or Hedstrom file.

Care must be exercised to avoid letting the patient swallow or aspirate the segment at this time.

With the fragment removed, the canal is prepared and filled and the surgery completed as described earlier.

REVERSE FILLING PROCEDURES

Indications.   For many years we thought that if there were any possibility for apical seal to be lacking, the canal should be reverse filled during the surgical procedure. We have had many excellent results following reverse filling cases (Figs. 11-35, 11-44, and 11-47) over significant periods, but have had other cases (Figs. 11-11 and 11-36) where the procedures should have succeeded and yet failed.

Currently, as a result of the reports of Dorn and Gartner and Frank et al., we have revamped our surgical procedure considerably and no longer employ amalgam as a material for canal reverse

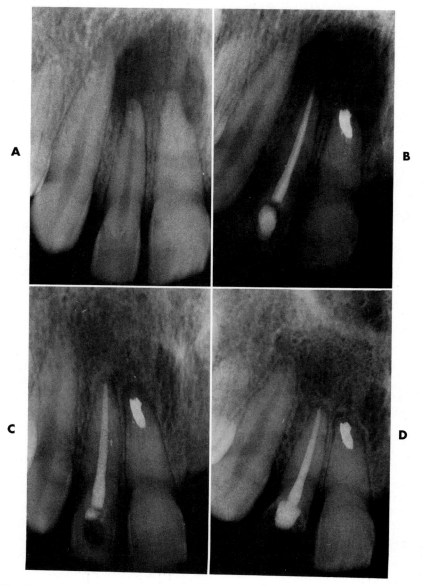

Fig. 11-35.   A, Preoperative radiograph of maxillary lateral and central incisors with large periapical lesion. There is no discernible canal in the central. **B,** Immediate postoperative film, after routine canal filling of the lateral, reverse filling of the central, and periapical curettage. **C,** Three years later, area has healed almost perfectly. **D,** Fourteen years after original treatment, area continues to look excellent.

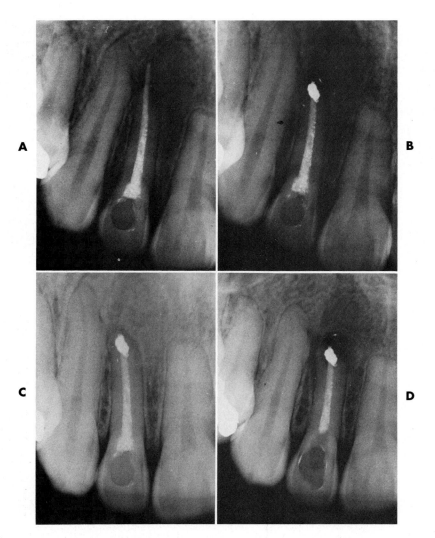

Fig. 11-36.   **A,** Radiograph of maxillary lateral incisor with gross overextension of canal filling material and apical sensitivity. **B,** It would have been better to remove the gutta-percha and refill the tooth, but curettage and reverse filling only were performed. **C,** One year later, lesion appears to have healed. **D,** Two years later, lesion has returned and there appears to be either apical resorption or fracture of the root tip.

filling. In fact, as stated earlier, we prefer not to reverse fill at all and attempt to replace a faulty canal filling by disassembling the coronal portion of the tooth in a failing case and then refiling and refilling the canal. Even if surgery becomes necessary, then the tip of the root may be trimmed down to solidly packed gutta-percha, and a reverse filling is not needed at all.

Had the case shown in Figure 11-36 been treated by refiling and refilling, rather than by reverse filling, I am certain that the tooth would still be in the patient's mouth. Teeth illustrated by Figures 11-13, 11-14, 11-27, and 11-37 were all

treated surgically, but into well-placed gutta-percha fillings requiring no reverse filling, and the cases were successful.

In instances where a reverse amalgam filling was used in one tooth adjacent to a tooth where a solid gutta-percha filling was employed, the healing of the gutta-percha filled apex was usually superior (Fig. 11-38).

Obviously in some instances it is impossible to place a gutta-percha canal filling through the canal, and there is nothing to do but rely on reverse filling procedures. The most common cases of this kind involve teeth with clinical and/or

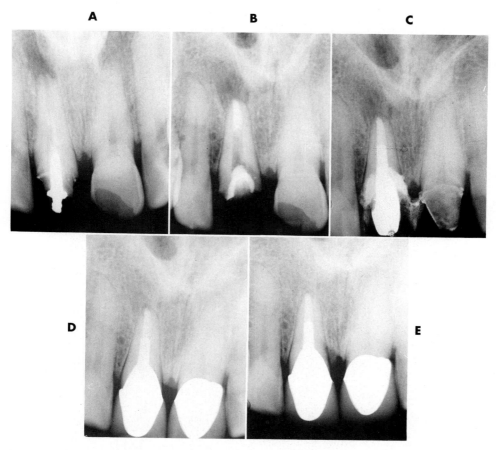

Fig. 11-37. **A,** Preoperative film of maxillary central incisor with post present, very poor canal filling, and periapical lesion. The patient was to leave the United States within several weeks, so surgical treatment was undertaken rather than merely re-treatment and observation. **B,** When the post was removed, a portion of the palatal tooth fractured off. The canal was prepared and filled with laterally condensed gutta-percha and Tubliseal, and the lesion was curetted. Post room was prepared, and the patient returned to the referring dentist for temporary restoration. **C,** Six months later, the patient returned to the United States and periodontal treatment was needed to expose more root margin. The periapical lesion is healing. **D,** Three years later. **E,** Six years after original treatment, area has healed perfectly and restorations look excellent. (Restorations by Dr. Edward LeMire, Chicago.)

radiographic symptoms and no negotiable canal, the presence of a well-fitting post and core that might cause root fracture during removal, a sectioned silver point, and an irretrievable broken instrument or filling material with lack of apical seal. Any of these situations may occur without clinical or radiographic evidence of damage being present. When this is the case, surgery is not indicated, but frequent recall examinations and evaluations should be conducted to ensure that no problems develop and then get out of hand.

Because of problems with previously reverse filled cases, some of these require re-treatment,

usually involving surgery. Discussion of such re-treatment will be presented at the end of this section.

Use of ultrasonic tips for reverse filling preparations. If any reverse filling is to be used, the root tip (or lateral root surface) must be prepared to receive the filling material. For many years, preparations were produced by the burs usually used for restorative dentistry—diamond stone and carbide burs (usually fissure and inverted cone types). Although these burs are still used to bevel the root tip (see next section), most of the preparation for the reverse filling itself is being

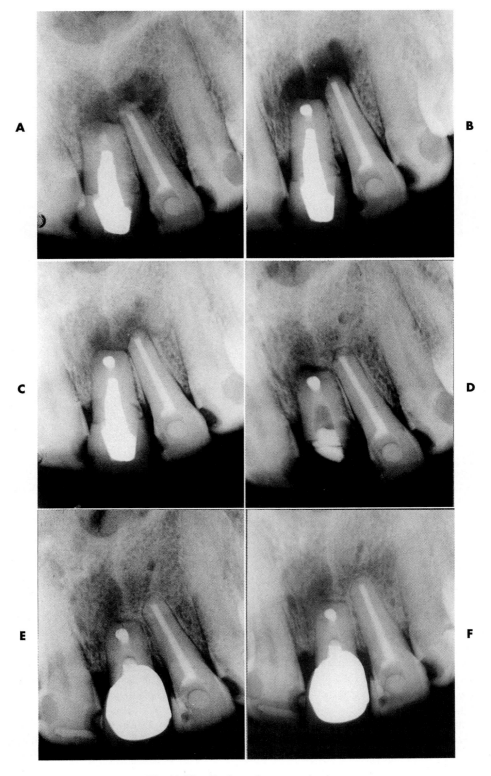

Fig. 11-38. For legend see opposite page.

performed with ultrasonic tips by more and more clinicians.

These tips (Fig. 11-39) are smaller than the burs that were formerly used, they conserve tooth structure and give more parallel preparations, they probably enhance the cleanliness of the prepared area, and the tip angles (Fig. 11-39, *B*) give better access. Rubinstein has indicated that a common site for remaining debris or old canal filling material is the most buccal portion of the preparation. It is difficult to cleanse this area with a handpiece-driven bur. However, the reverse angle of the ultrasonic tip allows more room to reach, and thus remove, these unwanted items. Ultrasonic preparation (see Chapter 7) has been used in routine endodontic therapy for several years to give better, cleaner preparations and remove unwanted materials. This application is now available for surgical treatment, as well.

The ultrasonic tip has allowed the operator to make very precise preparations because of the ease with which it removes old gutta-percha, in particular. It also will quickly widen and clean canals narrowed by reparative dentin to make an excellent shape for filling when no old canal filling is present (Figs. 11-40 and 11-41). However, don't cast aside the routine burs when surgery is necessary. Not only are these needed for root beveling, but also they are necessary to cut posts, silver points, and other metallic objects. The ultrasonic tips have little effect on cutting these metallic materials, although they may be used to loosen the materials from their hold in the canal.

Types of preparation. Two types of preparations have been in routine use for some time: the Class I and the slot, or Matsura, type. An additional preparation also has been described and is referred to as the figure-eight type of reverse fill preparation.

Before any preparation is begun, the root to be reverse filled must be beveled. Placing a filling in

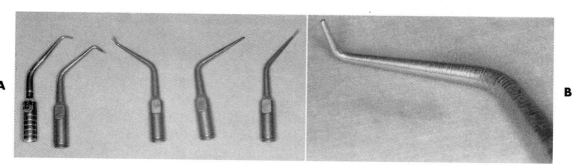

Fig. 11-39. Ultrasonic tips designed especially for preparations for reverse filling. **A,** These ultrasonic tips were specially designed for preparations to receive reverse fillings. Note several angles of tips provided to allow for preparation of roots with different apical inclinations. **B,** Closeup of tip on the right in **A,** for use in molar teeth.

Fig. 11-38. Relative healing between apex filled with gutta-percha and apex reverse filled with amalgam. **A,** Preoperative radiograph of maxillary anterior area, large periapical lesion associated with both central (left) and lateral (right) incisors, both teeth sore at the apex and mobile, history of previous surgery. Note that the portion of the lesion associated with the lateral is the larger. Because of the large cast core/post, it was decided to treat surgically only, probably reverse filling both apexes with amalgam. **B,** When the flap was raised, it was apparent that an incomplete fill was present on the lateral incisor. However, when the root was trimmed back, a solid gutta-percha filling was reached, so no reverse filling was performed. The central incisor had no apical seal whatsoever, so an amalgam reverse filling was placed. This film was taken immediately after the surgery. **C,** One year later, considerable healing, both teeth comfortable, and lateral incisor has better healing according to radiograph. **D,** Eighteen months after surgery, lateral incisor totally healed according to radiograph, slight radiolucency associated with central. **E,** Three years after original treatment, excellent healing and both teeth tight and comfortable. **F,** Six years after original treatment, all still looking excellent. (Restoration by Dr. Kerry Voit, Chicago.)

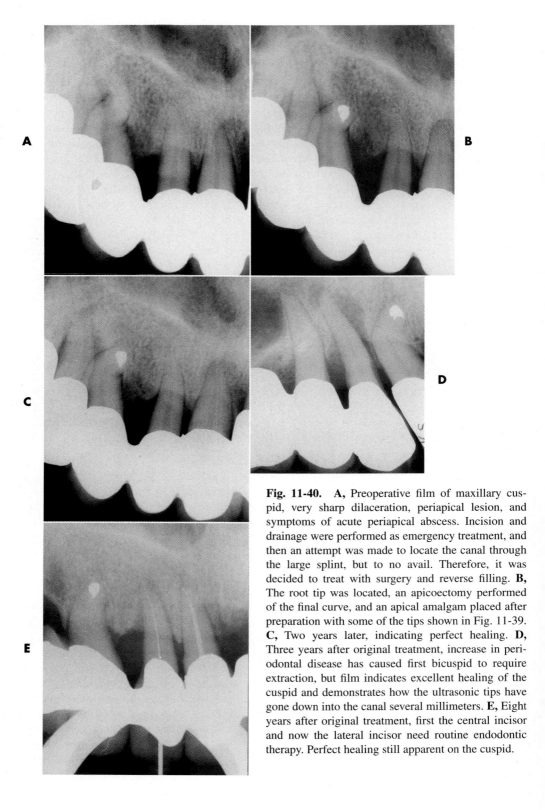

Fig. 11-40. **A,** Preoperative film of maxillary cuspid, very sharp dilaceration, periapical lesion, and symptoms of acute periapical abscess. Incision and drainage were performed as emergency treatment, and then an attempt was made to locate the canal through the large splint, but to no avail. Therefore, it was decided to treat with surgery and reverse filling. **B,** The root tip was located, an apicoectomy performed of the final curve, and an apical amalgam placed after preparation with some of the tips shown in Fig. 11-39. **C,** Two years later, indicating perfect healing. **D,** Three years after original treatment, increase in periodontal disease has caused first bicuspid to require extraction, but film indicates excellent healing of the cuspid and demonstrates how the ultrasonic tips have gone down into the canal several millimeters. **E,** Eight years after original treatment, first the central incisor and now the lateral incisor need routine endodontic therapy. Perfect healing still apparent on the cuspid.

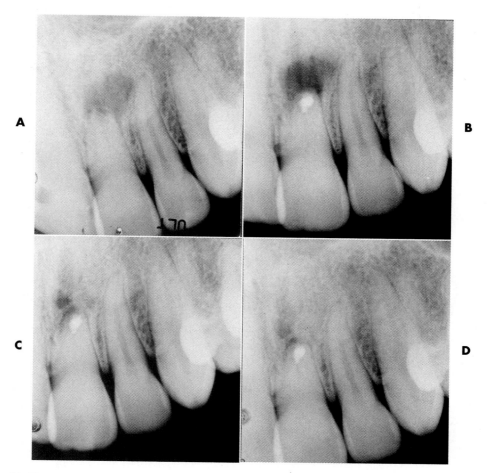

Fig. 11-41.   Reverse preparation with ultrasonic tips, reverse filling with SuperEBA cement. **A,** Preoperative radiograph of maxillary central incisor, very small canal space, apical resorption, apical soreness, some mobility, history of previous surgery but no canal filling. **B,** Area was flapped, root tipped curetted with regular ultrasonic tips, apical preparation made with tips shown in Fig. 11-39, several millimeters into canal. **C,** Six months after treatment, excellent healing, slight radiolucency still present. **D,** Eighteen months after treatment, lesion almost totally filled in. Radiolucency to upper left probably is an apical scar.

an unbeveled apex is similar to placing a filling at the point of a pyramid. No flat table would be present to pack against, and the filling material would merely fall down the sides and not seal the tip. Beveling on the tooth is obtained by using a fissure bur in the airotor or straight handpiece and cutting the root tip from mesial to distal surface at approximately a 45-degree angle to the long access of the tooth, allowing for visualization of the entire root face (Fig. 11-42). Teeth that have a palatal or lingual inclination may require a greater angle of beveling for ease of preparation and filling placement.

Beveling of the root tip may be accomplished without significantly reducing root length and thus retaining almost the same crown-root ratio. If the crown-root ratio is highly unfavorable, but the strategic importance of the tooth warrants its retention, the slot preparation should be made, which requires little, if any, root length reduction.

After beveling, the outline of the root face will have one of two configurations, either oval or figure eight. The most common shape will be a slightly irregular oval, with the canal having a smaller oval shape in the approximate center. The ideal reverse fill preparation for this shape is

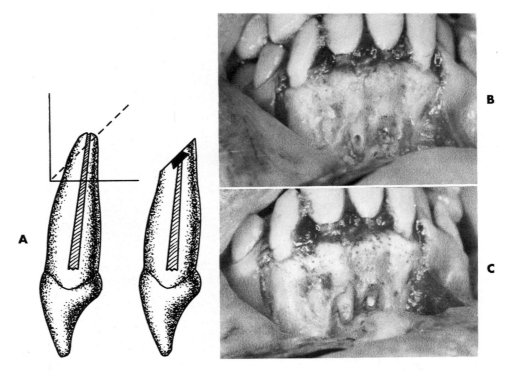

Fig. 11-42. **A,** Root tip must be beveled at an approximate 45-degree angle to provide complete visualization of entire root face. Only then may the operator prepare and place reverse filling. **B,** Lower anterior teeth have been beveled so entire root face is visible. Class I type of preparations were made with no. 33½ inverted cone bur. **C,** With this excellent exposure and access, it is no problem to place reverse fillings.

similar to the typical Class I occlusal amalgam preparation of operative dentistry, only in miniature. It is prepared by using a no. 33½ bur or ultrasonic tip down into the canal for a minimum of 1 mm but preferably at least 2 to 3 mm. It is important to remember that the bevel of the root face is at approximately 45 degrees and that if the preparation is made with the bur perpendicular to the root face, there is a good chance for perforation of the root lingually. Therefore the bur must come down along the long axis of the tooth and remain within the confines of the canal while the preparation is made. If insufficient room is available to come down the long axis, greater beveling of the root face or removal of periapical bone should be performed. If this is not desirable, the slot preparation should be utilized.

The other root face configuration developed after beveling is the figure-eight shape, with a long oval or slot canal in the center. This shape may be found when two canals are present in one root of a tooth, such as the mesiobucal root of a maxillary

first molar, maxillary and mandibular bicuspids, and mesial roots of mandibular molars and mandibular anterior teeth. When these roots have one canal in one root, the configuration of the root face after beveling will be oval.

The proper preparation for teeth having one root and two canals is the figure-eight preparation. A no. 33½ bur or ultrasonic tip is used and two round but touching preparations are made, with care taken to keep the bur along the long axis of the root. This type of preparation should be made in any one-rooted tooth when it is suspected that two canals may be present, even if only one canal was previously filled (Figs. 11-43 to 11-45).

The third type of preparation is the slot type, also referred to as the Matsura preparation, from the name of its early advocate. This should be used where it is inconvenient to utilize the other types of preparations that involve access along the long axis of the tooth. The slot preparation is made with the bur used perpendicularly to the long axis of the tooth and requires much less tooth and/or periapi-

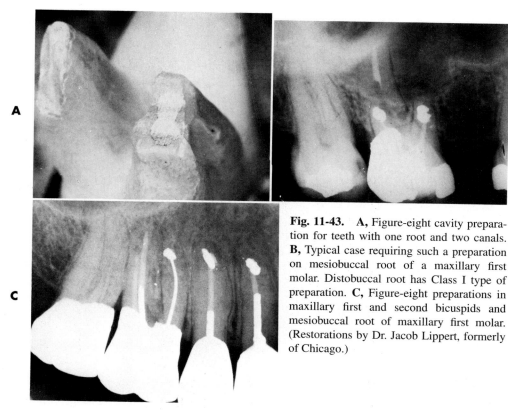

Fig. 11-43.   A, Figure-eight cavity preparation for teeth with one root and two canals. **B,** Typical case requiring such a preparation on mesiobuccal root of a maxillary first molar. Distobuccal root has Class I type of preparation. **C,** Figure-eight preparations in maxillary first and second bicuspids and mesiobuccal root of maxillary first molar. (Restorations by Dr. Jacob Lippert, formerly of Chicago.)

cal bone removal. The most common needs for the slot preparation are in those teeth where removal of root structure will lead to an inadequate crown-root ratio or removal of periapical bone sufficient to gain access will infringe on adjacent vital structures. Examples of the latter are maxillary bicuspids and molars near the maxillary sinus, mandibular molars near the mandibular canal, and maxillary anterior teeth near the nares. In addition, teeth with palatal or lingual inclinations, such as maxillary lateral incisors and mandibular anterior teeth, may be easier to prepare and fill by using the slot preparation.

The preparation is made by using a no. 700 bur in the straight handpiece or airotor. Starting at the apex of the tooth, the bur is brought toward the cervical margin approximately 2 mm, leaving a trough of tooth structure missing. Then a no. 33½ or 35 bur or ultrasonic tip is used to sharpen the corners of the preparation to afford undercuts for the retention of the filling material. When a slot preparation is used, much less root face beveling is

required, since the retention is obtained in the undercut areas near the base of the preparation (Figs. 11-46 and 11-47).

Types of filling materials.   Many filling materials have been suggested for reverse fills. Indium, a soft malleable metal, has been suggested with descriptions given for burnishing small segments into the cavity preparation. Gutta-percha cones and silver points, inserted from the apex rather than through the normal occlusal or lingual access, also have been used.

The requirements for an apically placed material are still the same as for a coronally placed intra-canal filling material. For many years that role was played with reasonable success by silver amalgam. Although other materials were suggested by some, amalgam remained dominant. Recently a number of studies have cast doubt on the efficacy of amalgam, and other materials are receiving attention.

The major problem in long-term follow-ups of amalgam reverse fills seems related to the fact that the root tip does not remain in a static condition.

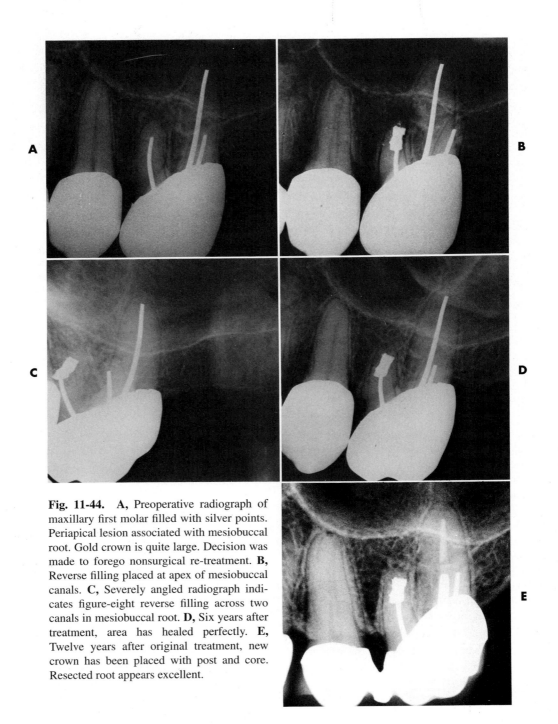

Fig. 11-44. A, Preoperative radiograph of maxillary first molar filled with silver points. Periapical lesion associated with mesiobuccal root. Gold crown is quite large. Decision was made to forego nonsurgical re-treatment. **B,** Reverse filling placed at apex of mesiobuccal canals. **C,** Severely angled radiograph indicates figure-eight reverse filling across two canals in mesiobuccal root. **D,** Six years after treatment, area has healed perfectly. **E,** Twelve years after original treatment, new crown has been placed with post and core. Resected root appears excellent.

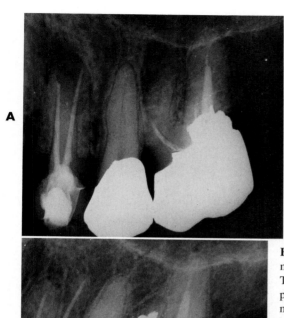

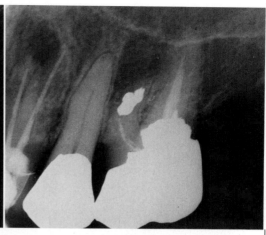

Fig. 11-45.   A, Preoperative radiograph of maxillary first molar. Periapical lesion associated with mesiobuccal root. The first bicuspid routine treatment had just been completed. **B,** Figure-eight type of reverse filling placed in mesiobuccal root. **C,** Four years later, all periapical lesions have healed.

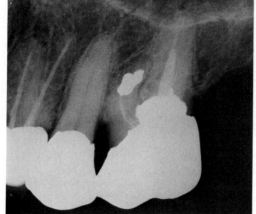

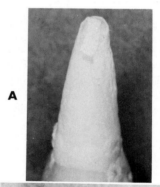

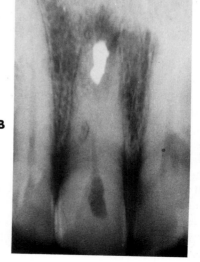

Fig. 11-46.   A, Slot-type preparation, made by small straight fissure and inverted cone burs. **B,** Slot preparation was needed in this case because of the absence of an apical radiolucency, limiting access to the apex. Attempt to locate canal through crown was fruitless, but tooth was symptomatic and required reverse filling.

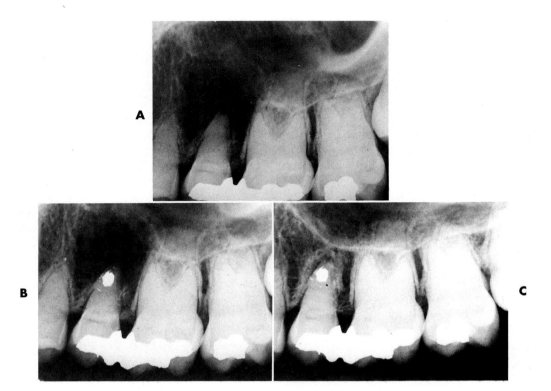

Fig. 11-47. **A,** Preoperative view of maxillary bicuspid and molar areas. Patient has a mesodermal dysplasia, which has caused taurodont molars and considerable diminution of root canal space, similar to dentinogenesis imperfecta. A large periapical lesion is present on the second bicuspid, and the floor of the sinus appears to be involved. **B,** Because of the shortness of the root, the preparation at the apex was made from the buccal, using the slot, or Matsura, preparation. The periapical lesion was curetted. **C,** Three years after original treatment, the bone has filled in very well, and the floor of the sinus appears regenerated radiographically. (Restorations by Dr. Robert Wheeler, Chicago.)

Rather, there is continuous resorption and apposition of cementum at that site, which can easily alter the face of the root that holds the reverse filling. When the marginal integrity is destroyed at the expense of the tooth-side margin rather than the restored segment, the result is still the same—loss of seal and potential apical percolation. This probably further contributes to the apical activity and potentiates the breakdown. With the solid mass of amalgam no longer held in place peripherally, the filling leaks badly and may even be exfoliated from the root tip (Fig. 11-10).

I fear that the newer choices in reverse filling materials, which will be listed later in this section, will suffer a similar fate even though they seem to be tolerated by the body better than amalgam. This is the major reason why I prefer to perform surgery with the philosophy of avoiding reverse filling whenever possible.

If reverse filling becomes necessary, I prefer a deep preparation into solid dentin, at least 2 to 3 mm, if possible. This can be accomplished more easily with the ultrasonic tips than merely with surgical burs, combined with canal filing from the apical end (see later in this section). I have found that reverse fillings placed deeply into solid dentin have had a good prognosis for success, even when filled with amalgam (Fig. 11-52). The additional retention developed in this manner will hold the material in place, even if some of the marginal integrity is destroyed by apical resorption.

A mixture of zinc oxide and eugenol may be used instead of silver amalgam as a reverse filling material. It has many of the same biologic properties as does amalgam but may be absorbable. Zinc oxide-eugenol (ZOE) has advantages in certain cases over amalgam. If amalgam is used to repair a labial perforation near the gingival areas of anterior teeth, a dark discoloration known as an amalgam tattoo may develop. When used for reverse filling a mandibular molar or bicuspid in the proximity of the mandibular canal, the bulk of the amalgam may cause damage to the mandibular vessels if excess filling falls. Being nonstaining, ZOE is used to seal the labial perforations that might result in unesthetic staining; being absorbable, that material would cause less lasting damage should it fall into the mandibular canal.

Two products similar to ZOE that are useful as reverse filling materials are IRM* and SuperEBA.† Both are reinforced ZOE cements (IRM with polymethylmethacrylate; SuperEBA with alumina) that have received excellent evaluations in studies by Dorn and Gartner, Beltes et al., and many others. As long ago as 1979, Oynick and Oynick cautioned against the use of amalgam and recommended the use of EBA-type cements.

IRM is a bit easier to use than SuperEBA. The latter requires experience in mixing and applying since it seems to be the correct consistency, but then thins further when preparing to insert. Once experience is gained with SuperEBA cement, it offers no serious problems in insertion (Fig. 11-41). IRM may be placed with the carriers shown in Fig. 11-25, but SuperEBA is best carried to the tooth with a plastic instrument. Both may be condensed with the miniature pluggers shown in Fig. 11-25.

No one is certain if these two ZOE hybrids are the answer to reverse filling problems. More research continues to clarify the value of other possible solutions. Several researchers have investigated the effectiveness of glass ionomer cements; some reports are very glowing, particularly concerning the biocompatibility of this material.

It will take time for the answers to be clear. Many of us thought that silver amalgam was an excellent reverse filling material. Aside from the antipathy of some clinicians to use a material containing a significant mercury content within the body, it was only after several long-term studies that amalgam was truly questioned in this regard. The important study by Frank et al. demonstrated many excellent cases 10 years and more after treatment. But they also showed cases that had healed completely, but then reversed to failures in the 10 years and greater time period. We will still need 10 years or more to investigate the long-term effects of IRM, SuperEBA, any glass ionomer cement, or any other reverse filling material. Judgments before that are premature.

Gutta-percha has gained increasing acceptance as a reverse filling material, although it is more difficult to manipulate than amalgam or ZOE. Studies by Tanzilli et al. and others indicate that cold-burnished gutta-percha has superior sealing qualities to amalgam when apically placed in a preparation.

There are several methods for gutta-percha use. It may be substituted for amalgam in a Type I or figure-eight preparation in either softened cone form or by an injectable method (see Fig. 11-54). Gutta-percha also may be used following apical filing (see Fig. 11-53).

Following placement, the gutta-percha should be packed down with pluggers or condensers and then cold burnished with any suitable instrument. Excess material outside the preparation is carefully removed with a scalpel.

Miniature carriers and pluggers. As mentioned in the discussion on armamentarium for surgery, reverse fillings require special carriers and pluggers. These instruments have miniature sizes when compared with those used in routine operative dentistry. The two sizes of carriers manufactured are approximately the widths of nos. 557 and 560 burs with the pluggers to match. Although these carriers may retain only a small fraction of the bulk of amalgam or other materials that the regular carriers do, it is more than sufficient for the extremely small preparations used in endodontic reverse fills. Two or three carriers will be adequate to fill the ordinary surgical preparations. It is important that no excessive flash material is left overlapping the outer portion of the barrel of the carrier. Excess filling cannot be packed into the preparation and generally falls adjacent to the root of the tooth and remains after surgery (Fig. 11-25, *B*).

If the regular carriers are used, an excess will be brought to the area and probably will lead to much superfluous material being packed into the adjacent bone and periodontal ligament space. Since these materials are well tolerated by periapical tissue, the excess as such will not cause a great problem. However, because they are radiopaque, excess material may prevent adequate radiographic evaluation of healing. Should excess material lodge in the adjacent bone and still be attached to the reverse fill in the tooth, bone remodeling or

*L. D. Caulk Co., Milford, Dela.
†Harry J. Bosworth Co., Skokie, Ill.

minor tooth movement may dislodge the filling from its preparation. Also, since the material is generally nonabsorbable, it prevents the ingrowth of new bone.

If one does not wish to purchase these instruments, the same function may be gained by heating silver solder into the barrel of an old amalgam carrier, almost obliterating the carrying area. When pushed against freshly prepared mixes, small chunks will attach to the solder and may be carried to the reverse fill preparations. For miniature pluggers, old pluggers or scalers may be ground to a smaller size and polished.

Reverse filling of a tooth with an incompletely formed apex. Reverse filling when the apex is incompletely formed is performed in two steps. With rubber dam applied, the blunderbuss canal is disinfected, enlarged, and filled. It is best to disinfect with phenol prior to filling, even if the tooth had not been left open for drainage, to decrease the seepage of fluids from the periapical tissues. The master cone used for filling must be of extremely large size and may even require hand rolling of multiple cones with a warm cement spatula to gain sufficient width. Lateral condensation is used, and the major objective of this filling is to gain as dense a fill as possible in the area of the narrowest canal constriction, which generally is found in the middle third of the root. It does not matter if excess material extends past the constriction or even into the periapical tissue, since the excess will be removed during the surgery.

After a temporary is placed in the access opening, the rubber dam is removed and the patient prepared for surgery. A suitable flap is reflected, exposing the root apex. The excess gutta-percha and sealer extending past the constriction are removed with a hot instrument, bur, or, even better, ultrasonic tip. When removing the gutta-percha, an undercut area occurs almost automatically. If it is not produced, an undercut will have to be prepared, usually with a no. 35 inverted cone, gaining an excellent result. The reverse filling material of choice—gutta-percha (condensed or thermoplastic) or reinforced ZOE—is packed into the preparation, with the previously placed gutta-percha and the root walls acting as a matrix to pack against. A radiograph is taken, and when all appears satisfactory, the area is closed (Fig. 16-11).

Reverse filling incompletely sealed cases. In any surgical case where a canal filling had been placed prior to surgery, the apical seal must be examined when the root tip is exposed. The short hook of the endodontic explorer (Fig. 11-23) is used to probe the margin between the canal wall and the filling for any voids. If an apicoectomy is to be performed, this examination must take place after the root tip has been removed and the beveling performed. A canal may be filled properly at the apex but not at some site away from that point. The apical portion of the remaining root that has been filled then becomes crucial to the case.

A thin layer of sealer always exists between the wall and the filling material but is often not even seen from the apex. The sealers used in endodontics will absorb if pushed into the periapical tissues due to an overextension but rarely will break down while in the canal.

It is wise to reverse fill failing silver point cases treated surgically (Figs. 11-42 and 11-48), since that material has a much less reliable sealing ability than does gutta-percha. This is especially important when the point is overextended or if the original canal shape was oval in cross section, because these canals cannot possibly be sealed by the round silver point.

Reverse filling of significant lateral canals. Lateral canals are frequently noticed in nonsurgical cases by extrusion of sealer during examination of the postoperative radiograph. Although there is considerable doubt as to whether these lateral canals are really sealed by the extruding sealer, there is a definite clinical impression that healing usually transpires.

Since some question remains as to the seal of these lateral canals, those of significant size should be reverse filled when surgery is performed. The Class I preparation is used, with the modification that the preparation is placed at the point where the lateral canal exits from the tooth substance. This is generally at a right angle to the long axis of the tooth.

When a radiolucency is present on the lateral portion of a root rather than at the apex, it is an indication that a significant lateral canal is present or that the apical foramen exits on the lateral portion of the root rather than on the apical portion. When surgery is performed in these cases, the portion of the root contacting the inflamed tissue must be examined to locate the canal in that area. When and if the canal is found, a reverse filling is placed (Fig. 11-49).

If a multiplicity of small lateral canals appears at the apex of a tooth to be treated surgically, it is

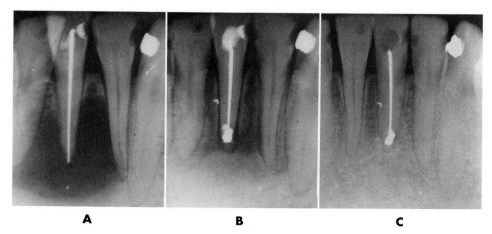

A   **B**   **C**

Fig. 11-48.   A, Preoperative radiograph of mandibular incisor. Routine endodontic treatment had been performed with a silver point placed 2 years earlier. When area failed to heal, curettage was performed but no apical canal filling was placed. Area became still larger, and the dentist thought that "cystic" cells had been left behind. **B,** An attempt was made to remove silver point, but it could not be done without severely cutting down the crown. Patient did not desire a replacement crown after such a long history of failure and requested another surgical treatment. At time of surgery, the root was beveled. Considerable space remained between silver point and canal walls. A reverse filling was placed. If curettage only were performed, it is doubtful whether healing would have occurred. This film was taken 1 year after surgery. **C,** Six years after surgery.

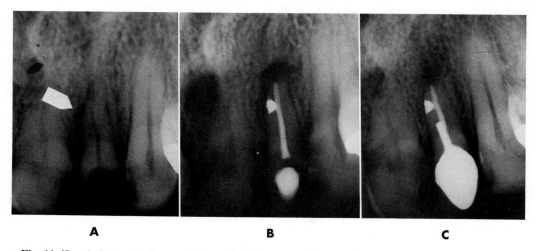

A   **B**   **C**

Fig. 11-49.   A, Lateral incisor requiring periapical surgery due to recurrent exacerbations. Note radiolucency on border of root *(arrow).* **B,** Canal was disinfected with phenol and filled with gutta-percha. At surgery, apicoectomy was performed and lateral canal toward radiolucency was reverse filled. **C,** Excellent healing 18 months later with new bone right up against silver amalgam. (Restorations by Dr. Steve Lynch, Chicago.)

best to trim the apical portion slightly with a fissure bur in the airotor. This removes any of the apical portion that may have some unfilled lateral canals that might perpetuate a lesion.

Reverse filling to seal perforation.   The sealing of small perforations is similar to the reverse filling of significant lateral canals. Heavy condensation procedures allow the root canal sealer to locate the position of these perforations, and the Class I type of preparation is used to retain the filling material. ZOE should be used when sealing labial perforations of anterior teeth to

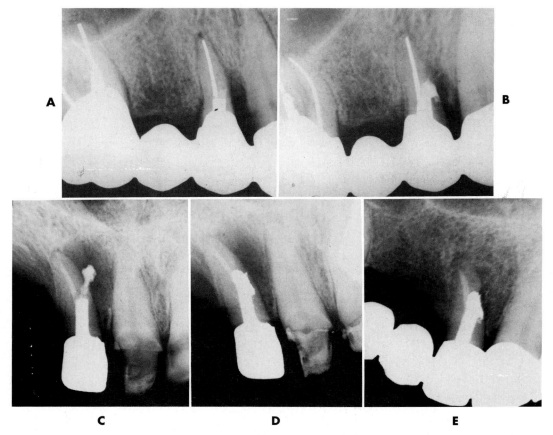

Fig. 11-50. Perforation repairs. **A,** Post preparation for maxillary first bicuspid led to root perforation and development of chronic draining sinus tract. **B,** Because perforation was to the buccal aspect, it was reverse filled with ZOE to avoid silver discoloration. **C,** Post perforation in maxillary lateral incisor resulted in large radiolucent area and periodic swelling. **D,** Reverse filling with amalgam. **E,** One year after surgery, healing is almost completed and tooth has been retained as abutment for a long span bridge. (Splint by Dr. Sheldon Bulwa, Evanston, Ill.)

prevent unesthetic amalgam tattooing (Fig. 11-50, *A* and *B*).

The sealing of larger perforations often requires considerable spontaneity. The true dimensions of large perforations, especially those from resorption, may not be revealed by the two-dimensional radiograph. Only after the area is flapped does the surgeon have a true picture of the degree of destruction. In most very large lesions a large round bur, no. 4 or 6, is used to clean out the necrotic material down to firm tooth structure in the same manner that large carious lesions are excavated. Ultrasonic tips usually are ineffective for preparation against metal. A no. 35 or 37 inverted cone bur is used to provide undercuts in sound dentin, and a no. 557 fissure bur removes

overhanging, badly unsupported tooth structure; then the preparation is filled (Fig. 11-50, *C* to *E*). When the lesion extends for some distance around the tooth, foil or bone wax may be placed against the bone to prevent a forcing of the filling material into the bony crevices.

Every case of treating large perforations is unique, and it is difficult to give a step-by-step procedure that will work in all cases. Two important points to remember are the following:

1. Be sure to remove from the walls of the defect any soft material that might harbor tissue to restart the resorptive process. Ultrasonic use may be effective here.
2. Be prepared for the unusual in size, shape, and depth of the lesion.

Large lesions due to resorption must be observed radiographically for a minimum of 2 years, since they show a high percentage of recurrence. It is not unusual for another surgical treatment to be required in such cases, even if a very careful surgical technique was observed.

Reverse filling when the most convenient access is from the apex.   Included in this category are cases requiring surgery when there is a well-fitting post and core, no apparent root canal, a sectioned silver point, or an irretrievable broken instrument or filling material. The surgery is a one-step proce-

dure, since no access through the normal occlusal or lingual opening is possible.

After the routine steps previously described for surgery, the root apex is exposed and beveled. Depending on the outline of the root face, either a Class I or a figure-eight preparation is made and filled. A radiograph is taken to verify that the apex has been properly sealed and the flap sutured (Fig. 11-7).

Filling when enlargement access is obtained from the apex.   A slight modification of the previously discussed types of cases, in which the access for fill-

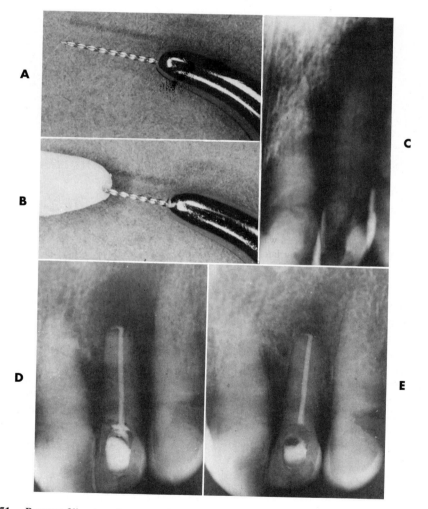

Fig. 11-51.   Reverse filing to gain preparation of entire canal. **A** and **B,** Segment of file placed in hemostat and used to enlarge canal from apex. **C,** Maxillary lateral incisor after referring dentist was unable to locate canal by way of lingual entry. Note that any further preparation would perforate through the labial of the tooth beneath the epithelial attachment. **D,** Decision was made to find and enlarge the canal by apical access. After the apex was beveled and enlarged, file was passed down canal until it protruded through lingual access. Case was completed with two open ends. **E,** Healing 1 year later.

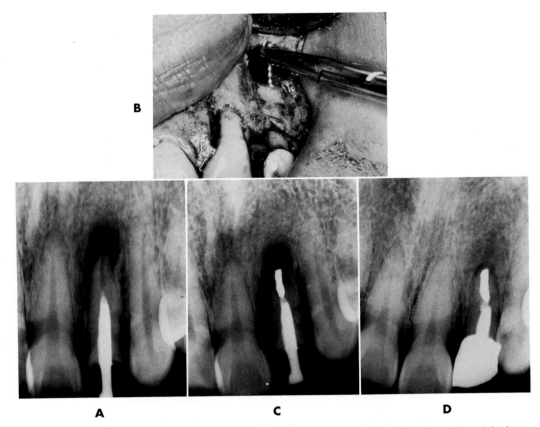

Fig. 11-52. Reverse filing and filling with amalgam. **A,** Preoperative radiograph of lateral incisor with large post, no canal filling, and a periapical radiolucency. **B,** Post could not be removed. After surgical exposure, apical portion of canal was reverse filed and reverse filled with amalgam. **C,** Postoperative view. **D,** Complete healing 1 year later. (Restoration by Dr. Sherwin Strauss, Chicago.)

ing was gained from the apex, is the situation wherein access for canal enlargement is from the apex as well. The typical case of this variety occurs when a definite but very sclerotic canal is present on a tooth requiring endodontic treatment. After attempts to uncover the canal orifice, it is determined that further exploration may lead to a perforation or to considerable gutting of the crown of the tooth or to both.

The answer is a surgical exposure of the apex of the tooth and a location of the canal from that vantage point. A 5 mm segment is cut from a small file, held in the beaks of a hemostat, and pushed into the apical foramen to widen that area (Fig. 11-51, *A* and *B*). A beveling of the apex in a manner similar to the beveling prior to reverse filling may aid in the location of the canal and the initial enlargement. Once the apical foramen has been discovered and enlarged with small files, it is no problem to file the canal serially to a desirable width.

If sufficient room exists, a regulation-length file may be inserted from the apex and forced through the canal into the lingual access opening. The case may be completed in the same manner used in the postresection filling technique (Fig. 11-51, *C* to *E*). This is quite an excellent way to complete the case because a well packed gutta-percha filling is placed and no reverse filling is needed.

If it is not possible to bring the canal into contact with the lingual opening, the entire enlargement and canal filling may be performed from the apical access (Figs. 11-52 to 11-54). Gutta-percha is used to fill the canal with any of the medium-setting sealers. Tubliseal would set too quickly and perhaps be adversely affected by any periapical moisture. The excess material is cut away with a sharp scalpel and the root face cold burnished.

In these still quite-small confines, gutta-percha cones may be difficult to manipulate. Therefore

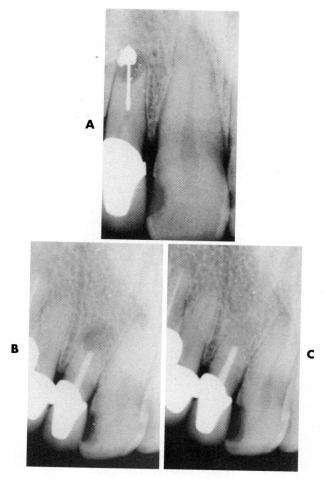

Fig. 11-53.   A, Preoperative radiograph of maxillary lateral incisor. Periapical surgery with reverse filling procedure had been performed 10 years earlier following flare-up from failing sectioned silver point treatment. There is considerable apical resorption, soreness, and swelling. The restoration was extremely esthetic, and the patient desired to keep the splint intact. Since periapical surgery had to be performed under any circumstances, it was decided to treat using reverse file and fill procedures. **B,** Accordingly, the area was flapped, the amalgam (no longer in the tooth) and the silver cone were removed, and the canal was prepared from an apical access. Filling was accomplished using lateral condensation of gutta-percha and Wach's paste. **C,** Thirty months later, a normal appearance is present. (Restorations by Dr. Ted Gordon, Chicago.)

the operator may prefer to use an apically performed preparation but reverse fill with injectable gutta-percha (Chapter 9). After making a preparation with the ultrasonic tips (Fig. 11-39), it is wise to use the no. 33½ bur to create some undercuts for the softened gutta-percha and sealer. The preparation is dried with air, aspirated with a miniature tip, and, if necessary, paper points. A suitable sealer is placed with the endodontic explorer, then any of the injectable materials inserted. Because of the problems of shrinkage, it is important to compact the softened gutta-percha with the miniature

pluggers (Fig. 11-25, A), then with the flat edge of the plastic instrument. Any excess is carefully trimmed with a scalpel (Fig. 11-54, B).

Handling of the surrounding tissues during reverse filling.   Ideally it would be wonderful if a rubber dam could be applied to the apex of a tooth and the reverse fill placed under the dry, clean conditions the dam affords. Unfortunately that method is rarely, if ever, available. An assistant's use of the miniature aspirator tip, fashioned from a cut-down 16-gauge needle, is mandatory to give completely unhindered visualization of the area.

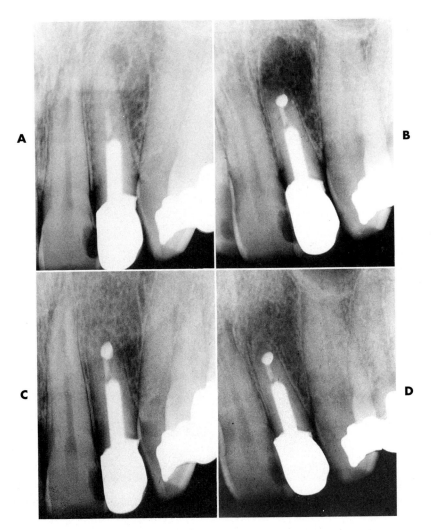

Fig. 11-54. **A,** Preoperative radiograph of maxillary lateral incisor with periapical lesion. A wide post was present that was considered to be too hazardous to remove for fear of root fracture or perforation. Therefore it was decided to treat with surgery. **B,** The surgical plan was to perform an apicoectomy to open up the apical portion of the canal, file, and then fill with condensed gutta-percha from the apex. Unfortunately the tooth had a considerable palatal inclination of the root, and I could not get files down the canal from the apical approach. Therefore I prepared the apex and filled with an injectable gutta-percha (Chapter 9) and Wach's paste. **C,** One year later. **D,** Three years after original treatment, the area has healed perfectly.

Constantly seeping blood vessels causing obstruction of view may be cauterized. The tip of a stellate plastic instrument is heated to cherry red and then placed into the area where the bleeding originates. Shreds of Horsley's bone wax, Glefoam, or Adaptic may be placed over the bone behind the root tip to aid in keeping the apex dry and preventing excess filling material from falling into the bone cavity. Cotton pellets may ade-

quately perform the same task. The use of high-concentration epinephrine should be avoided, since it may cause systemic vascular damage. Control of bleeding is better performed by the other methods mentioned.

The small aspirator tip is kept adjacent to the root tip during filling placement and condensation. Any excess material that falls from the preparation is quickly aspirated by the assistant before it adheres

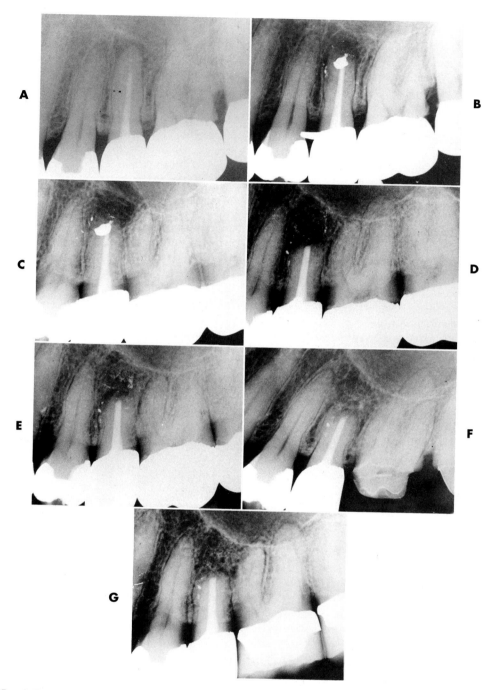

Fig. 11-55. **A,** Preoperative film of maxillary bicuspid region, poor canal filling present in second bicuspid and periapical lesion associated with the apex. I preferred conservative re-treatment, but the referring dentist convinced me merely to reverse fill. **B,** Three months after surgery, the tooth was symptomatic with soreness and mobility. I decided to refill the canal with a better laterally condensed filling. **C,** Refilling did no good; the lesion and symptoms remained. **D,** Therefore I went back in surgically, cut out the amalgam, and resected the root down to the well-condensed gutta-percha filling. **E,** One year later, healing is taking place. **F,** Two years later. **G,** Three years after initial surgery, no symptoms are present, tooth is tight, and lesion is healed radiographically. (Restorations by Dr. Lester Kaplin, Chicago.)

to the bone or adjacent tissue. Excess filling material may be trimmed and carved with the periodontal curette (Fig. 11-24, *D*). After the condensation is completed, the packing material is removed from the bony cavity. When it is known in advance that a reverse filling is to be placed in a tooth with a periapical radiolucency, the final tissue curettage of the area should be left until after the reverse filling is placed. In this way any excess filling material that eludes the aspirator and falls into the tissues will be removed when the curettage is completed.

Re-treating reverse filling failures. When confronted with failing cases with reverse amalgam fillings already in place, a number of evaluations must be made. The failure may be due to an improperly done reverse filling that might respond to nonsurgical re-treatment or correct periapical surgery. Generally an attempt at nonsurgical re-treatment is worth the effort if the canal is accessible (Fig. 11-55, *A*). A vertical root fracture may be present, in which case any attempt at retreatment will be unsuccessful. A missing root or canal may be present, which may be the cause of failure rather than the reverse filling. Such a condition may be remedied by nonsurgical re-treatment of the additional canal.

Should nonsurgical attempts meet with failure (Fig. 11-55, *C*), little has been lost because now a well-filled gutta-percha filling is in place to be reached with an apicoectomy. If sufficient root length is available, the reverse filling is cut away (Fig. 11-55, *D*) down to the site of the well-condensed gutta-percha and the periapical lesion is curetted. One hopes the area will heal in a desirable manner (Fig. 11-55, *E* to *G*).

SURGERY FOR ROOT FRACTURES

Importance of diagnosis. Diagnosis in cases involving horizontally fractured roots is most important. Some instances of root fracture require no endodontic treatment at all if the fragments remain in relatively close contact and pulp vitality is maintained. This must be verified periodically by radiographic evaluation and by thermal or electric pulp testing. If loss of vitality occurs and/or clinical symptoms develop, a chrome-cobalt alloy pin may be utilized to retain the segments if instrumentation can be carried out through the entire length of root. (See Chapter 10.)

However, if the root fractures into many splinters or if there is sufficient displacement of the segments to prevent the use of pin, surgery must be performed to retain the tooth.

Choices of surgical therapy. If surgery is necessary when the fracture occurs in the apical third of the root and sufficient root length is present, the therapy of choice is to remove the apical fragment after canal filling. On the other hand, if the root length available is insufficient or if the fracture occurs in the middle third of the root, the therapy of choice is removal of the apical fragment and placement of a chrome-cobalt pin through the prepared canal and into the tissues to restore the previous crown-root ratio.

Removing an apical fragment. Where possible, the canal should be prepared and a master gutta-percha cone obtained at the appointment prior to the surgery. On the day of surgery a typical two-step procedure is performed, with the rubber dam applied and the canal filled, using gutta-percha, Tubliseal, and a lateral condensation procedure. The patient is prepared for surgery in the routine manner and a suitable flap reflected.

The apex is uncovered, and the approximate extent of damage determined. It is important to remember that a root fracture which appears to be horizontal on a radiograph is horizontal from the mesial to distal aspect only. If seen in the proximal view, the fracture usually appears diagonal, with the lingual extent much closer to the cervical line than the labial extent (Fig. 11-56). This means that some portions of the root to be retained or the periapical bone will require removal to deliver the apical fragment. Unless there are vital structures in proximity, it is better to remove periapical bone that will fill in postoperatively and thus retain whatever root length is available. The bone on the lateral sides of the root also must be removed. The root tip may be removed with a spoon excavator or with surgical root picks.

A fissure bur is used to smooth the face of the remaining root portion. The canal filling is tested for apical seal and a reverse filling placed if necessary. A radiograph is taken, and if satisfactory, the flap is closed (Fig. 11-57).

Placing a chrome-cobalt alloy pin. Placing a pin is carried out in a manner similar to the postresection filling technique. Canal preparation may be performed at an appointment before the surgery, a minimal width of size 100 should be obtained. After routine surgical preparation, the apical portion of the root is exposed and the area examined. The apical fragments are removed using care to apply the knowledge that the fracture may be diagonal toward the lingual surface.

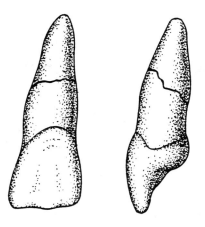

Fig. 11-56. From the labial view, as seen on typical radiograph *(left),* fracture site appears to be horizontal. If area could be visualized from proximal aspect *(as at right),* fracture usually would be seen to take a diagonal course through root that is close to gingival margin on lingual side.

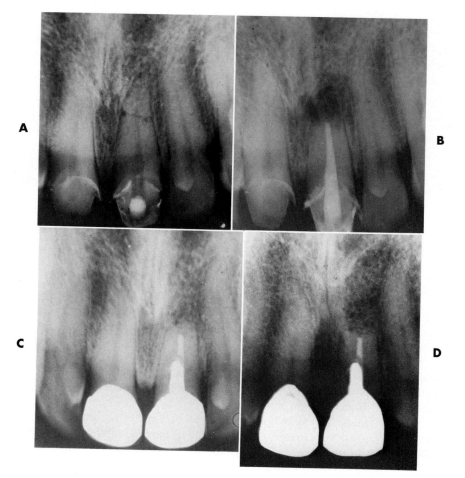

Fig. 11-57. **A,** Central incisor with root fractured in middle third and chronic draining sinus tract. Both segments could not be instrumented. **B,** Canal was filled to fracture line with gutta-percha, followed by surgical removal of apical segment. **C,** Seven years later, central incisors are restored but not splinted. Tooth operated on is firm and asymptomatic. **D,** Eighteen years after original treatment. (Restorations by Dr. Harold Laswell, Lexington, Ky.)

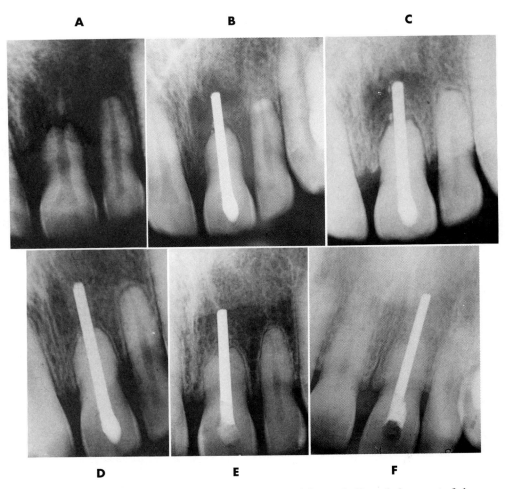

Fig. 11-58.   Treatment of root fracture by removing fractured tip surgically and placement of chrome-cobalt pin. **A,** Preoperative view of maxillary central incisor, indicating root tip separation, history of orthodontic movement. The tooth was mobile and sore to palpation near the apex. **B,** Immediate post-surgical film, apical segment has been removed and a chrome-cobalt pin has been placed to seal the apex and extend the root length. Note some excess sealer to the mesial of the pin. **C,** Three months after surgery, tooth is tightening. **D,** One year after surgery, the periapical bone has healed, and the tooth is firm and comfortable. **E,** Nine years after original treatment, tooth continues to do well. **F,** Nineteen years after original treatment, tooth looks excellent, is firm and comfortable. (Surgery by Dr. Alfred L. Frank, formerly of Los Angeles, Calif.)

A chrome-cobalt alloy pin is selected one size smaller than the largest instrument used and is placed through the opened lingual access cavity. Apically, the pin should reach the approximate position of the previously present root apex while still binding within the confines of the canal. If the pin binds prematurely within the canal and does not reach the desired length, the width of the canal is increased by using a larger file. If the pin reaches the desired length but does not bind within the canal, apical segments are removed from the pin until binding occurs.

The pin must not contact the bone in the periapical region, but a slight gap should be present between the two. If the pin butts against the bone, it may be prevented from gaining the desired degree of binding within the canal. It is important for the pin to bind within the canal and for it to be the binding rather than the periapical bone that prevents the pin from going any farther apically.

After the necessary adjustments are made to obtain the desired length and width of the pin, preparation for a procedure similar to a silver point twist-off is carried out. A no. 37 inverted

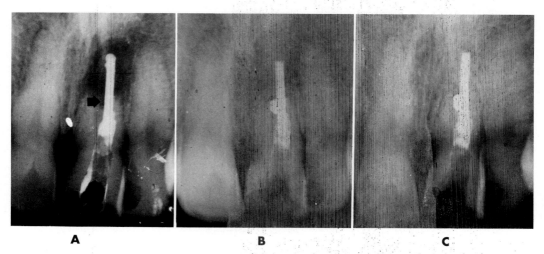

A **B** **C**

Fig. 11-59. **A,** Case similar to that in Fig. 11-58. However, when the pin as placed, a considerable open area around canal *(arrow)* was noticed and required reverse filling. **B,** Eighteen months postoperatively, tooth is firm without splinting. **C,** Seven years after treatment, tooth is firm and has healed perfectly. (Restoration by Dr. Joseph Krohn, Chicago.)

cone bur is used to weaken circumferentially the pin at the desired point of separation. This point should be well within the confines of the canal but be slightly short of reaching the cervical line. The pin may be weakened so greatly that only a thin sliver attaches the two segments. The metal used is strong and, since the width of the pin is much wider than the normal size of silver point, considerable apical pressure is still available.

Grossman's formula is used as the root canal sealer of choice. The canal is irrigated with 95% alcohol and dried with paper points. The sealer is mixed to a heavy but creamy consistency and applied to the canal walls with a reamer rotated counterclockwise. The portion of the pin that will remain within the canal is coated with sealer and placed into the canal with firm apical pressure. When the binding is obtained within the canal, the segment of pin protruding through the access opening is twisted, leaving the remaining portion within the canal and extending the correct length past the root (Fig. 11-58). The sealing of the canal is examined with the endodontic explorer. If a small void exists, the area may be packed with a mixture of zinc oxide and eugenol. If a large void is present, a preparation is made with a no. 33½ bur to include the full extent of the void and some surrounding solid dentin and is filled with amalgam for closure. A suitable temporary filling is placed, and the surgical site is closed (Fig. 11-59).

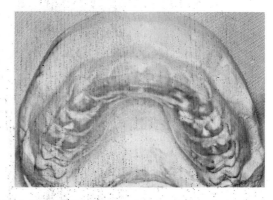

Fig. 11-60. During first few weeks after surgery, use of an acrylic overlay splint will aid in initial stabilization. Such an appliance may be removed for eating and for maintenance of oral hygiene.

It is hoped that the healing will allow new bone to conglomerate around the pin and stabilize the tooth. During the initial healing period, a splint may be utilized if more than minimal mobility is present postoperatively. Such a splint may be fabricated with acrylic, orthodontic wire, or orthodontic bands (Fig. 11-60).

USE OF THE OPERATING MICROSCOPE

Although used in medical surgery for a number of years, the surgical operating microscope (SOM) has been introduced into endodontics only recently. The use of loupes and magnifying glasses (2.5× to 5×) has been common among dentists for many years, particularly for those practicing fixed prosthodontics and surgery. But the SOM (Fig. 11-61), giving magnification of 25× and greater, has initiated a "new age" of surgical endodontics, providing the ability to perform procedures at a much higher level because of the vision and light imparted.

In addition to allowing us to do surgery better, the microscope has given us the ability to take photos of high quality and magnification for use in presenta-

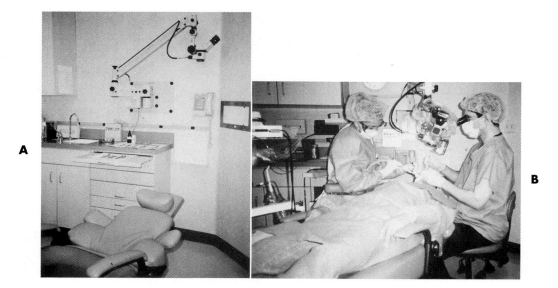

Fig. 11-61. **A,** Surgical operating microscope (SOM), by Urban Microscope, St. Louis, MO 63122, hanging on the wall. **B,** SOM being used during surgery. Dentist *(right)* and assistant *(left)* treating maxillary bicuspid (see Fig. 11-62). Draped patient is lying flat, operator's arms are comfortable as he looks through the microscope, and he is in a normal position relative to the patient. With magnifying glasses, usually the dentist must bend over to see the patient. This SOM has lens for operator only; some have set for the assistant, as well.

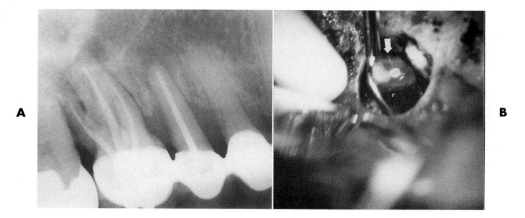

Fig. 11-62. Location of a fracture with the SOM. **A,** Preoperative radiography of maxillary posterior area. Endodontic treatment looks acceptable (perhaps, filling is a bit short), but a large periapical lesion is present and apical area is tender to palpation. **B,** Flap was raised, lesion curetted, and apex beveled. A crack is apparent *(arrow),* going from buccal to lingual. The tooth was extracted.

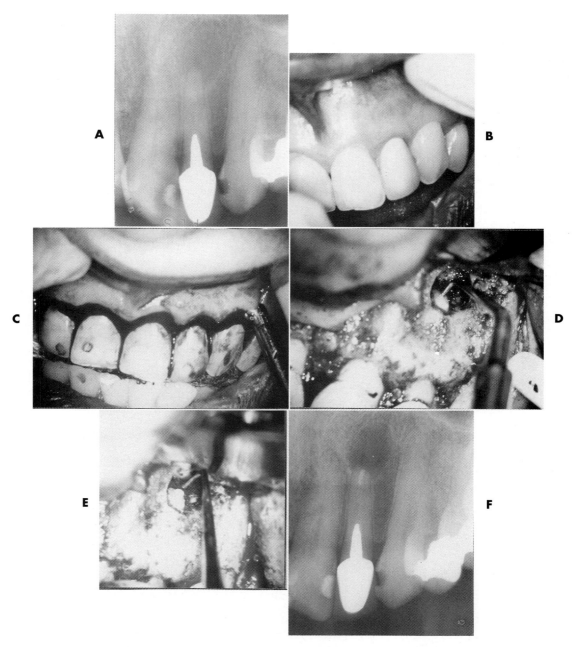

Fig. 11-63. Apicoectomy and reverse filling, using SOM. **A,** Preoperative radiograph of maxillary anterior area. Lateral incisor is restored with cast post-and-core porcelain crown. Removal for nonsurgical re-treatment would be very hazardous. **B,** Preoperative view of area, indicating esthetic restoration. **C,** Flap incision. **D,** Ultrasonic tip making reverse fill preparation. **E,** Packing apical preparation with SuperEBA. **F,** Postoperative radiograph. (Views through SOM, approximately 20×.)

tions and articles as well as providing us with documentation for referring dentists, insurance companies, dento-legal purposes, and patient education.

There can be no question that, for the most part, one can do better when one can see more and better. This is particularly significant in surgical procedures. Endodontics is one of the specific areas where magnification is so important, because of the small size of root tips (2 to 5 mm across, depending at the level of cutting) and canal fillings (.25 to 1 mm in diameter, at the widest) and the inherent darkness of the oral cavity.

Some common problems that have always bothered endodontic surgeons that are easily addressed when operating with a SOM are the following:

1. Should a reverse filling be placed, or is the existing filling sealed? (This is a very important question to clarify because of the less favorable prognosis of reverse fills.)
2. In mesial roots of mandibular molars and mesiobuccal roots of maxillary molars, is there a septum between the two major canals that should be addressed?
3. Is that line I see a fracture (Fig. 11-62)?
4. Is there an additional canal? (Common in many roots, particularly mesiobuccal of maxillary molars, mandibular incisors and first bicuspids, maxillary bicuspids.)
5. In evaluating a failing treatment, why has the therapy failed and what can I do to avoid another failure?
6. Should I take another radiograph to ensure that I have exposed the root? removed all excess filling material? kept my preparation within the root?

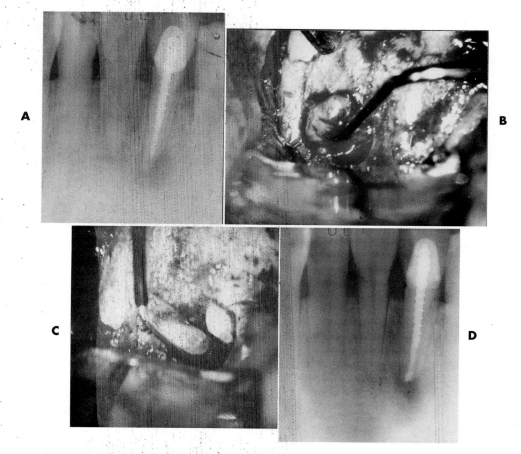

Fig. 11-64. **A,** Preoperative radiograph of mandibular incisor area, indicating lateral incisor with failing endodontic treatment. This tooth has a screw post and porcelain crown, hazardous materials to remove. **B,** Curettage of lesion. **C,** Miniature surgical mirror shows preparation for reverse filling made ultrasonic tips. **D,** Postoperative radiograph. (Views through SOM, approximately 20×.)

have sufficient bevel?, and many other similar questions (Figs. 11-63 and 11-64).

In addition to the help afforded in these cases, those using the SOM report less fatigue during surgery and increased enjoyment while performing it, even in such difficult cases as mandibular molars and bicuspids and palatal roots of maxillary teeth.

In view of all of the positive aspects of the SOM, it is difficult to present any arguments against it. However, I do wish to make some comments that may be construed as negative. In the initial portion of this chapter, I clearly stated all of the many types of endodontic problems that used to be treated surgically could now be treated without surgery. I tried to emphasize that we should always attempt nonsurgical treatment, particularly when treating failing cases, before we resorted to surgery, even in those instances when it seemed likely that surgery would probably be necessary. One major reason for the rise in stature of endodontic treatment among both practitioners and patients has been the minimal degree of pain both during treatment and post-operatively. Being able to avoid surgery in virtually every case has enabled us to reach this admirable goal.

There is no question that the SOM makes surgery easier and better. Financial investment in the equipment is considerable. It is very easy to guide the patient into surgical treatment rather than take the usually longer, not always successful, and generally less remunerative nonsurgical direction. We must avoid this pitfall.

Generally, it is in the best interests of the patient to attempt nonsurgical treatment or re-treatment. We should always cater to the patient's best interest above our own.

SUTURING

Adequate well placed sutures will aid in the healing process. Improper, insufficient, poorly placed sutures will diminish the rate of healing and may lead to uncomfortable or unesthetic scar or keloid formation. For placing sutures in the most desirable manner, the following suggestions are made.

1. *Digitally press the flap before suturing.* After the surgery is completed, the flap is returned to its original position, and firm but not overly forceful digital pressure is applied for 3 full minutes. This allows the fibrin network to begin its formation so that an adherence develops between the raised and underlying tissues.

2. *Never be skimpy with sutures.* The function of a suture is to keep the edges of the flap in contact during the period immediately after the surgery. In this way the tissues attach across the lines of incision, and optimal healing is gained. If the tissues are not apposed, granulation tissue will grow in, which is most undesirable. Also, the sutures prevent the underlying bone from being exposed to the oral environment and thereby lessen postoperative pain.

In order for these objectives to be accomplished, enough sutures must be placed to keep the edges of the flap in apposition. It is almost impossible to place too many sutures, and it is much better to err on the side of too many than too few. If any question arises as to the need for additional sutures after the surgeon observes the initially sutured flap, the answer is to place more.

3. *Take deep bites with the needle into the tissue.* Placing the sutures close to the incision lines may cause problems. It is difficult to avoid placing the knots over the lines of incision, and when the sutures are tightened, one side or the other may pull through the tissue. The answer is to take deep bites with the needle far enough from the lines of incision.

4. *Do not pull the stitches too tightly.* When deep bites are taken to place each suture, care must be exercised in tying the knot so that the edges are brought just into contact with each other and that no further tightening is allowed. There is room to tighten more, but this will cause a bunching of the edges and may lead to decreased blood circulation in the area.

5. *Avoid placing the knots over the lines of incision.* The knots of each stitch should be placed close to either of the puncture sites in the tissue rather than in the center. Leaving the knot in the center will place it right over the line of incision. The bulk of the knot, when pushed by the lip or cheek, will cause additional irritation and delay healing in the already inflamed areas.

If possible, the most desirable position for the knot is over the puncture site on the nonraised side of the incision, which is the most normal segment. If, after the suture is tied, it is noticed that the knot is over the line of incision, it can be moved easily. The knot is grasped by the teeth of the miniature

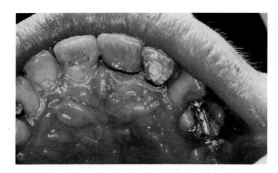

Fig. 11-65. Circumferential suture ties for surgery on a lateral incisor. Labial views are seen in Fig. 11-19, *A* and *B*.

hemostat and gently pulled toward the unflapped segment.

6. *Do not leave sutures in place for too long.* Individuals heal with different speeds, and it is impossible to predict with any accuracy the rate in a particular case. However, leaving sutures in place for too long always causes a local inflammation and may lead to overgrowth of tissue, embedding the thread. Therefore 5 days after the operation seems to be the average and thus ideal time to remove sutures, with the maximum being 7 days postoperatively.

7. *Be sure to schedule a suture removal appointment.* As ridiculous as it seems, in the exhilaration of a job well done, the surgeon may forget to schedule an appointment for suture removal at 5 to 7 days after surgery. Many patients have had resorbable sutures used in other surgical procedures and are not aware that the same type is not used in dentistry. Some weeks later the patient may call to complain of irritation in the area of the surgery, and an embedded suture is discovered, much to the chagrin of the surgeon. Similarly, the number of sutures placed must always be recorded on the patient's chart so the surgeon can be certain that no stitches have been left behind.

8. *Choose the type of suture material.* Many companies market packaged disposable presterilized suture material. There are a myriad of varying choices in thickness and type of material to replace the formerly used gut or silk material. Polyester fibers are woven and treated with a chemical that prevents oral fluids, bacteria, and other contaminants from being absorbed by the thread. It appears that

this foreign matter that accumulates within the suture material causes the local inflammatory response frequently noted. Suture material is also produced in a monofilament but is more difficult to tie. Both new materials, being so smooth, require the placing of three square knot ties to prevent unraveling.

Knots are no longer needed to attach the thread to the metal, but atraumatic needles are available so that a much smaller puncture hole is made. Individual packages are kept ready for the surgical procedure. When needed, the material is removed from its outer wrapper and dropped onto the surgical tray.

9. *Use a circumferential tie.* For use with vertical flaps, the circumferential tie, so named because of its similarity to the circumferential periodontal ligament fibers, is valuable. After the vertical incisions are sutured, the circumferential tie is used to bring the scalloped gingival margin to place (Fig. 11-65).

Assuming the most common condition of periapical surgery on a single tooth with one tooth on either side included in the flap, the circumferential tie is placed around the middle tooth. The surgeon inserts the needle approximately 3 mm apical to the gingival margin of the raised papilla on one side of the tooth and penetrates the tissue (Fig. 11-66, *C*). The thread is brought through the tissue to the inner surface of the flap, with a small tail remaining outside the flap. It is passed through the contact point in the manner for using dental floss (Fig. 11-66, *D*), looped around the lingual or palatal surface of the tooth, and brought through the other contact point (Fig. 11-66, *E*). No engagement of tissue occurs during this looping procedure. The needle is placed beneath the flap approximately 3 mm apically from the gingival margin of the raised papilla, pushed through the labial margin (Fig. 11-66, *F*), and the suture material is brought through. No further penetration of tissue will be needed to complete the tie. The thread is retraced through the closest contact point again (Fig. 11-66, *G*), looped around the lingual or palatal surface of the tooth, and brought through the other contact point (Fig. 11-66, *H*). The tie is completed by knotting this segment of thread to the tail of the suture that had remained from the first tissue penetration (Fig. 11-66, *I*).

It is remarkable how well the circumferential tie pulls the retracted tissue tightly around the gingival margins of the flapped teeth and leads to desirable healing. If the flap is very wide or if more

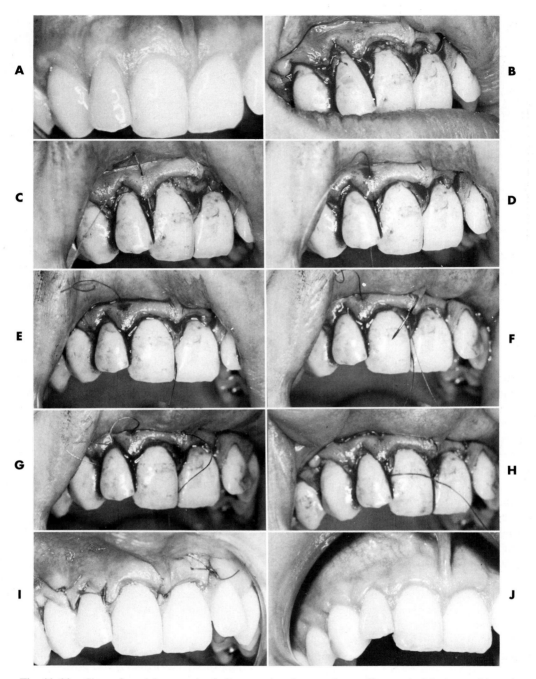

Fig. 11-66.   Circumferential suture tie. **A,** Preoperative photograph, maxillary central incisor and lateral incisor to have periapical surgery. **B,** After surgery, vertical incisions at distal of adjacent cuspid and distal of other central incisor are sutured. Gingival margins are free. **C,** Needle is inserted into papilla between lateral and central incisors approximately 3 mm apical to gingival margin and brought through to inner surface of flap. **D,** In the manner of using dental floss, suture material is brought through adjacent contact point to lingual surface. **E,** Thread is looped around lingual surface of central incisor and brought through mesial contact point to labial surface. **F,** Needle is placed from beneath flap into papilla approximately 3 mm apical to gingival margin. **G,** Suture material is brought back through between contact point of central incisors to lingual surface. **H,** Thread is looped around lingual surface and brought back through contact point between central and lateral incisors to labial surface. **I,** Three square knots complete the tie at original site of tissue penetration. **J,** Two weeks after surgery, tissue healing is quite advanced.

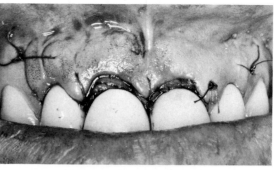

Fig. 11-67. **A,** Periapical surgery was performed on both maxillary central incisors. Because veneer crowns were to be remade, horizontal incision was placed in gingival sulcus. **B,** Circumferential tie was placed around both teeth with only three tissue penetrations. Initial needle insertion was in papilla to distal of the central incisor on right to the underside of flap, with the thread looped around lingual surface and penetration between the central incisors, looped around lingual surface, and the third and final penetration to distal of the central incisor on left. Suture material is passed back around lingual surface, interlaced under the suture between central incisors, passed around lingual surface again, and tied at the initial site of penetration.

than two teeth are central in the flap, more than one tooth may be involved in this type of suture or the circumferential ties may be interlaced for reciprocal retention with minimal tissue penetrations (Fig. 11-67).

This type of tie is so valuable because it does not involve penetration of the palatal tissues when maxillary teeth are treated. Because the palatal tissue is much more friable than the labial tissue, suture thread frequently tears through, causing blood seepage and lack of adaptation of the labial tissue to the underlying bone. In addition, since the thread in the circumferential tie remains snug on the lingual or palatal surface of the tied tooth, there is much less protruding to bother the patient's tongue and cause the constant manipulation that might cause displacement or loss of the suture.

POSTOPERATIVE INSTRUCTIONS

Printed postoperative instructions should be available and given to the patient after completion of the surgical procedure. Oral instructions may be forgotten or misunderstood, whereas the printed material is taken home and easily followed. After giving the patient the printed instructions, the surgeon should take a few minutes to go through the pertinent points with the patient. Even so, this method takes much less of the surgeon's time than does the recitation of oral instructions.

The following is an example of typical instructions to be given a patient. Similar sheets may be printed, mimeographed, or photocopied, with any desired additions or modifications that the surgeon wishes.

1. After leaving the office, go directly home.
2. Apply an ice bag, 10 minutes on, 20 minutes off, during the remainder of the day.
3. Do not lift your lip to examine the stitches. This may cause tearing of the tissues.
4. Brush your teeth in the normal manner, but be particularly careful near the area that has been surgically treated.
5. Tomorrow, rinse your mouth with mouthwash solution composed of ½ glass mouth wash to ½ glass warm water. Try to do this for 5 minutes every hour, if possible.

REFERENCES

Arens DE, Adams WR, DeCastro RA: *Endodontics surgery,* Philadelphia, 1981, Harper & Row, Publishers,Inc.

Beltes P, Zervas P, Lambrianidis T, Molyvdas I: In vitro study of the sealing ability of four retrograde filling materials, *Endod Dent Traumatol* 4:82, 1988.

Bhaskar SN: Diagnosis and treatment of common apical lesions, *Northwest Dent* 47:311, 1968.

Block RM, Bushnell A, Grossman LI, Langeland K: Endodontic surgical treatment—a clinical and histopathologic study, *J Endod* 5:101, 1979.

Chivian N: Surgical endodontics: a conservative approach, *JNJ Dent Soc* 40:234, 1969.

Dorn SO, Gartner AH: Retrograde filling materials: a retrospective success-failure study of amalgam, EBA, and IRM, *J Endod* 16:391, 1990.

Dorn SO, Gartner AH: Advances in endodontic surgery, *Dent Clin North Amer* 36:357, 1992.

Feldman M, Feldman G: Endodontic stabilizers, *J Endod* 18:245, 1992.

Finne K, Nord PG, Persson G, Lennartson B: Retrograde root filling with amalgam and cavit, *Oral Surg* 43:621, 1977.

Flath RK, Hicks ML: Retrograde instrumentation and obturation with new devices, *J Endod* 13:546, 1987.

Frank AL: Improvements of the crown root ratio by endodontic endosseous implants, *J Am Dent Assoc* 74:451, 1967.

Frank AL, Glick DH, Patterson SS, Weine FS: Long-term evaluation of surgically placed amalgam fillings, *J Endod* 18:391, 1992.

Friedman HI, Gerstein H: Effective endodontic suction apparatus, *J Endod* 5:371, 1979.

Friedman S: Retrograde approaches in endodontic therapy, *Endod Dent Traumatol* 7:97, 1991.

Garber FN: Surgical vs. non-surgical management of endodontic problems, *J Mich Dent Assoc* 46:246, 1964.

Grimes EW: A use of freeze-dried bone in endodontics, *J Endod* 20:355, 1994.

Grung B, Molven O, Halse A: Periapical surgery in a Norwegian county hospital: follow-up of 477 teeth, *J Endod* 16:411, 1990.

Gutmann J, Harrison JW: Posterior endodontic surgery: anatomical considerations and clinical techniques, *Int Endod J* 18:8, 1985.

Lalone ER, Luebke RG: The frequency and distribution of periapical cysts and granulomas, *Oral Surg* 25:861, 1968.

Luebke RG, Glick DH, Ingle JI: Indications and contraindications for endodontic surgery, *Oral Surg* 18:97, 1964.

Luks S: Root-end amalgam technic in the practice of endodontics, *J Am Dent Assoc* 53:424, 1956.

Madison S, Bjorndal AM: Clinical application of endodontic implants, *J Prosth Dent* 59:603, 1988.

Marshall FJ, Lane D, Domokos A: Endodontics surgery: criteria, indications, and procedures, *J Can Dent Assoc* 30:703, 1964.

Matsura SJ: A simplified root-end filling technic using silver amalgam, *J Mich Dent Assoc* 44:40, 1962.

Maxmen HA: The expanding scope of endodontics, *J Mich Dent Assoc* 41:125, 1959.

Moodnick RM, Levey MH, Bensen MA, Bordon BG: Retrograde amalgam filling: a scanning electron microscopic study, *J Endod* 1:28, 1975.

Olson AK, MacPherson MG, Hartwell GR, Weller RN, Kulild JC: An in vitro evaluation of injectable thermoplasticized gutta-percha, glass ionomer, and amalgam when used as retrofilling materials, *J Endod* 16:361, 1990.

Oynick J, Oynick T: A study of a new material for retrograde fillings, *J Endod* 4:203, 1978.

Patterson SS, Shafer WG, Healey HJ: Periapical lesions associated with endodontically treated teeth, *J Am Dent Assoc* 68:191, 1964.

Pissiotis E, Sapounas G, Spangberg LSW: Silver glass ionomer cement as a retrograde filling material: a study in vitro, *J Endod* 17:225, 1991.

Rossman LE: Endodontic surgery in posterior teeth—its role in maintaining arch integrity, *Compend Contin Educ Dent* 13:630, 1992.

Rubinstein R: New horizons in endodontic surgery, *Compend Contin Educ Dent,* accepted for publication.

Schlagel E, Seltzer RJ, Newman JI: Apicoectomy as an adjunct to diagnosis, *NY State Dent J* 39:156, 1973.

Simon JHS: Incidence of periapical cysts in relation to the root canals, *J Endod* 6:845, 1980.

Tanzilli JP, Raphael D, Moodnick RM: A comparison of the marginal adaptation of retrograde techniques: a scanning electron microscopic study, *Oral Surg* 50:74, 1980.

Tronstad L, Trope M, Doering A, Hasselgren G: Sealing ability of dental amalgams as retrograde fillings in endodontic therapy, *J Endod* 9:551, 1983.

Wais FT: Significance of findings following biopsy and histologic study of 100 periapical lesions, *Oral Surg* 11:650, 1958.

Weine FS: Preparación y obturación retrograda: un solucion ante problemas quirúgicos periapicales, *Rev Esp Endod* 2:69, 1984.

Weine FS, Frank AL: Survival of the endodontic endosseous implant, *J Endod* 19:524, 1993.

Weine FS, Healey HJ, Gerstein H, Evanson L: Canal configuration in the mesiobuccal root of the maxillary first molar and its endodontic significance, *Oral Surg* 28:419, 1969.

Weine FS, Patterson SS, Healey HJ: The effectiveness of phenol in endodontic immediate disinfection, *J Am Dent Assoc* 73:116, 1966.

12 Root amputations

Root amputation refers to the removal of one or more roots of a multirooted tooth while other roots are retained. Such procedures usually are more complicated than merely the extraction of the entire tooth. Therefore it might appear to be radical and complex at initial consideration, but often such is not the case. Grossman has referred to root amputation as dental proof of the old adage that half a loaf is better than none. I would like to amend the statement that with root amputation, half a loaf *may be* better than none. Unfortunately, I have seen some cases (Fig. 12-1) where great time, effort, and expense were invested, but wasted because aspects of treatment were not thought out or carried out properly.

Early in the 1960s, therapy involving root amputation was right on the cutting edge in both periodontics and endodontics. Classic papers by Hiatt and by Amen listed the indications and described the techniques for these procedures. Because of these and other reports, teeth were saved that, in similar situations, would have been thought to be hopeless and would never have been even considered for treatment. In reality, almost the exact same methods had been suggested by Black in the nineteenth century and also described by Sharp in the 1920s.

With improvement of techniques and materials in both periodontics and endodontics leading to more sophisticated therapy, marginal teeth increased in value to retain arch integrity. If only two-thirds or even one-half of a tooth was salvageable, its retention might add sufficient support to keep adjacent members of the arch. Also, since root amputations almost always involved molar teeth, and frequently the most posterior abutment or an aid to the posterior abutment, retaining even half a tooth could avoid the need for a removable prosthesis and enable the patient to use fixed replacement or a splint.

However, as with any valuable tool, root amputations have at times been performed incorrectly or in situations where they were not indicated. Patients were assured that if they accepted this form of treatment the involved tooth could be retained for a long time. Despite time-consuming and expensive therapy, certain types of failures began to crop up. Articles were written describing disaster cases, and some excellent practitioners even eliminated such treatment from their choices of therapy.

Causes of failure. Each of the molar teeth possesses a specific reason why root amputation procedures may fail, even assuming that the indications and treatment are correct. In the maxillary first molar, amputation of the distobuccal root has, by far, the most favorable outlook. The distobuccal root occupies much less area in the furcation than do the other two roots. The natural curvatures of the mesiobuccal and palatal roots will give resistance to all directions of stress without the distobuccal root. For this reason, the tooth need not be splinted to adjacent teeth—a fact not true in any other molar amputation. And, finally, the procedure is the easiest to perform among maxillary molar amputation procedures.

The long-term prognosis for distobuccal root amputation in the maxillary first molar is very favorable. My best cases, across many years, have been in this area. Fig. 12-2 demonstrates a maxillary first molar requiring a distobuccal root amputation. The endodontic, periodontal, and restorative phases of treatment were all performed properly, except that the palatal root was filed and filled incorrectly, causing a significant overextension of gutta-percha. As the years have passed, the gutta-percha has been gradually resorbed. In the 10-year postoperative film (Fig. 12-2, *C*), only a speck of gutta-percha remains, attesting to the considerable passage of time. Eighteen years after

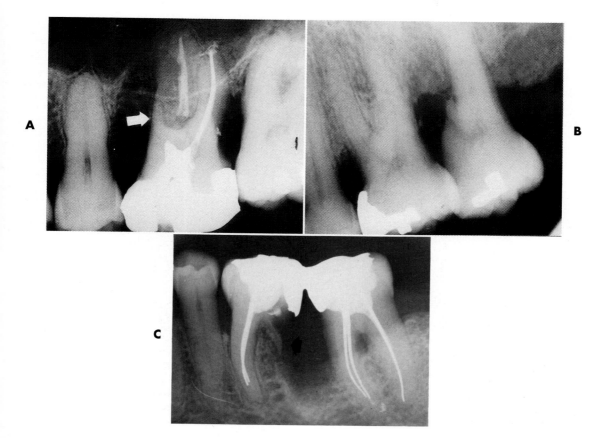

Fig. 12-1. **A,** Radiograph of maxillary first molar following amputation of mesiobuccal root. Canal filling was performed properly, but amputation procedure to eliminate pocket associated with mesiobuccal root is poorly done. Spike *(arrow)* of mesiobuccal root remaining is palatal portion because surgeon did not realize how wide buccolingually the root was. Now the periodontal problem is perpetuated instead of being eliminated. **B,** In this mesiobuccal root amputation on a maxillary second molar, the root was removed without any endodontic procedure being performed. The patient experienced severe pain and required emergency treatment of pulpal extirpation. **C,** In the mandibular first molar, a furcation problem was present, mainly associated with the distal root. An improper diagonal cut was used, leaving a spike *(arrow)* in the furcation area, making the chance of failure quite high despite an immense cost to the patient.

treatment (Fig. 12-2, *D*) no gutta-percha is left in the periapical tissue. This radiograph, demonstrating the time required for the body to remove the excess filling material, verifies that the course of treatment was correct and the tooth remains as an integral part of the dental arch.

Fig. 12-12 also described a very successful, long-term follow-up on a similar case.

Mesiobuccal and palatal amputations do not have anywhere near the long-term success enjoyed by the distobuccal removals. Both of these roots are quite large with retentive curvatures. Errors in surgery occur with palatal root amputations because the oper-

ators often think that the root is larger than it truly is. Conversely, surgical errors occur with mesiobuccal root amputations because the operators often think the root is smaller than it truly is. If either of these roots is removed, splinting to one or more adjacent teeth is mandatory. The restoration when either root is removed is very complex because of the shape of the remaining root in the furcation (Fig. 12-17, *F*).

Maxillary second molars have furcations at higher levels, roots closer together, and more differences in size and shape than do first molars. None of these situations bode well for amputations in the more posterior tooth.

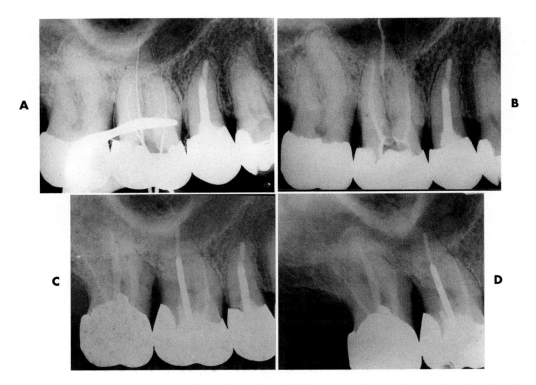

Fig. 12-2. **A,** Radiograph of maxillary first molar, with files in place for calculation of working lengths. Note extensive bone loss associated with the distobuccal root that will probably require an amputation of that root during the periodontal surgery that will follow the completion of the endodontics. **B,** Radiograph taken after filling the canals with laterally condensed gutta-percha and Wach's paste. Unfortunately, there has been a considerable overextension of gutta-percha beyond the apex of the palatal root. The distobuccal root amputation was performed a short time later. **C,** Ten years later, the area looks excellent. The first molar, without the distobuccal root, is functioning well and merely a speck of gutta-percha can be seen associated with the palatal root. The second molar also required endodontic treatment. **D,** Eighteen years after original treatment, both molars functioning well, and no gutta-percha can be seen periapically. Loss of the distobuccal root has not appreciably effected the longevity of the first molar. Restorations have been well contoured to allow for excellent home care. (Restoration by Dr. Richard Lamermayer, Kenilworth, Ill., and periodontal treatment by Dr. Harry Staffileno, Chicago.)

As to mandibular first molars, for may years few operators realized that the mesial root was larger, with deeper depressions and, hence, more retention than the distal root. If it could be saved, the mesial root could be vary valuable (Figs. 12-28 and 12-29). However, the mesial root was more difficult to treat endodontically, and periapical failures occurred. The root was difficult to restore, particularly when a post-and-core was placed. The distal root was easier to treat endodontically and restore, but it was much less retentive.

With maxillary second molars, again there were many more variants than for first molars, the furcation was further from the gingival line, and

the root apices were usually closer—all complications or outright contraindications to successful amputations.

Alternatives in periodontal therapy. The final blow to the selection of root amputation as the correct course of treatment has been the rather recent and quite successful periodontal procedure of guided tissue regeneration (GTR). Because it is a relatively new procedure, the long-term benefits have not yet been clearly analyzed. However, at this time, the procedure seems to have a multiplicity of advantages over root amputation. The types of cases that were most remarkably treated with root amputation were those with through-and through furcation involvement in both maxillary and mandibular molars. Root amputation did not fill in or grant healed bone. It simply allowed the patient the opportunity and access to keep the defect relatively clean. With GTR, the bone will fill in without any roots being removed and, if successful, the support of the roots remaining is much greater.

Also, GTR does not, in itself, require endodontic treatment, although a significant number of endodontists and some periodontists believe that the more serious defects are accompanied by pulpal degeneration and would profit by concomitant endodontic therapy.

This chapter will explain the advantages and disadvantages of root amputation, illustrate the correct uses and techniques for its use, and emphasize the limitations of the procedure.

INDICATIONS AND CONTRAINDICATIONS

Cautions to observe before starting amputation procedures. The techniques involved in root amputation in themselves are not terribly complex, particularly when a severe periodontal defect is present. In many cases the surgical procedure is well within the technical ability of most general practitioners. The greatest number of failures must be attributed to the inability of the dentist to restore the altered tooth form correctly or, in the absence of sufficient supporting structures, to retain the remaining portion of the tooth. Therefore, before any indications for root amputation are considered, it must be ascertained that these two more important considerations can be satisfied.

Root amputations are usually performed for reasons in one of two general categories. Either a severe periodontal defect is present or an endodontic or restorative problem is involved. Once it is determined that an indication for amputation is present, a careful evaluation must be made of the tooth segment that is to remain before any surgical procedures are performed.

Sufficient support available for the segment to be retained. When the indication for root amputation is a hopeless periodontal defect on one root, careful periodontal evaluation must be made of the segment that is to be retained.

Furcation involvements that require amputation do not always limit themselves to the surface of one root but often destroy the bony septum of the adjacent root as well. When one root is amputated, the neighboring retained root may still have a hopeless periodontal condition. This condition is found in mandibular molars with severe furcation involvement. Regardless of which root is amputated, the retained root may still have a severe periodontal lesion or insufficient bony support on the surface that had been adjacent to the furcation. This is particularly likely when the roots have little spread and thus minimal bone between them.

In any mouth in which periodontal disease is severe enough to require a root amputation, it is rare for the retained root to have little or no bone loss itself. That some periodontal therapy will be required is assumed. However, enough root must be available for use as an abutment. Therefore, before a root is retained, the existence of a satisfactory periodontal result and adequate crown-root ratio must be assured.

Proper restoration of retained segment practical. Another indication for root amputation is severe tooth destruction, often due to furcation caries. In these cases the retained segment must be restorable or else the entire procedure is doomed (Fig. 12-3).

In any amputation case a meticulous method of restoration must be followed. Step-by-step procedures for restoring various types of amputations will be found in Chapter 17. However, in general terms, after root amputation some type of post or coronal-root stabilization must be used, followed by a core that covers the entire root face. In most instances the remaining segment is not restored as a single unit, but rather splinted directly or by use of a pontic to one or more adjacent teeth.

If this regimen of post, core, crown, and probably splint is not practical or possible, the root amputation should not be performed. In certain cases the prognosis after amputation may be questionable, and the dentist is reluctant to place a complex prosthesis until the outcome is more certain. With this in mind, a temporary prosthesis may be fabricated but should be replaced by the more desirable restorative method when success is gained.

Periodontal indications for root amputation. The use of root amputation to retain teeth with serious periodontal involvements is indicated in the following conditions:

1. Severe vertical bone loss involving only one root of a multirooted tooth (see Fig. 12-12)
2. Through-and-through furcation destruction that may not be corrected by GTR or similar periodontal surgery

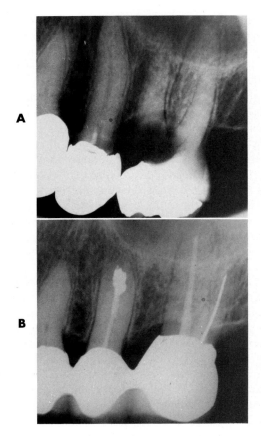

Fig. 12-3. A, Severe caries in furcation prevented maxillary molar from being restorable. **B,** However, once mesiobuccal root was amputated, a restorable two-rooted tooth was produced that preserved natural dentition of this segment of the arch and avoided need for a removable prosthesis. Radiograph taken 2 years after treatment. (Restorations by Dr. Stanley Martin, formerly of Chicago.)

3. Unfavorable proximity of roots of adjacent teeth, preventing adequate hygiene in maintenance of proximal areas
4. Severe root exposure due to dehiscence (Fig. 12-4)

Endodontic and restorative indications for root amputation. Although most root amputations are performed for periodontal reasons, there are many indications for amputations due to endodontic and restorative consequences. Among these are the following:

1. *Prosthetic failure of piers or abutments within a splint.* This indication may involve single-rooted or multirooted teeth and may be due to

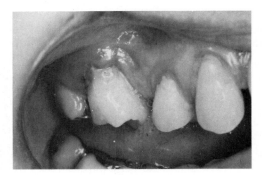

Fig. 12-4. Dehiscence of mesiobuccal root of maxillary first molar has produced a severe periodontal lesion. Note chronic inflammation of marginal gingiva.

severe loss of supporting structures, vertical root fracture, or endodontic failure. Instead of the entire bridge or splint being removed, if sufficient abutments remain, the root of the involved tooth is extracted, with the crown portion remaining in its casting to act as a pontic (Fig. 12-5).

2. *Endodontic failure.* When endodontic treatment has failed or is failing (Fig. 12-6) on only one root of a multirooted tooth, where re-treatment is impossible and apical surgery is impractical, amputation of the failing root may be useful to retain the successful portion. An excellent example of this would be a mandibular molar in which the distal root has healed after therapy but the mesial root now has a definite periapical radiolucency and the canals are filled with sectioned silver points. Since re-treatment of the mesial root is impossible, periapical surgery could be considered. However, in surgery on mandibular molars the thick cortical bone, proximity of the mandibular canal, and the problem of visibility make the procedure hazardous. Amputation of the entire root is usually preferable (Fig. 12-7).

In maxillary molars, particularly the first molar, periapical surgery is usually much easier to perform, and amputation of an endodontically failing root would be the second choice.

3. *Vertical fracture of one root.* The prognosis for a vertical fracture is hopeless. However, in a multirooted tooth, if the vertical fracture traverses one root while the other roots are unaffected, the offending root may be amputated and the remainder restored (Fig. 12-8).

4. *Severe destructive process (usually caries) making a portion of a multirooted tooth nonrestor-*

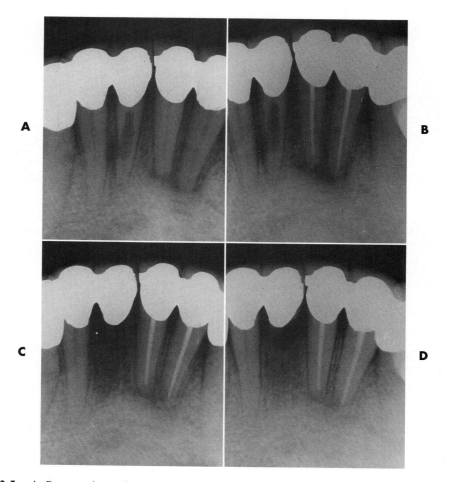

Fig. 12-5. **A,** Preoperative radiograph of mandibular anterior area. A periapical lesion involves both incisors to right (nos. 23 and 24), whereas central incisor to left (no. 25) has a severe internal resorption defect. Patient agreed to endodontics for nos. 23 and 24 but was unwilling to attempt recalcification procedures for no. 25 and requested extraction for that tooth. **B,** Endodontics completed for nos. 23 and 24. **C,** No. 25 root amputation from labial of root with a portion of crown remaining in splint, 3 months after surgery. **D,** One year later, areas have healed perfectly.

able. This may occur as a result of furcation or severe gingival caries, traumatic injury, large root perforation during endodontic therapy, or any other destructive process that causes severe destruction of a significant portion of a posterior tooth (Fig. 12-3).

Contraindications for root amputation. In addition to the absence of supporting bone and the nonrestorability of the retained segment, the following are contraindications for root amputation:

1. *Strong adjacent teeth available for bridge abutments as alternatives to root amputation.* The best consideration for the performance of a root amputation is to retain a posterior abutment and avoid a removable appliance. Another strong indication is to retain a root to aid weak adjacent abutments. However, if excellent potential abutments are available adjacent to the tooth with the need for amputation, it may be best to extract the entire tooth (Fig. 12-9). This consideration is stronger for mandibular teeth than for maxillary teeth, since in the former arch a fixed partial denture must always be fabricated to replace an amputated root, whereas in the upper arch a crown with altered shape may be sufficient as restoration.

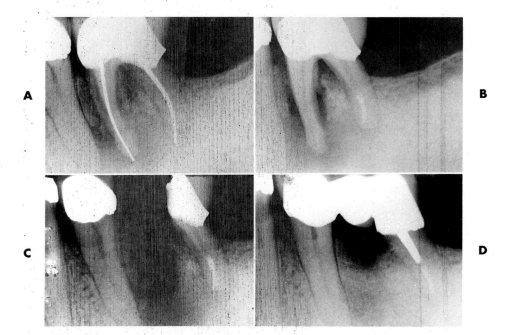

Fig. 12-6. Use of root amputation for predictable endodontic failure. **A,** Preoperative film of mandibular first molar. Tooth was treated previously 6 years ago, but was mobile and tender, with both buccal and lingual sinus tracts that traced to the mesial root. The silver points were removed rather easily and a second mesial canal located, but the sinus tracts persisted. Calcium hydroxide therapy was attempted (Chapter 16), but to no avail. It appeared that the mesial root was hopeless. **B,** Accordingly, the distal canal was filled with laterally condensed gutta-percha and post room prepared. The chamber was packed with zinc oxide-eugenol (ZOE). **C,** The mesial root was amputated easily by the vertical-cut method due to the minimal bony support around it. **D,** Eighteen month later, the area looks excellent, with the distal root acting as the distal abutment of a fixed bridge. (Restoration by Dr. Henry Gold, formerly of Chicago.)

2. *Inoperable canals in root or roots to be retained.* There is a belief among some practitioners that root amputation may be performed before endodontic treatment. After the surgical procedure is completed, the remaining canals are prepared and then filled. However, what happens to the case when it is determined that the canals in the retained roots are inoperable? Because of this question I believe that, whenever possible, root amputation should be performed only after the endodontic treatment is completed in the roots to be retained. If the canal is only partially negotiable, it may be filled to that extent and an apicoectomy performed to that depth or an apical filling used to seal the apex at the same surgical appointment. The same flap that allows the root amputation to be performed is deepened apically to allow the additional surgery. If the canal is inoperable

and surgery is impractical, the tooth must be extracted; although an alternative treatment plan must be utilized, the process of unnecessary amputation is avoided.

3. *Root fusion, making separation impossible.* This contraindication may be worked around and a successful case still preserved with meticulous surgical manipulation. However, preoperative radiographs must be carefully studied to determine if this condition is present so that proper planning can be made for the surgical procedure. For those with minimal experience in root amputation, it is unwise to tackle a case of this complexity. Among the teeth in which a fusion exists with some frequency are mandibular second molars with a "cow-horn" root, which may be open in the furca but fused at the apex, and maxillary second molars in which the buccal roots are fused or the

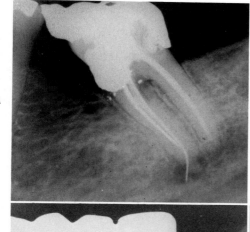

Fig. 12-7. **A,** Mandibular first molar has received endodontic treatment 1 year earlier. Although preoperative periapical radiolucency was decreasing around distal root, mesial root appeared to be failing, probably because of overfilling and overinstrumentation that had preceded it. Tooth was long (24 mm), and periapical surgery in area was considered hazardous. **B,** Mesial root was amputated, and area restored with a fixed partial denture. Distal root served as terminal abutment. Three years postoperatively, excellent healing. **C,** Eleven years after treatment, distal root is still functioning well. (Restorations by Dr. Arnold Wax, Chicago.)

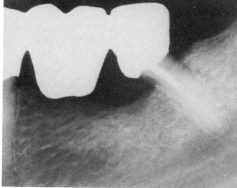

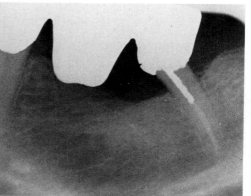

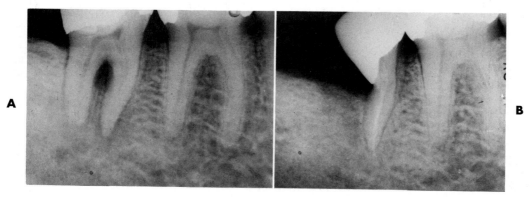

Fig. 12-8. **A,** Mandibular second molar received routine endodontic treatment for five appointments, but a chronic draining sinus communicating with distal root persisted. Decision was made to amputate distal root and retain mesial root. When crown was removed during amputation, a vertical fracture through furca was demonstrable. Distal root was removed. **B,** Four years later, area has healed very well. Mesial root is splinted to adjacent first molar and serves to prevent maxillary molars from supererupting. (Restoration by Dr. Stanley Martin, formerly of Chicago.)

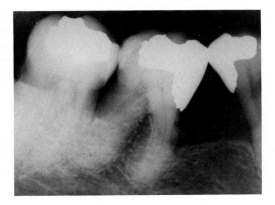

Fig. 12-9. Severe bone loss around mesial root of mandibular first molar was a good indication for mesial root amputation. However, general periodontal condition of the tooth plus the presence of excellent adjacent abutments contraindicated amputation in favor of extraction and replacement with a fixed partial denture.

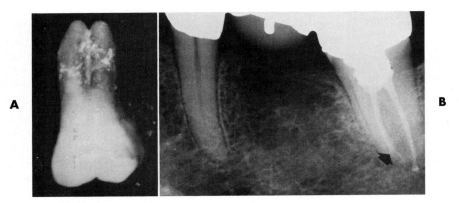

Fig. 12-10. **A,** Fusion of buccal roots of this maxillary second molar would make amputation of either root extremely difficult. **B,** Mandibular second molar was referred for treatment after a ledge had developed during preparation of mesial canal *(arrow)*. Chronic draining sinus from that canal was present during treatment and would not close, since the ledge could not be bypassed. Root amputation was considered but was contraindicated because of cow-horn shape and probable fusion of roots. Chloropercha technique was used to fill canals. Sinus healed immediately thereafter.

distobuccal root is fused to the palatal root. (See Fig. 12-10.) Also some mandibular molars may be C shaped or have fusion in the furca area, and the roots begin to divide only in the middle or apical third. Amputation of one root in these cases results in so much bone removal that the remaining segment is weakly supported.

ARMAMENTARIUM

If a flap is to be raised during the amputation procedure, all the instruments needed for periapical surgery as listed in Chapter 11 will be required, plus additional instruments. If a flap is not required, as in the case of many amputations due to periodontal problems, only the instruments shown in Fig. 12-11

will be required. However, in some cases the tooth that appears treatable without a flap suddenly becomes more complex during the procedure, and a flap is needed. Therefore the basic periapical surgery tray should always be available in a sterile condition during amputation procedures.

The instruments needed specifically for root amputation are as follows:

Surgical length or long shank fissure burs—sizes 700, 701, 557, and 558—used to separate roots and remove overlying bone

Long tapered fissure diamond stones—used to smooth retained tooth segment

Elevators—straight (wide and narrow tip); set of Potts or other angle elevators; apical elevators

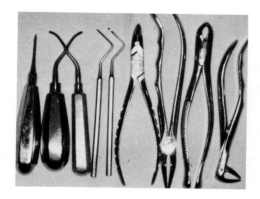

Fig. 12-11. Elevators and forceps used for root amputations. *(from left)* Straight elevator, set of Potts elevators, set of root-tip elevators, upper universal forceps, root-tip forceps, lower universal forceps, lower anterior forceps. To simplify identification, each Potts elevator has a different handle.

Forceps—upper and lower universal forceps and root-tip forceps, plus any other favorite forceps used for single-rooted teeth

GENERAL RULES FOR ROOT AMPUTATION

Importance of root anatomy. A knowledge of root anatomy is mandatory before any root amputation procedure is attempted. Just as the dentist performing endodontic therapy must know the typical position of canal orifices prior to preparing an access cavity, so must the practitioner performing root amputation be familiar with the most common configurations for the roots of the tooth to be so treated. For that reason, prior to describing the technique for root amputation of each molar, I will discuss the topography of the roots.

Endodontic therapy prior to root amputation. Whenever possible, canal fillings should be placed in the roots to be retained prior to the amputation. This may be accomplished either at a preceding appointment or at the same appointment but before the surgery.

Although the root to be amputated requires no canal filling to seal the apex, placement of a filling often facilitates the surgical procedure in aiding the location of the root. Therefore it is best to attempt to fill the root partway to the apex (usually half of the distance from the orifice to the apex is more than sufficient). The canal is enlarged to a minimum of size 60 and filled with gutta-percha by the lateral condensation method or enlarged to size 80 or more and filled with silver amalgam. If the latter method is used, the amalgam should be placed at the canal orifice with a small carrier and a Luks plugger used for condensation.

If the root is to be amputated at the same appointment during which the canals are filled, the chamber should be sealed with zinc oxide-eugenol (ZOE), accelerated with zinc acetate crystals. If the surgery will be performed at a later appointment, the chamber may be filled with silver amalgam or ZOE (Fig. 12-12). Amalgam is not used in the former case because it may not have set sufficiently by the time that the root is amputated, and a messy situation then develops.

Root amputation on periodontically involved teeth. As a general rule, when amputation is performed for a root with a severe periodontal lesion, there is no need to raise a flap. If either the vertical-cut or the crown-precontouring technique is utilized, the objective is still to separate the root to be amputated from the rest of the tooth at the furcation. That the separation has been obtained is determined by placing a straight elevator into the furca and giving it a slight rotatory movement. If separation is complete, the root being amputated will move in one direction while the portion of the tooth that is to remain will move in the opposite direction. If the entire tooth moves in one direction, further preparation of the furca must be performed.

After separation is verified, the root should not be delivered until the crown of the segment that is to remain has been reshaped. Any sharp edges that might cut the tongue or cheek are trimmed with the tapered diamond stone. The occlusal height is reduced to prevent strong occlusal contact during mastication of tough or chewy foods, and a modified preparation for the restoration to be placed may be performed. All this is done with the root to be amputated still in place to prevent amalgam, gold or temporary fillings, calculus, tooth, or other debris from being pushed into the socket, thereby retarding healing (Fig. 12-13).

The patient is instructed to rinse vigorously with mouthwash, and any remaining debris in the area is removed by suction evacuation. The angled elevators are used to loosen the root and may be sufficient to perform the compete root extraction. If a greater grasp on the root is required, suitable forceps are used.

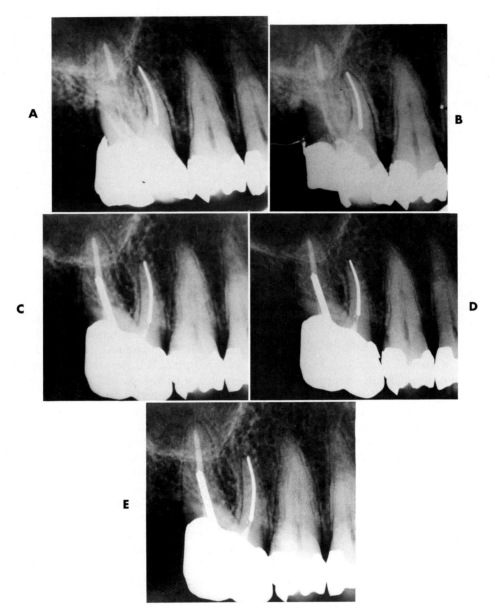

Fig. 12-12. **A,** Maxillary first molar required amputation of distal root for periodontal reasons. Palatal canal was filled with gutta-percha, and post room was provided; mesiobuccal canal was filled with a silver point. Distal canal was filled some distance with gutta-percha to provide a landmark during amputation. **B,** Distal root amputated. **C,** Four years postoperatively, area looks excellent. **D,** Twelve years after original treatment. **E,** Sixteen years after original treatment. (Restoration by Dr. Ascher Jacobs, formerly of Chicago, and periodontal therapy by Dr. Erwin Barrington, Chicago.)

Root amputation on teeth having normal periodontal support. In cases where there is relatively normal bone, a flap will be required to deliver the amputated root. All the rules for flap design as discussed in Chapter 11 must be followed.

Once the flap is raised, the object of the initial phase of the preparation is to produce a periodontal lesion. This is done by removing the bone around the root to be amputated, using a tapered fissure carbide bur with the airotor and water spray. Bone is similarly removed in the furcation area to allow direct visualization of the position where the root joins the rest of the tooth. Using the vertical-cut technique, which will be described for each molar later in this chapter, the operator separates the root to be amputated from the remainder of the tooth at the furcation. A straight elevator is used in the furcation to see whether separation has been accomplished, as in a periodontally involved case. Then an angled elevator is used to see whether sufficient bone has been removed to deliver the root. If the root does not appear to be loose in its socket, further removal of bone may be needed. For maxillary molars, only buccal bone must be removed; in mandibular molars, both buccal and lingual bone may require reduction.

There should be no hesitancy to remove alveolar bone closely surrounding a root to be amputated if the procedure then becomes much easier. This bone would undoubtedly resorb after the amputation anyway. For mesiobuccal roots of a maxillary first molar, which frequently have a distal curvature near the apex, it is often wise to remove all the buccal bone to the apex prior to using any elevation.

As with periodontally involved teeth, the crown of the remaining segment is trimmed prior to the amputation. Since a flap is used, sutures will be required after the root removal.

Vertical-cut method. The vertical-cut method utilizes a long shank, tapered fissure carbide bur in the airotor to section through the entire crown and root to the furca in gaining separation. Its use will be clarified for each molar tooth later in this chapter. Water is not needed while making this preparation on solid tooth structure, particularly on maxillary teeth where the spray would collect on the mouth mirror and interfere with vision. However, irrigation followed by suction evacuation is needed periodically to remove the tooth and temporary filling debris that tends to collect within the

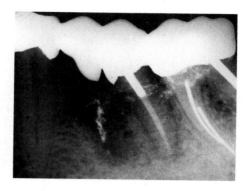

Fig. 12-13. Mesial root of mandibular first molar was amputated prior to trimming and recontouring of distal portion of tooth. Radiograph taken 6 months after surgery reveals that a considerable amount of debris and filling materials has remained in socket.

preparation and in the furcation area where bone should not be overheated.

It must always be remembered that both bifurcations and trifurcations are some distance from the occlusal surface of the tooth. Therefore a deep preparation is required before an elevator is used to see if separation is required before an elevator is used to see if separation is gained. If the elevator is used prematurely, a large section of crown may be snapped off, which might make subsequent restoration more complex, or the root may fracture at an undesirable angle. If doubt exists as to the depth of the cut, a radiograph can be taken for verification of position.

Advantages of the vertical-cut method include the following:

1. Direct visualization of the bur penetration to ensure that preparation will be in the correct position
2. Removal of that portion of the crown that is over the root to prevent undesirable postoperative occlusal forces
3. Position of each cut, based on the anatomy of the furca, to allow the root to cleave along desirable angles
4. Excellent visualization of the furca after amputation to allow for any needed trimming or smoothing with long shank, tapered fissure diamond stones

Presurgical crown-contouring method. As described by Kirchoff and Gerstein, this technique

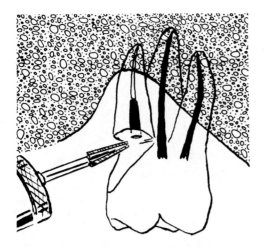

Fig. 12-14. In presurgical crown-contouring method, crown over root to be amputated is reduced with a fissure bur until entire root face is visible, marked by the root canal filling. It is then a simple matter to elevate the root.

is extremely useful in treating maxillary molars with periodontal defects. The presurgical crown-contouring method involves trimming the portion of the crown over the root to be amputated to gain separation. In this technique it is important that the root to be amputated have a canal filling prior to the surgery, since the gutta-percha or amalgam provides an important landmark.

A tapered fissure bur is used to trim back the crown over the root to be amputated, with the depth of the preparation being approximately at the cementoenamel junction. After some crown reduction has been accomplished, the face of the root will start to come into view to aid in further preparation. The position of the canal filling marks the center of the root (Fig. 12-14). As soon as the furcation is visualized, separation and extraction may be accomplished by the methods previously described.

Vertical as opposed to horizontal preparation. Amputation procedures have been described in which a horizontal cut is made through the tooth without the crown being altered in the preparation. Although this technique is used when removing one root or one tooth from under a splint, it is not the method of choice in most cases. Cutting the tooth in this manner leaves a deep trough between the crown and the alveolar mucosa, which is an obvious trap for food and debris. Also, since the crown has not changed in configuration, any

occlusal pressures over the amputated root will tend to put severe stress from an undesirable direction on the remaining roots.

With a vertical preparation, the crown over the amputated root is removed, and any occlusal stresses are dissipated along the long axes of the remaining roots. The restorative dentist is cognizant of the need for modified occlusal shape in a new crown, and there are no areas for collection of debris. The indication for root amputation may have been furcation involvement, and it is much easier for both the dentist and the patient to gain access for cleansing the new furca area without a bulky portion of the crown impeding the way.

ROOT AMPUTATION FOR MAXILLARY FIRST MOLAR

Root anatomy. The maxillary first molar has been involved in root amputation procedures because of the common finding of a deep pocket between the first and second molars or a dehiscence of either buccal root. Also, the bulky palatal root, often exhibiting a buccal curve, offers excellent anchorage either by itself or in combination with the mesial or distal root.

When the tooth is viewed from the buccal aspect, both buccal roots appear slender and fragile, with narrow mesiodistal dimensions of approximately equal width. The buccal groove is seen dividing in half the mesiodistal diameter at the cementoenamel junction (Fig. 12-15, *A*). This is the typical picture shown in the common intraoral radiograph, but it does not tell the true story of the anatomy of the buccal roots and the trifurcation area.

If the tooth is viewed from the proximal surface, an interesting new insight is gained into the configuration of the roots. The mesiobuccal root is wide as seen from the mesial aspect and takes up approximately two thirds of the buccolingual width of the tooth at the level of the furca (Fig. 12-15, *B*). The buccal portion of the mesiobuccal root is flat, but the palatal side has a slope from the apex to the furca. The palatal root is quite bulky and has a crescent shape, first curving away from the buccal area as it gently slopes away from the furca and then curving toward the buccal aspect in the apical area. This shape offers considerable resistance to pressures from almost any direction and explains why this root is so valuable.

The view from the distal aspect (Fig. 12-15, *C*) shows that the distobuccal root is much narrower than the mesiobuccal root and that the former has a generally conical shape, with minimal resistance to occlusal or lateral pressures. The buccolingual width of the root is approximately half the buccolingual width of the tooth at the height of the furca.

The view from the apex toward the furca lends further information (Fig. 12-15, *D* and *E*). The distal root demonstrates its conical shape, whereas the mesial root has a depression on both the mesial and the distal portions of the root. If bone is present in these areas, it will aid against either buccal or lingual movement of the root. This figure-eight shape also prevents torque of the root, whereas the conical distal root offers little resistance to that type of movement. The positions of the furca may be seen from the apical view. The trough between the distal and palatal roots extends distally; between the mesial and the palatal areas the separation points to the mesiolingual surface, whereas the space between the buccal roots points directly buccally. At its widest dimension, the buccolingual diameter of the tooth is much greater at the mesial surface than at the distal surface, since the crown has a rhomboidal shape. The buccal surface of the tooth slopes toward the palatal surface as it extends distally.

A diagrammatic representation of the furcation area of the maxillary first and second molars may be made, using a pie shape to represent the diameter at the furca (Fig. 12-16, *A*). The importance of this diagram will be stressed in the description of the root amputation procedures.

Amputation of the mesiobuccal root. The greatest problem in the amputation of the mesiobuccal root of the maxillary first molar is failure to recognize the considerable buccolingual width involved. The operator is fooled into thinking that the root is very slender, as indicated in the routine radiograph, and so the root is cut much too far buccally, leaving a spicule in the trifurcation. If the amputation was performed for periodontal reasons, this remaining root spicule would perpetuate the attraction and retention of debris in the furca and negate the effectiveness of treatment (Fig. 12-1, *A*).

The vertical-cut method is used to separate the lines of the furca, as depicted in the schematic drawing (Fig. 12-16, *B*).

It is usually a relatively simple matter to make a buccal cut, since the buccal groove correctly marks the position of the underlying furca. This cut is carried a few millimeters toward the center of the tooth. Next, the initial mesial cut is made at

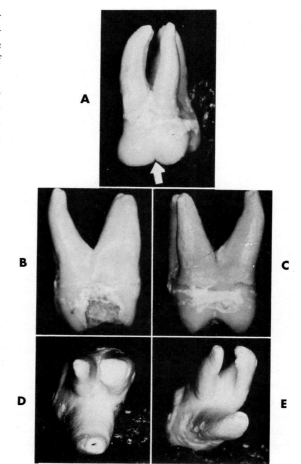

Fig. 12-15. A, Buccal view of maxillary first molar. Both buccal roots appear quite thin, with the buccal groove *(arrow)* dividing mesiodistal width of crown in half. **B,** Mesial view. Mesiobuccal root *(right)* is wide in buccolingual dimension and takes up approximately two thirds of buccolingual width of tooth at furcation level. **C,** Distal view. Distobuccal root is narrower than mesiobuccal root, taking up approximately half of buccolingual width at furcation level. Note that palatal root has a slight apical curvature toward buccal aspect. **D,** View from apex toward furca. Distobuccal root *(upper left)* is much smaller and more conical than mesiobuccal root. **E,** View toward furca at a slight angle. Depression on distal surface of mesiobuccal root is apparent, as is greater buccolingual width compared to distobuccal root.

a position approximately two-thirds the distance from the buccal surface of the crown to the lingual surface. This usually closely conforms to the position where the lingual extension of mesio-occlusal cavity preparation terminates. Again the cut is car-

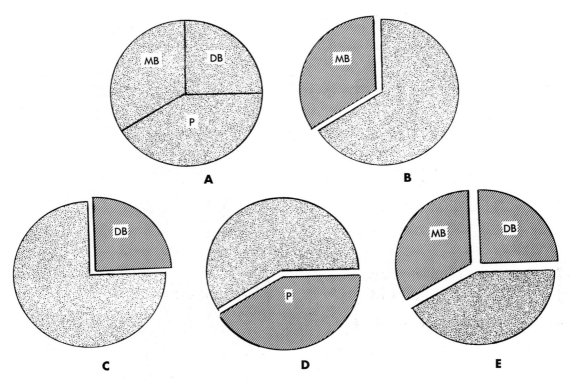

Fig. 12-16.   A, Diagram of furcation area of maxillary first and second molars. Mesiobuccal and distobuccal roots are divided by buccal groove. Mesiobuccal root *(MB)* takes up two thirds of mesial half of tooth, or one third of entire furcation area. Distobuccal root *(DB)* takes up half the distal half of tooth, or one fourth of entire furcation area, with palatal root *(P)* taking up the remainder. **B,** Vertical-cut preparation for mesiobuccal root amputation. Buccal groove gives position for buccal cut through to the furca. Mesial cut is made two thirds of distance toward palatal surface and brought to center of tooth. Then root may be delivered. **C,** Vertical-cut preparation for distobuccal root amputation. Buccal cut starts at buccal groove and is brought toward furca. Distal cut is made half the distance toward palatal aspect and brought to center of tooth, allowing separation of root and delivery. **D,** Vertical-cut method for amputation of palatal root. Mesial and distal cuts are made and extended to center of tooth to gain separation of palatal root and delivery. **E,** Vertical-cut method for amputating both buccal roots. Three cuts are used for amputation of these roots, and the roots are delivered separately.

ried a few millimeters toward the center of the tooth. These two cuts are joined with deep penetration of the fissure bur and should conform to the furcation position (Fig. 12-17).

As suggested in the rules for amputation, the separation is verified by a straight elevator. A snapping sound may occur when the elevator is used, and the operator may fear that the root has cracked in an undesirable position. On the contrary, cleavage generally will occur right through the furca to separate any portions that were not cut by the fissure bur. The remaining segment is trimmed and the root amputated, as outlined earlier in the chapter.

If the presurgical crown-contouring method is used, the entire coronal portion is trimmed back over the root until the furca is visualized.

However, as stated in the opening remarks of this chapter, amputation of the mesiobuccal root, in both the maxillary first and second molars, is strongly discouraged. Because of the difficult shape to work with, the need for the depression in the furcation area (Fig. 12-17, *F*), the need for splinting to an adjacent tooth, and the frequent errors in removal of this root (Fig. 12-1, *A*), I have seen many disasters when amputation was employed. If that is the only choice available, treatment should be undertaken. However, the patient

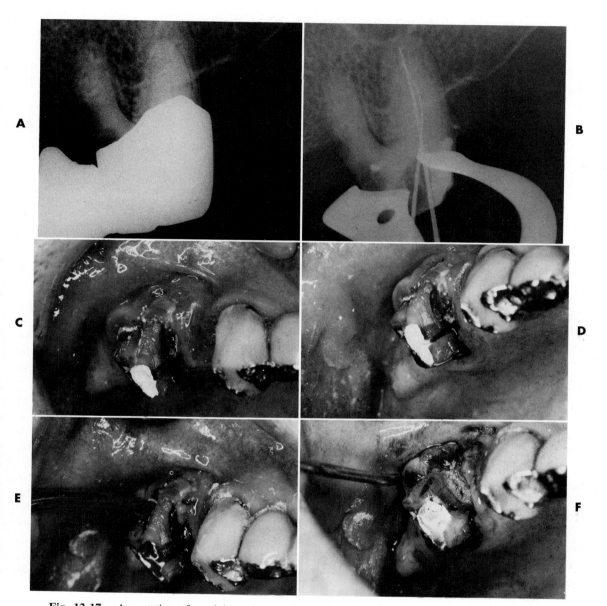

Fig. 12-17. Amputation of mesiobuccal root of maxillary first molar. **A,** Preoperative radiograph demonstrating large carious lesion on mesial of the mesiobuccal root, but the buccal bone loss is not apparent from the film. **B,** Files in place in distobuccal and palatal roots. Although I generally prepare and fill root to be amputated, deep caries made this almost impossible, so I merely packed orifice to the mesiobuccal canal with ZOE. Other two canals were filled with gutta-percha. **C,** Buccal cut and, **D,** mesial cut two thirds of distance between buccal and lingual portions of the tooth. Note severe buccal periodontal lesion apparent in these two clinical views. **E,** Cuts are joined, and separation is tested with an elevator. The Potts will then flick the root out. **F,** Note concave appearance of furcation area after mesiobuccal root has been correctly amputated. This is critical and must be restored with the identical shape.

Continued

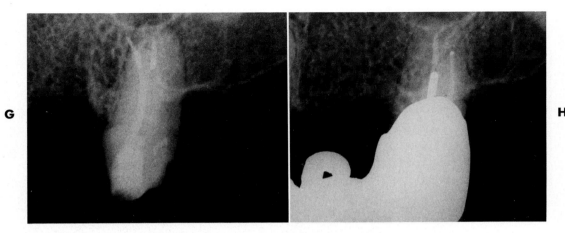

Fig. 12-17, cont'd. G, Radiograph following the amputation. Note smooth cut without an overhanging lip and the post room in the palatal canal. **H,** Four years later tooth still serves excellently as posterior bridge abutment. Excess gutta-percha past apex of distobuccal root has been resorbed and periodontal ligament spaces around the remaining roots are perfect. (Restoration by Dr. Harold Brill, Chicago.)

should be appraised as to the difficulty of therapy, the treatment plan must be carefully drawn, and the practitioners must perform their services on the highest possible level. Even then, the results may fall short of expectations.

Amputation of the distobuccal root. The buccal cut is placed in the same position as for amputating the mesiobuccal root. The distal cut is placed half the distance between the buccal and palatal surfaces of the tooth, and then both cuts are connected with deep penetration of the bur along the lines of the schematic drawing (Fig. 12-16, *C*).

Once separation is verified and the remaining crown contoured, the root is removed (Fig. 12-18).

The amputation of the distobuccal root unquestionably is the best tolerated of all the amputation procedures from a longevity standpoint (Fig. 12-12). The retained palatal and mesiobuccal roots are large and retentive and offer excellent support for the altered tooth. From a mesial view, the palatal root curves first to the lingual and then to the buccal (Fig. 12-15, *B*), whereas the mesiobuccal root from the buccal view curves first to the mesial and then to the distal (Fig. 12-15, *A*). Thus all directions of torquing are resisted.

Because of the strength of the remaining roots, it is not mandatory for the tooth so treated to be splinted to an adjacent abutment. In the other cases of root amputation on a maxillary molar, mesiobuccal or palatal, or any two roots, fastening to an adjacent tooth must be accomplished.

Amputation of a palatal root. Amputation of a palatal root is often a complicated procedure, even if a severe periodontal condition is present. In addition, restoring two buccal roots is a difficult problem. Therefore two buccal roots should be retained only when no other solution is available.

Unless the periodontal condition is so severe that a pocket reaches the apex of the palatal root, a flap should be raised for the amputation procedure. Otherwise the root's considerable length, width, and curvature often make it difficult to remove.

The mesial and distal cuts only are used to gain separation from the buccal roots. Care should be exercised in the use of the elevator to verify the separation because the thinner buccal roots may become loosened. A tapered fissure carbide bur is used to remove bone mesial and distal to the palatal root before any delivery is attempted (Fig. 12-16, *D*).

Amputation of both buccal roots. If both buccal roots are to be amputated, the mesial, distal, and buccal cuts are made as described earlier. The roots are delivered separately (Fig. 12-16, *E*). It is unwise merely to make the mesial and distal cuts and then attempt to remove the buccal roots in one section. The apical curvatures of these two roots often are toward each other, and any bone remaining between them may cause considerable problems.

Amputation of the palatal and distobuccal roots. Because of the considerable bulk of the

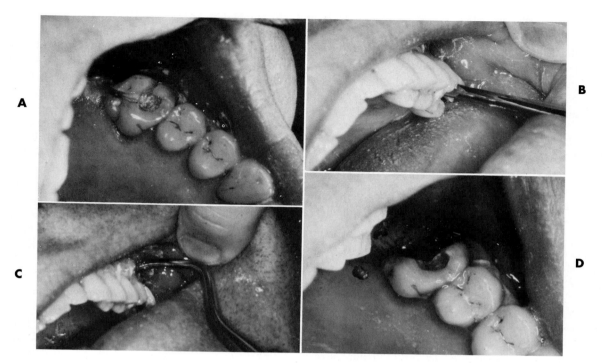

Fig. 12-18.   Amputation of distobuccal root by vertical-cut method. **A,** Occlusal view shows positions of vertical cuts extending toward furca. **B,** Straight elevator is placed in furcation area from occlusal aspect, and a slight turn is made to separate root to be amputated from rest of tooth. **C,** Then angled elevator is placed from buccal surface and used to lift separated root from its alveolar housing. **D,** Occlusal view shows distobuccal root amputated. Radiographs of a case similar to this are presented in Fig. 12-12.

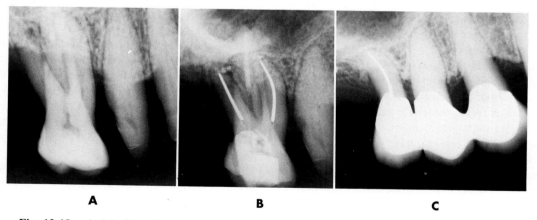

Fig. 12-19.   **A,** Maxillary first molar, in which treatment plan called for amputation of distobuccal root and separation but retention of both mesiobuccal and palatal roots. **B,** Endodontic treatment was completed prior to separation and amputation. When distobuccal root was amputated and remaining roots separated, palatal root was found to be very mobile. Therefore it was removed, too. **C,** Five years later, mesiobuccal root is tight and the splint functions well, thus avoiding need for a removable partial denture. (Restoration by Dr. Joseph Krohn, formerly of Chicago.)

mesiobuccal root (Fig. 12-15, *B*), it is possible to retain it alone in certain cases and amputate both the distobuccal and the palatal roots (Fig. 12-19 on p. 623). This should be done only in cases where there are no other molar abutments available and where there are sufficient anterior abutments to support and stabilize the mesiobuccal root.

ROOT AMPUTATIONS FOR MAXILLARY SECOND MOLAR

Root amputation for maxillary second molars should be avoided at an even higher level than those for the first molar. There are a number of reasons for this.

There are several variants in anatomy for this tooth, even though the most common condition is, similar to the adjacent maxillary first molar, three separate roots. However, even in this condition, root fusions of any combination (palatal to either buccal or two buccals to each other) may be present and are very difficult to diagnose prior to initiating the procedure. Attempting to amputate a fused root is frustrating and very difficult. Another condition, which occurs approximately 10% of the time (see Chapter 6), involves this tooth having only two roots, with the buccal root containing a single (most common) or two canals. Performing endodontic treatment prior to root amputation is very helpful in visualizing these conditions, since the canal fillings make the roots easier to identify on radiographs.

If only one buccal root is present, the difficulties encountered by surgical and prosthetic treatment contraindicate root amputation. Fortunately conditions requiring amputation with this root configuration rarely occur.

When three separate roots are present, the mesiobuccal root is very wide buccolingually with a higher than previously anticipated percentage of two canals (see Chapter 6), just as is that root in the first molar. Therefore, if the tooth is treated endodontically just to have an amputation of another root, unless a high percentage of two canals are located, the chance of endodontic failure will be high. When the mesiobuccal is the root to be amputated, problems with the buccolingual width and the position of the tooth being so far posterior make the surgical procedure quite difficult, even with a large periodontal defect and a flap.

As in the first molar, amputation of the mesiobuccal root in the second molar requires splinting.

Amputation of the distobuccal root is complicated by its posterior position, but has the advantage of usually not having a tooth behind it. With a large periodontal defect, the crown-contouring method works very well. Usually amputation of the distobuccal root will not require restoration with splinting to an adjacent tooth.

Amputation of the two buccal roots to keep a strong palatal root, particularly when the buccal roots are severely involved periodontally, is not complicated surgically (Fig. 12-20). However, restoring this root must involve splinting to an adjacent root. If the first molar is present, and not seriously involved periodontally, it would be better to extract the entire second molar rather than keep only a palatal root. Therefore, this procedure requires a restorable third molar to be adjacent.

Root amputation of the palatal root alone to keep the two buccals is a very rarely employed procedure.

Root anatomy. Since amputation is indicated only for the separate buccal roots, just the root anatomy pertinent to such therapy will be described.

Buccal roots are usually parallel to each other and often have a distal inclination. The roots have much less buccolingual spread than in the first molar, and the apex of each root usually lies well within the general circumference of the tooth.

Mesial and distal views reveal that the mesiobuccal root is slightly more narrow and the distobuccal root slightly wider buccolingually than in the first molar. However, the schematic drawing of the furcation is still similar to that for the first molar and is applicable to second molar amputation (Fig. 12-16).

Amputation of the mesiobuccal root. The buccolingual width of the mesiobuccal root is still quite wide compared to the mesiodistal width, even though it is not as wide as that root of the first molar. The amputation procedure is similar, however; a slight variation is that the mesial cut is placed slightly closer to the contact point between the first and second molars.

Amputation of the distobuccal root. The amputation of the distobuccal root of the maxillary second molar is very similar to that performed on the first molar. However, since the distal root may be slightly wider, the distal cut is placed slightly more to the lingual aspect.

Amputation of both buccal roots. As in the maxillary first molar, both roots of the second molar may require amputation. However, because

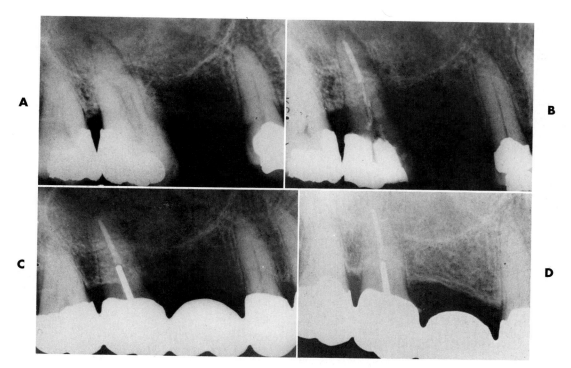

Fig. 12-20. **A,** Maxillary second molar has severe periodontal loss on both buccal roots and a periapical radiolucency associated with palatal root. However, third molar does not appear to be a satisfactory terminal abutment for a fixed partial denture; it requires an adjacent tooth or root for added support. **B,** Therefore palatal root was treated endodontically and filled with gutta-percha, whereas buccal roots were amputated. **C,** Four years later, complete healing of area and an excellent restorative result that could not have been accomplished without retention of palatal root. Excellent periapical healing of the palatal root. **D,** Eleven years after treatment. (Restorations by Dr. Jay Herschman, Chicago.)

of the smaller size of the palatal root compared with that of the first molar, such a procedure should be attempted only when adjacent support is available for splinting (Fig. 12-20). Use of the palatal root alone as a distal abutment is hazardous otherwise. For the amputation, as in the first molar, mesial, buccal, and distal vertical cuts are made and each of the buccal roots is removed separately.

Amputation of adjacent roots of the maxillary molars. A common site for a severe periodontal lesion is between the maxillary first and second molars. Surgical treatment for such a condition often will involve amputation of the distobuccal root of the maxillary first molar. Sacrifice of that root leaves the mesiobuccal and palatal roots, which are generally excellent retentive roots for the first molar (Fig. 12-12).

However, knowledgeable clinicians have cautioned against amputating the adjacent roots of these teeth, that is, the distobuccal root of the first molar and the mesiobuccal root of the second molar. They have stated that the teeth are complicated to restore, that the shapes developed are difficult for the patient to maintain in health, and that the patient might have speech difficulties.

On the contrary, I have found that the combination does not present serious problems (Fig. 12-21). As stated earlier, amputation of the mesiobuccal root of the maxillary second molar is more complicated than in the first molar. However, with the distobuccal root of the first molar removed, visualization of the mesial portion of the second molar is greatly improved. Consequently, when these procedures are necessary, the distobuccal of the first molar is amputated first, followed by the

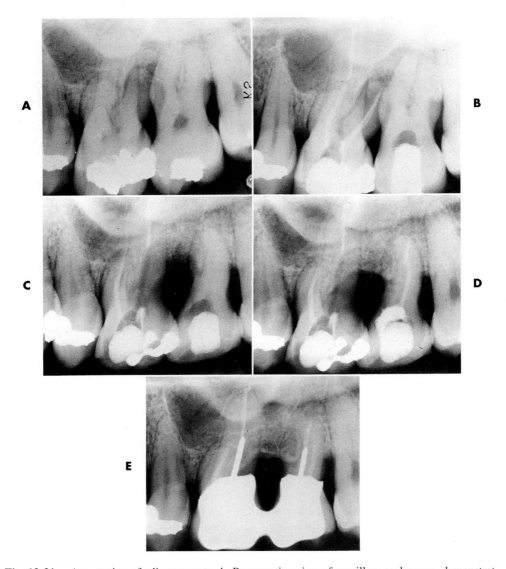

Fig. 12-21. Amputation of adjacent roots. **A,** Preoperative view of maxillary molar area, demonstrating hopeless periodontal condition of first molar distobuccal root and advanced bone loss associated with second molar. **B,** Accordingly, canals were enlarged and filled in the first molar. In the second molar, the pulps were extirpated and the access sealed with ZOE plus formocresol. The patient then was referred back to the periodontist. **C,** The distobuccal root of the first molar was amputated by the periodontist during surgery. He also determined that the mesiobuccal root of the second molar required amputation but that the remainder of the tooth was salvageable. With the distobuccal root of the first molar gone, amputation of the mesiobuccal root of the second molar is much easier to perform. **D,** Endodontic treatment was then completed on the second molar distobuccal and palatal roots. **E,** The teeth were restored with a splint, and 2 years later the area looks excellent. (Restoration by Dr. Steve Fishman and periodontics by Dr. Ken Krebs, both of Chicago.)

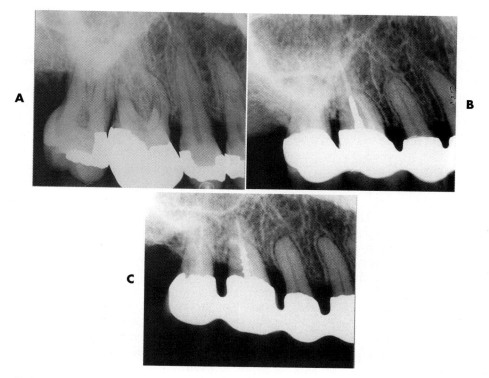

Fig. 12-22. Amputation of two distobuccal roots. **A,** Preoperative radiograph of maxillary molar area indicating considerable periodontal bone loss associated with distobuccal roots of both molar teeth. All canals were filled with gutta-percha and both distobuccal roots were amputated during periodontal surgery. **B,** Three years later, molars have been splinted to adjacent bicuspids. **C,** Sixteen years after original treatment, a new splint has been fabricated to give the patient a better opportunity to clean between the abutments. Some additional bone loss is seen as compared to the previous film, but the teeth continue to function well. (Restoration by Dr. Kerry Voit, and periodontal treatment by Dr. Harry Staffileno, both of Chicago.)

completion of the second molar surgery. If any question exists as to best access to the field of surgery, a flap should be raised. When the endodontist, periodontist, restorative dentist, and the patient work together to obtain proper diagnosis and treatment, efficient home care, and careful follow-up, the condition can be made quite favorable.

Amputation of the distobuccal root of both the first and second molars. This procedure is possible and does not lead to severely weakened teeth (Fig. 12-22) as would amputation of the mesiobuccal root of both molars. The schematic drawing of Fig. 12-16 is applied to both teeth, with the slight modification suggested above for the second molar.

The restorative procedures must be followed carefully to leave embrasures conductive to desirable home care (Fig. 12-22, *C*), and the result may last for a long period of time.

AMPUTATION PROCEDURES ON MANDIBULAR MOLARS

Root amputation procedures on mandibular molars are usually referred to as *hemisections*. Because of the two roots present, one half of the crown and one root is removed. In addition, another procedure, referred to as *bicuspidization,* may be performed on mandibular molars, in which a separation is made between the roots but neither is removed.

Root anatomy. Buccal and lingual views show that the typical mandibular molar has two separate roots of approximately equal length, with the mesial root usually slightly wider buccolingually (Fig. 12-23, *A*). Near the gingival third the mesial root curves mesially but then slopes distally to its apex. The distal root is less curved than the mesial root, but it has a definite distal apical inclination. A definite developmental depression starts at the cervical line on both the buccal and lingual aspect and extends to the furca area. The point of bifurcation is approximately 3 mm below the cervical line.

Neither of the two buccal grooves or the lingual groove on the crown of the molar conforms to underlying root structures. Therefore, unlike the buccal groove of the maxillary molar showing where the buccal cut should be made for root amputation, no clue is available to the root configuration seen on the crown of the mandibular molar. In rare instances an enamel projection may be present on a mandibular molar to indicate the position of the bifurcation. This anomaly is an extension of enamel from the crown into the furca area and is useful in amputation and bicuspidizing procedures (Fig. 12-24). Unfortunately it is absent in most cases.

Looking into the furcation from the distal aspect shows a depression on the distal portion of the mesial root (Fig. 12-23, *B*). The final mesial portion has a similar but smaller depression. This gives the

root a figure-eight shape in cross section, similar to the mesiobuccal root of the maxillary first molar. Because of these depressions and the greater curvature of the root, the mesial root probably has more resistance to stress than does the distal root and thus may be the better choice for retention when there is a question as to which root should be amputated in a mandibular molar. However, a key factor in such a decision must be the endodontic manipulation of the root canals, since the two canals of the mesial root are much more difficult to enlarge and fill than the single canal of the distal root.

Amputation of the mesial root. The vertical-cut method is excellent for amputation of either root of a mandibular molar. Because there are no clues on the crown as to the position of the furca, the use of a silver point placed in the bifurcation will greatly aid in the placement of the vertical cut. Since many molars have amputations because of the existence of furcation invasion, it is often simple to make a gentle curve in a size 40 silver point and insert it through the furca from the lingual to the buccal aspect (Fig. 12-25).

Even in cases where no furca damage is present, it is wise to remove bone in that area so the silver point can be inserted as a guide. If the cuts are not made in the correct position, too much tooth structure may be removed, making the restorative situation difficult, or the furcation problem may remain (Fig. 12-1, *C*).

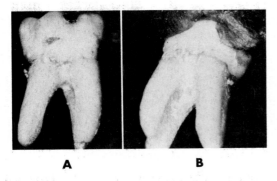

A   **B**

Fig. 12-23. **A,** Buccal view of mandibular first molar root configuration. Mesial root *(right)* and distal root are of approximately same length, but distal root is usually straighter. Developmental depression separates roots, and the furca is approximately 3 mm below cervical line. **B,** Lingual view of mandibular first molar, emphasizing interior anatomy of mesial root. Mesial root *(left)* has a definite depression on the distal portion. Similar but smaller depression on mesial portion gives the root a figure-eight outline in cross section.

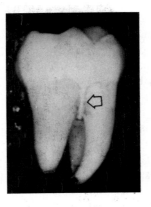

Fig. 12-24. Enamel projection *(arrow)* from crown gives an excellent guide to correct position of bifurcation between roots of a mandibular molar. Although this would be a useful landmark for placing the vertical cut for root amputation, the projection is not always present.

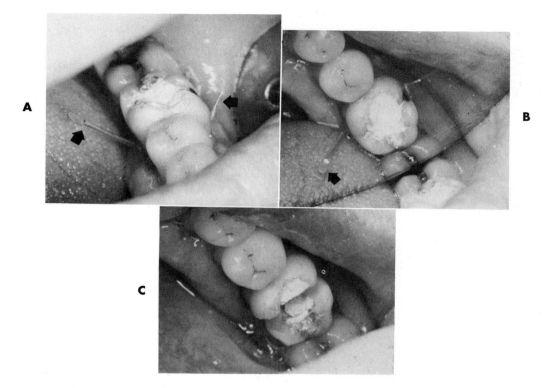

Fig. 12-25. Use of vertical-cut method for mandibular molar. **A,** Silver point *(arrows)* is placed through furca from lingual to buccal to indicate correct position for making vertical cut to amputate either mesial or distal root for tooth with severe furcation involvement. **B,** Occlusal view of silver point *(arrow)* through furcation. With this marking, it is a simple matter to use a tapered fissure bur and separate the two roots. When separation is completed, the silver point may be withdrawn occlusally. **C,** Occlusal view following completion of vertical cut.

It is then a simple matter to cut through the crown with a long shank, tapered fissure carbide bur in the airotor to the position indicated by the silver point. That complete separation has been gained is determined when the point may be removed occlusally through the preparation. Separation may be tested further by placing a straight elevator into the vertical cut and rotating slightly. The two roots will move in opposite directions if separation is completed.

Even when the silver point is used to indicate the area for making the vertical cut and in all cases where it is impossible to use such an indicator, radiographic verification should be made prior to cutting the crown in two. The fissure bur is used to cut deeply into the crown in the position that is assumed to be correct, but the cut is carried only approximately three fourths of the distance toward the furcation. At this point a radiograph is taken

with the film placed at a perfectly perpendicular position to the cut. The radiograph should verify that if the cut is extended, it will go directly between the two roots (Fig. 12-26). If the extension of the cut would go into a portion of the root, the proper alteration in direction must be made, carried deeper but not into the furca, and reradiographed to ensure the correctness of direction.

As with the maxillary molars, the distal portion of the tooth is trimmed and the area debrided. Lower universal forceps are used to extract the root, busing buccolingual rocking action. If the root is not delivered easily in a periodontally involved case, a flap should be raised and buccal bone removed until the root becomes looser. If a flap has already been raised and the root remains tight, it may be necessary to remove buccal and lingual bone almost to the apex. In many cases the bone that fills the depression on the mesial and

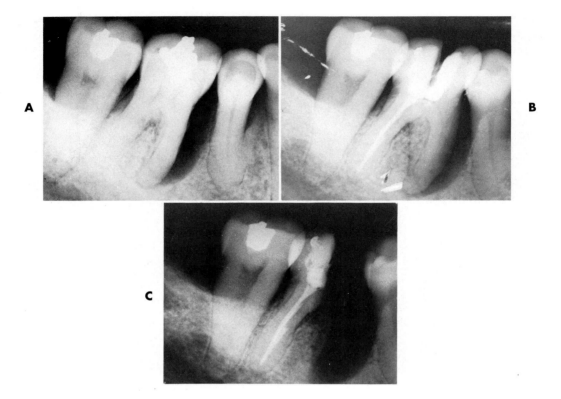

Fig. 12-26. **A,** Mandibular first molar that will require mesial root amputation because of severe periodontal lesion on mesial surface. Note absence of bone loss in furcation area. **B,** Distal canal has been filled, post room prepared, and chamber filled with ZOE. When vertical cut was approximately three fourths of distance toward the furca, a radiograph was taken to verify correctness of direction. **C,** Amputation completed.

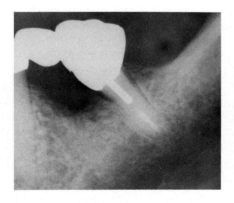

Fig. 12-27. Distal root has served as terminal abutment for this fixed partial denture for 6 years. Although mesial root was amputated for periodontal reasons, periodontal therapy and prosthesis have retained distal root in excellent condition. Contrast this with Fig. 12-1, *C.* (Restorations by Dr. Arnold Wax and periodontal therapy by Dr. Harry Staffileno, both of Chicago.)

distal surfaces of the root is sufficient to give retention. Penetration and bone removal to this depth may be required.

After root extraction the furcation area is trimmed with the tapered fissure diamond stone to ensure that no spicules are present to cause further periodontal irritation. Sutures may be needed to close the wound (Figs. 12-7 and 12-27).

Amputation of the distal root. The procedure is almost identical to that used for the amputation of the mesial root. The silver point is inserted and the vertical cut made into the bifurcation to gain separation. The distal root is usually easier to deliver, since it has a more consistently conical shape (Fig. 12-28).

As may be noted in Figs. 12-23 and 12-24, the mesial root of the mandibular first molar generally is wider and more retentive than the distal root. Many dentists do not realize this and think of the

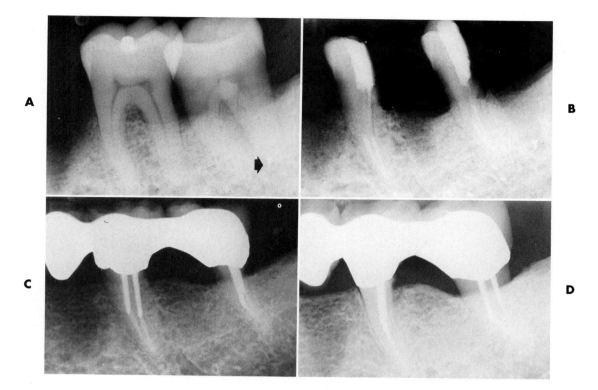

Fig. 12-28.   Amputation of distal roots of mandibular molars. **A,** Preoperative radiograph demonstrating severe bone loss around distal root of second molar and advanced bone loss associated with distal root of the first molar. Previous dentist had probed the second molar pocket with a gutta-percha cone. Portion of cone remains associated with apex *(arrow).* **B,** Endodontics completed and distal roots amputated. **C,** Three years later, area looks excellent. Double posts were placed in both mesial canals of each tooth due to difficulty of making long wide posts in mesial roots. **D,** Eight years after original treatment, both mesial roots are functioning well. (Restorations by Dr. Maury Falstein, formerly of Chicago.)

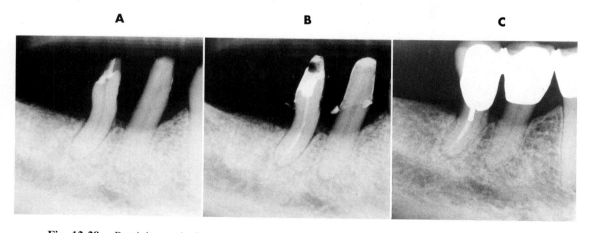

Fig. 12-29.   Retaining a single mesial root to prevent a removable partial denture. **A,** Preoperative view following amputation of distal root by restorative dentist and removal of pulp from mesial canals. **B,** Completion of endodontics. **C,** Two years later, the mesial root alone is serving as the distal abutment of a splint, thus avoiding the need for a removable partial denture.

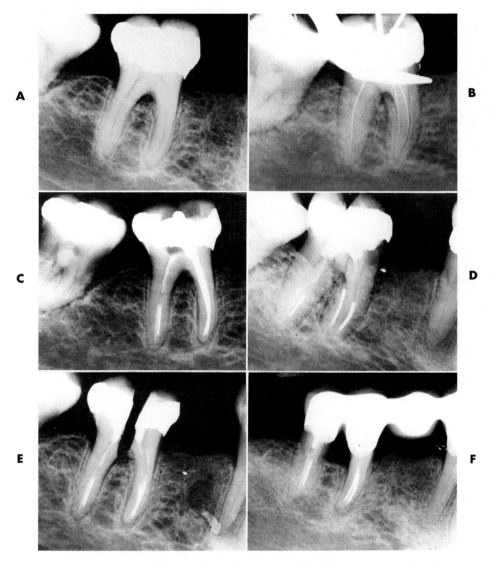

Fig. 12-30.   Bicuspidization with orthodontic separation of roots. **A,** Preoperative film of mandibular first molar with extensive restoration, early furcal invasion, and symptoms of pulpitis present. **B,** Film of initial files in place for calculation of working length. A second distal canal was located subsequently. **C,** Completion of endodontic treatment with distobuccal canal filled with laterally condensed gutta-percha, distolingual canal filled with silver point by twist-off technique (Chapter 9), and mesial canals filled with silver points extending into chamber. **D,** Four years later, the furcation area has worsened, although the tooth has been generally comfortable. It was decided to separate the two roots to open up the furcation for better home care by the patient. Accordingly, the silver points in the mesial canals were removed, the canals widened one full size, and new silver points placed by the twist-off technique. Angled view of this fill is shown. **E,** Using the vertical-cut technique with a silver point (Fig. 12-25), the two roots are separated. Because of the absence of adjacent teeth, the distal root could be uprighted orthodontically quite easily. **F,** Twenty years after original treatment and 16 years after bicuspidization, the area looks excellent. Because of the space between the separated roots, the patient is able to maintain the open furcation in a relatively healthy state. (Restoration by Dr. Rod Nystul, formerly of Park Ridge, Ill., and periodontics by Dr. Harry Staffileno, Chicago.)

distal as the larger root. Because of its size and the deep mesial and distal concavities that it contains, the mesial root is able to stand strongly in a splinted situation, either with the second molar (Fig. 12-28) or with the bicuspids anterior to it (Fig. 12-29).

This has been verified in articles by Gher and Vernino and Anderson et al. They demonstrated that the mesial root of the mandibular first molar has much greater circumferential surface area for potential periodontal ligament attachment than does the distal root.

A variant of the mandibular molar has two distinct distal roots, and such an occurrence may be verified by radiographs from mesial and distal angles. The additional root is lingual to the larger

distobuccal root and is often curved. If both distal roots must be amputated, both buccal and lingual flaps are required. Because of the curvature of the distolingual root when present and the excellent retention that it offers, it is usually best to amputate the single mesial root and retain the two distal roots to relieve a periodontal condition.

Bicuspidization. Through bicuspidization a single molar tooth can be converted into two bicuspids. Indications for the procedure are severe bone destruction in the bifurcation but excellent support on the nonfurca sides of each root (Fig. 12-30) or severe destruction of tooth structure in the furcation area. If both roots are to be retained, there should be a considerable spread between them for restorative procedures to be successful. If

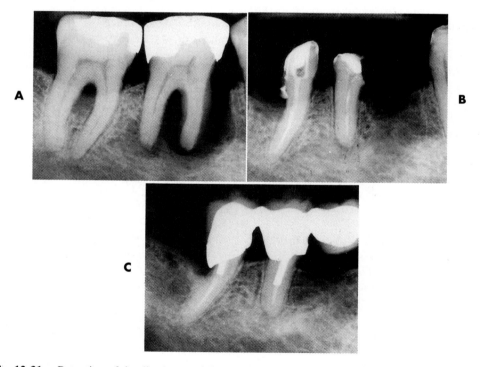

Fig. 12-31.   Retention of the distal root of the mandibular first molar and the mesial root of the second molar. **A,** Radiograph of mandibular molar area indicating massive bone loss associated with the mesial root of the first molar, a probable periapical abscess due to pulpal death on the distal root of the first molar, and a through-and-through furcation involvement of the second molar. Even though the mesial root is often more valuable than the distal root of the first molar, the bone loss is too great to retain the mesial root here. The distal root can be treated. By keeping the mesial root of the second molar, the roots to be retained will compliment each other in regard to retentive qualities. **B,** With this in mind, the two chosen roots were treated endodontically, post space created, and the unwanted roots amputated. **C,** Six years later, the retained roots function very well as a single molar created from two molars. But now the mesial root of the new molar is a distal root and the distal root of the new molar is a mesial root. (Restorations by Dr. Stephen Potashnick, Chicago.)

a greater spread is needed and there is room to the distal, orthodontic movement may be employed to spring the distal root distally (Fig. 12-30) and give a more desirable interfurcal area that allows for efficient patient home care. If the spread is minimal, it is best to amputate the poorer root and restore accordingly.

The procedure involves making the vertical cut after silver point placement. The crowns and furcation areas are trimmed with the diamond stone. The restoration will include two separate post-and-core crowns with a superstructure that allows for adequate hygiene in the area. (See Chapter 17.)

Retaining the distal root of the first molar with the mesial root of the second molar. As stated above, the mesial root of the mandibular first molar has considerably more area available for periodontal ligament attachment than does the distal root. When a furcation defect is present that affects both roots equally, it is far better to amputate the weaker distal root and retain the mesial root.

However, in some cases the periodontal condition is so bad for the mesial root that its retention is precluded (Fig. 12-31, *A*). If the second molar is very weak or missing, this distal root can act as a posterior abutment with proper restoration (Figs. 12-6, 12-7, and 12-27). If the second molar is strong, it probably would be best to extract such a first molar, rather than use this short, straight root as an abutment. In some cases, the second molar also is involved periodontally. If a furcation defect is present, a favorable situation may be created by amputating the distal root of the second molar.

The resulting combination of the distal root of the first molar and the mesial root of the second molar, splinted together and attached anteriorly to replace the removed mesial root of the first molar offers one of the most retentive conditions available following root amputation (Fig. 12-31). The result is another molar; only this time the mesial root of the new molar is really a distal root whereas the distal root of the new molar is really a mesial root. The new mesial root curves to the distal and then to the mesial, and the new distal root curves first to the mesial and then to the distal (Fig. 12-31, *C*). Since most mandibular first molars and virtually all second molars have roots that curve towards each other, the resultant molar created here has roots curving away from each other, producing a retentive combination superior to either of the original molars. Much more bone

is present between these two roots of the new molar than were present between the roots of the old molars (compare Fig. 12-31, *A* with *C*).

POSTOPERATIVE INSTRUCTIONS

If a flap has been raised, the same postoperative instructions should be given that were listed in Chapter 11. If the root has been amputated for periodontal reasons without a flap, postoperative discomfort is usually minimal, and instructions should be the same as those given for a simple extraction. In the latter case postoperative bleeding, common for periodontally involved teeth, may cause alarm to the patient. Therefore instructions should include a statement that hot liquids must be avoided for the first day after surgery.

TREATMENT PLANNING PROBLEMS IN ROOT AMPUTATION CASES

Difficulties encountered in determining when amputation is needed. It is most desirable to amputate a periodontally involved root after the canals of the roots that are to remain have been sealed. In most cases careful diagnosis and periodontal evaluation make it possible to ascertain in advance when a root will require amputation. However, in certain cases it becomes extremely difficult to determine whether a root amputation will be necessary or which root will require such a procedure prior to the retraction of tissue during periodontal surgery. Most often these situations occur in maxillary molars, in which trifurcations are more difficult to probe and radiograph than bifurcations.

If a question arises as to which root of a maxillary molar will be amputated during periodontal surgery, it is a simple matter to have all three roots filled in advance and to make the choice with the area surgically exposed (Fig. 12-32). However, it is not unusual for a serious defect to develop between the maxillary first and second molars that requires amputation of either the distal root of the first molar or the mesial root of the second molar. The final decision might require waiting until the time of surgical exposure for an unimpeded view of the area for best evaluation. In some cases periodontal defect is quite severe, and it is not certain that the affected tooth or teeth can be retained under any circumstances. To put the patient through the treatment time and expense of canal of canal fillings on all roots prior to surgery seems incorrect.

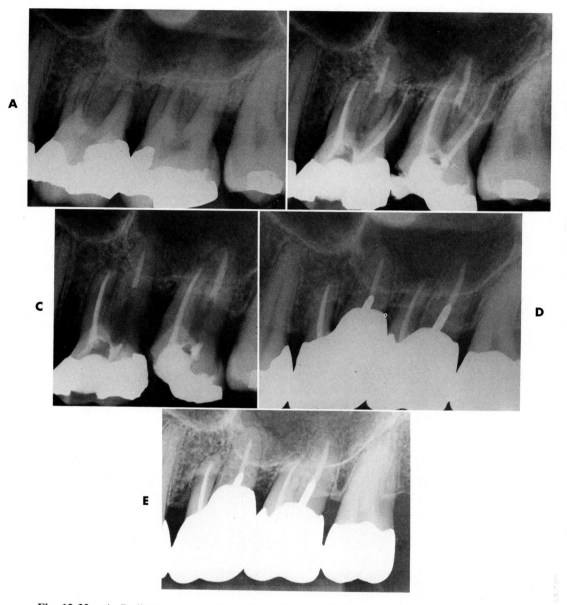

Fig. 12-32. **A,** Radiograph of maxillary left molar area. Considerable bone loss is associated with distal roots of first and second molars. Both teeth also have deep restorations. **B,** All canals were prepared and filled with laterally condensed gutta-percha, and post room was prepared. Case is now referred to the periodontist. **C,** During a flapped periodontal procedure, distobuccal roots were amputated. **D,** Four years later, area looks excellent. **E,** Eight years after original treatment. (Periodontics by Dr. Harry Staffileno and restoration by Dr. Irving Fishman, both of Chicago.)

To solve some of these problems when the exact course of treatment is undetermined prior to surgery, I suggest that the pulps in the involved teeth be extirpated and the canals measured prior to the surgical appointment (Fig. 12-33, *B*). This further verifies that the root or roots to be retained

are negotiable and treatable at a later date. It is very undesirable to have a retained root that proves to be untreatable endodontically when amputation procedures on that same tooth have already been performed. Following this initial endodontic therapy, the entire access cavity is

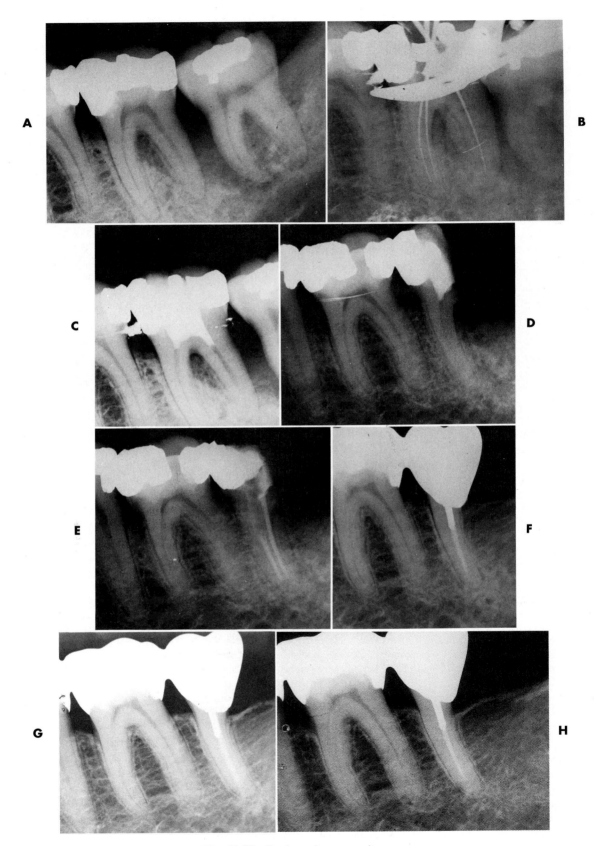

Fig. 12-33. For legend see opposite page.

closed with ZOE to which one drop of formocresol has been added (Fig. 12-33, *C*). This allows the periodontist to remove one root or extract the tooth with a minimal investment of time and finances (Fig. 12-33, *D*). If amputation procedures were performed, the endodontics is completed a short time later (Fig. 12-33, *E*) without the problems that attend retained vital tissues near the amputation site.

In come cases the periodontist may determine that all roots are to be retained (Fig. 12-34). The endodontist may regret that treatment was initiated at all, but I believe that a high percentage of such periodontally involved teeth have pulpal damage (Chapter 13) and so the treatment was merely performed earlier and the long-term outlook is favorable.

Under any circumstances some cases develop in which the amputation need is virtually impossible to ascertain prior to surgery. In these instances it is better to perform the amputation immediately with the vital pulp than to halt surgery, have the endodontics performed, and reenter later. I do recommend that endodontic emergency treatment be performed in these instances at the surgical appointment.

Problems of vital root amputation. Certain problems do occur if no pulpal treatment is performed at the time of the surgery. The exposed pulp may become inflamed and an acute pulpitis transpire, causing pain in addition to the postoperative discomfort that normally follows periodontal surgery. If a chronic pulpitis is present, as it might be in a periodontally involved tooth, the further trauma to the injured pulp might cause a severe exacerbation. Because of the close relationship between the pulp and the periodontal structures, the healing of the periodontal condition might be adversely affected by the inflamed pulp. Also, it might be more difficult to perform the endodontic

therapy with a severe contamination of the pulp by way of the open site due to the amputation.

To avoid these problems, it is suggested that endodontic emergency treatment be performed when a root is amputated from a periodontally involved but untreated tooth. The objectives of this emergency treatment would be to remove the part of the pulp that might initiate a painful condition and to seal off the portion of the tooth through which microorganisms might enter.

Technique for emergency treatment following vital root amputation. The instruments and supplies needed for this emergency procedure are those required for the initial access appointment and are listed in Chapter 5. The procedure given here applies to the maxillary molars, where the need is most frequent. Usually the amputated root in maxillary molars is either of the buccal roots. The modifications required for mandibular molars will follow.

It is necessary to provide for supplemental anesthesia to ensure the greater depth required for pulp tissue removal. Immediately following completion of the surgical procedure, a rubber dam is applied, using a routine maxillary molar clamp. The correct access for the tooth is prepared, and the orifices to the canals are located with the explorer. A small broach is selected and the pulp extirpated from the palatal canal. If sufficient width is present in the remaining buccal canal, a small broach may be inserted until just short of binding and the portion of the pulp that it reaches is extirpated. If the canal is too narrow, no instrumentation should be performed at this time, since partial canal enlargement might leave irritated pulpal remnants to cause postoperative discomfort.

A cotton pellet is dampened with formocresol and placed over the orifice to the roots that remain. A thick mix of ZOE, accelerated with zinc acetate

Fig. 12-33. **A,** Preoperative radiograph of mandibular molar area. Third molar is hopeless, and extensive bone loss associated with distal root of second molar makes that tooth extremely questionable. **B,** Pulp is extirpated, and working lengths are established. This verifies that it should be possible to complete treatment if a root amputation is utilized. **C,** No further therapy is performed, but chamber is completely sealed with ZOE plus a drop of formocresol. If tooth is extracted, there has been minimal investment of time and money by the patient. **D,** Distal root was amputated during periodontal surgery. Mesial canals were not contaminated because entire access was closed. **E,** Endodontics completed on mesial root. **F,** Four years later, area is restored by splinting of the mesial root to the first molar. **G,** Eight years after original treatment. **H,** Sixteen years after original treatment, entire area. (Periodontics by Dr. Henry Staffileno and restorations by Dr. Irving Fishman, both of Chicago.)

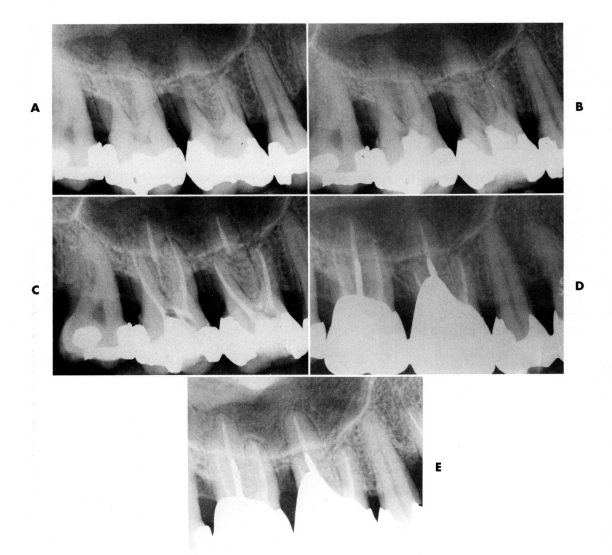

Fig. 12-34. **A,** Radiograph of maxillary right molar area. First and second molars had extensive bone loss associated with distobuccal roots. Deep restorations were present. **B,** pulps were extirpated, working lengths of all canals determined, and access cavities closed with ZOE plus formocresol. **C,** At surgical appointment the periodontist thought that all roots could be kept. Therefore the endodontics was completed. **D,** Four years later. **E,** Eight years after original treatment. Endodontics was required on the first bicuspid, and the periodontal condition soon may necessitate amputation of the distobuccal root of the first molar. (Periodontics by Dr. Harry Staffileno and restorations by Dr. Irving Fishman, both of Chicago.)

crystals, is prepared. The ZOE is placed in the access cavity in small quantities by using the plunger portion of the plastic instrument to pack the material into the opening caused by the amputation. When sufficient temporary filling has been placed to seal both the access cavity and the amputated root, the dam is removed and any excess that has extruded is trimmed. The patient may be safely rescheduled for completion of the endodontic therapy without fear of a painful episode due to the injured pulp.

Modification for mandibular molars. If a mandibular molar requires vital root amputation, the direct access to the pulp is usually present by virtue of the removal of one of the roots; but it may require enlarging for better visualization and instrumentation. The rubber dam is applied, using a bicuspid rather than a molar clamp. If the mesial half is removed, a broach is used to remove the pulp tissue from the distal canal. Care should be taken to examine the orifice to see if two canals are present. Removing the tissue from one canal but merely irritating the other distal canal may cause considerable postoperative pain.

If the distal root has been removed, the mesial canals are generally too narrow to permit broaching of the tissue. As with maxillary molars, a cotton pellet is dampened with formocresol and placed over the orifices. A mix of ZOE, accelerated with zinc acetate crystals, is prepared and used to close the access, and the patient is given another appointment.

REFERENCES

Amen CR: Hemisection and root amputation, *Periodontics* 4:197, 1966.

Anderson RW, McGarrah HE, Lamb RD, Eick JD: Root surface measurements of mandibular molars using stereophotogrammetry, *J Am Dent Assoc* 107:613, 1983.

Ash MM: *Wheeler's dental anatomy, physiology and occlusion*, ed 7, Philadelphia, 1992, Saunders.

Basaraba N: Root amputation and tooth hemisection, *Dent Clin North Am* 13:121, 1969.

Bergenholtz A: Radectomy of multirooted teeth, *J Am Dent Assoc* 85:870, 1972.

Black GV: In Litch W: *The American system of dentistry,* Philadelphia, 1866, Lea Brothers.

Black GV: *Descriptive anatomy of the human teeth,* ed. 4, Philadelphia, 1902, The S.S. White Dental Manufacturing Co.

Gher ME, and Vernino AR: Root morphology—clinical significance in pathogenesis and treatment of periodontal disease, *J Am Dent Assoc* 101:627, 1980.

Green EN: Hemisection and root amputation, *J Am Dent Assoc* 112:511, 1986.

Hiatt WH: Regeneration via flap operation and the pulpal periodontal lesion, *Periodontics* 4:205, 1966.

Hoag PM, Weine FS, Healey HJ: Measurements of the mesiobuccal of the maxillary first molar as related to the crown of the tooth. (Unpublished data.)

Kirchoff DA, Gerstein H: Presurgical crown contouring for root amputation procedures, *Oral Surg* 27:379, 1969.

Langer B, Stein SD, Wagenberg B: An evaluation of root resections: a ten year study, *J Periodontol* 52:719, 1981.

Sharp GC: The historical aspects of the pulpless tooth question, *J Am Dent Assoc* 24:1231, 1937.

Staffileno HJ: Surgical management of the furca invasion, *Dent Clin North Am* 13:103, 1969.

Weine FS, Healey HJ, Gerstein H, Evanson L: Canal configuration in the mesio-buccal root of the maxillary first molar and its endodontic significance, *Oral Surg* 28:419, 1969.

13 Endodontic-periodontal problems

The close relationship between endodontics and periodontics is firmly established. Endodontics may be thought of as periapical periodontics, since the maintenance of or the return to normal in the periapical tissues of the treated tooth is required. To explore further the close relationship, a consideration of the aspects of periodontal disease is necessary. Periodontal disease is defined as a disease of the supporting structures of the tooth. Those supporting structures are the alveolar bone, the components of the periodontal ligament, and the gingiva. It is obvious that these same structures—alveolar bone, components of the periodontal ligament, and gingiva—may be affected by pulpal disease.

Products of inflammation emanating from the pulp exit into the periodontal structures by way of the apical foramen and any existing auxiliary canals. Loss of or disease in the hard or soft tissues may cause inflammation in the periodontal ligament, affecting the vessels entering the apical foramen. Severe mobility in teeth may cause sufficient movement to crush or tear apical vessels, leading to alteration in the nutrition to the pulp. Certain procedures required for periodontal therapy may cause pulp damage.

Periodontal and pulpal diseases have some common clinical symptoms, most notably tenderness to percussion and swelling. Either disease may mimic the other, clinically or radiographically. Therefore an accurate diagnosis of the etiologic factors involved is needed for the correct course of treatment.

The basic area of dental treatment, that of restorative dentistry, is also closely involved. Aspects of periodontics are required in any of the restorative aspects of dentistry, from the simple Class II

I acknowledge the assistance of Dr. Harry Staffileno, Jr., Professor of Periodontics, University of Illinois College of Dentistry, Chicago, in the formulation of some of the philosophies stated in this chapter.

amalgam, which must have proper contour and contact, to the complex periodontal prosthesis. Similarly, any restorative procedure may cause some degree of pulp damage, which may be reflected by disease in the periodontal tissues.

Thus it may be seen that despite the segmentation of dentistry into the various areas of specialization, any dentist performing restorative dentistry, periodontal or endodontic therapy, either singly or in any combination, is automatically involved in all three.

CLASSIFICATION OF ENDODONTIC-PERIODONTAL PROBLEMS

Because of the close relationship between endodontics and periodontics, various classifications have been suggested to divide the types of cases that may require combined or single therapy. Just as in the delineation of pulpal diseases, much disagreement exists as to a correct classification that is consistent with histologic and clinical situations commonly encountered. I wish to suggest here a classification that is clinically oriented and that will be accurate in determining the correct method of therapy required.

Types of endodontic-periodontal problems. The classification is based on the fact that four types of endodontic-periodontal cases are commonly encountered. Divisions of the cases are based on the etiology of the disease, which determines the type of therapy required and the probable prognosis. The types are as follows:

Class I—tooth in which symptoms clinically and radiographically simulate periodontal disease but are in fact due to pulpal inflammation and/or necrosis

Class II—tooth that has both pulpal or periapical disease and periodontal disease concomitantly

Class III—tooth that has no pulpal problem but requires endodontic therapy plus root amputation to gain periodontal healing

Class IV—tooth that clinically and radiographically simulates pulpal or periapical disease but in fact has periodontal disease

Class I. The definition of periodontal disease just given states that the disease process occurs in the alveolar bone, components of the periodontal ligament, or the gingiva. If this definition is accepted, the teeth involved in Class I endodontic-periodontal problems are involved with periodontal disease. These teeth typically exhibit one or more of the following symptoms, all of which are suggestive of periodontal disease: mobility, bone loss in the furcation or adjacent to crestal bone, pocket depth, tenderness to percussion, chronic draining sinus tract (fistula), purulent exudate from the gingival sulcus, and foul taste.

The problem is that the definition given does not consider the etiology of the disease. In Class I endodontic-periodontal problems the etiology of the disease is from the pulp, and if periodontal therapy is performed without consideration of the pulpal problem, a desirable degree of healing will never occur. Only when the tissues and debris from the pulp canals are removed and a satisfactory canal filling is placed will the condition in the supporting structures be improved.

Because the more obvious clinical symptoms that these teeth manifest are typical of periodontal disease, diagnosis of the true problem is difficult unless a careful examination is performed. The most significant sign that an endodontic problem rather than a periodontal problem is present is that the patient does not have periodontal disease in other areas of the mouth. Because of the nature of the disease, it is rare that a severe periodontal lesion will be found involving only one isolated tooth, with all other areas relatively normal. When this occurs, examination for possible pulp damage must be performed before any periodontal therapy is instituted.

The presence of a pulpotomy, pulp capping, large restoration approximating the pulp, deep carious lesion, or considerable dimunution of the pulp canal space are all strong signs that an endodontic problem is present. The use of an electric pulp tester may be helpful but is not completely diagnostic, particularly if a multirooted tooth is involved. On the other hand, if a tooth with a severe periodontal lesion has no restoration or has one of only minimal size, is caries-free, has no fracture, and has a normal response to electric pulp testing, it must be assumed that periodontal therapy is required. As will be pointed out in the discussion on Class II endodon-

tic-periodontal problems, extensive periodontal lesions may cause pulp damage and require combined therapy, that is, endodontics and periodontics, to gain optimal results.

These defects probe with a periodontal probe identically to those of true periodontal defects. Some have suggested that in cases where the tissue depth is relatively normal for much of the periphery of the root but then suddenly a rapid plunge is discovered, the pocket is of endodontic origin. When there is a wide as well as deep pocket, extending for a considerable distance around the root, then the pocket is of periodontal origin. On the contrary, I have found many cases in which the pocket proved to be of endodontic origin when there was considerable measured depth of 180 degrees or more around the root, just as might occur in a purely periodontal defect (Fig. 13-1).

Unlike most periodontal lesions, Class I endodontic-periodontal problems are characterized by a rapid healing process and thus have an excellent prognosis. Often the clinical symptoms disappear after the initial canal debridement appointment. This is particularly impressive when a pocket depth of 8 to 10 mm present before treatment can be probed no more than 2 mm after only one appointment, a result rarely, if ever, found so rapidly in routine periodontal therapy. Also, in periodontal cases a result is considered acceptable when no further bone loss, as determined by radiograph and pocket probe, develops after therapy. In Class I endodontic-periodontal problems the bone damage, noted radiographically before treatment, is repaired and new mineralization is demonstrable routinely in postoperative x-ray films after 1 year or more. In fact, when a time lapse of 1 month or more takes place between the initial canal debridement and the completion of endodontic treatment in these cases, the radiographic appearance on the final canal filling film usually discloses a considerable improvement in the bone picture.

In summary, the Class I case looks as if periodontic therapy is needed but is really caused by pulp damage, requires endodontic therapy only, heals rapidly, and has an excellent prognosis (Fig. 13-2).

The longevity for these cases is quite excellent as well. In teeth with severe periodontal involvement the long-term outlook is guarded at best. However, in Class I endodontic-periodontal problems, once the lesion heals, the long-term prognosis is favorable. The reason for this is easily

Text continued on p. 646.

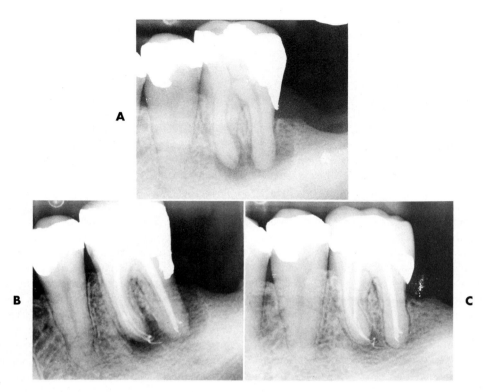

Fig. 13-1.   **A,** Preoperative film of mandibular molar, with pocket completely circling distal root from its buccal furcation around the distal to the lingual furcation. Pockets could be probed in multiple areas from 6 to 10 mm. Mesial root had periapical lesion; pulp was completely necrotic. **B,** Slightly angled view from the mesial, indicating canal filling with laterally condensed gutta-percha. Pockets could not be probed after appointment to prepare canals. **C,** One year later, distal root has healed beautifully, with bone returned all around the root and no probing possible. (Restoration by Dr. Ascher Jacobs, formerly of Chicago.)

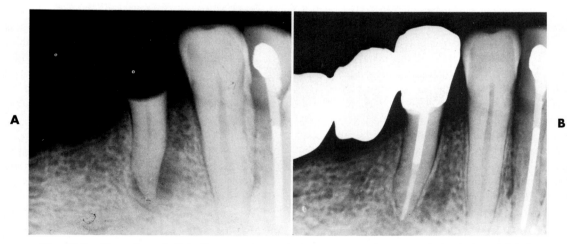

Fig. 13-2.   Examples of clinically appearing periodontal lesions that are endodontic in origin. **A,** Pocket to apex on mesial portion of a bicuspid. Patient was 87 years old. **B,** Four years later, after endodontic treatment, no periodontal treatment, and fixed bridge construction. (Restoration by Dr. Leon Rosenfeld, formerly of Chicago.)

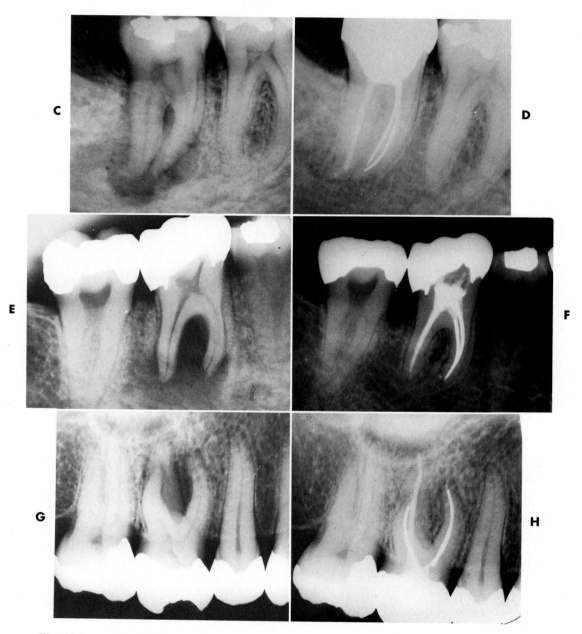

Fig. 13-2, cont'd.   C, Preoperative radiograph of mandibular second molar with a pocket to apex long distal root. **D,** Two years later, complete resolution after endodontic treatment and no periodontal treatment. (Restoration by Dr. W. Clinton Fisher, Chicago.) **E,** Bifurcation involvement of mandibular first molar. Tooth was mobile, and ball burnisher could be passed through furca. **F,** Three years later, after endodontic treatment only, complete healing has taken place. (Restoration by Dr. Sherwin Strauss, Chicago.) **G,** Trifurcation involvement of maxillary first molar. Pocket could be probed along buccal and mesiolingual surface of mesiobuccal root 8 to 10 mm. **H,** One year after endodontic treatment only.

Continued

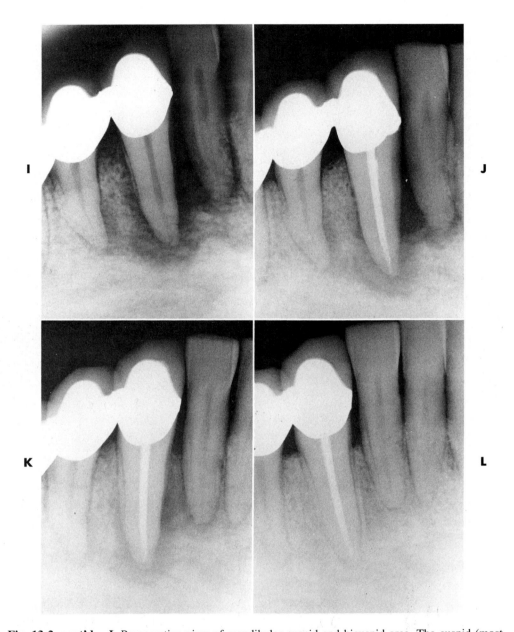

Fig. 13-2, cont'd.   I, Preoperative view of mandibular cuspid and bicuspid area. The cuspid (most mesial tooth in the splint) had a large periapical radiolucency, and the adjacent first bicuspid also seemed to have radiographic periapical involvement. The lateral incisor was quite mobile, but it was responsive to electric pulp testing. The cuspid and bicuspid could not be tested due to their veneer crowns. **J,** Endodontic treatment was completed on the cuspid, using routine procedures. The lateral tightened up immediately after the appointment for canal preparation on the cuspid. **K,** Three months later, the lateral was tight, no probing was possible between the two teeth, and it was decided that endodontic treatment on the bicuspid be postponed since the lesion appeared to be smaller. **L,** Four years after treatment, the periapical lesions have healed, and the lateral incisor remains without mobility.

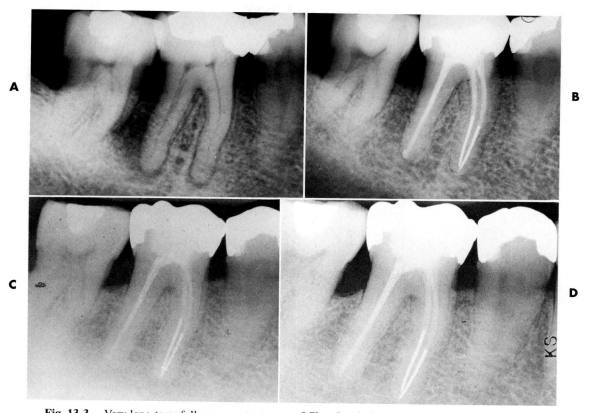

Fig. 13-3.   Very long-term follow-up on treatment of Class I endodontic-periodontal problem. **A,** Preoperative radiograph of mandibular molar area. Periodontal therapy had been performed on the distal root of the first molar for more than 1 year without any improvement. A pocket, probing 12 mm, surrounds the root from the mesiobuccal around the distal to the mesiolingual. The second molar also presents some periodontal bone loss. A response was obtained with an electric pulp tester, probably from the vital tissue in the mesial canals. Case was referred for endodontic treatment of the mesial root so that the distal root could be amputated. The retained mesial root would be used to help support the weak second molar. **B,** The distal canal was prepared at the first appointment without anesthetic, but the mesial canals were very vital and responsive to any manipulation. Therefore, the patient was seen 1 week later and given a mandibular block so that the mesial canals could be prepared. When the site where the distal pocket had been was probed, only a normal depth sulcus was present! Endodontic therapy was completed with no further periodontal treatment performed on this tooth. At the time of filling, I sectioned the silver points used to fill the mesial canals because I still feared a periodontal failure of the distal root and I wanted the availability of possible post room in the mesial canals should the distal root require amputation. The space above the silver points was filled with laterally condensed gutta-percha. This film was taken 18 months after treatment. Also note some excess gutta-percha and sealer extending to the radiographic apex of the distal root. **C,** Eleven years after original treatment, pocket depth has remained constant at between 2.5 and 3.5 mm. **D,** Seventeen years after treatment, bone level remains excellent.

Continued

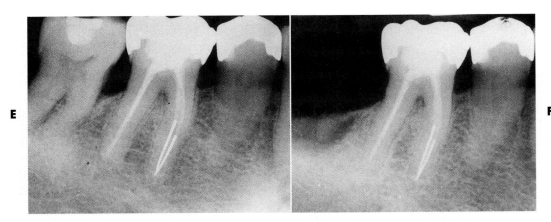

Fig. 13-3, cont'd.   E, Twenty-one years after original treatment, area still looks excellent. **F,** Twenty-six years after original treatment, the second molar had been extracted 1 year earlier for periodontal reasons, but the bone level is still quite acceptable on the distal surface of the distal root, compare with **A.** Also note that the gutta-percha filling in the apical portion of the distal root is now several mm shorter than it had been in **B,** due to sealer resorption and cementum apposition.

explained. These endodontic lesions will react in the same manner as a purely periapical lesion following proper endodontic therapy. The teeth shown in Figs. 13-3 and 10-6 are examples indicating healing and retained tissue normalcy of 20 or more years for such cases.

The major problem occurs when the dentist fails to identify the condition and incorrectly institutes periodontal therapy, assuming a periodontal problem (Fig. 13-3). If the roots are curetted and/or flap surgery is performed, it is possible that endodontic treatment, if later instituted, will be ineffective.

Class II.   Both pulpal and periodontal lesions may attack the same tooth. In these cases therapy in both areas is required to gain a satisfactory result (Fig. 13-4). Treating one phase and neglecting the other frequently retards the healing process for the area treated and may prevent any return to normalcy.

In combined lesions the prognosis for the periapical portion usually is superior to that for the periodontal portion. When a periapical lesion has healed after canal sealing, the incidence of recurrence is negligible. However, a periodontal lesion may recur after healing unless periodic maintenance treatment is carefully followed.

The criterion for diagnosis of Class II cases is that the patient *does* have periodontal disease in multiple areas of the mouth. If pulp damage or death occurs in a tooth already involved with a periodontal problem, a Class II situation has developed.

A high percentage of teeth that have two-thirds or more periodontal bone loss will also have pulp damage, even if no (or minimal) restorative work has been done. When periodontal therapy only is performed on these cases, the damaged pulp tissue may prevent the full degree of periodontal healing. Only when combined therapy is tendered will desirable healing transpire (Fig. 13-5). As will be discussed more fully later, the presence of a vital response to electric pulp testing does not ensure that a normal pulp is present in these cases.

It is a common practice among some dentists involved in reconstructive procedures on teeth with considerable periodontal damage to have endodontic therapy performed on mandibular anterior teeth with normal-appearing pulps prior to splinting. The chance is good that, prior to any treatment, some degree of pulp damage is present. By the time that periodontal flaps have been raised, roots scaled, crowns prepared, impressions taken, temporary fillings placed, and splints cemented, a considerably greater degree of pulp damage has occurred.

Should endodontic therapy become necessary after the splint is seated, because of either pain or the development or a periapical lesion, treatment is much more difficult than it would have been at the outset. Mandibular anterior teeth rarely have perfect alignment prior to being splinted, whereas the splints usually are constructed to make each abutment adjacent to its neighbor. Therefore there are no clues from the exterior topography of the crown as

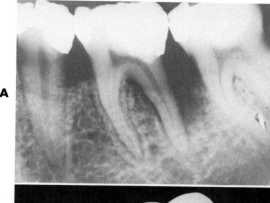

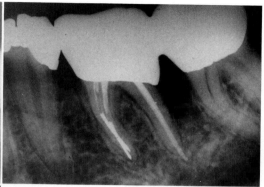

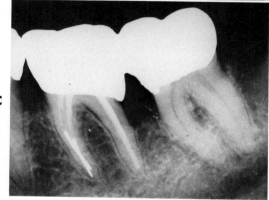

Fig. 13-4.   A, Preoperative radiograph of mandibular first molar with considerable distal bone loss. Pulp was responsive to electric testing, but periodontist insisted on both endodontic and periodontal therapy for optimal results. At the time of extirpation, pulp appeared to have little vitality. **B,** Two years later, periodontal treatment has restored a considerable portion of bone loss. **C,** Twelve years after original treatment, pocket depth has remained constant at 2 to 3 mm. Note complete resorption of excess gutta-percha that had been beyond distal apex. (Periodontal therapy by Dr. Erwin Barrington, Chicago, and restorations by Dr. Ascher Jacobs, formerly of Chicago.)

to the true position of the pulp canal. In an attempt to find the canal orifice, much gouging or ditching may be necessary, particularly if a chronic pulpitis has produced a considerable amount of reparative dentin. The weakening of the interior walls of the crown preparation may cause the treated tooth to break loose from the splint, become susceptible to recurrent decay, and lose periodontal support. Worse yet, during attempts to find the canal, a perforation into the periodontal ligament may occur, which would necessitate a surgical repair and leave a severely weakened member of the splint.

It is much easier on both the patient and the dentist to anticipate the possibility of future pulp damage and have endodontic therapy performed initially. Any inflamed or degenerating pulp tissue is removed, and the canals are sealed while access and vision are maximal. The severe tenderness to temperature changes frequently experienced during periodontal therapy is avoided. The teeth are prepared for crowns painlessly and splinted, with the pulp canals available for posts and cores should greater retention be required. The possibility of a painful pulpitis or periapicitis after splinting is similarly avoided (Fig. 13-6).

Summarizing Class II endodontic-periodontal problems, the diagnosis is dependent on determining that periodontal problems are present elsewhere in the mouth and that a pulpal pathosis is also present in the tooth in question. This pulpal problem may be coincidental to the periodontal lesion or may be due to the degree of periodontal damage. However, once the pulp has been sufficiently damaged in the latter case, relieving the periodontal problem will not result in pulpal healing. Thus it is similar to an irreversible pulpitis resulting from a carious lesion, operative procedure, or pulp exposure where the pulp has lost its recuperative powers and requires endodontic therapy to retain the tooth. In Class II endodontic-periodontal problems both endodontic and periodontal therapies are required to gain optimal healing. The prognosis for the endodontic portion of the problem may be slightly superior, since there is little if any chance for recurrence, whereas the periodontal problem must receive regular maintenance (Fig. 13-7). The exact methods for treating the three types of cases involving combined therapy will be discussed later in this chapter.

Class III.   The techniques for root amputations and the implications of the anatomy of the furcation region were discussed in the previous

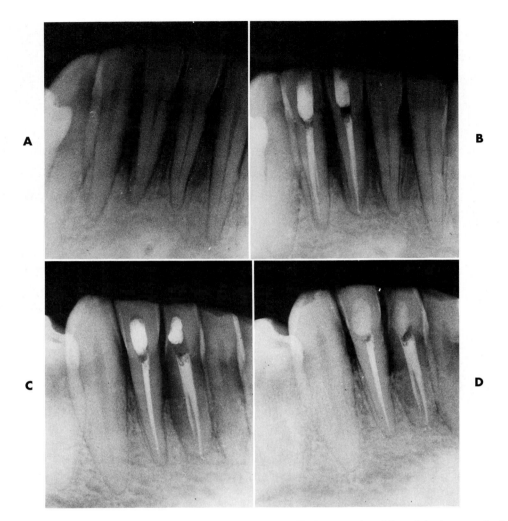

Fig. 13-5.   A, Extensive periodontal lesion between mandibular central and lateral incisors, probed approximately 8 mm, was unaffected by several forms of periodontal therapy. Both teeth responded to electric pulp testing. **B,** Endodontic therapy was performed, and two canals were located in each tooth. Pocket depth had not appreciably altered when endodontic treatment was completed. **C,** Further periodontal therapy was instituted, and pocket depth decreased to approximately 2 mm. Film taken 3 months after completion of endodontics. **D,** One year after completion, interproximal area has continued to heal. (Endodontics by Dr. Charles Neach and periodontics by Dr. Harry Staffileno, both of Chicago.)

chapter. In Class III endodontic-periodontal problems, endodontic therapy and root amputation are required to gain healing of a periodontal-only problem. That the use of an endodontic procedure produces healing of an area of periodontal disease only serves to emphasize further the important interrelationship of these two elements of dentistry.

The typical indication for root amputation is a severe periodontal defect around one root of a multirooted tooth while the other roots have healthy support. In these cases no further periodontal therapy may be required in the area after amputation of the involved root. The pulp may appear to be perfectly normal in these situations but must be sacrificed to retain the tooth. In actuality many pulps of teeth with this problem show some degree of pulpal inflammation when viewed histologically after extirpation. Even if the pulp were relatively normal at the time of removal, allowing the periodontal process to continue unimpeded by treatment would certainly cause an

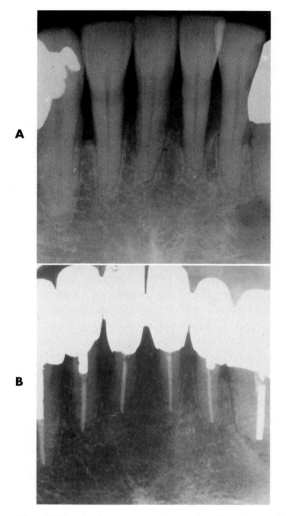

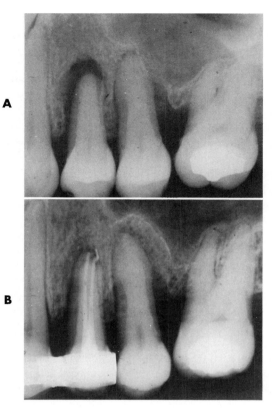

Fig. 13-7. A, Maxillary first bicuspid had a pocket around apex from mesial portion of root. Pulp was nonvital to electric testing. **B,** Endodontic treatment included debridement and filling of canals, but only minor periodontal treatment was performed. One year later, periapical portion of the lesion had healed but a 6 mm pocket persisted.

Fig. 13-6. A, Lower anterior teeth of patient with advanced periodontal disease in need of multiple complex dental procedures. Treatment plan called for provisional splinting, extensive periodontal surgery, and permanent splinting. Endodontic therapy was performed on incisors prior to any other treatment. **B,** Seven years later, the area looks excellent. (Endodontic therapy by Dr. Harold Gerstein, periodontal therapy by Dr. Harry Staffileno, Jr., and restorations by Dr. Jacob Lippert, all of Chicago.)

increased loss of bony support on the adjacent roots and probably pulp damage later.

Two theories exist concerning the timing of root amputation for periodontally involved teeth. One theory recommends that the amputation be performed at the same time that periodontal surgery is scheduled for that quadrant. In this way two surgical procedures need not be performed on one site, and the patient is limited to one postoperative recuperation period. The other theory suggests that the root amputation be performed prior to the periodontal surgery. Since many amputations are accomplished without the raising of a flap when a periodontally involved root is removed, the postoperative period is usually free of pain. After the amputation some degree of periodontal healing transpires, allowing for better evaluation when it is time for periodontal therapy.

In the introduction to the chapter on root amputations (Chapter 12), the diminishing role of root amputation among current dental procedures was discussed. Two factors were given for this change in therapy: (1) problems with long-term success of teeth treated with amputational therapy and (2) popularity and success, at least at this time, of guided tissues regeneration (GTR) procedures, which provided regeneration of lost periodontal structures without any root amputation and, often, without any endodontic treatment.

The prevailing view in periodontal therapy until recently was that periodontitis was not reversible, and the object of treatment was to halt destructive forces and prevent the disease from worsening. In few and far between cases, regeneration was claimed, but could not always be substantiated or anticipated in advance. Then, with the advent of GTR and the interest and research that has accompanied it, the objective of periodontal treatment has taken a remarkable, and very favorable, turn.

What the future will bring, no one can say, but it is my opinion that treatment of periodontal disease with root amputation, and, thus, Class III endodontic-periodontal problems, will continue to decline as a viable course of therapy. GTR appears to be an excellent alternative choice, being less destructive of existing tooth structures, being regenerative rather than adding to bone loss, and probably requiring less time and costs to patients. Considering that some of the amputational cases turned out less than desirable merely tips the balance further toward GTR.

Assuming that these views are accurate, I also might add that I believe that many more clinicians will find that teeth with advanced periodontal dis-

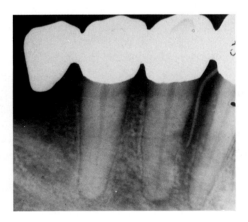

Fig. 13-8. Patient was referred with chronic draining sinus tract between mandibular cuspid and first bicuspid that appeared to be typical of periapical origin. Tract was traced with a gutta-percha cone to ascertain which tooth required endodontic treatment, since the splint prevented pulp testing. Cone went into a tortuous tract between the teeth and indicated a periodontal lesion. Periodontal therapy only was performed, and the area healed.

ease will have improved healing with GTR and endodontic therapy. Thus, the loss of Class III cases will, to some extent, produce more treatment of Class II endodontic-periodontal problems.

In summary, Class III endodontic-periodontal problems are those that require endodontic treatment plus root amputation to gain a periodontal result, even if no pulp damage is present in the involved tooth prior to treatment. (See Chapter 12.)

Class IV. The cases that fall into this classification are those that simulate an endodontic problem but in reality are due to periodontal disease. Although some of these cases might be considered Class II endodontic-periodontal problems for which both endodontic and periodontal therapy are required, Class IV endodontic-periodontal cases are those in which the periodontal condition is the only or the predominant problem. The difficulties occur when endodontic treatment only is performed without sufficient recognition of the periodontal disease. In the time required for completion of the endodontic therapy, the periodontal damage continues untreated.

Some of the symptoms of pulpal or periapical disease may be due to periodontal damage. A chronic draining sinus tract may lead to a periodontal pocket rather than a periapical lesion. As bone and soft tissue support is lost because of periodontal disease, affected teeth may become sensitive to changes in temperature, which might be misdiagnosed as an irreversible pulpitis. Tenderness to percussion, mobility, and swelling are other common symptoms of periodontal disease that may be confused with pulpal or periapical disease. Any of these clinical conditions might erroneously cause the initiation of endodontic therapy. Some of the symptoms might even be alleviated to some degree initially and reinforce the idea that a correct diagnosis has been made. However, unless periodontal therapy is simultaneously performed, the disease process will continue and cause further problems.

The diagnostic phase is extremely important since the etiology must be established prior to the institution of therapy. The mouth must be examined for the existence of periodontal disease in other areas. Its presence is an excellent indication that a Class II or IV endodontic-periodontal problem is involved.

If a chronic draining sinus tract is present, it must be traced by placing a gutta-percha cone into the tract's depth and taking a radiograph (Fig. 13-8). If the cone fails to point to or communicate with the apex, but rather falls into a periodontal pocket or cleft, the indication is of periodontal disease.

If a swelling is present, a pulp test is taken of the tooth in question. Although pulp vitality is not necessarily indicative of normalcy, nevertheless it is not a finding consistent with an acute periapical abscess and would strongly suggest the possibility of a lateral periodontal abscess. The gingival attachment should be probed and pocket depth examined. If a periodontal abscess is present, exudate will be expressed through the crevice.

Sensitivity to temperature changes is common in early stages of periodontal disease and after certain phases of therapy. When pulp damage is still reversible, this sensitivity usually diminishes in a few days, and a watch-and-wait attitude may be followed if the pain is not too severe. A desensitizing toothpaste may aid in a more rapid return to normal.

In contrast to the Class I endodontic-periodontal problem in which the postoperative radiograph indicates the initiation of healing, the Class IV case treated endodontically is characterized by a deteriorating condition. This is still another clue to the fact that the wrong avenue of therapy had been followed. The prognosis for the case is obviously poor unless periodontal therapy is started as soon as possible, assuming that sufficient periodontal support still exists.

In summary, the Class IV endodontic-periodontal problem appears to indicate the need for endodontic treatment but actually requires periodontal therapy. The clinical symptoms present at the start of therapy may be slightly improved after initial treatment but will soon return, and continued deterioration is noted

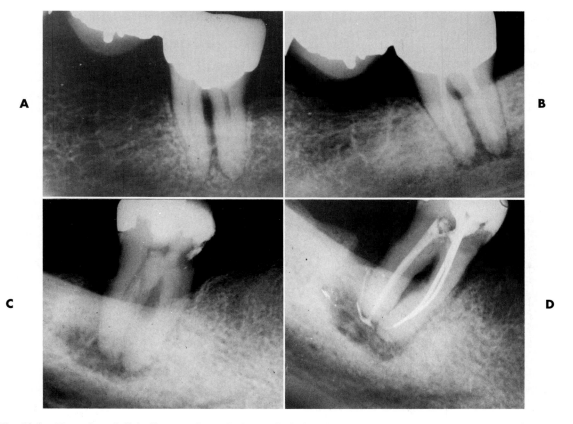

Fig. 13-9.   Examples of clinically appearing pulpal or periapical problems due to severe periodontal lesions. **A,** Patient referred for endodontic treatment of mandibular second molar with symptoms of sensitivity to temperature changes (really due to severe bone loss exposing root surfaces) and tenderness to percussion. **B,** Despite seemingly satisfactory canal fillings, the case deteriorated badly. Although patient exhibited pockets throughout the mouth, referring dentist refused to institute periodontal therapy until after the endodontic therapy was completed. Proper management would have included periodontal evaluation and initiation of treatment in all areas of periodontal destruction prior to completing endodontics. **C,** Periapical involvement of mandibular second molar was due to pulpal necrosis, but concomitant periodontal condition was hopeless. **D,** One month after therapy, endodontic treatment has not helped and tooth requires extraction.

as the case progresses. The prognosis is very poor unless periodontal treatment is also instituted. The key to solving the problem correctly is to make a correct diagnosis at the outset (Fig. 13-9 on p. 651).

EFFECT OF PERIODONTAL TISSUES ON PULP

A considerable portion of the literature has been devoted to a discussion of the effect of periodontal disease on the pulp. Among the papers are those by Cahn; Henrici and Hartzell; Seltzer, Bender, and Ziontz; Bender and Seltzer; Sinai; Mazur and Massler; Rubach and Mitchell (two papers); Stahl; and many others. A more complete bibliography appears at the end of this chapter.

Of all these papers, only two, those by Mazur and Massler and by Czarnecki and Schilder, disclaim any relationship of periodontal disease as a causative factor in pulpal disease. The others all state either that a relationship appears possible or that a definite correlation was found. Since the greater evidence appears to be on the positive side, until further and more definitive work to the contrary is published, it may be assumed that the interrelationship exists and must be taken into consideration in the treatment of patients with periodontal problems.

The following discussion will be concerned with the pathways and dynamics of such a relationship and followed by a discussion of the effects of the pulp on the periodontal structures.

Exposure or irritation through auxiliary canals. As periodontal disease extends from the gingival sulcus toward the apex, the inflammatory products attack the elements of the periodontal ligament and surrounding alveolar bone. If the tooth under attack has an auxiliary canal that is irritated by these inflammatory elements, pulpal inflammation may occur. More certainly, pulp damage will transpire if auxiliary canals are actually exposed to the oral environment as a result of loss of periodontal cloaking by extensive pocket depth. This type of exposure is just as serious as that caused by extensive caries (Fig. 13-10). In fact, because the diagnosis of a carious exposure is rather obvious on a radiograph, whereas this kind of exposure may be difficult to visualize, a frustrating clinical problem may develop. The tooth involved in the periodontal exposure may be caries free or restoration free, whereas the pocket may be tortuous and difficult to trace with a pocket probe. Yet the symptoms of a typical pulpitis may be unmistakable—tenderness to temperature change and percussion, particularly.

Only by meticulous examination is the truth discovered. Typically the patient will be able to pinpoint the involved tooth, and scratching of the root surface with an explorer evokes a severe response to the already inflamed pulp. If the auxiliary canal exists at a junction close enough to the gingival sulcus, it may even be directly located by probing.

If sufficient periodontal support remains, the tooth may respond favorably to endodontic and periodontal therapy and be classified as a Class II case. If the tooth has insufficient periodontal support, an extraction is indicated or an amputation of the root if a multirooted tooth is involved and there is a favorable situation available to retain the remainder of the tooth.

The irritation potential with a auxiliary canal may go in the other direction. If the pulp becomes necrotic in a tooth with a significant lateral canal in the cervical third of the root, a seemingly periodontal lesion may occur. Periodontal therapy will be ineffective because this again is a Class I type of condition. If endodontic therapy is correctly performed, the prognosis is good, and examination of the postfilling film probably will reveal sealer in the auxiliary canal (Fig. 13-11).

Furcation canals. The avenue of pulpal destruction by way of furcation canals is identical to that found with any type of auxiliary canal. In many instances the classical clinical symptoms of pulpal exposure will occur. In addition, some procedures involved in periodontal therapy such as ramping or use of pipe cleaners as debriders may further irritate any incipient inflammation or actually sever blood vessels communicating from the pulp to the periodontal ligament. If a patient with an open or closed furcation area displays the classic symptoms of a pulpitis, despite the absence of decay or extensive restoration, an endodontic procedure must be considered until another logical alternative is discovered.

Vital but not normal pulp. There is no doubt that the electric pulp tester is an important diagnostic tool, and its use in an endodontic evaluation is invaluable. However, when the pulp tester is used certain limitations of the instruments must always be considered before a final decision or treatment plan is made. Some of these limitations were discussed in Chapter 2.

Eliciting a response from a tooth with an electric pulp tester merely indicates that some vital nerve tissue probably is present within the pulp canal space. It may not be considered as any

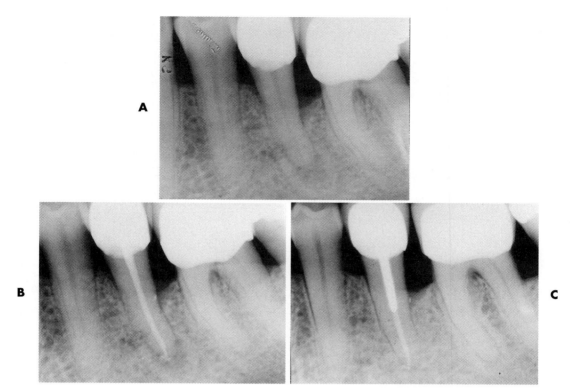

Fig. 13-10. Exposure via a lateral canal. **A,** Preoperative radiograph of mandibular bicuspid area indicating that the second bicuspid was restored with a porcelain-fused-to-metal crown, was quite mobile, and had a periapical lesion and a deep diagonal pocket on the distal. Because the patient did have other sites of advanced periodontal disease, endodontic treatment success did not appear very favorable. **B,** Nevertheless, treatment was instituted. The tooth tightened significantly and the pocket decreased in probing distance after the canal preparation appointment. This film was taken after canal filling with laterally condensed gutta-percha and Wach's paste, indicating a lateral canal at the distal in midroot, exactly to the site of the diagonal pocket. **C,** One year later, the tooth is firm, the periapical lesion has healed, and the pocket probes just to the site of the sealer in the lateral canal. It would appear that the pulp became exposed when the periodontal disease reached the lateral canal.

stronger statement than that, because some teeth with no vital pulp tissue but only gaseous material, as in a periapical abscess, have given positive responses.

Those who believe that pulp testing has considerable accuracy in disclosing the condition of pulp tissue recommend comparing the degree of current required to gain stimulation with the degree required to stimulate the conforming contralateral tooth. If less current is required, a hyperemic condition is present; if more current is needed, a degenerating condition is indicated; equal current requirements are said to suggest normalcy. There are obvious holes in this theory. The contralateral tooth itself may have degenerat-

ing tissue, considerable dentinal sclerosis, or a crown or other condition that would prevent or distort any comparison. A multirooted tooth may yield a response from a vital canal even when other canals are necrotic.

To clarify this matter further, an effort has been made by Weine et al. to determine the reliability of the electric pulp test in evaluating the pulpal condition of periodontally involved teeth. Over 200 teeth requiring endodontic treatment were selected, all of which responded positively within normal limits to the pulp tester when compared with a contralateral tooth. The pulps of these teeth were extirpated at the first appointment with a barbed broach and studied histologically. Approximately half of the

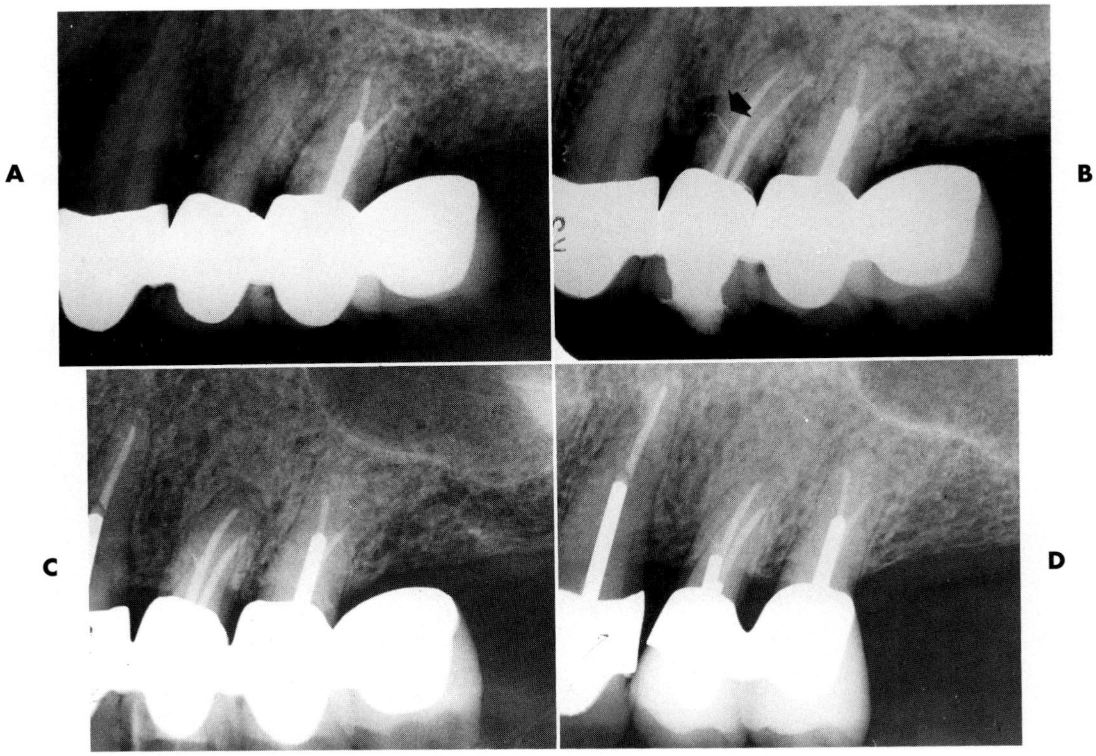

Fig. 13-11. **A,** Preoperative view of maxillary first bicuspid, referred for endodontic treatment because of periapical lesion. A 6-mm pocket could be probed on the mesial and appeared to be of periodontal origin. **B,** When the patient returned for her second appointment the pocket could not be probed. The canals were filled with laterally condensed gutta-percha and Kerr's Antiseptic Root Canal Sealer. This immediate postfilling film indicates sealer extruded through auxiliary canal *(arrow)*. **C,** Three years later, entire area looks excellent. **D,** Eleven years after original treatment, the area has retained normal appearance and no probing is possible. The wisp of sealer is still visible just apical and mesial to the post to the left. (Periodontal therapy by Dr. Harry Staffileno, Chicago.)

pulps examined exhibited varying degrees of pulpal inflammation, including chronic pulpitis, acute pulpitis, and necrosis (Fig. 13-12).

Because of these facts and because periodontal disease may result in pulpal disease, it may be possible for a relatively normal-appearing tooth to have a true pulpitis. Since pulpal disease similarly may cause periodontal disease, an untreated pulpal problem may prevent the optimal periodontal healing after seemingly correct therapy.

On the basis of these facts, Kramer and others have made the following suggestions relevant to the initiation of endodontic therapy on periodontally involved teeth:

1. If what appears to be a periodontal problem exists, perform periodontal therapy.

2. If the lesion does not heal to a desirable degree despite correct therapy, consider the possible presence of a pulpal problem.

3. If a considerable degree of bone loss is present or if a pulpal disease is likely, as evidenced by an extremely deep restoration, pulp capping, pulpotomy, or vague periapical lesion, perform endodontic therapy.

Effect of periodontal therapy on the pulp. Once it is determined that periodontal disease is present, some type of therapy is required. Among the instruments used to remove deposits from tooth surfaces are ultrasonics, vibrators, scalers, and curettes. Stanley has stated that if as little as 2 mm of remaining dentin thickness exists between the pulp and an irritating stimulus, there is little

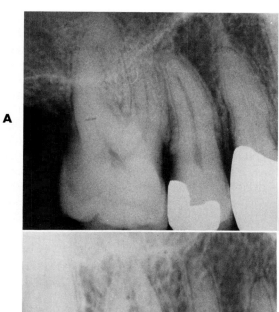

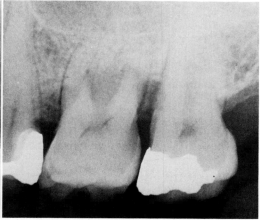

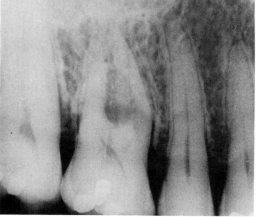

Fig. 13-12. Three maxillary molars, all with advanced periodontal disease but responsive to electric pulp testing, and all caries free. **A** and **B,** No restoration. **C,** Minimal peripheral restorations. Biopsies of pulps from palatal canals indicated massive destruction—**A** with advanced chronic pulpitis, **B** with calcific fibrosis, and **C** with necrosis. Causative agent for the advanced pulpal disease could only have been the periodontal disease.

chance of any pulp damage occurring. However, in some cases tooth configuration together with removal of a portion of the protective barrier, such as by crown preparation or curetting of necrotic cementum and dentin, may bring pulpal irritants well within the 2-mm limit.

Common sites of such intrusion are the proximal surfaces of the roots of mandibular anterior teeth, which are normally thin mesiodistally, and the furcation and buccal areas of the roots of maxillary and mandibular molars. Frequent periodontal procedures of lengthy duration may certainly cause pulp damage in this manner. Certain medications that have been advocated for chemical cautery of inflamed gingival tissues, such as formalin-containing solutions, may cause severe damage when coming in contact with pulp tissue.

Bender and Seltzer have reported that teeth with periodontal disease plus extensive restorations disclose a greater degree and more frequent examples of pulpal inflammation than those with either condition singly. If teeth with some degree of pulpal inflammation are further insulted by the irritational effects of some aspects of periodontal therapy, an irreversible condition may result. During the course of periodontal therapy, it behooves the dentist to watch for telltale signs of pulpal inflammation and to take whatever measures are needed to avoid pulp damage whenever possible. Such precautions should include the following:

1. Avoiding use of irritating chemicals when contact with root surfaces is unavoidable.
2. Minimizing use of ultrasonic and rotary scaling instruments when there is a strong possibility of less than 2 mm of dentin thickness remaining, particularly after removal of considerable depth of necrotic cementum and dentin.

3. Allowing minor pulpal irritations to subside before employing further procedures, which might cause more damage.
4. Recognizing the need for and instituting endodontic therapy when an irreversible condition has resulted.

None of these precautions should be misconstrued to imply that certain aspects of periodontal therapy are to be performed superficially. Deposits of calculus and debris, necrotic dentin and cementum, and areas with poor attachment potential must be removed. The plea here is to consider the possibilities for pulpal inflammation when performing the needed therapy and to take suitable steps to minimize the reaction. Just as a restorative dentist must consider the pulp within when preparing the coronal portion of a tooth for a crown or other restoration, so must the dentist performing periodontal therapy consider the pulp when altering the shape of the root.

EFFECT OF PULP ON PERIODONTAL TISSUES

Furcation canals—possible role in the development of Class I endodontic-periodontal lesions in molars. Rubach and Mitchell reported on several studies related to auxiliary canals, particularly those in the furcation area of molar teeth, and the effects of periodontal disease on the pulp. They showed histologically that the auxiliary canals in the furcation area led to the tissues of the periodontal ligament (Fig. 13-13, *A* and *B*).

Bender, Seltzer, and their research associates also stated that periodontal-endodontic combination problems were much more frequent in posterior teeth, particularly in molars, than anterior teeth because of the greater number of auxiliary and furcation canals present in molars.

Several authors have attempted to correlate teeth having greater numbers of auxiliary canals with increased presence of periodontal disease. Vertucci and Williams reported that 46% of mandibular first molars had auxiliary canals in the furcation region. In such cases, when pulpal inflammation begins within the coronal portion of the pulp and extends apically, the products of inflammation can cause damage in the periodontal ligament long before they reach the tissues at the root apex.

Such a reaction would give the typical radiographic appearance of the Class I endodontic-periodontal problem, where the furca is involved, as distinguished by a definite radiolucency in that area, whereas the periapical region shows minimal (Fig. 13-13, *C*) or no deviation (Fig. 13-2, *G*) from normal. The greater thickness of bone in the periapical region of mandibular molars compared with that in the area of the furca also tends to mask the radiographic visualization of the bone loss in the former while emphasizing the destruction in the thinner bone (Figs. 13-13, *C* and *E* and 13-14, *A*).

Moss et al. studied histologically the pulpal floor of primary infected and noninfected molars. They found that the floor of the pulp chamber of an infected molar was more permeable to methylene blue dye than was that of a noninfected tooth. Therefore, they concluded that there was a constant flow of material directly through the pulpal floor between the pulp and the adjacent tissues. No study has been made of the pulpal floor of permanent molars and the greater thickness as compared with that found in primary molars might be a sufficient barrier to prevent constant interchange. However, such a possibility does exist and might explain some of the Class I lesions where no furcal auxiliary canal is demonstrable (Fig. 13-14).

A high percentage of human primary molars have auxiliary canals in the furcation area. This accounts for the frequent finding of furcation radiolucencies noted with primary teeth whose pulps have become necrotic or where unsuccessful pulp capping or pulpotomy procedures have been performed. These teeth exhibit the classic clinical symptoms of the Class I endodontic-periodontal problem.

Moss et al. reported that auxiliary canals were found in the furcation area of 29% of the primary molars studied. Human molars also may have auxiliary canals in this area, but probably to a lesser extent. The most common site in permanent mandibular molars is the distal surface of the mesial root of the first molar (Fig. 13-13, *B, D,* and *F*) and, to a much lesser extent, to the mesial surface of the distal root of the first molar (Fig. 13-13, *G* and *H*). Very rare is an auxiliary canal extending from the floor of the chamber toward the furcation area vertically to the crest of the bone in mandibular molars. Although this condition has been described in histologic studies and confirmed by serial sectioning, I have yet to see this clearly established in a clinical case via extension of the sealer from chamber floor to periodontal ligament.

In view of these facts, the Class I endodontic-periodontal lesion in molars, which has cause so much confusion and misunderstanding for the

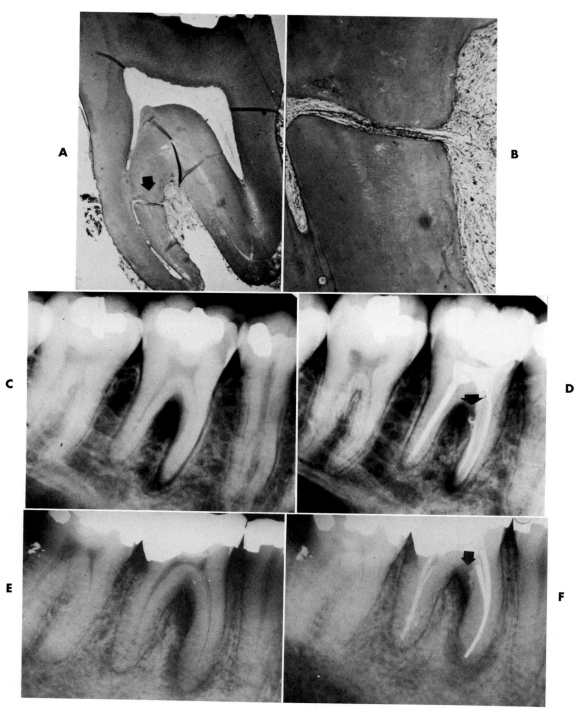

Fig. 13-13. Typical sites of furcation auxiliary canals. **A,** Photomicrograph of mandibular molar indicating communication of pulp tissue from the distal surface of the mesial root with the periodontal ligament. **B,** Higher power shows inflammatory infiltrate in both the pulp and the approximating periodontal ligament. (**A** and **B,** courtesy Dr. David Mitchell, formerly of Indianapolis.) **C,** Preoperative radiograph of mandibular first molar with typical Class I endodontic-periodontal problem. A large radiolucency is apparent in the furcation area and a smaller lesion is associated with the apical area of the mesial root. This difference may be due to thicker bone in the apical area than in the furcation area. A deep carious lesion is present on the mesial, and the adjacent proximal bone heights are normal. **D,** The canals were filled with laterally condensed gutta-percha and Kerr's Antiseptic Root Canal Sealer. Note the sealer extrusion exiting on the distal surface of the mesial root, exactly as shown in **A. E** and **F,** Similar situation on another mandibular molar, but this time the mesial canals were filled with silver cones and Kerr's Antiseptic Root Canal Sealer, extruded as in **A** *(arrow).* A large restoration was present in the tooth and the other bone levels were normal.

Continued

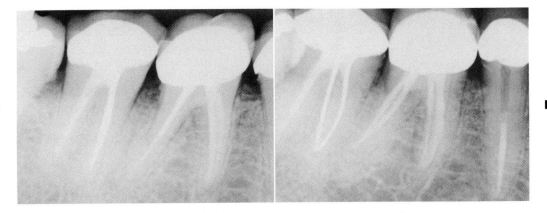

Fig. 13-13, cont'd. **G** (straight view) and **H** (angled view), of mandibular molar with four canals filled with laterally condensed gutta-percha and Kerr's Antiseptic Root Canal Sealer. The sealer is seen in a lateral canal on the mesial surface of the distal root, a less frequently found site.

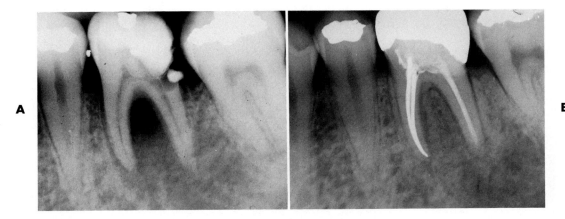

Fig. 13-14. **A,** Mandibular first molar with severe inflammatory process in furcation, althought minimal apical destruction was noted. Tooth was extremely mobile. **B,** Six months after endodontic treatment, area has healed. Pupal floor of chamber was packed, but no furcation canal was picked up with the sealer. (Restoration by Dr. Fred Hill, Cincinnati.)

dental population, becomes clear. The radiographic appearance of the furcation results from a pericanicular radiolucency of an auxiliary canal in the region or results from inflammatory products extending through the pulpal floor. The lesion suggests an inflammation of severe intensity due to the thinness of the bone and the normal presence of marrow spaces, which are susceptible to invasion in that area. The periapical area may appear normal radiographically because the inflammation has not yet extended through the tooth to that region and/or because a greater thickness of

bone is present to mask the destruction. Following endodontic therapy, with the toxic products removed from the pulp canal space, the dynamic healing potential of the bone brings about a return to normal. The speed of the radiographic change is similarly related to the thin bone of the furca, which allows for rapid visualization of the healing process.

Other types of Class I endodontic-periodontal problems. On occasion a recall radiograph will show a radiolucency on a lateral surface or in the furca of the treated tooth where no defect was present preoperatively. This lesion has the same features as the typical Class I endodontic-periodontal lesion, except that the root canals are filled, usually adequately. Those who are not in agreement with the pulpal etiology suggested for Class I lesions point to the cases of this type in repudiation.

Far from overturning the theory, these cases only serve to reinforce it by illustrating another situation in which the periodontal tissues are adversely affected by the pulp. The record of the preoperative condition of such teeth should be consulted. Invariably the diagnosis at that time was some type of pulpitis, indicating that most of the root canal was filled with vital tissue. By way of canal enlargement and frequent irrigation with hypochlorite, the inflamed pulp was removed from the canal proper and a dense root canal filling placed. However, inflamed tissue might have remained in any auxiliary canals present, relatively unaffected by the instrumentation and irrigation. After the canal filling, the remaining inflamed tissue undergoes necrosis and causes breakdown of the surrounding periodontal structures. This type

of failure is analogous to the root canal filing that does not seal an insufficiently debrided apex and allows for the development of a periapical radiolucency due to the breakdown of the tissue remaining within the canal.

The type of failure described may be successfully re-treated if the canal filling material adjacent to the radiolucency can be removed, with chloroform used to dissolve gutta-percha or a silver point removed with pliers or file. The canal is reprepared, enlarged a minimum of two sizes wider, and then refilled at a later appointment by any of the methods previously described in the chapters on canal filling. Since heavy condensation is most desirable when the existence of an auxiliary canal is anticipated, uses of gutta-percha with lateral or warm vertical condensation appear to be the techniques of choice. The postoperative radiograph will generally show sealer extruding from the canal toward the radiolucency (Fig. 13-15).

Similarly, whenever possible, posts should reach the depth of preparation to contact the canal filling material in the apical portion. In this

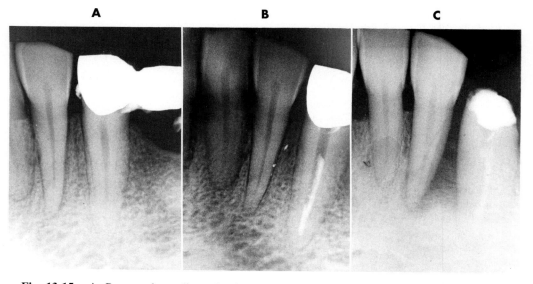

Fig. 13-15. A, Preoperative radiograph of mandibular cuspid area. A new bridge was to be constructed with the cuspid as anterior abutment, but recurrent caries under the old bridge caused a pulp exposure. **B,** Immediate postfilling film, with laterally condensed gutta-percha and Wach's paste used as canal filling materials at the second appointment and post room prepared. Treatment was uneventful. **C,** Ten weeks later, the bridge had not yet been remade, but the patient began to experience severe pain in the lateral/cuspid area. The lateral incisor was quite mobile, tender to percussion, and responded very weakly to electric pulp testing.   *Continued*

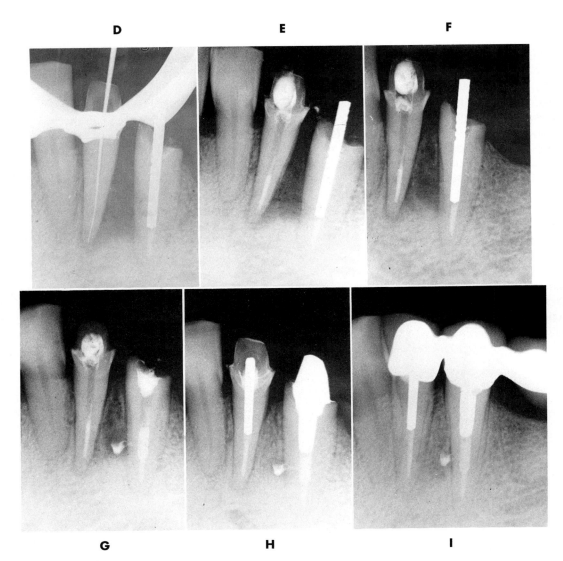

Fig. 13-15, cont'd.   D, Endodontic treatment was initiated on the lateral after a temporary splint was fabricated to halt the mobility. A temporary post was placed into the cuspid. It was decided that the position of this file in the lateral was too long. **E,** Endodontic treatment was completed on the lateral with filling by laterally condensed gutta-percha and Wach's paste and post room prepared. The tooth tightened following canal preparation. **F,** Ten weeks later, the area appears to be healing, but there is still a sore spot between the two teeth. **G,** On the chance that an unfilled lateral canal was present on the cuspid, the area made for post room was widened and reprepared, using heavy irrigation with sodium hypochlorite. The apical few millimeters of gutta-percha was left alone. At the next appointment the prepared site was filled with warm condensation of gutta-percha and Kerr's Antiseptic Root Canal Sealer. A significant lateral canal was demonstrated on the mesial, going exactly to the area of inflammation. **H,** Three months later, the area is healing, no pain is present, and neither tooth is mobile. **I,** After 18 months, the lesion is gone, the teeth are tight and comfortable, and a new bridge has been constructed.

manner the metal and cement will serve to close the area to bacteria, which might communicate to the periodontium.

RATIONALE FOR TREATMENT OF CLASS I ENDODONTIC-PERIODONTAL CASES

Many practitioners have difficulty believing the rapidity with which these Class I endodontic-periodontal lesions heal. Understanding that the classic severe periodontal lesion has a poor prognosis, with a very limited potential for a rebuilding of bone, these dentists have doubted the veracity of the case reports describing extensive healing. In lectures that I have given on the subject, I have been accused by some of showing preoperative films as postoperative results, and vice versa.

The healing of such cases as seen in Figs. 13-2 and 13-3 are quite spectacular, but there is nothing magical about them. One must understand that the lesions are *not* periodontal and, although their symptomatology is very similar, the difference in etiology accounts for the healing potential.

Similarity to a sinus tract.   Even though these lesions mimic periodontal defects, they are, in fact, much different. They are close to being chronic draining sinus tracts. Most dentists are familiar with the fact that chronic draining sinus tracts cause by pulpal necrosis heal readily after canal preparation. This is a routine process and requires no special treatment in addition to the intracanal procedures.

The defects of Class I endodontic-periodontal cases are also chronic draining sinus tracts (Fig. 13-16, *A*). When the canals are prepared properly, the defect heals quite readily and the "sinus tract" is gone by the next appointment. The case is finished in a routine manner (Fig. 13-16, *B*) and healing is quite predictable (Fig. 13-16, *C*).

Recording of the defect.   Because of the rapid and spectacular healing that immediately follows the canal-preparation appointment, the dentist may become confused when seeing a patient at the succeeding visit. Where was that pocket before? How deep was it? Was it on the buccal or lingual of the

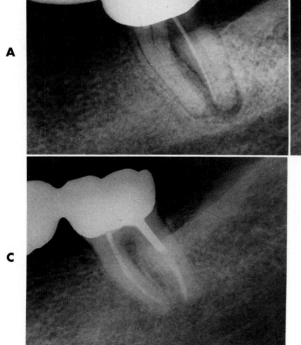

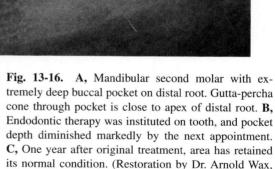

Fig. 13-16.   A, Mandibular second molar with extremely deep buccal pocket on distal root. Gutta-percha cone through pocket is close to apex of distal root. **B,** Endodontic therapy was instituted on tooth, and pocket depth diminished markedly by the next appointment. **C,** One year after original treatment, area has retained its normal condition. (Restoration by Dr. Arnold Wax, Chicago.)

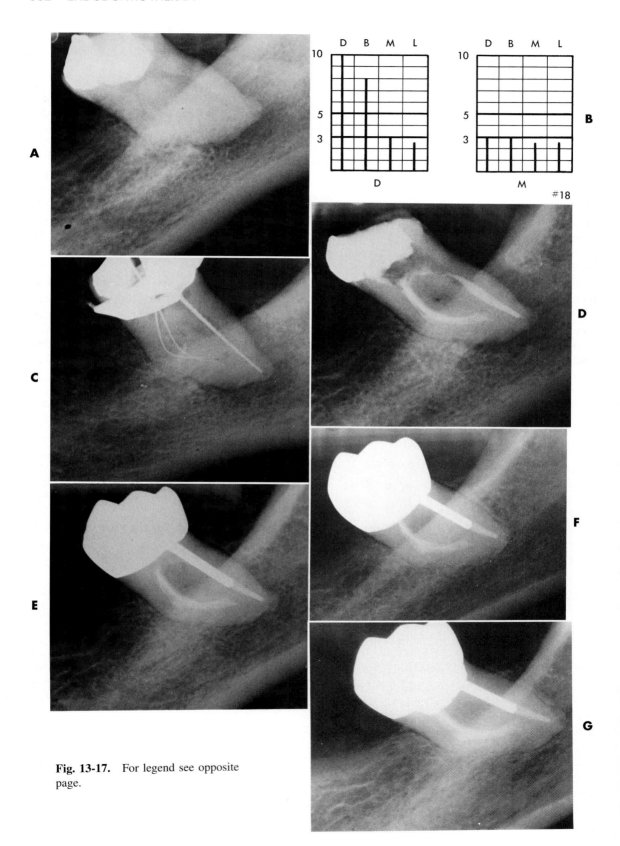

Fig. 13-17. For legend see opposite page.

Fig. 13-17.   Use of the "periodontal portrait" (courtesy Dr. John Melton, Las Cruces, N.M.) in recording periodontal configuration and pocket depth. **A,** Mandibular second molar with deep distal and buccal extension. **B,** Periodontal portrait accurately records pocket depth prior to treatment. Although distal portion of the lesion is obvious on the radiograph, buccal extent is not and thus there is no other
method for recording it. Portrait indicates that probings on mesial root are within normal limits. On
distal root, however, mesial and lingual probings are normal, although distal probed 10 and buccal
probed 8 mm. This remains part of permanent record and may be consulted in later evaluation of area
and for follow-up care. **C,** Files in place. **D,** Pocket depth decreased markedly immediately after
appointment for preparation, and canals were filled with laterally condensed gutta-percha and Wach's
paste. **E,** Eighteen months after treatment, healing is advanced. **F,** Six years after treatment, lesions
have healed and tooth is firm; no pockets probed. **G,** Seventeen years after treatment, periapical tissue
remains normal. (Restoration by Dr. Pete Feimer, Chicago.)

---

distal root? Attempting to reprobe incorrectly may
damage the sensitive healing tissue or injure the
normal areas.

Therefore, prior to initation of therapy on any
case that involves a periodontal defect, an accurate
recording of the preoperative conditions must be
made. I recommend the "periodontal portrait"
(developed by Melton, of Las Cruces, N.M.) as a
useful, easy-to-record, and accurate device for listing initial conditions and result of therapy. Obviously there are many other charting systems that
are acceptable, but this method is illustrated for
the case in Fig. 13-17.

When a Class I lesion is not a Class I lesion.
As shown in Fig. 13-9, the signs and symptoms of
these Class I lesions may be confused and the
incorrect treatment instituted. If what seems to be
a Class I lesion is started on a tooth and the pulp
appears to be essentially vital (even though not
normal) in the root associated with the periodontal
destruction, this is a reliable sign that endodontics
alone will not salvage the case. Perhaps that root
can be amputated or corrective periodontal treatment instituted, but the healing expected after
therapy on a Class I lesion will not occur.

TREATMENT OF COMBINED-LESION CASES

Combined-lesion cases all come under the category of Class II endodontic-periodontal problems,
that is, teeth with both pulpal or periapical disease
plus periodontal disease. Treatment of both problems must be met in order to gain optimal results.
In contradistinction to Class I cases, these patients
exhibit periodontal disease in a number of areas of
the mouth.

Three distinctly different types of lesions occur.
In the first the affected tooth has two separate

lesions, one endodontic and usually periapical and
one periodontal, with no communication between
each other. The second type contains those teeth
with a single lesion that involves both endodontic
and periodontal pathoses. The third type involves
teeth with periodontal and endodontic lesions that
were once separate but now communicate.

Separate and unrelated lesions.   Cases of this
type have separate lesions that coincidentally have
attacked the same tooth. The etiology of pulpal
damage is usually obvious—either a large restoration, deep caries, or vital pulp therapy.

The method for therapy is quite straightforward.
First, it must be determined that the periodontal
condition is treatable. Performing endodontic therapy on teeth with hopeless periodontal lesions is
disastrous (Fig. 13-9). Endodontic therapy is performed first (Fig. 13-18, *B*), and then periodontal
therapy follows. The healing of the periapical
lesion is unaffected by the periodontal therapy to
follow (Fig. 13-18, *C*).

**Single lesions with both endodontic and peri-
odontal components.**   Of all the conditions
described in this chapter, this is the most difficult
to treat successfully. My analysis of the method
for therapy is a point of controversy, and I wish to
forewarn the reader that my views are disputed by
a number of outstanding clinicians and academi-
cians. However, I have many cases that illustrate
this type of therapy, and those shown in Figs. 13-5
and 13-20 are merely three of many that validate
my position.

The involved tooth has a single lesion radiographically and probes just as a routine deep periodontal pocket would probe. The patient does have a
periodontal condition involving other teeth, and
there is a likely etiology for the endodontic condi-

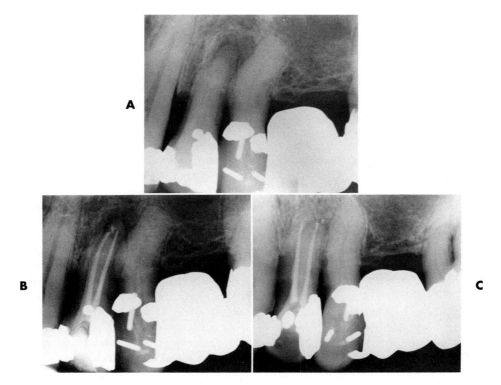

Fig. 13-18. **A,** Preoperative radiograph of maxillary bicuspid area. A periapical lesion is associated with the first bicuspid, and the pulp is necrotic in that tooth. The patient has a generalized periodontal condition present, but the periapical and periodontal lesions do not communicate. **B,** Canals filled with laterally condensed gutta-percha. **C,** One year later, periapical lesion has healed, even though there is no appreciable change in the periodontal picture.

tion; however, the cause may be more subtle than in Class I lesions and may, in fact, be due to the progress of a severe periodontal disease on the given tooth. Lateral canals frequently are culprits.

Generally periodontal therapy has been attempted and was not successful. Endodontic therapy is instituted, and pulp extirpation will reveal a pulp with a histologic condition similar to those shown in Fig. 13-12. Following completion of endodontic therapy (Fig. 13-19, *C*) the periodontal condition may improve but does not heal—clearly in opposition to Class I cases.

Then periodontal therapy is reinitiated. The same types of treatment may be performed (deep scaling, surgery, GTR, and so on) that were ineffective previously, but now healing will take place (Figs. 13-19, *D* through *F* and 13-20, *C*). Cases such as these are quite remarkable, but not consistently predictable, and the therapy suggested may lead to failure rather than success. When such

treatment is attempted, the patient must be forewarned concerning the doubtful prognosis.

Periodontal and endodontic lesions that have merged. This type of case is shown in Fig. 13-7. The patient has periodontal disease in other areas, and the pocket depth may have caused the pulp to become affected, periodontal therapy may have caused pulpal injury, or a more mundane etiology may be present (a large restoration or caries, for example). A periapical lesion results and merges with the periodontal pocket, even though separate lesions are present. That portion of the lesion extending from the apical area toward the crestal bone is periapical due to the pulpal damage, whereas the lesion from the sulcus extending apically is periodontal breakdown.

If endodontic treatment only is performed, the periapical lesion will heal to the site where the periodontal lesion begins (Fig. 13-7, *B*). If periodontal therapy only is performed, the crestal bone

A   **B**   **C**

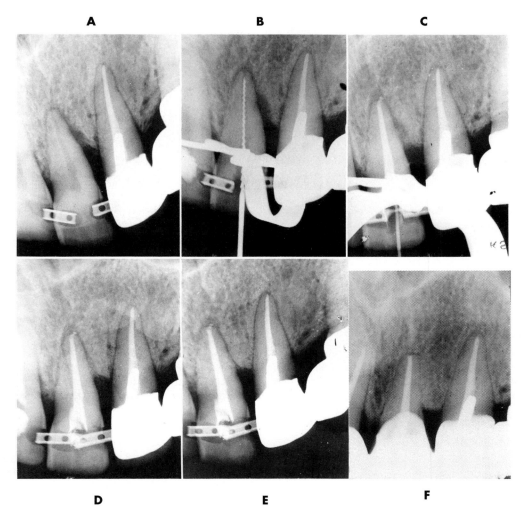

D   **E**   **F**

Fig. 13-19.   Elimination of lesion with both endodontic and periodontal components. **A,** Preoperative radiograph of anterior maxillary area. The patient has congenitally missing lateral incisors. The tooth with the existing endodontic treatment and post is a cuspid. The tooth to its left on the film is a central incisor that responds poorly to electric pulp testing and has a deep distal pocket to the apex. Periodontal therapy had been ineffective in this area although treatment had been successful in other sites for this patient. **B,** View of file in place to calculate working length. **C,** Film taken during canal filling with laterally condensed gutta-percha and Kerr's Antiseptic Root Canal Sealer. It was hoped that a lateral canal would be demonstrated in the area of defect, but this did not occur. **D,** The patient was returned to the periodontist who reinstituted similar periodontal therapy. Now it has been effective. This film was taken 6 months after treatment. **E,** Fourteen months after original treatment, with no probing possible on the distal of the central incisor. **F,** Eleven years after original treatment, area still looks excellent. (Periodontal therapy by Dr. Harry Staffileno, Chicago, and restorations by Dr. Richard Lamermayer, Kenilworth, Ill.)

A   **B**   **C**

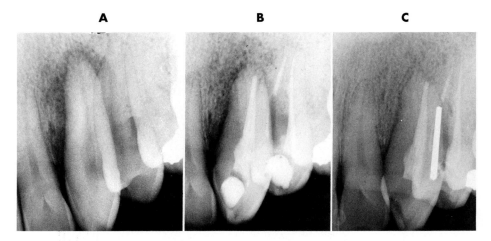

Fig. 13-20. **A,** Preoperative radiograph of cuspid with large, halolike radiolucency and a pocket to the apex on the mesial. Electric pulp test was negative. **B,** Endodontic treatment completed on both the cuspid and the adjacent first bicuspid. Pocket continued to probe to the apex during and after treatment. **C,** Two years later, the apical radiolucency is gone and the mesial pocket no longer probes. Periodontal therapy was instituted following completion of canal filling. (Periodontal therapy by Dr. Harry Staffileno, Chicago.)

may heal to where the periapical lesion begins. If the untreated lesion in either case is very active with considerable virulence, the treated lesion will not heal to its full potential because of continued irritation and inflammation from the untreated segment.

ENDODONTIC STABILIZERS

When the first edition of this textbook was being written, the use of implants was at its zenith. Books, periodicals, seminars, articles, postgraduate courses, and so on, were devoted to the use of pins, screws, blades, wires, casting, and other types of implants. At the time I though that the implant with the best chance for success was the endodontic stabilizer. Some implants fail because of an epithelial downgrowth at the neck of the implant, which eventually causes looseness and ultimately exfoliation. However, the endodontic stabilizer, with no communication between the oral cavity and the implant, appeared to have an outstanding chance for long-lasting effectiveness.

Unfortunately the endodontic stabilizer used to solve periodontal problems also proved to be a solution with a low percentage of success, and its use now is virtually nil. Of the 50 or more that I placed 15 to 22 years ago for periodontal reasons, only one still remains functional (Fig. 13-21). Others did last from 3 to 7 years, but more because of adjunctive restorative procedures than the effec-

tiveness of the implant. Interestingly, stabilizers I have placed surgically (Chapter 11) have had a good history of long-term retention.

The following description is presented for historical and informational use rather than as encouragement for treatment. Alternative methods of therapy are surely better. However, it should be mentioned that the early efforts of Frank in the United States and Orlay in Europe should still be applauded for their innovative and progressive thinking rather than derided because of the failures of treatment. Many of the failures of treatment were not the fault of these pioneers, but rather because implants were overused and misused (Fig. 13-22) in cases where the applicability and indications were grossly discarded.

Armamentarium. The basis for an endodontic stabilizer is the use of the chrome-cobalt pin as the implant material. This alloy is composed of 65% cobalt, 30% chromium, and 5% molybdenum. The nonelectrolytic, inert properties as well as the excellent tissue tolerance to the material have been verified by Bernier and Canby and others. These implants are available in standardized sizes, from 70 through 140, and have been manufactured by several companies.

The instruments and supplies needed for placing an endodontic stabilizer follow. The sterile tray setup is the same as previously described for filling canals with silver points. The irrigating

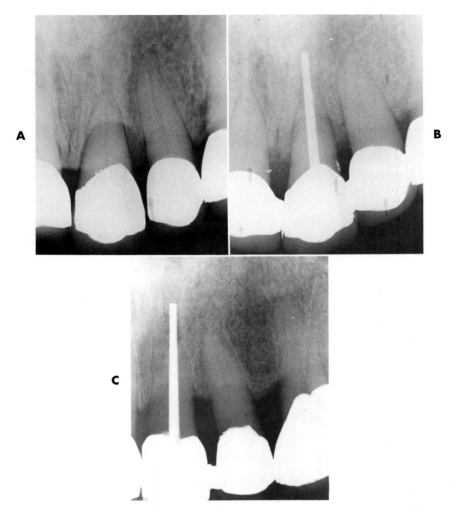

Fig. 13-21. A, Preoperative radiograph of maxillary central incisor with 12-mm lingual pocket and considerable mobility. The teeth are not splinted. **B,** An endodontic implant was placed, and a splint involving this tooth was constructed. **C,** Seventeen years after original treatment, periodontal condition has worsened somewhat, but the periapical areas appear normal. It is impossible to judge any mobility because of the splint in place. (Restorations by Dr. Leon Rosenfeld, Chicago.)

syringe for a one-sitting appointment or for the filling appointment in a multisitting treatment is filled with sterile distilled water to avoid the potential irritation of hypochlorite on periapical tissue. Supplies needed are the following:

Chrome-cobalt pins—two each of sizes 70 through 140, so that if one pin of a particular size is ruined in preparation or manipulation, no change in canal or bone preparation need be made before going to a larger size

Reamers—31 and 40 mm, sizes 10 through 140; the longer-length reamers are needed to gain the greater length required of the preparation; long-handled instruments are satisfactory for maxillary anterior teeth but useless in other areas

Intraosseous drill—to remove periapical bone when a hand reamer will not penetrate

Silver point forceps—to hold the pin and forcibly place it in its proper position

Joe Dandy disk—mounted on a straight handpiece mandrel, to be used to taper the pin and aid in the sectioning

Grossman's formula root canal sealer—powder and liquid, possibly replaced by Diaket or AH 26 as sealer of choice

Sterile paper points—to dry the canal

One-sitting as opposed to three-sitting treatment. Since many of the teeth that are treated by endodontic stabilization have no pulpal problem, a one-sitting technique usually works out satisfactorily. The entire treatment from lingual access to implant placement usually may be performed in 1½ hours or less. The postoperative pain after completion is generally minimal and can be alleviated by a prescription for moderate-strength analgesics. If two visits are taken to complete treatment, the first for canal and intraosseous preparation and the second for placement of the implant, the pain is not diminished.

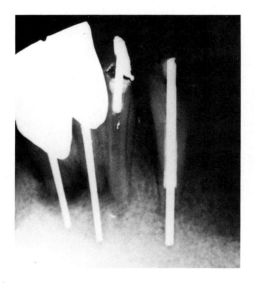

Fig. 13-22. Poor indications and techniques in using endodontic implants. Both mandibular central incisors as well as the lateral incisor and cuspid were implanted 6 months earlier. Both central incisors have large radiolucencies and are mobile despite extension of materials and splinting. Veneer crown had come off lateral incisor, and the implant came out with the core. Cuspid is firm, but radiolucency between canal space and implant indicates that canal is not sealed.

In fact, because of the mobility of the tooth, it may be impossible to relocate the preparation in the bone at the second appointment, and a new intraosseous reaming may be required.

However, if the tooth to be treated has a pulpitis with microbial activity or a periapical radiolucency due to pulp necrosis, a three-sitting procedure should be planned. The rationale for the three appointments is to rid the canal of irritants before entering the periapical tissues and forcibly injecting the normal bone with necrotic or infected material. Therefore, at the first appointment the contents of the canal are removed with enlargement to the radiographic apex. At the second sitting the effectiveness of the initial debridement is determined by examining the interior of the canal for debris. The third appointment is the longest, with all intraosseous preparation accomplished, followed by stabilizer placement.

Procedure for one-appointment treatment. A suitable local anesthetic is administered, with lingual (or palatal) anesthesia used in addition to the normal injections. The rubber dam is placed, and an access cavity is prepared. It is important that the access be placed as far labially (or buccally) as possible to give direct access to the apical tissues for the wider and stiffer reamers needed to complete enlargement and the rigid implant (Fig. 13-23, *A* and *B*). In mandibular anterior teeth the access is best placed at the incisal edge.

The vital contents of the canal are removed with a barbed broach and a size 10 reamer is placed through the apical foramen into the bone to a precalculated length. This length is an approximation of the tooth length, with the preoperative radiograph used as a guide, plus the desired length for the extension of the implant. The latter is generally 7 to 12 mm and depends on the proximity of adjacent vital structures and the amount of periapical bone. A radiograph is taken with the size 10 reamer in place to examine the position of the instrument within the bone relative to the apex and

Fig. 13-23.   **A,** In preparation of canal for stabilizer, entry must be placed more labially (or buccally) than normal. **B,** This allows direct access to periapical area for stiff, large-sized reamers. **C,** Working length for intraosseous preparation is approximately 8 mm past apical foramen. Rubber dam has been removed to ensure by digital examination that file does not perforate either the buccal or the lingual plate. **D,** Implant is firmly placed into tooth with silver point forceps. **E,** Radiograph is taken to confirm correctness of position. **F,** Stabilizer is weakened at a calculated position with no. 37 inverted cone bur and bent to gain separation. Portion retained in forceps will be used as plugger to force pin to reach correct position. **G,** Radiograph taken at the conclusion of the appointment. **H,** Three years later, tooth has been restored with a post, core, and telescope and is one abutment for an overdenture. **I,** Six years after implantation, the extension of periodontal disease has caused the loss of the other abutment, and considerable bone loss is now seen on the remaining abutment. Some mobility is present. (Reconstruction by Dr. Paul Chung, formerly of Chicago.)

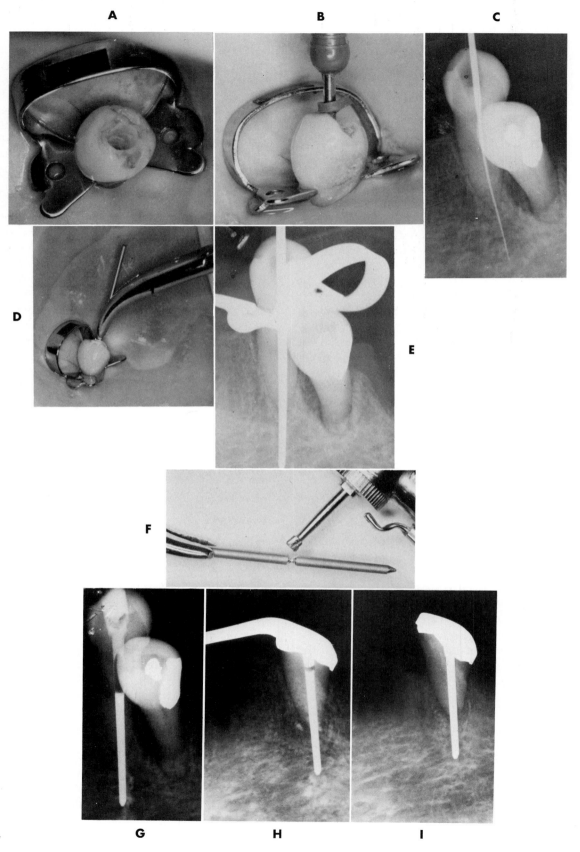

Fig. 13-23. For legend see opposite page.

to the adjacent structures. Any necessary adjustments in the working length are made at this time (Fig. 13-23, *C*).

If the reamer will not penetrate to the depth desired, the intraosseous drill may be used to gain greater length. Although this step is rarely required, the objective of the treatment is to increase the working root length by insertion of an implant, and it is important to reach the needed length. Prior to the use of the drill, the root canal is prepared with reamers through the apex to size 40 so the canal walls will exert no binding for the osseous preparation. The drill is mounted on a contra-angle handpiece and, at very slow speed, is carefully placed through the canal to prepare an opening through the bone of greater density.

After the desired length is established, the rubber dam is removed with the long reamer still in position. The labial and lingual (or palatal) tissues are carefully checked, both visually and with digital examination, to ensure that the reamer is not perforating into the soft tissue. Turning the reamer within the canal during the digital examination aids in the location if a perforation is present. If the reamer does exit from the bone into the soft tissue, the working length must be shortened to keep all preparation within the hard tissue. A perforation with a small instrument will cause no irreparable damage.

By use of reaming action only, the canal is enlarged at the calculated length to the desired width, with frequent irrigation of sterile distilled water. The ideal width to reach varies with the tooth to be treated and the type of case involved but must be a minimum of size 80. In mandibular anterior teeth and maxillary lateral incisors, sizes between 80 and 100 should be reached, whereas maxillary central incisors, cuspids, and mandibular bicuspids may be implanted with wider pins. The very wide sizes of 120 to 140 are ordinarily used in conjunction with a surgical treatment to replace a fractured root tip and are rarely used as stabilizers. If for some reason a compromise was made in the desired working length, usually due to the proximity of adjacent structures or the possibility of a perforation, a wider diameter than normally used should be reached.

A chrome-cobalt pin the same size as the largest reamer used in the preparation is selected and the tip shortened 0.5 mm and then beveled, using the Joe Dandy disk. While being held in the silver points forceps, with the forceps beaks acting as the incisal guide, the pin is placed into the salt sterilizer for 10 seconds, dipped into a disinfecting solution to cool, and then tried into the canal (Fig. 13-23, *D*). Because the pin was shortened, it should bind tightly at 0.5 to 1 mm short of the working length. The reason for this slight length discrepancy is the need for the binding in the canal and bone, preventing the pin from further penetration, rather than the tip of the preparation stopping it. If the latter occurs, it could be possible that the implant might not have good contact with the walls of the canal. This would not allow the implant to afford optimal stabilization; worse, it might prevent gaining apical seal. It must always be remembered that this is still an endodontic procedure, and wherever applicable, endodontic principles must be followed. Lack of apical seal is the most frequent cause of endodontic failure; and since the use of a stabilizer is a somewhat precarious situation, all possible protection against problems must be taken. Therefore it behooves the operator to take special precautions to gain apical seal of the canal.

Since the implants are manufactured to have a standardized taper, a segment from the tip may be removed with the Joe Dandy disk if the pin goes the full working length and thus does butt against the end of the preparation. The shortened pin is then retried for desired fit. This process of trimming may be repeated until the desired binding within the canal is obtained. If the pin does not go to the desired depth, further preparation must be performed.

Since the material is rigid, the chrome-cobalt pin must be completely severed rather than twisted off within the canal in the manner used for sectioning silver points. The position of sectioning must be calculated so that a 5- to 7-mm segment of the pin remains within the confines of the canal. This leaves sufficient room in the root for a post should one be required in the restoration of the tooth and still gives enough surface area of contact between the canal walls and the implant to provide stabilization. The pin is partially cut through from opposite sides with the Joe Dandy disk and then separated by bending (Fig. 13-23, *F*). This method is better than completely cutting through with the disk, which removes a portion of the pin and confuses the length calculations. Bending maintains the original length. All the while the incisal portion of the pin is held in the silver points forceps to retain the proper relationship to the incisal edge of the tooth.

Grossman's formula or the alternative root canal sealer of choice is mixed to a heavy consistency. The canal only is dried with sterile, absorbent paper points. The walls of the canal are coated by bringing the sealer into the tooth on the tip of a reamer that approximates the width of the canal, with a stop set to indicate canal length, and rotating counterclockwise. Usually two or three such applications are necessary to gain sufficient coating. The portion of the pin that will remain within the canal is also coated with sealer. The pin is grasped with a locking cotton pliers and inserted into the sealer-coated canal. The silver points forceps with the incisal portion of the sectioned pin are used as a plugger to push the apical portion to the desired depth into the intraosseous preparation. If the plugger portion is turned to right angles with the severed portion, a maximal contact is made to ensure correct seating of the pin. A radiograph is taken to verify the correctness of the pin position, and a suitable temporary filling is placed (Fig. 13-23, *G*).

Procedure for three-appointment treatment. If a radiolucency is present, no anesthetic is required for the first and second appointments. For pulpitis cases the same anesthetic that would be given for pulp extirpation in routine endodontic therapy is administered. A rubber dam is placed and an access cavity prepared, as before, as labially as possible for straight access to the apex.

A measurement is taken with a small-diameter file to establish the tooth length. This calculation is made to the radiographic apex of the tooth, not where it would ordinarily stop within the confines of the canal. The enlargement must purposely destroy the apical constriction but impinge on the periapical tissue to only a minimal degree. By enlargement to the radiographic apex, this is accomplished. If all the enlarging were performed within the canal and a tapered apical preparation placed in solid dentin, as in a routine case, it might be difficult to locate the apical foramen at the third appointment to initiate intraosseous preparation. The enlargement should be carried to approximately size 40, with heavy irrigation of hypochlorite. The canal is closed with zinc oxide-eugenol and the patient given another appointment.

At the second appointment the canal is examined for completeness of debridement. The tooth is considered ready for stabilization if it is no more than mildly tender to percussion. Because the contents of the canal are forced into the periapical bone when

an implant is placed, every effort should be made to gain a disinfected condition within the canal before proceeding to intraosseous preparation.

The third appointment requires the same anesthesia as the one-sitting technique. The rubber dam is placed and the access cavity opened. The procedure follows the same pattern as the one-sitting method, with determination of canal length, examination for possible perforation, intraosseous preparation, trial fit of the implant, and final placement with sealer.

Selection of cases. Careful selection of cases that would respond to therapy with the most predictability was considered paramount in placing stabilizers. Unfortunately, even with such care, the great majority of cases failed. Some of the considerations for selection were (1) long axis of tooth to be treated located over solid bone, (2) sufficient depth of bone available, (3) at last one-fourth bone support remaining, (4) use limited to one or at most two teeth in an arch, (5) apical foramen exiting along the long axis of the tooth, and (6) no medical history of bleeding.

Problems of canal enlargement. Emphasis has been placed on the fact that intraosseous and canal enlargement for stabilizers must be performed with reamers, using reaming action. The method of enlarging has been shown to have greater significance in determining the general shape of the canal than does the instrument used. To produce a preparation that is relatively round in cross section, reaming action must be used and filing action avoided. The use of the reamer rather than the file is not mandatory, and if the operator is more comfortable using a file, it may be substituted during the middle phases of canal preparation, provided it is used with reaming action. The reamer has good initial penetrating action and is certainly much safer to use than the intraosseous drill for that purpose. Also, the reamer is more effective than the file in removing debris from the preparation and therefore removes the dentin and bone shavings rapidly.

Even with careful use of reaming action, the preparation never achieves a truly round cross-sectional shape, whereas the implant used within it is round. As was shown in Chapter 9, canal eccentricities appear increased the farther one examines from the tip of the preparation. The apical foramen in a stabilization case occurs a minimum of 7 mm from the tip of the preparation. Therefore it is possible that a definite discrepancy will exist between the preparation and the

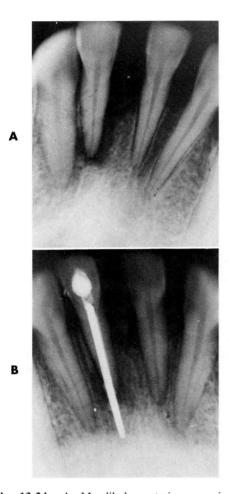

Fig. 13-24. A, Mandibular anterior area, indicating advanced periodontal disease, with pocket to the apex from the mesial on the central incisor to the left. The tooth was mobile, and the response to electric pulp testing was questionable. Diastemas were present between the incisors, and with only one tooth seriously involved and with extraction causing a very difficult restorative problem, it was considered a good indication for the use of a stabilizer. Upon entering the tooth, it was noted that no vital pulp tissue was present. Better judgment would have been to complete routine endodontic therapy with gutta-percha as the canal filling, but the implantation was carried out. **B,** One year later, the tooth has tightened and the pocket no longer probes along the mesial, but a small radiolucency may be noted near the apex. The tooth was lost 2 years later because of continued periapical, not periodontal, breakdown.

implant, which may lead to an inadequate apical seal and endodontic failure.

This may account for the success achieved in using implants to restore lost root length incorporated in a surgical procedure as opposed to stabilization cases. In the former instances the apical foramen is visible and the degree of seal is readily apparent. If an opening exists between the implant and the canal, that area may be reverse filled. In stabilization cases, since the root is not surgically exposed, there is no way to examine the adequacy of apical seal.

To compensate for this possible deficiency, an extremely thick mix of root canal sealer must be used and great care taken to ensure that the sealer adequately coats the canal walls before pin insertion. If a discrepancy does exist, it is hoped that the sealer will close the possible gaps. Routine use of a surgical approach to treat periodontally involved teeth to observe the effectiveness of apical seal is rejected because of the considerable loss of bone that might accompany the procedure. If a stabilizer is required, it is assumed that the tooth does not have a great deal of surrounding bone to spare.

Reasons for partial effectiveness yet ultimate failure of stabilizers. When stabilizer use was at its zenith and many seemingly favorable cases were reported, two prime reasons for success were responsible. A major factor was the great decrease in mobility that stabilizers afforded. With the pre-existing mobility eliminated, the other aspects of periodontal therapy could be instituted in a more favorable environment. A second reason was that in some cases the loss of bone and mobility were *not* purely periodontal, but rather of pulpal or combined etiology. With the pulpal factor eliminated by proper canal preparation, a degree of healing resulted, as seen in the typical Class I endodontic-periodontal problems; the tooth would be tighter for that reason rather than because of the implant. Fig. 13-24 demonstrates such a case where, in retrospect, it can be seen that the pocket to the apex was partially endodontic, which was verified when the canal was open and the pulp was necrotic. Instead of proceeding with the stabilizer, the canal should have been filled with gutta-percha. One year later (Fig. 13-24, *B*) the mesial pocket was well healed, but a periapical lesion was developing, which ultimately led to loss of the tooth several years later. The case failed because of the lack of apical seal, which was a frequent cause of stabilizer failure because of the difficulties involved in sealing an irregular space at the apex with a solid-core filling material.

The single major histologic investigation on the stabilizer indicated that the material was well tolerated by the adjacent bone. Unfortunately no study investigated the response at the junction of the root apex, the periapical tissues, and the implant on a long-term basis.

REFERENCES

Bender IB, Seltzer S: The effect of diseases of the periodontium on the human pulp. Presented at the Conference on Biology of the Human Pulp, Memphis, Sept. 1970.

Cahn LR: The pathology of pulps found in pyorrhetic teeth, *Dent Items Int* 49:598, 1927.

Czarnecki RT, Schilder H: A histological evaluation of the human pulp in teeth with varying degrees of periodontal disease, *J Endod* 5:242, 1979.

Frank AL: Directions for endodontic research, *Dent Clin North Am* 11:675, 1967.

Frank AL: Improvement of the crown-root ratio by endodontic endosseous implants, *J Am Dent Assoc* 74:451, 1967.

Frank AL, Abrams, AM: Histologic evaluation of endodontic implants, *J Am Dent Assoc* 78:520, 1969.

Gargiulo AV, Jr.: Endodontic-periodontic interrelationships: diagnosis and treatment, *Dent Clin North Am* 28:767, 1984.

Goldman HM: Therapy of the incipient bifurcation involvement, *J Periodontol* 29:112, 1958.

Goldman HM, Cohen DW: The infrabony pocket: classification and treatment, *J Periodontol* 29:272, 1958.

Gottlow J: Guided tissue regeneration using bioresorbable devices: initial healing and long term results, *J Periodontol* 64 (supp):1157, 1993.

Henrici AT, Hartzell TB: The bacteriology of vital pulps, *J Dent Res* 1:419, 1919.

Hiatt WH: Regeneration of the periodontium after endodontic therapy and flap operation, *Oral Surg* 12:1471, 1959.

Hiatt WH: Periodontal pocket elimination by combined endodontic-periodontic therapy, *Periodontics* 1:152, 1963.

Hiatt WH, Amen CR: Periodontal pocket elimination by combined therapy, *Dent Clin North Am* March 1964, p. 133.

Johnston HB, Orban B: Interradicular pathology related to accessory root canals, *J Endod* 3:21, April 1948.

Kramer G: Symposium on periodontic-endodontic treatment, Fourth International Conference on Endodontics, Philadelphia, April 1968.

Mazur B, Massler M: Influence of periodontal disease on the dental pulp, *Oral Surg* 17:592, 1964.

Melton JC: *The periodontal portrait and how to develop it,* Las Cruces, N.M., 1976, President.

Morris M: Healing of human periodontal tissues following surgical detachment and extirpation from non-vital pulps, *J Periodontol* 28:222, 1957.

Moss SJ, Addelston H, Goldsmith ED: Histologic study of pulpal floor of deciduous molars, *J Am Dent Assoc* 70:372, 1965.

Nyman S, Lindhe J, Karring T, Rylander H: New attachment following surgical treatment of human periodontal disease, *J Clin Periodontol* 9:290, 1982.

Orlay H: Splinting with endodontic implant stabilizers, *Dent Pract Dent Rec* 14:481, 1964.

Reynolds RL: The determination of pulp vitality by means of thermal and electrical stimuli, *Oral Surg* 22:231, 1966.

Rossman SR, Kaplowitz B, Buldinger SR: Therapy of the endodontically and periodontally involved tooth, *Oral Surg* 13:361, 1960.

Rubach WC, Mitchell DF: Periodontal disease, accessory canals and pulp pathosis, *J Periodontol* 36:34, 1965.

Rubach WC, Mitchell DF: Periodontal disease, age and pulp status, *Oral Surg* 19:482, 1965.

Seltzer S, Bender IB, Nazimov H: Pulpitis-induced interradicular periodontal changes in experimental animals, *J Periodontol* 38:124, 1967.

Seltzer S, Bender IB, Ziontz M: The interrelationship of pulp and periodontal disease, *Oral Surg* 16:1474, 1963.

Seltzer S, Soltanoff W, Bender IB, Ziontz M: Biologic aspects of endodontics. I. Histologic observations of the anatomy and morphology of root apices and their surrounding structures, *Oral Surg* 22:375, 1966.

Simon JHS, Glick DH, Frank AL: The relationship of endodontic-periodontic lesions, *J Periodontol* 43:202, 1972.

Simring M, Goldberg M: The pulpal pocket approach: retrograde periodontitis, *J Periodontol* 35:22, 1964.

Sinai I: The interrelationship of the pulp and the periodontal ligament. Presented at the American Association of Endodontists annual meeting, Atlanta, April 1970.

Stahl SS: Pulpal response to gingival injury in rats, *Oral Surg* 16:1116, 1963.

Stahl SS: Pathogenesis of the inflammatory lesion in pulp and periodontal tissues, *Periodontics* 4:190, 1966.

Stanley HR: Design for a human pulp study, *Oral Surg* 25:633, 1968.

Toto PD, Staffileno H, Weine FS, Das S: Age change effects on the pulp in periodontitis, *Annals of Dentistry* 36:13, 1977.

VandeVoorde HE: Combined endodontic-periodontic procedures, *J Tenn Dent Assoc* 56:57, 1976.

Vertucci FJ, Anthony RL: A scanning electron microscopic investigation of accessory foramina in the furcation and pulp chamber floor of molar teeth, *Oral Surg* 62:319, 1986.

Vertucci FJ, Williams RG: Furcation canals in the human mandibular first molar, *Oral Surg* 38:308, 1974.

Weine FS, Frank AL: Survival of the endodontic endosseous implant, *J Endod* 19:524, 1993.

Weinman JP: Progress of gingival inflammation into the supporting structures of the teeth, *J Periodontol* 12:71, 1941.

Wong R, Hirsh RS, Clark NG: Endodontic effects of root planing in humans, *Endod Dent Traumatol* 5:193, 1989.

Franklin S. Weine • Steven R. Potashnick

14 Endodontic-orthodontic relationships

The expanding role of endodontics into more phases of dental treatment is illustrated by the awareness of relationships with orthodontics. There are two major areas where endodontics and orthodontics share common ground. One is etiologic, because orthodontic treatment affects the tooth being moved and some of the response may be noted in the pulp tissue. The other, only recently presented as an entity of importance, is combined therapy, where orthodontic treatment is necessary to gain a desirable endodontic result.

EFFECT OF ORTHODONTICS ON THE TOOTH BEING MOVED

Orthodontic treatment is used to gain a much more esthetic appearance for the patient and is often further utilized to improve the occlusion. In the course of such therapy, certain changes may occur to the tooth being moved. The most common side effect of orthodontics is to blunt the root of the moved tooth, due to apical and sometimes lateral resorption.

Orthodontics as the etiologic agent for endodontics. Some teeth require endodontic treatment as a result of previous orthodontics. Because the action of the blunting of root tips usually occurs in the area where the apical blood vessels and nerves emerge, it can be seen that injury at this susceptible site could affect pulp vitality. Orthodontists suggest that this is not true and attempt to refute these statements with papers that describe the rotation of teeth 720 and even 1080 degrees without demonstrable pulp damage. However, the fact remains that I have treated a number of teeth in which the only possible etiologic agent for the loss of pulp vitality or damage to the pulp was via orthodontic therapy.

The most common situation is a maxillary cuspid that has been crowded out of position by the adjacent lateral incisor and first bicuspid, thus requiring orthodontic therapy to gain added eruption (Figs. 14-1 and 14-2, A). Because these teeth rarely have carious lesions or restorations and because symptoms are generally lacking, the initial signs that endodontic therapy is needed are discovered during the taking of routine periapical radiographs. The most frequent observation from the films is a periapical radiolucency (Fig. 14-1, A). However, another indication that pulpal damage has resulted may be seen when there is a considerable diminution of canal width (Fig. 14-2). This finding is similar to that seen when vital pulp therapy causes heavy deposition of reparative dentin. (See Chapter 16.)

The healing of these teeth follows the normal pattern (Fig. 14-1, B to E) and is not adversely affected in any way by the previously performed orthodontic treatment. However, it might be extremely difficult to locate and therefore treat teeth when the pulp space diminishes tremendously (Fig. 14-2), as does happen in some cases.

Resorptive defects. I have treated teeth with resorptive defects where the dental history included previous orthodontic treatment. Fig. 14-3 demonstrates an internal resorptive defect, whereas Fig. 14-8 illustrates a defect that could have originated internally or externally but eventually caused a communication between the pulp space and the periodontal ligament.

Whether it was the orthodontic therapy that caused the resorption is questionable under any circumstances. However, just as some pulpal changes include deposition of reparative dentin, resorption can also occur from pulpal injury that might have been initiated by orthodontic movement.

In another departure from routine circumstances, a recent report by Gruendeman (co-authored by two endodontists) described treatment of a preorthodontic lateral resorption on a maxillary lateral incisor that would be moved during orthodontic treatment. By applying the use of calcium hydroxide (Chapter 16) before orthodontic therapy, the resorption was halted, some calcification gained, and the case was able to reach a satisfactory conclusion, both in alignment and esthetics.

Necessary monitoring by the orthodontist and the general dentist. I strongly recommend that following orthodontic treatment a full set of radiographs be taken. These films should be scrutinized carefully by both the orthodontist and the general dentist for any incipient periapical lesions and any unusual changes in pulp canal shape. Furthermore, all teeth that have been moved, particularly those that were pulled into occlusion, should be monitored at least on a once-a-year basis via radiograph and careful clinical examination to verify normalcy of the pulp. If the pulp canal space does begin to diminish or get larger, endodontic therapy should not be delayed.

Treating teeth after orthodontic treatment. In my evaluation of teeth needing endodontic therapy that had previously received orthodontic movement, one observation is extremely frequent. There is a high percentage of overfills (Fig. 14-4, *B*). Because the apical dentin matrix development is a very important phase of the endodontic treatment that I espouse, this finding is disturbing to me because it indicates that no or insufficient matrix was present. I know that the chance of failure, although still quite small, increases when the master cones are demonstrable in the periapical tissues.

Of course, it seems quite obvious now but the cause of these overextensions is directly related to the orthodontic treatment, because the root end has been blunted by resorption. Therefore working length should be shortened when such teeth are being treated, and the customized master cone technique (Chapter 9) should be employed wherever possible to see whether a matrix is present.

Treating teeth during orthodontic treatment. Although I have had relatively few cases that fall into this category, some of the most complicated teeth that I have treated were those involved in simultaneous orthodontic movement (Fig. 14-5). Because of the conduction potential of the bands and archwires, electric pulp testing is impossible. Test cavity preparation is available; but it is diffi-

cult to drill into these teeth, which generally are noncarious and unrestored yet have large pulps, without absolute certainly that a necrotic pulp is present.

Apical and lateral radiolucencies and root resorption, which are common findings when endodontic therapy is needed, are found in these cases incident to orthodontics and do not necessarily indicate pulp damage. Evaluation of these teeth is most complicated and confusing.

Even when a correct decision is made in determination of therapy, some postoperative films may indicate the opposite (Fig. 14-5, *D*). It is extremely important to keep these patients under close supervision until complete healing is verified (Fig. 14-5, *F*) or further treatment is indicated.

ENDODONTIC-ORTHODONTIC COMBINED THERAPY

Endodontic-orthodontic cotreatment may become necessary to save teeth with advanced caries, traumatic destruction of the clinical crown (Fig. 14-6), lateral root perforation (Fig. 14-7), external or internal resorption near the alveolar crest (Fig. 14-8), or overzealous tooth preparation. Without such treatment these teeth may not offer sound tooth structure on which to place a restoration.

Isolated infrabony periodontal defects may also be amenable to forced eruption. Orthodontic therapy will improve the existing periodontal environment by modifying the osseous topography and minimizing the need to remove supporting bone on adjacent teeth. This occurs when movement of the tooth in an occlusal direction carries the connective tissue attachment in the same direction, modifying the osseous topography and pocket epithelium as they relate to the adjacent teeth. Movement of a tooth into an infrabony pocket rather than out of the pocket will eliminate the angular defect morphology but interposes epithelium between the root and bone. Such movement has no effect on the connective tissue attachment and is not advisable. Endodontic therapy in conjunction with eruption permits placement of a restoration that fulfills the periodontal and occlusal requirements of the tooth.

Lengthening the clinical crown by removing supporting bone to expose sound tooth structure or eliminate the existing periodontal defect is the solution usually recommended. Forced orthodontic eruption, in conjunction with endodontic, periodontal, and restorative therapy, is an alternative.

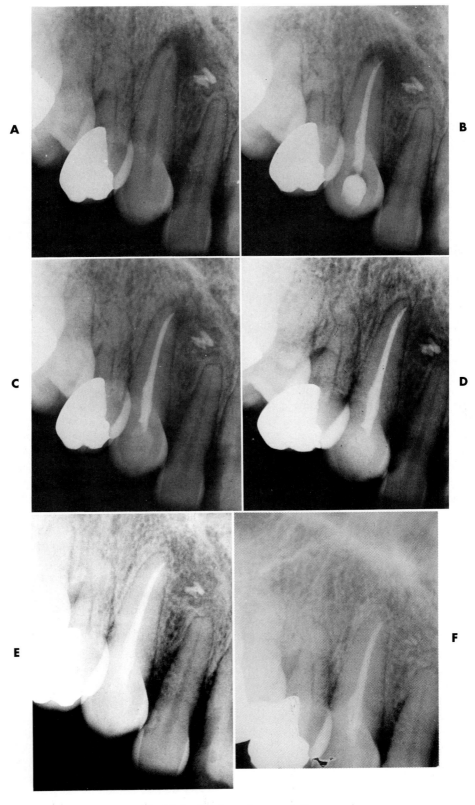

Fig. 14-1. For legend see opposite page.

Fig. 14-1. A, Preoperative view of maxillary cuspid periapical radiolucency. Tooth did not respond to pulp testing. Patient revealed that the tooth was erupting in an unfavorable position, and orthodontic movement was used to bring it into correct alignment. Radiopaque mass adjacent to the tooth is probably residual cement. **B,** Endodontics completed, canal is filled with laterally condensed gutta-percha and Wach's paste. **C,** Six months later, area is decreasing in size. **D,** One year later, periapical lesion is healed. **E,** Five years after treatment, periapical area remains normal, cement decreasing in size. **F,** Thirteen years after treatment, cement has been completely resorbed, periapical area associated with cuspid has healed perfectly. Periodontal condition on lateral incisor has worsened. (Restoration by Dr. Howard Paule, Highland Park, Ill.)

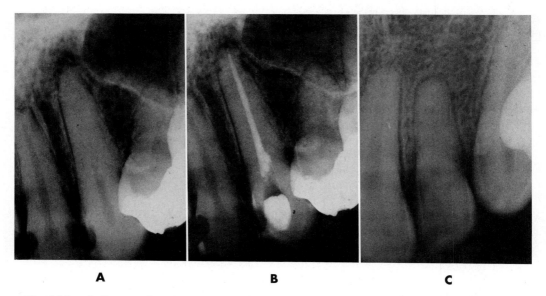

A   B   C

Fig. 14-2. A, Preoperative radiograph of maxillary cuspid with periapical lesion. Dental history of this case was identical to that of patient in Fig. 14-1. Canal is very narrow in apical portion but distinct in coronal portion, just the opposite of typical appearance of teeth with longstanding chronic pulpitis. This indicates that pulpitis initiated near apex and moved incisally. **B,** Endodontics completed. **C,** No apparent canal in maxillary lateral incisor. There was no history of trauma, but the patient reported that he had received orthodontic treatment for a large overbite and that maxillary anterior teeth had been moved (perhaps tipped) lingually. Note blunt apex of the tooth.

This multidisciplinary approach offers benefits not available with periodontal surgery alone.

The principles of forced eruption were documented in the dental literature by Angle before 1900. More recently they have been revived in the endodontic literature by Heithersay and in the periodontal literature by Ingber.

Basic periodontal principles for forced eruption. In health the alveolar bone mimics the rise and fall of the cementoenamel junction as it is followed around the tooth. The supra-alveolar tissue is comprised of sulcular epithelium, junctional epithelium, and gingival connective tissue. The biologic width has been defined as the combined dimension of supra-alveolar gingival connective tissue and the junctional epithelium, and in health it averages 2.04 mm. In a healthy periodontium the average dimension from the crest of the alveolar bone to the cementoenamel junction is 1.07 mm. This dimension measures the gingival connective tissue fibers from the alveolar crest to the base of the junctional epithelium. The average dimension

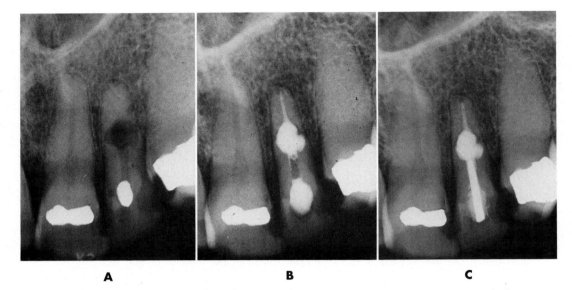

Fig. 14-3. **A,** Preoperative radiograph of maxillary lateral incisor with large internal resorptive defect and no apparent canal apical to the defect. Tooth has several large restorations that may have stimulated the resorption, but there was also a history of orthodontic movement. Note blunting of the apices of both central and lateral incisors and no apparent canal in the cuspid. **B,** Tooth treated according to Chapter 16, with placement of calcium hydroxide paste initially, waiting for some calcification, and then filling with vertically condensed gutta-percha and Kerr's Antiseptic Root Canal Sealer. **C,** Three years after original treatment, following reinforcement with an Endopost, tooth is asymptomatic and periodontal tissues around it have retained normal clinical and radiographic appearance.

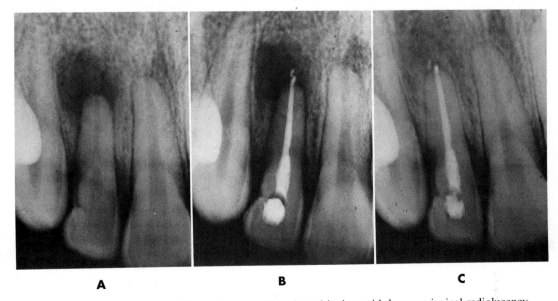

Fig. 14-4. **A,** Preoperative radiograph of maxillary lateral incisor with large periapical radiolucency. Tooth had a nonvital pulp of unknown origin, but trauma was probable cause since the young man was an amateur boxer. He had received orthodontic treatment several years earlier, and apices of both lateral and central incisors were blunted. **B,** Canal was prepared in a normal manner and filled with laterally condensed gutta-percha and Wach's paste. Although I thought I had an apical dentin matrix present, obviously I did not, for the master cone is pushed through into the periapical tissues. **C,** One year later, area is considerably reduced in size.

A   B   C

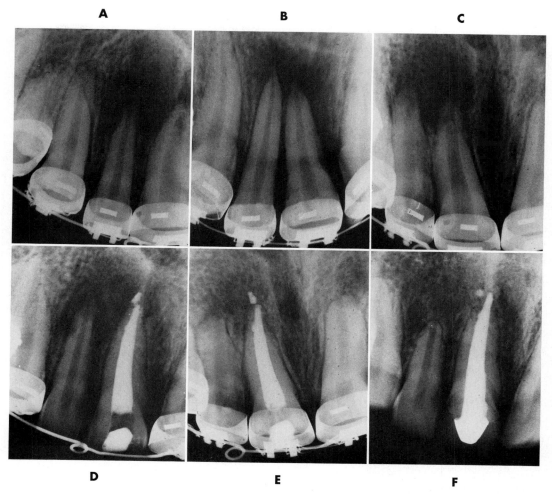

D   E   F

Fig. 14-5.   **A to C,** Preoperative radiographs of maxillary anterior area indicating a large radiolucency associated with lateral (no. 7) and central (no. 8) incisors. In **A,** lesion seems associated with no. 7 only; in **C** it seems predominantly associated with no. 8. **D,** Bands were removed from teeth in order to perform electric pulp testing. No. 8 was nonresponsive, whereas no. 7 responded normally. Accordingly, only no. 8 was treated. On receipt of this postoperative film, the referring dentist questioned my sanity. **E,** One year later. **F,** Two years after original treatment, excellent healing of lesion and return to a normal regular periodontal ligament on no. 7.

of the junctional epithelial attachment is 0.97 mm, with a range of 0.71 to 1.35 mm.

When the margin of a restoration is being placed below the gingiva, it is of utmost importance to maintain the health and integrity of the biologic width. A restoration that impinges on the biologic width will result in progressive periodontal disease. The initial response to this insult may be gingival recession, edema, or hyperplasia.

To avoid periodontal pathosis, the dentist must maintain the integrity of the biologic width. For this reason, an additional 1 or 2 mm of sound tooth structure must be available coronal to the epithelial attachment for placement of the margin of a restoration. The distance from the alveolar crest to the coronal extent of the remaining tooth structure should be a minimum of 3.5 to 4 mm. With any less tooth structure the clinician risks impinging on the junctional epithelium and connective tissue attachment in a subgingival preparation.

The biologic width of gingival tissue moves with the tooth as the tooth moves in health,

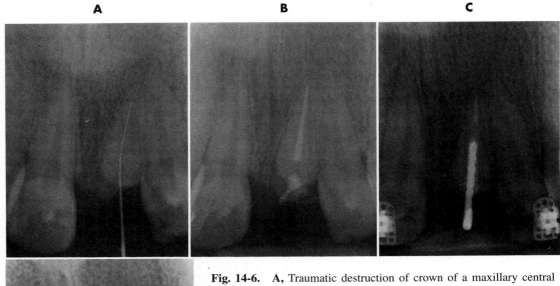

Fig. 14-6. **A,** Traumatic destruction of crown of a maxillary central incisor. Fracture extends to alveolar crest. File in place, locating the canal. **B,** Endodontics completed. **C,** Post-orthodontic therapy. Root was forcibly erupted approximately 3 mm. Note that alveolar crest has moved with tooth as the tooth moved in health. **D,** One year later.

maintaining its relationship to the tooth as the tooth is moved under controlled orthodontic force (Fig. 14-7). In the presence of inflammatory periodontal disease, tooth movement may contribute to the deepening of an existing osseous defect. Therefore controlled orthodontic movement must take place in a periodontal environment that is as healthy as possible. It must be maintained in health throughout the movement phase of therapy. This is achieved through gentle but thorough scaling, root planing, and soft tissue curettage on a biweekly basis as treatment progresses. Failure to control periodontal health during tooth movement may result in a less than optimal treatment response.

The traditional method of treating a tooth with advanced caries, resorption, or trauma extending apical or to the alveolar crest is to expose adequate sound tooth structure with periodontal surgery. In order to maintain a positive osseous architecture in which interradicular bone is coronal to radicular bone height, the operator must remove supporting bone from adjacent teeth. The adjacent alveolar crest to the tooth in question must be scalloped to form a smooth, harmonious contour from tooth to tooth. This reduces alveolar support on teeth other than the one in question, increases the crown-to-root ratio of these teeth, and compromises the esthetic appearance of anterior teeth (Fig. 14-8).

The scalloped gingival form associated with anterior teeth contributes to the difficulty in obtaining a cosmetic result when osseous surgery is completed on three or four teeth. The postoperative appearance of the surgically corrected area

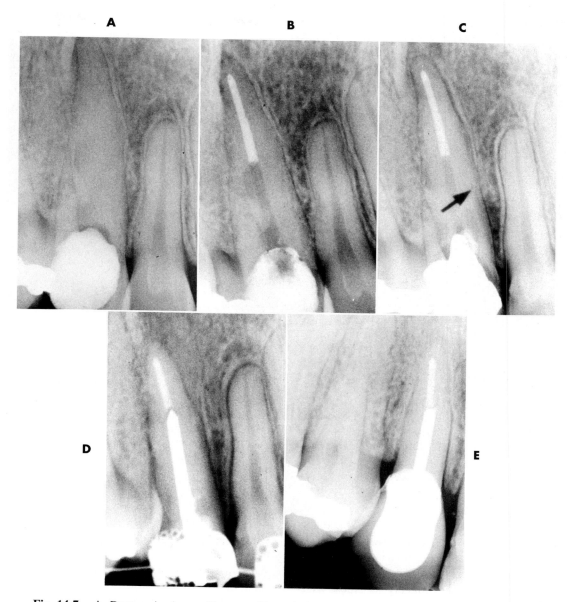

Fig. 14-7. A, Deep caries in maxillary cuspid requiring endodontic treatment. **B,** Canal filled with gutta-percha and post room prepared. **C,** Poor attempt at restoration, with perforation of the mesial wall *(arrow)* trying to change post preparation, lack of marginal fit, and resultant infrabony pocket. **D,** After forced eruption, mesial infrabony pocket has been eliminated by concomitant coronal movement of adjacent bone to where it could be managed surgically (see **H**). Notice the change in apical position of the cuspid as compared with the adjacent lateral incisor in **C. E,** Radiograph upon completion of restoration.

Continued

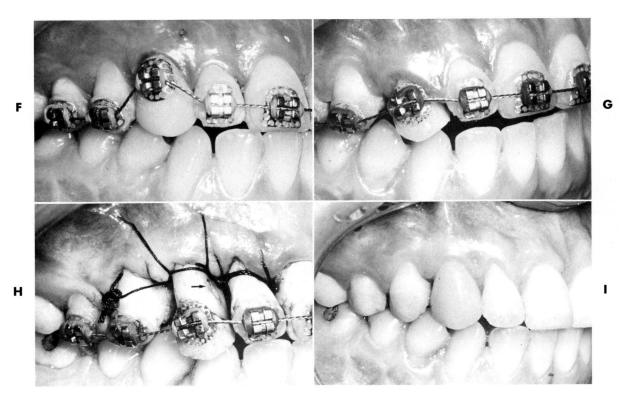

Fig. 14-7, cont'd. **F** through **I,** Clinical photographs. **F,** Initiation of forced eruption. **G,** Following forced eruption, note that the gingival margin has maintained its relationship to the orthodontic bracket throughout tooth movement. **H,** Gingival tissue and alveolar bone have been elevated to expose the perforation *(arrow)* and eliminate the residual periodontal pocket. Little bone had to be removed around the lateral incisor. **I,** Final restoration in place. (Endodontic treatment by Dr. Steven Sanders and final restoration by Dr. Sherwin Laff, both of Chicago.)

will present open interdental embrasures and teeth that seem longer than their neighbors (Fig. 14-9).

Orthodontically erupting the tooth with its attachment apparatus and gingiva may eliminate the need for periodontal surgery to expose sound tooth structure and reduce alveolar support on adjacent teeth. Surgery may be necessary to level angular interdental alveolar crests created by tooth movement and reposition the overlying soft tissue to its proper coronal level. Augmentation of the gingiva can be accomplished at the same surgery using soft tissue pedicle grafts of interproximal or edentulous ridge gingiva (Fig. 14-10). Periodontal surgery after eruption will restore form to the individual dental unit as it relates collectively to the adjacent teeth in the arch.

Exposing adequate sound tooth structure by periodontal surgery alone will lead to a shortened clinical root and a larger clinical crown as the tissues are positioned apically. The crown-to-root ratio of the tooth following surgery alone will exceed the crown-to-root ratio of the tooth that is first orthodontically erupted. There is thus a *relative* improvement in the crown-to-root ratio of the tooth undergoing orthodontic eruption followed by periodontal therapy that does not occur after a surgical procedure alone (Fig. 14-8).

The end result of forced eruption contributes to a more cosmetic and physiologic restoration. Osseous resection following forced eruption should be minimal on adjacent teeth (Fig. 14-11). The position of the gingival tissue margin will approximate

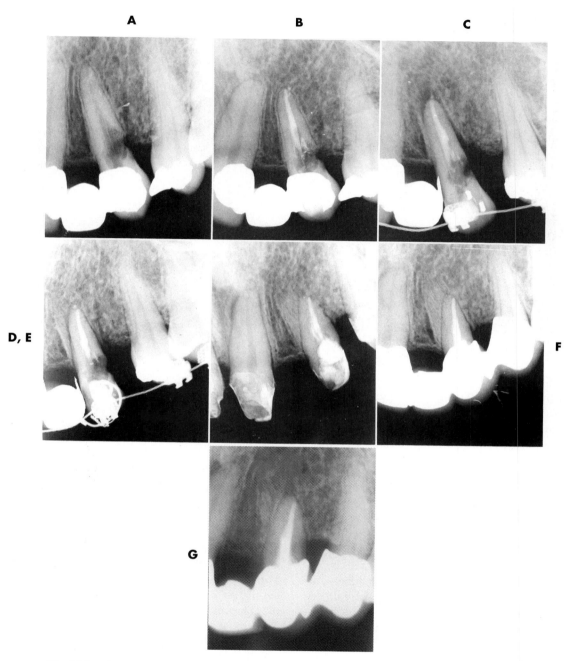

Fig. 14-8. **A,** Resorptive lesion at the alveolar crest causing an infrabony pocket. Patient had history of orthodontic treatment. **B,** Endodontic treatment completed and initial post room prepared for orthodontic movement. If only surgical treatment were employed to eliminate the pocket and expose the resorptive lesion, a crown-to-root ratio of 2:1 would result. By forced eruption and surgical exposure, a more acceptable ratio of 1:1 is obtained. The tooth also has poor axial inclination in this position. **C,** The tooth is erupted, and the alveolar bone and resorptive lesion are moved to a position more amenable to surgical exposure. **D,** An uprighting spring is placed to align the tooth for parallelism to adjacent teeth. **E,** Final tooth position. There is excellent bone fill and radiographic "ghosting" of the previously occupied socket. **F,** Final restoration, 2 years after original treatment. **G,** Six years after original treatment, "ghosting" has lightened, restoration looks excellent. Compare to **A.**

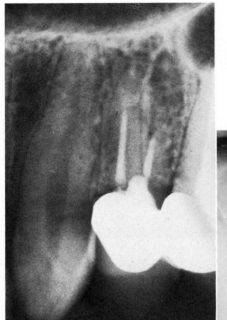

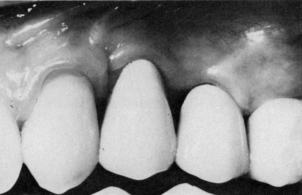

Fig. 14-9. **A,** Preoperative film of a maxillary first bicuspid with inadequate endodontic filling and advanced caries approaching alveolar crest. **B,** After endodontic re-treatment, periodontal surgery to expose sound tooth structure, and final restorative therapy completed. Tooth appears much longer than its neighbors.

A

B

its original level following the surgical procedure, and a relative improvement in the crown-to-root ratio will be achieved. This reduces the dimension of the esthetic deformities created by surgical management alone.

Basic endodontic principles for forced eruption. Teeth that are certain to require endodontic therapy should have such treatment completed prior to the initiation of tooth movement. In the case of an isolated periodontal defect, endodontic therapy should be completed before tooth movement if it appears that intentional extirpation will be required to restore the tooth after eruption. This decision is based on the morphology of the periodontal lesion and the amount of tooth movement required to modify it. Early endodontic treatment eliminates the problem of constantly changing working lengths as the tooth is erupted and the crown is adjusted to the opposing articulation. Teeth that have no pulpal problem and are undergoing eruption may have endodontic therapy completed in one sitting. Teeth that present with caries, resorptive or iatrogenic perforation, or posttraumatic destruction of the clinical crown will require a multisitting regimen.

A tooth with a subalveolar fracture may have endodontic therapy completed through the existing clinical crown if it can be stabilized to the adjacent teeth. This facilitates placement of a rubber dam, increases control of the working field, and reduces hemorrhage in the area.

At times endodontic therapy may become necessary after the initiation of tooth movement. In this case the pulpal tissue should be extirpated as completely as possible, the canal sealed, and the treatment completed as soon after tooth movement as possible. There is no contraindication to completing the endodontic therapy while the tooth is undergoing orthodontic movement (Fig. 14-12). The problems of treating a tooth in this situation are the presence of the orthodontic appliance and the changing working length.

Teeth with loss or destruction of the clinical crown must have endodontic therapy completed prior to tooth movement. Post preparation room of adequate width and length must be provided. A post may then be cemented into the tooth to allow for movement.

If the canal is hollowed out, as is the case with advanced caries, a customized post must be fabricated prior to cementation into the tooth. The temporary cements used to lute this post into the canal for tooth movement all contain eugenol. If a loose-fitting post is cemented into a canal and then

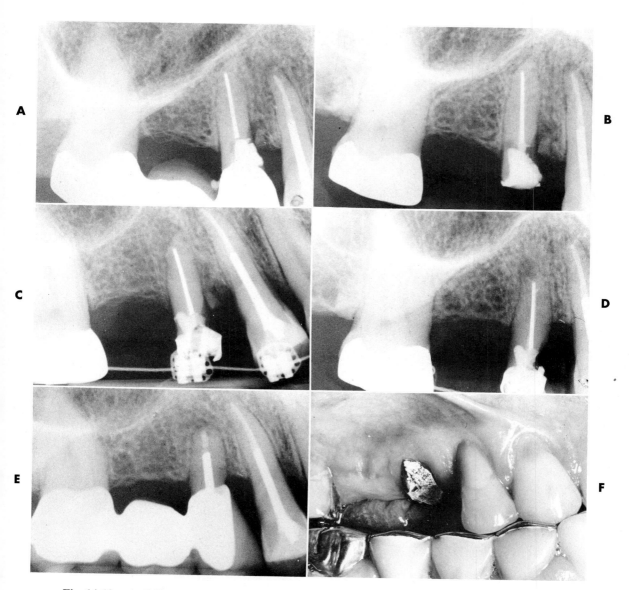

Fig. 14-10. **A,** Failing bridge, with lateral perforation and infrabony pocket on mesial of bicuspid. **B,** Bridge was removed, and in attempt to remove silver point to obtain adequate post room, a near perforation of the distal wall has resulted. **C,** After forced eruption, the mesial infrabony pocket has been eliminated, creating room to remove silver point. Tooth movement has created angular crests, which will be leveled without decrease of bone on adjacent bicuspid. **D,** Following surgery, the angular defects are eliminated and sound tooth structure created. The tooth is ready for endodontic therapy. **E,** Now it is much easier to remove the silver point, reprepare the canal, refill with gutta-percha and prepare long post room. This film was taken 18 months after original treatment. **F** through **K,** Clinical photographs. **F,** Appearance following removal of failing bridge and ineffective attempt to remove silver point, conforming to film **B.**

Continued

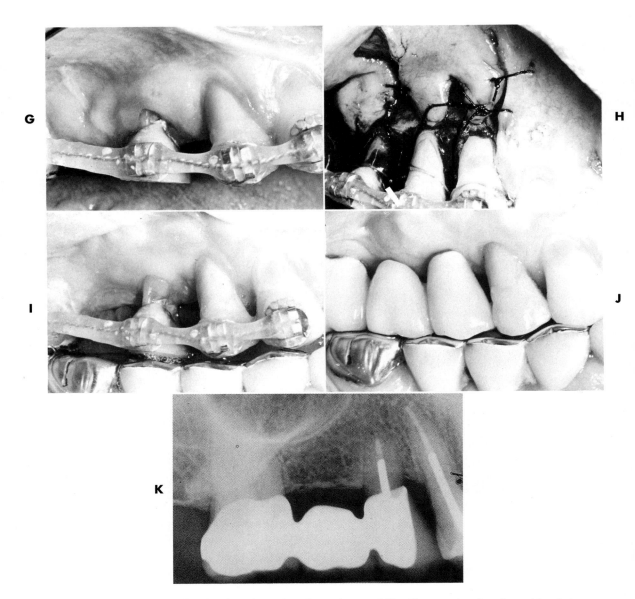

Fig. 14-10, cont'd. **G,** After forced eruption, the teeth are stabilized by covering the wire and bracket with autopolymerizing resin, creating a rigid splint. Note the narrow zone of masticatory mucosa on the bicuspids and cuspid. **H,** Laterally positioned pedicle grafts are completed following osseous surgery. The needs of the soft tissue can be addressed at the same time sound tooth structure is created, and infrabony periodontal pockets are eliminated. **I,** After periodontal surgery, exposing the perforation. Sound tooth structure is available for the new restoration and to remove the silver point. An adequate zone of attached gingiva has been created. **J,** Final restoration in place, 18 months after original treatment and 12 months after new bridge was placed. **K,** Radiograph taken 12 years after original treatment, compare to **B.** Lesion on first bicuspid is healed, lateral defect on second bicuspid has improved greatly, bridge looks excellent. (Final restoration by Dr. Joseph Krohn, formerly of Chicago.)

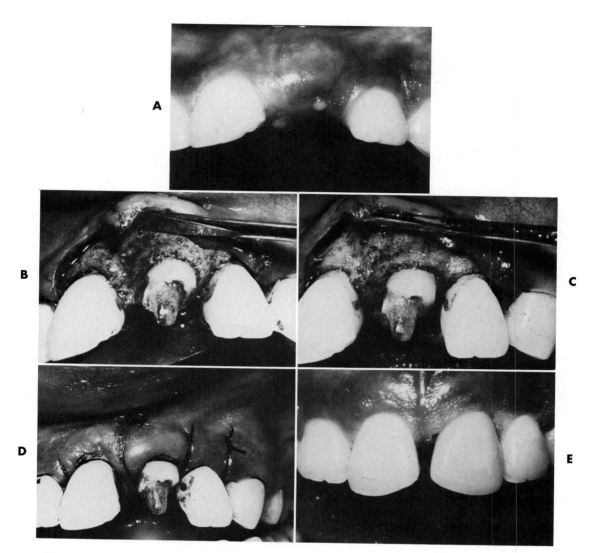

Fig. 14-11. A, Suppuration exiting from chronic draining sinus to remaining root segment of a fractured maxillary incisor. **B,** After orthodontic eruption, area is treated surgically to level the angular interdental alveolar crests. **C,** Angular crests are removed, and a horizontal interdental alveolar crest is formed. Alveolar bone is removed over radicular surfaces for sound tooth structure. There is no need to remove supporting bone over adjacent teeth. **D,** Gingiva is repositioned as close as possible to its original position at cementoenamel junction. **E,** Final restoration. Crown size and interdental soft tissue heights are within normal limits. Removal of root would have created difficult restorative problem in presence of naturally occurring diastema.

becomes loose during tooth movement, fabricating an acrylic post around a metal subcore may be more difficult. The eugenol from the cement will inhibit polymerization of the acrylic used to fabricate the customized post.

Gutta-percha is the filling material of choice for teeth undergoing forced eruption. The advantages

of semisolid filling materials and the criteria for readiness of the canal for filling are described in Chapter 9 and apply to this technique.

Filling the canal with solid materials such as silver points is contraindicated. The risk of dislodging a silver point during fabrication of a customized post, cementation, and post removal is

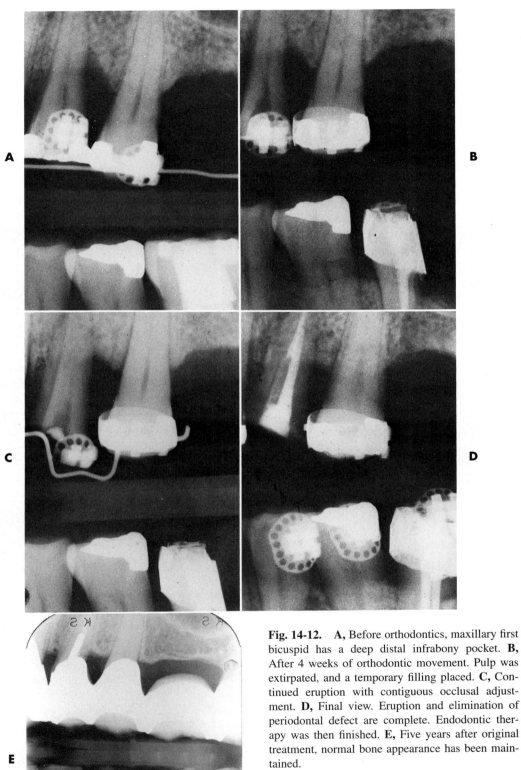

Fig. 14-12. A, Before orthodontics, maxillary first bicuspid has a deep distal infrabony pocket. **B,** After 4 weeks of orthodontic movement. Pulp was extirpated, and a temporary filling placed. **C,** Continued eruption with contiguous occlusal adjustment. **D,** Final view. Eruption and elimination of periodontal defect are complete. Endodontic therapy was then finished. **E,** Five years after original treatment, normal bone appearance has been maintained.

great. Contamination of the canal and silver point with saliva during these procedures risks slow, progressive oxidation of the silver point, leading to eventual endodontic failure.

On the contrary, the removal of a recalcitrant silver point may be aided by first erupting the tooth orthodontically (Fig. 14-10). Eruption allows the clinician to expose enough of the silver point to gain an adequate purchase and access for removal. This may be necessary when the silver point prevents the clinician from creating adequate post room or when the tooth requires re-treatment due to failure of endodontic origin.

Teeth requiring endodontic and orthodontic therapy should be restored following the principles described in Chapter 17.

Basic orthodontic principles for tooth movement. The patient must understand the indication for tooth movement and that endodontic therapy is essential or highly likely. The patient also must be aware that restorative dentistry will follow the endodontic-orthodontic cotherapy.

Prior to the initiation of treatment, an estimate of the amount of attachment apparatus remaining at the completion of tooth movement must be made. The tooth must have sufficient radicular attachment to assist in the support of a multiunit restoration or maintain its individual integrity while contributing to esthetics, phonetics, and function.

Single-rooted teeth generally narrow from the cementoenamel junction to the apex. Eruption of teeth with single roots brings a narrower portion of the root to the level of the cementoenamel junction

of adjacent teeth (Fig. 14-13). This improves the interdental environment if root proximity is present.

Posterior teeth, with their greater osseous support, root surface area, flatter interdental form, and esthetic requirements, are more amenable to osseous surgery than to forced eruption. Forced eruption risks bringing furcations closer to the level of the cementoenamel junction of adjacent teeth. This may result in furcation exposure.

The natural flaring of posterior roots increases root proximity problems when eruption is attempted. This is particularly critical between the distobuccal root of the maxillary first molar and the mesiobuccal root of the maxillary second molar.

Infection and inflammation must be controlled before tooth movement. Control of the inflammatory lesion by curettage of the soft tissue pocket wall and removal of the granulomatous tissue and gingival fibers to the alveolar crest must precede tooth movement. No tooth movement should be started unless the retention and stabilization phases have been fully planned.

Adequate anchorage must be available to produce only the movement specifically required. A minimum of two teeth on each side of the tooth to be erupted should be used, to resist their own displacement and to encourage movement of the tooth in question. Movement occurs in a vertical plane. Vertical movements are intrusion and extrusion. Intrusion is difficult to achieve and requires a greater force to be effective. Since there is no bone in the path of the erupting tooth, resorption is not a factor unless a tortuous root compresses

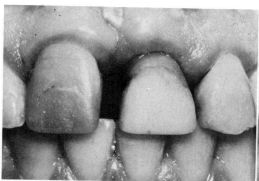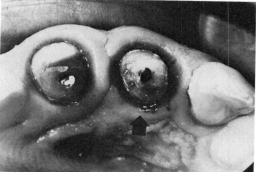

Fig. 14-13. **A,** Labial view, maxillary central incisor to left (no. 8) had received endodontic and some periodontal treatment. Incisor to right (no. 9) had received endodontic, periodontal, and orthodontic extrusion. **B,** In the preparation no. 9 *(arrow)* has oval cross-sectional area at level of soft tissue, whereas nonextruded tooth is larger and triangular at that level.

the ligament in an isolated area. Only light force is required when extrusive movement is being considered.

Conventional orthodontic appliances should be used whenever possible. Movement of a tooth to a wire or bar that is cemented or bonded to adjacent teeth limits the distance the tooth can be moved and reduces control by the operator. To replace or change a segmental archwire in orthodontic brackets takes very little time and offers flexibility that is not available with a stationary bar if additional movements are desired. Conventional mechanics allows for tooth movement in a mesial or distal direction for space distribution, rotation of roots for parallelism for use in a multiunit restoration, or for reduction of root proximity.

Situations of accelerated mesial drift and unfavorable tipping of teeth and axial tooth position may not lend themselves to forced eruption. Under these circumstances eruption may increase root proximity and obliterate interdental space. Uprighting and correction of axial tooth position may be necessary prior to eruption. All these movements are achieved with greater control when conventional orthodontic direct-bond brackets, bands, and archwires are used.

Removable orthodontic appliances are less exacting, depend on patient dexterity and cooperation, are bulky, affect speech, and cannot stabilize the tooth following eruption. Their advantage is to provide anchorage when an adequate number of natural teeth are absent. If possible they, too, should be avoided.

Unless very light force is used to extrude the tooth, a lag period occurs between movement of the tooth and movement of its attachment apparatus and surrounding gingiva. The attachment apparatus and gingival unit follow the tooth after it begins to erupt from the alveolus. Depending on the amount of eruption required, periodontal surgery may not be necessary. The amount of force used and the speed of eruption determine the lag time, because the faster the tooth is forcibly extruded the greater will be the lag between the movements of tooth and attachment apparatus (Fig. 14-14).

This may be used to the clinician's advantage. Early, rapid eruption may expose additional sound tooth structure and reduce the need for a surgical procedure later. The osseous and gingival margins are more likely to move with the tooth when slow, intermittent, light force is used. This is a consideration when I would like to align the gingival margin with the adjacent teeth to improve the overall esthetic result.

Our clinical impression is that the hard and soft tissues *always* move with the tooth. Whether they move as much as the tooth moves depends on the force applied over the course of treatment rather than the distance the tooth is moved. Our best results have followed a sequence of slow, progressive traction until the tooth demonstrates elevated mobility, followed by rapid, continuous force to bring the tooth to the desired final position.

Stabilization prevents the stretched periodontal ligament fibers from pulling the root back into the alveolus. An easy and fast technique to stabilize the tooth is to brush autopolymerizing resin over the sectional archwire and brackets to lock everything into position (Fig. 14-10). Another method is to place a passive archwire into the brackets.

The length of time a tooth needs to be stabilized will depend on the distance the tooth has been moved. A minimum of 6 weeks of stabilization generally is necessary. I use evidence of radiographic bone fill in the socket around the apex of the tooth as a guide. Stabilization is complete and relapse will not occur when the apical bone has filled the socket according to the radiograph (Fig. 14-8).

Forced eruption—methods and materials. With the advent of orthodontic direct-bonding brackets, adjunctive tooth movement such as forced eruption can be practiced efficiently and economically by the general practitioner.

With the clinical situation previously described, the technique of forcible eruption takes on one of two clinical protocols.

Tooth lacking a clinical crown. Endodontic therapy is completed immediately. Post room of adequate width and length is provided. Control of gingival inflammation by curettage is completed prior to tooth movement.

A 0.030- to 0.036-inch stainless steel wire is fit snugly to the post preparation. It may be notched to offer additional retention. If necessary, a customized post may be fabricated by adding cold-cure acrylic resin around a prefit post for maximum adaptation to the canal walls. The post should have a loop bend extending from the canal preparation. The wire may be cemented into the canal with semitemporary cement.

A snugly fit post will not be pulled or loosened from the canal during tooth movement, even when cemented with a temporary cement. The cement bond can be easily broken by rotating the wire in the

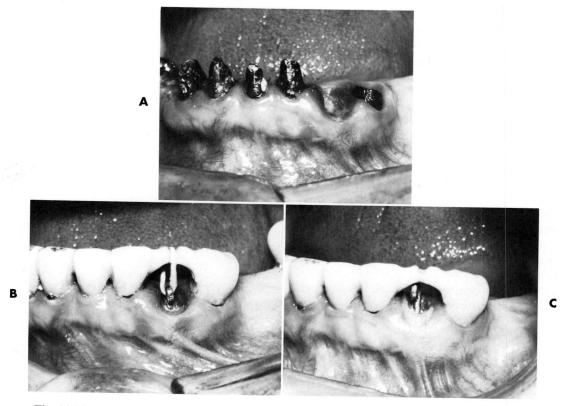

Fig. 14-14.   A, Preoperative view of a mandibular cuspid with advanced caries extending to attachment apparatus. **B,** Elastic ligature is tied from existing bridge to wire cemented into tooth. **C,** With rapid eruption, tooth is extruded from alveolus, exposing sound tooth structure. Some movement of attachment apparatus and gingival tissue did occur, as indicated by position of the soft tissue relative to the adjacent crowns. Compare **B** and **C.**

canal after tooth movement. The use of more permanent cements will increase the difficulty of removal. If the post loosens, escalating treatment with the use of more retentive cements may become necessary.

After successful completion of the endodontic and preparatory periodontal therapy, direct-bond orthodontic brackets are placed on a sufficient number of teeth on both sides of the tooth to be erupted for adequate anchorage.

The direct-bond orthodontic brackets should be placed as close to the incisal edge of the teeth as possible. They must not interfere with the opposing articulation. The channel in the brackets should be in the same horizontal plane so that a straight wire may be laid passively in all the channels. Placing the brackets as far to the incisal as possible increases the distance from the segmental archwire to the post cemented in the tooth.

A rigid 0.016-inch wire is ligated into the brackets. An elastic ligature cord is tied from the wire to the cemented post, activating tooth movement.

The tooth should be moved slowly into position over a period of 4 to 6 weeks. If necessary, a new segmental archwire bent to increase its distance from the erupting tooth may be placed.

The greater the force placed on the tooth, the more rapid will be its eruption from the alveolus. With slow, constant, light pressure, the alveolus and soft tissue will move with the tooth. *Do not be fooled into thinking that the tooth is not erupting if you do not see it extruding from the soft tissue.* If properly managed, the soft tissue will move with the tooth (Fig. 14-7).

Tooth having an intact clinical crown. A direct-bond bracket or orthodontic band is placed as far apical as is permissible.

Initially the tooth can be pulled to a segmental arch as previously described. As the tooth approaches the horizontal plane of the adjacent brackets, a multistrand flexible 0.015-inch wire may be placed. If deflected 2 or 3 mm, it will exert suitable extrusive force.

The use of a straight wire over a small interbracket distance may produce force greater than desired. By using narrow-gauge wire with vertical loops in the interbracket area, the operator can increase the working length of the wire. This will decrease the range of force applied as the wire is distorted into the bracket and should be considered when greater amounts of extrusion are desired over a longer time.

Care must be taken to adjust the occlusion and provide interarch space for movement. The bracket can be positioned apically if additional movement is required. A provisional restoration may be necessary to position an orthodontic bracket at a more apical level for further movement.

The tooth should be stabilized for a minimum of 6 weeks following orthodontic movement. Definitive periodontal and restorative therapy may be completed after that time.

REFERENCES

Amsterdam M: Periodontal prosthesis: twenty-five years in retrospect, *Alpha Omegan* 67:9, 1974.

Anstendig HS, Kronman JH: A histologic study of pulpal reaction to orthodontic movement in dogs, *Angle Orthod* 42:50, 1972.

Batenhorst KF, Bowers GM, Williams JE: Tissue changes resulting from facial tipping and extrusion of incisors in monkeys, *J Periodontol* 45:660, 1974.

Brown IS: The effect of orthodontic therapy on certain types of periodontal defects. I. Clinical findings, *J Periodontol* 44:742, 1973.

Copeland S, Green LJ: Root resorption in maxillary central incisors following active orthodontic treatment, *Am J Orthod* 89:51, 1986.

Ericsson I, Thilander B, Lindhe J, Okamoto H: The effect of orthodontic tilting movements on the periodontal tissues of infected and non-infected dentition in dogs, *J Clin Periodontol* 4:278, 1977.

Essig CJ: *The American textbook of prosthetic dentistry,* ed 2, Philadelphia, 1896, Lea Brothers & Co.

Garguilo AW, Wentz FM, Orban B: Dimensions of the dentogingival junction in humans, *J Periodontol* 32:261, 1961.

Goldman HM, Cohen DW: *Periodontal therapy,* ed 6, St Louis, 1980, Mosby.

Guilford HJ, Grubb TA, Pence DL: Vertical extrusion: a standardized technique, *Compend Contin Educ Dent* 5:562, 1984.

Gruendeman GW, Weine FS, Janik JM: Combined orthodontic-endodontic therapy: case report of orthodontic movement of a recalcified lateral incisor, *J Endod* 20:258, 1994.

Heithersay GS: Combined endodontic-orthodontic treatment of transverse root fractures in the region of the alveolar crest, *Oral Surg* 36:404, 1973.

Ingber J: Forced eruption. I. A method of treating isolated one and two wall infrabony osseous defects—rationale and case report, *J Periodontol* 45:199, 1974; 47:203, 1976.

Ingber JS: Forced eruption. II. A method of treating nonrestorable teeth—periodontal and restorative considerations, *J Periodontol* 47:203, 1976.

Ingber JS: Forced eruption: alteration of soft tissue cosmetic deformities, *Int J Periodont Restor Dent* 9:415, 1989.

Ingber JS, Rose LF, Coslet JG: The "biologic width"—a concept in periodontics and restorative dentistry, *Alpha Omegan* 10:62, 1977.

Kampfe LV: Endodontic considerations during orthodontic treatment, *J Prev Dent* 6:27, 1980.

Lindhe J: *Textbook of clinical periodontogy,* Copenhagen, 1983, Munksgaard.

Mandel RC, Binzer WC, Withers JA: Forced eruption in restoring severely fractured teeth using removable orthodontic appliances, *J Prosthet Dent* 47:269, 1982.

Maynard JG, Wilson R: Physiologic dimensions of the periodontium significant to the restorative dentist, *J Periodontol* 50:170, 1979.

Melsen B: Tissue reaction following application of extrusive and intrusive forces to teeth in adult monkeys, *Am J Orthod* 89(6):469, 1986.

Mostafa YA, Iskander KG, El-Mangoury NH: Iatrogenic pulpal reactions to orthodontic extrusions, *Am J Orthod Dentofacial Orthop* 99:30, 1991.

Ochsenbein C, Ross SE: A re-evaluation of osseous surgery, *Dent Clin North Am* 13:87, 1969.

Polson A, Caton J, Polson AP, et al.: Periodontal response after tooth movement into intrabony defects, *J Periodontol* 55(4):197, 1984.

Potashnick SR, Rosenberg ES: Forced eruption: principles in periodontics and restorative dentistry, *J Prosthet Dent* (in press).

Reitan K: Clinical and histologic observations on tooth movement during and after orthodontic treatment, *Am J Orthod* 53:721, 1967.

Ritchey B, Orban B: The crests of the interdental alveolar septa, *J Periodontol* 24:75, 1953.

Rosenberg ES, Garber DA, Evian CI: Tooth lengthening procedures, *Compend Contin Educ Dent* 1:161, 1980.

Simon JH: Root extrusion: rationale and techniques, *Dent Clin North Am* 28:909, 1984.

Simon JHS, Kelly WH, Gordon DG, Erickson, GW: Extrusion of endodontically treated teeth. *J Am Dent Assoc* 97:17, 1978.

Stern N, Becker A: Forced eruption: biological and clinical considerations, *J Oral Rehabil* 7:395, 1980.

Jerome V. Pisano • Franklin S. Weine

15 Microbiology of endodontics

There is some controversy concerning the efficiency and efficacy of cleansing and shaping techniques employed in root canal therapy. There are differences of opinion concerning types of filling materials and methods of filling root canals. There is one undisputed fact: Without microbial involvement in the pulp and associated periapical tissues there would be no need for endodontic therapy. More than 30 years ago Kakahashi et al. proved that without bacterial involvement, only minor inflammation occurred in exposed pulps. Pulpal abcesses, periapical lesions, swelling, and pain are the result of mixed microbial infections. Early studies attempting to identify these bacterial invaders were somewhat misleading because of flaws in sampling and culturing techniques that did not allow for the recovery and identification of anaerobic bacteria from infected pulps and periapical areas. Discovery of the anaerobic gramnegative rods and their relationship with other microbes in mixed infections points to the close relationship between basic science and clinical practice in the special field of endodontics. A thorough understanding of these organisms, including their destructive potential, their requirements for growth, their routes of entry, their sensitivity to pharmacotherapeutic agents, their synergistic dependence on each other, and their relationship to clinical symptoms is necessary to formulate a sound approach to root canal therapy.

The basics of endodontic therapy are much the same as those of wound debridement: thorough removal of diseased or necrotic tissue from the root canal. Included in this process must be an attempt to eliminate microbes, their end products, and substrate needed for their growth and to provide an environment that prevents reinfection. This environment, since no new tissue growth can take place in the canal space, must be filled with a bacteriostatic sealing agent.

Culturing has taken on new meaning and importance. This test, as it had been done to evaluate when a canal could be safely filled, is but a historical footnote. Modern anaerobic culturing techniques allow us to better understand from a scientific point of view the complex nature of the mixed infection often found in clinical cases. Culturing can, therefore, guide clinical therapy, but routine sampling is clinically impractical. Yet careful anaerobic culturing of stubborn space infections may be invaluable in determining appropriate antibiotic therapy as an adjunct to clinical procedures.

Increasing attention has been placed on sterilization procedures employed in all dental offices. Endodontic procedures demand the utmost of care in controlling the spread of infection, not only with attention placed on the individual case being treated, but also concern over cross contamination from patient to patient, patient to staff, and staff to patient. Although no concrete evidence has been presented to date documenting practitioner transfer of disease of any type to a dental patient, the unfortunate, unexplained case of a single dentist allegedly contaminating several patients with the human immunodeficiency virus (HIV) has brought public and governmental attention to the subject of patient and staff protection and the institution of barrier techniques and universal precautions. A thorough understanding of microbiologic principals is required to effectively protect all personnel.

ROUTES OF MICROORGANISM INGRESS

Microorganisms can reach the dental pulp by any of six routes. During operative, crown and bridge, and periodontal procedures these possible paths must be considered to prevent ingress. While endodontic therapy is being performed, these routes must be blocked to avoid contamination during treatment. Since the pulpal stump and periapical tissues are usually inflamed to some degree during endodontic procedures, these areas would be adversely affected if microorganisms were allowed access. After root canal obliteration, care must be taken to ensure maintenance of the occlusal and peripheral seal from oral contaminants. Microbes can reach the periradicular tissues through a root canal fill if exposed to oral fluids for extended periods of time.

Through the open cavity. The most obvious route for microorganism invasion is through an open cavity, as caused by dental caries. Enamel and dentin provide excellent layers of protection against pulpal inflammation while they are intact. These hard tissues will repel microorganisms and insulate against abrupt changes of temperature. However, once they are damaged by caries, this protection may be rapidly reduced until the underlying pulp is invaded. Even as the irritants approach the pulp, new protective layers of reparative dentin may be laid down to avert exposure. The rapidity and degree of this additional dentin deposition varies with individuals, but rarely can prevent microorganism entry without intervention by some type of caries excavation.

Traumatic injuries or operative procedures also may remove the protective dentin barrier and allow access to the pulp. To prevent contamination, only materials with good sealing ability should be used following operative procedures when any possibility of pulp exposure is present.

Through the dentinal tubules. Research has shown that microorganisms will penetrate into dentinal tubules and be able to reach the pulp. These invaders may enter the tubules from salivary contamination during operative procedures or through adjacent carious lesions.

The microorganisms able to penetrate after cavity preparation are usually low in number and virulence and rarely cause clinical symptoms of pulpitis. The pressure of impression materials, temporary restorative materials, acids, and cements may drive microorganisms from the surface of a preparation through tubules into the pulp. Phagocytic action by the defense cells of the pulp can frequently remove these invaders and retain a healthful environment. Even though irritation of this dimension may not cause clinical symptoms, protection for the pulp is available. Tubule sealants such as varnishes, sedative bases, or sedative cements should be used over exposed dentin in proximity to the pulp immediately after the completion of cavity or crown preparation.

However, when a deep carious lesion brings high numbers of microorganisms to tubules in proximity to the pulp, it has been shown that bacteria will penetrate to the pulp well in advance of the carious process. The pulpitis that may result occurs without direct pulp exposure.

Through the gingival sulcus or periodontal ligament. As discussed in Chapter 13, microorganisms and other irritants from the periodontal ligament may reach the pulp through the vessels in the apical foramen or any auxiliary foramina present. Also, in some teeth auxiliary canals may be present some distance from the apex of the root, toward the crown of the tooth. If periodontal disease destroys the protecting bone and soft tissues to a sufficient degree, the canal may be exposed to microorganisms present in the gingival sulcus. Pulp exposure occurs without caries or trauma, but with heavy ingress of irritants.

Through the bloodstream. A transient bacteremia may occur for any number of reasons during the normal day of a healthy individual. Studies have been undertaken to determine whether bacteria present in the blood would be attracted to the dental pulp following trauma or operative procedure that produced inflammation without causing pulp exposure. This attraction is known as anachoresis and has been described in classic studies of inflammation. Hypotheses concerning this anachoretic effect were given to explain the finding of a periapical lesion with bacterial contamination in connection with a tooth in which the pulp became necrotic due to trauma. To clarify this, research by Burke and Knighton and by Smith and Tappe demonstrated that trauma to teeth could attract bacteria in the absence of pulp exposure. Robinson and Boling and Gier and Mitchell collected injected organisms in the unexposed pulps of teeth in which a pulpitis was induced through operative procedures. Just as when microorganisms enter the pulp though cut dentinal tubules, the invaders attracted to a mild pulpitis are probably effectively eliminated by phagocytic cells. However, if the degree of trauma or the operative procedures are sufficient to cause considerable damage, the repair cells may have too great a task to restore the pulp to a healthy condition and repel the microorganisms. The damaged pulp offers excellent culture media for continued growth of the microorganisms.

Through a broken occlusal seal or faulty restoration of a tooth previously treated by endodontic therapy. Controlled studies by Torabinejad et al. have proved that salivary contamination from the occlusal aspect can reach the periapical area in less than six weeks in canals obturated with gutta-percha and sealer. If there is a delay in restorative procedures following endodontic therapy and the temporary seal is broken, if the tooth structure fractures before final restoration, or if the final restoration is inadequate or becomes inadequate due to subsequent decay, bacteria may gain access to the periapical tissues and result in infection. This problem is often compounded by hydrophilic composite cores placed under cast restorations that begin to leak with time, absorb contaminants, and serve as a reservoir of bacteria. Unused post space further complicates the situation in a leaking restorative system acting as an incubator for anaerobic bacteria, inviting them to travel to the periradicular tissues through the apex. Microbes traveling around only 4 to 5 millimeters of gutta-percha and sealer—or through the much shorter route of contamination, lateral canals—are causing an increasing number of endodontic failures over extended periods of time.

Through extension of a periapical infection from adjacent infected teeth. There is considerable question whether or not bacteria from a periapical area will enter an adjacent, noninfected tooth. Large periapical radiolucencies may appear to encompass the roots of multiple teeth, yet be caused by pulp necrosis of only one tooth. This occurs with greatest frequency in the lower anterior teeth. Only the causative tooth is treated endodontically, and the entire radiolucency heals. Despite the presence of the granulomatous tissue and multiple colonies of microorganisms, the nerves and blood vessels can safely penetrate and course through the lesion.

Of course, if a pulpitis or trauma severely affects a tooth and its neighbor does have an infected periapical area, the microorganisms may easily reach the newer problem by the interlacing blood and lymph systems, by physical extension, or by pressure. In a process similar to the anachoretic effect, the injured pulp is invaded, and the proximity of the source of microorganisms may yield a high number of organisms.

MICROORGANISMS FOUND IN ROOT CANALS AND ASSOCIATED PERIRADICULAR LESIONS—HISTORIC AND CURRENT

There has always been a strong correlation between the basic science of microbiology and the clinical science of endodontics. Gram-negative anaerobic microorganisms currently are the sub-

ject of extensive basic science research and clinical studies as the main causative agent of endodontic infections, the severity of such infections, and the resultant clinical symptoms associated with these infections. These anaerobic invaders are not found clinically in pure culture because of their synergistic nature requiring specific nutrients for growth and the presence of other organisms to supply some of these products necessary for survival. Therefore, attention to these newly studied organisms should not detract completely from the classical early microbiologic investigations by early researchers that searched for a cause-and-effect relationship between specific microbes and endodontic infections. Since any microorganisms of the oral cavity, upper respiratory tract, sinus area, nasopharynx, or gastrointestinal tract can gain access to the root canal system, the genera and species that must be dealt with could be vast. This is not the case. Invaders of the endodontic complex may not reproduce in the root canal environment or may not be pathogenic in their new oxygen and nutrient limited setting. On the other hand, many species that are normal, nonpathogenic residents of the oral cavity, including the gingival crevice, become invasive, destructive members of a community of microbes producing toxins and enzymes that cause inflammation, tissue necrosis, and infection.

Aerobes and their significance. Table 15-1 summarizes five important studies from 1947 to 1968. These research efforts were well-controlled, involved large numbers of cases, and were supportive of each others' results. Alpha-hemolytic streptococci were the most commonly recovered organisms. *Streptococcus mitis* and *Streptococcus salivarius,* referred to as the viridans group in some classical studies, are numerous in the oral cavity and numerous, as well, in infected root canals. *S. mitis* is of particular importance in that it is frequently cultured from heart valves after attacks of subacute bacterial endocarditis, therefore proving its pathogenicity in a site remote from the root canal. Beta-hemolytic and less pathogenic nonhemolytic *Streptococcus* were also cultured in large numbers in early research efforts. There is still great significance in the presence of *Streptococcus* organisms because of their cell wall components. Peptidoglycans and lipoteichoic acids give structural rigidity to the cell wall. Lymphokine production, such as the osteoclast-activating factor, as well as prostaglandin production, are a

Table 15-1.   Historic review of microorganisms thought to be found in root canals prior to 1969

	Slack (%)	Shay (%)	Grossman (%)	Winkler and van Amerongen (%)	Leavitt et al. (%)
Streptococcus					
Alpha	25	5	29	23	45
Beta	3	7	1	4	35
Gamma	23	45	5	1	8
Enterococci	NR	NR	5	19	NR
Anaerobic	NR	NR	NR	4	16
Staphylococcus		19		17	
aureus	12		0.4		13
albus	12		16		54
Pneumococci	2	NR	13	NR	7
Lactobacilli	5	5	0.3	6	35
Bacillus subtilis	1	7	5	NR	30
Diphtheroids	2	NR	0.5	5	40
Neisseria	7	NR	0.2	NR	6
Escherichia					
coli	2	NR	5	NR	6
Pseudomonas	0.6	NR	0.1	NR	2
Monilia	5	2	17	NR	16
Miscellaneous	1	4	5	20	50
Number of miscellaneous strains	3	7	5	NR	10
Total canals studied	514	709	1017	Over 4000	154

NR, Not reported.

result of peptidoglycan action. Both mediators enhance the pathogenicity and symptoms of infectious disease of the periapical tissues. Immunologically, peptidoglycans activate, complement, and stimulate B lymphocytes. Lipoteichoic acids enhance the destructive process as well by inducing bone resorption and, immunologically, by activating the complement cascade.

Enterococci, commonly residents of the digestive tract, were also commonly recovered in endodontic cultures. Some species such as *Streptococcus faecalis* are difficult to eliminate from endodontic infections because of their resistance to many antimicrobial agents, and they can become stubborn invaders in selected cases. In summary, the contribution made by the organisms isolated in aerobic cultures to the disease process that we know of as endodontic infection is significant, yet a basic flaw in that culturing and incubation process overlooked what we know now to be the predominant microbes in endodontic infections, the anaerobic gram-negative rods.

Anaerobes—disease production and symptoms. In 1976 a landmark complex dissertation was published by Sundqvist of Sweden on the potential role of anaerobic bacteria in endodontic infections. A relatively small number of 32 cases were evaluated, but most important, an anaerobic glove box and "mobile anaerobic laboratory" were used to collect and process microbiologic samples and ensure as close to an anaerobic laboratory situation in a clinical setting as possible. Of the 32 cases, 18 positive cultures were incubated. Table 15-2 summarizes the findings. All eighteen teeth had periradicular destruction; only one tooth with a periapical lesion yielded a negative culture. Seven teeth exhibited painful symptoms, and 11 were asymptomatic. The striking discovery was that black-pigmented anaerobic rods were only present in all 7 symptomatic cases and could not be detected in the 11 teeth without pain. Even though criticized at that time because of its small sample size, this pioneering effort led us to the literature now replete with substantiating research (see Table 15-3). Com-

Table 15-2.   Bacteria found by Sundqvist in teeth without and with pain

Microorganism	Number in samples of 7 teeth with pain	Number in samples of 11 teeth without pain
Bacteroides melaninogenicus	7	0
Other *Bacteroides* strains	1	3
Actinomyces	3	2
Arachnia propionica	1	1
Campylobacter sputorum	5	1
Eubacterium	5	3
Fusobacterium	5	4
Lactobacillus	6	3
Peptostreptococcus	6	3
Streptococcus mitis	1	2
Others	3	3

Adapted from Sundqvist G: Bacteriological studies of necrotic dental pulps, *Umea University Odontological Dissertations*, no 7, 1976.

Table 15-3.   More recent studies reporting anaerobic growth in teeth with necrotic pulps

Author (year)	Number of teeth	Anaerobic growth (%)	Number with Bacteroides (Porphyromonas-Prevotella)	Number with Peptostrepto-coccus	Number with Actinomyces
Bergenholtz (1974)	84	76	48	15	NR
Kantz and Henry (1974)	24	72	8	7	15
Wittgow and Sabiston (1975)	40	84	27	9	1
Keudell and Ernest (1976)	55	64	11	2	2
Labriola et al. (1983)	50	86	12	8	1
van Winkelhoff et al. (1985)	28	93	26	NR	NR
Pantera et al. (1988)*	119	49–86	69	NR	NR
Sundqvist and Johansson (1989)	72	90	22	12	1

NR, Not reported.
*Immunofluorescent study.

plicating the interpretation of the literature is the fact that there have been several taxonomic name changes for these organisms over the past several years. To better interpret the literature of the last 15 years, Table 15-4 has been adapted from work by van Winkelhoff et al. and shows the former and current designation of genus and species of the black-pigmented anaerobic gram-negative rods. The *Bacteroides melaninogenicus* and "other *Bacteroides* strains" of Sundqvist's original work have been biochemically differentiated over the years into two major genera, *Porphyromonas* and *Prevotella*. These asaccharolytic bacteria have been cultured, isolated, compared, and contrasted as to their virulence, pathogenicity, antimicrobial sensitivity, and serology and have even been DNA fingerprinted. It may be helpful to refer to Table 15-4 when interpreting current literature and the remainder of this chapter.

A major work by Bystrom was the next step in unravelling the mystery of these newly discovered anaerobic bacteria from root canals with necrotic tissue and periapical areas of bone destruction. His larger sample size of 140 teeth showed again an 80% presence of anaerobic strains with *Bacteroides (Porphyromonas)* and *Peptostreptococcus* being the most common. Sampling methods were similar to those of Sundqvist. Since culturing took place at different stages of treatment, certain other assumptions were made. The closed root canal system appears to be a very efficient incubator for bacteria between visits, and the best method for

Table 15-4. Comparison of old and new nomenclature used in the identification of human oral black-pigmented anaerobic rods

Former	Present
Black-pigmented *Bacteroides*	Black-pigmented anaerobic rods
Bacteroides gingivalis	*Porphyromonas gingivalis*
Bacteroides endodontales	*Porphyromonas endodontales*
Bacteroides intermedius	*Prevotella intermedius*
Bacteroides melaninogenicus	*Prevotella melaninogenicus*
Bacteroides denticola	*Prevotella denticola*
Bacteroides loescheii	*Provotella loescheii*

Adapted from van Winkelhoff A, van Steenbergen M, de Graaff J: *J Endod* 18:431, 1992.

controlling this microbial reproduction was shown to be 0.5% sodium hypochlorite as an irrigating solution and the placement of calcium hydroxide in the canal as an interappointment dressing.

Comparing the symptoms associated with endodontic infections and specific bacteria has been the subject of a significant collection of recent literature. The work of Griffee et al. in 1980 was the first significant published report in this area. They found such symptoms as pain, foul odor, sinus tracts, sensitivity to percussion, and localized swelling statistically greater in cases where *Bacteroides* (*Porphyromonas* and *Prevotella*) were present. Later in 1987, Yoshida confirmed Griffee's findings culturing *Bacteroides* (*Porphyromonas* and *Prevotella*) and *Peptococcus* species from clinically symptomatic teeth. Anaerobic infections often produce pain, swelling, and a febrile state. A purulent, foul, swelling discharge indicates the present of anaerobic bacteria metabolites such as ammonia, urea, indole, and amino acids. Further studies by Hahn et al. (1993), Hashioka et al. (1994) and others have shown a definite relationship between the spread of symptomatic endodontic infection and enzyme production by anaerobic bacteria such as *Eubacterium, Prevotella, Peptococcus,* and *Porphyromonas.* These enzymes include collagenase, chondroitinase, and hyaluronidase. Some investigators have even tried to correlate symptoms such as thermal sensitivity, percussion sensitivity, and periapical lesion size to specific genera and species of microbes cultured from symptomatic cases. Most studies, because of their small sample size, are of great interest, but are not such that sweeping conclusions can be drawn.

Porphyromonas endodontalis is one species almost exclusively isolated from endodontic infections. It differs from the other *Porphyromonas* species, *intermedius* and *gingivalis,* in that it appears to

be less proteolytic and much more oxygen sensitive. What is common to all *Porphyromonas* species and other gram-negative bacteria is the presence of endotoxins in their cell walls. Schein and Schilder, Yamasaki et al., Horiba et al., and others have shown how significantly destructive lipopolysaccharide is in periapical infections and necrotic pulps. Inflammation, bone destruction, pain, swelling, and fever are all a direct or indirect effect of lipopolysaccharide (LPS) induction. LPS can stimulate B lymphocytes and activate the complement cascade initiating an immune response. Endotoxin (LPS) enhances virulence by causing the release of collagenase and induces fever by stimulating the release of interleukin from macrophage cells. Production of pain mediators such as bradykinin, histamine, and prostaglandins is enhanced by LPS.

Yet with all these strong indicators that specific bacteria exhibit specific traits and capabilities of component parts of the disease process, it is clear that no one microbe can be responsible for endodontic infections. A synergistic relationship exists between the prime bacterial players and the support microbes that overcome the body's defense mechanisms and cause the disease state. Low-oxygen environment, specific growth factors affecting virulence, such as succinate and hemin, and the predisposing influence of the original invaders (the gram-positive aerobic forms) are all necessary before the clinical endodontic infection as we see it can exist. Sundqvist (1989), Griffee, van Winkelhoff, and others demonstrated that the mixed cultures obtained from infected root canals show similar combinations of a number of species of several bacteria and suggest this essential synergistic system. Included in this repetitive pattern of support players are *Streptococcus, Peptostreptococcus, Eubacterium, Fusobacterium,* and *Actino-*

myces. To quote Sundqvist, "In the root canal, substrate limitation and a build up of metabolic growth inhibitory products give rise to the diverse community of primary and secondary nutrient utilizers with a variety of bacterial interactions. Endodontic treatment interferes with this system."

Some brief attention should be placed on the unique genus of microorganisms called *Actinomyces*. Baumgartner, Gohean, O'Grady, and others have demonstrated with increasing frequency the presence of this unique organism in root canals and periapical lesions and in some cases of persistent stubborn infections resistant to control by standard endodontic clinical procedures and routine antibiotic therapy. *Actinomyces* are anaerobic or microaerophilic gram-positive filamentous bacteria. They are common nonvirulent inhabitants of the oral cavity from the nasopharynx to the gingival crevice. An actinomycotic infection classically produces a suppurative exudate of "sulfur granules," which are actually colonies of the microorganisms. Routine biopsy of periradicular lesions is an easy way to identify this bacteria; their unique acid-fast staining branching filamentous form is distinctive on microscopic examination. Usually, surgical curettage is sufficient to eliminate the contamination, but persistent postsurgical infection by this organism may require surgical reentry and aggressive oral antibiotic therapy for a month or longer.

SIGNIFICANCE OF MICROORGANISMS IN ENDODONTIC THERAPY

A great deal has been thus far presented showing the possible routes of entry for potentially pathogenic bacteria, and several types of bacteria have been singled out as to their ability to cause the disease process we call endodontic infection. How can we apply all this basic scientific information to clinical practice?

We are all aware that teeth with large periapical lesions caused by pulp necrosis are often symptom free. However, in some cases these teeth exacerbate after initial canal preparation. There have been many suggestions as to how to avoid these most unpleasant occurrences, running the entire gamut of treatment modalities. Some clinicians have suggested complete instrumentation, whereas others favor minimal enlargement at the first visit; some recommend interappointment medicaments, while others claim them to be unnecessary and possibly a complication. Some authors advocate intentional overinstrumentation, while others decry such a

practice. Yet microbes bring all diverse opinions together in that the specific combination of bacteria present is far more important than which form of therapy is employed to eliminate them. Any clinical procedure, any opening or closing of a root canal, accidental innoculation of necrotic substrate or bacterial toxin or by-product into the periapical area, any introduction of oxygen into the root canal, any number of other controllable or uncontrollable iatrogenic procedures may alter the delicate balance that exists between invader and host—that determines health or disease process.

Hobson in 1965 first described this equation in the endodontic literature:

$$\frac{\text{Number of MO*} \times \text{Virulence of MO*}}{\text{Resistance of Host}} = \begin{array}{c}\text{Severity}\\\text{of}\\\text{Disease}\\\text{Process}\end{array}$$

All the factors of this equation, except for the number of microorganisms, are qualitative in nature. Host resistance depends on many factors and can even vary significantly from host to host. Disease severity can be only qualitatively compared on factors such as pain, swelling, and tissue destruction. Comparative virulence of bacteria can be discussed but not measured. For example, *Porphyromas endodontalis* possesses a capsule that offers resistance to phagocytosis and produces significant serum sensitivity. *P. endodontalis* also has proteolytic capability that causes degradation of immunoglobulins G and M and complement factors C3 and C5. Even toxic metabolic products such as butyrate and propionate are produced to enhance the virulence of this important resident of many endodontic infection sites.

Considering all the bacterial influences and their overwhelming capability of causing tissue destruction and pain, how can endodontic therapy best combat their influence? We can return to a hypothesis proposed by Torneck in the late 1960s that stated:

1. Among the causes in the prevention or delay of healing are the actions of microorganisms. However, they are not effective unless other irritating factors such as overinstrumentation, overmedication, unfilled root canal space, or periodontal disease have already elicited an inflammatory response.
2. Not all microorganisms can influence periapical repair. The type and number of microorganisms present are of major significance in each individual case.

*MO = microorganisms.

These original assumptions seem consistent with more recent research and support the objectives and clinical procedures of endodontic therapy as practiced today. Thorough cleansing and shaping of the root canal system with adjunctive use of sodium hypochlorite as an irrigant not only removes bacteria, but their substrate as well. Oxygenating a canal simply by opening it is detrimental to strict anaerobic bacterial forms, and the use of oxygenating agents such as gly-oxide further enhances the introduction of oxygen to these oxygen nontolerant microbes. The operator must take care to avoid inoculating oxygenating agents past the apex into the periapical tissues where inflammation and pain may result. This attempt at creating an oxygen-rich environment should not be used as an excuse for leaving teeth open to drain or to "air out." The introduction of other oral cavity microorganisms into the canal and therefore to the periradicular tissue is contraindicated and compounds an already complex combination of synergistic bacteria.

Yang, Farber, and Seltzer in separate papers summarized the work of other researchers and stated that the variety of microorganisms cultured from canals left open to drain was quite great, resembling the entire flora of the oral cavity. Those canals kept closed and similarly cultured had a flora that was predominantly anaerobic. This observation, which may seem obvious, should be carefully considered when there is a choice to leave open or close an endodontic canal system. If possible a tooth that exhibits serous, purulent, or hemorrhagic drainage should be allowed to drain with the protection of the rubber dam in place for a period of time under supervision. Other patients may even be attended to during this extended visit as long as the patient is closely monitored and not left unattended. The tooth may then be irrigated, dried, and closed. Evaluation of the need for antibiotic therapy can be made at this time. Thorough cleansing and shaping combined with effective use of an antibacterial irrigant that serves as a necrotic tissue solvent is still the best assurance of a successful case.

Another weapon used to combat the bacteria that may stubbornly persist is our armamentarium of modern antibiotics. Before the discovery of the predominance of black-pigmented anaerobic rods in infected root canals, antibiotic therapy was designed to eliminate mainly *Streptococcus* and *Staphylococcus* microorganisms. Penicillins including Potassium Penicillin G, ampicillin, amoxicillin, cephalosporins, and, for those patients allergic to these more popular medications, erythromycin have been and are still used extensively. Clindamycin has been proven to be an effective alternative or even primary medication when dealing with endodontic and other oral infections. Its affinity for bone and its favorable, rather wide spectrum of effectiveness has earned it new popularity. According to Hargreaves, the unfair stigma of this medication being responsible for pseudomembranous ulcerative colitis limited its use for a time. It has been proven that most any oral antibiotic can upset the flora of the gastrointestinal tract leading to this serious complication. Care must always be taken to monitor patients under prescribed medication and encourage a call at any time if any adverse side effects occur. In fact, clindamycin is now an accepted alternative recommended by the American Heart Association for premedication in cardiac-compromised patients who exhibit an allergic history to amoxicillin.

Since it is well known today that obligate anaerobic bacteria are most frequently found in root canals and periradicular areas of teeth with acute apical periodontis, why have we been so successful when selecting antibiotics targeted specifically for aerobic and facultative forms? It certainly could be that the synergistic balance required for the strict anaerobes' survival requires the presence of such organisms as *Streptococcus, Peptostreptococcus,* and *Eubacterium,* all effectively controlled by our original antibiotics of choice. We upset the balance, deny the anaerobes their by-products and growth requirements, and eliminate the infection. Yamamoto et al. in 1989 performed a well-controlled laboratory study of the antimicrobial susceptibilities of several organisms with special emphasis on anaerobic genera such as *Bacteroides* (*Porphyromonas* and *Prevotella*). Minimum inhibitory concentrations of several antibiotic types were calculated for these forms (Table 15-5.) These results confirm that antibiotics commonly used in the past are quite effective against the newly identified culprits that have always been present. Our antibiotic drug therapy need not undergo a major revision to accommodate the newest discoveries.

The formula for success is debridement, antibacterial irrigation, the judicious use of canal medicaments and oxygenating agents, the careful selective prescribing of antibiotics, and finally the

Table 15-5. Minimum inhibitory concentrations (MIC) in microgram per milliliter sample for three bacterial types (90% kill rate)

Type	Penicillin	Ampicillin	Amoxicillin	Erythromycin	Gentamicin
Eubacterium	6.3	1.6	1.6	100	100
Peptostreptococcus	6.3	3.1	1.6	12.5	100
Black-pigmented anaerobic rods	0.2	0.2	0.1	25	100

Adapted from Yamamoto K, Hisanori F, Heronori T, Herosuke S: *J Endod* 15:112, 1989.

three-dimensional obturation of the root canal system to avoid the creation of a very efficient bacterial incubator.

Assuming we have a formula for success, can this equation be substantiated by analyzing failure? Lin and co-workers attempted to answer this very question. More than two hundred failing endodontic cases were evaluated. None of these cases involved advanced periodontal disease, post perforations, or crown or root fractures. Furthermore, there were nearly an equal number of cases that were filled short, filled flush, or that had an overextended fill. Surgical samples were stained for bacterial colonies, and nearly 70% demonstrated the presence of microorganisms in the periradicular tissues or segments of unfilled root canals. Also demonstrated was the fact that cases with preoperative periapical radiolucencies had a higher than 70% higher failure rate compared with those without demonstrable periradicular bone destruction. Research clearly shows the presence of bacteria in these lesions. It should also be noted that canals apparently well filled from a radiographic standpoint were incompletely cleansed and obturated. Canal curvature, complex canal configuration, and our inability to evaluate these morphological variances affect the influence of overall microbial involvement.

In summary, our philosophy remains unchanged in light of new and convincing endodontic microbiologic research. We still maintain: *The presence of microorganisms does not ensure endodontic failure nor does the absence of microorganisms guarantee success. However, the presence of microorganisms, particularly those of certain types, provides an additional source of irritation that the body must overcome to gain optimum results. Therefore, the control of microorganisms and possible substrate must be an objective in every endodontic case.*

TROUBLESHOOTING

As has been indicated, pain, swelling, and fluid production are all indicators of the presence of microorganisms. Continued tenderness to percussion after cleansing and shaping the root canal system is an indication that at least periapical inflammation and possibly bacterial contamination still persists. The following common errors should be checked when encountering a case with suspected microbial involvement: a faulty seal, the presence of an additional root canal, a canal configuration that lends itself to insufficient debridement or miscalculation of working length.

A faulty interappointment seal is the most likely cause of persistent discomfort or fluid production. Teeth with multiple interlocking restorations, or teeth where even one large restoration is present through which access has been made, are susceptible to leakage. A heavy mix of zinc oxide–eugenol cement accelerated with zinc acetate crystals or IRM-type material is recommended to seal the tooth after all previous restorations and decay have been removed. A preformed crown may be cemented with a more permanent type of cement such as carboxylate or zinc oxyphosphate to ensure a seal on a tooth exhibiting excessive coronal destruction. Access preparation through these crowns plus the negative forces caused by rubber dam placement can be responsible for loosening these intermediate restorations. It may be helpful in some cases, where healthy adjacent teeth are present to "clamp around" the tooth undergoing treatment when placing the rubber dam to minimize this problem. In cases where a splint or bridge is present, the abutment being treated may have a loose coronal restoration that may go undetected because of excellent retention of other abutments. If suspected, and if practical, the entire bridge or splint should be removed, a separate seal placed, and the bridge temporarily re-seated. However, one must weigh the danger of fracturing the firmly attached abutment when attempting bridge removal. Cases will present themselves for which the prudent approach will be to sacrifice the bridge and section it adjacent to the healthy abutment. Once done, these cases often reveal an abutment with significant decay that would have required total replacement of the bridge span anyway.

Additional unprepared canals may be discovered by taking radiographs at various angles (Chapter 2). Ribbon-shaped canals may be present in single or multirooted teeth that have canals with a wide buccolingual dimension, such as mandibular anterior teeth and first bicuspids, maxillary bicuspids, and mesiobuccal roots of maxillary molars. Despite significant enlargement, some sections of these canals have been shown to have fins or slits of uncleansed canal space harboring necrotic debris and bacteria. Re-preparing these canals with a flare or step-preparation and filing with a rasping action in a buccolingual direction may succeed in gaining adequate debridement. (See Chapter 7.)

Incorrect length determination may result in filing short of the apical constriction and leaving debris and viable microorganisms in the anaerobic sections of the root canal. Filing past the minor diameter of the canal will certainly produce periapical inflammation. Recalculation of working length by taking radiographs at various angles should rectify this problem.

In cases where severe canal curvature or canal dilaceration limits the safe enlargement of the root canal, other techniques should be emphasized. Repeated sodium hypochlorite irrigation during filing and leaving the canal damp with residual sodium hypochlorite upon sealing is an effective method of minimizing bacterial interappointment growth. This attention to irrigation and the use of a heavy condensation technique will yield the best possible apical seal and poorest possible environment for bacterial multiplication. Finally, it should be emphasized that an asymptomatic tooth with a dry canal system is no guarantee of a microbial-free environment. The techniques described above can be and should be considered in all cases whether symptomatic or not to give every case the best chance for success.

THE CULTURE—HISTORIC AND CURRENT PERSPECTIVES

An asymptomatic tooth, exhibiting a dry canal and one, two, or three negative cultures were all required at one time before final filling of the root canal was allowed. Now that our knowledge of bacteria present in the root canal has grown to include more anaerobic organisms, it is time to reevaluate the necessity, practicality, and accuracy of routine culture tests. There is no doubt that determining the presence and identification of microorganisms in infected root canals and adjacent areas of soft and hard tissue may be invaluable, and the elimination of these invaders is of paramount importance in endodontic therapy. In fact, the aseptic technique practiced during modern endodontic therapy was adopted partially because of routine cultures taken in endodontic cases in dental schools to attempt to ensure quality care. Yet the days of requiring two successive negative cultures in the educational setting before allowing the obturation of a root canal system are but a historical footnote.

Bender and Seltzer, Morse, and others have thoroughly discussed the fallibilities of all culture techniques. When the difficulties of sampling and culturing obligate anaerobes is considered, along with all the false-positive and false-negative results, it no longer seems desirable to culture routine endodontic cases. However, the academic environment must still stress the value of aseptic technique, and students should still be taught the sophisticated materials and methods now necessary to gather accurate information from a culture test. Without this basic scientific background intelligent interpretation of the endodontic and microbiologic literature is impossible.

Culture media. When culturing is done, whether for scientific purposes or for clinical information, a proper media must be used that will properly support the growth of aerobic and anaerobic organisms. Even if a common media could be developed, the incubation conditions are considerably different, therefore, it is practical to choose a different media for each incubation process. A classical and still very useful aerobic culture broth was developed by Brewer. This media supplies nutrients and conditions when incubated with oxygen present to support the growth of aerobes commonly found in endodontic infections. It even supports the growth of some less strict anaerobic types. The ingredients of this readily available broth and their function can be found in Table 15-6.

As mentioned previously, culturing strict anaerobes demands considerably different ingredients as well as an incubation environment free of oxy-

Table 15-6.   Ingredients of Brewer's thioglycolate broth and their uses

Constituent	g/L	Function
Trypticase	15.0	Enrichment
Cystine	0.5	Essential amino acid
Dextrose	5.0	Carbohydrate
Yeast extract	5.0	Vitamin and growth factor
Sodium chloride	2.5	Keeps solution isotonic
Sodium thioglycolate	0.5	Reducing agent; keeps oxygen level low
Resazurin	0.001	Dye that shows oxygen presence with red band
Agar	0.75	Prevents oxygen diffusion

gen. Blood agar, trypticase soy, or brain/heart infusion media base may be fortified with defibrinated blood. Hemin, sodium lactate, and vitamin K are added to any of the base media mentioned, and most of these media are incubated in chambers with flowing gas mixtures of almost pure carbon dioxide with less than 5% hydrogen or mixtures of oxygen-free gases such as 80% nitrogen, 10% hydrogen, and 10% carbon dioxide.

Methods for taking cultures.   Accurate routine culturing of all endodontic cases in the office or undergraduate clinical setting is not practical and in most cases impossible. The equipment and materials necessary to yield a culture truly representative of the anaerobic flora present are available only in the laboratory environment or only in settings where mobile anaerobic equipment is available. To perform these scientifically invaluable tests, the canal orifice must be flushed with nitrogen gas during sampling. Sterile, charcoal-impregnated, absorbent points are used to anaerobically transfer the sample to media enriched with the growth requirements already discussed and then incubated in an oxygen-free atmosphere. Most of the data reviewed in these pages was gathered using a similar technique.

Notwithstanding all the limitations governing the taking of routine cultures, one must not overlook the responsibility of culturing acute exacerbations resulting in tissue space infections. These cases are often encountered after careful cleansing and shaping of the root canal space and after the administration of what is supposed to be the appropriate antibiotic. A challenging dilemma presents itself in the nonresponsive patient with increased swelling and pain in facial tissue spaces. All experienced practitioners have experienced the frustration of the patient who suffers the puzzling predicament of persistant swelling of the canine space invading the infra-orbital region or other

facial spaces prone to the spread of infection such as the buccal, submandibular, and submental areas. Careful sampling of exudate from these closed spaces can yield very helpful information that leads to an intelligent adjustment in antibiotic therapy. Stubborn actinomycotic and pseudomonas induced infections, as well as other infections caused by antibiotic resistant strains of more common aerobic and anaerobic strains have been diagnosed in this manner. Sampling is not difficult. The fluctuant space abcess is pulpated, and the most dependent part of the swelling is determined; the surface of the mucosa in that area should be thoroughly disinfected with alcohol before needle penetration of the space. An empty, sterile syringe and attached needle is used to aspirate a fluid sample from the area. Samples of this type are often very accurate; the sample is never exposed to room air, and the closed tissue space still exhibits a mixed culture of organisms that has not been contaminated with additional oral flora by any other operative or surgical procedure. The sample in the syringe, or after being inoculated into an appropriate transfer media, is sent immediately to a microbiologic laboratory or hospital that has suitable facilities for growing both aerobic and anaerobic organisms. Strict anaerobes not only require an atmosphere devoid of oxygen, but also require substances for growth described earlier that are not found in simple broths and agars used for aerobic forms. Both identification and sensitivity should be requested from the laboratory; these results should be requested as soon as possible via phone to facilitate proper antibiotic choice and dosage in the unresponsive patient. A written, complete follow-up lab report must become part of the patient's permanent record.

Other microbiologic identification techniques. Someday even our newest culturing techniques may be discovered in a sealed time capsule to convey to future generations how bacteria were identified in the days of early scientific methodology. Techniques such as indirect immunofluorescence and DNA fingerprinting are on the horizon and are the wave of the future as accurate state of the art analysis options in bacteriologic identification. Pantera et al. demonstrated in detail the use of indirect immunofluorescence for the detection of *Bacteriodes* species (now *Porphygromonas* and *Prevotella*) in the human dental pulp. This less time-consuming, less expensive analytical method is already being used to routinely detect organisms such as *Haemophilus influenzae* in meningitis cases and *Legionella* species in legionnaires' disease. For endodontic application, smears of processed pulp samples were reacted with species-specific polyclonal antisera or monoclonal antibodies. Resultant conjugates were then tested by immunofluorescence for cross-reactions against a broad selection of Gram-positive and Gram-negative oral microorganisms. In more than one hundred samples, a higher percentage of anaerobic black-pigmented rods were discovered than by anaerobic culture techniques alone.

DNA fingerprinting may prove to be the most accurate method of bacterial identification available. Glickman and van Winkelhoff et al. have demonstrated the application of genetic code analysis to bacterial identification. DNA from one infection can be compared with DNA from other infections, and relationships can be confirmed. A technique called PCR (polymerase chain reaction) that multiplies or amplifies the genetic code has been particularly useful in bacterial typing. Only a few bacterial cells are required for accurate identification with this method, but accuracy is such that several strains of the same *species* of bacteria can be identified and compared—all having common indicators of that specific species. *Porphyromonas endodontalis* has been analyzed in this way. Although time consuming and expensive, this technique will likely evolve to become the most efficient method of bacterial identification.

STERILIZATION AND DISINFECTION

Sterilization is no longer just a concern of ensuring clinical success in endodontic therapy. Certainly carrying nonpathogenic bacteria from the oral cavity into the canal or innoculating another patient's pathogenic or nonpathogenic bacteria into an altered environment can cause

these forms to become virulent, disease-producing invaders. Public and governmental concern has shifted to the potential danger of transferring from patient to patient, or health-care worker to patient or vice versa, both bacteria and viruses that are causative agents for life-threatening and debilitating diseases such as HIV, hepatitis, multidrug resistant strains of tuberculosis (MDR-TB), and herpes. Dentistry, and endodontics in particular, have been leaders in promoting aseptic conditions and sterile techniques in clinical practice. A proactive report by the ADA in 1978 authored by the then Council on Dental Materials and Devices recognized the importance of patient and health-care-worker protection. Several subsequent publications by the Centers for Disease Control and Prevention (CDC) concerned with the protection of the patient and health-care worker and documents made public by the Occupational Safety and Health Administration (OSHA) addressed the same issues. In 1986, the CDC published a report entitled "Recommended Infection Control Practices for Dentistry." This report was supplemented in 1987 and updated in 1988 and 1993. Finally, in 1991 OSHA printed its "Standard on Occupational Exposure to Bloodbourne Pathogens" in the *Federal Register* with compliance required in 1992 by all health-care providers. The OSHA regulations simply mandated most of the practices already employed in dental offices.

Office infection control.   A summary of these recommendations and regulations as they apply to dentistry in general and endodontic practice in particular will be helpful. First the use of barrier protection and personal protective equipment (PPE) is at times cumbersome, but essential. Protective eye wear with side shields, long-sleeve, fluid-resistant, washable or disposable gowns, fluid-proof masks, and, most of all, disposable gloves are required as protection against blood-borne pathogens. (Fig. 15-1). In fact, these measures, part of what are considered "universal precautions" afford protection against pathogens that may be contaminants of blood and other body secretions including saliva. It is *not* possible to determine which patients may be carriers of hepatitis, human immunodeficiency virus or other infectious diseases. Histories may be inaccurate, or the patients may be unaware of their infected state; all patients must unfortunately be considered a risk. Wrapping exposed and potentially contaminated surfaces with disposable materials or disinfecting these surfaces are essential to a

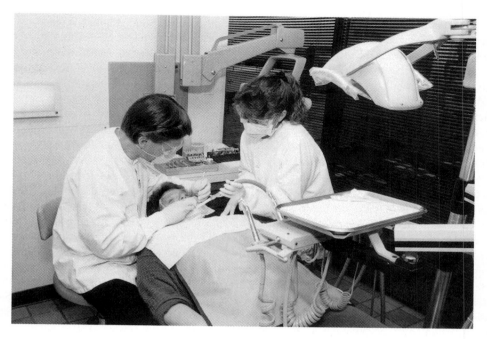

Fig. 15-1.   Barrier protection: gloves, masks, glasses, gowns, and rubber dam.

program of breaking the chain of possible transfer of microorganisms.

The use of latex or vinyl gloves being required no doubt makes endodontic therapy more difficult; practice and fine tuning of tactile skills are required before the precision handling of files necessary to cleanse and shape canals returns to your hands. This makes the use of the rubber dam more important than ever. Use of the rubber dam has universally been required to prevent contamination of oral cavity contaminants into the root canal and, of course, to eliminate the possibility of aspiration or ingestion of small endodontic instruments. It assumes a more important role today in greatly minimizing atomization of possibly contaminated oral fluids and now acts as a critical barrier against an errant file dropped by an operator now wearing gloves for all procedures. In fact, there is great credibility in the resurgence in the use of the rubber dam for other than endodontic procedures for protection of the patient and the health-care team as well. Aseptic technique, so often referred to in endodontic education, has spread to all disciplines of dentistry and clinical health care. The use of personal, protective, equipment-surface decontamination, effective handwashing, immunization

against hepatitis-B, and efficient record keeping are all requirements of a mandated infection-control program, but all are no more important than effective sterilization procedures.

Sterilization procedures. Infection control involves either reducing the spread of contamination or eliminating pathogens once contamination has occurred. The latter involves techniques of sterilization. Disinfection cannot be confused with sterilization. Sterilization by definition involves any process that kills not only all microbes, but also kills high numbers of bacterial spores. Inhibition or destruction of disease-producing microorganisms can be accomplished by disinfection, but spore forms are unaffected. Chemical agents are employed in disinfection procedures, and some glutaraldehyde solutions are capable of sterilization if materials are subjected to certain concentrations of these agents for longer than ten hours. Sterilization is more commonly accomplished by steam autoclave, dry-heat sterilization, and, a less popular method, unsaturated chemical vapor. But, before sterilization can be achieved, instruments must be clean.

The CDC states that "cleaning is the basic first step of all decontamination"; OSHA regulations include the statement "all equipment and environmental and working surfaces shall be cleaned . . ."; the ADA has taken the published position that "patient debris and body fluids must be removed from the instruments and surfaces before sterilization or disinfection." The message is clear, instrument cleaning is the first and most often ignored step in the process of sterilization. Endodontic instruments present a special challenge to clean; the flutes and spirals of endodontic hand instruments become clogged with pus, blood, and organic and inorganic debris. Allowing these by-products of intracanal preparation to dry on the instruments makes their removal even more difficult. Immediately placing them in soap and water is an effective, quick-holding method until time for the next cleaning step is available. Ultrasonic cleaning is ideal to remove debris in that the instruments are placed in a basket and cleaning is automatic; excessive instrument handling and therefore potential cuts or puncture wounds are minimized. Scrubbing by hand of small or large instruments is more dangerous in this regard, and splattering of debris can be a problem. If manual brushing of instruments cannot be avoided, it should be done under running water, and heavy rubber gloves should be added to the usual PPE for additional protection. No matter what method is used, cleaned instruments should be rinsed in clear water before they proceed to the next step of true sterilization.

No matter what method is used, it should be noted that the materials to be sterilized must be kept at the desired temperature for a specific period of time for each method. The time required to reach this optimal temperature must be added to the recommended time of heat exposure (Table 15-7). The steam autoclave (Fig. 15-2) is the backbone of any infection control program. It destroys all microbial forms including spores by protein denaturation. Heat of 250° to 273° F for 20 to 30 minutes is imposed under 15 pounds of pressurized steam to speed up the process, which would take far more time if boiling water were used. "Flash sterilization" at the higher temperature requires only 3 to 10 minutes of time and requires that the instruments remain unwrapped. Flash sterilization is not recommended for everyday office routines because the instruments must then be handled and stored aseptically to avoid recontamination. It may be used in emergency situations to sterilize an "only instrument" required for a procedure that may have been dropped or otherwise contaminated. Packaging for the 20 to 30 minute process should be in paper/biofilm, self-sealing packets, nylon tubing, sterilization wrap, wrapped closed perforated trays, or thick paper bags, which all allow steam penetration (Fig. 15-3). All of these options allow storage of sterilized instruments ready for use and patient scrutiny. It should be noted that the CDC, ADA, and Federal Drug Administration (FDA) all require sterilization of

Table 15-7. Methods and times required for sterilization for endodontics

Type	Temperature (°F)	Time	Instruments and Materials	Packaging
Steam autoclave	250	20–30 min	Handpieces, non-intracanal hand instruments, paper/cotton materials	Paper/biofilm packages, nylon tubing, sterilization wrap, paper bags, perforated wrapped trays or cassettes
Steam autoclave	273	3–10 min	Same	None
Dry heat	320	60–120 min	Intracanal instruments, burs, hand instruments, sharp instruments of any kind	Closed metal or composite heat resistant boxes
Chemical vapor	270	20 min	All instruments except handpieces	None

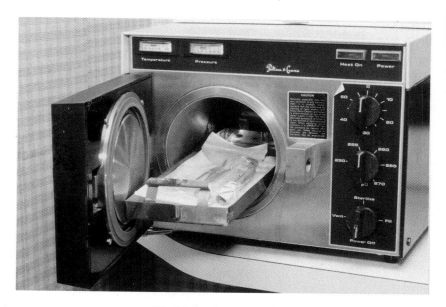

Fig. 15-2.   Steam autoclave.

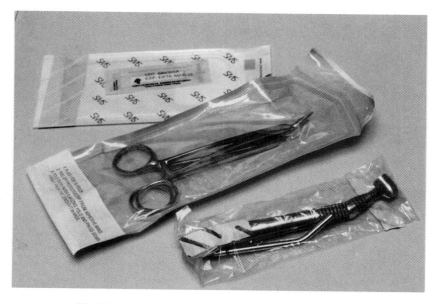

Fig. 15-3.   Steam autoclave packaging and spore test strip.

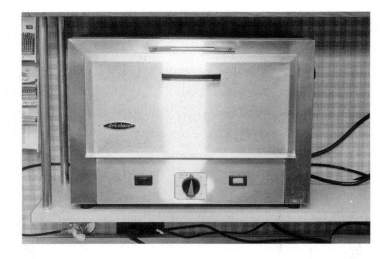

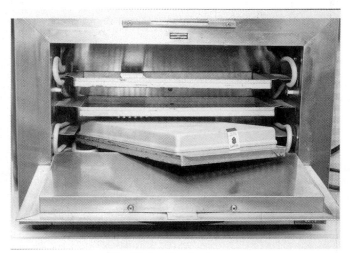

Fig. 15-4. Dry heat ovens.

dental handpieces, and steam sterilization is usually the only practical option as rubber and plastic components of these precision devices are unharmed by this method, whereas dry heat or chemical vapor can cause serious damage. Unfortunately, steam autoclaving dulls sharp points and edges of cutting instruments including files and reamers. Endodontic instruments tagged for re-use are better sterilized by high dry heat.

Dry-heat ovens (Fig. 15-4) with sustained temperatures of 320°F or higher for at least 60 minutes are also sporicidal and virucidal. Advantages include the fact that instruments remain sharp and can be sterilized in closed metal or composite boxes

that remain uncontaminated in storage for lengthy periods of time if unopened (Fig. 15-5). The obvious main disadvantage is the time required to process instruments, which requires a greater inventory of instruments. Care must be exercised to avoid heat higher than 350°F because plastic handles may melt or solder joints on other instruments may be weakened. Excessive heat also causes scorching or burning of paper or cotton products that are better sterilized by the steam method.

Unsaturated chemical vapor sterilization is not widely employed, but is a time-efficient method of true sterilization that requires only 20 minutes of exposure. Special solutions for predipping, ade-

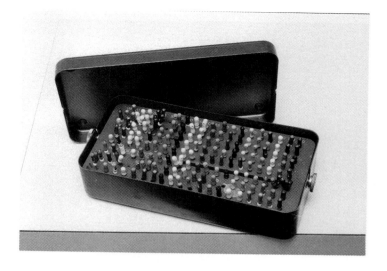

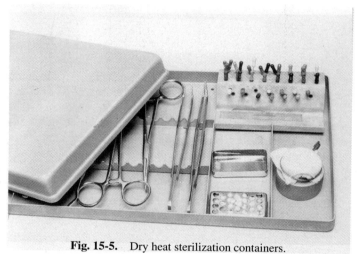

Fig. 15-5. Dry heat sterilization containers.

quate ventilation, potential damage to both rubber and plastic, and the requirement of open containers are sufficient encumbrances to cause one to consider one of the other methods, if possible.

Bead sterilizers, which should be converted to hot-salt sterilizers, are of particular interest to endodontic practitioners. Although unacceptable as a true sterilization process because only the working end is immersed and sterilized, it is a valuable chairside adjunct to aseptic technique. Glass beads should be replaced by table salt to eliminate the accidental transfer of a glass bead adherent to a file into a root canal, which could form an impenetrable barrier. If inadvertently car-

ried into the canal, salt may be dissolved or flushed away by water or sodium hypochlorite irrigation. Temperatures of 450°F are reached, which will sterilize the metallic immersed portion of a clean file in 5 seconds (Fig. 15-6). This device not only provides a convenient method of decontaminating a file exposed to oral fluids or infected canal material so that it can be safely reintroduced into another canal, but also provides an aseptic method of passing a premeasured intracanal instrument from dental assistant to operator.

Disinfecting solutions. Disinfectants are compounds such as quaternary ammonium products, mercurials, phenolics, glutaraldehydes, and sodium

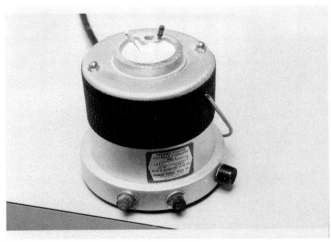

Fig. 15-6.   Hot salt sterilizer.

hypochlorite solutions. They should not be confused with, and are not recognized as acceptable sterilization alternatives. Ritchie studied the use of glutaraldehyde solutions as a disinfectant to eliminate quickly many common organisms found in the root canal. If glutaraldehydes are to be expected to be sporicidal, overnight immersion is required, and even conforming to this time requirement is not acceptable as an alternative option to steam or dry-heat sterilization as outlined by the CDC and FDA. Uses for these solutions include the disinfection of endodontic items such as rubber dam frames that do not enter the oral cavity, but are nondisposable. Many of these agents have been modified for use as counter and surface wipes for interpatient room decontamination.

Sterilization monitoring.   The CDC and other agencies recommend weekly monitoring of sterilization systems. Heat indicators incorporated into autoclave tape and dry-heat-indicator labels that change color during the sterilization process are not accurate indicators that the sterilization system is actually destroying all virus and spore forms. These indicators show that a certain temperature has been attained and are a good benchmark test for each package or cassette being processed, but periodic processing of spore strips, vials or ampules, and their subsequent culturing will assure proper operation of sterilizing equipment. Commercial spore testing packets (Fig. 15-3) of nonpathogenic *Bacillus stearothermophilus* or *Bacillus subtilis* spores are available and offer valuable verification by an outside agency of sterilizer functions. After reviewing all the precautions and efforts employed to eliminate microbes during endodontic therapy, there is no safer procedure in dentistry than root canal therapy for either the patient or health-care provider.

REFERENCES

ADA Workshop: Sterilizing dental handpieces, *J Am Dent Assoc* 123:45, 1992.

Baumgartner J, Falkler W: Bacteria in the apical 5 mm of infected root canals, *J Endod* 17:380, 1991.

Bence R, Madonia JV, Weine FS, Smulson MH: A microbiologic evaluation of endodontic instrumentation in pulpless teeth, *Oral Surg* 35:676, 1973.

Bender IB, Seltzer S: The probability of error of the negative culture with the use of combinations of antibiotics in endodontic treatment, *Oral Surg* 7:1311, 1954.

Bender IB, Seltzer S, Turkenkopf S: To culture or not to culture, *Oral Surg* 18:527, 1964.

Bergenholtz G: Micro-organisms from necrotic pulp of traumatized teeth, *Odont Rev* 25:347, 1974.

Bergenholtz G: Pathogenic mechanisms in pulpal disease, *J Endod* 16:98, 1990.

Besic FC: The fate of bacteria sealed in dental cavities, *J Dent Res* 22:349, 1943.

Borssen E, Dundqvist G: Actinomyces of infected root canals, *Oral Surg* 51:643, 1981.

Burke GW, Knighton HT: The incidence of microorganisms in inflamed dental pulps of rats following bacteremia, *J Dent Res* 39:205, 1960.

Bystrom A: Evaluation of endodontic treatment of teeth with periapical periodontitis, *Umea University Odontological Dissertations* 27:5, 1986.

Carlsson J, Sundqvist G: Evaluation of methods of transport and cultivation of bacterial specimens from infected dental root canals, *Oral Surg* 49:451, 1980.

Faecher R, Thomas J, Bender B: Tuberculosis a growing concern for dentistry? *J Am Dent Assoc* 124:94, 1993.

Farber R, Seltzer S: Endodontic microbiology. 1. Etiology, *J Endod* 14:363, 1988.

Fulghum RS, Wiggins CB, Mullaney TP: Pilot study for detecting obligate anaerobic bacteria in necrotic dental pulps, *J Dent Res* 52:637, 1973.

Gier RE, Mitchell DF: Anachoretic effect of pulpitis, *J Dent Res* 47:564, 1968.

Glickman G: On the horizon. . . DNA fingerprinting with PCR, *Endodontics, Colleagues for Excellence,* AAE Publication Fall/Winter 1994.

Gohean R, Pantera E, Schuster G: Indirect immunofluorescence microscopy for the identification of Actinomyces sp. in endodontic disease, *J Endod* 16:318, 1990.

Griffee MB, Patterson SS, Miller CH, et al: The relationship of Bacteroides melaninogenicus to symptoms associated with pulpal necrosis, *Oral Surg* 50:457, 1980.

Grossman LI: The treatment of infected root canals, *Int Dent J* 2:371, 1952.

Grossman LI, Oliet S: Correlation of clinical diagnosis and bacteriologic status of symptomatically involved pulps, *Oral Surg* 25:235, 1968.

Hahn C, Falkler W, Minak G: Correlation between thermal sensitivity and microorganisms isolated from deep carious dentin, *J Endod* 19:26, 1993.

Hargreaves K: Successful management of pain and infection in the dental office, presented before the E.D. Coolidge Endodontic Study Club, Chicago, Sept 1994.

Hashioka K et al: Relationship between clinical symptoms and enzyme-producing bacteria isolated from infected root canals, *J Endod* 20:75, 1994.

Hedman WJ: An investigation into residual periapical infection after pulp canal therapy, *Oral Surg* 4:1173, 1951.

Herweijer J, Loos B, Neiders M: Characterization of total membrane proteins of Porphyromonas endodontalis, *J Endod* 18:620, 1992.

Hobson P: The bacteriological problems of root-canal therapy, *Dent Pract* 16:43, 1965.

Horiba N et al: Cytotoxicity against various cell lines of Lipopolysaccharides purified from Bacteriodes, Fusobacterium, and Veillonella isolated from infected root canals, *J Endod* 15:530, 1989.

Kakehashi S, Stanley HR, Fitzgerald RJ: The effects of surgical exposures of dental pulps in germ-free and conventional laboratory rats, *Oral Surg* 20:340, 1965.

Kantz WE, Henry CA: Isolation and classification of anaerobic bacteria from intact pulp chambers of nonvital teeth in man, *Arch Oral Biol* 19:91, 1974.

Keudell K, Ernest M: Microorganisms isolated from pulp chambers, *J Endod* 2:146, 1976.

Labriola JS, Mascaro J, Alpert B: The microbiologic flora of orofacial abscesses, *Oral Surg* 53:711, 1983.

Leavitt JM, Naidorf IJ, Shugaevsky P: The bacterial flora of root canals as disclosed by a culture medium for endodontics, *Oral Surg* 11:302, 1958.

Lin L, Skribner J, Gaenzler P: Factors associated with endo-

dontic treatment failures, *J Endod* 18:625, 1992.

Miller C: Cleaning, sterilization and disinfection: basics of microbial killing for infection control, *J Am Dent Assoc* 124:49, 1993.

Molinari J: Practical infection control for the 1990s: applying science to government regulations, *J Am Dent Assoc* 125:1189, 1994.

Morse DR: The endodontic culture technique: a critical evaluation, *Oral Surg* 30:540, 1970.

Morse FW, Yates WF: Follow-up studies of root canal filled teeth in relation to bacteriologic findings, *J Am Dent Assoc* 28:956, 1941.

Myers JW, Marshall FJ, Rosen S: The incidence and identity of microorganisms present in root canals at filling following culture reversals, *Oral Surg* 28:889, 1969.

Naidorf I: Clinical microbiology in endodontics, *Dent Clin North Am* 18:329, 1974.O'Grady J, Reede P: Periapical actinomycosis involving Actinomyces israelii, *J Endod* 14:147, 1988.

Palmer GR, Lazzarotto JR, Weine FS: Paper point transfer of minimal numbers of microorganisms from a prepared canal in vitro, *Oral Surg* 42:824, 1976.

Pantera E, Zambon J, Shih-Levine M: Indirect immunofluorescence for the detection of Bacteroides species in human dental pulp, *J Endod* 14:218, 1988.

Perez F, Cala P, de Falguerolles A, Maurette A: Migration of a Streptococcus sanguis strain through the root dentinal tubules, *J Endod* 19:297, 1993.

Ritchie GM: Glutaraldehyde as a cold sterilizing agent for endodontic instruments. Master's thesis, Loyola University, 1971.

Robinson HBG, Boling LR: The anachoretic effect in pulpitis. I. Bacteriologic studies, *J Am Dent Assoc* 38:268, 1941.

Schein B, Schilder H. Endotoxin content in endodontically involved teeth, *J Endod* 1:19–21, 1975.

Serene TP, McDonald ED: Endodontic culturing: a statistical study, *J Am Dent Assoc* 78:1013, 1969.

Shay DE: The selection of a suitable medium for culturing root canals, *J Dent Res* 26:327, 1947.

Shearer B: MDR-TB another challenge from the microbial world, *J Am Dent Assoc* 125:43, 1994.

Shovelton DS: The presence and distribution of microorganisms within non-vital teeth, *Br Dent J* 117:101, 1964.

Slack GL: The bacteriology of infected root canals and in vitro penicillin sensitivity, *Br Dent J* 95:211, 1958.

Smith L, Tappe GD: Experimental pulpitis in rats, *J Dent Res* 47:17, 1962.

Sommer RF, Crowley M: Bacteriologic verification of roentgenographic findings in pulp involved teeth, *J Am Dent Assoc* 27:723, 1940.

Sundqvist G: Bacteriological studies of necrotic dental pulps, *Umea University Odontological Dissertations,* no 7, 1976.

Sundqvist G: Ecology of the root canal flora, *J Endod* 18:427, 1992.

Sundqvist G, Johansson E: Prevalence of black-pigmented Bacteroides species in root canal infections, *J Endod* 15:13, 1989.

Sundqvist G, Reuterving C: Isolation of Actinomyces israelii from periapical lesion, *J Endod* 6:602, 1980.

Tani N, et al.: Immunobiologic activities of bacteria isolated from the root canals of postendodontic teeth with persistant periapical lesions, *J Endod* 18:58, 1992.

Torabinejad M, Ung B, Kettering J: In vitro bacterial penetration of coronally unsealed endodontically treated teeth, *J Endod* 16:566, 1990.

Torneck CD: An aseptic approach to endodontic practice, *Dent Clin North Am,* 11:567, 1967.

Torneck CD: The role of microorganisms in endodontic disease, *Alpha Omegan,* 62:180, 1969.

van Steenbergen TVM, et al: Bacteroides endodontalis sp. nov., an asaccharolytic black-pigmented Bacteroides species from infected dental root canals, *Int J Systemic Bacteriol* 34:118, 1984.

van Winkelhoff AJ, Carlee AW, de Graaff J: Bacteroides endodontalis and other black-pigmented Bacteroides species in odontogenic abscesses, *Infect Immun* 49:494, 1985.

van Winkelhoff A, van Steenbergen M, de Graaff J: Porphyromonas (Bacteroides) endodontalis: its role in endodontal infections, *J Endod* 18:431, 1992.

Wayman B, Murata S, Almeida R, Fowler C: A bacteriological and histological evaluation of 58 periapical lesions, *J Endod* 18:152, 1992.

Wesley R, Osborn T, Dylewski J: Periapical actinomycosis: clinical considerations, *J Endod* 3:352, 1977.

Winkler KC, van Amerongen J: Bacteriologic results from 4,000 root canal cultures, *Oral Surg* 12:857, 1959.

Wittgow WC, Sabiston DB, Jr: Microorganisms from pulpal chambers of intact teeth with necrotic pulps, *J Endod* 1:168, 1975.

Yamamoto K, Hisanori F, Heronori T, Herosuke S: Antimicrobial susceptibilities of Eubacterium, Peptostreptococcus, and Bacteroides isolated from root canals of teeth with periapical pathosis, *J Endod* 15:112, 1989.

Yamasaki M et al: Endotoxin and gram-negative bacteria in the rat periapical lesions, *J Endod* 18:501, 1992.

Yang P: The role of microorganisms in endodontic disease, *Univ Tor Dent J* 5:13, 1992.

Yoshida M et al: Correlation between clinical symptoms and microorganisms isolated from root canals with periapical pathosis, *J Endod* 13:24, 1987.

Zeldow BJ, Ingle JI: Correlations of the positive culture to the prognosis of endodontically treated teeth: a clinical study, *J Am Dent Assoc* 66:23, 1963.

16 Alternatives to routine endodontic treatment

Improvements in the field of endodontics in the past few decades have raised the quality of treatment and the prognosis to new all-time highs. Even the most complicated cases will yield excellent long-term results from correct treatment. Even so, some dentists continue to use alternatives to routine endodontic therapy when pulp exposure or periapical pathosis caused by pulpal necrosis occur.

Some dentists prefer to use vital pulp therapy—pulp capping or pulpotomy procedures—for exposed pulps, rather then extirpate and perform routine treatment. For many years clinicians in some European countries have treated both vital and necrotic pulps with deep pulpotomy procedures, as described by Baume, in preference to complete filing and filling. Also used in various forms in Europe has been the Sargenti technique, employing paste filling. This technique received some acceptance on several different occasions from dentists in the United States, as well, but currently, for reasons that will be explained later in this chapter, usage has dwindled down to a faithful few.

Pulpotomy and other similar procedures for root development may be used with routine therapy to follow in certain cases, such as incomplete root development with pulp exposure, or resorptive defects.

This chapter will describe the advantages, disadvantages, and treatment modalities of these procedures.

VITAL PULP THERAPY

Why vital pulp therapy? There seem to be three main reasons why dentists select vital pulp therapy rather than routine endodontic treatment for teeth with exposed vital pulps.

1. *The limited endodontic skill of the practitioner.* Unfortunately, the education of many dentists included little, if any, teaching of endodontic skills. Also, the methods taught in some schools were so taxing and complicated that many competent operators were "turned off" by the complexities of treatment.

2. *Anatomic difficulties offered by some teeth.* Some dentists may perform routine endodontic therapy on most anterior and bicuspid teeth, but they may not treat molars or teeth with severe curvatures and/or dentinal sclerosis because of the difficulties and great time requirements necessitated by these more complicated cases (Fig. 16-1).

3. *Limited financial resources of the patient.* Because of the considerable time and effort involved in endodontic treatment of some teeth, particularly molars, a fee that is only a fair remuneration for the dentist may be excessive for the patient (Fig. 16-2).

If these reasons are present and if referral to a general dentist who enjoys endodontic treatment or to a specialist is not available or practical, only vital pulp therapy remains to avoid extraction of an involved tooth.

History and review of the literature. There are few areas of the dental literature that have been more written about than vital pulp therapy. Among materials that have been suggested to be applied to the exposed pulp are starches and steroids, coal tar products and antibiotics, and phenolics and alcohol derivatives.

In the infancy of endodontics the objective of treatment for the exposed vital pulp was its retention because of the severe pain involved in pulp removal. Many endodontic treatments administered in the nineteenth and early twentieth centuries were pulp-capping procedures. Many materials were described at this time for use, including thin lead

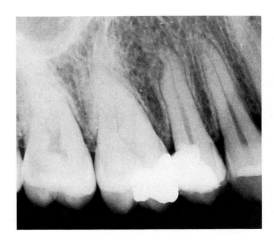

Fig. 16-1. Because of sharp distal dilaceration, which would make routine endodontic treatment difficult, vital exposure of maxillary second bicuspid was treated with pulp capping. Dressing is in place over the exposure and is covered by zinc oxide–eugenol.

leaf covered by gold foil, goose quill, parchment paper, gold leaf, asbestos, essential oil, creosote, phenol, and cologne. I cannot fail to mention also the now famous description of Hunter, who in 1883 stated that he mixed English sparrow droppings with sorghum molasses, applied it to the exposed pulp, and reputedly enjoyed 98% success.

During the late 1920s, a number of pulp amputation investigations took place in Germany, and Hermann first introduced the use of calcium hydroxide. Teuscher and Zander reported on the action of the material used in pulpotomies, describing the formation of a dentinlike layer beneath the site of exposure and above a layer of odontoblasts. This was called the dentin bridge, corresponding to the frequent radiographic appearance of a radiopaque line apical to the dressing in a tooth treated with vital pulp therapy.

In a follow-up report the next year, Zander described the action of calcium hydroxide alone and in combination with other salts. He attempted to justify its use on a biochemical basis, theorizing that the calcium ions in the medication would cause a precipitation of calcium salts from the blood to gain the calcified material for the dentin bridge.

It was not until 1964 that Pisanti and Sciaky and Stark et al., using labeled radioactive calcium, established the exact source of the calcium in the

bridge. When radioactive materials were used in the medication, none was found in the dentin bridge. However, when labeled calcium was injected intravenously, the radioactive ions could be demonstrated in the bridge. They concluded that the calcium in the dentin bridge came from the bloodstream only and that the medication merely created a suitable condition for bridging rather than entering in its formation. Although evaluated only on a clinical basis, many reports described and modified the use of calcium hydroxide, usually describing a high degree of success.

However, Via surveyed 103 out of more than 800 patients treated with calcium hydroxide at the children's clinic of the University of Michigan. Under an average observation period of 24.9 months he judged 68.9% to be unsuccessful, mostly due to internal resorption. Ostrom and Lyon and Quigley also reported series of failures, noting that some pulps treated with calcium hydroxide showed dentin bridges and also pulpal degeneration in the same teeth.

Mitchell and Shankwalker described the extensive osteogenic potential of calcium hydroxide. Clinical observations of others have been that pulps treated with it often present problems if endodontic treatment later becomes necessary because of heavy deposition of secondary dentin that takes place even if the tooth involved develops a necrotic pulp.

For these reasons, other medications were used in vital pulp therapy that did not produce the potentially harmful extensive bridging. Mixtures of zinc oxide and eugenol plus other additives have been described with excellent results by some, and areas of necrosis, abscess formation, and inflammatory infiltration have been described by others.

Formocresol has been widely used as a pulpotomy dressing and extensively described, usually compared with the action of calcium hydroxide or zinc oxide and eugenol. Sealed over the exposed vital pulp stump, formocresol produces chemical fixation of the tissue contacted and contiguous middle third of the root. Berger, Doyle et al., Law and Lewis, and Spedding et al. all described the vitality of the apical pulp and the normalcy of the periapical tissues after its use. Heavy deposition of irritation dentin was not seen.

Another type of vital pulp therapy involves the use of a corticosteroid, generally in combination with an antibiotic, which results in tremendous

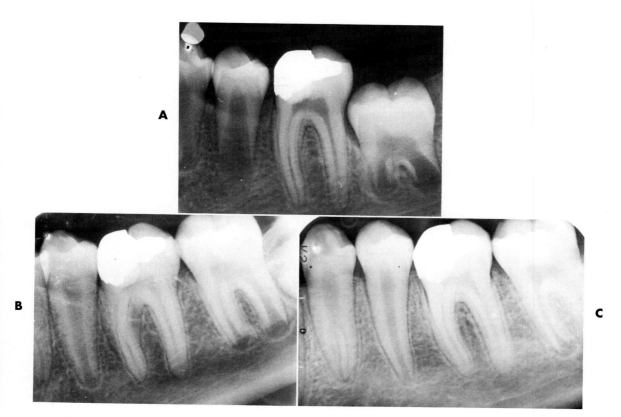

Fig. 16-2. **A,** Pulp capping after pulp exposure of mesiobuccal horn of mandibular first molar. This treatment was instituted because of the limited financial resources of the patient's parents. **B,** Two years after treatment. **C,** Three years after treatment, tooth is comfortable and radiographically normal. Because pulp capping was performed with zinc oxide–eugenol, if endodontics should be necessary later and the patient could afford the fee, excessive dentinal deposition would not occur.

deposition of dentin, as described by Baume. However, an illuminating study was reported by Lawson and Mitchell, followed by Mullaney et al. and Compton and Mitchell. Results of a double-blind experiment with a corticoid and two antibiotics as a pulp-capping agent on human subjects suffering with symptomatic pulpitis indicated that 100% success after 3 months dissipated to less than 20% in 5 years.

In evaluating the histologic sections, Mullaney et al. illustrated the importance of examining serial sections in pulp studies, since some areas showed considerable dentinoid bridging, whereas others in the same tooth showed the absence of complete bridging and sites of necrosis. They also pointed out the fallacy of determining success on the basis of radiographs alone, which could not possibly show if the dentin bridge had been complete (Fig. 16-3).

Consequences of calcium hydroxide pulp cappings. Most of the studies seem to agree that calcium hydroxide will give the highest percentage of pulp-capping success. Unfortunately, if such therapy fails and the tooth becomes symptomatic, it may be difficult, if not impossible, to treat with routine endodontics because of the severe calcifications in the root canal. Perforations may occur during attempts to follow the canal sclerosis to gain patency to the apex (Fig. 16-4).

When examining teeth treated by vital pulp therapy in general and those treated with calcium hydroxide in particular, the dentist must not only examine by radiograph the periapical areas for signs of incipent breakdown, but also must observe any indication of potential increase or decrease in the size of the pulp canal space. If that area becomes much narrower, it indicates a

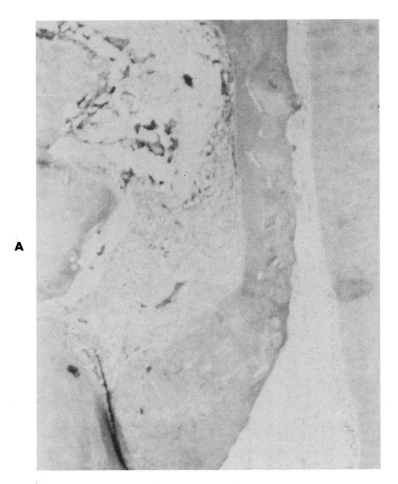

Fig. 16-3. **A,** Photomicrograph of monkey mandibular incisor pulp exposure treated with corticoid-antibiotic mixtures. Apparently complete dentin bridge. (From Mullaney TP, Lawson BF, Mitchell DF: *Oral Surg* 21:479, 1966.)

low-grade chronic inflammation of the pulp, which may lead to diminution so that the canal is smaller than the smallest endodontic instrument. This would make any further nonsurgical treatment impossible. Similarly, if the pulp space becomes increasingly wider, particularly in one area, the existence of an internal resorption defect may make any subsequent endodontic treatment highly complicated (Fig. 16-5).

Pulp capping as opposed to pulpotomy. In my opinion, pulpotomy procedures, particularly in anterior teeth after trauma, should be used rather than pulp capping. In many cases certain young people seem to be accident prone and repeatedly suffer blows to their face and jaws. In pulp cap-

ping the dressing is placed over the edge of the pulp exposure and a temporary covering provided. Any subsequent trauma will easily loosen or dislodge the temporary, displacing the dressing and probably resulting in pulpal contamination and resultant necrosis. The pulpotomy dressing is placed more deeply in the canal with a cement covering that will prevent loss of the dressing even if the temporary cover is lost.

Best indications for successful vital pulp therapy. Recognizing the potential problems that might occur, it is suggested that the following types of cases of exposed vital pulps would appear to give the best indications for alternatives to routine endodontic treatment:

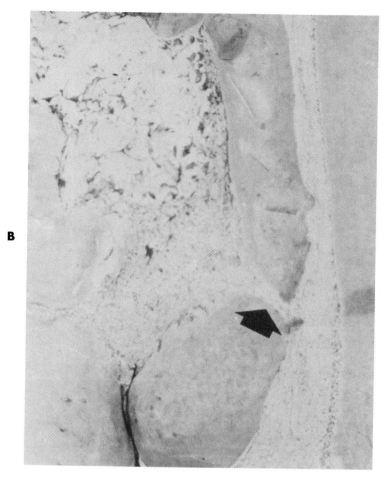

Fig. 16-3, cont'd. B, Serial section of the same tooth showing pulp tissue extending through the incomplete bridge *(arrow)*. (H & E; ×32.)

1. *Teeth with incomplete apical development.* This is an excellent indication for pulpotomy because the prognosis for routine endodontic therapy would be doubtful due to the lack of apical constriction needed to pack the root canal filling. Pulpotomy procedures will usually keep the apical portion of the pulp vital and allow for relatively normal root development and closure, at which time routing therapy can be accomplished.
2. *Primary teeth.* Various types of vital pulp therapy have been used for many years to retain primary teeth until the normal time of exfoliation. Calcium hydroxide and zinc oxide-eugenol (ZOE) as capping agents and calcium

hydroxide and formocresol as pulpotomy agents have been reported with great success in the primary dentition. In fact, routine endodontic therapy is difficult to accomplish on these teeth because of the common finding of thin and curved canals, multiple lateral canals and ramifications, and resorbing roots that prevent the preparation of an apical dentin matrix.

3. *Teeth that would be difficult to treat endodontically.* Obviously, this indication varies from one practitioner to another, since someone with considerable endodontic skill could treat a tooth that would be nearly impossible for someone with lesser ability. Generally,

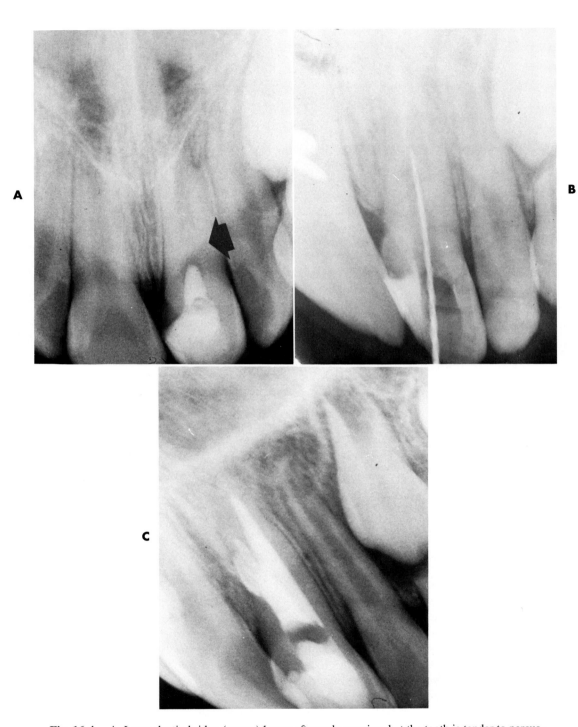

Fig. 16-4.   **A,** Large dentin bridge *(arrow)* 1 year after pulp capping, but the tooth is tender to percussion. **B,** In the attempt to penetrate through dentin bridge, the file appears to be leaving canal. **C,** Final angled radiograph after canal filling shows the site of perforation. (Courtesy Dr. Edward P. Theiss, Boulder, Colo.)

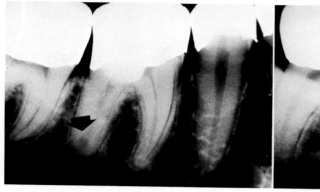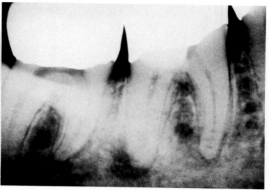

Fig. 16-5. Internal resorption after Ca(OH)$_2$ pulpotomy. **A,** One year, no periapical changes. Area of internal resorption in distal root *(arrow)* was not noted at that time. **B,** Two years, periapical area broken down and resorptive defect much larger, making prognosis less favorable. At this time the earlier radiograph was reexamined and the defect noted in retrospect. For completion of this difficult case, see Fig. 9-28.

teeth with sharp apical dilacerations, extremely long multirooted teeth, and third molars with unusual root shape or number of roots might be considered for vital pulp therapy if exposure occurs.

4. *Teeth involved in simple restorations.* If a pulp exposure does occur on a tooth that is surrounded by sound adjacent teeth, vital pulp therapy may be performed knowing that the consequences of failure would not involve the jeopardizing of a complex prosthesis.

5. *Teeth with pulpal inflammation confined to a small segment of the coronal pulp.* Vital pulp therapy should not be considered when the tooth has been percussion sensitive, which indicates apical spread of pulpal inflammation (Chapter 5), or when a long history of pain is reported, indicating a long-standing, chronically inflamed pulp. In these cases either pulp capping or pulpotomy would probably leave much inflamed pulp tissue remaining in the canals, and recovery would be problematic. If, however, only a small segment of the pulp is inflamed, probably adjacent to the site of exposure, either pulp capping or pulpotomy could remove it, and the recuperative potential of the pulp might lead to success.

Contraindications for vital pulp therapy. In the following cases it is advised that vital pulp therapy not be considered for the exposed vital pulp but rather that routine endodontic treatment be performed.

1. *Teeth in which the canal space could be well utilized to hold a post and core.* In some instances trauma, decay, or operative procedures result in little clinical crown with a tiny pulp exposure. The tendency here might be to retain the vitality of the pulp by vital pulp therapy and then to build up the crown with pins or screw posts in restoration. Unfortunately, should the pulp become necrotic later and/or radiographic changes develop, it might be extremely difficult to locate the canal through the mass of restorative materials with little crown guidance as aid. In actuality, restoration of the tooth probably would have been easier if the pulp had been removed at the time of the exposure, with routine endodontic therapy performed through the easy and direct access of little crown and no covering being present, and later restoration with a post and core (Fig. 16-6).

2. *Splint, bridge, and precision partial denture abutments.* If a tooth that is to be used as a splint, fixed bridge, or precision partial denture abutment is exposed, it probably should undergo routine endodontics initially. This would avoid the necessity of having to go through and weakening a complicated prosthesis, perhaps removing much internal tooth

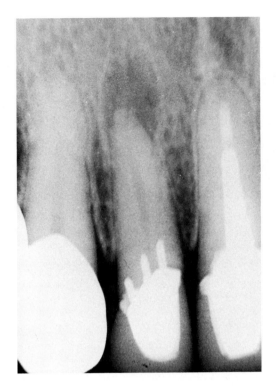

Fig. 16-6. Crown of maxillary lateral incisor had broken off at gingival line 2 years earlier, but no exposure was noted. Multiple pins were placed, a core was built up, and a new jacket crown was placed. Now radiograph indicates periapical involvement. Root canal space would have been better used to hold post and core. If nonsurgical therapy is performed now, there is a strong chance of ruining the crown.

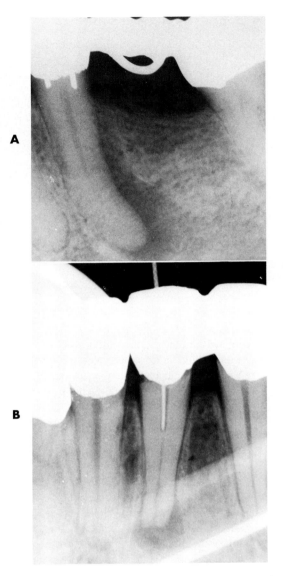

Fig. 16-7. Pulp-capping failures under complex restorations. **A,** Multiple pins were used to build up a pulp-capped mandibular second bicuspid in an effort to avoid endodontic treatment 12 months earlier. Large sinus tract is now present. **B,** Mandibular incisor was pulp capped 18 months earlier to avoid endodontic treatment on this splint abutment. Large dentin bridge is present that complicates gaining access to the apex, but a large radiolucency at the apex required treatment.

structure and possibly perforating if endodontic therapy is required after restoration. In these situations it would be best to complete routine endodontic therapy prior to any restoration. The treated tooth then is utilized as an abutment after restoration with a post-and-core type of crown (Fig. 16-7).

3. *Teeth involved in complex periodontal therapy and resultant periodontal prostheses.* As stated in Chapter 13, it is my opinion that pulpal inflammation will often accompany severe periodontal lesions. Therefore I believe that a definite number of teeth involved in complex periodontal treatment already have some degree of pulpal inflammation, probably of the more chronic type. If these teeth are flapped and the roots are scraped and curetted during periodontal treatment, prepared for splinting, temporized, and crowned in restoration, it is obvious that any pulpal inflammation present will increase. In addition, teeth that were free of

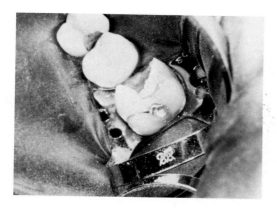

Fig. 16-8. Exposure was anticipated, so rubber dam was placed in advance. Because of severe decay on mesial aspect, exposure occurred. A thin mix of ZOE was applied as capping agent.

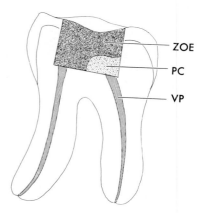

Fig. 16-9. Diagram of pulp capping of posterior tooth. Vital pulp *(VP)* was exposed and is covered by medication *(PC)*. Access is closed with a temporary covering *(ZOE)*. At next appointment, occlusal portions of temporary covering will be removed, and a restoration will be placed without disturbing areas closer to the pulp.

pulpal inflammation prior to treatment might indeed be insulted sufficiently to cause pulpal damage. Many teeth involved in periodontal prostheses, particularly mandibular incisors, are caries free and restoration free, but receive crown preparation prior to splinting. Attempting to gain parallelism of abutments might lead to exposure of the vital pulp. Endodontic treatment at this time would be simple, but the operator might consider vital pulp therapy. Should such treatment fail, it might be extremely difficult to locate and prepare the entire canal, resulting in need for periapical surgery or extraction.

Pulp capping of posterior teeth. When a pulp exposure is anticipated, it would be well for the dentist to place a rubber dam for the excavation. This is not always possible because decay may extend deeply into unanticipated areas or exposure may be due to operative procedures. Once the exposure occurs, the desired medicament is placed over the pulp without pressure (Fig. 16-8). A thin mix of ZOE is placed over the medicament; then a thick mix of ZOE accelerated with zinc acetate crystals is prepared and used to close the entire preparation (Fig. 16-9).

It is recommended that the final restoration not be placed at the same appointment. The least possible operative manipulation after the exposure would be most conducive to healing. If an amalgam restoration is condensed, the pulpal dressing may be loosened or impacted into the pulp chamber, with disastrous results. In addition, if the tooth becomes symptomatic and requires complete endodontic treatment, the restoration would have to be partially destroyed during access cavity preparation.

By leaving the tooth closed with the ZOE temporary covering, the dentist may restore the tooth 1 to 4 weeks later if it is symptom free. A new cavity preparation is made at that time, leaving the pulp capping as covering plus some additional portions of the temporary covering in place as a base.

The same procedure is followed in both primary and permanent teeth. In the former dentition a metal crown may be utilized as the restoration of choice and only the periphery of the tooth is trimmed, with most of the ZOE temporary covering remaining.

Formocresol pulpotomy for posterior teeth. Studies indicate that one-sitting pulpotomy procedures are as effective as those performed in two appointments. Rubber dam placement aids in accomplishing the objectives of treatment, and a local anesthetic is mandatory.

When the exposure is found, the roof of the chamber is removed. A sharp, sterile, no. 4 round bur is used to remove the coronal pulp tissue so the bleeding pulpal stumps only are seen at the floor of the chamber. Sterile cotton pellets are used to absorb hemorrhage. After hemostasis is achieved, a

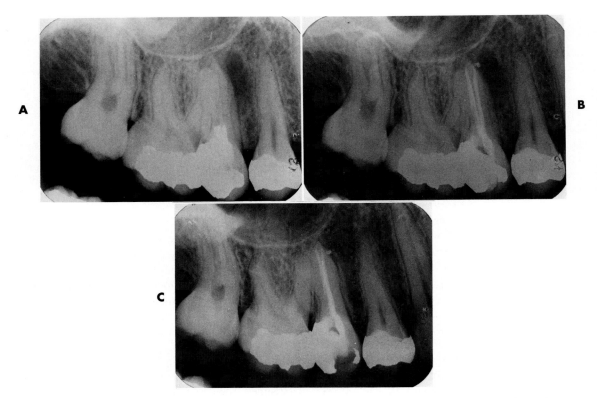

Fig. 16-10. Failing pulpotomy procedure, successfully re-treated by routine therapy. **A,** Radiograph of maxillary second bicuspid treated with a pulpotomy 3 years earlier. The pulp had been vital at the time of vital pulp therapy, but a large lateral radiolucency is now present. The dentist who had done the original therapy strongly objected to the re-treatment, advising the patient that his treatment was successful since the tooth was not causing any pain. **B,** Canals were quite wide, and it was no problem to prepare and fill them with laterally condensed gutta-percha. **C,** Excellent healing only 4 months later. The referring dentist did not even have time to place a more permanent restoration and the lesion had healed.

cotton pellet is lightly dampened with formocresol and applied to the pulp stumps for 3 minutes.

A thin mix of formocresol and zinc oxide is prepared and placed on the fixed pulp. A thick mix of ZOE accelerated with zinc acetate crystals is placed to provide occlusal seal. The tooth may be restored if symptom free from 1 to 4 weeks later.

One of the best reasons for using formocresol rather than calcium hydroxide as a pulpotomy medication is the implication for further treatment if the pulp therapy should fail. It is generally easy to perform endodontic therapy on teeth treated with formocresol. The periapical lesion present allows for treatment without local anesthetic, and usually the lesion heals without difficulty (Fig. 16-10). On the other hand, calcium hydroxide may

cause reparative dentin formation and result in considerably diminished pulp canal space.

Pulpotomy treatment of anterior teeth. Because of the ease of performing complete endodontic treatment on anterior teeth, it is recommended that vital pulp therapy not be used except in cases in which apical development is not yet completed. Accordingly, such cases will be discussed in the segment of this chapter dealing with treatment of the open apex.

Follow-up after vital pulp therapy. After vital pulp therapy, radiographs should be taken and clinical symptoms evaluated at regular 6-month intervals. Ideally the treated tooth should remain comfortable with no sinus tract development. Radiographically, the periapical areas should remain normal. In addition to x-ray examination of the periapical tissues, the dentist must be certain to examine the interior of the tooth and specifically the shape of the canals as well.

If the canal suddenly starts to decrease in size greatly, the dentist should consider routine endodontic intervention while a patency to the apex still exists. If the canal shows a sudden enlargement in a specific area, indicating internal resorption, routine endodontics must be initiated immediately, before the defect becomes too large and mitigates against successful treatment. This examination of the canal shape is at least equal in importance to following the progress of the periapical regions.

When evaluating primary teeth, the dentist should further see that the tooth is resorbing at a relatively normal rate, comparing it to the contralateral tooth. If it is resorbing at an accelerated pace, which is not unusual after vital pulp therapy, the permanent successor should be erupting more rapidly to take its place earlier. For some time it was believed that bicuspids that erupted with pitting of the enamel were adversely affected by vital pulp therapy. However, Kaplan et al. showed that this is not the case and indicated that such pitting probably is due to a periapical abscess developing from the primary molar, but not from the vital pulp therapy.

The finding of a dentin bridge does not always indicate success by itself and negate the need for any further evaluation.

TREATMENT OF TEETH WITH INCOMPLETE APICAL DEVELOPMENT

For many years patients with teeth that were incompletely developed or had open apices and pulpal or periapical involvement offered dentists a most difficult condition to treat. These patients usually were young and had suffered trauma only shortly after the injured tooth had erupted, causing pain to the child, mental anguish to the parents, and a perplexing treatment problem to the dentist.

Problems of the open apex. The open apex case occurs when trauma or decay causes pulpal exposure and/or periapical involvement prior to the completion of root development. An open apex refers to the absence of sufficient root development to provide a conical taper to the canal and is referred to as a "blunderbuss" canal. This means that the canal is wider toward the apex than near the cervical area. Since it is necessary to seal the

apex to gain endodontic success, it is physically impossible to achieve this objective through ordinary procedures in open apex cases.

For many years, the problem of the blunderbuss apex, particularly if the pulp was necrotic and a periapical lesion was present, was treated surgically (Fig. 16-11). The tooth was opened and prepared as well as these wide, irregular canals could be cleaned, and then packed with gutta-percha (Fig. 16-11, *B*). Rarely could a true seal be achieved, but then the apex was flapped, the lesion curretted, and some type of apical filling placed (Fig. 16-11, *C*).

Flapping teeth on youngsters is not easy and the time taken for the procedures, even with a well-behaved or possibly sedated patient, made cooperation dubious. Psychological problems towards dentistry could develop following such efforts, even though it was the only way to conserve the injured tooth at that time.

The preferable solution is to allow the apex to complete development. If a pulp exposure occurs while the tissue within the canal remains vital, a pulpotomy procedure will permit the apex to develop. However, for many years it was thought that apical development could not be completed if the pulp was necrotic. Fortunately, work by Frank and many other authors, some listed at the conclusion of this chapter, has provided nonsurgical treatment for this condition as well, referred to as *apexification*.

Treatment of open apex with vital pulp. A pulpotomy procedure is indicated in the tooth with an open apex to allow completion of apical closure, as long as the apical pulp remains vital. This is referred to as *apexogenesis*. If there is any chance at all that the apical portion of the pulp is vital, the pulpotomy procedure should be attempted. When the apical pulp can be retained in a vital condition, the root end and canal usually will assume a relatively normal size and shape. However, when the pulp is completely nonvital and apexification procedures must be employed, the root end often develops in a short blunted condition, whereas the canal remains rather wide.

The pulpotomy procedure for anterior teeth (Figs. 16-12 and 16-13) is almost the same as previously described for posterior teeth and is accomplished in one sitting. After anesthetic administration and rubber-dam application, the coronal pulp is amputated to approximately the cervical line with a sharp, sterile, no. 4 bur. Sterile cotton pellets

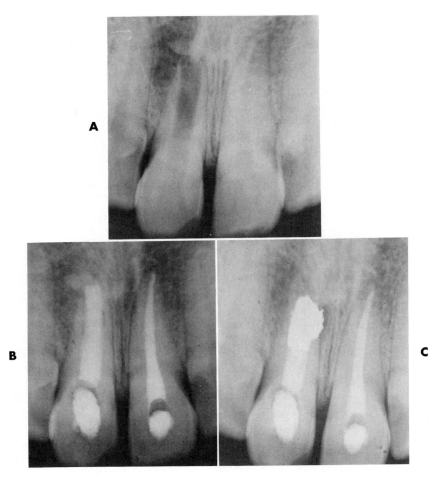

Fig. 16-11. **A,** Preoperative radiograph of maxillary central incisor area; patient is a 15-year-old man; history indicates several episodes of trauma to the teeth. Central incisor to the left has an open apex and a periapical lesion, indicating that the injury to the tooth occurred when the patient was approximately 7 years old. The central incisor to the right has a fully formed apex, a slightly decreased canal size for his age, and a periapical lesion, indicating that the causation of the pulpal damage had occurred several years earlier. Both teeth were nonresponsive to temperature testing. **B,** These teeth were treated prior to the use of apexification procedures, and the blunderbuss apex at that time required surgical intervention. Accordingly, both teeth were prepared and filled with laterally condensed gutta-percha and Tubliseal. The filling is well done for the fully formed apex, but, obviously, no seal has been obtained in the open apex case. A flap was raised, the areas curetted, and an apical amalgam filling placed on the tooth with the open apex. **C,** One year later, the areas have healed well. However, the incisor to the left has been shortened, the canal is quite wide, and there may be some reaction to the amalgam (compare with Figs. 16-17, *G* and *H* and 16-18, *G*). Because the youngster was 15 years old at the time of treatment, he tolerated the procedure relatively well. Similar surgical treatment on younger patients for open apex repair often leads to poor emotional reactions to further dental treatment.

A   B   C

D   E   F

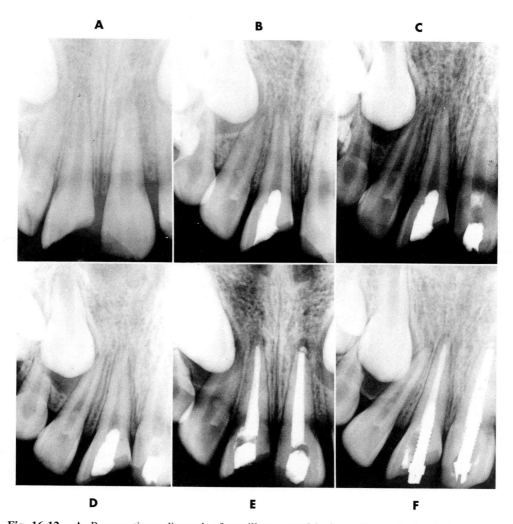

Fig. 16-12.   A, Preoperative radiograph of maxillary central incisors. Traumatic incident 4 months earlier had caused crown fracture to both centrals. The incisor to the right on the film did not respond to electric or temperature tests, and a radiolucency was present at the apex. The incisor to the left was acutely sensitive to both hot and cold temperatures. It was decided to treat the right central with apexification procedures and attempt to allow apical development on the left central with apexogenesis, keeping the apical pulp vital. **B,** Pulpotomy performed on left central, with formocresol placed and ZOE temporary closure. **C,** Six months after treatment, apex is forming. **D,** By 9 months after treatment, the apex has formed sufficiently to complete treatment. **E,** Canal filled with laterally condensed gutta-percha and Wach's paste. The apex had formed sufficiently on the other central to complete therapy on it as well. **F,** Two years after original treatment. Compare apical appearance to **B.** (Restorations by Dr. Lynn Ballard, formerly of Chicago.)

are used to absorb hemorrhage, and a cotton pellet lightly dampened with formocresol is applied to the pulp stump for 3 minutes.

A thin mix of formocresol and zinc oxide is prepared and placed on the fixed pulp. A thick mix of

ZOE accelerated with zinc acetate crystals is placed to provide a seal to the canal and is followed by a suitable temporary covering (Fig. 16-12, *B*).

The tooth so treated is radiographed at 6-month intervals (Fig. 16-12, *C*). When apical closure has

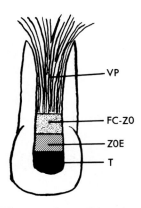

Fig. 16-13. Diagram after pulpotomy to allow vital pulp complete apical closure. A thick mix of formocresol and zinc oxide *(FC-ZO)* is placed over pulp stump *(VP)*. This is followed by *ZOE* and a suitable temporary seal *(T)*.

occurred, routine endodontic treatment is undertaken (Fig. 16-12, *D*). If the pulp becomes necrotic and development halts, apexification procedures are required.

Apexification procedures—treatment of open apex with nonvital pulp. (Fig. 16-14). Apexification requires two sittings, with anesthesia usually not needed for either. At the first appointment the rubber dam is applied and the access cavity prepared. The working length is established (Fig. 16-14, *A*) and the canal debrided. Often the largest file is too narrow to fit snugly in the canal. However, a large Hedstrom file may be used to rasp the walls of the canal with heavy irrigation. The canal is dried with sterile paper points, although it is acceptable to have some moisture remain, since the open apex teeth often have continuous weeping of the periapical tissues. A sterile, dry cotton pellet is placed in the chamber, and the access is closed with ZOE.

The second appointment is scheduled 1 to 2 weeks later. The rubber dam is again applied and the cotton removed. The canal is irrigated, the walls again rasped to remove debris, and the canal dried. Similar criteria for canal filling of routine cases (Chapter 9) are applied here to determine readiness to complete the initial phase of treatment. It is most important that the treated tooth must be free of tenderness to percussion. Although it is usually impossible to open these teeth with wide apices and find a perfectly dry canal, still there must be no active exudation present.

Because of the considerable width and unusual shape of the canal, preparation of such cases is often very difficult. It is extremely doubtful whether these canals can ever be truly debrided as compared to narrow canals. However, for this very reason, considerable time and effort must be expended in order to gain better canal preparation.

For irrigation, it is wise to alternate between sodium hypochlorite and hydrogen peroxide. The effervescence thus obtained will gain more physical debridement and help rid the crevices of debris that might not be removed by filing and rasping alone. Also, the oxygen liberated in the reaction between the two chemicals will kill any anaerobes that might later cause problems. An ultrasonic unit (Chapter 7) may aid the cleanliness obtained during the preparation.

For increased physical debridement, in addition to the Hedstrom file, a cotton-wrapped instrument may be used. A large broach or file is placed in the center of a cotton roll and turned clockwise until it is completely wrapped in the cotton fibers. It is then dipped into the salt sterilizer for 10 seconds and used to wipe the canal walls at the conclusion of canal preparation. Care must be taken to turn the instrument only clockwise within the canal to accomplish this, or the cotton will spin off into the canal and cause great difficulty in removal. It is interesting to see the accumulation of debris that is removed by this instrument after the canal is assumed to be relatively clean.

Frank described the placing of a thick paste composed of calcium hydroxide and CMCP in the debrided canal (Fig. 16-15). The paste must reach the apical portion of the canal to stimulate the tissues to form a calcific barrier. Therefore a Jiffy tube or syringe may be used to ensure proper depth of placement. Calcium hydroxide in a methyl cellulose paste* is available in a syringe (Fig. 16-14, *B*). If this is used, a stop is placed on the needle portion at the proper working length (Fig. 16-14, *C*), and a uniform paste is easily delivered to the correct position in the canal. Although this material contains no parachlorophenol or similar medicament, the calcium hydroxide is the activating member of the mixture and its presence is of prime importance in gaining the desired result.

*Pulpdent Corporation, Brookline, MA 02147.

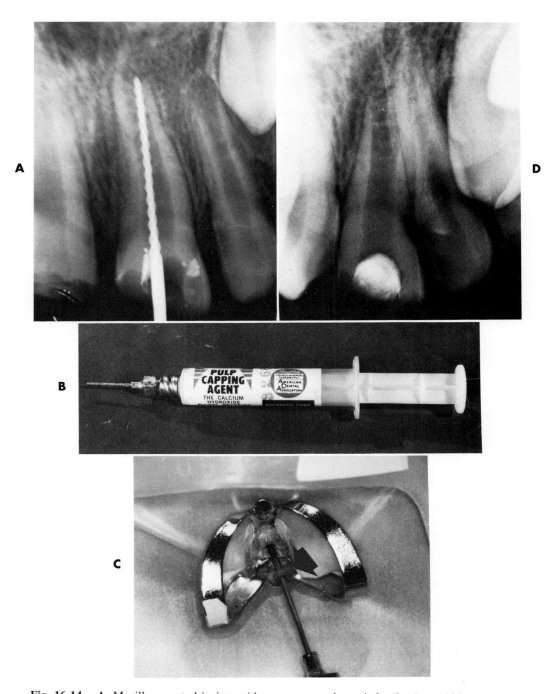

Fig. 16-14. A, Maxillary central incisor with open apex and nonvital pulp. A no. 120 reamer is in canal at a working length of 20 mm, but no stop is present and the instrument could have been pushed many millimeters past apex. **B,** Calcium hydroxide in methyl cellulose paste is available in a syringe. **C,** Working length is marked on syringe tip with rubber stop *(arrow),* and calcium hydroxide is placed in canal. **D,** Radiograph taken 1 year later indicates that some apical calcification has taken place, but it was decided to wait another 6 months before instituting routine therapy. Note root development of adjacent lateral incisor.

Continued

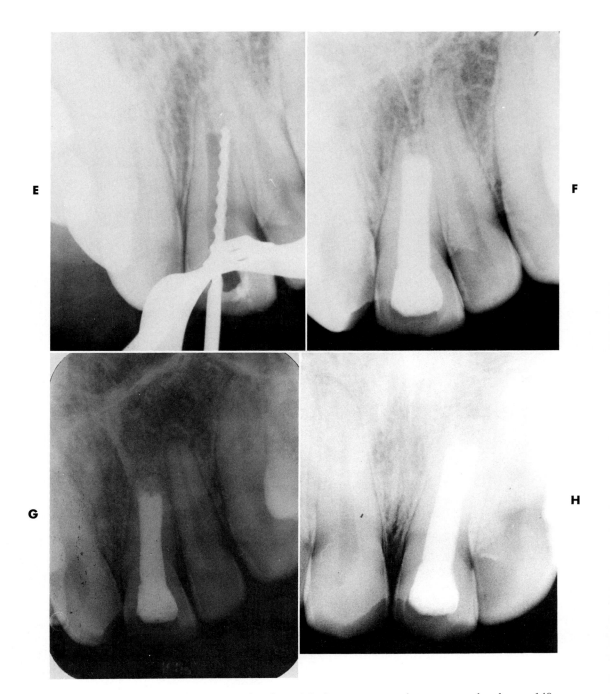

Fig. 16-14, cont'd. **E,** Eighteen months after original treatment, canal was reopened and a no. 140 reamer placed at 20 mm hit a "dead" stop. **F,** Final canal filling with laterally condensed gutta-percha completed the case. This film was taken 2 years after final filling. **G,** Nine years after final filling, after 3 years of orthodontic treatment, which was responsible for some root tip blunting. **H,** Fifteen years after original treatment.

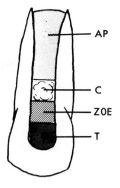

Fig. 16-15. Diagram after apexification procedures to complete apical closure with a nonvital pulp. Apexification paste *(AP)* is composed of calcium hydroxide and CMCP or calcium hydroxide in methyl cellulose and is placed into the canal as close as possible to the apex. A cotton pellet *(C)* is placed in the chamber, followed by ZOE, and a suitable temporary seal *(T)*.

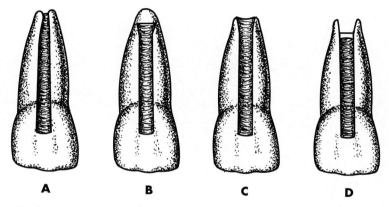

| A | B | C | D |

Fig. 16-16. The four successful clinical results of apexification procedures. **A,** Continued closure of canal and apex to a normal configuration. **B,** Apex closes, but canal remains with a "blunderbuss" configuration. **C,** No radiographic change, but a thin osteoid-like barrier provides a definite stop at or near the apex. **D,** Radiographic evidence of a barrier short of apex.

Another technique for paste placement has been described by Teplitsky and others, using the compactor, as originally used by McSpadden for canal filling (Chapter 9). Although rarely used in the gutta-percha condensation technique any longer, it reputedly delivers a very thick mix of the calcium hydroxide pastes. One of the problems with the instrument has been a tendency to fracture when attempting to fill narrow, curved canals. This is not a problem in the extra-wide canals treated with apexification procedures.

Cotton is placed in the chamber, followed by a thick mix ZOE and a suitable temporary cover or cement. It is most important that the access be sealed during the observation period that follows to avoid dislodgement of the dressing or contamination of the canal, which probably would result in failure.

At 6 months the patient is recalled for radio-graphic examination (Fig. 16-14, *D*). One of the following five apical conditions will be found (Fig. 16-16):

1. No radiographic change is apparent; but if an instrument is inserted, a blockage at the apex will be encountered.
2. Radiographic evidence of a calcified material is seen at or near the apex. In some cases the degree of calcification might be extremely extensive (Fig. 16-17). In other cases it is minimal.
3. Apex closes without any change in the canal space.
4. Apex continues to develop with closure of the canal space.
5. No radiographic evidence of change is seen, and clinical symptoms and/or development of a periapical lesion occur.

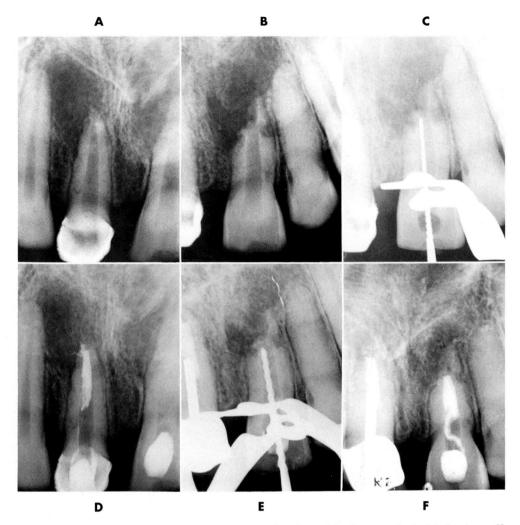

Fig. 16-17. **A,** Preoperative film of maxillary central incisor with a larger periapical lesion but sufficient apical closure to complete therapy in a routine manner. **B,** Preoperative film of maxillary central to the right of tooth shown in **A,** with a larger periapical lesion that has caused considerable apical resorption and possible root fracture. The adjacent lateral incisor has no apparent canal but no periapical lesion. There was a history of trauma to the face and jaws. **C,** Radiograph of file in place to calculate working length, with no stop present for incisor to the right on film. Canal was debrided and calcium hydroxide placed. **D,** Meanwhile, the central incisor to the left on the film was debrided and filled with laterally condensed gutta-percha and Wach's paste. **E,** Nine months later, a solid stop is present with a size 90 reamer placed to working length. **F,** Canal filled with laterally condensed gutta-percha and Wach's paste. **G,** One year later, radiolucency healing on central incisor to the left. Compare to **A.** **H,** Two years after original treatment, radiolucencies have healed and teeth are tight and well restored. There has been no change at the apex of the lateral incisor. (Restorations by Dr. Robert Kimbrough, Chicago.)

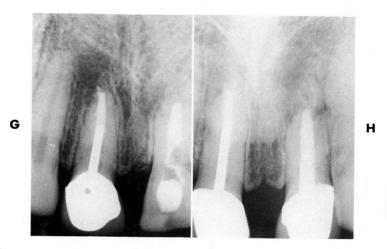

Fig. 16-17, cont'd. For legend see opposite page.

If any of the first four conditions occur, routine endodontic treatment may be carried out, with the canal filled to the newly formed apex or calcific stop (Fig. 16-14, *E*). If the fifth condition develops, apexification should be reattempted.

Canal filling after completion of apexification. With the solid stop to pack against, there is rarely any problem in filling the canal after apexification is completed. Gutta-percha is obviously the filling material of choice because it can be packed into the irregularities that are present in these large canals (Fig. 16-14, *F*). When the master cone is developed with the customized technique (Chapter 9), the solid dentin matrix is readily visualized by examining the apical portion of the imprint. In some cases the canal will remain wide, and it may be necessary to invert the master cone so the normally apical portion is to the incisal edge and the widest area is customized.

After radiographic verification, the sealer is introduced, the master cone inserted, and condensation procedures performed, as described in Chapter 9. Even with very heavy condensation there will be little, if any, excess materials extruded if the matrix has been verified. The restoration of choice then is placed at the filling appointment or soon thereafter (Figs. 16-18 and 16-19).

Mechanisms of apexification. There have been many articles written about apexification, with various descriptions of the induced apical depositions, including cementum, bone, osteocementum, osteodentin, cementoid, among others. After exper-imentally induced apexification, both gross and microscopic evaluations of this phenomenon indicates that the new apical formation is not solid but maintains a Swiss cheese configuration.

It has been stated by some that Hertwig's epithelial root sheath is not completely destroyed when the pulp becomes nonvital in the forming tooth. Thus the apexification procedures stimulate further function of the sheath to continue apical development. Others maintain that the osteogenic potential of calcium hydroxide, possibly because of the high pH of the material, creates a calcific mass adjacent to it, resulting in the closure, without relationship to the previously present root sheath. However, techniques besides those using the high-pH materials have yielded excellent closure, too.

Under any circumstances a mineralized barrier is formed that gives a clinically acceptable means for packing the root canal that had been previously unattainable. The root development after apexification procedures generally results in a somewhat different shape than the configuration of the root after normal development. The root may be shorter, the canal wider with thin lateral walls, or even inversely tapered (Fig. 16-20). *If there is thus any chance that the pulp has vitality in a tooth with incomplete apical development, it is preferable to attempt a pulpotomy.* If after a suitable observation period the desired result fails to occur, the apexification procedures can be utilized.

It is interesting to note that radiographs of some patients are seen with root configurations typical

Text continued on p. 736.

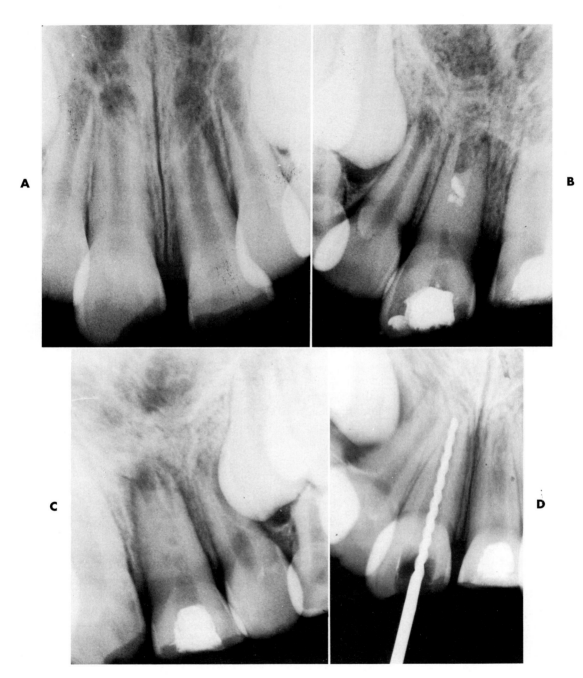

Fig. 16-18.   Typical apexification cases on anterior teeth. **A,** Preoperative radiograph, nonvital pulps of central incisor on left (no. 8) and central on right (no. 9) due to trauma. Apices in both teeth are incomplete, and periapical radiolucencies are present. **B,** Apexification paste placed in no. 8. I would have preferred material to be closer to radiographic apex. **C,** Paste placed in no. 9. **D,** One year later, working length calculation for no. 8. A solid stop existed at this length. Note how much calcification resulted, with apical curvature to the distal.

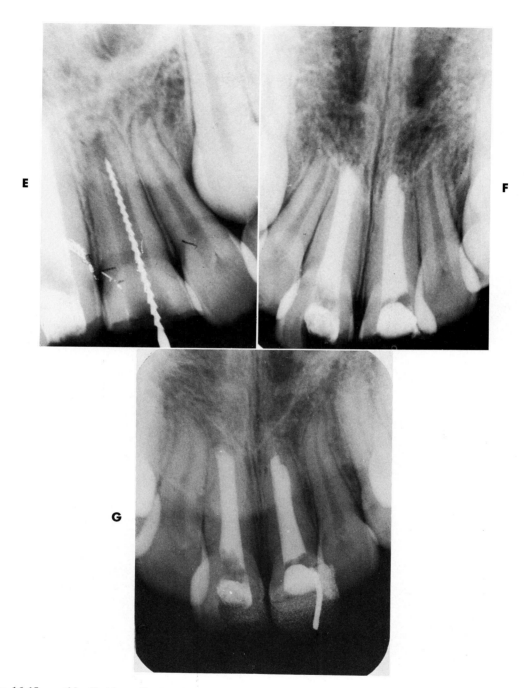

Fig. 16-18, cont'd. E, Also at 1 year after apexification was initiated, working length calculation for no. 9 at a point where the patient felt sensitivity. An anesthetic was administered and some degenerating tissue removed at 2 mm longer than indicated length, where a solid stop was felt. **F,** Canals were filled with gutta-percha and lateral condensation. Note the absence of periapical lesions. **G,** Three years after filling and restoration, roots have continued to develop and periapical area are normal.

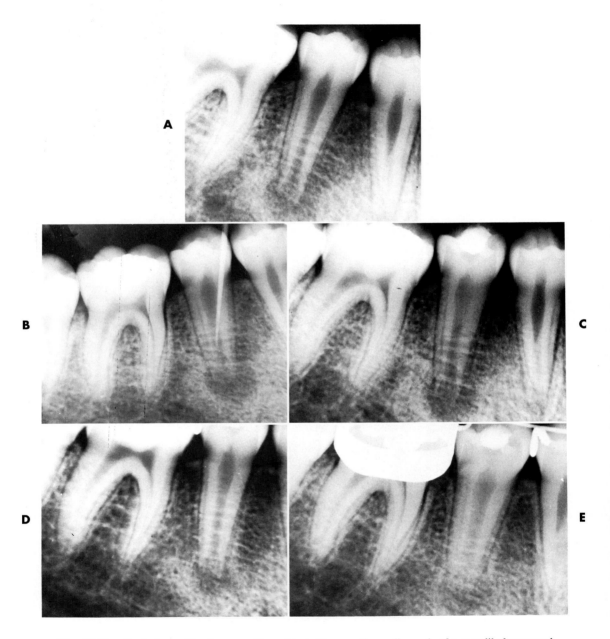

Fig. 16-19.   Typical apexification on a bicuspid. **A,** Preoperative radiograph of a mandibular second bicuspid with incomplete apex and periapical radiolucency. Deep fissural groove was carious, and pulp became involved within a year of eruption. **B,** Chronic draining sinus tract traced with gutta-percha cone. **C,** Apexification paste placed. No radiopaque agent had been used. **D,** Six months later, apex starting to develop and radiolucency diminishing. **E,** One year after initial treatment, apex has continued to develop. **F,** Canal was filled with gutta-percha and lateral condensation. **G,** Six years after initial treatment. **H,** Eleven years after initial treatment. **I,** Nineteen years after initial treatment. Compare apex to **A** and **F.** (Restoration by Dr. Alvin Altman, Highland Park, Ill.)

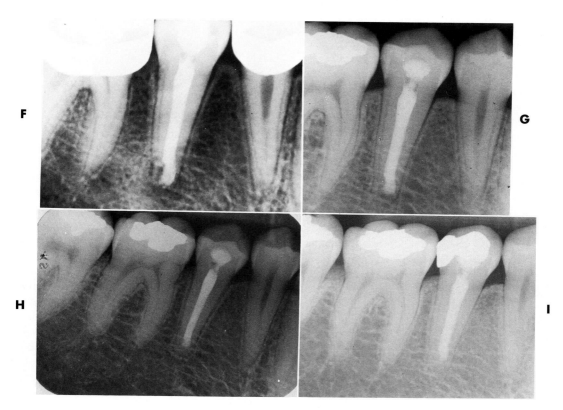

F   G

H   I

Fig. 16-19. cont'd.   For legend see opposite page.

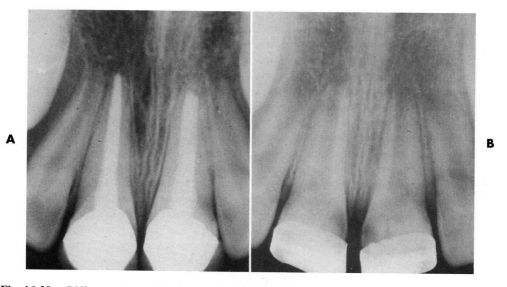

A   B

Fig. 16-20.   Difference in root development between pulpotomy and apexification treatment. **A,** Preoperative radiograph after trauma 5 months earlier. Central incisor to left (no. 8) had a nonvital pulp, so apexification procedures were employed. Pulp in central to right (no. 9) remained vital, and a pulpotomy was performed. **B,** Eighteen months later, treatment has been completed in both teeth by guttapercha fillings with lateral condensation. Root development in no. 9 appears normal from standpoint of width, shape, taper, and apical configuration. In no. 8, canal is much wider by comparison and seems to come to a dead stop a few millimeters short of radiographic apex. (Restorations by Dr. Alvin Altman, Highland Park, Ill.)

of those produced by apexification. However, the patient may state that he had never been to the dentist, or it can be seen that the tooth had never received treatment (Fig. 16-21).

Ham et al. reported that the finding of a negative culture gave a much better prognosis for continued apical development. However, some cases of apexification have been seen in which the canal was obviously contaminated. Still, it seems much more logical to consider that healing would transpire more readily in the absence of contamination by microorganisms. Therefore, if an intratreatment seal is lost, the apexification paste or the canal filling, as the case may be, should not be attempted; rather, the canal again is debrided, irrigated, and reclosed so the intended treatment can be accomplished at the next appointment.

Long-term results of apexification. I have followed a number of my apexification cases for 10 or more years (Figs. 16-14, *H,* and 16-19, *I*) and found them to be extremely successful. Some authors have reported that a seemingly successful apexification broke down a few years later and

required re-treatment or surgery. The cases that break down seem to be those with the apical portion of the canal still quite wide even though an apical stop is present (Fig. 16-16, *B* and *C*). These canals are difficult to cleanse thoroughly and then obliterate, which leaves open spaces that later may harbor bacteria and tissue breakdown products. Since the apical calcification barrier itself may be porous, the potential for failure is present.

Because of the simplicity of gaining excellent results, apexification success has been taken for granted. This may be the cause for some of the failures. Considerable care must be taken during the initial and final canal preparation procedures, even acknowledging that these canals may be virtually impossible to cleanse perfectly. Wiping the walls with cotton-wrapped broaches, alternating hydrogen peroxide and sodium hypochlorite irrigants, and utilizing ultrasonic preparation are encouraged for optimal canal cleaning. Canal filling should be performed so a deep penetration of the spreaders with numerous wide auxiliary cones is effected.

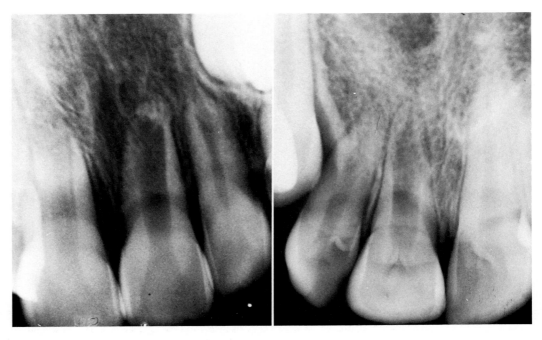

Fig. 16-21. Both central incisors had history of trauma and root development similar to those seen after apexification procedures. However, neither patient had ever been to the dentist prior to this radiographic survey appointment. Note that no restorations are present.

If the case requires re-treatment later, the old canal filling may be removed with a suitable solvent. Canal preparation must be performed even more diligently, and then the best possible filling placed in the canal.

Apexification in molars. There is no contraindication to apexification procedures according to a patient's age or tooth designation. In most cases the teeth treated are those affected by trauma, which generally involves anterior teeth. However, Fig. 16-19 describes therapy on a mandibular bicuspid where caries caused pulpal necrosis shortly after eruption. Fig. 16-22 involves a maxillary molar where previous caries followed by failed vital pulp therapy left the palatal root undeveloped. It was determined that the buccal canals could be treated routinely, but apexification procedures were instituted for the palatal canal. Accordingly, the buccals were prepared and filled with gutta-percha, whereas calcium hydroxide paste was placed into the palatal canals (Fig. 16-19, *B* and *C*). As time went on, the palatal canal was eventually filled with gutta-percha, too (Fig. 16-19, *E* and *F*).

Such partial treatment is very acceptable in a multirooted tooth. It would have been foolish to use calcium hydroxide pastes in the buccal canals to hold them until the entire case could be filled with gutta-percha. By the same token, it would not have been possible to fill all the canals successfully with gutta-percha shortly after the case was started (Fig. 16-19, *B*).

Treatment of perforating internal resorption. An interesting application of apexification procedures was reported by Frank and Weine in nonsurgical treatment of perforating defects due to internal resorption. Usually this type of problem requires some type of surgical intervention, such as sealing of the defect with amalgam after flap retraction and location of the point of perforation. Because of the absence of predictability in locating these resorptive defects, surgical treatment in these cases is often complicated and not necessarily successful.

However, cases were reported in which the canal was debrided, the calcium hydroxide–CMCP paste placed, and the tooth observed for healing. At subsequent appointments the canal is reprepared and filled with heavy lateral and vertical condensation of gutta-percha. Excellent healing was demonstrated without any surgical treatment needed (Figs. 16-23 and 16-24).

Treatment of aggressive external resorption. External resorption is one of the most difficult dental conditions to treat properly. Frank recently wrote an excellent paper attempting to put sense into treatment of this most perplexing problem.

Attempting to perform endodontic therapy (treatment within the tooth) for every condition of external resorption (problem on the periphery of the tooth) is futile. The soft tissue problem for external resorption is periodontal, as opposed to pulpal problems addressed by endodontic therapy.

Frank described specifically that in two types of cases, endodontic therapy must be used to treat external resorption—when perforation of the pulp canal space occurs because of the advancement of the resorptive defect from the outside and when the only access to the resorptive defect is through the pulp canal space.

Another condition that requires alternative treatment with calcium hydroxide therapy, followed by routine endodontic treatment ultimately, is that involving aggressive external resorption that threatens to put the affected tooth in severe jeopardy. Such a case typically displays a tooth with a normal root shape (Fig. 16-25, *A*) that begins to indicate a site of external resorption (Fig. 16-25, *B*). As the resorption continues to enlarge in proximity to the pulp, it becomes obvious that allowing this defect to continue untreated could cause irreparable damage to the tooth (Fig. 16-25, *C*). This condition is best treated by pulp extirpation (Fig. 16-25, *D*) and an interim canal filling with calcium hydroxide, preferably with the syringe (Figs. 16-14, *B,* and 16-25, *E*). An observation period of 6 to 12 months should demonstrate clearly that the resorption has been arrested (Fig. 16-25, *F* and *G*). Then the canal may be filled by routine methods (Fig. 16-25, *H*). Hopefully, follow-up observations will indicate a retention of this favorable condition (Fig. 16-25, *I* and *J*).

The initial waiting period with the canal not yet filled with gutta-percha should be observed in case the resorption continues. If so, further preparation and replacement of the calcium hydroxide is mandatory in the hope that the resorption can be made to cease.

The cause of such cases is unknown, but may be related to trauma or problems of occlusion. The latter may have been responsible for the problem shown in Fig. 16-25.

Text continued on p. 745.

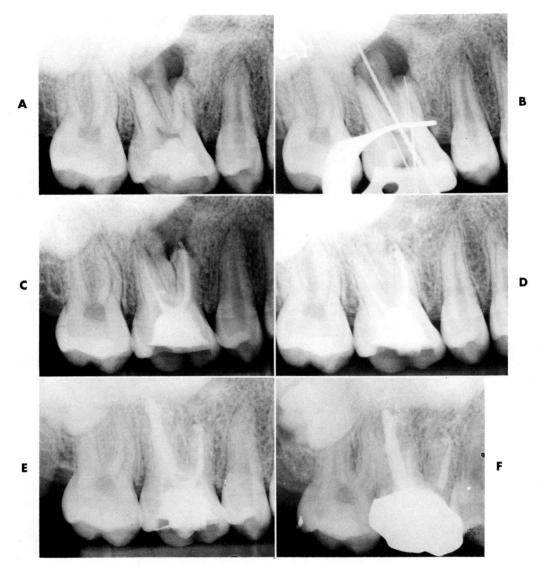

Fig. 16-22. **A,** Preoperative radiograph of maxillary first molar of 13-year-old female. A large peri-apical lesion was associated with the palatal root and smaller lesions around the buccal roots. Some type of vital pulp therapy had been performed several years earlier. **B,** The apices were well formed in the buccal canals, but a size 80 file passed through the palatal canal without binding. Therefore it was decided to debride and fill the buccal canal routinely and use apexification procedures for the palatal canal. **C,** Two canals that merged were debrided in the mesiobuccal root and one in the distobuccal root, all filled with laterally condensed gutta-percha and Wach's paste. The palatal canal was debrided and calcium hydroxide paste placed. **D,** One year later, the radiolucency appeared to be gone, and the palatal canal was reprepared. **E,** The palatal canal was filled with laterally condensed gutta-percha using a customized cone (Chapter 9) and Wach's paste. **F,** Three years after original treatment. (Restoration by Dr. Sherwin Strauss, Chicago.)

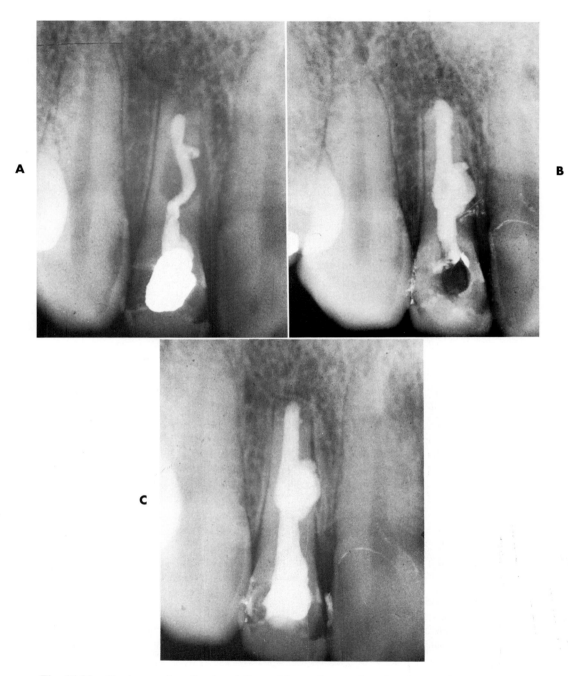

Fig. 16-23. Treatment of perforating defects of internal resorption. **A,** Large perforating resorptive defect on mesial aspect of lateral incisor with failing endodontic treatment. **B,** After calcium hydroxide placement, gutta-percha was packed with heavy lateral condensation. **C,** One year after treatment, excellent healing. (From Frank AL, Weine FS: *J Am Dent Assoc* 87:863, 1973.)   *Continued*

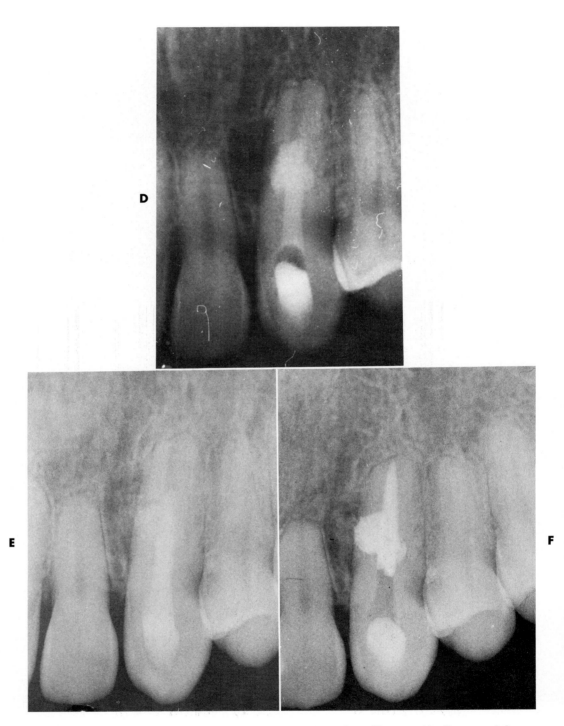

Fig. 16-23, cont'd.   **D,** Large radiolucency on mesial surface of maxillary cuspid adjacent to defect. Chronic draining sinus tract was present, too. Canal has been packed with calcium hydroxide. In apical portion, pulp had remained vital. **E,** Six months later, sinus tract is closed and lateral radiolucency appears to be closing down. **F,** Canal packed with gutta-percha and heavy lateral condensation.

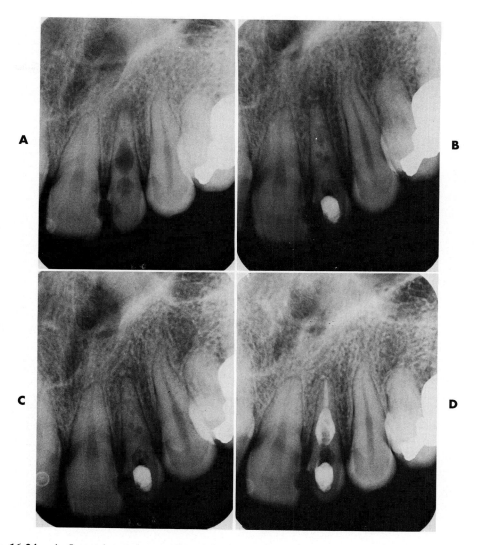

Fig. 16-24. **A,** Large internal resorption defect with perforation to buccal surface. During canal preparation, heavy bleeding occurred periodically. Tooth seemed almost hopeless. **B,** Two weeks later, canals had been cleansed as well as possible, and calcium hydroxide mix was placed with a syringe. Note periapical lesion. **C,** Two months later, periapical lesion had decreased considerably. **D,** Canal was reprepared and filled with laterally condensed gutta-percha and Wach's paste as sealer. Post room was prepared. (Original therapy by me, second canal preparation by Dr. Charles Neach, Chicago, and restoration by Dr. Sherwin Strauss, Chicago.)

Continued

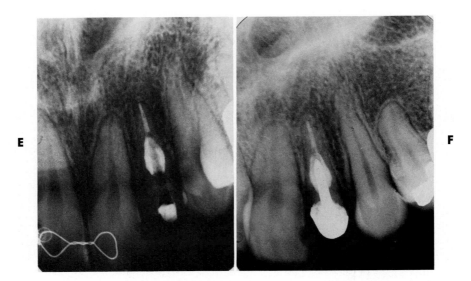

Fig. 16-24, cont'd. E, Nine months after canal filling, area has retained desirable appearance and tooth is quite comfortable. **F,** Post and core placed and followed by an acrylic jacket crown, which will be replaced when this youngster is older. Film taken 3 years after initial treatment.

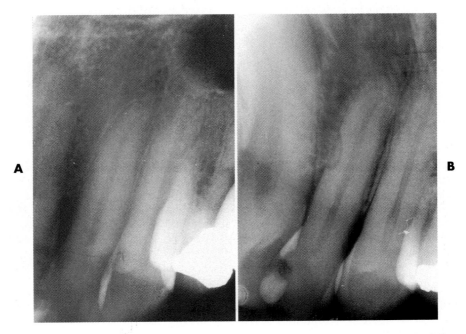

Fig. 16-25. Treatment of aggressive external resorption. **A,** Radiograph taken as part of a full-mouth series in 1982, indicating a lateral incisor with a normal root shape, a mesial composite filling, slightly overlapping the adjacent central incisor and cuspid. **B,** Four years later, again from a routine full-mouth series, an area of resorption is now clearly seen on the mesial surface in midroot. After 1 year of observation, the lesion was again seen to enlarge, and the case was referred to me.

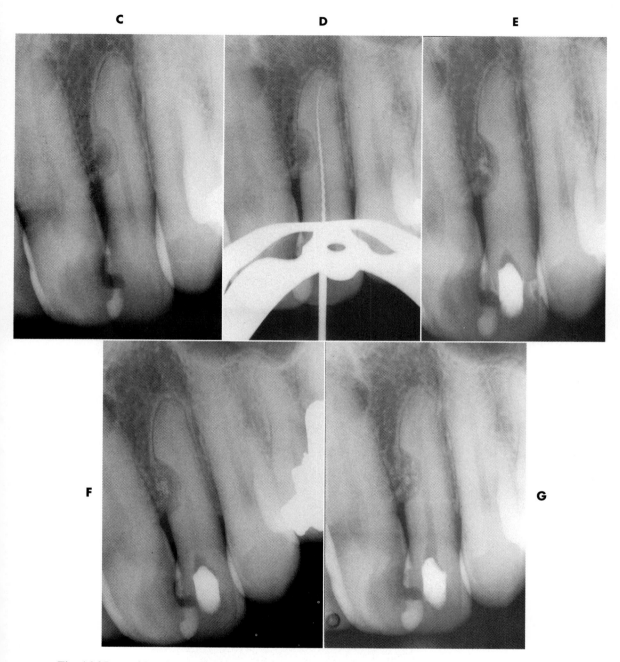

Fig. 16-25, cont'd.   C, My preoperative film, taken in 1988, indicating that the resorptive defect has continued and now is almost to the pulp canal space. **D,** The tooth was entered and pulp extirpated. The pulp was vital but definitely not normal—very shreddy and bleeding. The working length was calculated at 24 mm. **E,** At the second appointment, the canal was enlarged to size 40 and a calcium hydroxide/methyl cellulose paste was placed. The access was closed with a sterile cotton pellet and ZOE. **F** and **G,** Six months and 1 year after placement of the paste, indicating arresting of the active resorption.

Continued

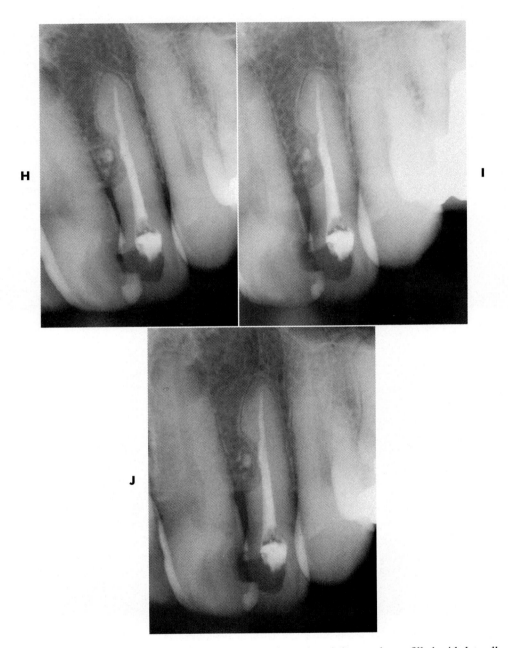

Fig. 16-25, cont'd.   H, Minimal preparation was performed, and the canal was filled with laterally condensed gutta-percha and Wach's paste. It appears that some sealer has escaped into the defect and, perhaps, some gutta-percha has been packed into the resorbed area. **I,** One year after completion of canal filling. **J,** Thirty months after completion of filling, 5 years after **C,** indicating no increase in active resorption and, perhaps, some remodeling of the defect wall. The tooth is firm, comfortable, and symptomless. (Restoration by Dr. John Lilleberg, Park Ridge, Ill.)

THEORY OF REPEATED TRAUMAS

In regard to accidents to the face and teeth, youngsters seem to fall and injure themselves in one of four places. These are (from superior to inferior), the forehead, the nose, the teeth, or the chin. Those who fall and injure their foreheads will continually injure their foreheads; those who fall and injure their teeth will continually injure their teeth, and so forth.

This is a significant situation to consider from two important standpoints when treating a traumatic injury to the teeth. The first is that when treating dental trauma, the dentist must always consider that the accident being evaluated and treated might not be the first incident to the affected area and that the damage noticed might be due to a previous event or even several previous events. Fig. 11-59 illustrates a case of trauma caused by a blow to the teeth from a ski-lift. Both the referring dentist and I were shocked to notice that the damaged tooth with a midroot fracture displayed a radiographic absence of a pulp canal space even though the accident had occurred only a few days earlier. Questioning the patient elicited the information that he had suffered a similar ski-lift accident to the same tooth 25 years earlier!

Fig. 16-11 describes a situation where the patient suffered an injury to the teeth initially at approximately 7 years old, and again received a serious blow to the dentition at approximately 12 to 14 years old.

The second consideration is to realize that whatever treatment is rendered, including stabilization, temporization, and/or restoration, it must address the possible need to withstand further traumatic events. Therefore, the insertion of any fillings over temporary paste placements must be sufficiently strong and well-packed to withstand another accident. If another blow to the teeth should occur, the patient must be seen in the dental office to ascertain any possible damage or dislodgement of the previously placed materials.

Youngsters, particularly males involved in contact sports, should wear protective devices for their teeth when participating in any athletic endeavor, even one that is not particularly prone to causing an accident. Somehow, these patients who are often involved in accidents seem to attract traumatic incidents even when contact is minimal.

Anyone who watches professional baseball and college and professional basketball and football will notice how common it is to see the athletes wearing various types of mouth guards and protectors. With this in mind, it would not be too difficult for the dentist to suggest to these accident-prone young men how they can mimic their favorite players by wearing similar devices.

The patient demonstrated in Fig. 16-26 was injured initially approximately at age 7, when one central incisor received a midroot fracture. A radiograph several years later indicated severe closure of the pulp canal space of the adjacent central incisor, caused by the same, or possibly a subsequent, trauma. Several years later another accident caused breakdown of the healed fractured tooth, which had been treated successfully with surgery. Even though his parents did provide a protective device for the young man (now in college) to wear during athletic events, he did not insert the protector when playing in a pick-up basketball game. The result was a blow to the teeth that avulsed and pulverized the shortened tooth (Fig. 16-26, *H*).

PASTES AS CANAL FILLING MATERIALS

Pastes have been used as canal filling materials for well over 100 years. Walkoff pastes were used for many years in Europe, and pastes with arsenic were used in America and Europe until shortly after World War II. Pastes are still used with great frequency in eastern Europe as canal filling materials and often cause problems in re-treatment because of not having a known solvent. Much of the poor reputation of endodontic treatment early in the twentieth century was due to the high failure rates of the pastes.

Improvements in the use of pastes for filling canals have occurred during the last few years. Maisto, Krakow, and Sargenti have all written considerably on methods and criteria for the use of pastes. The pastes are generally similar in physical and chemical properties to root canal sealers, which were discussed in Chapter 9. Pastes may be introduced into the canal by using a Lentulo spiral by hand or engine, by syringe or similar forcing device, or, if thickly mixed, by packing with a condenser.

Disadvantages. Despite the statements of adherents of this method, it is difficult to visualize how a creamy pasty material can possibly obliterate a canal with the same degree of efficiency as a solid-core material plus a sealer. Since the sealing of the apical portion of the canal is most important, it would appear that the use of a solid core,

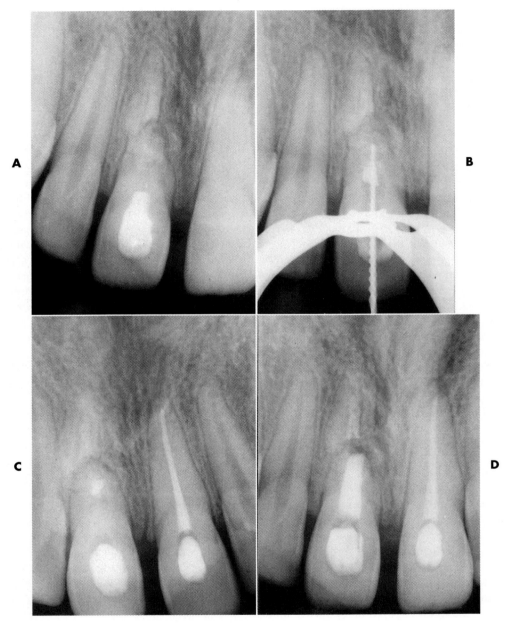

Fig. 16-26. Example of multiple injuries to the teeth. **A,** A young man, 15 years old, was referred to me by Dr. M. Levin, of Washington, D.C., for completion of treatment for the central incisor to the left (tooth no. 8). A midroot fracture had occurred following trauma to the face and teeth, with pain and displacement and mobility of the coronal segment, treated with calcium hydroxide for approximately 1 year. This radiograph was my preoperative film, indicating reestablishment of a regular periodontal ligament space for no. 8, which is tight and comfortable. The apical segment of no. 8 is some distance palatally. However, note that the adjacent central incisor (tooth no. 9) displays only a small canal in the apical few millimeters radiographically. **B,** I opened the access for no. 8 and a size 50 file came to a dead stop at the length indicated (16 mm). However, the inside of the canal had much debris present, so I decided to reprepare the canal and place calcium hydroxide/methyl cellulose paste. A small periapical lesion seemed to be present. **C,** After preparing access for no. 9, I did locate the canal, which I enlarged and then filled with laterally condensed customized gutta-percha and Wach's paste at a second visit. Note the small lesion at the apex of no. 8. **D,** I completed the canal filling for no. 8 with laterally condensed customized gutta-percha and Wach's paste.

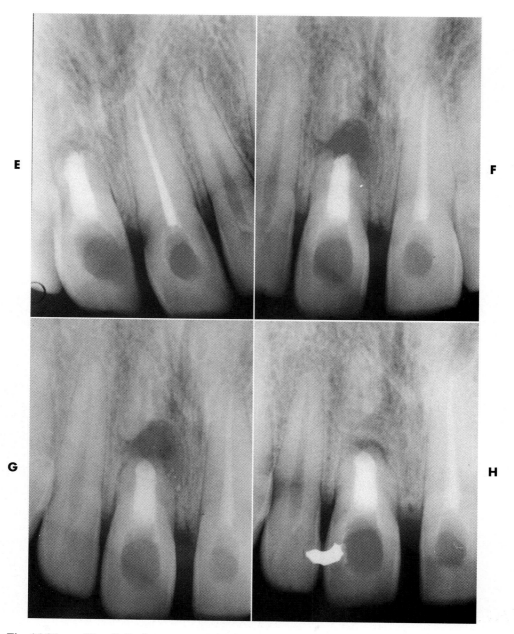

Fig. 16-26, cont'd.   **E,** Radiograph taken 6 months later, indicating healing of the periapical lesion of no. 8. **F,** By now the patient had entered college and had been involved in another accident to his teeth. Tooth no. 8 is now mobile, tender to percussion, and a large lesion is present at the apex. **G,** I flapped the tooth, curetted the inflammatory tissue at the apex, and placed Super EBA (see Chapter 11) at the apex. **H,** One year later, 4 years after I started treatment, the periapical lesion is almost completely healed, the tooth is comfortable again, and no. 9 is normal. Because of the shortness of the coronal segment of no. 8, his dentist placed a metal device with bonding to give it additional support. Although he had a plastic protector made for his teeth to wear during athletic activities, 1 year later he became involved in a pick-up basketball game where he was elbowed in the mouth. The tooth was knocked out and someone stepped on it, breaking it into many pieces! He now wears a flipper, waiting to have a fixed bridge in the future. Tooth no. 9 seems fine, but one can only speculate on how long before it, too, will be reinjured.

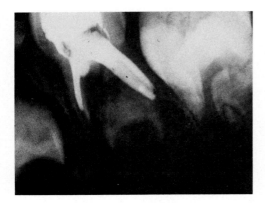

Fig. 16-27. Canals of this primary molar are filled with a paste containing zinc oxide, eugenol, and formocresol.

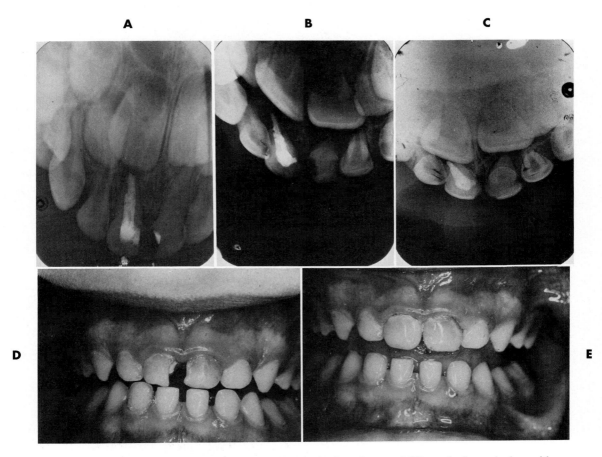

Fig. 16-28. **A,** Radiograph taken with periapical projection after canal filling of primary incisor with ZOE-formocresol paste in a patient 3½ years old. Child was a model, and his parents were very conscious of his appearance. He injured his teeth in a tricycle accident and developed a periapical abscess. The parents did not want him to lose the teeth prematurely and insisted on endodontic therapy. **B,** One year later (occlusal projection). **C,** Twenty-one months after original treatment (occlusal projection). Note relatively normal eruption of permanent tooth. **D,** Original appearance. **E,** Restorations with Ion crowns.

such as gutta-percha or silver points, as a plunger set to the required depth is more dependable than spinning or packing in a paste.

Most of the pastes used are radiopaque, and radiographs give the impressions that the paste has filled the canal. Since radiographs are only two dimensional, however, they are unable to distinguish between having paste on the canal walls and actual obliteration of the space.

Indications. Despite these apparent deficiencies, there are definite indications for the use of pastes. Pastes are usually absorbable and may be used when complete endodontic therapy is performed on primary teeth in cases where pulpotomy by formocresol or similar methods is contraindicated. The canal filling will be absorbed along with the roots and will leave no bulk material at exfoliation (Figs. 16-27 and 16-28). Pastes have been suggested when replantation is performed and the canal is to be filled before reinsertion. This is not the method advised at this time (Chapter 5).

Technique. A suitable paste for the suggested indications may be developed by mixing zinc oxide and eugenol with one additional drop of formocresol to the mass. Sufficient zinc oxide powder is added so the paste is thick enough to be packed with a root canal condenser. Small portions are introduced on the condenser tip or with a wide-mouthed amalgam carrier into the canal to be filled and then packed toward the apex. Since this paste is radiopaque, an x-ray film should be taken to determine whether the desired depth has been obtained. The paste should be packed as close to the radiographic apex as possible and should have uniform thickness throughout the canal, with the material terminating slightly above the floor of the chamber. Some packing should be done on the chamber floor, since auxiliary canals are frequently present in the furcation area of primary teeth. A suitable temporary seal is then placed until a final restoration is fabricated. Usually stainless steel crown forms are most desirable for treated primary molars.

The N2-Sargenti technique

The term *N2* was coined by Sargenti to describe the *second nerve,* that placed during treatment. The red color of the filling material he also used to coincide with the color of the pulp. N2 is presently used to mean both the technique and the canal filling material, although other formulation names are also available.

The Sargenti technique, relying heavily on a formaldehyde-containing paste, was originally introduced to American dentists in the early 1960s but met little acceptance due to the unpredictable and unscientific method with which it was used. Further development and refinement followed, as well as some basic science investigations, and a revised N2 was reintroduced to American dentists 10 years later. This time many adherents were gained. The American Endodontic Society (AES), composed of dentists who had taken courses in the technique, was

Table 16-1. Clinical treatment differences between Sargenti and traditional methods

Clinical situation	Sargenti method	Traditional method
Canal preparation	Uses engine-driven reamers or giromatic full length of preparation	Generally hand instruments exclusively; may use engine-driven instruments in coronal half of canal
Use of sodium hypochlorite or other intracanal irrigants	No	Heavy use to dissolve necrotic debris, lubricate walls, and foam debris
Radiographic verification of working length	No	Always used
Filling materials	Paste with paraformaldehyde to give off constantly nascent formaldehyde; often has lead salts	Solid core of gutta-percha plus sealers
Solvent for filling materials	No known solvent	Xylene or chloroform for gutta-percha and sealers
Frequency of changes in filling materials	Multiple changes since 1960	Same formulas used for many years
Surgical treatment	Fistulator used to complete "gangrenous teeth" in one sitting; other indications	Rarely, if ever, needed

formed to promote the philosophies of Sargenti among general dentists in the United States.

Sargenti method. Briefly, the technique employed canal preparation with engine-driven instruments, no intracanal irrigant, and canal filling with a formaldehyde paste (either with or without lead). There was no standard theoretic ideal for determination of length control, and one-sitting treatment was strongly endorsed. Artificial fistulation was recommended in certain cases but with-

Table 16-2. Basic science research with N2

Author (year)	Other materials tested	Site, animal	Results
Guttuso (1963)	AH-26, Riebler's resin, Diaket, Rickert's sealer, Tubliseal, Procosol, PBSC, Microside A	Rat connective tissue	N2, Riebler's resin, and Tubliseal provoked consistently severe responses.
Rappaport et al. (1964)	Rickert's sealers, AH-26, Mynol cement, Diaket, Kloropercha Procosol, ZOE	Rat subcutaneous tissue	Only N2 still had severe response at 35 days.
		Tissue culture (HeLa cells)	Only N2 and Diaket were still toxic at dilutions of 0.2%.
		Versus common canal contaminants	ZOE inhibited all microorganisms; N2, Diaket, and Mynol inhibited all but one microorganism.
		Rabbit eye (conjunctival sac)	N2 liquid, powder, and medicament and Procosol only were irritating at 24 hours.
Feldman et al. (1967)	Pure silver	Spheres in rabbit mandibles	Capsule thickness was greater around N2, indicating higher degree of irritation and greater number of exudative cells around N2.
Langeland et al. (1969)	None	Pulp and periapical tissue of human, monkey, and swine teeth	Pulp tissue in contact with N2 showed disintegration and multiple abscess formation; periapical tissue responses still severe at 652 days.
Spangberg (1974)	Riebler's resin (also a paraformaldehyde paste)	Paste implants in mandibles of guinea pig	Extensive bone necrosis present at 3 days, sequestration at 12 weeks; heavy infiltration of lymphocytes and plasma cells.
Brewer (1975)	Overfills with gutta-percha and Procosol	Overfills in monkey periapical tissue	Only N2 preparation caused ankylosis, root resorption, and bone necrosis in almost all specimens; both caused moderate to severe inflammation, but N2 still had severe reaction at 118 days, much milder with gutta-percha preparation.
Oswald and Cohn (1975)	—	Through cuspids of cats	Liver, kidneys, adrenal glands, and spleen showed high concentrations of labeled lead.
Brown et al. (1979)	Gutta-percha, laterally condensed	Radioisotopes	Numerous voids in RC2B fills; canals prepared with Giromatic and filled with RC2B had more leakage than did GP fills after hand preparation.
Newton et al. (1980)	Controls were infected, but untreated, teeth	Periapical tissue of monkeys	No difference between untreated necrotic controls and those treated with RC2B; all had severe periapical inflammation with areas of necrosis and some indications of osteomyelitis.

out raising a flap. Some of the basic differences between N2 and traditional endodontics are listed in Table 16-1 (see p. 749).

Opposition by American endodontists. The great preponderance of basic science articles on the N2 method indicated that the materials employed had many undesirable properties (Table 16-2). There never was a study in any prestigious American dental journal that encouraged its use. For this reason, endodontists of the United States were very vocal in their opposition to N2 as well as to all other lead or formaldehyde pastes. The AES attempted to circumvent some of these criticisms by removing lead from the formula in the RC2B paste.

The use of artificial fistulation, called apical fenestration by Sargenti, was another point of severe disagreement on the part of endodontists—particularly his use without any type of flap, thus robbing the operator of the needed visualization of the area. I always believed that the use of such treatment as encouraged by Sargenti was incorrect. In the more than 18,500 cases that I have treated in my private practice, many very complicated, with referral only after several unsuccessful attempts by the originating dentist, I used a fistulation procedure only twice. The other cases could be controlled by nonsurgical intervention, antibiotics, or

apical curettage with a flap to allow for full visualization.

This in itself does not make fistulation wrong, but the procedure is prone to misuse. I have seen several cases where the apical fenestration led to disastrous results (Fig. 16-29). For these reasons, I never recommended fistulation on anywhere near a routine basis, particularly without a flap, and much of the endodontic community has agreed with me.

Presently, N2 users present no serious problem to those who have chosen legitimate forms of endodontic treatment. Occasionally a tooth treated with N2 is seen when viewing full mouth radiographs of a patient new to a practice. Many of the teeth treated in the 1970s and 1980s by advocates of N2 required extraction or re-treatment because of incomplete debridement or incomplete seal (Fig. 16-30, *A*). This was not unexpected by endodontists who understood the inherent weakness of any paste filling, since there was little chance to seal the canal (Fig. 16-31).

A number of the N2 treatments where preparation was carried out close to the apex and the canal was filled reasonably well seem to be successful. But cases are still seen with damage caused by fistulation (Fig. 16-29) or strange looking overfills (Fig. 16-32). The claims of simplicity, ease, and reliability by the N2 method proved to be hollow

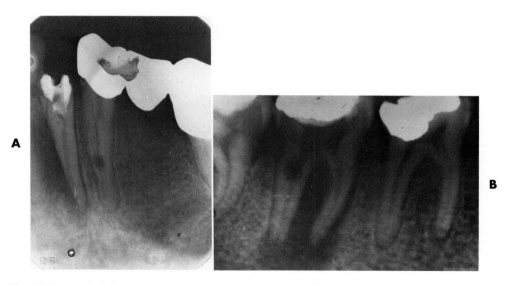

Fig. 16-29. Apical fenestrations that led to disaster. **A,** Mandibular cuspid treated by an advocate of the Sargenti method. Dentist was having considerable difficulty and attempted an apical fenestration; but without a flap to delineate clearly the area of suppuration, he drilled into adjacent first bicuspid. **B,** Sargenti advised fistulation of mandibular molars to be placed in bone in the furcation. However, misdirection of fistulator caused perforation into the distal root. (Courtesy Dr. Stephen F. Schwartz, Houston.)

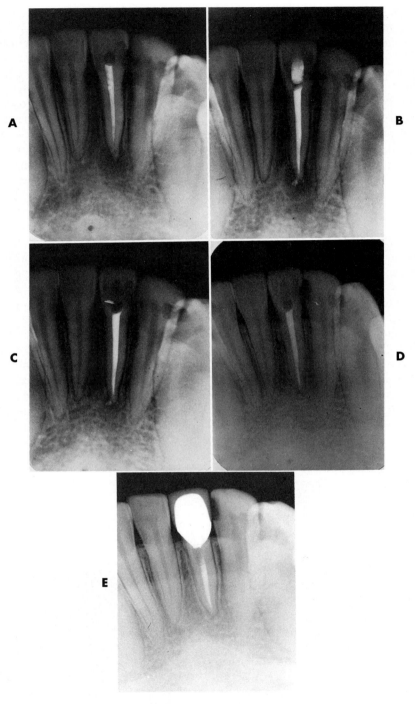

Fig. 16-30.   Re-treatment of an N2 case. **A,** Preoperative radiograph of mandibular incisor. Paste fill is several millimeters short of desirable length. Patient reported that fistulation was also performed at the canal filling appointment, 1 year earlier. A small, pimplelike sinus tract developed near mucogingival junction. **B,** Canal was reprepared and filled with laterally condensed gutta-percha. Sinus tract healed immediately after the preparation appointment. **C,** Two years later, area is much smaller, but a small apical radiolucency persists. **D,** Five years after original treatment, lesion is almost gone. Persisting radiolucency is probably a fibrous scar from the fistulation. **E,** Twelve years after original treatment. Compare to **A.**

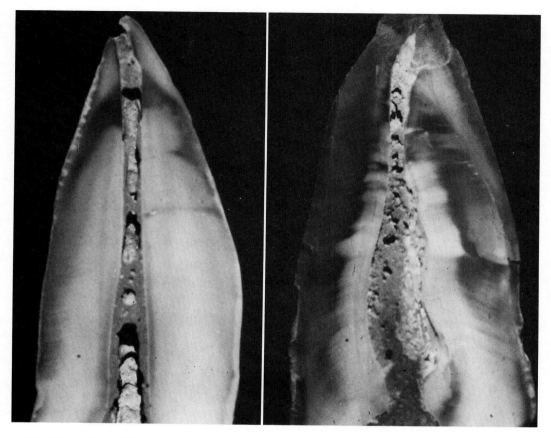

Fig. 16-31. Paste fills placed in canal after treatment suggested by Sargenti. Teeth cut in long section. Note that paste attaches to many portions of the walls, but there is no bulk to obliterate the canal space. (Courtesy Dr. B.D.K. Brown, Ft. Wayne, Ind.)

Fig. 16-32. Maxillary first molar was treated using the N2-Sargenti paste. The palatal canal was overprepared due to failure to confirm working length by radiograph with a file in place. With no apical stop present, the paste was forced into the periapical tissues and the adjacent maxillary sinus. The patient experienced severe and constant pain that eventually spread to the opposite sinus due to the irritating contents of the N2 paste. The patient sued the dentist for malpractice, and the jury found in favor of the plaintiff.

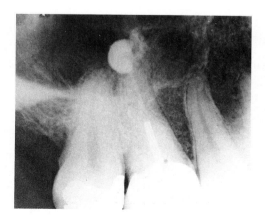

indeed and failed to stand the test of time.

Some initial endorsers of N2 have gone on to other techniques of dubious value. Others have been attracted by some of the newer thermoplastic techniques for canal filling, which were similar to the injection of the pastes.

Other former advocates were scared off the use of Sargenti materials and techniques by several large settlements levied against users of N2 in malpractice suits (Fig. 16-32). Because the procedure standards were vague, particularly in determining canal length, some serious overextensions of filling material resulted. Of course, this may happen in conventional treatment too, but due to the high inflammatory potential and toxicity of the N2 materials, when such overextensions caused fillings to be placed in and around the maxillary sinus or mandibular canal, the results were far more serious than when the more traditional filling materials were used.

Re-treatment of failing N2 cases. A key problem in attempting to re-treat N2 cases is that the paste has no known solvent. However, fortunately the very poor N2 cases, which are the most frequent to require re-treatment, are generally relatively easy to penetrate and bypass with careful use of endodontic files. With heavy irrigation and rasping to remove material on the outstroke, the chunks of set paste are carefully removed.

A correct working length is verified by radiograph and the canal reprepared. The filling is placed at a subsequent appointment (Fig. 16-30, *B*). Cases that have been fistulated may never heal perfectly radiographically; a small radiolucency often persists (Fig. 16-30, *C*), which is probably fibrous tissue and a normal remnant of the surgical entry.

REFERENCES

Vital pulp therapy

Anthony LP, Grossman LI: A brief history of root-canal therapy in the United States, *J Am Dent Assoc* 32:43, 1945.

Baume LJ: Diagnosis of diseases of the pulp, *Oral Surg* 29:102, 1970.

Baume LJ, Fiore-Donno G: The effects of corticosteroids on the dental pulp, *Adv Oral Biol* 4:151, 1970.

Baume LJ, Holz J, Risk LB: Radicular pulpotomy for category III pulps. Part II. Instrumentation and technique, *J Prosthet Dent* 25:525, 1971.

Berger JE: Pulp tissue reaction to formocresol and zinc oxide–eugenol, *J Dent Child* 32:13, 1965.

Compton DE, Mitchell DF: Pharmacologic treatment of painful pulpitis: a five year report, *J Dent Res* 49:183, 1970.

Doyle WA, McDonald RE, Mitchell DF: Formocresol versus

calcium hydroxide in pulpotomy, *J Dent Child* 29:86, 1962.

Hermann BW: Dentinobliteration der Wurzelkanalel nach Behandlung mit Kalzium, *Zahnaertzl Rundsch* 21:887, 1930.

Hume WR: The pharmacologic and toxicological properties of zinc oxide–eugenol, *J Am Dent Assoc* 113:789, 1986.

Hunter WC: Saving pulps, a queer process, *Dent Items Interest,* 1883, p. 352.

Kaplan NL, Zach L, Goldsmith ED: Effects of pulpal exposure in the primary dentition on the succedaneous teeth, *J Dent Child* 34:237, 1967.

Koecker L: *Principles of dental surgery,* London, 1826, T & G Underwood.

Law DB, Lewis TM: Formocresol pulpotomy in deciduous teeth, *J Am Dent Assoc* 69:601, 1964.

Lawson BF, Mitchell DF: Pharmacologic treatment of painful pulpitis: a preliminary controlled, double-blind study, *Oral Surg* 17:47, 1964.

Mitchell DF, Shankwalker GB: Osteogenic potential of calcium hydroxide and other materials in soft tissue and bone wounds, *J Dent Res* 37:1157, 1958.

Mullaney TP, Lawson BF, Mitchell DF: Pharmacologic treatment of pulpitis: a continuing investigation, *Oral Surg* 21:479, 1966.

Ostrom CA, Lyon HW: Pulpal response to chemically treated heterogenous bone in pulp capping sites, *Oral Surg* 15:362, 1962.

Patterson SS, Van Huysen G: The treatment of pulp exposures, *Oral Surg* 7:194, 1954.

Pisanti S, Sciaky I: Origin of calcium in the repair wall after pulp exposure in the dog, *J Dent Res* 43:641, 1964.

Quigley MB: A critical history of the treatment of pulpal exposures, *J Dent Child* 23:209, 1956.

Quigley MB: Effect of blood clotting on hamster pulp exposures, *Oral Surg* 10:313, 1957.

Spedding RH, Mitchell DF, McDonald RE: Formocresol and calcium hydroxide therapy, *J Dent Res* 44:1023, 1965.

Stark MM, Myers HM, Morris M, Gardner R: The localization of radioactive Ca-45 over exposed pulps in the rhesus monkey: a preliminary report, *J Oral Ther* 1:290, 1964.

Tagger M, Tagger E: Pulp capping in monkeys with Reolit and Life, two calcium hydroxide bases with different pH, *J Endod* 11:394, 1985.

Teuscher GW, Zander HA: A preliminary report on pulpotomy, *Northwest Univ Bull* 39:4, 1938.

Via WF: Evaluation of deciduous molars treated by pulpotomy and calcium hydroxide, *J Am Dent Assoc* 50:34, 1955.

Zander HA: Reaction of the pulp to calcium hydroxide, *J Dent Res* 18:373, 1939.

Apexification

Binnie WH, Rowe AHR: A histological study of the periapical tissues of incompletely formed pulpless teeth filled with calcium hydroxide, *J Dent Res* 52:1110, 1973.

Bouchon F: Apex formation following treatment of necrotizing immature permanent incisor, *J Dent Child* 33:378, 1966.

Bystrom A, Claesson R, Sundqvist G: The antibacterial effect of camphorated paramonochlorophenol, camphorated phenol and calcium hydroxide in the treatment of infected root canals, *Endod Dent Traumatol* 1:170, 1985.

Cooke C, Rowbotham TC: Root canal therapy in non-vital teeth with open apices, *Br Dent J* 108:147, 1960.

Dumsha TC, Gutmann JL: Clinical techniques for the placement of calcium hydroxide, *Compend Contin Educ Dent* 6:482, 1985.

Dylewski JJ: Apical closure of non-vital teeth, *Oral Surg* 32:82, 1971.

Frank AL: Therapy for the divergent pulpless tooth by continued apical formation, *J Am Dent Assoc* 72:87, 1966.

Frank AL, Weine FS: Nonsurgical therapy for the perforative defect of internal resorption, *J Am Dent Assoc* 87:863, 1973.

Frank AL: Extracanal invasive resorption: an update, *Compend Contin Educ Dent* 16:250, 1995.

Gutmann JL, Fava LRG: Periradicular healing and apical closure of a non-vital tooth in the presence of bacterial contamination, *Int Endod J* 25:307, 1992.

Ham J, Patterson SS, Mitchell DF: Induced apical closure of immature pulpless teeth in monkeys, *Oral Surg* 33:438, 1972.

Harrison JW, Rakusin H: Intracanal cementosis following induced apical closure, *Endod Dent Traumatol* 1:242, 1985.

Heithersay GS: Stimulation of root formation in incompletely developed pulpless teeth, *Oral Surg* 29:620, 1970.

Heithersay GS: Calcium hydroxide in the treatment of pulpless teeth with associated pathology, *J Br Endod Soc* 8:74, 1975.

Koenigs JF, Heller AL, Brilliant JD, et al: Induced apical closure of permanent teeth in adult primates using a resorbable form of tricalcium phosphate ceramic, *J Endod* 1:102, 1975.

McCormick JE, Weine FS, Maggio JD: Tissue pH of developing lesions in dogs, *J Endod* 9:47, 1983.

Michanowicz JP, Michanowicz AE: A conservative approach and procedure to fill an incompletely formed root using calcium hydroxide as an adjunct, *J Dent Child* 32:42, 1967.

Ostby BN: The role of the blood clot in endodontic therapy, *Acta Odontol Scand* 19:323, 1961.

Rivera EM, Williams K: Placement of calcium hydroxide in simulated canals: comparison of glycerin versus water, *J Endod* 20:445, 1994.

Smith JW, Leeb IJ, Torney DL: A comparison of calcium hydroxide and barium hydroxide as agents for inducing apical closure, *J Endod* 10:64, 1984.

Steiner JC, Dow PR, Cathey GM: Inducing root end closure of non-vital permanent teeth, *J Dent Child* 35:47, 1968.

Steiner JC, Van Hassel HJ: Experimental root apexification in primates, *Oral Surg* 31:409, 1971.

Stuart KG, Miller CH, Brown CE, Newton CW: The comparative antimicrobial effect of calcium hydroxide, *Oral Surg Oral Med Oral Pathol* 72:101, 1991.

Teplitsky P: McSpadden compactor: vertical condensation technique to deliver calcium hydroxide, *J Can Dent Assoc* 52:779, 1986.

Torneck CD, Smith JS, Grindall P: Biological effects of endodontic procedures on developing incisor teeth, *Oral Surg* 35:541, 1973.

Van Hassel HJ, Natkin E: Induction of root end closure. *J Dent Child* 37:57, 1970.

Webber RT: Traumatic injuries and the expanded endodontic role of calcium hydroxide. In Gerstein, H, editor: *Techniques in clinical endodontics,* Philadelphia, 1983, Saunders.

Webber RT: Apexogenesis versus apexification, *Dent Clin North Am* 28:669, 1984.

Paste canal fillings

Block RM, Lewis RD, Sheats JB, Fawley J: Cell-mediated immune response to dog pulp tissue altered by N2 paste within the root canal, *Oral Surg* 45:131, 1978.

Brewer DL: Histology of apical tissue reaction to overfill, *J Calif Dent Assoc,* Feb 1975, p 58.

Brown BDK, Kafrawy AH, Patterson SS: Studies of Sargenti technique of endodontics—autoradiographic and scanning electron microscope studies. *J Endod* 5:14, 1979.

Cohler CM, Newton CW, Patterson SS, Kafrawy AH: Studies of Sargenti's technique of endodontic treatment: short-term response in monkeys, *J Endod* 6:473, 1980.

Feldman G, Nyborg H, Conrado CA: Tissue reactions to root filling materials. I. A comparison between implants of the root filling material N2 and silver in the jaws of rabbits, *Odontol Rev* 18:387, 1967.

Garcia-Godoy F: Evaluation of an iodoform paste in root canal therapy for infected primary teeth, *J Dent Child* 54:30, 1987.

Gregory WB, Brown BW, Goodman A: Paraformaldehyde-containing pastes in endodontic therapy, *NC Dent Soc J,* Aug. 1974, p. 16.

Grossman LI: Paresthesia from N2: report of a case, *Oral Surg* 46:700, 1978.

Guttuso J: Histopathologic study of rat connective tissue responses to endodontic materials, *Oral Surg* 16:713, 1963.

Horsted P, Hansen JC, Langeland K: Studies on N2 cement in man and monkey—cement lead content, lead blood level, and histologic findings, *J Endod* 8:341, 1982.

Langeland K, Guttuso J, Langeland LK, Tobon G: Methods in the study of the biologic responses to endodontic materials: tissue response to N2, *Oral Surg* 27:522, 1969.

Lewis BB, Chestner SB: Formaldehyde in dentistry: a review of mutagenic and carcinogenic potential, *J Am Dent Assoc* 103:429, 1981.

Montgomery S: Paresthesia following endodontic treatment, *J Endod* 2:345, 1976.

Muruzabal M, Erausquin J: The process of healing following endodontic treatment. In Grossman LI, editor: *Transactions of the Fifth International Conference on Endodontics,* Philadelphia, 1973, University of Pennsylvania.

Newton CW, Patterson SS, Kafrawy AH: Studies of Sargenti's technique of endodontic treatment: six-month and one-year responses, *J Endod* 6:509, 1980.

Oswald RJ, Cohn SA: Systemic distribution of lead from root canal fillings, *J Endod* 1:59, 1975.

Rappaport H, Lilly GE, Kapsimalis P: Toxicity of endodontic filling materials, *Oral Surg* 18:785, 1964.

Rowe AHR: A histologic study of the healing of pulp remnants under N2 root canal sealer, *Br Dent J* 117:27, 1964.

Sargenti A: *Endodontics,* Locarno, Switzerland, 1973, Endodontic Educational Service.

Serene TP, McKeluy BD, Scarmella JM: Endodontic problems from surgical fistulation: report of two cases, *J Am Dent Assoc* 96:101, 1978.

Snyder DE, Seltzer S, Moodnik R: Effects of N2 in experimental endodontic therapy, *Oral Surg* 21:635, 1966.

Spangberg L: Biologic effects of root canal filling materials: the effect on bone tissue of two formaldehyde-containing root canal filling pastes: N2 and Riebler's paste, *Oral Surg* 38:934, 1974.

Steven R. Potashnick • Franklin S. Weine •
Sherwin Strauss

17 Restoration of the endodontically treated tooth

The overwhelming success of endodontic therapy has allowed for the retention of more teeth than ever before in the history of dentistry. Following endodontic therapy, the restorative dentist is faced with the dilemma of deciding how to restore treated teeth for use as individual units or as abutment supports for fixed or removable restorations in a predictable long-term manner (Fig. 17-1). The techniques and guidelines of how and when to restore endodontically treated teeth have evolved from clinical tradition and anecdotal descriptions. Research on the biomechanics of posts and cores over the past decade has replaced many of our traditional ideas with data that more clearly direct the restorative dentist as to how and when to best restore these teeth. Although any number of post designs or no post at all may be used in a clinical situation, success can only be achieved when the technique choice best meets the needs of the individual clinical diagnosis—specifically, the needs of the individual diseased tooth and the clinical use for which it is intended.

PHILOSOPHY OF RESTORING TEETH AFTER ENDODONTIC THERAPY

Endodontic treatment removes the vital contents of the canal, leaving the tooth pulpless and resulting in teeth with calcified tissues that contain significantly less moisture than that of vital teeth. Are these teeth more fragile because of this? Substantiated in vivo and in vitro studies of dessication with a subsequent reduction in elasticity and increase in brittleness are sparse. Rather, the variables of remaining tooth structure, root and pulp morphology, periodontal support, and occlusion are of far greater importance when evaluating restorative needs.

Need for posts. It is the manipulation of the pulp chamber that leads to the greatest weakness of a treated tooth. The roof of the pulp chamber has the configuration of an arch, which is a shape extremely resistant to pressure and stress. When the roof of the chamber is removed for endodontic access, the inherent resistance of the treated tooth is greatly reduced. This weakening leads to the need for strong interior as well as exterior support.

Canal enlargement removes a portion of the inner substance of the tooth and decreases the dentin in the root. The amount of tooth structure that remains following endodontic therapy with or without post preparation is of prime importance. The canal filling, even when silver points are used, does not in any way return strength to this area.

The motivation for placing a post should not be exclusively for reinforcement. Studies of posts used to reinforce treated teeth offer mixed results regarding success. Intact endodontically treated teeth show little difference in their resistance to fracture when compared with untreated teeth, whereas studies testing the concept of reinforcement have shown decreased, no different, and increased resistance to fracture when a post was placed. Teeth with the smaller of two posts demonstrated greater resistance to fracture than teeth having larger posts. These studies lend credence to the contention that the strength of the remaining dentin around the post provides strength and resistance to fracture rather than the post itself.

Anterior teeth fared no better when a post or full-coverage restoration was placed than when this was not done. The rate of clinical success was significantly improved with coronal coverage of maxillary and mandibular premolars and molars. It appears that the location of the tooth in the arch and the amount of remaining tooth structure are also important factors when determining restorative requirements for longevity and function.

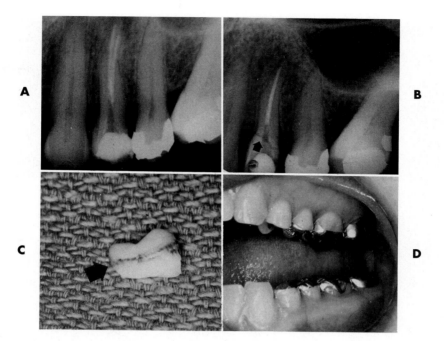

Fig. 17-1.   A, Radiograph taken after completion of endodontic therapy for a maxillary first bicuspid. Canals were filled with gutta-percha, and room was provided in both canals for parallel posts. Note periapical radiolucency. **B,** Four months later, the patient returned, complaining of a sharp pain in the area. Radiograph revealed that the periapical radiolucency had healed but a fracture of the crown *(arrow)* beneath gingival attachment had occurred. Restorative dentist had decided to wait and see if healing would occur prior to placing of final restoration, a costly procrastination. **C,** When crown fracture occurs, usually it extends far beneath gingival line *(arrow)*, resulting in an extremely difficult restorative problem. **D,** Multiple endodontically treated and restored teeth. All posterior teeth, both maxillary and mandibular, except for maxillary first bicuspid, were treated endodontically. Restorations provided full cuspal coverage over post and cores to prevent fracture. (Restorations in **D** by Dr. Jacob Lippert, formerly of Chicago.)

The weight of available evidence suggests that an endodontically treated tooth with a minimal loss of sound dentin is not more likely to fracture than a vital tooth and probably does not need a post. Teeth with minimum decay and/or restorations do not require endodontic therapy. It is those teeth with large restorations, recurrent decay, bridge abutments, or periodontal problems requiring unusual crown preparation that are candidates for treatment. The primary function of a post is to aid in retaining a core to restore lost tooth structure for retention of a restoration and not to provide strength or resistance to fracture.

Possible overuse of posts.   Recent information indicates that posts probably have been overused rather than underused in the past. Also, more problems occur from improper selection of posts and their incorrect use than the failure to use them (Figs.

17-2 through 17-4). For many years there has been a broad recommendation that any tooth following endodontic treatment requires a post for restoration. The sole exception to this was the anterior tooth with no prior restoration requiring therapy due to trauma. We no longer hold to these views.

Each tooth must be analyzed as to post requirement prior to preparation for final restoration of the treated tooth. Anterior teeth with minimal or no prior restorations not involved in bridges or splints probably do not require posts and often do not need complete coronal coverage. Many molar teeth may be similarly restored without post systems, too. Molar teeth with intact buccal and lingual walls requiring routine access preparation and not involved in extensive complex restorations in combination with other teeth probably are best restored without posts. Closure of the pulp chamber of such

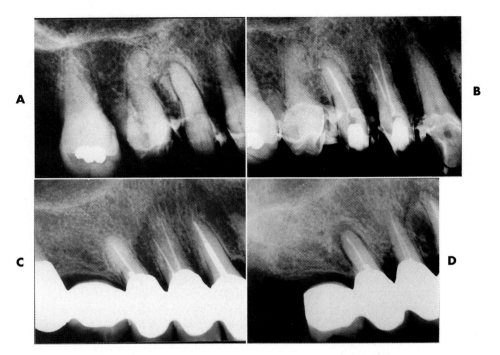

Fig. 17-2. **A,** Preoperative radiograph of maxillary posterior area, indicating that all molars and bicuspids were periodontally involved. The bicuspids and first molar required endodontic therapy, but only the bicuspids could be treated, so the first molar was extracted. **B,** Endodontic therapy completed on bicuspids. **C,** One year later, fixed bridge constructed to replace first molar, teeth splinted for periodontal reasons. Posts quite short in bicuspids. **D,** Six years later, the second molar was failing periodontally, so it was extracted and the molar pontic was allowed to exist as a cantilever. That, plus the short post, created sufficient torque to cause a fracture of the second bicuspid, noted by the considerable increase in periodontal ligament space all around the root.

a tooth may be accomplished with amalgam, composite, or other materials. Bicuspid teeth also may be restored without posts when involved in single restorations and when extensive access cavity preparations were avoided.

Even if posts are not required, it is our firm belief that *all posterior teeth require full cuspal coverage following endodontic therapy* (Fig. 17-1, D). Most of the teeth pictured in this chapter have been restored with posts because many are involved in combination with other teeth. This is not to infer that all treated teeth require posts.

The remainder of this chapter describing post use assumes that the indication for post use has been carefully considered and verified.

BIOMECHANICAL PRINCIPLES OF POST SELECTION

The retention of a post and distribution of stress to the surrounding root depends on the length,

design, diameter, and surface texture of the post. The clinician may choose from prefabricated or custom-made post systems of various lengths and diameters. Posts are designed with tapered or parallel sides. Their surface configuration may be smooth, serrated, or threaded. The shaft of the post may be hollow, solid, or split and may or may not be vented.

Types of posts. For many years, posts were cast in gold, either separately or in combination with their cores. Then, gradually, cast post use decreased with the introduction of the prefabricated post systems. At first, only a few types were available, but then, with their advantages so obvious, the prefabricated posts took over virtually the entire market.

Currently there are well over 100 different prefabricated post systems available. It may seem that every dental school and prominent prosthodontist has their own pet technique with an associated

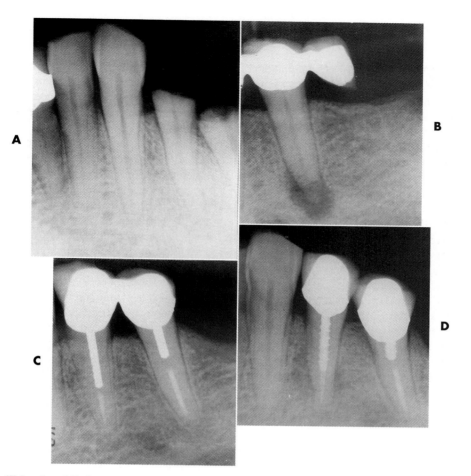

Fig. 17-3. **A** and **B,** Preoperative radiographs of mandibular bicuspid area. Failing fixed bridge (film **B,** removed for **A**), had allowed severe decay resulting in large periapical lesion for second bicuspid and pulp exposure of first bicuspid. Both teeth were symptomatic. **C,** Endodontic treatment and excellent restorations have brought favorable condition to the area. Periapical lesion has resolved. **D,** Four years later, patient changed to a new dentist who decided to replace restorations, preferring threaded posts. Unfortunately, now the first bicuspid has two lateral radiolucencies, indicative of a crack, verified following extraction.

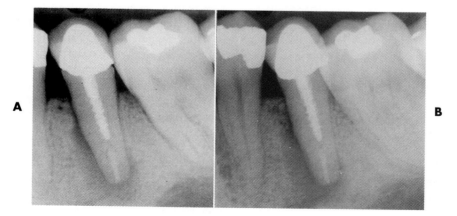

Fig. 17-4. **A** (straight) and **B** (angled), views of mandibular second bicuspid. Excellent endodontic therapy had been performed with post room prepared. Posts with threads were turned into the canal to increase retention, resulting in crack, apparent by noting considerable increase in periodontal ligament space starting in midroot on the mesial, encircling the apex, and extending almost to cervical area on the distal.

post. Even so, despite the claims of some authors and manufacturers, there is no perfect post system that will cover each and every type of clinical situation. It is incumbent upon the restorative dentist who restores many endodontically treated teeth to be conversant with several different types of systems and be able to handle a wide variety of clinical conditions.

Even with this huge number to select from, there are really only five basic systems of prefabricated posts that are commercially available. Other prefabricated systems are variations of these five basic designs. The basic post designs are the following:

1. *Tapered, smooth-sided post systems* are cemented into a channel prepared with endodontic files or reamers of matching sizes. An example is the Kerr Endopost.

2. *Parallel-sided, serrated, and vented post systems* are cemented into a matched channel prepared with a twist drill of matching size. An example is the Whaledent Parapost.

3. *Tapered, self-threading post systems* are screwed into a channel prepared with matched reamers. An example is the Dentatus screw.*

4. *Parallel-sided, threaded post systems* engage the dentin wall by self-threading or with use of matched taps. Examples are the Radix anchor,[†] which is self-tapped, and the Kurer anchor,[‡] which is first tapped and then threaded into dentin.

5. *Parallel-sided, threaded, split-shank post systems* engage the dentin wall in a channel prepared with matched reamers. An example is the Flexipost.[§]

Parallel posts are more retentive than tapered posts. As the angle of convergence exceeds 3.5 degrees, surface area of the post and resistance to displacement decrease dramatically. Tapered posts crate a wedging effect, with the greatest stress created at the coronal shoulder, whereas smooth-sided parallel posts generate their greatest stress at the apex of the preparation. Parallel posts resist tensile shear and torquing forces better than tapered posts and distribute stress more evenly along their length during function, providing greater protection against dentin failure. It is inter-

esting to note that when dislodged, cement adheres to the parallel-sided serrated posts as opposed to tapered posts, in which failure occurs at the post-cement interface.

Because parallel posts in tapered roots risk perforation and weakening of the dentin wall, parallel posts with tapered ends have been developed. Parallel-sided posts are more retentive than parallel posts with tapered ends. The dual-design posts create higher wedging stresses than parallel-sided posts, in which more uniform stresses are observed. Therefore parallel posts with tapered ends offer no advantage over parallel posts alone.

Surface texture has a dramatic effect on retention and stress distribution. Retention decreases as one progresses from threaded to serrated to smooth surface configurations. The desire for added retention prompted the development of the threaded post designs.

Normal-length threaded posts create the greatest radicular stress in loaded and unloaded states, followed by smooth-tapered and parallel-serrated post designs.

Of the threaded designs, the tapered screw creates the greatest wedging effect and highest stress levels. Tapped, parallel-sided, threaded posts generate far less stress than the tapered systems. However, the taps can generate very high stress levels if not completely withdrawn and if the tapped flutes are not thoroughly cleaned after every two turns. Extreme care must be observed in the tapping process to prevent dentin fracture.

Threaded posts with shoulder countersinks also generate very high stress levels when the countersink is fully engaged. These extreme stress levels can be reduced by counterrotation of the post one-half turn. Placing a split in the shank of a tapered threaded dowel creates stresses that are comparable in magnitude to parallel-sided serrated post systems. The threaded screw post offers the best distribution of stresses at short lengths of approximately 4 mm. However, at this length retention is severely compromised. The parallel-sided threaded post is the most favorable type utilizing mechanical retention.

Of the five basic post designs, the parallel-sided, serrated, vented post produces stresses that are distributed most evenly along its length and is best able to protect the dentin. Retention must be weighed against stress distribution for the given case. Tapered self-threading screws are the most likely to cause stress fractures and cannot be recommended. Parallel-sided threaded posts that are

---

*A.B. Dentatus, Hagersten, Sweden.
[†]Maillefer, Ballaigues, Switzerland.
[‡]Union Broach, Co., Long Island City, N.Y.
[§]Essential Dental Systems, New York, N.Y.

tapped may be used when additional retention is needed. The parallel-sided, threaded, split-shank design may reduce stress to even lower levels, but additional clinical and laboratory data are needed before this design can be recommended on a more universal basis. Results of available data are extremely promising, and future studies should be followed with interest.

Importance of post length. The factors influencing retention are dowel design and depth of placement, in that order. Increasing post length has a direct affect on retention regardless of the post system used (Fig. 17-5). Parallel-sided threaded posts have the greatest retention, whereas parallel-sided, serrated, cemented posts have intermediate retention. Tapered, smooth-surface posts are the least retentive.

In addition to retention, increasing post length has a significant effect on stress distribution. A reduction of compression and shear concentrations occurs with increased post length. Accompanying the increased reduction in stress is an increased resistance to fracture. The longer the post, the greater is the retention and support and the better is the stress distribution. Therefore post length should be as long as possible without jeopardizing the apical seal or risking perforation of a narrowing or fluted root. At the very least, the post should equal the length of the clinical crown.

The greatest advantage of the prefabricated post systems was the ability to provide long posts to gain these important properties of retention and stress distribution. The cast posts were limited by the length that wax could be placed into a relatively narrow root canal space. Attempting to widen this space to allow deeper placement of wax weakened the dentin walls and could contribute to root fracture. Being able to cast to a preformed post provided the length and strength needed.

Short posts are especially dangerous and often lead to root fracture because of their failure to be completely surrounded by periradicular bone (Fig. 17-5). This may be compounded by changes in the other elements of the restorations, as seen in Fig. 17-2.

Our recommendation for maximum length takes into consideration the fact that all studies evaluating stress replicate a relatively normal crown-to-root ratio with the alveolar crest at or near the cementoenamel junction. The fulcrum point of a short post is closer to the occlusal table in a healthy situation and may not be located in a portion of the root supported by alveolar bone in a patient with a

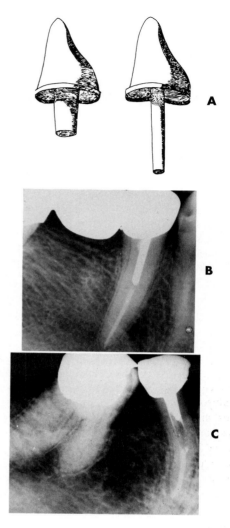

Fig. 17-5. **A,** Post retention is proportional to contact between outer area of post and walls of canal preparation. Therefore longer, thinner post with greater circumferential area is preferable to shorter, wider post. **B,** Long post is placed in preparation encompassed by both tooth and periradicular bone. Pressures applied to restoration will be distributed through cervical half of root and surrounding bone. (Restoration by Dr. Robert Wheeler, Chicago.) **C,** Short, fat post contacts little tooth structure and does not go beneath level of bone. Stress would tend to fracture root at this level. Note that sufficient post room length was provided by the endodontist but not utilized by the restorative dentist. (Endodontic therapy by Dr. Leonard Evanson, formerly of Chicago.)

Table 17-1. Suggested widths of post preparations[*]

Tooth	Enlarge to size
Maxillary	
Central incisor	80 to 100
Lateral incisor	70 to 80
Cuspid	80 to 110
Bicanaled bicuspid	80
Single-canaled bicuspid	80 to 100
Molar, palatal canal	80 to 110
Mandibular	
Incisors	70 to 80
Cuspid	80 to 100
Single-canaled bicuspid	80 to 100
Molar, distal root	80 to 110
Immature teeth	
Maxillary anterior	110 to 140
Mandibular anterior	90 to 110

[*]Widths may vary according to width of root and preoperative width of canal. Length of post room equals one to one and a half times length of clinical crown.

history of periodontal bone loss. In those patients with alveolar bone loss due to periodontal disease, the post should move the fulcrum point as far from the occlusal table as possible. To achieve this, the post needs to be as long as possible.

Individual figures for post lengths are not helpful because they do not allow for individual clinical conditions and variations. As a general rule, the post should be as long as possible, conform to the shape of the root canal, lie within the long axis of the tooth, and be of a minimum diameter to maximize preservation of remaining dentin.

There is little support for the contention that an increase in post diameter results in increased retention or helps to reinforce the root. On the contrary, increasing the diameter of the post has little effect on retention. An increase in post diameter does increase stress levels in the apical portion of the root. Reducing post diameters has the favorable effect of increasing fracture resistance. Suggestions for post diameters are listed in Table 17-1, indicating apical widths.

The type of cement used also has little effect on retention. Cement type does affect retention of tapered smooth-sided posts. In this case zinc phosphate cements were the most retentive, with carboxylate cements exhibiting intermediate retention.

Cementation. Cementation is more dependent on operator technique than the material used. The objective is to lute a post in place with minimum film thickness between the dentin and post. Vertical vents in the post design reduce hydrostatic back pressures that build up during cementation and reduce film thickness. Minimum film thickness is attained when parallel-sided vented posts are used.

Post cementation using unfilled BIS-GMA resins offers promise. The smear layer is an ultramicroscopic layer covering the dentin surface. It is composed of mostly inorganic debris left by instrumentation. This layer covers the dentin and acts as a barrier covering the dentinal tubules. EDTA, followed by sodium hypochlorite (NaOCl) as well as citric acid, phosphoric acid, and polyacrylic acid (polycarboxylate liquid), has been shown to remove the smear layer and open dentinal tubules. Studies have demonstrated the ingress of low-viscosity resins into the dentinal tubules when the resin is placed on such a cleaned surface. The use of this technique increases retention when the clinician is forced to use a short post.

This technique may also be extended to use with etched nonprecious metal posts, as in Maryland-type bonded bridges. Sandwiching the post, resin, and dentin together in this manner may strengthen the root system in addition to increasing post retention. Additional research is needed to clarify the mechanics of retention and stress characteristics for posts placed in this manner.

It is known that greater tensile and shear forces are required to unseat restorations placed with luting agents having higher compressive strengths. Unfilled BIS-GMA resins have compressive strengths that are approximately two and one-half times greater than luting agents meeting the ADA specification no. 8 for compressive strengths of cements. Adhesion of cementing agents is more important than their resistance to shearing forces, and this can be increased with elimination of the smear layer prior to cementation and use of unfilled resins.

Other considerations. Sharp angles and countersinks at the post shoulder produce high levels of stress during loading. If sound dentin remains, it should be included within the core. Preparations with residual coronal tooth structure have stresses that are more evenly distributed. The use of reverse bevels or the ferrule principle will reduce stress. Sharp angles that can generate fracture planes within the root should be avoided. The use of grooves and keyways as antirotation devices are acceptable as long as their internal aspects are smooth and rounded.

The fully cast post is the only system that can achieve accurate adaptation to all root canal configurations. From a biomechanical perspective, it is the least retentive of all post systems and generates high levels of wedging stress. The fully cast post system is indicated when the canal system has been overprepared or for teeth in which root development is incomplete.

Posts are available in wrought precious and nonprecious alloys. They can be used with a variety of direct and indirect techniques. The ability to cast to a wrought post eliminates the problem of obtaining an accurate impression of the canal system. However, the risk of corrosion when dissimilar metals are used may result in weakening at the post-core junction and may lead to eventual failure.

No one post system satisfies all criteria for success under all clinical situations. The clinician must judge the situation on its individual merits and select a system that fulfills the needs of the case while maximizing retention and minimizing stress.

CHOICES FOR RESTORATION

The endodontically treated tooth may be restored as a single unit within the arch, as an abutment within a fixed restoration, or as an abutment for a removable prosthesis. For the tooth to function satisfactorily in any of these categories, careful planning must be given to the restorative procedure.

The endodontically treated tooth must be fortified in such a way that it will withstand both vertical and lateral forces and not be subject to fracture. Amalgam, as routinely used to restore a tooth, is not considered the best choice, since the cusps (already undermined by endodontic preparation) are left unprotected and are subject to vertical fracture. An inlay, insofar as it also is an intracoronal restoration, leads to the same weakness as does the amalgam.

Clinical success is not solely dependent on the presence or absence of a post. A root-filled tooth with a minimal loss of dentin is no more likely to fracture than a tooth with a vital pulp. However, the few clinical studies on the success rates of post crowns suggest that the major predictor of success for premolars and molars is complete occlusal coverage.

The success rates of teeth with and without intracoronal reinforcement without crowns were similar for single teeth. The success rates of single teeth with coronal coverage were greater in those teeth that did not have post reinforcement. Although pulpless teeth with custom-cast posts failed more frequently than comparable teeth without posts, parallel-sided serrated posts prolonged tooth longevity.

Clinical studies suggest that the need for intracoronal reinforcement increases as the clinician progresses from an individual crown to an abutment for a fixed restoration and to an abutment for a removable prosthesis. Post placement significantly improved the prognosis of teeth used as abutments for removable prosthesis. Posterior teeth do benefit from full-coverage protection. The need for intracoronal reinforcement is more a factor of whether the tooth is supporting a fixed or removable restoration than whether it is a mandatory part of our restorative process.

The clinician must have a more flexible approach to the placement of intracoronal reinforcement. Anterior teeth with a minimal loss of tooth structure can be restored with conventional restorative materials, and full-coverage restorations are not mandatory. The decision to use a post depends on the need to restore lost coronal tooth structure with a core. The retention of cores has been shown to be improved significantly when a post is used to assist in retention of cores in both crowned and uncrowned posterior teeth.

If there is any question at all, we prefer to use a crown over an endodontically treated tooth, with additional intracoronal reinforcement. Further reduction of already undermined walls may render the treated tooth subject to horizontal fracture at or near the gingival line. The core should therefore be supported and retained by a properly fit post.

To reinforce the treated tooth and protect against vertical fracture, some type of stabilization is required that will fasten the restoration to the remaining tooth structure. This is accomplished by using a post, preferably with a core or coping and a crown or onlay as superstructure to give coronal-radicular stabilization.

Certainly the potential damage resulting from the use of a particular post system must be considered when an intracoronal method of reinforcement is chosen. The operator must also keep in mind when selecting a system that retention is important but resistance to fracture is crucial.

Endodontic and restorative therapies must be directed at the preservation of tooth structure to provide strength and resistance to fracture of the endodontically treated tooth. The need for continuous analysis of post crowns, the materials used, and the techniques advocated is essential if we are to continue to modify our skills as we learn what factors contribute to clinical success and failure.

PREPARATION OF POST AND CORE

The preparation for the post room is best made at the same appointment when canal filling is completed. The angle and lengths of the roots are well known at this time, and the correct length of post room is easily calculated. The risk of disturbing the apical seal later is reduced when post space is made at the time of obturation. The root canal may be sealed with any of the acceptable methods. If a solid-core filling is used, the sectional technique must be employed. (See Chapter 9 and 10.)

When post length equals or exceeds crown length, the clinical success rates increase significantly. Success rates approaching 100% have been reported for dowel lengths that exceed crown lengths. Therefore the length of the post must be one to one-and-a-half times the length of the clinical crown. Such a calculation is easily made by measuring either the incisogingival length of the coronal portion of the tooth or the desired length if all or a portion of the crown is missing. The length of the post should approach the maximal one-and-a-half times the clinical crown length as long as the apical seal is not jeopardized. Leaving 3 to 5 mm of apical filling intact is sufficient to ensure a seal at the apex.

If gutta-percha was used as a canal filling (Fig. 17-6, *A*), a heated root canal plugger is placed in the canal to begin the preparation for the post (Fig. 17-6, *B*). On removal, portions of the softened filling will adhere to the instrument. This is repeated until the desired penetration is reached. Root canal reamers are used to widen the canal serially by reaming action to ensure a relatively round preparation (Fig. 17-6, *C*). Canals to be prepared for prefabricated post systems with their accompanying reamers or twist drills should have the canal widened to a size approaching that of the rotary instrument chosen. The reamers and twist drills are used to *shape* the canal and follow the direction and depth created by hand instrumentation. They are not to be used to remove filling materials. When used, engine-mounted instruments are run under low speed in 10:1 gear reduction handpieces. The instruments should never be forced and should merely be allowed to

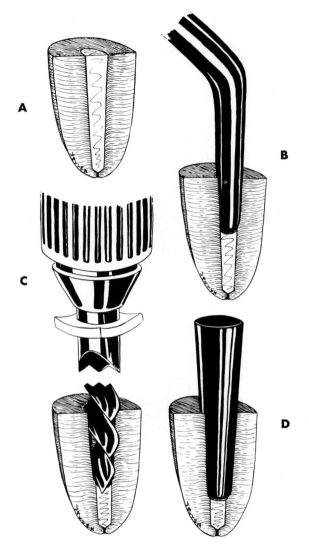

Fig. 17-6. Preparation of post room. **A,** Canal filled with gutta-percha. **B,** Hot plugger placed into canal removed filling material from cervical portion of root, leaving apical portion intact. **C,** Hand reamers are used serially to widen canal so post will contact solid dentin rather than canal filling material. No root perforation is possible when hot pluggers and hand reamers are used to correct depth. **D,** After completion of post preparation, an Endowel or Endopost is inserted to verify correctness of fit. At this point, further shaping may be needed to prepare for some post system other than the Endowel or Endopost. (Courtesy Star Dental, Valley Forge, PA 19482.)

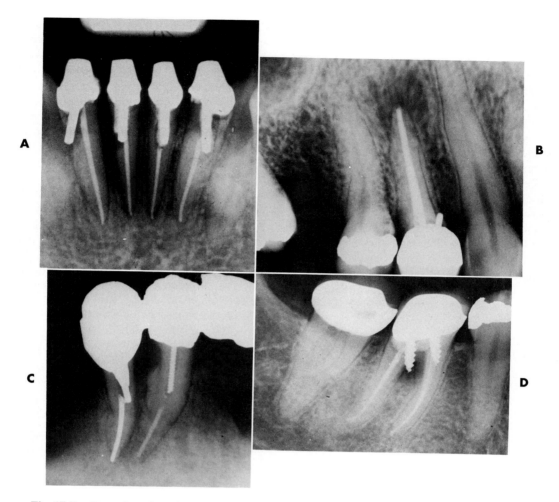

Fig. 17-7.   Examples of canals prepared for posts by using rotary instruments. **A,** Mandibular anterior teeth with endodontic treatment ruined by perforating post preparations. **B,** Maxillary first bicuspid had large radiolucency prior to treatment, which appears to be healing extremely well in this film made 6 months later. Attempt to prepare pin room with a bur led to perforation, placing entire tooth in jeopardy. **C,** Poor posts. First bicuspid *(left)* has near perforation and a canal that is much wider than the post. Cuspid *(right)* has a post with poor fit within the prepared canal. **D,** Perforation of furcation in mandibular molar for placement of a screw post. (Endodontics in **A** by Dr. Samuel Patterson, formerly of Indianapolis.)

follow the course of the canal previously established. When properly prepared and executed, very little hand pressure is needed. The instrument will direct the operator rather than the clinician directing the instrument. Stops should be placed on engine-mounted instruments at the desired depth as an added safety precaution. Burs and engine-mounted instruments may penetrate and gouge the dentin, cause undesirable vertical angulation of the preparation, or, even worse,

perforate the root if great care is not exercised (Fig. 17-7).

Hot pluggers and hand reamers will only remove materials and tooth structure from the canal and the areas adjacent to the canal walls (Fig. 17-6). If the canal is sclerotic and enlargement becomes tedious, the use of a canal irrigant or chelating agent will be helpful. (See Chapter 7.) Non–end cutting instruments such as Gates-Glidden drills can be used carefully to widen the canal in preparation for reamers, twist drills, or taps. The same rules regarding the use of 10:1 gear reduction handpieces—light pressure without forcing and depth stops—apply to these instruments as well. When increasing canal size with these instruments, the next larger instrument should not be used until the last instrument can enter and exit the canal without any resistance at all. The smallest possible canal diameter consistent with fit of the prefabricated system should be chosen to preserve the inherent strength of the root.

Post retention is proportional to the contact between the circumferential area of the post and the inner surface of the canal. For this reason, dowel length is more important than dowel width (Fig. 17-5, *A*).

In addition, the placement of a short post may increase the possibility of root fracture (Fig. 17-2).

As stress is applied to the superstructure, the post is forced against the root. A long post distributes the stress throughout the root that it contacts, which is well surrounded by bone. The short dowel distributes more stress on less root surface, some of which may not be surrounded by bone (Fig. 17-5, *B* and *C*). Should a wide but short dowel be involved, the root segment weakened to allow for the wide preparation will be even more subject to fracture.

PREPARATION OF THE ORIFICE

In most maxillary anterior teeth and mandibular bicuspids, the post preparation around the orifice leads to a symmetric shape. Orientation of the post and core can be difficult, since proximal, buccal, and lingual views all look the same. Also, such a situation will offer no resistance to twisting of the core, since the post is round. Therefore, in addition

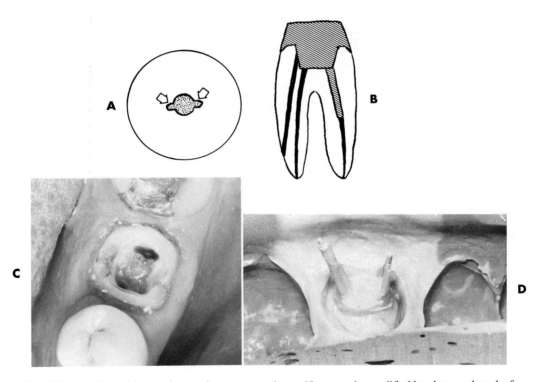

Fig. 17-8. **A,** To avoid a purely round post preparation, orifice must be modified by slots or cloverleafs placed with a tapered diamond stone or carbide bur. Addition of slots *(arrow)* will aid in seating of casting and will resist torque. **B,** Teeth with large pulp chambers are handled differently. An occlusal inlay preparation is developed within chamber to gain torque resistance for the casting. **C,** Badly decayed mandibular molar with little remaining coronal tooth structure. The tooth is prepared to bulk sound tooth structure and pulp chamber prepared to give an inlay effect. **D,** Plastic Endowels, fit to each canal, are picked up in impression material. The Endowels support the material and reduce likelihood of tearing. The pulp chamber and divergent canals are well represented in the impression material.

to the preparation of the needed depth and width to allow for post placement, attention to the configuration of the area at the orifice and extending a few millimeters toward the apex are necessary.

Regardless of the type of post and core used, all internal designs should be smooth and rounded to reduce the creation of fracture planes. Unsupported dentin, caries, and old restorations are removed, and the gingival seat is flattened to reduce apical pressure and wedging stress by the post during function. A thin, pointed, tapered diamond stone or no. 557 carbide bur is used to notch or cloverleaf the orifice area (Fig. 17-8, *A*).

Further modification of the orifice depends on whether a cast or prefabricated direct post system is used. For cast cores the rotary instrument is held at a 45-degree angle and inserted 2 to 3 mm into the canal. A blunt-end tapered diamond stone is ideal to trim the walls to give a slight divergence toward the occlusal surface, being certain that all

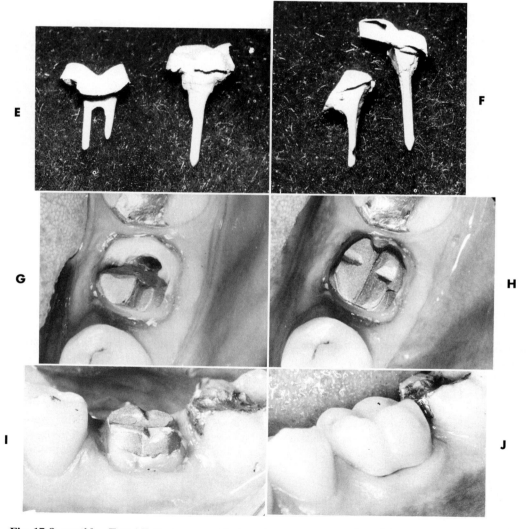

Fig. 17-8, cont'd.   **E** and **F,** Posts are cast in two pieces to accommodate divergent mesial and distal canals. Castings have extensions and projections that conform to the preparation of the orifice and canals. **G,** Mesial post-core in place. **H,** Distal post engages over the mesial core. **I,** Final posts and cores assembled and cemented. **J,** Final restoration. See Fig. 2-24 for radiographs of case.

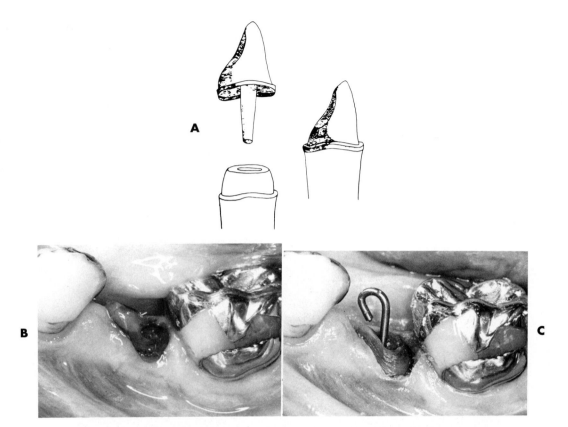

Fig. 17-9. **A,** Full coping is most desirable core. It utilizes an apron that grips entire root face and periphery to distribute forces and afford maximum protection to remaining tooth structure. **B,** Mandibular premolar with the barest minimum of remaining sound tooth structure above the gingival margin. **C,** Tooth is prepared, modifying the pulp chamber orifice and fitting an Endopost. Finish line is placed as dictated by the remaining sound tooth structure and level of gingival attachment. Circumferential tooth structure is prepared with common path of insertion to the Endopost. The Endopost is crimped to a cane configuration for better pickup by the impression.

undercuts are eliminated. For teeth with large pulp chambers, such as maxillary bicuspids or molars, the chamber is handled as for an occlusal inlay preparation, while increasing the general eccentric shape of the chamber, orifice, or both to afford excellent additional retention (Fig. 17-8, *B*). The occlusal portion of the preparation is given a bevel with a fine, tapered diamond.

When the casting is completed, the post will have fins, extensions, bulges, or other shapes to conform to the preparation at the orifice. These additions will aid in the seating and retention of the casting and afford resistance of the entire core against torque (Fig. 17-9, *C* to *J*).

The orifice is prepared differently when a core is built directly around a prefabricated post, whether the core material is composite resin or amalgam. The orifice is notched and tapered along the post toward the apex. The notches need not have a common path of insertion and are intentionally undercut to each other to add extra resistance to displacement. This will also increase the strength of the core by increasing the volume of material at the post-core-tooth interface. Even badly mutilated posterior teeth can be restored by using the interior portion adjacent to the canal to aid in the retention of the cast or prefabricated post systems. With the cervical portion of the canal prepared for the post, attention must now be directed to the preparation of the remaining tooth structure for the core or coping.

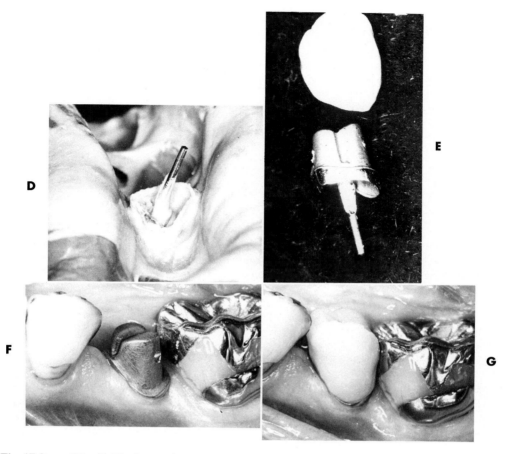

Fig. 17-9, cont'd. **D,** The impression must accurately reflect the fit of the Endopost to canal, preparation of canal orifice, remaining tooth structure, and preparation finish line. **E,** One-piece post-coping providing a ferrule effect. The collar is highly polished where it contacts the soft tissue. The coronal portion is sandblasted with prepared grooves to assist in metal-to-metal crown retention. **F,** Post-core-coping in place. The margin on the coping for the overcase ends just coronal to the gingival margin. No more than one margin must be placed in the gingival sulcus if gingival health is to be preserved. **G,** Final restoration.

TYPES OF CORES

The type of core depends on the amount of remaining sound tooth structure. The success of the post and core greatly depends on whether a ferrule is placed in the core/coping or in the overlying crown. A ferrule is defined as a metal ring or cap placed around the end of a cane or tool, giving it added strength. The ferrule around the circumference of the tooth strengthens it by increasing resistance to wedging forces.

When less than 3 mm of circumferential sound tooth structure remains, the most desirable core is a full-cast coping, which incorporates a casting to go over the entire root surface with an apron of metal. This gripping of the entire root face and periphery equally distributes the forces directed against the overlying crown, incorporates the ferrule as part of the core coping, and thus gives maximum protection to the remaining tooth structure (Fig. 17-9). The risk of the post and core loosening or the tooth fracturing is greatly increased when the margin of the overlying crown functions as the ferrule around less than 3 mm of sound tooth structure. The reason for this is that any breakdown of the cement bond at the margin around the minimal sound tooth structure results in a transfer of energy to the surface area in greatest contact with the internal surface of the crown. That area is the core contacting the inside of the crown, with the resulting stresses being directed to

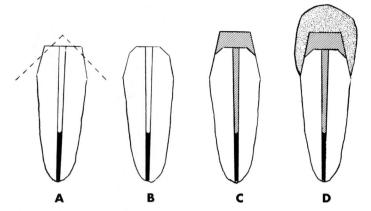

Fig. 17-10. Core preparation when adequate clinical crown is present. **A,** Forty-five-degree angled bevels are placed at occlusal or incisal edges. **B** and **C,** Core portion of casting will cover these bevels and afford protection against occlusal forces. **D,** Superstructure fits over the cemented post and core to grip supragingival tooth structure and protect against lateral forces.

the post and root with minimal dissipation or protection by the ferrule effect at the margin.

The other type of core frequently used is really an extension of the diminished crown in conjunction with the post. It is used when some bulk of tooth structure remains after endodontic therapy but greater height is required for crown retention (Figs. 17-8, *I,* and 17-10). The entire root face and periphery is covered by the casting of the crown rather than by the core. This core may be cast, or made of amalgam or composite resin.

In planning for which type of core to use, the clinician can be fooled by what appears to be adequate axial walls of sound tooth structure surrounding a crater-like void, created by caries, in the body of the remaining root. In preparing the tooth, the restorative dentist must chase the margin in an apical direction until an adequate volume of sound tooth structure is reached. What appears at first to be a tooth with adequate sound tooth structure that is badly hollowed out by caries, but that can be restored with a prefabricated post-and-core system, may quickly become a tooth with a minimum of sound tooth structure that then requires a cast-post–coping for proper restoration. Recognition at the diagnostic phase will avoid this pitfall by removing caries and evaluating the length and thickness of the remaining axial walls before endodontic therapy is completed.

CAST VERSUS PREFABRICATED POST AND CORES

Prefabricated post-and-core systems share several common advantages and disadvantages. Their advantages are that they (1) are relatively simple to use, (2) are less time consuming, (3) can be completed in one appointment, (4) are easy to temporize, (5) are cost effective, and (6) are remarkably strong. The major disadvantages of these systems are that (1) the root is designed to accept the post rather than the post being designed to fit the root; (2) their application is limited when considerable coronal tooth structure is lost; (3) chemical reactions are possible when the post and core materials are made of dissimilar metals; and (4) attachments for removable prostheses cannot be applied to the post and core unless a separate casting is fabricated to be placed over it.

Advantages of cast post systems are that they (1) are custom fit to the root configuration, (2) are adaptable to large, irregularly shaped canals and orifices, (3) can be adapted to be used with wrought posts and prefabricated plastic patterns, (4) are strong, and (5) have considerable documentation to support their effectiveness. Their disadvantages are that (1) they are expensive; (2) they require two appointments; (3) they are less retentive; (4) temporization between appointments is more difficult; (5) corrosion can occur due to the casting process or because of the use of dissimilar alloys; (6) there is a risk of casting inaccuracies; and (7) they may require the removal of additional coronal tooth structure.

CAST POST AND CORES

With the intracanal preparation for the post and the root-face preparation for the core completed, it is time to place the post prior to fabrication of the casting by either direct or indirect methods.

Types of materials available for fabricating posts. For many years post length, so important for strength and retention, was compromised because of difficulties encountered in taking an impression of the interior of a prepared canal or making a long, thin, direct wax-up. Posts that were long usually resembled a thin toothpick and rarely gave any semblance of fitting the prepared canal. Wider posts did offer some retention but usually were far short of the desirable length and led to root fractures. However, there are three materials currently available for the fabrication of a post that allow for maximum length with superior accuracy of fit:

1. *Endopost.** This high-fusing precious metal alloy, manufactured in sizes corresponding to standardized endodontic instrument sizes 70 through 140, may be cast with gold or other precious metals. It was the first of the practical manufactured aids to post fabrication that consistently and reliably afforded post length and fit.

2. *Endowel.†* Described by Weine et al., this plastic pin is available in standardized sizes 80 through 140. When incorporated in a pattern, it will burn out of the investment to yield a casting of one metal with very reasonable expense (Fig. 17-11).

3. *Parapost.‡* Unlike endodontic instruments, it has no taper and requires the use of rotary instruments for canal preparation. Currently it is not available in sizes corresponding to the standardized endodontic system.

Tooth with an adequate clinical crown. In preparing a post and core for a tooth that has an adequate clinical crown, the dentist should reduce the occlusal or incisal height to a point where the walls surrounding the prepared canal are of suffi-

*Kerr Dental Manufacturing Co., Romulus, MI 48174.
†Syntex Dental Products, Valley Forge, PA 19482.
‡Whaledent Corp., New York, NY 10001.

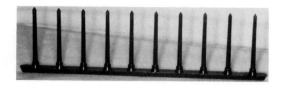

Fig. 17-11. The Endowel is a plastic pin manufactured to correspond to standardized endodontic instrument sizes 80 through 140, with ten posts of same size per stick. Pin will burn out of an invested pattern far below casting temperature with no residue to yield a casting of one metal.

cient bulk. This ensures a strong working model and minimizes possible chipping or fracture of the preparation when trying in, adjusting, and cementing the completed post-and-core restoration. The occlusal or incisal height should also be reduced adequately to ensure a core that is at least 2 to 5 mm long for convenient handling and casting purposes. This adequate reduction may be checked by eye or by a wax interocclusal record if the restoration is in the posterior part of the mouth where the interocclusal distance is difficult to visualize.

When the occlusal or incisal heights have been reduced, the remainder of the preparation is a standard crown preparation with or without shoulder. Although different operators favor different sequences and instruments, a discussion of sequence and instrumentation is offered here for reference and perspective.

If a single tooth is involved with adjacent teeth present, the contacts are most conveniently broken by use of a thin, pointed, tapered diamond. Then gross reduction is accomplished with the use of a heavy, blunt, tapered 6- to 7-mm diamond. The occlusal, lingual, and buccal or facial surfaces all may be reduced with the use of this rotary tool. The occlusal surface is reduced first and then the buccal and lingual surfaces.

If no shoulder is needed, the proximal, lingual, and buccal or facial surfaces are connected and finished, and a bevel is imparted to the occlusal or incisal portion of the preparation with the same thin, pointed, tapered diamond used to break the contacts. The simplicity and speed of using only three rotary instruments is considered a convenience in this procedure.

If a facing is desired for the full-coverage restoration, a slender, tapered, blunt-end diamond should be included in the armamentarium to

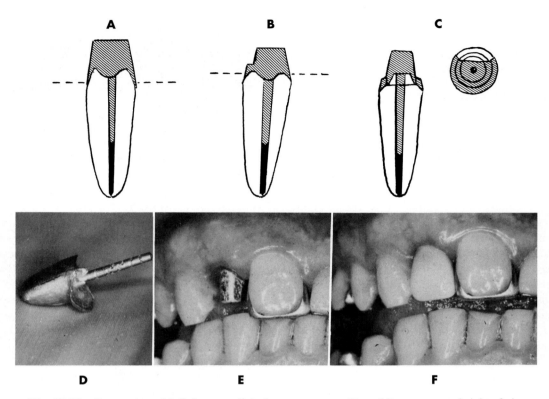

Fig. 17-12.   Preparation with little or no clinical crown present. (*Dotted line* represents height of gingiva.) **A,** Tapering of gingival margins, keeping walls as nearly parallel as possible, improves retention of casting. **B,** Shoulder placed entirely in core portion. **C** *(left),* Front view of root and core with labial portion cut away to allow for improvement of esthetics. *(right)* Top view of core and tooth showing core cut away to allow crown to butt directly against tooth structure. **D,** Post and core with shoulder absent at labial surface but present on proximal and lingual surfaces. **E,** Core cemented over preparation. **F,** Veneer crown placed over core.

accomplish the shoulder preparation, and the preparation is finished with the thin, pointed, tapered diamond as just stated.

Imparting a bevel to the occlusal or incisal portion of the preparation guards the preparation against fracture from lateral forces of mastication, since the casting will incorporate and hold in the top portion of the preparation (Fig. 17-10, *A* to *C*).

The full-crown prosthesis placed over the cemented post and core will impart the final maximum protection from vertical and horizontal forces (Fig. 17-10, *D*).

Tooth with an inadequate clinical crown.   The second category for discussion is the endodontically treated tooth with little or no clinical crown. In such a case additional retention and support are more difficult to attain, and careful planning is of prime importance.

In treated teeth with little or no clinical crown, not only the canal and pulp chamber can be depended on for retention but the extracoronal portion of the tooth as well. This is attained by tapering the remainder of the preparation with a thin, pointed, tapered diamond as in full-crown preparation (Fig. 17-12).

The surfaces of the tooth are connected and finished by placing the thin, tapered diamond 1 to 2 mm subgingivally. The circumferential tapered finish line should be as close to parallel as possible to afford maximum retention.

Additional retention may be gained in teeth having little or no clinical crown with the use of well preparations in the occlusal portion of the tooth. Wells may not be used if their preparation will leave thin unsupported walls and may only be used if sufficient bulk is available in the cervical area. When adequate tooth structure is available, a series of 2-mm preparations may be placed in the occlusal table with the use of a no. 701 carbide bur to increase the surface area and enhance retention.

Additional considerations in post-and-core procedures for a tooth with little or no clinical crown. See the following list of variations:

1. *Accommodation for facing is needed.* In such a case a shoulder or chamfer is prepared on the buccal or facial surface, as in a routine veneer crown preparation, and the post and core is shaped accordingly to allow room for facing. A blunt-end tapered diamond is used to prepare the shoulder, which is carried one third of the way into the approximal region to afford maximum esthetics. The shoulder should be carried 1 to 2 mm beneath the crest of the gingiva so there will be little or no metal showing, and it should be beveled with a fine, thin, tapered diamond. If used, the chamfer is attained in the same manner except that a round-tipped tapered diamond is used.

2. *Facing is desired, but the tooth has inadequate buccal or facial bulk.* In cases where a facing is desired but there is inadequate buccal or facial bulk, the shoulder may be placed entirely in the core portion (Fig. 17-12, *B*). This is accomplished by cutting the shoulder in the core pattern at the time of wax-up and placing the shoulder one third of the way into the interproximal space from the buccal surface. Even though the gingival band is kept as thin as possible, esthetics is usually compromised by a thin line of metal.

3. *Facing is desired, and esthetics is an important consideration.* In anterior restorations involving endodontically treated teeth with little or no supragingival tooth structure, often severe demands are made for maximum esthetic results. In these cases a band of metal, or even a darkening of gingiva due to subgingival metal, is incompatible with the desired result. To avoid these problems, the faciogingival portion of the casting of the post and core will be eliminated one third of the way into the interproximal areas. This allows sufficient room for the facing only to be seen above the gingiva.

The facial portion of the post and core is cut away in the wax-up of the core portion so that no metal will rest on the labial shoulder up to a third of the way into the interproximal space. Some retention is sacrificed in this procedure; therefore the operator must carry the proximal and lingual

portions 1 to 2 mm subgingivally, use well preparations, if possible, and use a long post to gain retention in other areas of the root face (Fig. 17-12, *C* and *D*).

When the core and crown are cemented, there will be no metal showing above the shoulder (Fig. 17-12, *E* and *F*). The operator should be sure to opaque any porcelain jacket restorations to mask the metal of the core and, if using an acrylic or porcelain veneer, be sure that the metal band is tucked subgingivally.

4. *Use of two parallel endodontic posts in bicanaled roots.* In certain cases two endodontic posts may be used in a single root in which little or no clinical crown remains, as long as the two canals present are parallel or can be prepared to be parallel. Usually this will occur in maxillary bicuspids, but the mesial root of a mandibular molar (Fig. 17-8) and a buccolingually wide mandibular cuspid may be other candidates. This type of post system may also be used in bicanaled teeth when minimal post length is available, as in very short-rooted bicuspids and molars or when the canals have been filled with nonsectioned silver points.

The tooth is prepared to include a figure-eight configuration in the chamber for maximum retention. It is important that the preparation of the canals will ensure that both are parallel, because the impression might pull with nonparallelism, but attempting to seat the casting could lead to root fracture.

5. *Use of two nonparallel endodontic posts in multicanaled teeth.* When the roots are not parallel, an overlapping two-piece cast core can be fabricated by the laboratory. This is a simple way of restoring post and cores to a tooth with multiple but divergent canals without the problems of paralleling complex keyways to the parallelism of the post sections. A combination of the techniques described in points 4 and 5 is also possible (Fig. 17-8).

Another technique to overcome this problem is the use of cemented prefabricated post systems. Each post is individually cemented into each divergent canal, and the posts are linked together within the body of a composite or amalgam core (Fig. 17-13).

Selection and setting of post. When the preparation within the root for the post is made at the time of canal filling, it is important that the correct length and width be recorded on the patient's

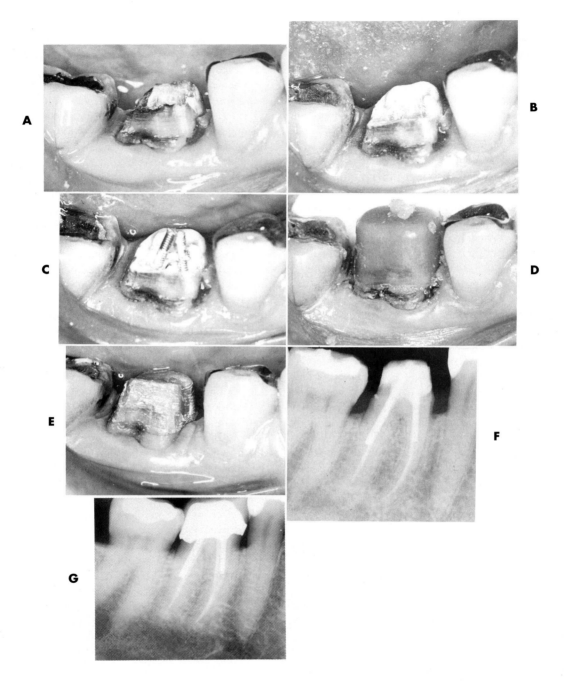

Fig. 17-13. A, Mandibular molar with divergent canals requiring additional coronal preparation height. **B,** Caries removed and orifice prepared and undercut to increase retention of composite resin core. **C,** Paraposts cemented into divergent canals to height of core preparation. Sequence of placement is determined prior to cementation to prevent interference of second post by the first post placed. **D,** Composite resin is injected into the orifice, and core is built up with a matrix form. **E,** Excess composite resin is removed as the final crown preparation is completed. **F,** Radiograph of final post core. Note post length, divergent canals, and height of posts to the coronal extent of the core. **G,** Nine years after restoration, everything looks excellent. Endodontic treatment is seen in Fig. 6-47, *A* through *E.*

chart. When the preparation is performed by an endodontist, these dimensions are sent to the referring dentist in a report, along with any other pertinent information. The report may specify, for example, Mrs. Jones—tooth no. 30; mesial canals filled with silver points and distal with guttapercha, post room in distal 14 mm, size 90; cotton and cement over canals.

The example given means that the post preparation is in the distal canal, that it extends 14 mm from the occlusal plane, and that a size 90 file was the largest used to that depth. This does not mean that a size 90 Endopost or Endowel will immediately and accurately seat to the desired length, since variations in manufacture may occur. Therefore verification is required before the impression is taken.

A file the same size as the largest used is selected, and a stop is placed to mark the correct length. This instrument is placed in the prepared portion of the canal to ensure its patency. Canal filling material, cotton, cement, or other debris may accumulate or pack the area after the prepa-

ration and prevent the post from reaching the desired position. A post corresponding to the same file size is selected. If the Endopost is used, a gentle bevel is placed by using sandpaper or a Joe Dandy disk. The Endowel is manufactured with an apical bevel. Without an additional bevel, the flat tip might catch or snag on the smooth parallel walls and not allow complete seating. Also, because the canal-enlarging instrument comes to a point, the preparation for the post is not flat (Fig. 17-14).

A desirable fit is obtained when the post is seated to the correct length and resists removal with the fingers. If the post is too loose, 1-mm segments of the apical portion should be removed, the tip again beveled, and the post retried for fit. Because the post has taper, such a procedure slightly increases the diameter at the tip until the correct circumference is obtained. If the post does not go to the correct length before binding, segments of the tip of the file should be removed and further preparation afforded to widen the preparation slightly.

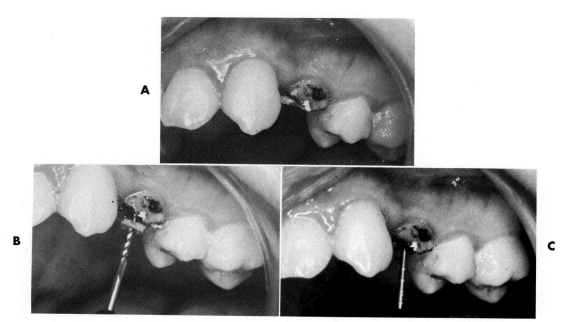

Fig. 17-14. Trial placement of a post. **A,** Patient has returned from endodontist with canals filled and post room prepared in buccal canal of a maxillary bicuspid to depth of 13 mm and width of size 80. **B,** Size 80 file with stop set at 13 mm placed in canal to remove any debris or filling materials. This is done prior to preparation of remaining tooth structure so reference point for depth of post will be available to measure from. **C,** Post is placed into canal to correct length and resists removal with fingers, verifying desirable fit. It is removed and set aside until remaining tooth structure and orifice are prepared.

The occlusal end of the post may be bent to a cane shape with pliers or a clasp bender so it will be picked up more easily by the impression material (Fig. 17-9, *C*). If elastic impression materials are used, adhesive may be painted on the portion of the post that protrudes. The risk of not picking up a tight-fitting post in the impression is great if the post is not bent to the cane shape and is left protruding straight out of the tooth.

TAKING IMPRESSION FOR POST AND CORE

The following is a step-by-step technique for the taking of the impression to fabricate the post and core.

1. The portion of the post that will be within the canal is lightly painted with a lubricant to allow for easier removal of the tightly fitting post. The post is firmly placed to its seat (Fig. 17-15, *A*). If rubber-base impression material is to be used, adhesive may be placed on the exposed portion of the post.

2. Gingival retraction is gained by the method of choice. If an Endopost is being utilized, rubber-base or elastic impression material is used rather than the more fragile hydrocolloid. Any of these impression materials may be used for the Endowel.

3. A syringe is used to place the impression material into the orifice portion of the preparation. A gentle stream of air is used to blow the impression material into the orifice and around the post. This reduces the risk of trapping air bubbles or creating a void in the impression. Additional material is then placed with a syringe around the preparation. This is an extremely important segment of the procedure, since the picking up of the orifice portion of the preparation is necessary for increased retention of the core. The remainder of the impression is taken as desired, allowing for proper length of time for set. The post should pick up cleanly with the impression (Fig. 17-15, *B* and *C*).

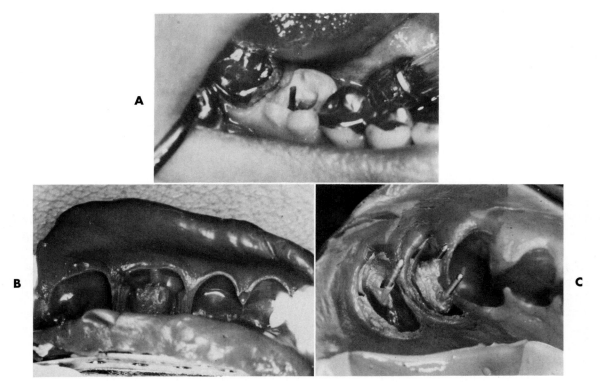

Fig. 17-15. Impressions for post and core construction. **A,** Endowel placed in distal canal of mandibular molar. **B,** Hydrocolloid impression with Endowel in place. **C,** Rubber-base impression of Endoposts in maxillary bicuspids. Second bicuspid *(left)* had one post; first bicuspid had two parallel posts. Note that orifice portions of preparations are picked up by impression materials.

4. Opposing arch impression and bite registration are taken if the post and core and crown are to be constructed from one working model. If complex reconstruction is being performed, with some abutments endodontically treated, it is best to make the cores initially. Then the preparations in the arch are completed and impressions taken for the prosthesis so that suitable mounting procedures are followed, as needed.

TEMPORIZATION

Temporization may be handled by any suitable method. The objective is not to protect the pulp, as in nontreated teeth, but to keep tooth-to-tooth relationships from being altered while the laboratory procedures are performed and to prevent gingival tissues from creeping over the margins.

In the cases for temporization where little clinical crown remains, the Endopost is ideal for fabricating a sturdy provisional restoration. It is preferable that an alginate impression of the endodontically involved tooth be taken prior to treatment and a model poured. A plastic template is made on the model, including the teeth adjacent to the treated tooth. If the tooth on the model is badly broken down, it should be built up with Clayette or similar material prior to fabrication of the template. The plastic template is made with the use of an Omnivac.*

An Endopost is prepared in the same manner as for the impression to fabricate the post and core. The nonworking end of the post is bent to a cane shape so it will fit within the coronal portion of the template. This may be judged by seating the template to place before proceeding. If the cane portion is too long, it may be further bent or cut until it does fit within the template. With the Endopost in place, a creamy mix of quick-setting acrylic is prepared and poured into the coronal portion of the template. Before the template is inserted to place, a portion of the acrylic is painted on the cane portion of the post by means of a camel's-hair brush. The template is seated to place and the patient instructed to close gently into the occlusal surface of the template. The excess acrylic is used as a gauge for setting time. When the acrylic reaches a rubbery consistency, the patient is instructed to open, the template is removed (the temporary restoration usu-

ally comes out with this removal), and the temporary restoration with the post is separated from the template by means of a plastic instrument. This is done carefully to avoid distorting the soft acrylic. The gross flash is cut off with the small scissors. While still in a soft state, the restoration is reinserted into the preparation and allowed to set. On setting, the restoration is removed by hand or with a heavy hemostat. The remainder of the flash is removed with a heavy carbide acrylic bur, and the restoration is polished with pumice and whiting. It is seated with any suitable temporary cement.

This procedure may be modified on anterior teeth with the use of an Ion crown.* In this technique, the Ion crown is selected to correspond to the original tooth size (Fig. 17-16, *A*) and adjusted for contact and gingival fit with the use of the laboratory carbide acrylic bur. When the adjustments have been completed, the Endopost is selected, prepared in the aforementioned manner, and bent into a cane shape in the nonfitting end with a clasp adjuster so it will fit within the coronal portion of the Ion crown (Fig. 17-16, *B*). If the nonfitting end cannot be bent in such a way as to fit within the crown portion of the Ion crown, the post may be cut off and notched so the notched portion is embedded in the acrylic. A creamy portion of quick-setting acrylic is prepared, the Ion form filled to the top of the mass, a portion painted on the nonfitting end of the post, and the form pushed to place with gentle pressure (Fig. 17-16, *C*). The excess may be removed in its soft state with an explorer while the acrylic is setting. In both of these techniques the use of a small amount of Vaseline is indicated as a separating medium to be painted on the prepared tooth with a camel's-hair brush. If little tooth structure remains, a small amount of saliva is adequate as a separating medium.

When the acrylic is set within the Ion crown form, the form, along with the Endopost, is removed from the preparation, the remaining flash is trimmed, and the temporary crown is polished (Fig. 17-16, *D*). The crown is returned to the mouth so occlusal adjustments may be made, if necessary. Then the temporary restoration is seated to place with a suitable temporary cement (Fig. 17-16, *E*).

---

*Buffalo Dental Manufacturing Co., Brooklyn, NY 11207.

*3M Dental Products, Irvine, CA 92704.

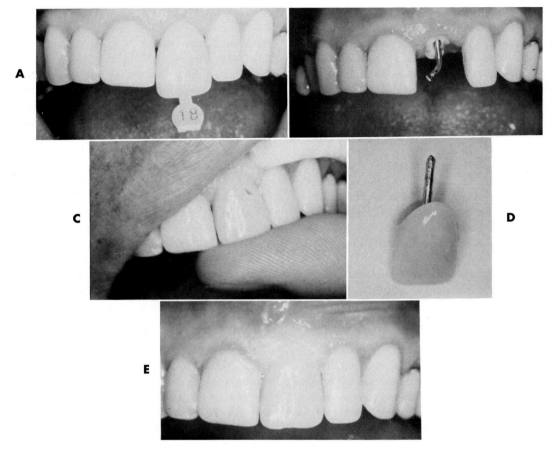

Fig. 17-16.   Use of an Ion crown form to construct a temporary crown for an individual retainer. **A,** Ion crown selected with approximately correct tooth size and shape. **B,** Endopost placed into post preparation, with the nonfitting end bent. **C,** Quick-setting acrylic is mixed, placed in crown form, and carried to preparation with the post in place. **D,** Trimmed and polished temporary crown. **E,** Temporary crown cemented.

LABORATORY TECHNIQUES FOR INDIRECT POST AND CORE FABRICATION

The step-by-step procedure for the laboratory technique involved in the fabrication of the post and core follows:

1.   The portion of the post protruding from the rubber-base impression is carefully painted with Mucolube or some other appropriate separating material.

2.   A plastic toothpick (or an old Endowel) is attached with sticky wax to go from the buccal or facial flange of the impression toward the post and is painted with separation medium (Fig. 17-17, *A*). After the model is poured, this pin will be removed; but it will produce a channel in the model to the apical portion of the post. When the post is reinserted into the model during the waxing

and polishing phases of the technique, this channel will aid in the verification that the post has reached its apical seat (Fig. 17-17, *B*).

3.   The impression with the lubricated post and pin in place is poured up in a hard crown and bridge stone.

4.   When the stone is completely set, the model is separated from the impression first with the post being removed by the impression material. This should be done carefully and with knowledge of the direction of the post so a fracture does not occur at the junction of the post and the stone.

5.   The plastic pin leading to the tip of the post is removed. If a fine wall of stone prevents the visualization of the tip of the post, it is broken through with an explorer tip.

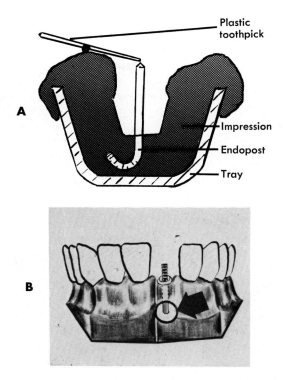

Fig. 17-17. Laboratory procedures for indirect post and core fabrication with an Endopost. **A,** Cross section through a rubber-base impression showing plastic toothpick or old Endowel attached with sticky wax to buccal flange of impression and extending to apical tip of the Endopost. **B,** After model is poured, toothpick is removed, leaving a channel *(arrow)* in the model to use for verifying that the Endopost is in its correct apical position. In some cases incisal portion of Endopost will protrude farther than desired incisal length of core. It is best to allow this excess to remain to aid in handling of wax-up. After casting, excess is trimmed with a heatless stone. (Courtesy Kerr Dental Manufacturing Co., Romulus, MI 48174.)

6. The post and orifice portions of the preparations are painted with separating medium. The post is reinserted into its position on the model and inlay wax applied, with great care being taken to ensure that wax is placed in the critical orifice portion of the preparation.

7. The post attached to the wax core is carefully withdrawn from the model, sprued, invested, and cast in the accepted manner. With the Endopost, a reducing investment is required to gain a bond between the core and alloy post. Any investment is acceptable with the Endowel.

8. After casting, the ring is allowed to cool for at least 30 minutes for proper heat treatment. After separation from the investment, the casting should be pickled by boiling in hydrochloric acid rather than by heating and then dropping into the acid.

9. Any excess post is trimmed, and the core portion of the casting is polished to a satin finish. The post portion should not be altered except to remove any bubbles or obvious excess material.

10. If the superstructure is to be fabricated on the same model, the procedures to accomplish that portion are now undertaken (Fig. 17-18).

FABRICATION OF POST AND CORE BY DIRECT METHOD

Both the Endopost and the Endowel are adaptable to direct techniques using either inlay wax or dipolymer acrylic resins for the development of the core.

The post and orifice preparations are developed and the suitable post selected as described earlier. Wax or resin is applied directly to the

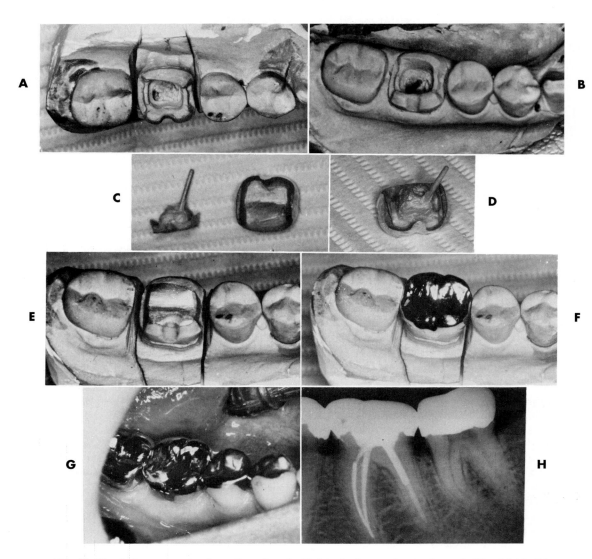

Fig. 17-18. Laboratory procedures for using the Endowel. (Impression is shown in Fig. 16-12, *B.*) **A,** Stone model of impression. **B,** Interior of impression is painted with separating medium, and Endowel is inserted into post preparation. **C,** Two castings made from the model: post and core *(left)* and superstructure *(right).* **D,** Castings interlock for maximum retention and protection of underlying tooth structure. **E,** Core on model. **F,** Superstructure on model. **G,** Castings in place on tooth. **H,** Radiograph of completed endodontic treatment and restoration. (Restoration by Dr. Arnold Wax, Chicago.)

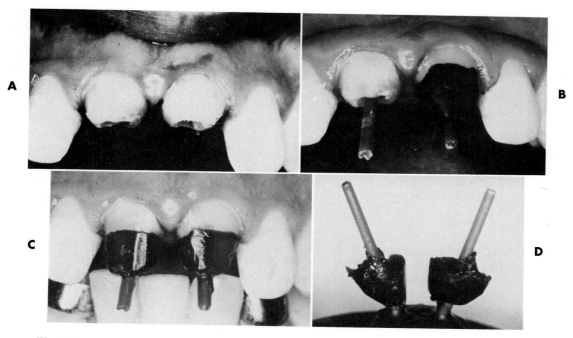

Fig. 17-19. Post and core construction by direct method using the Endowel. **A,** Preparations completed. **B,** Endowels inserted, waxing completed in central incisor *(to right).* **C,** Both wax-ups completed. Note that extension of the Endowel through the wax is available to aid in handling of patterns. **D,** Patterns are placed in base former, with Endowel extensions used as sprues. (Courtesy Dr. Gary Taylor, La Grange, Ill.)

post and lubricated tooth structure, with care taken to compress material into the orifice preparation. Necessary adjustments and trimming are performed in the mouth. The portion of the post protruding through the core is grasped with a hemostat to remove the completed wax-up. If an Endowel is used, the protruding portion of the pin may be used as the sprue. Investing and casting are performed as in the indirect method (Fig. 17-19).

CEMENTATION OF POST AND CORE

1. The temporary restoration is removed, and the canal is cleaned out thoroughly with the size file corresponding to the prepared canal.

2. The area is isolated and is dried with air and paper points. The use of paper points is important in drying the canal, since air will not dry the apical portion of the post preparation.

3. The post and core is tried in, and adjustments are made for adequate clearance of opposing teeth. If the coronal portion has already been made, this will be unnecessary since there is adequate clearance on the working model.

4. A creamy mix of crown and bridge cement is prepared and inserted into the canal with Lentulo spiral filling instruments or a Jiffy tube. The post and core is painted with crown and bridge cement and gently seated to place by hand pressure. Hammering and tapping the post and core to place are *absolutely* unacceptable, since the hydraulic pressure built up within the canal could lead to root fracture. The Endowel has built-in vents to allow for escape of excess cement.

5. From this point the tooth is handled as a routine abutment.

It should be noted that a gold-to-gold cementation is not as strong as gold-to-tooth cementation. To ensure better retention when the superstructure is cemented, the addition of grooves and wells in the core portion is advised. This is accomplished with a no. 700 or 701 tapered fissure bar. A series of three or four grooves may be placed buccally and lingually if there is adequate room. A well

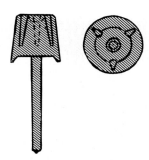

Fig. 17-20. To aid in retention of gold-to-gold cementation, grooves and wells are placed in core. Front *(left)* and top *(right)* views of core demonstrate ideal areas for placement.

may be placed occlusally or incisally with the same bur if room is available (Fig. 17-20).

METAL POST AND COMPOSITE RESIN COMBINATION

Improvements in materials and techniques have been introduced that make the restoration of endodontically treated teeth with a metal post and composite resin combination extremely practical. Without question this technique has gained in popularity due to its simplicity. Adequate tooth structure must be available for this method, and the margins of the final crown must be placed no less than 2 mm apical to the junction of composite resin and dentin to protect against leakage at this interface.

The advantages of using a composite buildup versus an amalgam buildup are not only ease and speed but also that the tooth is ready for final preparation at the same sitting. In addition, the strength and physical properties of composite are very similar to those of amalgam. The failure of post and cores due to corrosion when two dissimilar metals are used is a problem that is eliminated with the use of composite against the metal post.

After endodontic therapy has been completed, the temporary stopping is removed and the canal is cleansed and shaped to accept the prefabricated post following the manufacturer's instructions (Fig. 17-21, *A* and *B*). A parallel-sided, serrated, vented post is the system of choice, but a gold Endopost or an Endowel cast in precious or nonprecious alloy can be used as well. The orifice is prepared as previously described and as much coronal tooth structure as possible is retained to which to bond. The

use of auxiliary pins is avoided when possible by notching and undercutting the core relative to the path of insertion of the post.

The post is tried in the tooth and is tested for a snug fit (Fig. 17-21, *C*). The length of the post is adjusted so it does not exceed the height of the final crown preparation while maximum length is maintained (Fig. 17-21, *D*). If necessary, the coronal portion of the post may be bent at the cervical line to remain within the confines of the finished preparation. When more than one post is to be placed, as in a mandibular molar, the clinician should test to see which post should be inserted first and adjust the posts so they do not interfere with one another on insertion or when fully seated. Adjustment of the post should be complete before cementation. There is the risk of disturbing the cement bond when adjustments are made to the post following cementation and before the core is placed, and this should be avoided (Fig. 17-21, *E*).

After the posts are adjusted, a matrix to hold the composite resin is selected and festooned for maximum fit (Fig. 17-21, *G*). The Coreform* kit comes in approximately 20 assorted sizes and has been found useful in most situations. If a Coreform cannot be found to fit the tooth, a copper band can be used as a matrix.

Cementation follows the technique described for cast posts, with the prefabricated post held lightly in place with a large, serrated-end amalgam condenser. An alternative to cementation with zinc phosphate cement is the use of a low-viscosity composite cement such as opaque Compspan. The canal must be absolutely clean and dry when composite cements are used. Moisture in the canal will inhibit adhesion of composite cement to the dentin wall.

Excess cement is removed from the retention portion of the post, orifice notches, and coronal undercuts after the cement has set (Fig.17-21, *F*). The assistant should have all materials and supplies laid out on the work surface and ready to use in a stepwise fashion for the core buildup. The operator will need a 37% phosphoric acid gel to decrease the smear layer, a C-R syringe, the Coreform previously chosen, a dentin-bonding resin, and a core resin. Although it was once necessary to add vegetable dye or indelible pencil scrapings to the resin to create a contrasting color that could be differentiated from the dentin, composite resins

---

*Kerr Dental Manufacturing Co., Romulus, MI 48174.

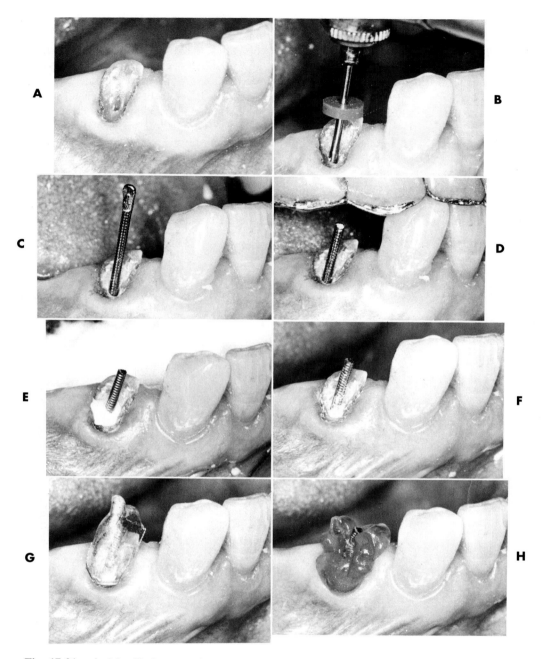

Fig. 17-21.   A, Mandibular premolar with temporary stopping removed. **B,** Canal is cleansed and shaped. Orifice is notched. Stops are used to prevent overpreparation when shaping canal. **C,** Parapost tried in for snug fit. **D,** Post is reduced in height prior to cementation, reducing risk of dislodgement later. **E,** Post cementation. **F,** Excess cement carefully removed from retention and notched areas. **G,** Coreform fit and festooned. **H,** Smear layer removed and dentinal tubules opened with phosphoric acid gel etch.   *Continued*

are now manufactured for this purpose and come in colors such as blue, stark white, and gray. The tip of the C-R syringe can be cut, allowing for easier injection of the core composite.

The coronal dentin is then etched with the 37% phosphoric acid gel for 1 minute (Fig. 17-21, *H*). The tooth is washed for 30 seconds and thoroughly air dried with blasts of warm, dry air until the dentin-bonding resin is applied with a fine brush (Fig. 17-21, *I*). The excess resin is blown off, and a second coat is immediately applied and again blown off. While the operator is applying the dentin-bonding resin, the assistant mixes one of the small-particle–size composite resins specifi-

cally designed for this purpose. Enough resin is mixed to allow the assistant to fill the injection syringe and the Coreform. The core material is immediately injected around the post and into the antirotation notches and undercuts (Fig. 17-21, *J*). The loaded Coreform is immediately placed over the post and held in the position decided at the try-in stage (Fig. 17-21, *K*). The area is kept dry while the composite resin is allowed to set for 10 minutes. The tooth is now ready for final preparation and temporization (Fig. 17-21, *L* and *M*).

Composite resins are affected by zinc oxide–eugenol cements. Their stability with regard to carboxylate and glass ionomer cements are

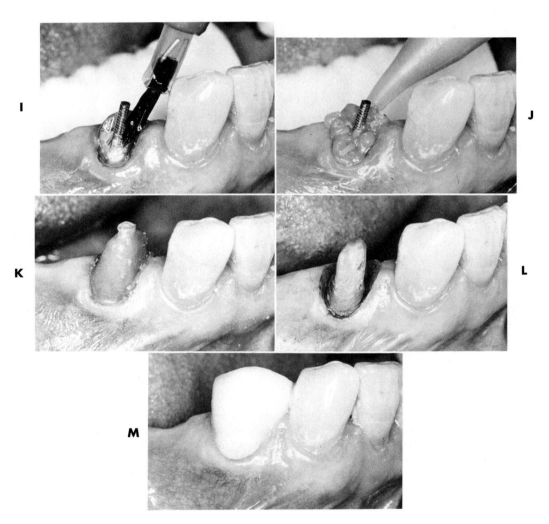

Fig. 17-21, cont'd. **I,** Placement of autopolymerizing dentin-bonding agent. **J,** Composite core resin carefully injected around post and into retentive notches. **K,** Loaded Coreform placed and held in correct axial position until resin has set. **L,** Final preparation. **M,** Provisional restoration.

unknown. Care should be taken to use zinc phosphate or composite cements in these cases. Temporary restorations should be cemented with non–eugenol containing cements, and the final restorations should be cemented with zinc phosphate cement as well.

After undergoing endodontic treatment, teeth with individual crowns or bridge abutments often can be satisfactorily strengthened and retained by a parallel-sided, serrated post cemented into the prepared canal. The pulp chamber can then be etched, and a dentin-bonding resin and core composite applied to bond and strengthen the axial walls. After the composite has set, a Class I amalgam preparation can be prepared to close and seal the endodontic access cavity through the crown and the occlusion can be adjusted. An otherwise extensive and expensive repair or remake thus can be avoided.

SCREW POST METHOD FOR REBUILDING TREATED TEETH

A method for rebuilding endodontically treated teeth incorporates the use of screw posts. After the posts are screwed into prepared canals, composite resin as previously described or silver amalgam is compactly condensed around the protruding coronal portion using a copper band or suitable matrix around the tooth. We favor newer split-shank screw post designs in this family of posts (Fig. 17-22). For the sake of completeness, this section describes

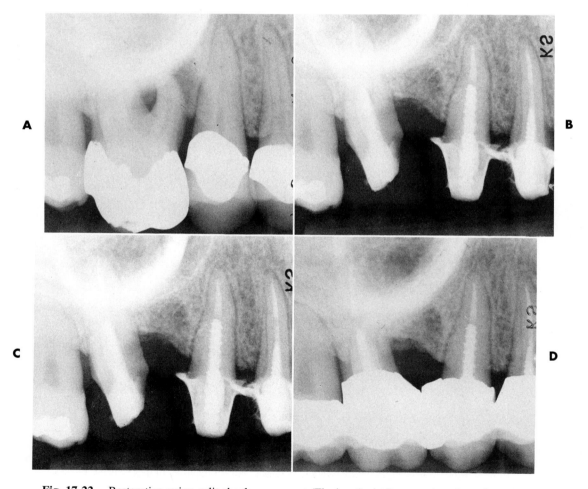

Fig. 17-22. Restoration using split-shank screw post (Flexipost). **A,** Preoperative view of maxillary molar and bicuspid areas. First molar has hopeless periodontal condition around mesiobuccal root. **B,** Bicuspids required endodontic treatment as well. Endodontic therapy performed on first molar, and mesiobuccal root amputated. **C,** Split-shank posts placed. **D,** One year after final restoration. (Restorations by Dr. Kerry Voit and periodontal therapy by Dr. Harry Staffileno, both of Chicago.)

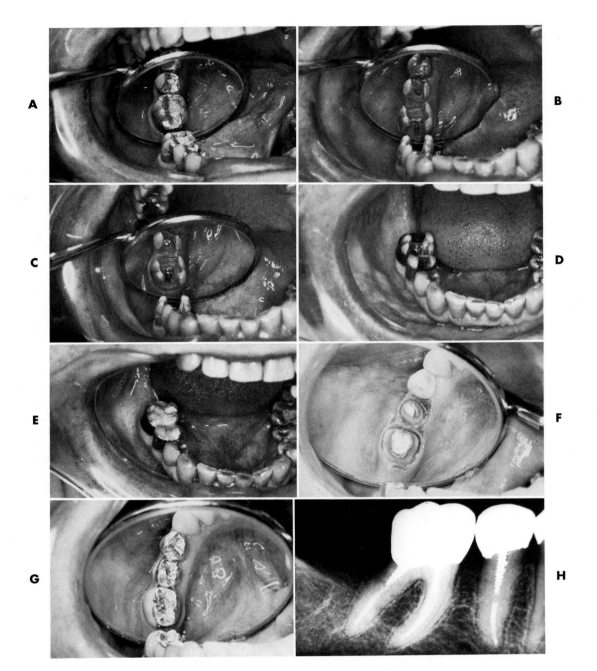

Fig. 17-23. Technique for placement of screw posts, amalgam buildup, and restoration. **A,** Patient returns from endodontist following treatment of mandibular second bicuspid and first molar with access cavities closed by zinc oxide–eugenol. **B,** All filling materials are removed, and pulp chamber is widened. **C,** Screw posts are placed. **D,** Copper band matrices in place, festooned to gain tight adaptation at gingival margin and cut down so occlusion will not have any interferences. **E,** Amalgam condensed into canals, around screw posts, and into preparation. **F,** Final preparation prior to taking impressions. **G,** Final restorations. **H,** Final radiograph. **I,** Twenty-two years after original treatment, both teeth look excellent; no further treatment required.

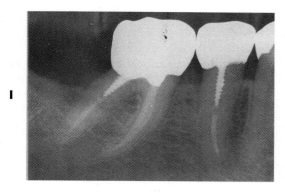

Fig. 17-23, cont'd.   For legend see opposite page.

the use of screw posts with an amalgam core. The mechanical retention achieved between the tooth, post, and silver amalgam provides a suitable core of sufficient bulk and strength to be prepared in the usual manner and covered with a crown.

Advantages and disadvantages. There is no middle road in regard to screw posts—clinicians either love them or despise them.

The screw post method has many advantages. It is convenient, easy to use, and relatively inexpensive. There is minimal or no discomfort to the patient, and therefore no anesthesia and little chair time are required. The technique is simple and atraumatic. Multiple posts ensure nonparallelism of the canal and enhance retention; the result is a strong, rigid, retentive core on which a crown can be placed for maximum permanence. Nonparallelism is a serious problem with cast cores for molars, necessitating the use of only one canal of the available three or requiring a complicated interlocking of nonparallel posts.

The disadvantages are less numerous but nevertheless significant. Care must be exercised in post placement since overtwisting can result in breaking off the retentive head in several of the available systems. Even worse, overtwisting can result in root fracture. Because of its initial fragility, it is unwise to prepare or take an impression of a screw post amalgam placement within 24 hours of insertion.

Following endodontic treatment (Fig. 17-23, *A*), all temporary filling material, decay, and foreign material are removed from the tooth until sound tooth structure is reached. The occlusal portion of the remaining tooth surface should be free of sharp angles, and the pulp chamber is widened to lend as much bulk to the central core as possible (Fig. 17-23, *B*).

Posts should be as long and as thin as possible. A minimum of one third of the root length is essential for adequate strength and retention. Multiple screw posts are preferred where possible. Try-in of the posts for size (Fig. 17-23, *C*) and checking by radiographs are advised. Before final insertion, the posts should be removed and any debris thoroughly cleaned from around the threads. They may then be replaced and cemented to place.

After the posts are cemented, the operator adapts a copper band around the remaining tooth structure, making certain that it does not cut the epithelial attachment and does not interfere with the occlusion but does fit tightly at the gingival margins (Fig. 17-23, *D*). The area is isolated with cotton rolls or a rubber dam, and the tooth is dried with air.

The silver amalgam is condensed compactly into all crevices within the copper band matrix, root canal, and chamber and around the screw post (Fig. 17-23, *E*) and placed to the height of the band. The occlusion is adjusted to avoid any occlusal interferences, and any sharp edges of the band are smoothed with a tapered diamond stone. The patient should be cautioned about favoring this tooth until the following day.

At the next visit, the copper band is removed and the amalgam buildup prepared for impression taking (Fig. 17-23, *F*). It is preferable to crown such a tooth for maximum permanency (Fig. 17-23, *G*).

ENDODONTICS PERFORMED AFTER FINAL PREPARATION OF THE TEETH

Occasionally during the preparation of teeth, particularly those that were periodontally involved and had extensive periodontal therapy, the further insult of restorative treatment may cause pulpal inflammation or pulpal necrosis. The timing of this occurrence may be inconvenient to the operator in that it could transpire after the final restoration and/or fixed prosthesis has been fabricated but before the final preparation and/or fixed prosthesis has been cemented. If this series of circumstances presents itself, endodontics may be performed on the prepared tooth or teeth as long as such treatment does not involve the finishing line and does not lead to gross depletion of the existing morphology. If treatment is being performed by a general dentist and an endodontist, careful communication between them is essential in order to guard against any of these problems.

If the prerequisites for this type of endodontics can be maintained, the endodontist performs the treatment making certain that the insult of entry is as small as possible. Post room is prepared, and the case is returned to the general dentist. These teeth, like any other endodontically treated teeth, need protection from fracture due to vertical and horizontal forces. In placing an Endopost, the operator follows the same series of procedures, making sure that there is no insult to the preparation when removing the temporary or provisional splint and when cleansing the preparation. The temporary stopping is removed, and the canals are cleaned with the appropriate file.

The canals are dried with paper points, and the appropriate Endoposts are selected corresponding to the last file used and cut off with a Joe Dandy disk to fit just inside the endodontic preparation. A smooth, weak mix of zinc-oxyphosphate cement (not watery) is prepared and inserted into the

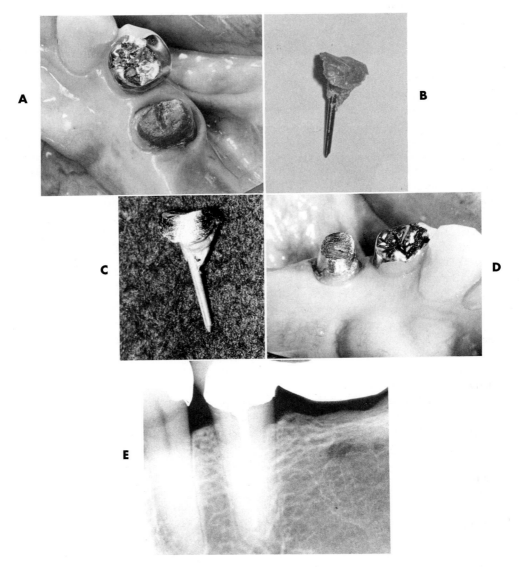

Fig. 17-24. **A,** Core is formed around plastic post using the lubricated crown as a matrix. Flash is avoided at marginal area to prevent crown from seating completely. **B,** Plastic pattern is removed and trimmed. **C,** Cast pattern with sprue removed from occlusal surface. **D,** Casting is adjusted to fit the tooth and overcase. **E,** Final radiograph of post, core, and overcase permanently cemented to place.

canal(s) with a Lentulo spiral drill. The prepared Endoposts are immediately seated to place with an amalgam condenser. The same mix may be slightly thickened if desired in order to seat the final restoration or fixed prosthesis. With this technique the necessity of remaking the final restoration has been avoided.

Fabrication of a post and core to fit an existing bridge may become necessary when a bridge abutment loosens and endodontic therapy becomes necessary due to chronic irritation or recurrent caries. If the bridge can be removed and the margins of the abutment tooth remain sound, a post and core can be made to fit the existing restoration, preventing a costly remake of the restoration.

Endodontics is completed, post room is made, and the patient returns to the general dentist. The temporary stopping is removed, and the canal is cleaned with the appropriate file. A plastic Endowel of the appropriate size is fit to the canal and shortened to fit under the existing crown. The Endowel is removed, and the remaining coronal tooth structure is lightly lubricated with a silicon separating medium such as Masque.* The inside of the abutment that will accept the core is also lightly lubricated. The Endowel is replaced into the canal, and red Duralay† inlay resin is carefully placed around the Endowel using a brush-on technique. The bridge is placed over the abutment teeth, and the patient is instructed to close to be certain the bridge is fully seated and the occlusion is at the correct position. The resin is allowed to set for 5 minutes, and the bridge is removed. Voids in the core are carefully filled in with small amounts of additional resin, and the procedure is repeated. In this way the abutment castings are used as a matrix for the underlying core (Fig. 17-24, *A*).

The plastic pattern of the post and core is removed, trimmed, and cast (Fig. 17-24, *B* and *C*). Spruing of the pattern should be done at its top so that adjustment of the casting will have a minimum effect on the axial walls and on retention to the overcasting.

The casting is tried in and adjusted to seat completely in the tooth (Fig. 17-24, *D*). The operator must be certain that the new post and core do not prevent the bridge from going completely to place. This can be checked by using a low-viscosity sili-

con pressure paste such as Fit-Checker.* Pressure spots are adjusted and the fit is confirmed with the use of radiographs. The post and core and bridge are then cemented permanently (Fig. 17-24, *E*).

RESTORATION OF TEETH AFTER ROOT AMPUTATION

As described in Chapter 12 root amputation has greatly aided in the retention of certain posterior teeth when severe involvement of only one root jeopardized the entire tooth. It is necessary to emphasize that the elimination of one root or more considerably alters the shape of the restoration to be used for a tooth so treated. Failure to allow for such a deviation from routine will probably lead to loss of the tooth despite otherwise excellent endodontic and surgical treatment.

The retention of single roots of multirooted teeth may add great stability to adjacent splint abutments. As a posterior abutment, a single root may be the difference between a fixed and a removable prosthesis. When careful restorative measures are followed, teeth that have had root amputation may serve this purpose as successfully as noninvolved teeth.

Indications for root removal include furcation control, severe carious destruction, control of tight embrasures due to tight root proximity, and endodontically untreatable roots. Indications for root separation with the maintenance of both roots include the need to control the environment of a furcation, the desire to separate the prognosis of the roots of a given tooth, and the need to eliminate caries that invade a furcation area.

The remaining roots require full-coverage restoration and generally must be splinted to an adjacent tooth or teeth. They are rarely strong enough to function alone.

Mandibular molar—retaining the distal root. In cases where severe periodontal involvement of the mesial root or a furcation is present and the involved tooth is the distal abutment, or where further stability is required for a distal abutment, the distal root becomes a critical root to retain (Fig. 17-25). For the restorative dentist the distal root is usually the easier root to retain because it is the straightest, has the widest canal, and will accommodate the largest and deepest post. Being the distal root, it is more posterior and gives a greater

---

*Harry Bosworth Co., Skokie, Ill.
†Reliance Manufacturing Co., Worth, Ill.

*G-C International Corp., Scottsdale, Ariz.

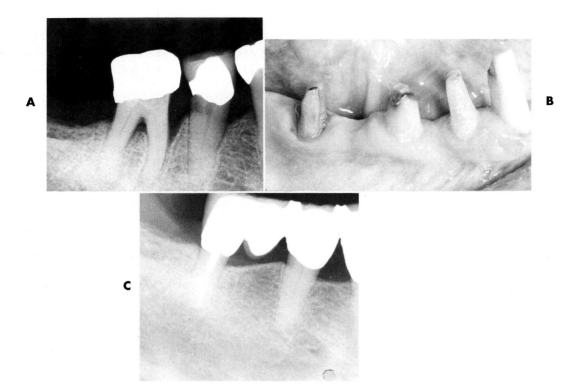

Fig. 17-25. Root amputation retaining distal root. **A,** Severe periodontal involvement of mandibular molar with through-and-through furcation and mesial infrabony defect. The tooth is the most distal in the arch, making the distal root a critical abutment. **B,** Following hemisection, root removal, and endodontic and periodontal therapy. **C,** Final restoration. Furcation and infrabony defects are eliminated. Periodontal health restored to normal. Mesial root replaced with small bicuspid pontic, 5-year postoperative radiograph. (Endodontics by Dr. Charles Neach, Chicago.)

arch length than the mesial root being retained. In cross section the mesial and distal surfaces are concave, but the concavities are not as deep as on the mesial root and are easier to follow when placing a finish line as compared to the mesial root.

The distal root is wider in a buccolingual than mesiodistal direction and is handled like a bicuspid in its preparation for a post and core. When the distal root has two canals, the distobuccal canal is usually the larger and should receive the post. The orifice of the single distal canal is oval or kidney shaped, and the preparation to widen this area should be made in a buccolingual rather than mesiodistal direction to avoid perforation of the mesial portion of the root.

The space vacated by the amputation is replaced with a small bicuspid pontic, allowing for adequate embrasures for cleanliness of the retained root.

Mandibular molar—retaining the mesial root. The mesial root of either the mandibular first or second molar should be retained when (1) the periodontal support is greater; (2) the distal root cannot be salvaged for endodontic, periodontal, or restorative therapy; or (3) maintenance of the distal root jeopardizes the adjacent root and/or tooth. The retention of the mesial root rather than the distal root is more difficult from an endodontic and restorative standpoint, although the mesial root has more total circumferential area for potential attachment.

The mesial root usually has two small curved canals, which are certainly much more complicated to prepare and fill than the wider straight distal canal. Also, neither mesial canal is as ideal for post retention as the distal canal. In most instances the straighter mesial canal, the mesi-

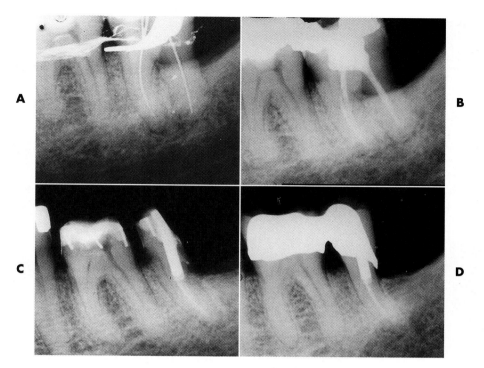

Fig. 17-26.   Amputation of the distal root of a mandibular second molar, retaining the mesial root. **A,** Film of files in place of mandibular second molar with furcation involvement. The pulp was necrotic and small periapical lesions were present, so it was hoped that the periodontal condition was related to the pulpal problems (Chapter 13). However, no periodontal healing occurred after canal preparation or after (**B**) competion of endodontic therapy. **C,** The distal root of the second molar was amputated, the mesiolingual canal was posted, and a temporary splint was fabricated to ensure healing. **D,** Eleven years later, the area looks excellent, and only minimal bone loss has occurred subsequently. (Restoration by Dr. Dan Mackey and periodontics by Dr. Harry Staffileno, both of Chicago.)

olingual canal, is prepared to hold a single post. Some greater retention may be gained by using a small preparation at the orifice of the unused canal with the inlay type of effect for a cast post and core and a locking effect for a direct post and composite buildup. Because of the curved nature of these canals, care must be exercised not to make the posts so long that they deviate from the prepared canal shape and head toward a perforation in the naturally occurring mesial and distal concavities along the sides of the root (Fig. 12-31, *D*).

Both mesial canals can be used for twin posts. They must be parallel in the cervical third of the canal if a cast post is used but can deviate if prefabricated cemented posts are used. The total retention here is equal to the sum of the post lengths, which is considerable, without going too

deep in either canal. This is desirable in very curved roots in which post length is difficult to obtain.

With the restoration of the mesial root by the post and core, the tooth is now treated as a bicuspid (Fig. 17-26). If the mesial or distal root of a first molar is used in conjunction with the mesial root of the second molar, a small pontic with adequate embrasures replaces the lost root when adequate room is present.

Mandibular molar—retaining the mesial and distal roots.   Retention of both mesial and distal roots of the same molar is difficult to achieve even when both roots are equally good candidates for management. It is rarely possible to create a satisfactory environment for future cleaning around both roots because the two roots are usually not divergent enough to gain a sizable interproximal

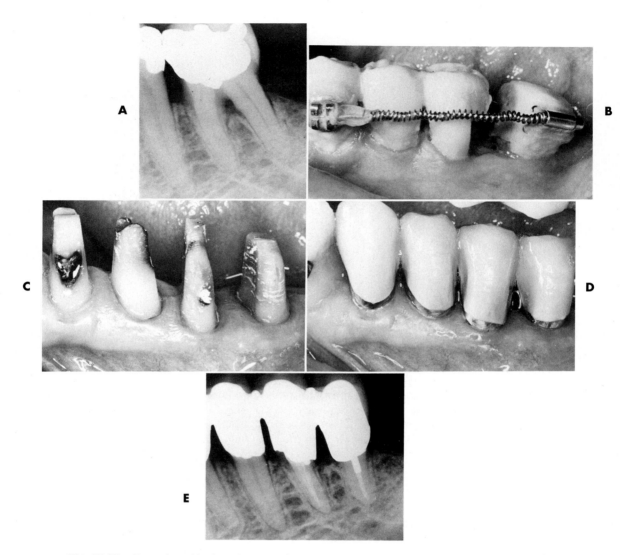

Fig. 17-27. Retention of both molar roots. **A,** Mandibular molar with through-and-through furcation. The bone in the furcation is horizontal, and both roots have comparable attachment. **B,** Following endodontics and root separation, the distal root is tilted back, increasing embrasure space. The area of interest is at the gingival margin. Rotation of the root around a fulcrum below the gingiva makes movement at the occlusal table appear to be more than needed. Movement at the gingival margin, where needed, is far less than rotation at the occlusal table, where it appears excessive. Provisional restoration used as anchorage; open coil spring drives root backward along guidewire in buccal tube. Distal root is taken out of occlusion to allow for rapid movement. **C,** Individual roots following endodontics, separation, minor tooth movement, post placement, periodontics, and repreparation for final restoration. **D,** Final restoration is a four-unit splint designed as four bicuspids. **E,** Radiograph of final restoration. Note excellent embrasure form between molar roots and horizontal bony topography. (Periodontics by Dr. Douglas Gorin, Chicago.)

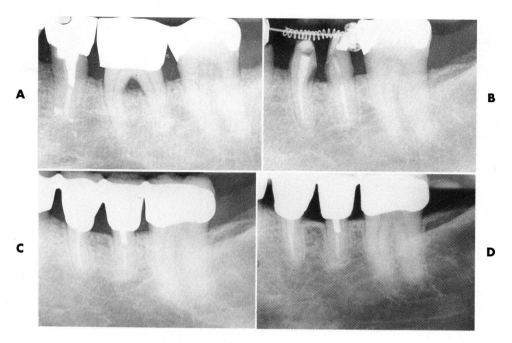

Fig. 17-28. Retention of both molar roots and second molar. **A,** Through-and-through furcation defect on first molar with horizontal crestal bone, minimal periodontal involvement of second molar. Patient desires to save all teeth while creating an optimal environment. Inadequate room between the roots of the first molar to create embrasure room for cleaning by patient. **B,** Second molar and distal root of first molar are moved distally and uprighted, increasing space between first molar roots. Movement is begun following completion of endodontic therapy. **C,** Final restoration. Roots of first molar and second molar are paralleled and optimal interradicular space created for restoration and daily plaque control removal. **D,** Eight years after completion, note that crestal bone between separated roots has remained at the same level due to excellent home care by the patient, and planning of case design. (Endodontics by Dr. Paul Ashkenaz, Chicago.)

space where the furcation had been located. If the anatomy of the tooth allows such a procedure, however, both roots are prepared for post and cores and the separate roots individually handled as previously described.

A solution to the problem of inadequate space is minor orthodontic tooth movement (Fig. 17-27). If the distal root is the most distal abutment, it can be tipped distally to increase the space between it and the distal surface of the mesial root, creating a restorable and cleanable embrasure form. When the distal root is not the last root in the arch, the distal root and the second molar behind it can be moved to distribute and create a restorable amount of space, overcoming the problem of root proximity. Although individual distal root tipping can be completed rapidly and in a matter of weeks, moving several teeth and roots

is a more time-consuming and difficult task (Fig. 17-28).

Maxillary molar—retaining the mesiobuccal or distobuccal and palatal roots. Post room is prepared in the palatal root. Preparation of the areas adjacent to the retained roots is critical because as much of the trifurcation formed by the missing and two remaining roots should be eliminated to prevent the residual furcation from acting as a shelf and forming a food and plaque trap that cannot be cleaned (Fig. 17-29).

The preparation at the gingival margin resembles a figure-eight shape as the preparation is barreled into the area of the furcation between the remaining two roots (Fig. 17-30, *A*). The shape of the final restoration at the gingival margin will depend on the horizontal depth of the concavity created between the two roots. The greater the

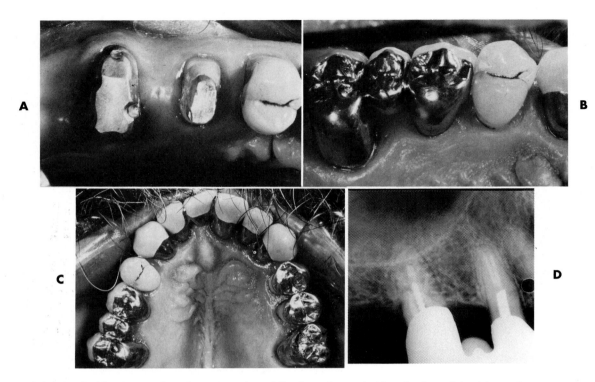

Fig. 17-29. Restoration after amputation of distobuccal root. **A,** Note that buccal *(top)* is much more narrow than palatal and that wells are placed on the buccal and mesial for added retention of gold-to-gold superstructure. **B,** Bridge seated. **C,** Occlusal view of completed prosthesis. Note that terminal abutment molar *(lower right)* is much wider at buccal than the tooth with the amputation *(lower left)*, even though palatal widths are approximately equal. **D,** Twelve years after treatment, the remaining roots are functioning well. (Restoration by Dr. J. Schulz-Bongert, Dusseldorf, Germany.)

concavity deviates away from an imaginary line drawn from the most convex surface on the proximal side of the palatal root to the most convex surface on the proximal side of the remaining root, the greater will be the concave form at the gingival margin. The alternative is to replace the ceiling of the furcation chamber in the restoration, creating a flatter proximal surface but one that replaces a portion of the shelf that was removed (Fig. 17-30, *B* and *C*). Flatter contours with mild concavities are more easily cleaned and are preferred. This type of contour creates a narrower sulcus around the tooth with less area to become a depository for debris (Fig. 17-30, *D* and *E*). The final coronal restoration for this preparation has an occlusal configuration similar to that of a molar, but with the mesiobuccal or distobuccal portion reduced to lessen occlusal stress over the area where no root is present. At the gingival margin there is a large embrasure where the amputated root formerly resided (Fig. 17-30, *D*).

Following amputation of the distobuccal root of a maxillary first molar, a single nonsplinted restoration may be used, as shown in Fig. 17-30. The distobuccal root represents less than 25% of the total surface area of the tooth at the furcation level. The remaining roots are quite retentive, because the mesiobuccal root curves initially to the mesial and then to the distal, whereas the palatal root curves initially to the palatal and then to the buccal (Chapter 12).

However, retention of the distobuccal and palatal roots following the amputation of the mesiobuccal is more complicated. The mesiobuccal represents at least 33% of the tooth at the furcation level, and the retained distobuccal root is not nearly as retentive. Therefore, when the mesiobuccal root is amputated, the remaining roots must be splinted to either or both of the adjacent teeth (Fig. 17-31).

Maxillary molar—retaining the buccal roots. In rare cases the palatal root is amputated and the

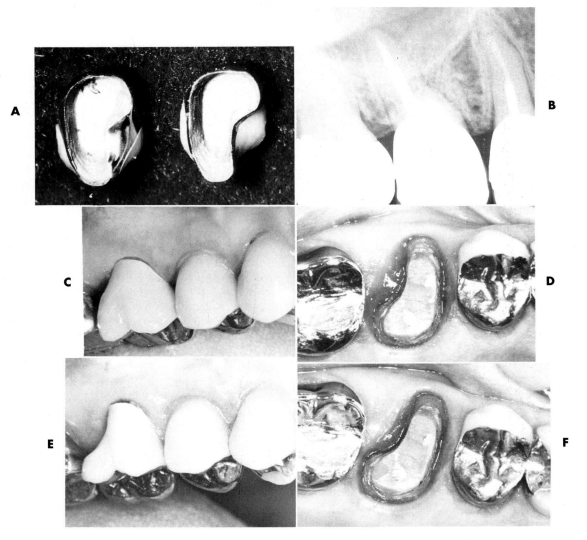

Fig. 17-30.   Crown contour after amputation of distobuccal root. **A,** Crowns made from same die with different gingival contours. Both show concave finish line in area of distobuccal root removal. Crown contour *(left)* replaces ceiling of trifurcation removed in tooth preparation with convex contour. Crown contour *(right)* follows finish line, with mild concavity between palatal and mesiobuccal roots. **B,** Radiograph of final restoration, with post placed in palatal root. **C,** Crown with convex contour in place. **D,** Inflamed sulcus corresponding to crown contours of **C. E,** Crown with concave proximal contour in place. Note embrasure previously occupied by distobuccal root and normal occlusal configuration. **F,** Healthy narrow sulcus corresponding to contour of crown in **E.** Sulcus is less likely to be a depository for debris and is more easily cleaned. This is the contour of choice for the final restoration.

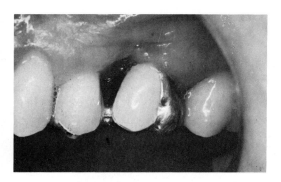

Fig. 17-31. Restoration following mesiobuccal root amputation. The occlusal configuration is similar to a maxillary molar, with the mesiobuccal portion reduced to lessen the occlusal stress over the site of amputation. The crown is contoured at the gingival margin of the mesial to allow for a large embrasure and is splinted to the adjacent second bicuspid.

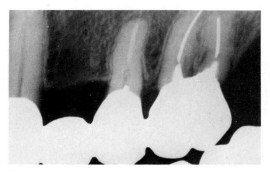

Fig. 17-32. Maxillary molar restored after palatal root amputation. Tooth resembles a bicuspid lying sideways. (Endodontic therapy by Dr. Harold Gerstein, Chicago.)

buccal roots are retained. In this configuration the distobuccal root is usually the choice for the post in that it is the straighter of the two retained roots. A small preparation at the orifice of the unused root may be used for extra retention. This configuration is treated as a bicuspid lying sideways (Fig. 17-32). The trifurcation between the buccal and palatal roots is eliminated by preparing out the ceiling of the furcation chamber connecting these roots on the palatal aspect. The coronal restoration in this configuration is narrow buccolingually to eliminate stress and must be placed exactly over

the retained roots rather than over the center of the preoperative configuration. Care must be exercised to avoid a palatal shelf over the straight palatal surfaces of the mesial and distal roots, which would collect debris and perpetuate periodontal disturbance.

Maxillary molar—retaining the palatal root. In the configuration where only the palatal root remains, a fairly ideal restorative situation exists. The palatal root is the widest of the maxillary roots, and circumferential concavities on its palatal surface are far more subtle than concavities on the other maxillary molar roots. The canal is most ideal for constructing a post and core (Fig. 17-33).

The divergence and curvature of the palatal root presents special problems of tooth preparation, restoration, and occlusal design. This single remaining root must be used in conjunction with another tooth or teeth, since it is usually not strong enough to function alone. The natural buccal curvature of the palatal root creates a severe undercut on its straight buccal surface relative to the preparation of adjacent teeth. A beveled shoulder preparation of the buccal surface of the palatal root is required to parallel it with adjacent teeth and allow preparation of the undercut margin. This naturally narrows the buccolingual width even further. The superstructure must necessarily be narrow buccolingually and placed exactly over the segment. Often this will place the occlusal table in a crossbite relationship to the mandibular occlusal table (Fig. 17-33, *E*). The final splint should resemble abutments over the adjacent teeth and a pontic type of casting over the retained root. Adequate mesial and distal embrasures must be created for cleanliness.

In certain cases the palatal root is retained with either the mesial or distal root, but the roots must be separated from each other. This might be due to periodontal disease or perforation of the chamber floor. The retained roots are treated as separate roots at the gingival margin with individual posts, tooth preparation, and embrasure form between them. Often they require telescopic copings for parallelism (Fig. 17-34, *A*), either to each other or the other teeth to which they will be splinted. The overcase may treat each root as a separate unit with individual form and occlusal morphology (Fig. 17-34, *B*), or the occlusal surface may be recontoured to resemble a single unit that would follow a root amputation.

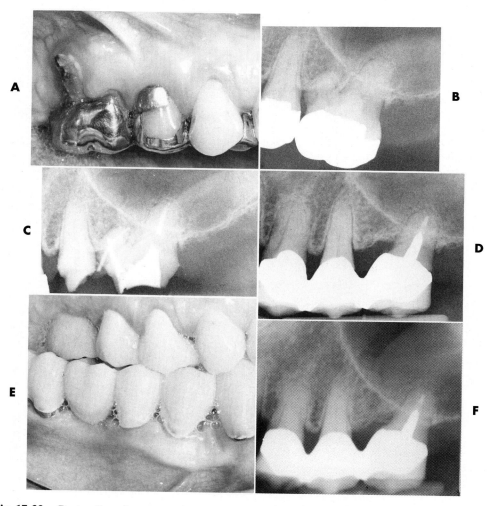

Fig. 17-33.   Restoration after amputation of both buccal roots. **A,** Preoperative view of maxillary first molar with dehiscence of distobuccal root. **B,** Preoperative radiograph. **C,** Distobuccal root removal. Attempt to save mesiobuccal root failed; gutta-percha point traces fistulous tract to apex of mesiobuccal root. Only the palatal root could be retained. **D,** Radiograph 6 years following placement of splint. **E,** Final restoration. Palatal root is contoured and placed in crossbite relationship to direct forces to the apex. **F,** Eight years after original treatment, area looks excellent, slight bone loss on mesial. (Clinical photographs are mirror shots and appear reversed.)

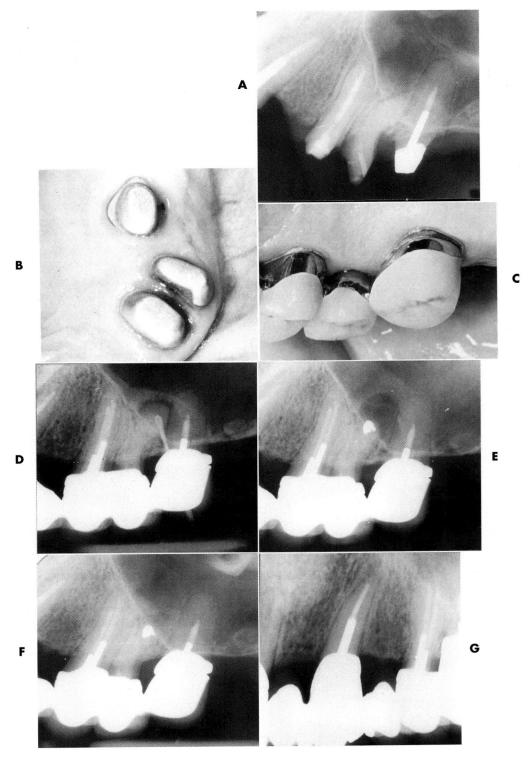

Fig. 17-34. For legend see opposite page.

Fig. 17-34.   Restoration of individual roots in a splinted case with periodontal conditions present. **A,** Radiograph of maxillary posterior area. An endodontically treated second bicuspid is present, but the adjacent molars both had severe periodontal defects. The distobuccal root of the second molar was hopeless periodontally, so that root was amputated. On the first molar, only the distobuccal root was salvageable. All of the amputations were performed by the periodontist during surgery, before the patient saw the endodontist. When opened by the endodontist, no canal could be located in the mesiobuccal root of the second molar, and the palatal canal stopped several millimeters short of the apex. Since the case was planned for copings, it was decided to keep the roots from the second molar until the endodontic condition worsened. **B,** Parallel telescopic copings were placed on the remaining roots, with posts in the distobuccal and palatal roots. **C,** Posterior segment of completed restoration over telescopic copings. Each root was treated as a separate tooth, with individual contour, considerable embrasure space for cleaning, and occlusal design. Note that the margins of the splint meet the copings at or above the gingival line. **D,** Three years later, a chronic draining sinus tract is noted, tracing to the apex of the mesiobuccal root of the second molar. Although the root tip appears to be within the maxillary sinus, unquestionably it is buccal to the sinus and surgery is relatively safe. **E,** Apical curettage, apicoectomy, and reverse filling with amalgam of the mesiobuccal root of the second molar. There was no communication with the sinus. **F,** Four years after surgery, 8 years after starting treatment, entire area looks excellent, bone level looks good around the amputations. Please note that the posterior abutment is a simulated molar tooth, with a mesiobuccal root (which really is a distobuccal root), a distobuccal root (which really is a mesiobuccal root), and a palatal root. **G,** Anterior segment of the splint. (Periodontics by Dr. Douglas Gorin, Chicago.)

OVERLAY DENTURE

In some terminal cases in which a few stray abutments remain in an arch where severe periodontal disease has been present and where fixed prosthesis is no longer a consideration, an overlay denture may be utilized. The repeated insertion and removal for the denture causes far less damage to the retained teeth than would a removable denture with clasps that were constantly moving the involved teeth.

There are many advantages to an overlay denture compared with a prosthesis for a completely edentulous patient. Just a few abutments, even with some support lost because of a periodontal disease, offer much improved retention to the denture. Teeth retain alveolar bone. In addition, by receptors in the periodontal structures, they provide proprioception to the patient for the prosthesis that has been shown to be superior to those fully supported by tissue only. Retaining the teeth prevents the loss of alveolar bone, which would resorb after extraction and reduce the basal bone for full denture support. Should any abutment reach the stage where lost support makes it a liability, it may be cut loose from the other teeth and extracted. The resultant space in the denture is filled by processing acrylic.

The importance of communication is essential when the restorative dentist and endodontist manage a patient with these problems. The endodontist should be aware of the plans for a final restoration. How much of the remaining tooth will be reduced in size, whether post space will be needed, and whether an intraradicular or root surface attachment will be used will guide the endodontist in the preparation of space for a post.

Often teeth to be used for overlay dentures have gone through considerable periodontal and previous restorative therapy. Knowing that the final restoration includes decoronalization of the tooth lets the endodontist decapitate the tooth in search of canals that may be extremely difficult if not impossible to find due to retreat of the original canal from previous trauma.

Recently implants have been utilized as abutments for overdentures instead of the few, stray, periodontally involved teeth, and several reports have indicated that they functioned quite well. Mericske-Stern compared studies that evaluated overdentures supported by teeth with those involving implants. She concluded that the implant studies indicated slightly better results, even though the length of time for their evaluation was shorter. Closer analysis of the data reveals some important considerations that were not addressed.

Mericske-Stern listed the later need for endodontic treatment to be a source of failure, which

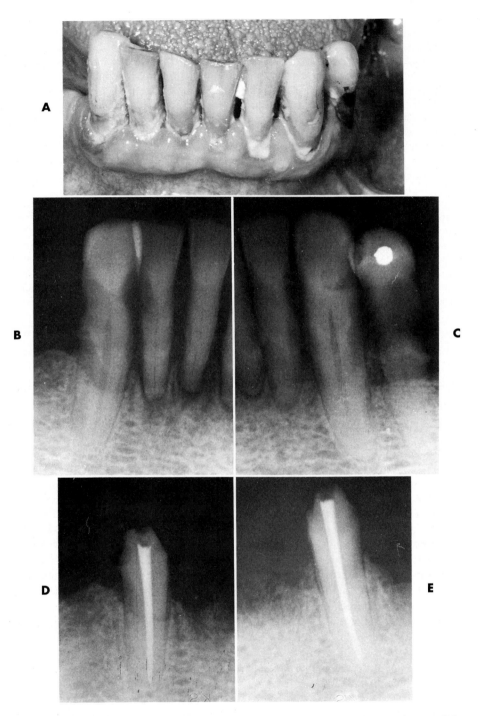

Fig. 17-35. Overdenture with minimum restoration of abutments. **A,** Preoperative condition of remaining mandibular teeth. **B** and **C,** Preoperative radiographs. **D** and **E,** Postoperative radiographs after endodontic treatment and closure of access preparations with composite. **F,** Abutment teeth after treatment. **G,** Dentures in place. **H,** Tissue side of overdenture. (Endodontic therapy by Dr. Edward Theiss, Boulder, Colo., and prosthetics by Dr. Hardy Ensing, formerly of Maywood, Ill.)

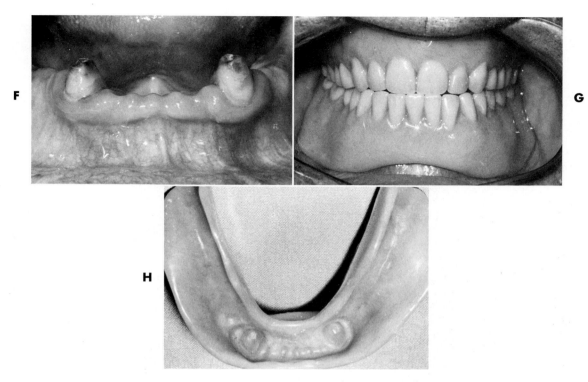

Fig. 17-35, cont'd.   For legend see opposite page.

should not be so. Many authors have suggested endodontic therapy for these teeth prior to prosthesis construction. Since the involved teeth generally are anteriors with severely reduced crown length, the endodontic treatment is quite simple, even if needed subsequently. The loss of the tooth (or the implant) is the failure that should be considered as crucial, and applying this factor to the statistics more than balances the results of these studies toward tooth retention, when possible.

We certainly agree that implants may be useful with overdentures, and, in cases where the abutments may be weak periodontally, they may be superior to the teeth available. However, if, in the opinion of the dentist, the potential abutments offer acceptable root length, number, and periodontal condition, they are preferable to implantation.

Minimum restoration of abutments.   There are many techniques available to utilize the remaining teeth to support the overlay denture. In the simplest form the teeth to be retained are reduced in height and treated endodontically, and the access

preparations are closed with amalgam or composite. The overdenture is fabricated in the routine manner (Fig. 17-35).

Restoration of abutments with telescopes. A much more complex method of building up the teeth to be retained involves the use of telescopes. After endodontic treatment the abutments are cut down, and small post and cores are fabricated. The smallness of the preparation and the post and core must be emphasized because these abutments must accommodate individual or splinted copings, which in turn will aid in the retention of a removable prosthesis. If remaining teeth are adjacent, additional stability may be gained by splinting these teeth with soldered copings. Because of the periodontal conditions that are generally present in these cases, the copings are fabricated over the cemented post and cores and soldered together in such a way as to allow for adequate embrasures. After cementation of the superstructures, the overdenture is constructed in the routine manner (Fig. 17-36).

Other techniques, such as those involving bars

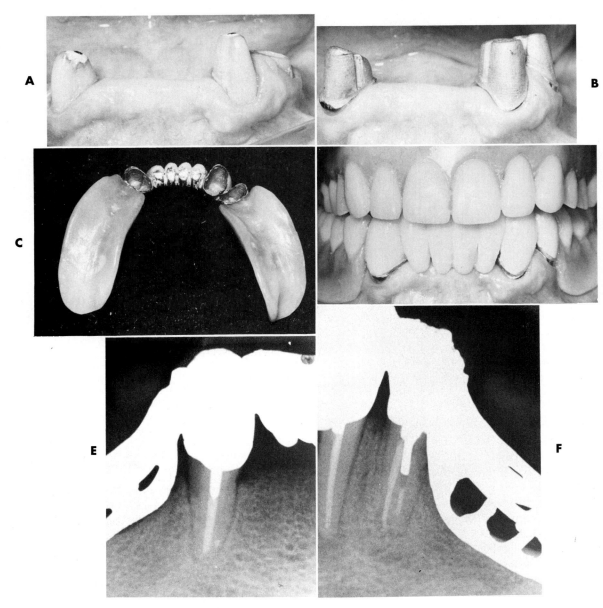

Fig. 17-36. Overdenture over parallel telescopic copings without anterior flange. **A,** Preoperative condition of remaining three mandibular teeth. **B,** Parallel telescopic copings in place. Grooves are placed to increase surface area and frictional retention to removable overcase. **C,** Tissue side of overdenture. Metal extension arms on which to process the posterior saddle areas are soldered to the anterior segment. **D,** Maxillary denture and mandibular overdenture in place. Elimination of anterior flange improves esthetics by reducing distortion of lower lip. **E** and **F,** Postoperative radiographs with posts, copings, and overcase in place. (Endodontic treatment by Charles Neach, Chicago.)

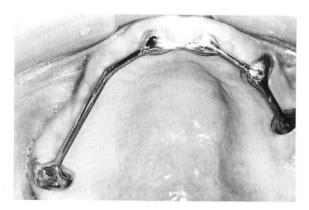

Fig. 17-37. Overdenture with bar and clip retainer. Preservation of five remaining teeth following endodontics, periodontics, and coping and bar placement. Overdenture fits over the coping and bar. Preservation of these roots maintained the alveolar bone to afford maxillary denture retention greater than with construction of a full denture or without the bar.

between remaining teeth or attachments directly into treated roots, may be used in these cases (Fig. 17-37). As long as teeth remain to prevent the loss of the precious alveolar bone, the prognosis for overdenture cases is much better than for the completely edentulous patient.

BLEACHING

Bleaching was not discussed in the first two editions of this textbook. However, in the third edition a section in this chapter was included with directions for bleaching endodontically involved teeth as well as those with stains and vital pulps. This was done to satisfy increased interest in the subject at that time.

Recently a number of papers have been published indicating the possible dangers of resorption following bleaching. For this reason, we do not believe that we can endorse and encourage bleaching at this time. It may be that the frequency of resorption following bleaching is so low that it has no true impact. If so, further investigations will clarify this situation and indicate predictability. Subsequent editions may include more information on the subject, but this current text does not.

REFERENCES

Abrams L, Trachtenberg D: Hemisection—technique and restoration, *Dent Clin North Am* 18:415, 1974.

Anusavice KJ, deRijk WG: Performance of dental biomaterials: conference report, *Dent Mater* 6:69, 1990.

Assif D, Bleicher S: Retention of serrated endodontic posts with a composite luting cement: effect of cement thickness, *J Prosthet Dent* 56:689, 1986.

Baraban DJ: The restoration of pulpless teeth, *Dent Clin North Am,* Nov. 1967, p. 633.

Brewer AA, Morrow RM: *Overdentures,* St Louis, 1975, Mosby.

Colley IT, Hampson EL, Lehman ML: Retention of post crowns, *Br Dent J* 124:63, 1968.

Cooney JP, Caputo AA, Trabert KC: Retention and stress distribution of tapered and endodontic posts, *J Prosthet Dent* 55:540, 1986.

DeSort KD: The prosthodontic use of endodontically treated teeth: theory and biomechanics of post preparation, *J Prosthet Dent* 49:203, 1983.

Frank AL: Protective coronal coverage of the pulpless tooth, *J Am Dent Assoc* 59:895, 1959.

Gelfand M, Goldman M, Sunderman EJ: Effect of complete veneer crowns on the compressive strength of endodontically treated posterior teeth, *J Prosthet Dent* 52:635, 1984.

Gerstein H, Burnell SC: Prefabricated precision dowels, *J Am Dent Assoc* 68:787, 1964.

Goerig AC, Mueningoff LA: Management of the endodontically treated tooth. I. Concept for restorative design, *J Prosthet Dent* 49:340, 1983.

Goldman M, DeVitre R, White R, Nathanson D: An SEM study of posts cemented with unfilled resin, *J Dent Res* 63:1003, 1984.

Goldman M, Devitre R, Tenca JI: A fresh look at the anatomy of the prepared post space, *Compend Contin Educ Dent* 6:628, 1985.

Gross MJ, Turner CH: Intraradicular hydrostatic pressure changes during the cementation of post-retained crowns, *J Oral Rehabil* 10:237, 1983.

Gutmann JI: Preparation of endodontically treated teeth to receive a post-core restoration, *J Prosthet Dent* 41:163, 1977.

Guzy GE, Nicholls JI: In vitro comparison of intact endodontically treated teeth with and without endo-post reinforcement, *J Prosthet Dent* 42:39, 1979.

Healey HJ: Coronal restoration of the treated pulpless tooth, *Dent Clin North Am,* Nov. 1957, p. 885.

Helfer AR, Melnick S, Schilder H: Determination of the moisture content of vital and pulpless teeth, *Oral Surg* 34:661, 1972.

Hoag PE, Dwyer TG: A comparative evaluation of three post and core techniques, *J Prosthet Dent* 47:177, 1982.

Johnson JK, Sakumura JS: Dowel form and tensile force, *J Prosthet Dent* 40:645, 1978.

Kayser AF, Leempoel JB, Snoek PA: The metal post and composite core combination, *J Oral Rehabil* 14:3, 1987.

Krupp JD, Caputo AA, Trabert KC, Standlee JP: Dowel retention with glass-ionomer cement, *J Prosthet Dent* 41:163, 1979.

Kurer HG, Combe EC, Grant AA: Factors influencing the retention of dowels, *J Prosthet Dent* 38:515, 1977.

Lloyd PM: Fixed prosthodontics and esthetic considerations for the older adult, *J Prosthet Dent* 72:525, 1994.

Lloyd PM, Palik JF: The philosophies of dowel diameter preparation: a literature review, *J Prosthet Dent* 69:32, 1993.

Mericske-Stern R: Overdentures with roots or implants for elderly patients: a comparison, *J Prosthet Dent* 72:543, 1994.

Mericske-Stern R, Wedig A, Hofman J, Geering AH: In vivo measurements of maximal bite force and minimal pressure threshold on overdentures supported by implants or natural teeth: a comparative study, part I, *Int J Oral Maxillofac Implants* 8:641, 1993.

Montgomery S: External cervical resorption after bleaching a pulpless tooth, *Oral Surg* 57:203, 1984.

Mosen PJ, Nichols JI, VanHassel HJ: An in vitro comparison of retention between a hollow post and core and a solid post and core, *J Endod* 10:91, 1984.

Musikant BL, Deutsch AS: A new prefabricated post and core system, *J Prosthet Dent* 52:631, 1984.

Portell FR, et al: The effect of immediate versus delayed dowel space preparation on the integrity of the apical seal, *J Endod* 8:154, 1982.

Preiskel HW: Precision attachments in dentistry, ed 3, St Louis, 1979, Mosby.

Rosen H, Gitnick PJ: Separation and splinting of the roots of multirooted teeth, *J Prosthet Dent* 21:34, 1969.

Ruemping DR, Lund MR, Schnell RJ: Retention of dowels subjected to tensile and torsional forces, *J Prosthet Dent* 41:159, 1979.

Sorensen JA, Martinoff JT: Clinically significant factors in dowel design, *J Prosthet Dent* 52:28, 1984.

Sorensen JA, Martinoff JT: Intracoronal reinforcement of coronal coverage: a study of endodontically treated teeth, *J Prosthet Dent* 51:780, 1984.

Sorensen JA, Martinoff JT: Endodontically treated teeth as abutments, *J Prosthet Dent* 53:631, 1985.

Standlee JP, Caputo AA, Hanson EC: Retention of endodontic dowels: effect of cement, dowel length, diameter, and design, *J Prosthet Dent* 39:401, 1978.

Standlee JP, Caputo AA, Holcomb JP: The Dentatus screw: comparative stress analysis with other endodontic dowel designs, *J Oral Rehabil* 9:23, 1982.

Standlee JP, Caputo AA, Holcomb J, Trabert KC: The retentive and stress-distributing properties of a threaded endodontic dowel, *J Prosthet Dent* 44:398, 1980.

Standlee JP et al: Analysis of stress distribution of endodontic posts, *Oral Surg* 33:952, 1972.

Weine FS, Wax AH, Wenckus CS: Retrospective study of tapered, smooth post systems in place for 10 years or more, *J Endod* 17:293, 1991.

Weine FS et al: The use of the standardized tapered plastic pins in post and core fabrication, *J Prosthet Dent* 29:542, 1973.

Yalisov IL: Crown and sleeve retainers for removable partial prostheses, *J Prosthet Dent* 16:1069, 1966.

Zamikoff II: Overdentures—theory and technique, *J Am Dent Assoc* 86:853, 1973.

18 Endodontics following complex restorative procedures

As indicated in Chapter 2, endodontic therapy should be completed whenever possible prior to restorative efforts. This concept is well accepted, with near unanimous agreement, but what happens when pulpal or periapical disease signs or symptoms appear after the completion of complex restorations? Then the horse comes after the cart, and some serious problems may result. When one considers the trauma that a healthy pulp must absorb during the course of some complicated procedures—overheating of teeth, impressions and bite registration, temporization, cementations, time in splints, permanent cementation, and adjustments—it probably is a minor miracle that the need for endodontics later is a rare entity.

This chapter will discuss some of the problems that may occur when the need for endodontics is discovered after the completion of complex restorative procedures and the appropriate solutions.

PREVENTING POSTRECONSTRUCTIVE PROBLEMS PRIOR TO RECONSTRUCTION

Some of the problems that occur from an endodontic viewpoint after reconstruction could have been prevented if certain steps had been taken earlier in the treatment plan.

Utilize the pulp canal space to retain the post. When little or no coronal tooth structure remains, it is better to introduce an endodontic procedure than attempt to avoid the pulp with pins, exotic buildups, or compromised use of abutments (Figs. 16-6 and 16-7, *A*). If this is done, the pulp canal space is available for use of a post, and the entire procedure goes more smoothly. It is much easier to treat the tooth without a complicated casting to penetrate than after the reconstruction is in place.

Avoid vital pulp therapy for abutments. As stated in Chapter 16, the percentage of success with vital pulp therapy is much lower than with routine endodontic therapy. When a tooth has a minimal pulp exposure without previous history of symptoms, the temptation to pulp cap is present. However, if the tooth involved is an abutment for a bridge, partial, or splint, it is probably better to invest in the greater effort required by complete endodontics.

If the pulp capping had been successful, all would be fine; but what if the capping has resulted in failure? Now the casting must be penetrated, and thus weakened, to make the access cavity preparation. It may be much more difficult to locate the canals; if calcium hydroxide or a corticosteroid has been used as a capping agent, the canals may have become partially obliterated with reparative dentin. A potential failure is imminent in these conditions.

Again, it is simply more predictable to go ahead with the endodontics in the first place.

Recognize the potential endodontic-periodontal relationships. As stated in Chapter 13, some percentage of teeth with advanced periodontal involvement also have a pulpal problem as well. This is true even if the tooth responds to an electric pulp tester or to thermal stimulation, because a vital pulp does not guarantee pulpal normalcy.

The etiologic agent for many reconstructions is moderate to advanced periodontal disease. The abutment teeth in these cases already have some periodontal damage and thus at least some possibility of pulpal damage. Such cases will probably require initial preparation, temporary stabilization, advanced periodontal procedures, repreparation, impressions, retemporization, casting try-ins, and final cementation. All these procedures—necessary as they are—may cause additional pulpal damage (Fig. 18-1). Everything considered, it is surprising that more teeth involved in periodontal reconstructions do not require endodontic treatment.

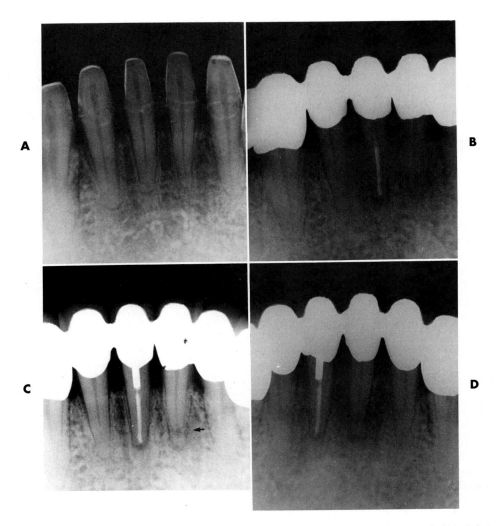

Fig. 18-1. **A,** Radiograph of mandibular anterior teeth after temporization prior to periodontal therapy. Moderate bone loss was present, and periodontist recommended that endodontic therapy be carried out on incisors prior to final reconstruction. Restorative dentist disagreed, and castings were seated. **B,** Less than 1 year later, one central incisor developed a periapical area and required endodontic treatment. **C,** Three months later, treated central was healing and post had been placed. However, adjacent central seemed to be developing an area several millimeters from the apex *(arrow)*, and periapical sensitivity was present. **D,** Three additional months later, the periapical area was definite and treatment was undertaken. **E,** One year later, areas healing well. However, splint was weakened during therapy, and some sensitivity was present in the area. **F,** Eighteen additional months later, and 4 years after original treatment, areas on treated teeth have healed perfectly. However, transient sensitivity is still present, and further therapy is anticipated.

Therefore, in evaluating teeth prior to final preparation, recognize the incipient symptoms of pulpal inflammation and undertake proper therapy. Typical of these symptoms are diminished pulp canal space, temperature sensitivities that do not decrease markedly after periodontal treatment, episodes of relatively brief but nevertheless intense pain, and persistence of periodontal defects following seemingly correct treatment. If any of these conditions are present, judicious use of endodontic therapy will greatly enhance the long-term result.

Be certain to re-treat endodontic failures and potential failures prior to reconstruction. When an endodontic case is obviously failing (Fig. 18-2), there should be no question as to the need for re-treatment prior to completion of the entire recon-

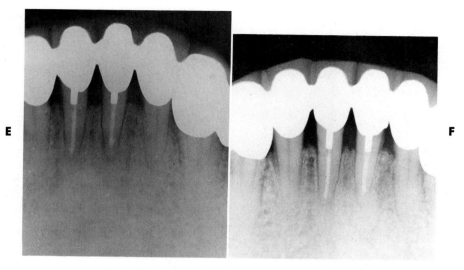

Fig. 18-1, cont'd.   For legend see opposite page.

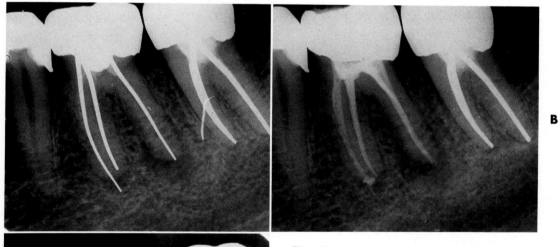

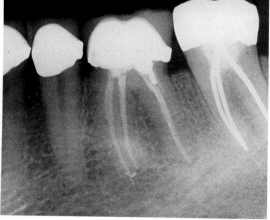

Fig. 18-2.   A, Radiograph of mandibular molars whose canals had been filled with silver points approximately 3 years earlier. Both teeth had had vital exposures then. Second molar was fine and was left alone. First molar was in need of re-treatment prior to the remaking of multiple posterior porcelain-fused-to-gold crowns. **B,** Silver points were removed, and canals reprepared and filled with laterally condensed gutta-percha. Overfill of mesiolingual canal was due to severe overextension of the silver point. **C,** One year later, periapical lesions on both roots had healed well. Second molar continued to present normal appearance. (Restorations by Dr. Rod Nystul, formerly of Park Ridge, Ill.)

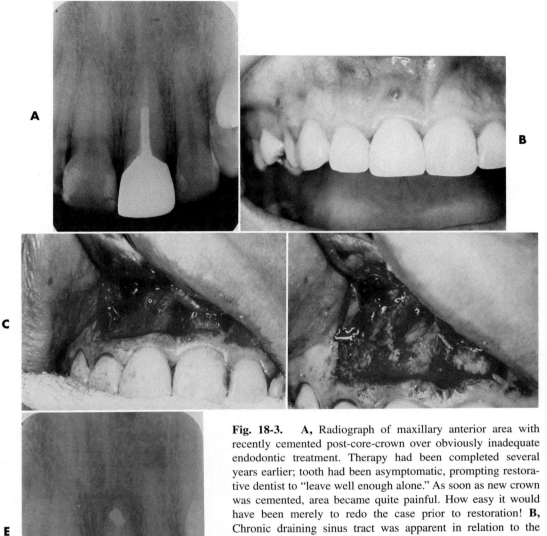

Fig. 18-3. **A,** Radiograph of maxillary anterior area with recently cemented post-core-crown over obviously inadequate endodontic treatment. Therapy had been completed several years earlier; tooth had been asymptomatic, prompting restorative dentist to "leave well enough alone." As soon as new crown was cemented, area became quite painful. How easy it would have been merely to redo the case prior to restoration! **B,** Chronic draining sinus tract was apparent in relation to the tooth. Crown was quite esthetic. **C,** Flap raised for surgery was of the Oschenbein-Luebke type to try to keep marginal gingiva intact. **D,** Root was beveled deeply because I feared a possible perforation during post preparation. Lesion was entirely at apex, however, and an apical amalgam was placed after curettage. **E,** Postoperative radiograph.

struction. However, when a poor endodontic result is found even without radiographic or clinical symptoms, strong considerations to early re-treatment should be given. Those inadequately treated cases may become symptomatic after the final cementation is made, and thus the case becomes extremely complicated. How much better it would have been merely to re-treat the tooth initially, verify that the canal was well cleansed and well filled, make adequate post room, and restore. I have seen a number of teeth with inadequate endodontics that had been asymptomatic suddenly blow up after cementation of a casting. Then the necessary procedure often becomes surgical (Fig. 18-3), with the attendant discomfort and trauma that the procedure induces.

SOLVING PROBLEMS IN POSTRECONSTRUCTIVE ENDODONTICS

Difficulty in diagnosis on postreconstructive cases. Because of the large restorations present in postreconstructive cases, carious lesions often do not show up on radiographs until they are quite deep and in proximity to the pulp. This is certainly a disadvantage of crowns and large onlays. Determining the need for endodontic treatment after reconstruction that is apparent by radiograph in the form of deep caries or a periapical lesion offers no great problem in diagnosis. However, diagnosis of the etiology of pain after completion of a complex restorative case often is quite difficult. It is common for temperature sensitivity (usually to cold) to occur after placing a casting, and, if multiple castings are placed, a single tooth that is more sensitive may cause considerable difficulty in location. Even if the sensitivity becomes severe, as long as it remains bearable, there is the tendency to want to wait out the discomfort rather than drill into a new crown or onlay. The dentist hopes that the pain will diminish or fears that the incorrect abutment might be entered when seeking relief.

Determiniation of pulp vitality, as discussed in Chapter 2, is more complex for highly restored teeth than for teeth with minimal or no restoration. False negatives may be obtained because considerable reparative dentin was laid down, electrical tests may not be applicable with full coverage, and deep bases may keep the teeth insulated from the stimulus. False positives may be reported by nervous patients or, when using temperature tests, if hot or cold strikes an adjacent, more responsive tooth by accident.

Usually, the best action in these cases when the offending tooth cannot be identified positively is inaction. Eventually the tooth requiring treatment will become more painful and will be directly discernible, or the tooth will start to lose vitality and lapse into painlessness for a while until a positive symptom occurs in the form of a periapical lesion, a chronic draining sinus tract, acute tenderness to percussion, or swelling. If decay is present, it will increase in size sufficiently so that it will be seen beneath the radiopaque restorative metal (Fig. 18-4). At that time the culprit is easily identified, and the correct treatment may be instituted. Now there will be no fear of starting an incorrect tooth, and the patient usually appreciates the dentist's conservative attitude.

Be aware of pulpal damage indicated by lateral canals. Since carious lesions may become quite deep and not be seen easily in radiographs following placement of extensive restorations, a careful diagnostician must use other factors for evaluation of pulpal or periapical damage in these cases. A valuable indicator may be present as hints of lateral canal lesions.

Lateral sinus tracts may be present associated with endodontic or periodontal lesions (see Chapter 13). Fig. 13-8 indicates a mandibular cuspid/ bicuspid area with an interproximal defect that was of periodontal origin on a patient with other sites of periodontal breakdown. However, the patient illustrated in Fig. 18-5 did not have any appreciable periodontal problems. She came to my office with soreness between the cuspid and adjacent lateral incisor. It was not possible to determine the vitality of the cuspid, although the lateral was responsive to temperature tests. The soreness diminished in several days, but several weeks later, she reported the presence of a sinus tract (Fig. 18-5, B). Another radiograph, just a month later (Fig. 18-5, C) indicated the presence of a periapical and a lateral lesion. Even though the lateral lesion was above midroot, it was the type generally associated with a lateral canal. The sinus tract healed immediately following the appointment for canal preparation, and the filling film verified the presence of the lateral canal.

Fig. 13-10 demonstrates another type of lateral canal lesion. The patient was referred for treatment of the mandibular second bicuspid with an obvious periapical lesion. Examination indicated that she had several sites of periodontal breakdown. The tooth in question was quite

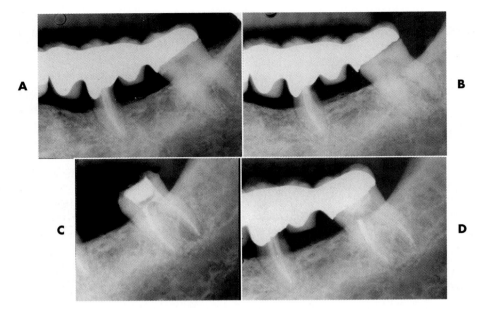

Fig. 18-4. **A,** Well-constructed complicated splint has been present for 4 years in posterior mandibular area, with anterior abutments being bicuspids (not shown), mesial root of second molar as a pier abutment, and third molar as posterior abutment. Patient now has recurring pain in the area, sometimes sensitive to temperatures, sometimes to pressure, but never seemingly in the exact same place. In this radiograph both teeth seem normal, no periapical lesions or signs of decay (same true of bicuspids). The pain was transitory and bearable, so the patient was encouraged to continue the status quo. Radiographs were taken for several 3-month periods without change. **B,** One year later, radiograph of third molar indicates decay on distal beneath the crown and a small periapical lesion associated with the distal root. The splint was removed and decay was found on the third molar, exposing the pulp. **C,** Endodontic therapy was completed. Discomfort vanished immediately after the appointment for canal preparation. **D,** One year later, the periapical lesion has healed following endodontic treatment, the decay was removed, and the bridge refitted. (Restorations by Dr. Kerry Voit, Chicago.)

Fig. 18-5. Pulpal damage indicated by lateral canal lesion. **A,** Mandibular cuspid and bicuspid area of patient with soreness and a small swelling between the cuspid and adjacent lateral incisor. The patient was advised to wait until further symptoms developed. No periodontal disease was identified for this patient. **B,** Two weeks later, she returned and a chronic draining sinus tract was present, draining from the mesial surface of the cuspid, indicated by a gutta-percha cone tracing. No more pain was present, and she was scheduled for appointments to begin several weeks later. **C,** At that time, another radiograph was taken which indicated a periapical and lateral *(arrow)* lesion. **D,** Canal filling with laterally condensed gutta-percha and Wach's paste, with puff of sealer exactly to the site of the lateral canal lesion. **E,** One year later, periapical lesion is healed.

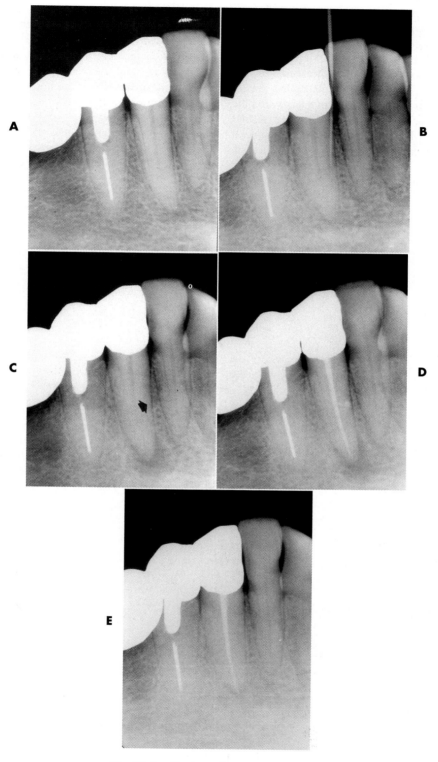

Fig. 18-5.   For legend see opposite page.

mobile, more than expected with the degree of bone loss present (Fig. 13-10, *A*). The treatment plan was to treat the tooth endodontically and then periodontally.

After the appointment for canal preparation, the tooth tightened remarkably. When filled, sealer exited exactly to the periodontal breakdown on the distal (Fig. 13-10, *B*). Evidently the periodontal pocket on the distal had opened up the lateral canal and caused a pulpal exposure at that site. Conceivably, the crown and restorative efforts did not cause the injury to the pulp. A follow-up film (Fig. 13-10, *C*) indicated advanced healing and a relatively tight tooth.

Problems related to locating canals. One of the most serious obstacles in treating teeth after complicated restorative procedures is the difficulty involved in locating canals. The castings on the teeth often have no relationship whatever to the roots beneath and therefore not only give no clue to the location of the canals but may, in fact, give false and misleading clues.

I strongly recommend that initial entry into any splint or bridge abutment be performed with no rubber dam in place (Fig. 18-6, *B*). Then, once the roof of the chamber has been penetrated or one canal located, the dam may be applied. The degree of canal contamination that results will still be quite

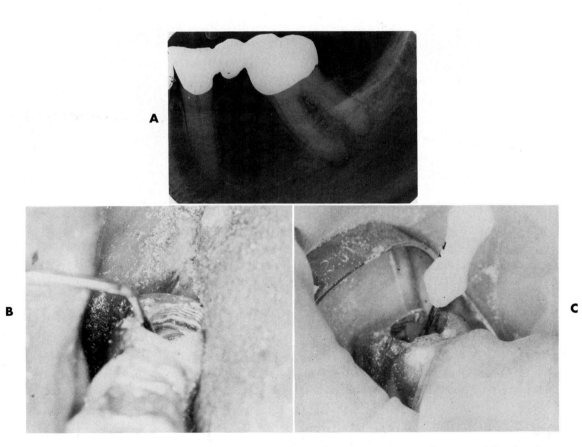

Fig. 18-6. **A,** Radiograph of mandibular posterior area in need of endodontics on mesially tipped second molar, a posterior bridge abutment. **B,** Initial entry is made without rubber dam in place so as to have maximum area of visualization, unobstructed by the dam. Crown of tooth itself gives little clue to underlying anatomy. **C,** After one canal is located, dam is placed and a file inserted into that canal. **D,** Radiograph indicates that canal located is the distal. Radiopaque flash is grindings from gold casting. **E,** Now that I am certain what canal I am in, it is a simple matter to open up toward the mesial and locate another canal. **F,** This is verified to be the mesiolingual. **G,** The mesiobuccal is also verified. Exact lengths are not significant at this point, merely canal location and identification.

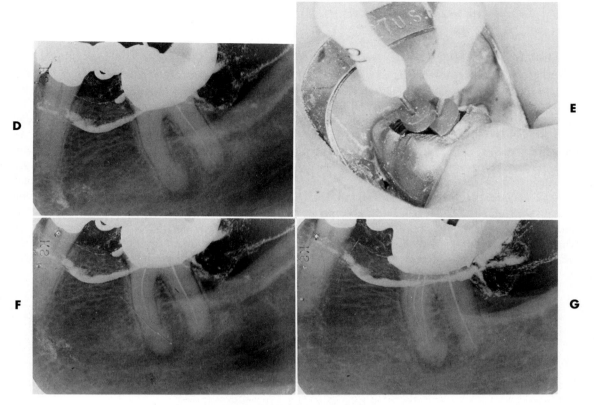

Fig. 18-6, cont'd. For legend see opposite page.

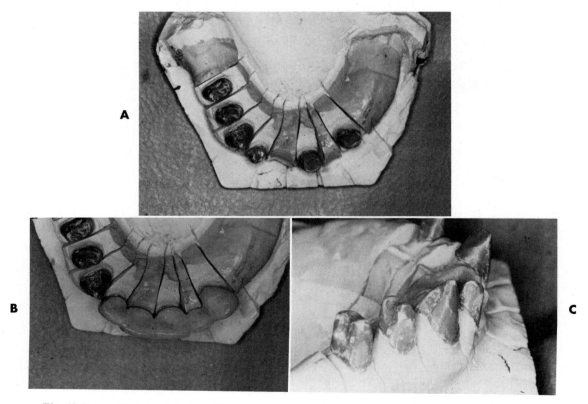

Fig. 18-7. **A,** Study model of maxillary teeth of reconstructed case completed several years earlier. **B,** Anterior temporary splint worn while the patient was originally treated is kept over abutments and stored. **C,** First bicuspid and cuspid now require endodontic therapy. Examining the model aids in access cavity preparation.

minimal and surely will be strongly reduced by the irrigation and canal preparation that soon follow.

Aid in location of canals may be gained from the study and intratreatment models used during the construction the castings (Fig. 18-7, *A*). These may be stored in boxes and used to hold the temporary splints. If a facing cracks or chips from the final reconstruction and requires removal and reglazing of the splint, the temporary thus retained may be used as an interim replacement (Fig. 18-7, *B*). Careful examination of the preparation on the stone model (Fig. 18-7, *C*) will show where the greater amounts of tooth structure are present and where the deeper portions of the

preparation have been made. These observations greatly aid in determining access cavity preparations and areas to avoid when going through the castings.

Attempting to locate narrow canals in tipped and rotated teeth is very hazardous (Fig. 18-8, *A*). Even careful attempts may result in perforations into the lateral periodontal spaces (Fig. 18-8, *B*). The correct procedure in these last-ditch efforts is to scribe a line on the radiograph with a felt-tip pen to correspond to the directional axis of the canal extended through the crown (Fig. 18-8, *B*). This film is held just labial to the tooth, and the felt-tip pen is used to transfer this line to the tooth

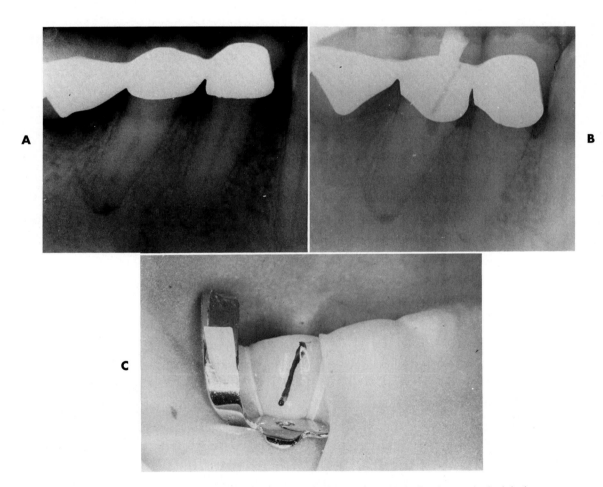

Fig. 18-8. Mandibular bicuspid area. **A,** Preoperative radiograph indicating periapical lesion on mesially tipped second bicuspid with an extremely receded canal. **B,** After two appointments, no canal had been located. Radiograph was taken and showed that access was too far to mesial and about to perforate. A line made on radiograph with a felt-tip pen indicates correct axial inclination of the canal. **C,** When the radiograph is held over labial surface of the tooth, this line is transferred to facing of the crown. Handpiece held to coincide with this line should locate the canal.

itself. (Fig. 18-8, *C*). A razor blade, or bur, may be used to cut out the line on the film, and then the pen just goes through this slot onto the tooth, in the precisely correct angulation. Once this directional aid is apparent on the crown, the long-shank bur in the handpiece may locate the canal (Fig. 18-8, *D*). Obviously this method may lead to perforation in either the buccal or the lingual direction, but at least the mesiodistal angulation will be correct. With this aid the tooth may be completed uneventfully (Fig. 18-8, *E* and *F*).

Problems in identifying canals. When working through complicated bridges and splints, you can never be certain—even when you find a canal in a posterior tooth—which canal you are in. A maxillary bicuspid may be in severe lingual ver-

sion prior to reconstruction. However, the crown inserted puts all the teeth in that area in seemingly correct alignment. If you locate a canal that is toward the palatal, you might assume that you must prepare to the buccal to locate the other canal. However, further preparation will lead to perforation.

One must understand that the casting on a tooth may have minimal relationship to the structures beneath it. The laboratory technician making the casting has no knowledge of the interior anatomy of the tooth in the model being worked upon. Sometimes it seems that the main function of the crown on the restored, capped tooth is to confuse the operator searching for canals should the tooth require endodontics.

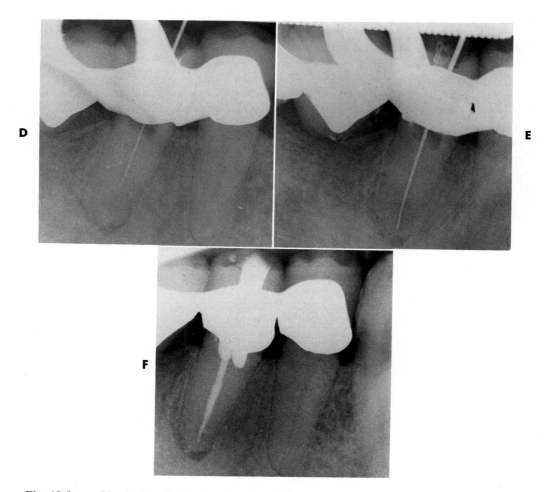

Fig. 18-8, cont'd. **D,** By altering the direction of the access cavity, the dentist is able to find the canal. Note file within canal confines. **E,** Exact determination of working length. **F,** Conclusion of treatment.

Canals *MUST* be located one at a time, as demonstrated in Fig. 18-6. In these cases, until one canal is positively identified, attempting to locate another is absolutely fraught with danger. In many cases, I have located what I thought was the mesiobuccal canal of a maxillary molar, only to find that after radiographic identification I had located the distobuccal. Similarly, in mandibular molars it might be assumed that the orifice to one particular mesial canal had been entered, but later it is identified to be the other mesial canal. In tipped abutments, as seen in Fig. 18-6, *A*, it might be the distal located when it was assumed to be one of the mesial canals.

Tipped mandibular molars also may make identification complicated (Fig. 18-6). When one canal has been located, apply the rubber dam, insert a file in that canal (Fig. 18-6, *C*), and take a radiograph (Fig. 18-6, *D*). If this canal is found to be a mesial, then go to the distal. If it is a distal, open up to the mesial and locate another canal (Fig. 18-6, *E*), verifying this by radiograph (Fig. 18-6, *F*) prior to going to the third (Fig. 18-6, *G*).

In maxillary molars similar procedures are followed. Attempt to locate the largest canal (i.e., the palatal) so that it can lead you to the buccals, which are more difficult to uncover. Once one buccal canal has been located, identify it by taking a film with files in the palatal and the discovered buccal canals. Do not attempt to locate the other buccal until a positive identification is made for the canal already found.

Even in maxillary biscupids, canal identification might cause a problem through a splinted abutment (Fig. 18-9). The proper procedure is to attempt to uncover one canal. When this is accomplished, put a file in that canal and take an angled radiograph (Fig. 18-9, *C*). Do not even attempt to assume which canal has been located without radiographic verification. Once one canal has been identified positively, the correct direction for preparation to locate the other canal becomes obvious (Fig. 18-9, *D*). The case then becomes much easier (Figs. 18-9, *E* and *F*).

When working through abutments for precision cases, understand that the crown is much bulkier to allow for the insertion of the male attachment. This means that the access cavity probably should be made mesiodistally wider than normal (Fig. 18-10).

Problems related to sheared crowns. Single crowns of a reconstructed case may shear off at or near the gingival margin, often without a pulp exposure. Attempting to recement these members, with virtually no supragingival tooth structure, is next to impossible. Attempts to avoid the pulp with pin buildups usually will cause perforation into the pulp or the periodontal ligament (Fig. 16-6).

It is much better to perform a one-sitting endodontic treatment for the tooth. Post room is made and an Endopost is fit that will utilize most of the room in the root yet fit within the confines of the crown. The coronal portion of the post is bent for additional retention, and the crown is filled with quick-cure acrylic and reinserted over the post. After initial set the crown-post is removed and may be recemented as a temporary while a new crown is constructed. Fig. 19-4 illustrates such a case.

Problems related to bombed abutments. Attempting to perform endodontic therapy through bombed abutments rather than removing the superstructure almost always leads to disaster (Fig. 18-11). It is much better to remove the existing splint or bridge, commit yourself to remaking the prosthesis, and perform the endodontics in the most desirable manner. Even if the canals could be properly located in Fig. 18-11, they would become badly contaminated during treatment and surely cause a painful episode after the filling appointment.

Once it has been established that the prosthesis over a bombed abutment will be remade (Fig. 18-12, *A*), cut the splint between the tooth to be treated and the next natural tooth rather than leave a pontic as cantilever. Remove the decay and uncover the canals. Some slight peripheral decay may remain to help retain the rubber dam clamp (Fig. 18-12, *B*). Then measure and debride the canals.

Temporization between appointments is always a problem in these cases. Attempts to place cotton pellets with or without medication will not leave sufficient bulk for the zinc oxide–eugenol (ZOE) cement. However, if something is not placed over the orifices, the cement may clog the canal and block access to the apices. The solution to this problem is to place short, blunted paper points in each orifice, extending for approximately half the distance to the apex. Medication may be placed on the points if you wish (Fig. 18-12, *C*). Then the entire access is closed with ZOE (Fig. 18-12, *D*).

At the next appointment, carefully trim the ZOE and remove each paper point by ensnaring with a broach. Do not irrigate until the points have been removed; the liquid will cause the points to swell and make removal very complicated. The treatment is complicated as with any other typical case (Fig. 18-12, *E* and *F*).

Text continued on p. 821.

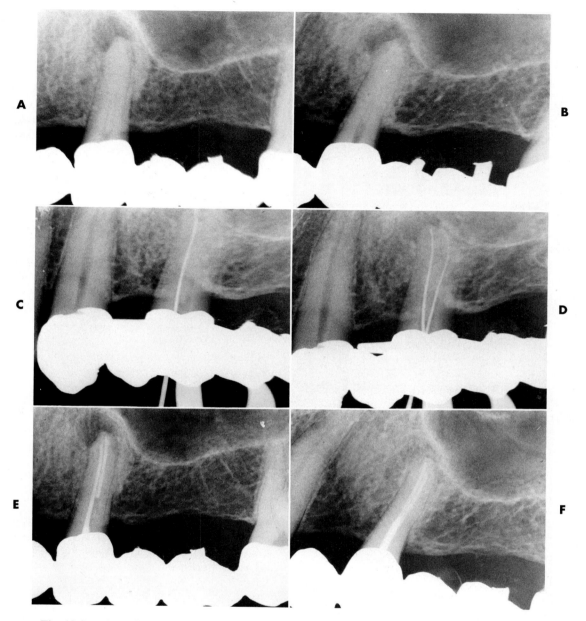

Fig. 18-9.   **A** and **B,** Preoperative radiographs taken from straight and angled positions of maxillary second bicuspid acting as pier abutment, with periapical area and necrotic pulp. Two canals and two roots seem to be present. The restored crown of pier abutments rarely resembles the original preparation crown shape, and determination of canal relationship is very difficult. **C,** I opened up a fairly wide buccopalatal access and located one canal that seemed to be more toward the buccal portion of the tooth, but I was unsure which canal I had found. Accordingly, I took a sharply angled view from the mesial with a file in the located canal. Determination of length was unimportant; only canal identification was significant. Since the view was from the mesial, the canal with the file is obviously the palatal. Had I assumed the located canal to be the buccal, further preparation to the palatal would have led to a perforation. **D,** Angled view after location of the other canal to determine working length. **E,** Canals filled with gutta-percha and post room prepared. **F,** Two years later, periapical lesion has healed and bridge remains functional according to this angled view. (Restorations by Dr. Joseph Krohn, Chicago.)

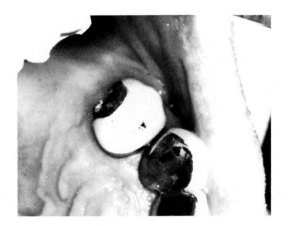

Fig. 18-10. When a crown is used as an abutment for a precision attachment, it must be assumed that the crown is wider than normal mesiodistally to allow for the keyway. Consequently, endodontic treatment of such teeth requires a larger access preparation than routine, as demonstrated on this maxillary first bicuspid.

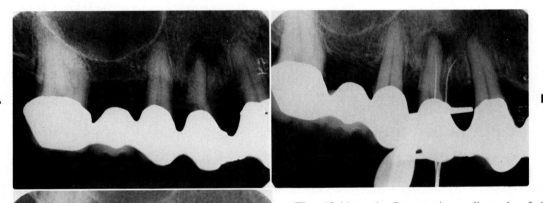

Fig. 18-11. **A,** Preoperative radiograph of first bicuspid with periapical lesions, but there is recurrent decay on both mesial and distal areas. Referring dentist insisted that tooth could be treated through the splint. **B** and **C,** Straight and angled films of files in place indicate perforations in attempts to locate the canals.

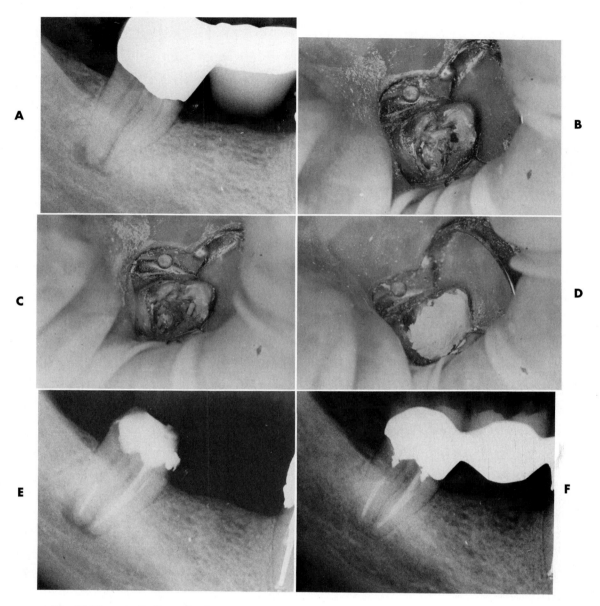

Fig. 18-12.   A, Radiograph of mandibular second molar, posterior bridge abutment, with recurrent decay at the distal and buccal involving the pulp; periapical lesion also present. Referring dentist agreed to remove the crown, cutting the bridge at the distal of the next anterior abutment. **B,** Coronal portion of the tooth has decay removed and canals located (mesial is to *left*). There is very little room for placement of a cotton pellet. **C,** Short paper points are placed into orifices of canals to keep them patent. **D,** ZOE is used to close the preparation. **E,** Completion of treatment, with post room made in both distal and mesiobuccal canals. **F,** Two years later, complete healing of periapical lesion and new bridge in place. Radiolucency on mesial near crown is cervical radiolucency and not new area of decay. (Restoration by Dr. Maury Falstein, formerly of Chicago.)

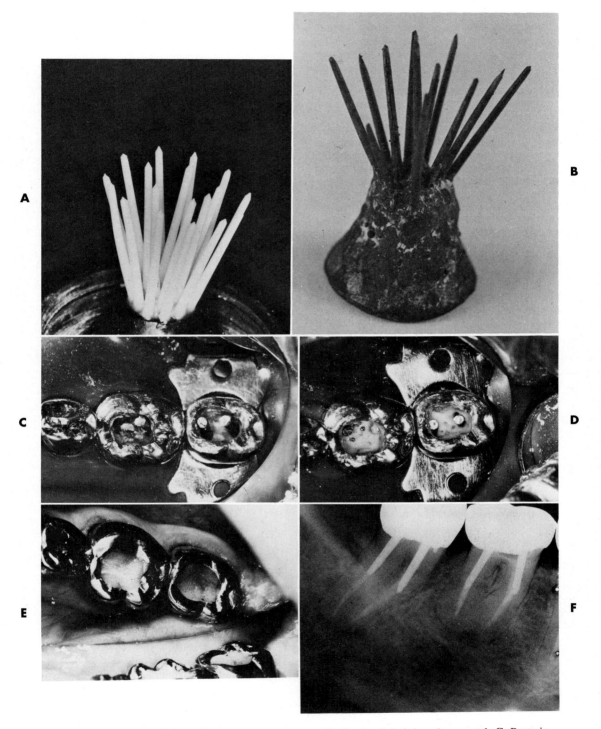

Fig. 18-13. **A,** Endowels sprued prior to investment. **B,** Casting in semiprecious metal. **C,** Posts in preparations. **D,** Durelon is placed in canals and access cavity around castings. **E,** Restorations completed. **F,** Final radiograph. (Courtesy Dr. Scott B. Schellhammer, Canton, Ohio.)

Problems related to coronoradicular stabilization. When the abutment to be treated is not bombed, the objective of both the endodontist and the restorative dentist should be to retain the casting and merely repair the damage made in the access cavity opening. However, when only the occlusal (or lingual) is merely refilled, there is no stabilization developed between the crown and root. When possible, coronoradicular stabilization is a positive and desirable objective because it prevents fracturing of the crown off the root and distributes occlusal forces through the root to the alveolar bone.

Such stabilization may be gained by placing a premade or precast post or screw in the coronal portion of the root canal space and then filling up the remainder of the access with a suitable restorative material.

An easy-to-use and inexpensive method involves the plastic Endowels. (See Chapter 17.) After the completion of endodontic therapy, post room is prepared. In molar teeth room should be made in more than one canal (i.e., the distal and mesiolingual of the mandibular and the palatal and distobuccal of the maxillary). The preparation need not be quite as deep as in a routine case but should reach into the middle third of the root. As in a routine case, the width is made to at least size 80 in the smaller canals and to 100 in the larger canals.

A supply of Endowels should be available cast in semiprecious metal (Fig. 18-13, *A* and *B*). As compared to the price of Endoposts and other preformed posts, the cost of these is quite low; but they are extremely versatile and useful in this situation. A mix of Durelon is prepared, to which is added blue food color. The cast posts are placed in the canals (Fig. 18-13, *C*) and the prepared mix is inserted to fill the access to the occlusal (Fig. 18-13, *D*). Were the food color not used, it would be impossible to distinguish between the Durelon and the dentin of the tooth at a later date should any of the work need to be redone. As it is, the tint of the food color is quite sufficient to make the distinction. The occlusals are polished (Fig. 18-13, *E*) and the case completed (Fig. 18-13, *F*). An otherwise complicated and costly procedure is quickly and relatively inexpensively accomplished.

19 Endodontic timetables

Successful endodontic therapy requires that a pre-determined plan of treatment be carefully followed. As in most dental techniques, to reach the desired goal one step must follow another in a pre-arranged sequence. This chapter will propose definite step-by-step procedures to be followed for the treatment of single-canaled, bicanaled, and molar teeth (Tables 19-1 to 19-3). A separate timetable for the treatment of teeth that have been left open at some time is included (Table 19-4), since this differs from the other situations.

References for the steps of treatment. Each step of treatment is indicated in the tables, together with the correct timing for its performance. When further information is needed to clarify any phase, the appropriate portion in this text should be consulted. For this reason, pertinent chapter numbers are indicated in the timetables adjacent to each step of treatment.

Need for having predetermined objectives. It is important to have a blueprint to follow to accomplish a definite amount of work at each appoint-

Table 19-1. Timetable for treating teeth with one canal

Treatment (chapter reference)	First appointment (steps)	Second appointment (steps)
Diagnosis and treatment plan (2)	1	
Administer anesthetic, if needed* (6)	2	1
Initial access	3	
Apply rubber dam	4	2
Complete access (6)	5	
Intracanal treatment procedures (7)		
Irrigate canal	6	4
Broach canal	7	
Establish length	8	
Obtain apical enlargement plus flare		
Minimal (size 25)	9 (curved canal)	
Moderate (size 30 to 40)	9 (straight canal)	5 (curved canal)
Maximal (size 50 to 60)		5 (straight canal)
Dry canal	10†	7
Seal with zinc oxide–eugenol	11	
Seal with cement		9
Remove dressing and temporary seal		3
Canal filling procedure (9)		
Fit and verify master gutta-percha		6
Condense canal		8
Take final radiograph		10
Time required for appointment (hours)	½ to 1	½ to 1¼
Time until next appointment	1 to 2 weeks	Wait a week or more before restoring

*Use anesthetic for teeth with vital pulp, optional for filling appointment. May be used for teeth with nonvital pulp when clamp impinges on tissue.
†When no medicament will be used, some residual irrigant may remain in the canal.

ment. It is easy to procrastinate in the course of treatment. Because further appointments have been scheduled, the dentist may believe that it makes little difference if minimal treatment is accomplished at any one sitting, since there will be time to make it up at the next. Unfortunately, this is rarely the case. As a result of such an attitude, more time is required to complete the tooth, and thus there will be more opportunities for the temporary material to be dislodged or an exacerbation to occur.

Another common error in treatment is to enlarge a small, but vital, canal to size 20 or smaller at a particular appointment. This enlargement is insufficient to allow a broach to reach the apex, and thus much tissue is packed in that area in an inflamed condition. It would be better to avoid any enlargement whatsoever if a canal cannot be broached to the apex at the conclusion of the appointment.

Obviously, not all the desired treatment will be accomplished at every appointment. However, the objectives for each sitting must be known in advance so the clinician will be aware of the amount of work that should be performed.

Degree of canal enlargement. The tables in this chapter list the desirable width of canal enlargement to be obtained at each appointment. These specifications should be considered only as guides and not used absolutely in every case. Obviously, in young patients canals usually require much greater enlargement to remove debris properly, prepare canal walls, and facilitate the filling procedures. Also, such conditions as tooth length, root curvature, and dentinal sclerosis may militate against the suggested enlargement in specific cases.

As a general rule, most canals will be minimally prepared by enlarging three sizes wider than the largest instrument that initially binds near the apex. For example, if a size 15 instrument is the widest that will reach the full working length of a given tooth, that canal should be enlarged to size 30 or more. Ribbon-shaped canals such as those found in maxillary bicuspids and the distal roots of mandibular molars usually require greater enlargement than a three-size increase to gain cleansing of the entire width as well as length.

Table 19-2. Timetable for treating teeth with two canals

Treatment (chapter reference)	First appointment (steps)	Second appointment (steps)
Diagnosis and treatment plan (2)	1	
Administer anesthetic, if needed* (6)	2	1
Initial access	3	
Apply rubber dam	4	2
Complete access (6)	5	
Intracanal treatment procedures (7)		
Irrigate canals	6	4
Broach canals	7	
Establish length	8	
Obtain apical enlargement plus flare		
Minimal (size 25)	9	
Moderate (size 30 to 40)		5
Flare canals		6
Dry canals	10†	8
Seal with zinc oxide–eugenol	11	
Seal with cement		10
Remove dressing and temporary seal		3
Canal filling procedure (9)		
Fit and verify master gutta-percha		7
Condense canals		9
Take final radiograph		11
Time required for appointment (hours)	½ to 1	¾ to 1½
Time until next appointment	1 to 2 weeks	Wait a week or more before restoring

*Use anesthetic for teeth with vital pulp, optional for filling appointment. May be used for teeth with nonvital pulp when clamp impinges on tissue.

†When no medicament will be used, some residual irrigant may remain in the canal.

Table 19-3. Timetable for treating molars

Treatment (chapter reference)	First appointment	Second appointment	Third appointment
Diagnosis and treatment plan (2)	1	1	1
Administer anesthetic, if needed* (6)	2		
Initial access	3	2	2
Apply rubber dam	4		
Complete access (6)	5		
Intracanal treatment procedures (7)			
Irrigate canals	6	4	4
Broach canals	7 Maxillary, palatal Mandibular, distal(s)	7	
Establish lengths	8 Maxillary, palatal Mandibular, distal(s)	5 Maxillary, buccals and recheck palatal Mandibular, mesials and recheck distal(s)	
Obtain apical enlargements plus flare			
Size 25 to 35	9 Maxillary, palatal Mandibular, distal(s)	6 Maxillary, buccals Mandibular, mesials	5 Complete enlargement
Size 30 to 45		8 Maxillary, palatal Mandibular, distal(s)	
Flare canals		9	6
Dry canals	10	10	8
Medicate (optional)†	11	11	
Seal with zinc oxide—eugenol	12		
Seal with cement		3	10
Remove dressing and temporary			3
Canal filling procedure (9)			
Fit and verify master gutta-percha cones‡			7
Condense gutta-percha			9
Take final radiographs			11
Time required for appointment (hours)	¾ to 1½	1 to 2	1 to 2
Time until next appointment	1 to 2 weeks	1 to 2 weeks	
Comments		If time permits, may fill largest canal (Fig. 19-1)	Wait a week before restoring

*Use anesthetic for teeth with vital pulps, optional for filling appointment. May be used for teeth with nonvital pulps if clamp impinges.
†When no medicament is used, some residual irrigant may remain in canals.
‡If using Thermafil, see Chapter 10 for filling.

Table 19-4. Timetable for treating teeth to be left open* or those already left open[†]

Treatment (chapter reference)	First appointment, emergency treatment*	Second appointment[†]	Third appointment
Diagnosis (2,3,5)	1		
Administer anesthetic, if needed‡ (6)	2	1§	
Initial access	3		
Apply rubber dam	4	2	1
Complete access (6)	5		
Intracanal treatment procedures (5,7)			
Broach canals	6	6	3,6
Irrigate canals	7 (sterile warm water/ saline)	3 (heavily with NaOCl)	2,5 (alternate H_2O_2 and NaOCl)
Establish lengths	8	4 (if not already done)	
Obtain apical enlargements plus flare			
Minimal (size 20 to 30)	9 (through apex if needed to get drainage)		
Moderate (35 to 40)		5	
Dry canals			4,7
Leave open	10‖	7	
Seal with zinc oxide–eugenol			
Time required for appointment (hours)	¼ to ¾	¼ to 1	½
Time until next appointment	2 to 7 days	1 to 3 days	2 to 7 days¶

*If leaving tooth open with acute periapical abscess present.
[†]If tooth already had been left open, start with second appointment.
‡Generally a block anesthetic is used because infiltration would not be indicated with acute periapical abscess.
§Only needed if vital tissue is still present or if clamp impinges on tissue.
‖Best to allow for drainage and reclose (Chapter 5).
¶For teeth with one canal, complete according to Table 19-1, start at second appointment; for teeth with two canals, complete with Table 19-2, start at first appointment; for molars, complete with Table 19-3, start at second appointment.

Even more significant at the first appointment for any tooth is the initiation of flaring (see Chapter 7) as soon as practical. Widening the orifice portion eliminates curvatures at the entrances to the canals, thus providing more direct access to the apex. This makes apical preparation, particularly in curved canals, more effective by retaining original canal shape more easily. Also, the intracanal irrigants can reach sites deeper in the canal to dissolve necrotic tissue and eliminate microorganisms. All of these conditions are very favorable and improve endodontic results.

Time requirements. The time requirement for each appointment is indicated so the operator will have a general idea for scheduling purposes. A wide range of time is listed because there are many variables in each tooth and among individual dentists. Also, experience has a great deal to do with the time needed to perform any given step. In general, time should be subjugated to quality. If more time is needed than indicated on the chart for the work to be performed, the dentist should allow for it. However, if the maximum time listed is much too short for almost every situation, the dentist should reevaluate the methods of treatment to see whether inefficiency is creating the problem.

The ideal time period between appointments is presented. Again it is not necessary to conform perfectly to the suggestions. However, treatment will be smoothest if the appointments are set up to fall well within the given time. When appointments are too close together, periapical tissues do not have an opportunity to recover from their mild inflammation, which always occurs, before they are reirritated at the next sitting. If the appointments are too far apart, the problems of displacement of temporary seal, chance for exacerbation, and ingrowth of chronically inflamed tissue occur.

Filling canals of molar teeth at different appointments. It has always been assumed in endodontics that all canals of each treated tooth are to be filled at the same appointment. Whereas this has been the general treatment for many years, there is no reason to conform rigidly to this

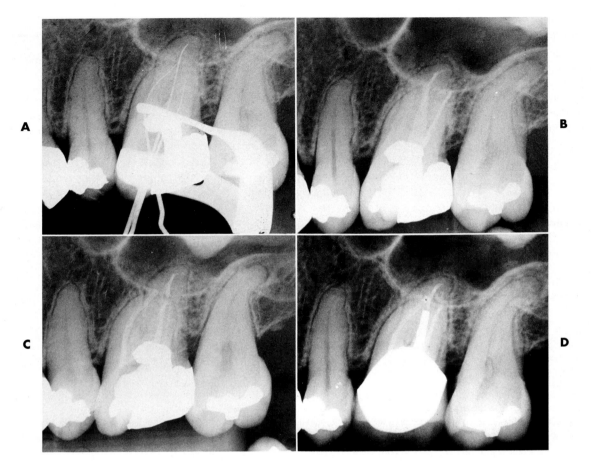

Fig. 19-1. **A,** Radiograph of maxillary first molar with files in place to determine working lengths. The palatal canal has a sharp apical curvature, and the file in the mesiobuccal canal is too long. **B,** The canals were relatively easy to prepare, despite the curvature, and sufficient time was available to fill the palatal and distobuccal canals at the second appointment with laterally condensed gutta-percha and Wach's paste. **C,** At the third appointment, the mesiobuccal canal was completed and post room prepared in the palatal canal. **D,** One year after treatment. (Restoration by Dr. Robert Wheeler, Chicago.)

practice when alternative scheduling would be better from the standpoint of both dentist and patient.

When treating molar teeth, long appointments should be scheduled—from 1 to 2 hours (Table 19-3)—so that a considerable amount of work is performed at each sitting. More appointments of shorter duration merely extend the total treatment period, require more total injections, and allow more time for intratreatment problems.

At the end of the second appointment it is possible that the canals are well cleansed, prepared, and flared. If there is sufficient time remaining and the conditions required for canal filling have been met (Chapter 9), it is perfectly permissible to fill the

largest canal of the tooth at that time—the palatal canal of maxillary molars or the distal canal of mandibular molars. In maxillary molars it is acceptable to fill the distobuccal canal as well, if time permits (Fig. 19-1). This leaves the entire third appointment available for completing the mesiobuccal root, which often has a second canal and is the most complicated root in maxillary molars.

When two canals are present in the same root (in either a Type II or III alignment), it is best to fill those at the same appointment. The exact relationship may prove to be other than anticipated, which could lead to a blocking out of the unfilled canal in an unfavorable position. Therefore, in mandibular molars it is best to fill both mesial canals at the same appointment. If two canals exist in the distal root, it is best to fill both of them at the same appointment as well.

In some very difficult cases treatment may extend for several more appointments than normal, usually due to difficulty in locating some or all of the canals, or extreme canal narrowness or curvature of the canals (Fig. 19-2). As preparation of one canal is completed, prior to the other canals being ready for filling, it is recommended that the first canal be filled (Fig. 19-2, *C*). This gets that portion of the tooth out of the way, and thus the available time for succeeding appointments can be spent exclusively with the more difficult canals.

Leaving teeth with acute abscesses open versus keeping them closed.   For many years teeth with an acute periapical abscess were treated by gaining drainage and being left open. This regimen was advocated in the first three editions of this textbook. However, newer views have indicated the advisability of keeping all teeth closed whenever possible. The full ramifications for this view are presented in Chapter 5.

Despite this desire for closure, some teeth are still left open when emergency treatment is rendered for a tooth with an acute periapical abscess. In addition, in some cases a dentist initially sees patients who have had a tooth already left open anywhere from several days to several months earlier. Incorrect treatment for such teeth will cause continued problems and recurrent flare-ups. For these reasons, Table 19-4 is presented as an advisable, tried-and-true method for treating such cases with minimal problems resulting.

Third appointment when treating teeth left open.   In Table 19-4 the plan for the third appointment lists several numbers beside the steps listed as irrigating, broaching, and drying canals. The intent of these listings is to indicate that at this appointment, when the tooth is to be closed without filing, the canal is irrigated heavily, broached, and dried several times. Although this sequence is listed twice, it may be gone through three, four, or more times to verify proper handling prior to closure.

Fourth appointment when treating teeth left open.   In teeth with single canals it is probable that complete canal preparation and filling of the tooth can be accomplished successfully at this appointment. If some residual exudate is present, or not all symptoms have disappeared, it is best merely to complete preparation with heavy irrigation, reclose,

and reappoint for filling at another sitting. For bicanaled and molar teeth, I prefer not to fill at this fourth appointment but merely to complete preparation and schedule the filling 1 to 2 weeks later. This regimen has worked best for me in the long run.

Timetables necessarily subject to change by the clinician.   Tables 19-1 to 19-4 are presented merely to act as a guide during therapy. As the operator becomes more proficient in the required techniques, certain steps may be merged or altered. As new and improved methods are learned through publications or postgraduate courses, they should be substituted accordingly. The type of scheduling suggested, as originally presented by Healey, has been used with considerable success in many endodontic cases. Although following it will not guarantee success, it will aid in the avoidance of frequent problems and pitfalls.

One-sitting endodontic treatment.   No tooth or pulp condition is presented to be completed in only one appointment. Although a tooth with a radiolucency may be filled and have apical curettage at one appointment (Chapter 11), nonsurgical single-sitting treatment is discouraged. Many operators claim high rates of success with one-sitting endodontic therapy, particularly when their patients come great distances and would be considerably inconvenienced by return trips.

I believe, however, that if a patient's tooth is worth saving it is also worth his returning for a second appointment for completion. In vital pulp cases the pulpal stump bleeds after amputation. Just as no inlay should be cemented or any amalgam packed in a bay of blood or saliva, so should the cementation of a root canal filling be accomplished in a dry environment. If the pulp is necrotic and the canal is filled at the first appointment, facultative anaerobes may multiply in the new environment and cause an exacerbation. It is much easier to open a tooth for relief of pain if there is no canal filling present.

An ability to relieve pain quickly and efficiently is the major reason for not completing endodontic treatment in one sitting. According to Clem, at least 25% of patients undergoing endodontic therapy will experience moderate to severe pain, most frequently after the canal preparation appointment, whether the pulp is vital or necrotic. If the tooth is prepared but unfilled, the pain has probably resulted from overinstrumentation and relief is usually obtained rapidly through the canal. (See Chapter 5.) However, if the tooth is filled at the

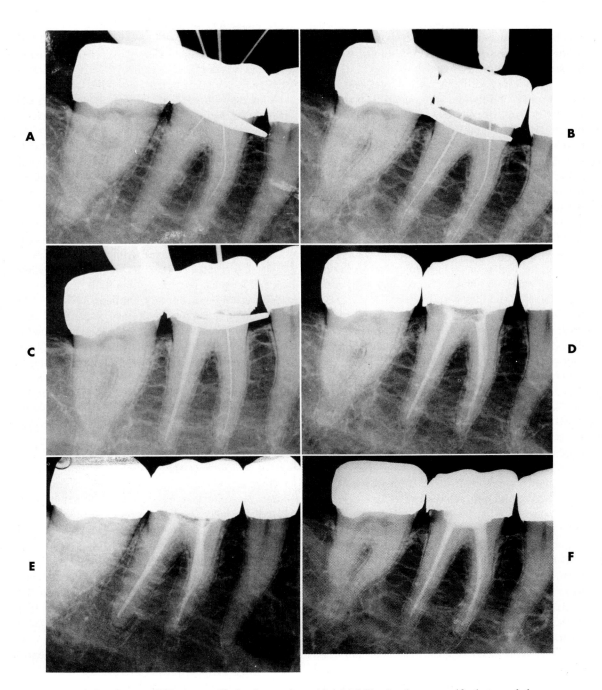

Fig. 19-2.   A, Very difficult mandibular first molar, with initial files in place to verify that canals have been located. The canals are quite long (25 mm) and very narrow. **B,** It took two full appointments to reach this point—files in place in distal and mesiobuccal canals to determine working lengths. **C,** By the end of the next appointment, film shows that the distal canal could be completed and the file is in the mesiolingual canal. **D,** Two more appointments were required to complete the case. Final film after canal filling with laterally condensed gutta-percha and Wach's paste. **E,** Angled view. **F,** Six years of treatment, the periapical lesions appear normal, tooth is comfortable. Decay on the distal has been reported to the referring dentist for repair or replacement of the crown. (Restorations by Dr. Stanley Martin, Chicago.)

first appointment, the filling must be removed to gain relief through the canal or analgesics must be prescribed, with more time for discomfort present. When gutta-percha is the filling material, chemical dissolution and removal with instruments frequently increase apical inflammation. When silver is the filling material, removal may be extremely difficult or even impossible, particularly when a sectional technique has been employed.

A few dental schools are currently teaching one-sitting treatment in every case, and some are teaching it in selected cases. A number of practitioners regularly perform therapy in this manner, but this seems to have a geographic tendency, that is, in certain areas of the United States it is very popular; in other areas it is used only rarely. In general, European dentists use it more frequently then do those from the United States.

Those encouraging this method state that the number of patients with postoperative pain is no greater than following multiple-visit cases. Furthermore, they state that the healing rate of the two types of treatment will not vary with any significance. My own belief relating to degree of pain is that even if the number of cases with pain is no greater with one-sitting, it is still much easier to treat postoperative pain without the canal filling. As far as the degree of success, all of the articles on this subject seem to indicate that there is no difference in long-term success.

Several advocates of one-sitting treatment say that they present the possibilities to the patient at the case presentation, and then they allow the patient to choose between single- and multiple sittings. I have a lot of problems with this philosophy. If, in fact, one-sitting treatment is best for that operator, then that method should be used in any and all applicable cases. If, on the other hand, the dentist is uncomfortable with single-sitting treatment, it should not be used. It should never be left to the patient to make this choice.

When I intend to perform one-sitting treatment, particularly for prosthetic reasons, I inform the patient of the *possibility* for this type of therapy, but I indicate that as treatment goes on, it may or may not be practical to do so. Thus, if some problem transpires, I am not locked in to a direction where I am uncomfortable with treatment modalities.

There are certain conditions that might force the operator to complete a tooth in one appointment. Typical is the prosthetic indication in which an anterior tooth fractures near the gingival line without apparent pulp exposure (Figs. 19-3 and 19-4)

and thus no microorganism ingress. Most frequently this will occur on a tooth that has been restored with a jacket crown (Fig. 19-4, *A*). Because of the esthetic problem, patients will not accept waiting a few days without a tooth so the normal schedule of endodontic treatment can be completed and a temporary jacket fabricated. A flipper type of partial denture could be constructed as a temporary restoration to replace the crown of the single fractured tooth, but some patients have difficulty talking or eating with the palate covered. Also, it still requires at least 1 day to produce such a temporary restoration.

In these cases one-sitting endodontics is acceptable as long as no apical radiolucency is present, the tooth is not tender to percussion (indicating absence of prior apical inflammation), and there is no open exposure to cause pulpal infection. It is even more important to confine all endodontic preparation procedures to the canal and prevent overinstrumentation than in routine cases (Figs. 19-3, *C*, and 19-4, *A*) because of the inability to grant relief through the canal. If it is discovered during the preparation that much overinstrumentation has occurred by error, the tooth should not be completed in one appointment. Instead, prophylactic use of a corticosteroid antibiotic as an apical medicament (Chapter 5) is advised, and the patient may be rescheduled at least a few days later for completion.

For one-sitting cases, I do make some variations from routine procedures. Case selection is quite important to rule out teeth with preoperative apical periodontitis because they are more prone to postoperative problems (Figs. 19-3, *A*, and 19-4, *A*). I prefer to have a quite clean complete pulp extirpation with a broach, hopefully quite close to the apical constriction (Fig. 19-3, *B*). In some routine multiple-visit cases I have had difficulty gaining a clean extirpation because of pulp inflammation or failure to impale the soft tissue properly. The canal may subsequently be enlarged to adequate size, and all soft tissue is removed. At the next appointment, however, I often remove large chunks of soft tissue that has broken down due to the medicament, irrigants, or removal from apical blood supply. If I had attempted to fill the canal at the previous appointment, this mass of macerated material would surely have prevented an optimal apical seal and might have led to failure.

An accurate working length is determined and verified by radiograph (Figs. 19-3, *C* and 19-4, *A*). This is an extremely important step in any endodontic case; but it has special significance in the

Text continued on p. 834.

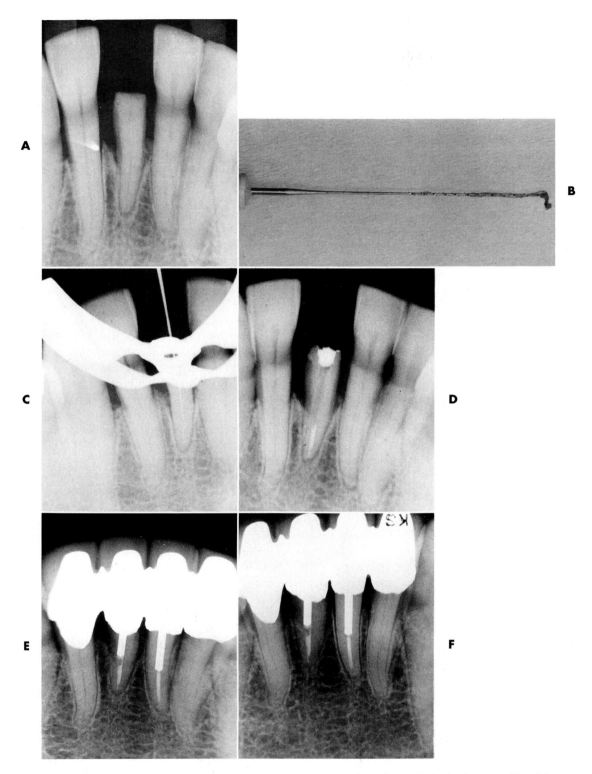

Fig. 19-3. Good indication for one-sitting treatment. **A,** Preoperative film of mandibular incisor area. The right central incisor has fractured slightly above the gingival line due to severe labial erosion, but no exposure is present and there never has been a history of pain. Endodontic therapy must be performed for restorative purposes. **B,** The pulp was extirpated seemingly en masse close to the apical constriction. **C,** Film of file in place to determine working length, verifying that the canal has not been overinstrumented. If it had, I would not have completed the tooth in one sitting. **D,** Canal filled with laterally condensed gutta-percha and Wach's paste, post room prepared. The patient experienced no pain after completion of the tooth in one visit. **E,** The adjacent central also required treatment. Post-and-core crowns were made for the treated teeth and crowns for the adjacent lateral incisors. **F,** Four years after original treatment, everything looks good. (Restorations by Dr. Asher Jacobs, formerly of Chicago.)

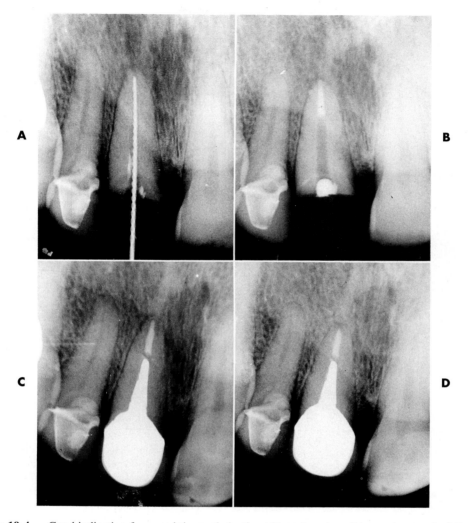

Fig. 19-4. Good indication for one-sitting endodontics, although patient did experience pain follow-ing treatment. **A,** Maxillary central incisor had been restored with jacket crown that fractured near the gingival margin, with no pulp exposure and no previous symptoms. Endodontic therapy had to be per-formed in one sitting for esthetic reasons. Pulp was extirpated similarly to that shown in Fig. 19-3, *B*. File in place would indicate that no excessive apical preparation had taken place. **B,** Radiograph taken after canal filling with laterally condensed gutta-percha and Wach's paste, post room prepared. Despite my attempt to confine the preparation within the canal, the canal filling did reach the periapical tissues, as indicated by being flush with the radiographic apex. Patient had periapical pain for several days, which was controlled by analgesics. The old crown was used as a temporary. **C,** Tooth restored with a post-and-core crown; note mild increase in periodontal ligament space. **D,** Five years later, area looks excellent. Note that apical extent of filling is now short of radiographic apex, probably due to addi-tional deposition of cementum. (Restoration by Dr. Morton Schreiber, Highland Park, Ill.)

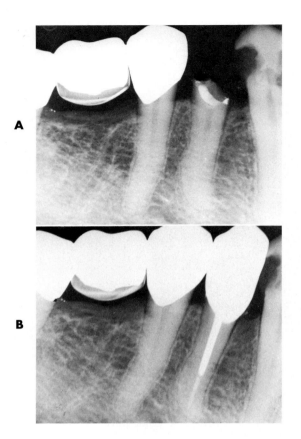

A

B

Fig. 19-5. Poor indication for one-sitting endodontic treatment. **A,** Esthetics was no problem in this mandibular bicuspid. Two-sitting treatment is safer, particularly in posterior teeth, in which apical surgery would be so much more difficult to perform if initial treatment should fail. Pulp was extirpated and canal prepared at the initial appointment. At second sitting the canal was filled with gutta-percha and lateral condensation. **B,** One-year postoperative view. This is same type of restoration as shown in Fig. 19-4. (Restoration by Dr. Irving Fishman, Chicago).

Fig. 19-6. **A,** Radiograph of mandibular first molar indicating a lesion associated with the distal root, extending laterally towards the crestal bone. A small increase in periodontal ligament width may be present on the mesial root. A canal is quite distinct in the distal root, but only barely visible in the mesial root, not unexpected in a first molar with a large metal crown. A sinus tract was present, extending from the distal lesion. **B,** The access cavity was prepared, and the distal canal located. Even with a deep preparation at the first appointment, no mesial canals were found. The lesion extending crestally on this film is even more apparent than on the preoperative view. **C,** Further efforts to locate the mesial canals did not meet with success. However, the sinus tract healed after canal preparation of the distal canal only. With no other clinical symptoms apparent, the distal canal was filled with laterally condensed gutta-percha and Wach's paste. Sealer is seen extending up the distal root crestally, following the direction of the healed tract. **D,** Radiographs were taken at 6-month intervals, but by 18 months postoperatively, the mesial root displayed an obvious lesion. Note that the lesion on the distal root has now filled in quite well. Accordingly, it was decided to reinitiate search for the mesial canals. If that effort did not meet with success, periapical surgery with apical filling would have been employed to retain the tooth. **E,** Deeper penetration indicated that the mesial canals were treatable, according to this view from the mesial. **F,** and **G,** Mesial canals filled with laterally condensed gutta-percha and Wach's paste, as seen in these angled and straight views taken immediately after filling. **H** and **I,** Angled and straight views taken 9 months after completion of the mesial canals, indicating considerable healing associated with that root and almost total healing associated with the distal root. The tooth is comfortable, and the prognosis favorable.

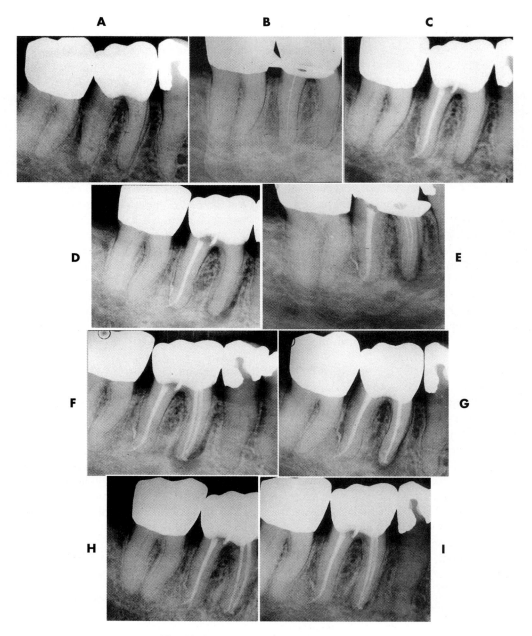

Fig. 19-6.   For legend see opposite page.

single-visit treatment, when overinstrumentation must be avoided. Anterior teeth, which are easier to radiograph, offer a better chance for one-visit success than do molar teeth. The canal is prepared to a maximal size consistent with retaining the original canal shape. This width of enlargement is necessary to ensure the removal of the predentin layer and any residual soft tissue tags that might decrease the chance for optimal seal.

The canal is filled with gutta-percha in a condensation technique (Chapter 9), and post room is prepared (Figs. 19-3, *D* and 19-4, *B*). (See Chapter 17.) Any necessary reshaping of the root face is performed, and impressions are taken to construct a post-and-core type of crown.

Temporization is simplified if a previously made jacket crown is available. A metal post is placed in the canal so it protrudes through the access but does not prevent complete seating of the crown; then the crown is filled with composite and seated. If no jacket is available, the tooth may be temporized as described in Chapter 17. The final restoration is completed according to normal procedures (Figs. 19-3, *E*, and 19-4, *C*). Long-term follow-up should be maintained on these teeth, just as with every endodontic case. In most instances the area remains normal, and the restored teeth function in good condition for many years (Figs. 19-3, *F*, and 19-4, *D*).

If a similar situation occurs on a posterior tooth, even without symptoms and in the absence of pulpal exposure, it is advisable to complete the case in two appointments (Fig. 19-5).

Even in molar teeth it is permissible to deviate from Table 19-3 and complete in two sittings by lengthening the time for each appointment if distance is a problem. In these cases the treated tooth must be kept closed between appointments and be asymptomatic at the time of filling.

Filling roots of molar teeth several years apart. At the other end of the spectrum from one-sitting treatment is the multiyear treatment, which, when necessary, generally is used for molar teeth. Also this method is not used by design, but rather out of necessity.

The typical scenario involves a molar tooth with symptoms, such as pain to percussion or the presence of a draining sinus tract (Fig. 19-6, *A*), indicating apical spread of inflammation. The radiographs reveal the canals to be quite narrow, suggesting that it might be difficult to locate them (Fig. 19-6, *B*). After opening into the tooth, not all the canals can

be penetrated to the apex, and, in some cases, some canals cannot be found at all (Fig. 19-6, *C*). If a periapical lesion is present, it is associated with the root that can be prepared acceptably.

The canal or canals that can be instrumented are enlarged to acceptable sizes, and the symptoms cease, that is, the tooth is no longer tender to percussion or the sinus tract has closed. The prognosis for this tooth has now improved, and probably it is worth continuing treatment.

The canals are filled according to Chapter 9, and if a large restoration was entered for access, this entrance is repaired. If the tooth requires a crown or similar restoration, an acceptable temporary should be fabricated that will last for several months to one year. The patient is put on a definite recall regimen of not less than every 3 to 6 months and advised of the necessity to keep these evaluation appointments.

Periodic radiographic and clinical evaluations are made. If, after one year the tooth remains comfortable and no symptoms or periapical changes are noted on the untreated root or roots, a final restoration may be considered. If this occurs, the periodic evaluations should still continue.

If periapical breakdown is noted (Fig. 19-6, *D* and *E*) or symptoms occur, further attempts to locate the canal or canals of the untreated root or roots should be considered. In some cases, this location, so difficult to find at the first attempt, may be found with less difficulty. If so, canal preparation and filling are performed (Fig. 19-6, *F* and *G*). If the recalcitrant root or roots cannot be instrumented, periapical surgery with reverse filling (see Chapter 11) or root amputation (see Chapter 12) are the only choices left for retaining the tooth.

Hopefully further follow-ups will indicate a successful conclusion to this very long-term treatment (Fig. 19-6, *H* and *I*).

REFERENCES

Ashkenaz PJ: One-visit endodontics, *Dent Clin North Am* 28:853, 1984.

Clem WH: Posttreatment endodontic pain, *J Am Dent Assoc* 81:1166, 1970.

Fox J, Atkinson JS, Dinin AP, Greenfield E, et al: Incidence of pain following one-visit endodontic treatment, *Oral Surg* 30:123, 1970.

Landers RR, Calhoun RL: One-appointment endodontic therapy: an opinion survey, *J Endod* 6:799, 1980.

Pekruhn RB: The incidence of failure following single-visit endodontic therapy, *J Endod* 12:68, 1986.

Soltanoff W: A comparative study of the single-visit and the multiple-visit endodontic procedure, *J Endod* 4:278, 1978.

Franklin S. Weine • Jeffrey L. Wingo

20 Drug therapy useful in endodontics

AUTHOR'S NOTE: In the last decade there has been an explosion in the field of pharmacology; thus it is impossible for any clinically oriented dentist to be conversant in all the applicable medications for dental treatment. The tables in this chapter should not be construed by the reader as complete, but merely some of the most commonly used drugs in the classifications listed. A number of other substances may be substituted with equal success. Also, the reader should not construe the listing of any drug as an endorsement by us of that preparation. However, we have prescribed every drug listed in this chapter at one time or another, and we believe that each has efficacy in the context described.

Patients receiving endodontic therapy may need the prescription of drugs for any of three common problems. Because of the connotation of "nerve" removal or complex dental treatment in general, endodontic patients may suffer from mild to severe apprehension. When this reaches a degree that produces alteration of physiologic and/or psychologic functions, preoperative sedation is required, usually in the form of sedatives or tranquilizers. The pain from a pulpitis or apical periodontitis that produces the need for endodontic therapy may be unbearable without analgesics. Also, a similar degree of pain may follow appointments in which the canals are enlarged or filled, particularly when the apical constriction is violated or following a surgical procedure. Infections requiring antibiotic control may occur prior to the initiation of therapy, and exacerbations characterized by microorganism fulmination may happen after treatment is begun.

It should be emphasized that in many cases the need for drugs would be eliminated with proper endodontic treatment. A firm and efficient, while still empathetic, attitude of the dentist will do much to relieve anxiety and tension in the fearful patient. However, if the clinician is bumbling, appears unsure of the course of therapy, and is rough in tone and treatment, even the most sedate individual will feel fear.

Analgesics may be necessary before an emergency appointment, but if correct diagnosis is made and treatment indicated in Chapter 5 is performed, pain relief is almost immediate in virtually every instance. When accurate measurement radiographs are taken and the canal preparation is terminated in solid dentin, minimal postoperative pain results.

Except in the cases where extremely virulent microorganisms are present or the resistance of the host is low, infections requiring antibiotic administration during therapy are rare. When the canals are properly debrided in a minimal number of appointments with a desirable length of time allowed between sittings (Chapter 19), the chance for intratreatment infection is greatly diminished. Exacerbations are most frequent when extra appointments must be scheduled because of inability to gain the desired objectives at regularly scheduled visits, or when visits are scheduled excessively far apart. Even when the patient seeks treatment while suffering an acute periapical abscess, most incision and drainage procedures will be effective without antibiotic coverage, particularly when drainage is obtained through the canal.

However, in addition to the pharmacologic effectiveness of drugs, many people may have a positive psychologic reaction to a prescription. Reports have been made indicating that some individuals will recover faster with a prescription for a placebo than with no prescribed medication. Typical among this group are older retired individuals, homemakers with much spare time, and persons with hypochondriac tendencies.

This is not to suggest that prescription should be given for either actual or placebo medications on just the slightest indication. However, in the treatment of a patient who has one of the backgrounds mentioned, when no drug prescription is indicated, this information should be emphasized to the patient, lest he or she infer that optimal treatment is not being received. Furthermore, it is wise to call personally or have the receptionist call the patient the next day to verify that the patient is doing well. Should the condition then indicate the need for pharmacologic assistance, a prescription may be given.

IMPORTANCE OF MEDICAL HISTORY

Included as a part of the medical history for every patient is possible allergy to any drug and a listing of any disease or condition that might cause impairment of the organ in which a particular drug is detoxified (Chapter 2). No drug should be prescribed without a consideration of the patient's medical history to ensure that the desired prescription will be safe. If doubt exists, the *Physicians' Desk Reference* should be consulted for indications, contraindications, and possible side effects for the drug. If the patient has a sizable medical history, it is best to consult with his or her physician before prescribing.

Even in the absence of patient sensitivity to a drug, further interrogation should be pursued before prescribing any drugs with a high level of reactions, such as the antibiotics. It is wise to say, "I am going to prescribe____(drug)____for your (infection, pain, anxiety). You did say that you have never had any untoward reaction to drugs of that type; is that not correct?" It is strange, but patients may not think of all classes of drugs when a dentist takes a medical history and may mention only those he thinks are involved in dental treatment. This prior statement of the type of drug and its general action will serve to refresh the patient's memory in case a possible allergy has been overlooked.

Most drugs have alternate prescriptions that are equally able to produce the desired effect. There should be no problem in making a substitution when any drug appears to have contraindications on an allergic or systemic basis.

ANALGESICS

Relief of pain is a basic objective of any phase of dental treatment. The pain may have occurred in the past, may be immediately responsible for the patient's presence in the dental office, or may occur in the future unless definitive treatment is provided. In any case the dentist must make the comfort of the patient an overriding factor in determining treatment procedures.

In endodontics many patients requiring therapy have a great deal of chronic inflammation present in either the pulp or the periapical tissues. Even if pain is not a factor initially, the change in environment produced by any treatment may result in an acute reaction. The resultant need for analgesics is an almost constant condition in endodontic therapy for enabling the patient to overcome the usually short but often present postoperative discomfort.

Tables 20-1 and 20-2 list the commonly used drugs for relief of mild to moderate to severe pain. These tables will be useful in prescribing for relief when an emergency or an unexpected degree of pain is encountered.

Usually the clinician learns to prescribe according to the degree of trauma induced. Therefore Table 20-3 lists the types of analgesics for certain endodontic conditions. Since most analgesics have greater effectiveness when they are taken prior to development of pain sensation of severe intensity, suitable prescriptions should be given to the patient at the conclusion of the appointment if postoperative pain is anticipated. The analgesic then can be taken either while the local anesthetic is still effective or, if no anesthesia was used, as soon as possible after the treatment. When a local anesthetic is used and an analgesic is prescribed, the dentist must calculate the anticipated duration of remaining anesthesia effectiveness. The analgesic should be ingested 30 to 60 minutes prior to the wearing off of the anesthetic so the drug will have sufficient opportunity to take effect. The dentist must remember that highly nervous or fidgety patients may metabolize rapidly, and thus the anesthesia lasts for less than the anticipated duration.

It is impossible to gain accurate information by asking the patient whether he has mild, moderate, or severe pain. To most patients their pain seems severe, and any attempt to minimize the intensity may cause antagonism. Therefore, when a patient calls the office or home requesting a prescription for pain relief and no analgesic has been prescribed, an inquiry should be made as to what, if anything, is being taken presently for relief. Usually aspirin, Tylenol, Darvon, or some drug containing codeine, all often present in the household medicine cabinet as prescribed for previous

Table 20-1. Analgesics for relief of mild to moderate pain.

Drug	Adult dosage	Comments
Acetylsalicylic acid (aspirin, ASA)	300 to 1000 mg every 3 to 4 hr	Most widely used analgesic in use today—the standard of comparison, used in combination with many other drugs, literally trillions of doses taken; also has antipyretic and antiinflammatory (needs higher dose, 3× analgesic dose) actions; problems are infrequent but serious potential side effects: GI disturbances and prolonged bleeding times (blood-thinning effect used for those susceptible to heart attacks)
Tylenol (acetaminophen) regular strength—325 mg	1 to 2 tablets every 4 to 6 hr (total dose not to exceed 4000 mg/day)	Popular ASA substitute for patients with GI or bleeding problems, antiinflammatory action much less than ASA
Fiorinal 50 mg butalbital 325 mg ASA 40 mg caffeine	1 to 2 tablets every 4 hr (total dose not to exceed 6/day)	Butalbital is a short- to medium-acting barbiturate, combining anxiolytic and muscle relaxant properties; this coupled with ASA are synergistic and give relief for headache associated with dental treatment
Darvocet Darvocet-N-50 50 mg propoxyphene 325 mg acetaminophen Darvocet-N-100 100 mg propoxyphene 650 mg acetaminophen	1 tablet every 4 hr, as needed for pain	Derived from Darvon-type drugs, once very popular, then suspect to any efficacy beyond ASA content and due to addictive potential; must not be prescribed for anyone suicidal or addiction prone and with caution to those taking antidepressants or tranquilizers or users of alcohol in excess; is an alternative drug to people without above problems, but with allergies to other analgesics
Nonsteroidal antiinflammatory analgesics (NSAIDs)		
Motrin (ibuprofen)—300, 400, 600, and 800 mg	400 mg every 4 to 6 hr, not to exceed 3200 mg per day	NSAID with antipyretic and analgesic properties, supposedly nonaddictive, all good for treatment of chronic or acute pain; often taken by patients for relief of tendonitis
Dolobid (diflunisal)—250 and 500 mg	1000 mg loading dose, then 500 mg every 8 to 12 hr	Requires loading dose to be taken before treatment, as in predictably painful procedures such as periapical surgery or extirpation of symptomatic molar; is salicylic acid derivative, thus having side effects similar to ASA
Nalfon (fenoprofen)—200, 300, and 600 mg	200 to 400 mg every 4 to 6 hr	Actions and reactions similar to Motrin
Naprosyn (naproxen)—250, 375, and 500 mg, suspension 125 mg/5 ml	250, 375, or 500 mg twice daily	Reason for development and main advantage is rapid absorption, works quickly requiring no multihour loading dose, peak plasma levels reached in 2 hours
Anaprox (naproxen sodium)—275 mg, Nanprox DS—550 mg	550 mg starting dose, then 275 mg every 6 to 8 hr, maximum daily dose is 1375 mg	Sodium salt allows even faster absorption (within 1 hour); must not be given concomitantly with Naprosyn, long-term administration may lead to renal pathosis
Ansaid (flurbiprofen)—50 and 100 mg	200 mg starting dose, 300 mg total daily dose	Long-acting, very effective when administered preoperatively

Table 20-2. Analgesics to relieve moderate to severe pain

Drug	Adult dosage	Comments
Empirin with codeine—325 mg ASA plus No. 2—15 mg codeine No. 3—30 mg codeine No. 4—60 mg codeine	1 or 2 every 4 hr	Excellent for relief of moderate to severe pain, well tolerated and widely used; thus patients will already know degree of effectiveness and possible history of allergy; action of ASA for its 3 properties adds to effectiveness of codeine
Tylenol with codeine—300 mg acetaminophen plus No. 2—15 mg codeine No. 3—30 mg codeine No. 4—60 mg codeine (also available in elixir)	1 or 2 tablets every 4 hr Maximums: codeine, 360 mg/day; acetaminophen, 4000 mg/day	Very popular compound for patients who cannot take aspirin or barbiturates
Phenaphen with codeine—325 mg acetaminophen plus No. 2—15 mg codeine No. 3—30 mg codeine No. 4—60 mg codeine	1 or 2 capsules every 4 hr	Formula changed recently, dropping phenobarbital, phenacetin, aspirin and substituting acetaminophen; now almost exactly the same as Tylenol with codeine, but with slightly more acetaminophen
Lortab tablets each Lortab tab contains 500 mg acetaminophen plus: 2.5/500—2.5 mg hydrocodone 5/500—5 mg hydrocodone	1 to 2 tablets every 4 to 6 hr (do not exceed 8/day)	Basically the same as Vicodin, but has additional dose forms, including liquid, which may be very handy in certain situations
7.5/500—7.5 mg hydrocodone	1 tablet every 4 to 6 hr (do not exceed 6/day)	
Lortab liquid contains 2.5 mg hydrocodone 120 mg acetaminophen 7% alcohol per 5 ml (1 tspn)	1 tspn every 4 hr (do not exceed 6 tspn/day)	
Meperidine (Demerol) 50 mg tablets 100 mg tablets syrup—50 mg/5 ml (1 tspn)	50 to 150 mg every 3 to 4 hr (may be given IM)	For relief of severe pain; very effective when pain is due to pressure build up, as in acute periapical abscess prior to swelling occurring or for severe cases of acute pulpitis with apical periodontitis; classically, it is the strongest analgesic prescribed by dentists; Schedule II narcotic analgesic with action similar to morphine, but less smooth muscle spasms, constipation, or cough suppression
Fiorinal with codeine No. 3—30 mg codeine 50 mg butalbital 40 mg caffeine 325 mg ASA	1 or 2 capsules every 4 hr (do not exceed 6/day)	See Fiorinal in Table 20-1; useful when sedation is needed in addition to pain relief, or for headaches associated with dental treatment

Table 20-2.   Analgesics to relieve moderate to severe pain—cont'd

Drug	Adult dosage	Comments
Synalgos DC 356 ASA 30 mg caffeine 16 mg drocode	2 capsules every 4 hr	Drocode is dihydrocodeine, a semisynthetic narcotic related to but with less undesirable side effects than codeine; principal therapeutic action is analgesia along with some relaxation of CNS and smooth muscle components; use with care on active individuals doing potentially hazardous tasks (using machinery, heavy driving), elderly or debilitated patients, or children below the age of 12
Talwin NX 50 mg pentazocine HCl 0.5 mg naloxone HCl	Initial dose 1 tablet every 3 to 4 hr, may be increased to 2 tablets when needed (do not exceed 12/day)	Pentazocine is a potent analgesic in 50 mg oral dosage which is equivalent to 60 mg of codeine; has rapid onset of 15 to 30 min; must not be given to patient with history of seizures or to children below the age of 12; due to chances for chemical dependency, is a Schedule IV controlled substance
Vicodin 5 mg hydrocodone 500 mg acetaminophen	1 or 2 tablets every 4 to 6 hr (do not exceed 8/day)	Hydrocodone is a semisynthetic narcotic with analgesic and antitussive actions similar to those of codeine; it has less serious side effects than codeine (less emesis and constipation), but this varies greatly; it is a Schedule III drug with some abuse potential; do not use with patients who have prostate problems
Vicodin ES 7.5 mg hydrocodone 750 mg acetaminophen	1 tablet every 4 to 6 hr (do not exceed 5/day)	

Percodan and related drugs
Percodan
    325 mg ASA
    4.88 mg oxycodone
	1 tablet every 6 hr	Oxycodone is semisynthetic narcotic similar to morphine requiring Schedule II prescription; risks are: may cause dependency, impair ability to drive car or perform other difficult tasks, cause CNS depression; very effective for severe acute pain

Percodan-Demi
    325 mg ASA
    2.44 mg oxycodone
	1 to 2 tablets every 6 hr	

Percocet
    325 acetaminophen
    5 mg oxycodone
	1 tablet every 6 hr	

Toradol (Ketorolac) 10 mg	1 tablet every 4 to 6 hr, limited duration	New and probably most effective for severe pain of the NSAIDs; 10 mg of Ketorolac is equivalent to 50 mg of Demerol and 6 mg of morphine; because it is not addictive, it may be used for patients with abuse potential; due to severe side effects (GI disturbances), should not be given for more than 5 days for dental problems

nonrelated pain, has already been taken. If that drug has been ineffective, the next stronger class of analgesics should be prescribed.

For many years one of the frequent objectives of pharmacologic research has been the finding of a replacement for aspirin as an analgesic for mild to moderate pain. Aspirin does have two potentially serious side effects—gastrointestinal (GI) disturbances and prolonged bleeding. There are several viable and effective alternatives available for patients who have these problems (Table 20-1). However, much recent clinical research seems to enforce the efficacy for using aspirin and, if anything, has enhanced its reputation. In addition to its analgesic properties, aspirin has antiinflammatory potential, although at a higher dosage than that used for relief of pain, which is very helpful in the aftermath of many endodontic procedures. Several popular pain relievers of the 1960s (e.g.,

Darvon Compound) have been found to be no more effective than their aspirin content allows them to be. In other words, for the pharmacologic effectiveness, it was the aspirin content alone that gave the analgesic effect.

Davron has gone through hard times in the past 15 years, although we prescribed it frequently and thought from a clinical standpoint it was effective and reliable. In addition to the studies that questioned the necessity of its propoxyphene content, other problems have arisen. Propoxyphene can be dangerous when taken in combination with tranquilizers, sedatives, antidepressants, and antihistamines. Dentists frequently distribute a small number of pain relievers to their patients at the conclusion of a dental appointment, in case of anticipated immediate pain. *If a Darvon product is the analgesic, the patient must receive an insert warning of the potential dangers.*

Table 20-3. Suggested analgesics after certain endodontic procedures or conditions

	Initial choice	If more needed
Canal debridement	Aspirin, Tylenol, or NSAID	Analgesic with ¼ g codeine or Synalgos DC
Canal debridement where considerable overinstru-mentation has occurred*	Analgesic with ¼ g codeine or Synalgos DC	Analgesic with ½ g codeine or equivalent
Canal filling where over-filling has occurred and periapical tissue is normal	Analgeisc with ¼ g codeine or Synalgos DC	Analgesic with ½ g codeine or equivalent
Root amputation without flap	Nothing	ASA, Tylenol, or NSAID
Periapical or amputational surgery with minimal trauma	ASA, Tylenol, or NSAID	Analgesic with ½ g codeine or equivalent
Extensive surgery with considerable trauma	Analgesic with ½ g codeine or equivalent	Demerol, Vicodin, Percodan or Percocet, or Toradol
Call after office hours with moderate pain	Analgesic with ½ g codeine or equivalent	Toradol, Vicodin, or Vicodin ES
Call after office hours with severe pain	Demerol, Percodan or Percocet, Toradol, or Vicodin ES	

*Use corticosteroid-antibiotic combination prophylactically. Give patient prescription, but advise taking it only if pain occurs.
Note: ½ g codeine=30 mg. ¼ g codeine=15 mg.

Recently an additional group of analgesics for the relief of mild to moderate pain was introduced—the nonsteroidal antiinflammatory analgesics (NSAIDs). They were developed to give an alternative to aspirin and the milder opiates, with the hope that the side effects would be fewer and less severe. In truth, however, some of the side effects were so severe that several of the drugs had to be removed from the marketplace. Suprol (suprofen) caused alteration of kidney function (flank pain syndrome), and Zomax (zomepirac), which had wide acceptance shortly after introduction, was responsible for several anaphylactic deaths.

These drugs all work similarly and are antipyretic and antiinflammatory in addition to being analgesic. Their similarity to aspirin is further emphasized by their mechanisms of action and their possible side effects. Aspirin and NSAIDs afford pain relief by inhibiting prostaglandin synthesis, although the exact mechanism by which this happens is not completely understood. The NSAIDs may cause gastric irritation and bleeding, as may aspirin. Aspirin is listed as one of the top ten allergenic drugs, with 0.25% to 1% of the population of the United States showing sensitivity.

Because the NSAIDs have not been used for nearly as long as aspirin, their total allergenic potential has not yet been determined accurately. However, if a patient advises an allergy to aspirin ingestion, NSAIDs are not the answer and should *not* be prescribed as a substitute.

Even so, NSAIDs are valuable adjunctive medications to handle endodontically caused conditions. Some patients benefit psychologically from newer medications even if minimal dosage forms are used. Dolobid (diflunisal) requires a loading

Table 20-4.   Types of penicillin for use during endodontic therapy

Drug	Adult dosage	Comments
Potassium penicillin V (V-Cillin-K, Pen-Vee K, Veetids, Betapen-VK)	250 to 500 mg 4 times/day	Specifically developed for oral administration; very high levels of penicillin developed; has had extremely wide and successful use for 20 years
Aminopenicillin, ampicillin (Polycillin, Omnipen, Unasyn)	1 to 4 g divided and given every 6 hr	Not penicillinase resistant, but has a wider spectrum than potassium penicillin V
Amoxicillin (Amoxil, Wymox, Trimox)	250 to 500 mg every 8 hr	Advantage over K penicillin V and ampicillin is that it may be used in 3 rather than 4 doses and gives high blood levels for longer periods; replaces other penicillin forms for SBE prevention drug of choice according to American Heart Association (AHA) guidelines; also comes in liquid suspension form
Penicillinase-resistant penicillins		Effective against penicillinase producing microorganisms, but weak against others; only appropriate use is vs. staphylococci penicillinase-producing bacteria
Cloxacillin	250 to 500 mg every 6 hr	
Dicloxacillin	250 to 500 mg every 6 hr	
Beta-lactamase inhibitors Augmentin		Wide spectrum against gram-positive and gram-negative anaerobes; also, due to clavulanate portion, is effective against betalactamase producing microorganisms which are usually resistant to penicillin and cephalosporin
Amoxicillin and calvulanate potassium	250 mg every 8 hr (tablets, chewables, and oral suspensions do not have equivalent amounts of each chemical; see instructions for use)	

dose that is taken prior to treatment and may be given before an endodontic procedure that will predictably cause postoperative pain, such as periapical surgery or treatment of a mandibular molar with a diagnosis of acute pulpitis along with acute apical periodontitis. Motrin (ibuprofen) and Nalfon (fenoprofen) are similar drugs that have already developed a track record for relieving mild to moderate dentally related pain.

NSAIDs have value in treatment of toothaches because of the loading dose phenomenon that many possess. Patients may call your office in the morning with pain that you know is pulpal or periapical, but your schedule will not permit you to see them conveniently until much later in the day for emergency endodontic treatment. In such a case, an appropriate NSAID is prescribed, to be started as soon as possible, and several additional doses taken, if necessary, prior to treatment.

In many cases, the patients do well and will wait until you have sufficient time in your schedule to treat the tooth properly. This will work out much better than trying to fit the patient in between regularly scheduled appointments earlier and not being able to administer best therapy. The problems that may occur are that the patient, now free from pain, cancels or fails the emergency appointment or that differential diagnosis between several possible teeth becomes difficult.

Analgesics are the most susceptible prescription products to overdosage abuse by the patient in a dental situation. Sedatives and tranquilizers may be abused similarly, but usually these are prescribed in such a small number that the patient rarely can cause serious damage. On the other hand, analgesics are usually prescribed at least 10 in number, and perhaps as high as 25 at a time.

The patient may delay the initial administration until after moderate to severe pain is present. Then, the normal dosage may be insufficient to give complete relief, or the pain returns quickly. Further pills are taken and, if the patients fear the return of pain, too many pills are quickly ingested. This scenario may cause serious consequences.

As may be noted in Tables 20-1 and 20-2, many of the analgesics are combinations of several substances. To guard against taking too much of these drugs, the maximum daily dose is indicated when pertinent. This may be added to the instructions

that the pharmacist will place on the label to help minimize an inadvertent overdose.

Acetaminophen is a frequent drug used alone, or in combination, for analgesia. This drug may cause severe liver damage if more than 4000 mg are ingested in a single day. Therefore, in all drugs with acetaminophen present, the maximum allowable daily dosage is calculated so that no more than 4000 mg may be taken and is so listed.

ANTIBIOTICS

Tools for the control of infections in modern dentistry are usually provided by antibiotics. However, because endodontic therapy now emphasizes the importance of debridement procedures and the elimination or reduction of microorganisms and their substrate, infections of serious nature rarely occur. Even when they do transpire, drainage is generally established easily through the canal space. It is only when the drainage becomes difficult to obtain, or when the host resistance is low or attacker virulence is high, that pharmacologic aid is required.

A common error in antibiotic therapy is to prescribe too little or for too short a duration. Unfortunately such a schedule will kill off the weaker organisms, thus leaving more substrate available for those with greater virulence to become entrenched. Most antibiotics are given at least four times a day. When prescribing prophylactically to prevent an infection, the dentist should specify a minimum of 2 to 3 days for keeping up the therapy. When dealing with an already present infection, therapy should be continued for at least 6 days or for a minimum of 2 days after the infection appears to be under control.

One of the recent major advances in prescribing antibiotics has been the increase in dosage by many practitioners. It has been found that insufficient dosage as well as insufficient time on the antimicrobial has killed off the weaker organisms and led to newer, stronger breeds of bacteria. Due to this impetus, many antibiotics that were available as a maximum in 250 mg forms are now standard in 500 mg forms per dose.

The 500 mg dosage form, although constant for most penicillin-type antibiotics, is not followed for the nonpenicillin drugs listed in Table 20-5; all those antibiotics have dosage forms other than 500 mg. Vibramycin (doxycycline) is a tetracycline derivative but has a much lower dosage form than most other tetracyclines. If too much is prescribed,

Table 20-5.   Nonpenicillin antibiotics for use during endodontic therapy

Drug	Adult dosage	Comments
Erythromycin	250 to 500 mg 4 times/day	Depending on microorganism type and drug concentration, is either bacteriocidal or bacteriostatic; most commonly used alternative for penicillin-allergic patients, named by AHA as substitute in SBE/rheumatic fever patients, good antibacterial spectrum; only serious problem is that many patients experience serious gastritis, even when ingested orally with empty stomach; also available in oral suspension form
PCE (erythromycin particles in tablets)	333 mg every 8 hr or 500 mg every 12 hr	Due to special coating to inactivate gastric acidity, is absorbed in small intestine rather than stomach and causes less stomach upset; although it may be taken without regard to meals, optimal blood levels are obtained in fasting state (½ to 2 hr before meals); 500 mg dosage form allows less frequent administration
Clindamycin (Cleocin)	150 to 300 mg every 6 hr; for serious infections, 300 to 450 mg every 6 hr	Broad spectrum antibacterial with greater effectiveness against gram-negative anaerobes (including *B. melaninogenicus*) than erythromycin; serious side effect is pseudomembranous colitis, occuring with diarrhea, so should only be used when antibacterials with similar spectrum are ineffective
Vancocin HCl (vancomycin HCl)	500 mg IV every 6 hr or 1000 mg IV every 12 hr; no more than 10 mg/min	Useful for patients who are allergic or have infections resistant to penicillin; used, sometimes in combination with other antibacterials, against SBE, given IV
Cephalosporin classifications: 1st generation (Keflex) 2nd generation (Ceclor) 3rd generation (Cefobid)	250 mg every 6 hr 250 mg every 8 hr 1 to 2 g every 12 hr, IV or IM	Very popular broad spectrum antimicrobial; check for patient sensitivity to penicillin, because there is a 10% to 15% crossover sensitivity to the cephalosporins; as you go to the newer generations, gram-negative antibacterial effects increase, but gram-positive antibacterial effects decrease; has effectiveness against bone infections, so has good use in endodontics; because they are powerful antimicrobials, the cephalosporins may be overused when less expensive antibiotics would be just as effective
Note: there are many more examples for each generation		
Tetracycline (Achromycin, Sumycin)	250 to 500 mg 2 to 4 times/day	Bacteriostatic, not bacteriocidal, but with a broad spectrum; has many side effects and should be used only after sensitivity testing; not best drug of choice in endodontic infections
Doxycycline (Vibramycin)	100 mg every 12 hr for 1st day, 100 mg/day thereafter	Tetracycline with more convenient dosage form; must adhere to dose regimen or more serious side effects occur; more useful in endodontic and periodontic infections
Minocycline (Minocin)	200 mg initially, then 100 mg every 12 hr	Another form of tetracycline with similar dosage form to doxycycline, similar problems may result, but effect against broad spectrum of microbials
Fluoroquinolone Ciprofloxacin (Cipro)	250 to 500 mg every 12 hr	Broad spectrum with convenient dosing schedule; very expensive, but works well against many gram-positive and gram-negative species; do not use on children and pregnant and nursing women

Continued

Table 20-5. Nonpenicillin antibiotics for use during endodontic therapy—cont'd

Drug	Adult dosage	Comments
Metronidazole (Flagyl)	Loading dose: 1 g IV Maintenance dose: 500 mg every 6 hr; both to be infused not faster than 1 hr Oral dose: 500 mg every 6 hr, not to exceed 4 g/day	Oral synthetic antiprotozoal and antibacterial agent with antibacterial spectrum very effective against *Bacteroides* species and other gram-negative anaerobes; good drug to give along with penicillin for coverage against both gram-positive and gram-negative bacteria; vomiting occurs when alcohol is ingested while taking this medication

Table 20-6. Sedatives and tranquilizers useful during endodontics

Drug	Adult dosage and comments
Sedatives, barbiturates	Use Schedule II prescriptions
Pentobarbital (Nembutal)	Hypnotic dose is 100 mg at bedtime; dosage for elderly or debilitated patients shoud be reduced because of increased sensitivity to barbiturates
Secobarbital (Seconal)	50 mg night before appointment and 50 mg 30 minutes before appointment
Sedatives, nonbarbiturates	Use Schedule IV prescriptions
Flurazepam (Dalmane)	Hypnotic dose is 15 to 30 mg before retiring, 15 mg for elderly or debilitated patients
Triazolam (Halcion)	0.125 to 0.25 mg for most adult patients will be sufficient; for unusual cases where the higher dose does not give sufficient effect, 0.5 mg may be tried, but not exceeded; not to be taken when alcohol has been ingested; some disturbing adverse reactions have been cited; however, most of these have been after long-term usage and would not be involved with dental treatment
Tranquilizers	
Diazepam (Valium)	Schedule IV prescription; very commonly taken drug for many types of conditions, including alcohol withdrawal, management and relief of anxiety, skeletal muscle spasms; dosage has wide variations, depending on patient and condition; for dental use, 5 or 10 mg tablets, 1 tablet night of appointment and 1 tablet 1 to 2 hours before appointment
Chlordiazepoxide (Librium)	5 mg capsules, 1 capsule 3 times day before appointment, 1 capsule morning of appointment
Oxazepam (Serax)	Schedule IV prescription. 10 to 30 mg capsules and tablets, 1 taken at bedtime night before appointment and 1 taken 1 to 2 hours before appointment; has no hang-over effect

serious side effects might occur. Therefore, if any question exists as to the correct dosage form required, or when prescribing a drug not in your normal list, be certain to consult *Physicians' Desk Reference* of a current year.

In addition to effective coverage against infections, antibiotics are used during endodontic therapy prophylactically for patients with a history of rheumatic heart disease and other systemic conditions. (See Chapter 2.) Tables 20-4 (see p. 841) and 20-5 list the antibiotics commonly used in endodontics.

SEDATIVES AND TRANQUILIZERS

Dentistry in general and endodontics in particular have long been victims of a "bad press." As a consequence of erroneous and often false tales heard from others and based on rare past traumatic encounters, certain patients enter the office in a state of such nervousness or agitation that they find the taking of a radiograph almost unbearable. Even some of those who outwardly appear normal are suffering from severe inner torment. Before even suggesting suitable prescriptions, we shall emphasize that this behavior is beyond the control of some individuals and should not be taken as a personal affront against the dentist. Ridicule, scorn, or other insults will serve no useful purpose. Rather, a kindly supportive, and understanding attitude, together with suggestion for control of such feelings, will be greatly appreciated and usually yield acceptable response.

Sedatives and tranquilizers as groups contain drugs that are central nervous system depressants and decrease cortical excitability. Both have similar actions reducing abnormal excessive response to environmental situations that produce agitation, tension, and anxiety. The major difference between the groups is that sedatives in high enough dosage will produce general anesthesia or sleep, whereas tranquilizers will not. The latter also serve effectively to block hostile or overly aggressive reactions used as a cover for fear. Sedatives and tranquilizers useful in endodontics are listed in Table 20-6.

Ambulatory patients for whom sedatives are prescribed must be warned to have someone with them who can drive home at the completion of the appointment. Because of the differences in tolerance and metabolism of individuals, a sedative dosage normally considered relatively low may depress the central nervous system of a patient to

such an extent that motor skills and judgment are impaired.

Therefore the use of tranquilizers is excellent in endodontic therapy. They usually require no accompaniment to the office, eliminate the more objectionable types of patient defense reactions and produce acceptable skeletal muscle relaxation. Both sedatives and tranquilizers potentiate the action of local anesthetics.

Although tranquilizers in themselves will not produce sleep, they may relax patients to such a degree that extreme drowsiness will develop and the patient will go to sleep. This is particularly true if tensions or other emotional factors have caused recent lack of sleep. Therefore tranquilizers should be prescribed in their lower dosages for patients without prior experience of ingestion until some indication as to the degree of relaxation produced by a given dose is determined. If the smaller dosage is sufficient, it should be maintained for succeeding appointments. If more relaxation is necessary, a larger dose is prescribed. If there is any question as to the ability of this patient to react properly at the conclusion of the appointment, arrangements should be made for a companion to drive home.

The short-acting barbiturates and their substitutes are excellent for use with endodontic therapy. The initial dose should be given the night before the appointment to ensure a restful night, with another taken 30 minutes before the patient is seated in the operatory. Patients requiring sedatives should be seen in the morning so that they will have less opportunity to mull over the distasteful prospects of treatment.

Many drugs in each classification are often used intravenously or intramuscularly. For most endodontic procedures oral dosage is adequate. Because of the potential danger, other routes should be used only when postgraduate study or hospital experience has properly prepared the practitioner.

DRUGS FOR CHILDREN

Children are usually excellent endodontic patients, particularly when their parents have not preconditioned them negatively and when they are unaccompanied in the operatory. However, almost any of the drugs mentioned for adults may be used on children, but only after appropriate change in dosage.

The usual alteration in dosage may be computed by Clark's rule. It states that the full dosage should be given to an adult of 150 pounds, and the child's dosage is calculated on the basis of the child's weight as a ratio to a full dose.

$$\frac{\text{Child's weight}}{150} = \text{Fraction of adult dose to be given}$$

Because of the frequency of upper respiratory and other infections in youngsters, almost every antibiotic has excellent dosage forms for children. Tablets (or capsules) are available in 125 mg form, and many antibiotics are manufactured so that syrups may be compounded by the pharmacist of 125 mg per teaspoon.

Some drugs may be given to adults but not to children. Therefore the *Physicians' Desk Reference* should always be consulted for contraindications before a prescription for children is written.

REFERENCES

Ciancio SG, Bourgault PC: *Clinical pharmacology for dental professionals,* ed 3, St Louis, 1989, Mosby.

Desjardins PJ: The top 20 prescription drugs and how they affect your dental practice, *Compend Contin Educ Dent* 8:740, 1992.

Gilman AG et al: *Goodman and Gilman's the pharmacologic basis of therapeutics,* ed 8, New York, 1990, McGraw-Hill.

Gurney BF: Anesthesiology and pharmacology in endodontics, *Dent Clin North Am* 11:615, 1967.

Holroyd SV: Clinical pharmacology of antibiotics of dental importance, *Dent Clin North Am* 14:697, 1970.

Miles M: Anesthetics, analgesics, antibiotics, and endodontics, *Dent Clin North Am* 28:865, 1984.

Pallasch TJ, Kunitake LM: Nonsteroidal anti-inflammatory analgesics, *Compend Contin Educ Dent* 6:47, 1985.

Physicians' desk reference, ed 47, Oradell, New Jersey, 1993, Medical Economics.

Reynolds DC: Pain control in the dental office, *Dent Clin North Am* 15:319, 1971.

Small EW: Preoperative sedation in dentistry, *Dent Clin North Am* 14:769, 1970.

Index